SYNTAX	PHONOLOGY
	0-2 mo—vegetative sounds 2-4 mo—cooing, laughing 4-6 mo—quasi-resonant nuclei, vocal play 6-10 mo—canonical, reduplicated babbling-CV syllables
	Jargon babble with intonation contours of language being learned
	First 50 words •Most often have CV shape •Use same consonants used in early babbling •Use of reduplication, syllable deletion, assimilation, and final consonant deletion is common •Words are selected or avoided for expression based on favored and avoided sounds
Brown's Stage I: Basic Semantic Roles and Relations Two-word utterances emerge Word order is consistent Utterances are "telegraphic" with few grammatical markers	By 24 mo, 9-10 initial and 5-6 final consonants are used Speech is 50% intelligible 70% of consonants are correct CVC and two-syllable words emerge
Brown's Stage II: Grammatical Morphemes Early emerging acquisition: -*ing* in, on, plural /s/ Use of *no, not, can't, don't* as negation between subject and verb Questions formed with rising intonation only Sentences with semi-auxiliaries *gonna, wanna, gotta, hafta* appear	Awareness of rhyme emerges
Brown's Stage III: Modulation of Simple Sentences Present tense auxiliaries appear (*can, will*) *Be* verbs used inconsistently Overgeneralized past-tense forms appear Possessive ('s) acquired	Speech is 75% intelligible at 36 mo Ability to produce rhyme emerges
Brown's Stage IV: Emergence of Embedded Sentences First complex sentence forms appear Auxiliary verbs are placed correctly in questions and negatives Irregular past tense, articles (*a, the*) acquired	Use of reduplication, syllable deletion, assimilation, and final consonant deletion is less common Use of stopping, fronting, cluster reduction, and liquid simplification continues
Brown's Stage Late IV–Early V Early emerging complex sentence types, including the following: •Full prepositional clauses •*Wh-* clauses •Simple infinitives •Conjoined	Use of cluster reduction decreases
Brown's Stave V Later developing morphemes acquired, including the following: •*Be* verbs •Regular past •Third person /s/ Past-tense auxiliaries used Later-developing complex sentences emerge, including the following: •Relative clauses (right branching) •Infinitive clauses with different subjects •Gerund clauses •*Wh-* infinitive clauses Basic sentence forms acquired	Speech is 100% intelligible Ability to segment words into syllables emerges Use of most simplification processes stops; errors on /s/, /r/, /l/, *th* may persist

Milestones of Later Communication Development

TYPICAL AGE	PRAGMATICS	SEMANTICS
5-7 yr	Narratives are true "stories" with central focus, high point, and resolution	Reorganization of lexical knowledge from syntagmatic (episodic) to paradigmatic (semantic) networks Average expressive vocabulary size is 3000 to 5000 words
7-9 yr	Stories contain complete episodes with internal goals, motivations, and reactions of characters; some multiple-episode stories appear Language is used to establish and maintain social status Increased perspective-taking allows for more successful persuasion Provide conversational repairs by defining terms or giving background information Begin to understand jokes and riddles based on sound similarities Can perform successfully in simple referential communication tasks	School and reading experience introduce new words not encountered in conversation Pronouns used anaphorically to refer to nouns previously named Word definitions include synonyms and categories Some words understood to have multiple meanings Capacity for production of figurative language increases
9-12 yr	Stories include complex, embedded, and interactive episodes Understand jokes and riddles based on lexical ambiguity	Vocabulary used in school texts is more abstract and specific than that used in conversation Students are expected to acquire new information from written texts Can explain relationships between meanings of multiple-meaning words Begin using adverbial conjuncts (4% of utterances contain them) Most common idioms understood
12-14 yr	Expository texts used in school-sponsored writing Most academic information is presented in expository formats Understand jokes and riddles based on deep structure ambiguity	Abstract, dictionary definitions given for words Use of adverbial conjuncts increases Can explain meaning of proverbs in context
15-18 yr	Language is used to maintain social bonds ("just talking") Persuasive and argumentative skills reach near-adult levels	Average vocabulary size of high school graduate is 10,000 words

Adapted from Chapman, R. (2000). Children's language learning: An interactionist perspective. *Journal of Child Psychology and Psychiatry, 41,* 33-54; Nippold, M. (1998). *Later language development: The school-age and adolescent years.* Austin, TX: Pro-Ed; Westby, C. (1999). Assessing and facilitating text comprehension problems. In H. Catts and A. Kahmi (Eds.), *Language and reading disabilities* (pp. 154-223). Boston, MA: Allyn & Bacon.

Milestones of Literacy Development

TYPICAL AGE	LITERACY SOCIALIZATION	PHONOLOGICAL AWARENESS	PRINT KNOWLEDGE
0-2 yr	Enjoys joint book-reading Learns to hold book right-side up Learns to turn pages Answers questions about pictures, characters	Exposure to rhyme initiates rhyme awareness	Learns to distinguish print from pictures
2-5 yr	Learns the need to turn page to get to next part of story Learns left-right progression of print • Learns print is stable; anyone reading a book reads the same words	Can segment sentences into words Can segment words into syllables Can recognize/produce rhymes Can recognize/produce words with same beginning sound Can segment/blend words by onset/rime (s+un=sun)	Learns alphabet song Learns to recognize and name letters Learns letters "have" sounds Learns clusters of letters separated by space form words
5-7 yr	Reads picture books for pleasure, with assistance (e.g., audiotaped book) Reads picture books for pleasure, independently	Can identify (name) first sound in word Can list words that start w/ same sound Can count sounds in words Can blend 3-4 sounds to make a word (/h/+ /æ/+/n/+ /d/=hand) Can segment words into 3-4 phonemes (hand= /h/+ /æ/+/n/+ /d/) Can manipulate sounds in words (What's hop without /p/? [/ha/])	Learns alphabetic principle: Words are made up of sounds; sounds can be represented by letters Learns all letter names, letter sounds for consonants Learns sounds for vowels Can match letters to sounds
7-9 yr	Reads "chapter books" for pleasure independently May read non-fiction for pleasure, as well	Can play with sounds in words, as in pig latin and other secret codes	Begins to learn conventions for punctuation, capitalization, other conventions of print
9-12 yr	Reads for information as well as pleasure		Continues improving knowledge of writing conventions Errors in these decrease
12-18 yr	Develops study skills to retain material read		Masters basic rules for punctuation, capitalization, etc.

Adapted from Kaderavek, J., & Justice, L. (2004). Embedded-explicit emergent literacy intervention II: Goal selection and implementation in the early childhood classroom. Language, Speech, and Hearing Services in Schools, 35, 212-228; Kamhi, A. & Catts, H. (2005). Reading development. In H. Catts & A. Kamhi (Eds.), *Language and Reading Disabilities.* 2nd Ed. (pp.26-49.) Boston: Allyn & Bacon.

SYNTAX / PHONOLOGY/METALINGUISTICS

SYNTAX	PHONOLOGY/METALINGUISTICS
Use and understanding of passive sentences emerges Mastery of exceptions to basic grammatical rules begins	Last residual speech errors overcome Ability to segment words into phonemes emerges Understand concept of "word" separate from its referent
Literate language syntax needed for academic participation develops A few errors in noun phrases ("much bricks") persist	Articulation is mostly error-free Some difficulty with complex words may persist (*aluminium*) Phonological knowledge is used in spelling Sound manipulation in activities such as pig latin is seen
Syntax used in school texts is more complex than that used in oral language Use of word order variations increases in writing ("Around the house we put a fence)	Morphophonological knowledge develops and is used in spelling Metacognitive skills emerge
Use of perfect aspect (*have/had* + [verb]) increases Syntax used in writing is more complex than that used in speech	Knowledge of stress rules (*yellow*jacket vs. yellow *jacket*) is acquired
Sentence length and complexity in written language is greater than in spoken Rate of modal auxiliary use increases Full adult range of syntactic constructions reached	Knowledge of morphophonological rules reaches adult level

READING / WRITING

READING	WRITING
May pretend to read when others are reading	Learns to hold crayon, scribble
Learns to recognize name in print May recognize environmental print (reads "McDonald's" sign)	Begins representational drawing Learns to write name Distinguishes drawing from writing Learns to write some letters May use invented spelling to label drawings
Learns to decode by identifying sounds for printed letters and synthesizing sounds across letters to form words Learns some words by sight	Learns conventional spelling for some words Learns to spell by segmenting words into sounds and writing letters for sounds Makes errors based on phonetic correspondences Writing is simpler than speech Writing begins to be more common than drawing
More words recognized by "sight" More phonic patterns are recognized to increase automaticity of decoding (e.g., "silent e rule") As reading becomes more automatic, more attention is focused on comprehension Reading moves toward fluency	Learns spelling patterns (e.g., -*ight* pattern words) Increases vocabulary of known spellings Makes fewer spelling errors Uses writing to send messages Begins school-sponsored writing, such as book reports Writing resembles level of complexity in speech Oral and literate styles are mixed in writing Narrative writing predominates
Reading is fluent Decoding is efficient and automatic Comprehension is focus; reads to learn	Learns morphophonological rules and patterns in spelling (e.g., *photograph* has two 'o's, you can hear them both in *photography*) Writing has a more consistently literate style; more subordinate clauses Persuasive and expository writing is introduced in the school curriculum
Begins to develop critical reading/thinking skills Learns to distinguish fact from opinion in writing Can construct knowledge from print sources using reasoning, analysis, synthesis and judgment	Level of complexity in writing begins to be greater than in speech More low frequency syntactic forms appear in writing than in speech Persuasive and expository writing continue to improve beyond high school, given adequate experience and opportunity

LANGUAGE DISORDERS
from INFANCY THROUGH ADOLESCENCE

ASSESSMENT & INTERVENTION

RHEA PAUL, PhD, CCD-SLP

PROFESSOR, COMMUNICATION DISORDERS
SOUTHERN CONNECTICUT STATE UNIVERSITY
NEW HAVEN, CT

With a Contribution From
Courtenay Norbury, DPhil
Nuffield Foundation New Career Development Fellow
Language and Cognitive Development
Department of Experimental Psychology
University of Oxford
Oxford, England

Photographs by
Pamela Bruni and Ayub Balweel

THIRD EDITION

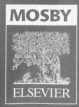

MOSBY

ELSEVIER

MOSBY
ELSEVIER

11830 Westline Industrial Drive
St. Louis, Missouri 63146

LANGUAGE DISORDERS FROM INFANCY THROUGH ADOLESCENCE:
ASSESSMENT AND INTERVENTION, THIRD EDITION

ISBN 13: 978-0-323-03685-6
ISBN 10: 0-323-03685-6

ISBN 13: 978-0-323-03685-6
ISBN 10: 0-323-03685-6

Publishing Director: Linda Duncan
Editor: Kathy Falk
Developmental Editor: Melissa Kuster Deutsch
Publishing Services Manager: Patricia Tannian
Project Manager: John Casey
Book Designer: Jyotika Shroff

Printed in United States of America

Last digit is the print number: 9 8 7 6 5 4 3 2 1

*To the memory of **my father**,*

who was the kind of teacher I have always tried to be,

*and of **my sister**,*

whose too-short life was devoted to helping handicapped children.

A Note to the Instructor

This book attempts to tell students everything they ever wanted to know—and then some—about child language disorders. It covers the entire developmental period and delves into many additional concepts that are important to the practice of child language disorders, including prevention, syndromes associated with language disorders, and multicultural practice.

Like the last revision, this one attempts to incorporate new trends in the practice of language pathology. In reviewing the last 5 years of research and writing on child language disorders, one of the most encouraging developments has been the emphasis on evidence-based practice. Many of the assessment and treatment approaches that have been used in our field, mostly as a result of clinical intuition and experience, have been subjected to empirical research, and some now have impressive amounts of evidence to support their use in practice. I've tried to incorporate this new evidence in the discussions of methods and procedures throughout this edition.

As before, this book is short on theory and long on clinical application and concrete procedures. My goal in writing it was to provide a broadly based, practical introduction to the field of language pathology to students planning a career as clinicians in speech-language pathology, students who need to know what to do that first Monday morning of their clinical career, but who also need to develop the ability to think critically and creatively about the myriad kinds of clinical problems they would encounter in the course of their practice.

My hope is that students will use this book during their introductory language disorders course and will also find it a helpful reference as they progress through their clinical education and even into their professional practice. For this reason, students reading the book for the first time may feel that it is too comprehensive, that they cannot possibly absorb all the information in it in one or two terms. They are probably right. My hope is that their instructors can help them to understand that they can return to the book later and not only refresh their memories, but also take in more of it as their experience broadens and they have more background information and more clinical savvy with which to approach it. Helping students understand that they do not have to master the entire volume the first time through, that they will have opportunities as their career goes on to assimilate more of the material, can help alleviate their anxiety. What they should get from reading the book the first time is knowledge of the basic concepts and vocabulary used in the field, an overview of its issues and controversies, an understanding of the scope of communicative difficulties that make up child language disorders, and a sense of how a language pathologist approaches the processes of assessment and intervention.

To provide this sense, case studies and vignettes are included throughout the book. These are meant to serve as examples of applying the material in the text to some real-life situations. In using the case studies in class presentations, one approach might include having students work in groups to come up with alternative approaches to the ones given in the book for dealing with the cases presented. This can help students develop a sense that there is no one "right" way to deal with a client and that several different approaches might be equally appropriate, so long as each takes the client's needs into account. Another way to use the case studies is to have some students present their own clients as case studies for the chapters that apply to them. They can use the case studies in the book as models for applying the principles discussed in the chapter and use a similar approach to come up with an assessment or intervention plan for a client being presented. If the students work on the case in a cooperative learning arrangement, with several groups of four to six students working independently to come up with a plan for the case to present to the whole class, the diversity of possibilities for addressing a client's needs can again be illustrated.

As the Preface of this book states, much of the material contained here represents the author's opinion or point of view. In fact, in this third edition, I have changed my mind on several positions I took in the first two. Instructors who have used the first edition may be surprised to find that, for example, I have de-emphasized cognitive referencing in defining language disorders and have become more tentative on the Communication Needs model for determining when AAC is needed. These and the other changes in this edition reflect what I perceive as a change in the consensus in the research literature. I have made every effort to include modifications like these in the third edition so that it represents as closely as possible the current state of knowledge and best practice in our field.

Still, many instructors who teach courses in child language disorders will find themselves in disagreement with some aspects of the book's content. My hope is that instructors will let students know when this happens and give them that alternate point of view. As I've tried to emphasize throughout the book, language pathology is not a field in which there are long-established sets of accepted premises and practices. Our field is lively with controversy and differing opinions about how to conceptualize, organize, explain, assess, and treat child language disorders. Students should be aware of this ferment. The best way to give them this awareness is for an instructor to focus on points of disagreement with the text, to elaborate and explicate the differences, and to argue an alternative point of view. Students exposed to opposing points of view from two authoritative sources—their teacher and their textbook—have a good chance of becoming critical thinkers about the material in their coursework and later in their professional practice.

This book is organized into 14 chapters, which could correspond roughly to the 14 weeks of a typical semester. If the book is being used to teach a one-semester course, one chapter of the book could be covered during each week of the term. Increasingly, though, programs in speech-language pathology are expanding their language curriculum to cover two terms rather than one. Some programs divide the curriculum into assessment and intervention portions. Others divide along developmental lines, teaching early assessment and intervention during a first term and language learning disorders in school-age children the second. If this book is used over a two-term sequence using an assessment/intervention structure, the chapters could be covered in the following order:

Term 1	Assessment
Chapter 1	Models of Child Language Disorders
Chapter 2	Evaluation and Assessment
Chapter 6	Assessment and Intervention in the Prelinguistic Period
Chapter 7	Assessment and Intervention for Emerging Language
Chapter 8	Assessment of Developing Language
Chapter 11	Assessing Students' Language for Learning
Chapter 13	Assessing Advanced Language

Term 2	Intervention
Chapter 3	Principles of Intervention
Chapter 9	Intervention for Developing Language
Chapter 10	Language, Reading, and Learning in School: What the Speech-Language Pathologist Needs to Know
Chapter 12	Intervening at the Language-for-Learning Period
Chapter 14	Intervention for Advanced Language
Chapter 4	Special Considerations for Special Populations
Chapter 5	Child Language Disorders in a Pluralistic Society

If, on the other hand, the sequence is organized along developmental lines, the chapters could be covered as follows:

Term 1	Early Assessment and Intervention
Chapter 1	Models of Child Language Disorders
Chapter 2	Evaluation and Assessment
Chapter 3	Principles of Intervention
Chapter 6	Assessment and Intervention in the Prelinguistic Period
Chapter 7	Assessment and Intervention for Emerging Language
Chapter 8	Assessment of Developing Language
Chapter 9	Intervention for Developing Language

Term 2	Working with Language Learning Disabilities
Chapter 10	Language, Reading, and Learning in School: What the Speech-Language Pathologist Needs to Know
Chapter 11	Assessing Students' Language for Learning
Chapter 12	Intervening at the Language-for-Learning Period
Chapter 13	Assessing Advanced Language
Chapter 14	Intervention for Advanced Language
Chapter 4	Special Considerations for Special Populations
Chapter 5	Child Language Disorders in a Pluralistic Society

Finally, if an undergraduate course is included in the child language curriculum, the first section of the book, Topics in Child Language Disorders, could serve as the text for the undergraduate course, and Chapters 6 through 14 could be covered in the graduate curriculum.

Most of the chapters on assessment contain detailed procedures for doing analyses of various communicative behaviors. Some of these contain sample transcripts or other material on which students can try the analyses being presented. The best way to learn these analyses is by doing them, either on the transcripts given in the book or on others provided by the instructor. Having students work in groups, again, reduces their anxiety and provides more heads addressing the problem. Using class time to practice some of the analyses, or assigning students to do them as group projects outside of class, can be an effective way to be sure that students "get their hands dirty" with the nitty-gritty of analyzing communication. Having done so will give them more confidence to try some on their own and, we hope, to continue using communication analyses in addition to testing as part of their professional practice.

As stated in the Preface, the answers to the exercises given in the book are, like all language sampling results, subject to disagreement. If disagreements with the answers given to the exercises occur, this is an excellent opportunity to discuss the reasons for the disagreement and to probe the justification for the opposing judgments. It may be that the instructor and class together will decide that their answer is better than the one given in the text. This kind of exercise, too, helps students realize the subjectivity involved in most communicative analyses and brings home the point that as long as analyses are thorough, thoughtful, and careful, they do not always have to be in exact agreement to be useful in intervention planning.

Each chapter contains a study guide at the end to help students review the material. Some instructors may wish to use the study guides to structure discussion of the topics in class. Students also can be encouraged to form study groups and discuss the questions in the guide together. Taking questions from the guides to elicit essay responses on examinations is another way to use them. Students can be encouraged to study the guides for a particular set of chapters on which they are to be tested, and can be told that examination questions will be chosen from among the questions in the guides. I have found this method to be an effective way of getting students to study the full range of material covered, and still have a reasonably small number of questions for them to answer on a 1- or 2-hour examination.

It is my hope that instructors will find using this book helpful in preparing their students for practice in child language disorders. In some ways, having a comprehensive text should make this job easier. It will no longer be necessary to gather reams of reprints and handouts to copy and distribute in order to cover all the material that needs to be covered. It should no longer be as difficult to find case examples and transcripts with which to illustrate points made in class; at least a starter set is provided here. Teaching child language disorders, though, will continue to be a challenge. It requires helping students begin to assimilate the vast amount of information that has been accumulated and letting them know that it won't all stick with them after just one pass. It includes helping students to accept the degree of flux and tension over ideas in the field and teaching them by example to find a way to develop their own point of view on controversial topics. It means imparting the skills to master many specific procedures and concepts without losing sight of the need to remain flexible, creative, and attuned to the needs of each client. While it is hoped that this book can help instructors to meet these challenges, it is certain that teaching child language disorders will remain an exciting and demanding endeavor.

PREFACE

One thing you will notice right away as you read this book is that it is written in first person. It's cranky, preachy, and personal. Many of the positions taken here will be debated by others in the field. Your instructor, in fact, may disagree with some of the material in the book. It is this lack of consensus among experts in language pathology that prompted me to write this book as I did, in a style that constantly reminds the reader that a lot of what it contains is opinion rather than established fact. Language pathology is a relatively young field, and many of its tenets, assumptions, and paradigms are still in the process of being established. Given this state of affairs, it would be premature to suggest to students that there is a broad consensus about its basic issues. It's just not true, although it is more true now than it was when the first edition of this book appeared, and changes in this edition of the text reflect these changes that have occurred in our field. Still, a range of opinion exists, and I've given you my perspective on it. Your instructor's point of view may differ, but my hope is that when it does, you will be exposed to both sets of thinking and be in a better position to establish your own view. While it may seem confusing at first to be told that your textbook does not contain the last word on every question, learning to live with this kind of "creative confusion" is part of what it takes to develop into a thoughtful and critical professional, one who evaluates information rather than merely "consuming" it.

Creative confusion reigns even in the text's practice exercises. The chapters on assessment contain several example transcripts on which you can try the analysis methods discussed in each chapter. Answers to these practice exercises are given in the appendices to these chapters. I've called these "my" answers, rather than the "right" answers. That's because you and your instructor may disagree with some of them. Language pathology is not an exact science. There are no laboratory tests or firmly established quantitative measures. Many of the analyses we do in our business involve a considerable amount of judgment, and even careful judges can sometimes disagree. Again, the important thing is not to decide which answer is right, but to think each decision through. If you or your instructor disagree with a judgment I've made about a transcript, consider the opposing positions and try to evaluate the data in light of each. You may come to the conclusion that your analysis is correct and mine is in error. That's OK. The important thing is to develop a consistent set of criteria that you will apply reliably to all the analyses you do, whether or not it conforms to mine. If you have a good justification for your position, stick with it. Developing a clearly delineated set of criteria for analyzing the language you study is the goal of these exercises.

The book is organized into three sections. The first deals with some issues in the practice of language pathology with children that cut across developmental levels. These issues have to do with how we define and organize language disorders, and the basic principles we will try to follow in assessing and intervening with children at any developmental level. Some other topics that apply to children of any age include knowing something about the various syndromes and conditions that often accompany language disorders in children and developing techniques for working with children who come from cultural or linguistic backgrounds that differ from our own.

The next two sections of the book look in detail at the communicative issues that are specific to each developmental level from birth through adolescence and give assessment and intervention methods targeted for each level. The levels should be thought of as developmental rather than age- related. Because of developmental disabilities, children of widely varying ages could perform at any of these levels, so it is better to try to think of them as representing stages of functioning rather than chronological age. For this reason I have given them labels that do not refer to age.

Section II deals with development from birth to the point at which basic language skills are acquired. In the child language literature, the acquisition of these basic language skills is often indexed by stages introduced by Roger Brown (1973). I have labeled the end of this period with the highest of Brown's stages of early language development, Brown's Stage V. Essentially, this section covers the period of development that normally occurs between birth and the end of the preschool period, at about age 5. It includes information on what is usually considered "early" assessment and intervention and is divided into three periods: the "prelinguistic" stage (corresponding to the first year and a half of normal development), the "emerging language" stage (corresponding to developmental levels from 18-36 months), and the "developing language" phase (corresponding to developmental levels from 3 to 5 years). Again, though, some developmentally delayed clients who need the methods discussed in this section will be older than preschool age.

Section III deals with children who have acquired basic oral language skills but have trouble with the linguistic demands of the academic curriculum. They will be at least school age; that is, older than 5 years, though not all clients older than 5 will have skills commensurate with this level. The section divides later language development into two broad periods: "language for learning," which comprises what normal children acquire during the elementary school years, and the "advanced language period," which deals with skills typically learned in adolescence and used in the secondary school curriculum.

Because such a large amount of information is covered in each chapter, I've tried to help students assimilate it by providing a study guide for each one. The guide essentially lists, in question form, all the major topics introduced in the chapter. For the information that is more or less factual, the questions ask you just to recall or review it. For portions of the chapter that are more conceptual or debatable, the study guide encourages you to discuss or argue the issues. The point of the study guide is to supply an outline to use in reviewing the material in the chapter and to help you organize the information in your own mind. Answering the questions literally is not the most important goal. It's more fruitful to use the guide as a way of thinking back through all the issues raised in the chapter. Because studying this material often involves mastering concepts and understanding issues rather than memorizing facts, many students find that using the guides in study groups is more helpful than doing them alone.

In order to bring the discussion down from an abstract to a more concrete level, I've included many vignettes and case studies in the text to illustrate the points being made or to serve as examples of how the principles discussed in the book can be applied in real practice. All the vignettes and case studies are drawn from my own clinical experience, although they are usually embroidered to illustrate a particular point in a short time period. Their purpose is to breathe some life into the text and to show how the methods can be integrated in working with a single child. As case studies, though, they are limited in scope and are not meant to represent the only way to implement the procedures in the text. They are just an example of one way.

Many of the problems that I've raised here—the youth of our field, its lack of a firmly established knowledge base, the fluidity of development that makes age a poor indicator of functioning level—can make the study of language disorders in children seem a daunting task to beginning clinicians. But these same problems are what make our field so fertile and exciting. There is so much to learn, so much room for growth and acquisition of new knowledge, and so much opportunity for each clinician to contribute unique information and develop innovative methods that really address children's needs. I hope you'll try, as you struggle through the sense of being overwhelmed that inevitably accompanies learning a lot of new things in a short time, to keep those possibilities in mind.

ACKNOWLEDGMENTS

There are so many people whose help and encouragement made possible the completion of this book in its original form that I hesitate to begin naming them, for fear of being unable ever to complete the list. First, I must thank my colleagues at Portland State University, particularly Mary Gordon-Brannan, Ellen Reuler, and Joan McMahon, for their unflagging willingness to "take up the slack" in department chores to allow me to concentrate on the writing, and for their continuing support and friendship. Second, I want to express my gratitude to my colleagues at the Yale Child Study Center, the late Dr. Donald Cohen and Dr. Fred Volkmar, for their long-standing friendship and support. My thanks also go to teachers Carol Chomsky, Robin Chapman, Jon Miller, Larry Shriberg, and Jean Chall, who taught me most of what I know and how to learn the rest. Much appreciation goes to the people who reviewed early drafts of this work and provided insightful suggestions for revision, including Melanie Fried-Oken, Christine Dollaghan, Anne van Kleeck, and Pat Launer. I am grateful, too, to the students at Portland State University who struggled through early versions of the book and were so patient and accepting of its many imperfections. I am indebted, as well, to the assistants who worked on the first two editions, Nanette Dieterle, Sara Rosenbaum, Nicole Midford, Dave Andrews, Anne Cole, and John Hanlon. Thanks also to Brent Schauer and his staff at the PSU Graphic Arts Department for their help with figures and tables.

In preparing the third edition, Susan DeWitt was an invaluable help in all aspects of preparation. Thanks also go to Pat McMahon for her help with computer graphics. Again, I want to express my deepest thanks to Sandra Holley-Carter, Dean of Southern Connecticut State University's School of Graduate Studies and First Lady of the Connecticut State University system, for making it possible for me to complete this edition back home in New England. I am deeply grateful to colleagues including Linda Swank, Denise Rini, Althea Marshall, Wendy Marans, Sherri Ellis, Deb Selden, and Nancy Lebov both for their love and encouragement, as well as for the clinical insights they shared with me. Special thanks go to Southern Connecticut State University's Center for Communication Disorders Director, Kevin McNamara, for his unfailing generosity in helping not only with this book, but with every aspect of my role at SCSU. I am grateful to my children, Will, Marty, and Aviva Isenberg for coping so graciously with their working mother. Finally, I want to express gratitude to my late husband, Charles R. Isenberg, for the love he always gave so freely and the pride he took in all my endeavors.

CONTENTS

LIST OF BOXES AND TABLES

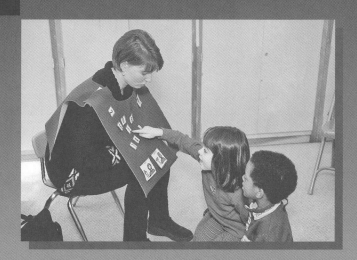

TOPICS IN CHILD LANGUAGE DISORDERS

MODELS OF CHILD LANGUAGE DISORDERS

Rhea Paul, PhD
Courtenay Norbury, PhD

CHAPTER OBJECTIVES

Readers of this chapter will be able to do the following:
- Discuss several definitions of child language disorders.

- Give a brief history of the field of language pathology.
- Define terms associated with child language disorders.

As a beginning graduate student in communication disorders, one of us took a seminar on language disorders in children that was required of all graduates. We were a lively, argumentative group, and we spent our class periods debating the "hot" issues in the field circa 1977. During one session in the middle of the term, though, we got onto the topic of defining just what we meant by *child language disorders*. After a good deal of discussion, it became clear that no one (including the professor) had a really good definition, and most of the ways of defining it came down to saying what it was not. Some of the students were shocked. They confronted the professor in dismay: "You mean we've spent this whole term talking about something, and you don't even know what it is?"

It is easy to understand these students' frustration. Unfortunately, things have not changed all that much today. You may be surprised to learn that defining *child language disorders* is not a simple matter or even one about which everyone in the field agrees. You can see this for yourself in Jamie's story.

When 6-year-old Jamie was referred for language evaluation in September because he failed his kindergarten screening, Ms. Reese conducted an intensive assessment and found that he was functioning at a 4-year-old level in terms of receptive and expressive language. The school psychologist also tested Jamie and found that he functioned in the borderline range on an IQ test, not low enough to be placed in a special classroom or to be identified as developmentally delayed. Ms. Reese, the school's speech-language pathologist (SLP), decided to include Jamie in her caseload because her testing confirmed that he was clearly functioning below chronological age level in his language skills.

Ms. Reese was transferred in October to a middle school, and Mr. Timmons took over her caseload. Mr. Timmons reviewed Ms. Reese's testing and the school psychologist's report. He concluded that Jamie was functioning at the language level to be expected, based on his mental age, which the psychologist had reported as 4 years 2 months. Mr. Timmons dropped Jamie from the caseload and put him on monitoring status.

Who's right? Does Jamie have a language problem, or doesn't he? Even his SLPs do not know for sure. Yet that is one of the major functions of the speech-language clinician—to decide who requires services for communication disorders. What goes into making this decision?

DEFINITIONS OF CHILD LANGUAGE DISORDERS

The American Speech-Language-Hearing Association (ASHA) has defined *language disorder* as an impairment in "comprehension and/or use of a spoken, written, and/or other symbol system. The disorder may involve (1) the form of language (phonologic, morphologic, and syntactic systems), (2) the content of language (semantic system), and/or (3) the function of language in communication (pragmatic system), in any combination" (1993, p. 40).

This definition is useful in that it is quite broad, covering not only spoken but also written language. However, it does not help the clinician decide just what constitutes the "impairment" in acquisition. Some definitions, such as Fey's (1986), emphasize the notion of a standard against which the child's performance is measured. According to Fey, a language disorder is "a significant deficit in the child's level of development of the form, content, or use of language" (p. 31).

Still, the clinician needs to determine what a significant deficit is and relative to what.

We'll throw our hat into the ring with yet another definition, because it will allow us to discuss some of the important issues in making decisions about children with language problems. Children can be described as having language disorders if they have a significant deficit in learning to talk, understand, or use any aspect of language appropriately, relative to both environmental and norm-referenced expectations for children of similar developmental level.

Let's take this definition apart and see what its contents are.

NORMATIVE OR NEUTRALIST?

The definition involves a significant deficit relative, in part, to environmental expectations. In common-sense terms that means a deficit big enough to be noticed by ordinary people such as parents and teachers—not just language-development experts—and one that affects how the child functions socially or academically in the world in which he or she lives. The deficit, in other words, has to have some adaptive consequences. Fey (1986) refers to this as a "normativist" position.

The definition goes a step further, though. It says that the deficit also must exist relative to "norm-referenced expectations." That means that in addition to being noticeably handicapped in the ability to use language forms and meanings to communicate in everyday life, the child with a language disorder also must score significantly below expectations on some standardized or norm-referenced tests. Fey (1986) refers to this standard as a "neutralist" position. Both the *Diagnostic and Statistical Manual of Mental Disorders*, fourth edition (DSM-IV; American Psychiatric Association, 2000), and the *International Classification of Diseases* (ICD-10; World Health Organization, 2005)—the systems used by medical and mental health professionals worldwide to classify disorders—require that both of these criteria (the normativist, or adaptive dysfunction criterion, and the neutralist, or standardized criterion) be met for a child language disorder to be diagnosed. In this text, we adopt this position and say that a child must both score significantly low on standardized testing *and* be perceived as having a communication problem, as evidenced by either parent complaint or teacher referral, to be labeled as language disordered.

There are certainly reasons to quarrel with this position, and many readers no doubt will. One very legitimate reason is that standardized tests with adequate psychometric properties —such as validity; standard errors of measurement; and large, representative norming samples—are not always available for testing all of the age levels, from toddlers to adolescents, or all the aspects of language, from phonology to pragmatics, that we would like to have tested (Adams, 2002; Plante & Vance, 1994). This issue is discussed more fully in Chapter 2. For now, suffice it to say that many tests in the language area are not constructed as well as they might be and that many age levels and areas of language are very sparsely covered, if at all, by standardized measures.

This situation has led some in the field to advocate use of informal or naturalistic assessment (e.g., Dunn, Flax, Sliwinski, & Aram, 1996; Lund & Duchan, 1993), because of its greater ecological validity (goodness-of-fit with the real world) and greater ability to assess dynamic, integrative aspects of language use without cultural biases (Gillam, Pena, & Miller, 1999; Gutierrez & Peña, 2001). As we will show when discussing the principles guiding the assessment process, describing language functioning in a child certainly necessitates such valid, dynamic evaluation. As Tomblin, Records, and Zhang (1996) point out, though, there are difficulties in establishing reliability for these naturalistic assessments. In addition, the limited task of identifying that a child's language performance is significantly below that of peers is not the same as specifying the components of that problem in detail. Sometimes this limited task can be accomplished more efficiently with the use of norm-referenced testing. Finally, most educational agencies require that some form of norm-referenced criteria be met in order for a child to qualify for publicly funded services. For these reasons, most clinicians find that they need to resort to standardized assessments, at least in the initial phase of an evaluation.

Still, real problems certainly exist with standardized tests, particularly if the child is developmentally very young; primarily disabled in an area such as pragmatics, in which few tests are available (Adams, 2002); or is from a culturally different background. One solution currently in vogue is to assess children on measures that are not reliant on cultural or linguistic knowledge (Campbell, Dollaghan, Needleman, & Janosky, 1997). These measures typically assess underlying "processing-dependent" skills, such as the ability to repeat nonsense words, which are thought to play a causal role in language disorder (see 'The Specific Disabilities Model' section in this chapter). While these measures appear to reliably distinguish language difference from language disorder (Rodekohr & Haynes, 2001), they do not provide the clinician with a picture of the child's linguistic capabilities, making them of limited use in planning intervention.

The solution advanced in this text and elaborated in Chapter 2 is that it is the clinician's obligation to be familiar with the psychometric properties necessary to make a test fair. The fairness of a test is established by its ability to demonstrate high levels of *reliability* and *validity* (see Chapter 2 for definitions). In addition, Dollaghan (2004) emphasizes the importance of choosing tests that are *accurate*. By this, she means that tests must provide empirical evidence of adequate *sensitivity* (the ability of a test to correctly identify children who have a disorder—the rate of false-negative results) and *specificity* (the ability of a test to correctly identify children as *not* having a disorder—the rate of false-positive results). The clinician's responsibility then becomes evaluating all available tests for properties of fairness and accuracy and choosing tests that come closest to meeting the necessary criteria. The more closely the tests used to identify language disorders approach these standards, the fewer additional assessments that should be necessary to establish a disorder. Conversely, the weaker the test's properties, the more necessary it is to supplement its score with data from other tests or from criterion-referenced or informal measures.

HOW LOW CAN YOU GO?

A second reason for quarreling with the proposed definition is that it gives no standard for deciding how low a score on a standardized test needs to fall to qualify a child for services. This problem, too, has not been resolved within the field. Clearly, an age-related criterion will not be helpful, because a 1-year delay in a 2-year-old represents a much more severe problem than a 1-year delay in an 8-year-old (Bishop, 1997; Plante, 1998). A more promising guideline would be a standard score cutoff such as 1, 1.5, or 2 standard deviations (SDs) below the mean, or a percentile score level, such as below the 10th percentile for the client's expected level of functioning. Again, of course, our confidence in the validity of the test is an important issue. But even if we can place a high degree of credence on the score, how low must it go?

In some agencies or school districts, cutoff scores for eligibility for services are mandated and the clinician must abide by them, having leeway only in choosing which instruments to use to measure performance. In other cases, this decision is made on the basis of caseload considerations. If, for example, a clinician were to accept into the caseload all the children who score more than 1 SD below the mean on a standardized test (about 17% of that particular population), the results might be chaos and rapid burnout. Restricting eligibility too narrowly, though, to children who score more than 2 SDs below the mean, for instance, would result in serving fewer than 2% of the population. This restriction would probably leave stranded many youngsters who genuinely need help. Unfortunately, clinicians often must decide what cutoff score to use without much guidance from any source.

We would suggest adopting the criterion used by Fey (1986) and Lee (1974) of below the 10th percentile, corresponding approximately to a standard score of 80 (about 1.25 SDs below the mean), as a middle-ground position. There are some limited empirical data to support this criterion (Tomblin, Records, & Zhang, 1996), at least for the kindergarten age group. However, it is important to point out that a score more than 1.25 SDs below the mean on only one measure of language performance would not be sufficient to identify a disorder. Tomblin, Records, and Zhang (1996) found that a child needed to score below the 10th percentile on at least two of a battery of language assessments to meet clinical criteria for impairment.

ASPECTS AND MODALITIES OF LANGUAGE

The third piece of our definition has to do with the range of communicative behaviors it encompasses. Both Bloom and Lahey (1978) and Lahey (1988) discussed language as comprising the following three major aspects, which are schematized in Figure 1-1:

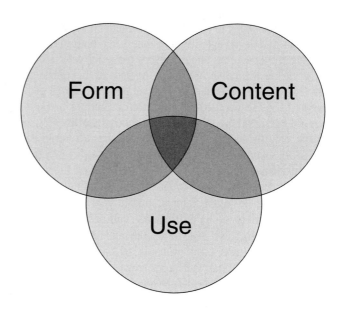

FIGURE 1-1 ✦ Bloom and Lahey's taxonomy of language. (Adapted from Lahey, M. [1988]. *Language disorders and language development.* New York: Macmillan.)

1. *Form*: including primarily syntax, morphology, and phonology
2. *Content*: essentially made up of the semantic components of language—knowledge of vocabulary and knowledge about objects and events
3. *Use*: the realm of pragmatics, which consists of the goals or functions of language, the use of context to determine what form to use to achieve these goals, and the rules for carrying out cooperative conversations

Lahey (1988) discussed and defined *language disorders* in terms of the interaction of these three aspects.

Chapman (1992), Miller (1981), and Miller and Paul (1995) talked about language in terms of its two primary modalities—comprehension and production—integrating each of the three aspects previously listed within these two modalities. From their viewpoint, *language disorders* would be defined according to the modalities primarily affected; the aspects or domains affected within these modalities are used to describe the language disorder once it is identified. Both *DSM-IV* and *ICD-10* also define language disorders primarily on the basis of the modality or modalities affected. Whether it is the domains and their interactions or the modalities of language that are used to define disorders, the important point is that disorders be defined broadly. We certainly want to be able to identify clients who fit the traditional idea of a child with a language impairment (LI) (the one who has trouble learning to put words together to make sentences), but we also want to be able to identify and therefore help the child like Tommy, who is described in the following text.

Tommy was a very easy baby. His mother remembers that he was happy to lie in his crib for hours on end, watching his mobile. By age 2 Tommy was using long, complicated sentences and knew the name of every model of vehicle on the road, as well as the names of most of the parts of their engines. At age 4 he took apart the family lawn mower and put it back together. However, his preschool teacher was concerned about him. He took almost no interest in the other children, choosing, when he spoke, to speak only to adults. When he did talk, he invariably asked complex but inappropriate questions on his few topics of interest, such as mechanical objects. He dwelled incessantly on a few events that were of great importance to him, such as the time the family car doors would not open. Tommy seemed very bright in many ways and did well on an IQ test that was part of his kindergarten screening. But in social settings, he just did not know how to relate, and his language was used primarily to talk about his own preoccupations rather than real interactions.

Tommy might be considered a child with Asperger syndrome (see Chapter 5), but the primary manifestation of his disorder is in social communication, not in the understanding or production of sounds, words, or sentences. It is important that a definition of *language disorder* allow a child such as Tommy to qualify for services, even though his problem is confined to the use of language for communicative purposes, with formal aspects of language relatively unaffected. So we want a definition of language disorders to include the notion that a deficit in any aspect or modality, no matter how broad or limited, will result in that child's receiving help.

DISCREPANCY-BASED CRITERIA

The last part of the definition to be considered is the idea of relating language deficits to the child's developmental level. Let's consider what this means. One way to describe children with developmental disabilities is to say that their developmental level is significantly lower than their chronological age. (This description is by no means complete; other conditions are necessary for a child to be diagnosed as having mental retardation, for example.) Mental age is an index of developmental level; it is an age-equivalent score derived from a standardized measure of cognitive ability.

In using mental age to diagnose language disorders, we try to use cognitive tests that do not involve the production or understanding of speech, or that do so as little as possible. We do not want to evaluate the cognitive ability of children with LIs on the basis of their language abilities. We already know that these children's language skills are not likely to be very good or they would not have been referred in the first place. Most intelligence tests use language-based items extensively, because in normal development, language and general intellectual level are very highly related. But some tests of cognitive skill are designed to assess aspects of thinking and problem solving that minimize the involvement of language. These tests are discussed in Chapter 2. For now, we simply need to be aware that procedures exist to assess a child's cognitive level by primarily examining nonverbal abilities.

Why might we want to use mental age, rather than chronological age, as a reference point to decide whether a child has a language disorder? For one thing, we usually would not expect a child's language skills to be better than the general level of development. Should a child functioning at a 3-year level overall be expected to achieve language skills commensurate with his chronological age of 8 years? Miller (1981) suggests that language level very rarely exceeds nonverbal cognitive level in the developmentally delayed population, even though the relationships between language and cognition are more complex and variable in normal development (Krassowski & Plante, 1997; Miller, Chapman, Branston, & Reichle, 1980; Notari, Cole, & Mills, 1992; Rice, Warren, & Betz, 2004). The *DSM-IV* also adopts nonverbal mental age as a reference point for language skills in identifying language disorders.

A second reason that discrepancy-based criteria for identifying language disorders have evolved is related to the needs of researchers who study language problems in children. Stark and Tallal (1981) set the stage for the widespread use of a discrepancy-based approach in research. They proposed defining specific language impairments (SLIs) according to a set of criteria involving IQs within the normal range, with language age scores at least 6 to 12 months less than the mental age found on the basis of the IQ test. They chose this approach to accomplish two goals: (1) to restrict the study of SLI to children with normal intelligence and (2) to "devise a standard approach to the selection of children with SLI" (p. 114) so that studies of this population could be consistent across various researchers in terms of their subject descriptions. This approach became the standard for researchers in child language disorders, and since no compelling alternative existed, it naturally spilled over into use in clinical settings.

Is the use of nonverbal mental age as a yardstick against which to measure language skill a matter of universal agreement? You probably guessed the answer! It's not. Lahey (1990) was perhaps the first to stake out a position against mental-age referencing. She pointed out that many psychometric problems are associated with measuring mental age. For one, it is not psychometrically acceptable to compare age scores derived from different tests of language and cognition that were not constructed to be comparable, were not standardized on the same populations, and may not have similar standard errors of measurement or ranges of variability. Second, there are fundamental problems in using age-equivalent scores at all to determine whether a child's score falls outside the normal range. These issues are discussed further in Chapter 2. Lahey also emphasized the theoretical difficulties of assessing nonverbal cognition, centering her argument on the justification for deciding which of the many possible aspects of nonlinguistic cognition ought to be the standard of comparison. For all of these reasons, Lahey suggested that chronological age is the most reliably measured and viable benchmark against which to reference language skill to identify language disorders.

Bishop (1997) offered a further argument. She pointed out that, in some cases, the linguistic skills in children with developmental disorders (such as William's syndrome or autism) have exceeded their cognitive levels, as demonstrated by Bellugi, Marks, Bihrle, and Sabo (1998) and Tager-Flusberg and Joseph (2003). It is therefore at least theoretically possible that language could lead cognitive development. If language intervention were offered, then, to all individuals with developmental disabilities, some might improve in cognitive performance as well as a result of the boost given by advancing language skills. Many clinicians would embrace this position, if only because it gives all children with developmental disabilities the possibility of being eligible for speech-language services, regardless of whether language skills were more poorly developed than other aspects of their functioning.

Remember Jamie? The two clinicians involved in his case differed on precisely this point. While the debate is still an active one, a consensus has begun to emerge on this point. ASHA (2000) argued strongly against "cognitive-referencing" in making decisions about eligibility for services. A major criticism is that different combinations of tests can yield different eligibility recommendations for the same student. How can this be? Often, young children with LI show an uneven language profile, with severe deficits in morphology and syntax and relative strengths in vocabulary knowledge (Abbeduto & Boudreau, 2004; Rice, 2000, 2004). Therefore, we might expect vocabulary scores to be more in line with nonverbal IQ scores, while tests of morphosyntax might result in a very large discrepancy. A second criticism is that longitudinal studies of children with language disorders have reported a drop in nonverbal IQ scores over time (Botting, 2005; Stothard, Snowling, Bishop, Chipchase, & Kaplan, 1998). It is unlikely that this reflects an actual loss in ability but rather that nonverbal assessments are rarely "pure" measures of nonverbal ability. The majority of nonverbal tests incorporate verbal directions, and many linguistically able children use verbal strategies to help them reason out the answers. This puts the child with LI at a distinct disadvantage. Third, the degree of discrepancy between verbal and nonverbal abilities does not necessarily predict a child's responsiveness to intervention. Research has shown that children with generally depressed nonverbal scores can still benefit from therapy (Fey, Long, & Cleave, 1994). Finally, a categorical denial of services to children because of generally depressed nonverbal IQ scores is not consistent with the ethos of the Individuals with Disabilities Education Act (IDEA Amendments of 1997, Public Law 105-17), which stipulates that services be determined on an individual basis (Whitmire, 2000).

But even if we do not use mental age-based discrepancy criteria to identify children with language disorders, mental age still provides us with some guidelines to help in determining the goals of intervention. By getting a general idea of a child's developmental level, through standardized tests as well as through instruments that measure adaptive behavior, we can determine what behaviors are reasonable to target in an intervention program. We would not expect a child with retardation, for example, to work on language goals appropriate for his or her chronological age, even if that age were used as the reference point to identify the need for language intervention. Instead, we would want to evaluate at what level the child is functioning currently and target language behaviors closer to overall developmental level. Using what Fey (1986) called *intralinguistic profiling* (see Figure 2-2), we can graph the child's skills in a range of areas, including semantics, syntax, phonology, nonverbal mental age, and motor skill. We can then make a comparison among these areas and target language skills that are currently most depressed, attempting to bring them more into line with overall developmental level. This strategy is discussed in more detail in Chapters 2 and 3.

The use of nonverbal mental age as a reference point for defining language disorders may not be agreed on by all SLPs, as we have seen. Still, all language pathologists today could agree that some such reference point should be established. But it hasn't always been so. Only recently have children with a wide range of language disorders associated with a variety of neurological and physiological conditions been considered to have something in common that requires the services of a specialist in language and its disorders. Let's talk a little about how this change has taken place.

A Brief History of the Field of Language Pathology

Descriptions of the syndrome of disorders of language learning in children date back to at least the early nineteenth century. Gall (1825) was perhaps the first to describe children with poor understanding and use of speech and to differentiate them from the mentally retarded. Subsequently, a great many exciting new discoveries about the relations between the brain and language behavior were made by neurologists such as Broca (1861) and Wernicke (1874). The disorders Gall first identified were thought to be parallel to the aphasias these neurologists were studying in adults. For the first century of the existence of the study of language learning and its disorders, neurologists dominated the field, focusing attention on the physiological substrate of language behavior.

The neurologist Samuel T. Orton (1937) can perhaps be thought of as the father of the modern practice of child language disorders. He emphasized the importance not only of neurological but also of behavioral descriptions of the syndrome and pointed out the connections between disorders of language learning and difficulties in the acquisition of reading and writing. In the 1940s and 1950s, other medical professionals, such as psychiatrists and pediatricians, took an interest in children who seemed to be unable to learn language but did not have mental retardation or deafness. Gesell and Amatruda (1947) were pioneers in developmental pediatrics; they devised innovative techniques for evaluating language development and recognized the condition they called "infantile aphasia." Benton (1959, 1964) provided the fullest descriptions of children with this syndrome and is credited with evolving the concept of a specific disorder of language learning that is structured by excluding other syndromes, rather than by parallels to adult aphasia.

At about the same time as these medical practitioners were refining notions of language disorders, another group of workers also was advancing concepts about children who failed to learn language. Ewing (1930), McGinnis, Kleffner, and Goldstein (1956), and Myklebust (1954, 1971) were all educators of the deaf and, as such, had developed a variety of techniques for teaching language to children who did not talk or hear. They all noticed that some deaf children's language skills were worse than could be expected on the basis of their hearing impairment alone. This observation led them to focus more interest on the LI itself and to attempt to develop more effective methods of remediation for children who did not succeed with the standard approaches that were used to teach language to other children with hearing impairments.

However, until the 1950s, no unified field of endeavor addressed the problems of the language-learning child, considered these problems to be disorders of language itself, rather than a result of some other syndrome ("infantile aphasia" or deafness, for example), or treated language disorders in children regardless of whether the disorder was caused by deafness, mental retardation, or presumed neurological dysfunction. Aram and Nation (1982) give credit to three individuals for developing this new field: Mildred A. McGinnis, Helmer R. Myklebust, and Muriel E. Morley. These pioneers integrated the information currently available on language disorders in deaf and "aphasic" children and devised educational approaches that could be used to remediate the language dysfunctions demonstrated by these children.

McGinnis (1963) developed the "association method" for teaching language to "aphasic" children. This method was very influential in the development of the field of language disorders, providing the first highly structured, comprehensive approach to language intervention. McGinnis also was one of the first to distinguish between two types of language problems seen in children: what she called expressive, or motor, aphasia (what we today would call *specific expressive language disorder*) and receptive, or sensory, aphasia (what we would term *receptive language disorder*).

Morley (1957) was instrumental in applying information on normal language development to the problem of treating children with a language disorder and was one of the first individuals from a speech pathology background to push language and its disorders into the purview of the "speech therapist." She fostered the use of detailed descriptions of children's language behavior in making diagnoses and planning intervention programs. She also was important in providing definitions that allowed clinicians to distinguish language from articulation disorders.

Myklebust (1954) went, perhaps, the furthest in establishing a new and distinct field of study and practice, which he dubbed "language pathology." Like Morley and McGinnis, he was interested in differential diagnosis. He developed schemes for classifying language disorders in children, which he called

"auditory disorders," and for differentiating them from deafness and mental retardation. But Myklebust, like Orton, also was concerned with the continuities between disorders of oral language acquisition and their consequences for the acquisition of literacy skills. In founding the new discipline of language pathology, Myklebust pointed the way toward considering language disorders in this broad context, including difficulties not only in producing and comprehending oral language but also in the use of written forms of language.

At about the same time that the field of language pathology was being established, the study of language itself was being revolutionized by the introduction of Chomsky's (1957) theory of transformational grammar. This innovation led to an explosion in research on child language acquisition that the new discipline could use. In the 1960s and 1970s, as child language research expanded in focus from syntax to semantics to pragmatics and phonology, language pathology followed in its footsteps, broadening our view of the relevant aspects of language that needed to be described and addressed in clinical practice. The vast amount of new information on normal development being compiled made it possible for language pathologists to describe a child's language behavior in great detail and to make specific comparisons to normal development on a variety of forms and functions. Further, the large database on normal acquisition provided a blueprint of the language development process that could serve as a curriculum guide for planning intervention. As we shall see when we talk about models of language disorders, this possibility has greatly influenced how language pathology is conceptualized and practiced today.

■ TERMINOLOGY

The changes over the years in how language disorders are conceptualized also have influenced the terms used to label them. A variety of names have been given to the problems we have been discussing, including *language impairment, language disability, language disorder, language delay, language deviance,* and *childhood* or *congenital aphasia* or *dysphasia.* At certain points in the history of language pathology, some terms have predominated, whereas others were used less commonly, if at all. The terms in use today differ somewhat from the terms used even 10 or 15 years ago. However, language pathologists still disagree to some degree about which terms are most appropriate.

The use of terms to label a problem is neither arbitrary nor trivial. It usually reflects something about the beliefs and assumptions of the people who use the terms. For example, people who favor making it illegal for a woman to voluntarily terminate a pregnancy refer to their movement as "pro-life." Those who support this right refer to their opponents as "anti-abortionists" and to themselves as "pro-choice." Clearly, the use of these labels reflects very differing attitudes toward the same set of positions. Let's see how the terms used to talk about language problems also can reflect attitudes and assumptions.

Perhaps the oldest term used to label a language disorder is *childhood* or *congenital aphasia*. As we've seen, this term has been used since the 19th century to describe children who, in the absence of other disorders, failed to learn language normally. This type of language disorder, the kind not associated with other known primary handicapping conditions, is only a subset of the disorders of language learning now treated by SLPs. But its identification shaped the field of language pathology.

The use of the term *childhood* or *congenital aphasia* grew out of the belief that developmental disorders of language paralleled those seen in adults with acquired aphasias. As we will see, the evidence for comparable brain damage in children with LI is lacking. For this reason—because language disorders in children do not seem to have the same root in localized brain lesions as do adult aphasias—the terms *aphasia* and *dysphasia* seem too weighted toward neurological explanations of dubious value. Most SLPs no longer use them.

The terms *language delay* and *language deviance* carry assumptions, too, although of a somewhat different nature. Language delay seems to imply that the client's language is just like that of a younger child and that the "delayed" child will, like someone delayed by a missed bus, eventually arrive at the desired destination—normal development. The term *language deviance*, on the other hand, suggests that the child's language development is not just slower than normal but is different in some important, qualitative way. What is the evidence for the positions these terms imply?

A variety of studies (Aram, Ekelman, & Nation, 1984; Bishop, Price, Dale, & Plomin, 2003; Paul, 1993b; Paul & Cohen, 1984; Rescorla, 2005; Snowling, Adams, Bishop, & Stothard, 2001; Snowling, Bishop, & Stothard, 2000; Stothard, Burns, & Griffin, 1998) reported that language disorders identified in the preschool period tend to persist in a majority of children, often resulting in diminished ability to acquire written forms of language. Although it is difficult to know for any particular preschooler whether the ultimate destination of normal functioning will be reached, it is clearly safe to say that a preschooler with a language-learning difficulty is at risk for chronic language and academic problems.

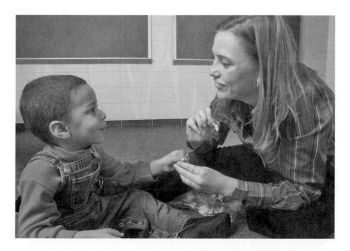

Young children with language impairments are often labeled "language delayed."

Using the term *delayed* seems to make a prognostic statement that is not necessarily justified by the evidence available.

There has been a long-running debate in the literature about whether children with language disorders show *deviant* acquisition patterns—patterns unlike those seen in younger normal children—or whether they exhibit a slowed-down version of normal development. Early studies (Lee, 1966; Menyuk, 1964) reported that there were qualitative differences in the linguistic systems of normal and disordered children. But more recent research, summarized by Leonard (1989, 1997) and Rice (2004), suggests that children with language disorders do resemble younger normal speakers in the general nature of their linguistic systems and in most aspects of the order of acquisition.

If we were to compare children, then, on the basis of some measure of linguistic maturity such as mean length of utterance (MLU) rather than on the basis of age, we would generally find that the structures used by children at similar language levels were similar. A 4-year-old with an MLU equal to that of a normal 2½-year-old would use language structures very similar to those used by the younger child with normal language function. But there would be a few differences. Certain forms—particular grammatical morphemes, for example—are especially difficult for children with language learning problems to acquire. These difficult forms are acquired by children with language problems later than other forms learned contemporaneously by normally developing children. For example, "-ing" marking is produced in normal development at about the same time as the plural /s/ marker. But children with LIs typically use the plural /s/ considerably later than "-ing." If we compared the language production of our 4-year-old with a LI to our 2½-year-old with normal language function and with the same MLU, we would probably find that both used "-ing" marking but only the younger child used plural /s/.

Does this mean that the language development of the child with an impairment is deviant, or is it simply slower than normal? The answer to this question seems to be, "It depends." It depends on whether we mean that the system of a child with a disorder is an exact slow-motion version or one that would clearly be recognized as such, with a few subtle differences. The answer to this question, though, may be less important than knowing that in general, with a few exceptions, a child who has trouble learning language will follow the normal sequence of development. This knowledge has important clinical implications. It can be taken to suggest that the normal sequence can serve as a reasonable guide in deciding the order in which to target language forms and structures in intervention. We'll talk more about this implication when we discuss models of language disorders.

The implications of the terms *language deviant*, *language delayed*, and *developmental* or *congenital aphasia* or *dysphasia* lead us, then, to believe that their use ought to be avoided. It seems important to use only those terms whose assumptions we have examined carefully and can accept with confidence. For the terms in question, this standard has not, in our opinion, been met.

Another limitation of these labels is that they imply that all of the challenges faced by the child with language learning difficulties originate within the child and his or her "faulty" development. The variation we see in children with language disorders immediately suggests that this is not the case. Two children with the same diagnosis may have very different levels of functioning in everyday life, just as two children with similar levels of functioning may have quite different speech and language profiles. In explaining these differences and figuring out what to do about them, we need to consider environmental factors as well as child-specific factors.

The World Health Organization (WHO, 2001) provides a framework for considering the strengths and needs of the child in a more holistic fashion. This framework is provided in Box 1-1. Like the *ICD-10,* the framework begins with a consideration of *Body Structures and Functions.* These involve physical or psychological (including language) impairments experienced by the child. This component of the framework is neutral with respect to cause or severity. It simply states that the child is different in some respect to his or her peer group.

Activities and Participation requires us to consider the impact of the child's impairment on activities of daily living, including communication and education. The focus is on both strengths and restrictions and gives us a better picture of the child's communication needs in everyday situations, especially the classroom.

Finally, *Contextual Factors* are those additional factors that impact on the child's situation. These include environmental factors such as people in the child's environment, the use of technology, social policies, and attitudes. Here we are referring to the ways in which we can work not only with the child but also with the people in the child's environment to maximize participation and success. In using this concept, we will be invoking what we refer to a little later as the *systems model* of communication problems. This model looks not only at what's wrong with the child but also at what the environment contributes to the child's difficulties. Further, it looks for ways to change both the child and the environment to alleviate some of these problems.

This framework moves away from labeling individuals and focuses instead on building a profile of strength and needs. This is likely to be more useful to us in planning our interventions, but labels do have a role in helping us communicate with other professionals and in evaluating research focused on the populations we see. With this in mind, *language impairment, language disorder,* and *language disability* are the terms we generally use to talk about the differences and difficulties with which our clients must cope.

Kamhi (1998) has suggested one additional distinction in terminology that may be useful for us. Researchers generally try to study the nature of language disorders in children with "pure" language disabilities, those uncontaminated by mental retardation or other kinds of deficits. The children in their studies are typically referred to as having specific language impairment (SLI), meaning that their problem is more or less confined, or specific, to language (although, as you might guess, there are some debates on that point, too!). Kamhi argues that these children with "pure" language disorders are relatively rare compared to the population of children treated by working speech-language clinicians. This larger population, who he refers to as having *developmental language disorders (DLDs),* includes children with lower IQs and more concomitant problems. The distinction between research subjects in studies of SLI and the broad range of children with DLD may be important for us to keep in mind as we evaluate the results of research that we read in this field and attempt to apply it to our clinical work.

We need to say one more thing about terminology. Since the Americans with Disabilities Act of 1990 (Public Law 101-336, 1997) was passed by Congress, it has been recommended that we use "people-first" language in referring to our clients. This means putting the person before the problem in the label; saying, for example, *children with language impairments* instead of *language-impaired children* or *children with autism* instead of *autistic children.* This somewhat awkward diction is supposed to focus our attention on seeing our clients as people who have problems, rather than focusing on the problem in isolation from the person.

ETIOLOGY OF SPECIFIC LANGUAGE DISORDERS

Although we occasionally hear in the media about the detrimental effects of television or working mothers on children's language development, it is generally agreed that language acquisition is too robust and deeply ingrained in our biological

---

BOX 1-1	**Terminology Defined by the World Health Organization**

Body Structures and Function—Impairments are problems, such as significant deviation or loss, in the anatomical parts of the body (organs, limbs and their components) and/or the physiological functions of the body, including psychological functions.

Activities and Participation—Any restriction in a person's ability to address the needs of daily living or execute specific tasks; these can change in different situations or stages of life.

Contextual Factors—The physical, social, and attitudinal environment in which people live and conduct their lives. Thus, an individual may be affected not only by his or her own impairment or disability but also by the attitudes and biases of others with whom the person comes in contact.

Adapted from the *International Classification of Functioning, Disability and Health.* Geneva: The World Health Organization, 2001 (accessed from www3.who.int/icf/).

equipment to be easily derailed (Locke, 2005; Pinker, 1994). Instead, research investigating the causes of SLI has capitalized on our knowledge of the brain regions important for language and the observation that LIs (both spoken and written) tend to run in families (see Leonard, 1998; Newbury & Monaco, 2002; Ullman & Pierpont, 2005, for review).

Investigations into the brain basis of SLI stemmed from the early neurologists' conviction that difficulties in children's learning language were analogous to the loss of language seen in adults with acquired aphasias. This notion evolved from observations that "aphasic" children often appeared quite bright and able in other aspects of development. They also seemed to have normal affective bonds to the people around them and were not emotionally disturbed. Their inability to acquire language normally was attributed to some sort of neurological dysfunction thought to be comparable to localized brain lesions that resulted in aphasia in adults.

A multitude of studies that attempted to identify these neurological lesions in children with language deficits (see Webster & Shevell, 2004, for review) failed to find brain structure or function differences that were either common to all the children studied or specific to children with language disorders. Furthermore, children with focal lesions of the type that lead to severe aphasia in adults do not show long-lasting LI of the kind seen in SLI (Bates, 2004). This is not to say that children with language disorders do not have neurological involvement but simply that the involvement they do have does not appear to be similar to the localized pathology seen in adults with aphasia.

More subtle differences in brain structure and function may become apparent thanks to advances in brain imaging techniques. Although few studies currently exist, these studies provide some evidence for differences in the development of the brain. Galaburda, Sherman, Rosen, Aboitiz, and Geschwind (1985) studied postmortem brains of four individuals with language and literacy impairments. These individuals had an increase of ectopias (excess cells in the wrong area of the brain) and dysplasias (disoriented large cells that disrupt the layered structure of the brain). Typically, individuals have asymmetrical brains; language structures (such as the planum temporale) tend to be bigger in the left hemisphere. However, children with SLI have generally smaller and more symmetrical brain hemispheres (Leonard, Lombardino, Walsh, Eckert, Mockler, Rowe, Williams, & DeBose, 2002). Studies of adults with language difficulties have revealed that they were more likely than individuals with no history of LI to have an extra sulcus (one of the grooves on the brain) in Broca's area, in either brain hemisphere (Clark & Plante, 1998). It is important to realize that no one pattern of brain architecture has been consistently shown in all individuals with LI. Instead, these structural differences appear to act as risk factors for language difficulty. What is interesting about these studies is that they all point to prenatal influences on early brain development that might affect how the regions of the brain are connected to and communicate with one another, increasing the risk for LI.

SLI tends to run in families, suggesting that genetic factors may be involved in the etiology of language disorder. However, families share environments as well as genes; we therefore need more convincing evidence of a genetic effect. Throughout the 1990s, a number of studies of twins raised together were published that provided such evidence. The logic of a twin study is as follows: monozygotic (identical) twins are genetically identical and share the same family environment. Dizygotic (fraternal) twins also share the same home environment, but they share only 50% of their polymorphic genes. (Polymorphic genes are simply genes that show variation from person to person and so can explain individual differences, such as eye color.) Therefore, if identical twins resemble each other more in terms of language behavior than do fraternal twins, then we assume that this similarity is genetically mediated. This is indeed the case (see Bishop, 2002, for review). More important, certain language tasks have been shown to be highly "heritable," meaning that we can identify aspects of language functioning that are influenced by genetic factors. These include non-sense word repetition (Bishop, Adams, & Norbury, 2005; Bishop, North, & Donlan, 1996) and marking tense (past tense -ed; third person singular -s; Bishop, Adams, & Norbury, 2005).

The mapping of the human genome has resulted in great optimism that we will be able to find the specific gene (or genes) involved in language disorder. Unfortunately, progress to date has been slow, not the least because of the heterogeneity of the disorder. However, in 2001, researchers in England identified a gene, *FOXP2*, that caused a severe form of speech and language impairment in a three-generational family, the KE family (see Bishop, 2002; Marcus & Fisher, 2003, for a review). This gene was trumpeted as the "gene for grammar" by the popular press but, of course, the reality is much more complicated than that. First, the KE family does not have a typical profile of LI. They present with a severe oromotor dyspraxia that results in articulation deficits as well as more pervasive impairments with vocabulary and grammar. Second, systematic searches for genes in more typical clinical populations have not identified *FOXP2* as a risk factor (SLI Consortium, 2002). Third, *FOXP2* is not specifically associated with grammar—it is expressed not only in the brain but also in the heart, lungs, and gut. It is also expressed in other species, including mice, and we have yet to find a talking mouse!

So what does this gene have to do with language? The short answer is we are not entirely sure and geneticists are working hard to find out. What we do know is that *FOXP2* acts as a "chief executive officer" (Marcus & Fisher, 2003) in that it is involved with controlling the genetic programs of cells. Therefore, one hypothesis is that *FOXP2* is important in the embryonic development of brain structures associated with language. This hypothesis is supported by brain imaging studies of the KE family showing subtle abnormalities in brain volume and activation (Vargha-Khadem, Gadian, Copp, & Mishkin, 2005).

One final point should be made before leaving this section. Few clinicians share our enthusiasm for etiological studies that highlight genetic and neurological origins of LI, reasoning that if the problem is in the brain or in the genes, then surely we are powerless to do anything about it. But this is not true. For a start, although identical twins resemble one another on language tests, the resemblance is not perfect, suggesting that environmental factors influence the severity of impairment. Second, it is possible to influence the development of areas of the brain through increased environmental input and training (Tallal, Miller, Bedi, Byman, Wang, Nagarajan, Schreiner, Jenkins, & Merzenich, 1996). Finally, as Bishop (2002) points out, once we understand how a gene acts, it is often possible to intervene with positive outcomes (diet restrictions used to combat the effects of phenylketonuria, which is now identified through newborn screening, is an excellent example). Studies of genes and brains do not suggest that the environment is unimportant, nor do they make any predictions about how individuals will respond to environmental interventions.

MODELS OF CHILD LANGUAGE DISORDERS

A model is simply a way to represent how we think something works. Like a label, a model usually embodies some of our beliefs and assumptions about the thing being represented. The way we conceptualize the model influences what we choose to do about the thing it represents. For example, if we believe that language disorders arise from faulty neurological functioning, we treat them very differently than if we believe they arise from inadequate input from the environment. That's why being aware of the model being used is important when discussing a language disorder. It is quite possible for professionals to disagree about what model best represents the phenomenon of language disorder; in fact, there is no one model to which every professional in the field subscribes. But it is not possible to discuss how these differences influence clinical practice unless the models and assumptions are clear in our minds. Let's look at some of the models that have been used to discuss language disorders in children.

THE SYSTEMS MODEL

Viewing a language disorder from a systems perspective means that we do not assume that all of the communication problems are "in" the child but, rather, are in the relationship between communication partners. This implies that not all the solutions involve changing the child; some involve changing the environment (Nelson, 1998; Prizant & Wetherby, 2005). Although at first glance this model may not seem relevant to the SLP, it does have some applications that are important for extending our thinking about language disorders in children, especially our thinking about how to overcome a child's handicaps or barriers to mainstream participation.

First, this model is important in deciding what constitutes a language disorder, as opposed to a language difference. If a child speaks a dialect other than that used by the teacher or other conversational partners, the child may be viewed as having

a problem or disorder. In truth, though, the disorder may be in the mismatch between the child's speech style and that used in the particular school or day-care center. To consider the child as having the disorder would imply that the child was in need of "remediation" or should be taught the dominant language or dialect. To see this problem, instead, as a mismatch between the client and the context means that some change may need to take place in the child, but some change in the communication environment also may be necessary. Perhaps individuals in the environment simply need to be made aware of the dialectical variations that are operating, or perhaps it may be that the teacher needs to discuss the concept of register variation with the student (see Chapter 6). The teacher can help the student to identify appropriate contexts for different language forms so that the child can see that it is possible, and at times preferable, to talk differently at home and at school. In any case, the problem is seen as one of interaction, rather than as residing solely in the client. Because a systems model suggests that the interactive environment should be the focus of change, it also is helpful when deciding on a management strategy for a culturally different client. In this case, the problem may not be so much in the client's communication as in the reaction it gets from others. A systems perspective allows us to work both with the client and with the communication partners to make the interaction more effective.

Cultural and dialectical differences are not the only context in which a systems model can be useful. When working with clients who have severe disabilities, it often helps to think about how the environment can be changed to facilitate the communication or to reduce handicapping conditions rather than focusing solely on what the clients need to learn to communicate. For example, perhaps a nonverbal client with autism is frustrated because he cannot get people to understand that he wants to watch a certain television program. This frustration leads to aggressive or self-abusive behavior. Although it is true that the problem of being unable to get his message across is "in" the individual with autism, perhaps the

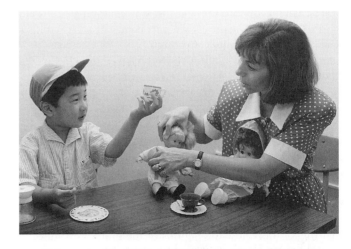

Systems models aid in understanding cultural differences in language use.

environment can be modified so that the boy can communicate, using the means at his disposal, to short-circuit the cycle of frustration and aggression. Perhaps a switch with pictures that label different channels that the boy can operate himself can be attached to the television, obviating the need for assistance. Perhaps the adults in the environment can learn to recognize the client's signal for assistance and respond before he reaches the level of frustration that leads to the maladaptive behavior. This would eliminate the mismatch between the form of communication and the signals expected by the environment.

An important implication of the systems perspective is that it does not require that "normal" or "standard" levels of language use be the target. This model often is an especially sensible approach when thinking about intervention for clients with severe or profound disabilities, when chronologically age-appropriate language skills are not the goal, and when we are concerned with finding some way for the client to send and receive messages to important people in his or her life. It is wise to remember that the environment must be responsive for communication to be rewarding for any client. Even if we believe that the disorder is "in" the client, we can always ask how the environment might make communication more meaningful and profitable for children, to encourage their best efforts and to reduce their handicap in any given situation. In these ways, the systems perspective can be a beneficial adjunct to our thinking about any language disorder.

THE CATEGORICAL MODEL

This approach to classification organizes language disorders on the basis of the syndromes of behavior they accompany and is basically a medical model. It attempts to identify the best categorical or diagnostic label to apply to a child who is not using language as well as would be expected for the age level; it attempts to identify similarities among children with similar diagnoses; and it implies that the diagnostic categories used play a causal, or etiological, role in the language disorder. In this model, language disorders are classified on the basis of the known medical conditions—or lack of them—that they accompany. They could be identified as those associated with mental retardation, hearing impairment, autism, other behavioral or emotional conditions, and known neurological damage and those with no known concomitant, which were referred to as "developmental aphasia or dysphasia" in older literature or as "specific language impairment" in more recent sources.

This approach has many advantages. It is a readily understandable and common-sense way to identify the kind of problem a child has, and it quickly summarizes how a client is different from other children. Also, these category labels are often necessary for the child to qualify for services from schools and other agencies.

However, this orientation to language disorders is not without difficulties. Bloom and Lahey (1978) were the first to discuss the problems associated with this model. Their work and that of Lahey (1988) pointed out that although the categories

are assumed by the model to be causative of the language delay, it is often difficult to see how this can be so. For example, here are capsule descriptions of two 12-year-olds, Sam and Max, each with an IQ of 50.

Sam is a little charmer. When he meets you, he walks right up to you, shakes your hand, and says, "Hi, I'm Sam. What's your name?" In school, he gets reading and writing instruction and does well on the primary-level readers that have been adapted for his use. Sam is in a special vocational training program in which he works in his middle school's cafeteria each lunch period, helping to refill the steam trays. All of the cafeteria workers are fond of him and look forward to hearing him tell them what he did in class each morning when he comes in for work at noontime. Sam follows the cafeteria staff's directions easily and cheerfully and doesn't get confused when he is told to do a new task, as long as it is explained slowly with some demonstration.

Max works with Sam in the cafeteria at lunchtime and does a good job at the tasks that he's practiced for some time. He seems quiet, though, and rarely talks spontaneously. Even when spoken to, he answers in one or two words, which are often so misarticulated that the cafeteria workers don't understand what he says. Max's teachers and parents have worked hard to try to improve his social communication and to increase his spontaneous speech, but it's an uphill battle. He just doesn't seem to have much to say to anyone, and even when he does, he can't seem to put more than two or three words together to say it.

Did Max's mental retardation cause his language problem? How can it be so when Sam, with the same IQ, has language skills that are far superior? Clearly, the categorical label cannot always explain the level of language performance we see in a given child. Then, too, talking about causality is a slippery business. For example, we may say that a child's language disorder is caused by mental retardation, but what caused the retardation? It could be a chromosomal abnormality, such as Down syndrome; a metabolic disorder, such as phenylketonuria; birth trauma; or a postnatal infection, such as meningitis. Mental retardation itself is really just a description of a group of behaviors that we infer to be the result of some form of central nervous system damage caused by something that we may or may not be able to identify. And even if we could identify what caused the retardation at one level, we can always ask for a deeper explanation. If we know it was caused by Down syndrome, for example, we still don't know how a person's having one extra chromosome results in either mental impairment or language disorder.

The example of Sam and Max highlights another difficulty with the categorical system. Sam and Max are clearly very different children, with different language abilities, despite having the same diagnostic classification of moderate mental retardation. Although diagnostic categories are often thought to be useful because they describe similarities among clients, in fact two clients with the same diagnosis are often as different as night and day. Take Sharon and Elizabeth, for example.

Sharon is an 8-year-old girl with a 60-dB bilateral hearing loss. The loss was discovered before she was 2 years of age, primarily because a history of hearing impairment in the family made the parents very sensitive to the issue. When it was diagnosed, she was immediately fitted with hearing aids, which her parents very conscientiously made sure that she wore. She entered a mainstream preschool program at age 3 and received consultative services from the state's hearing impairment program. She started kindergarten at age 6 and has been able to function in a mainstream classroom ever since. Her teachers have consistently received support services from the state's aural rehabilitation specialists. Sharon's language is marked by some features of "deaf speech" but is intelligible to those who know her, and with amplification, she can understand much of the oral language she hears. She is very popular among her classmates and is often invited to their homes to play after school. She keeps up with the current slang, describing her music teacher as "awesome." She performs just slightly below grade level in reading and language arts.

When Elizabeth was 2, she had not yet started to talk, but because she was the fourth child in the family, people told her mother it was just because everyone else talked for her and she didn't need to learn. It wasn't until Elizabeth was 3 that her mother mentioned to her family doctor that Elizabeth wasn't talking. The doctor recommended a hearing test and discovered that Elizabeth had a bilateral loss of 60 dB. The audiologist prescribed hearing aids, but by then Elizabeth's mother was pregnant again and just couldn't manage the aids along with everything else. Elizabeth wore them sporadically until she was 5. At that time, she failed a kindergarten screening. After a thorough evaluation, it was decided to enroll her in a special school for the deaf. The teachers there saw to it that she wore her aids at least during school hours. By age 8, Elizabeth was producing some three- and four-word sentences with moderate intelligibility and had an expressive vocabulary of 300 to 400 words. She was beginning to receive some reading instruction but could not yet read any words spontaneously.

Sharon and Elizabeth both have the same degree of hearing loss but very different profiles of language skills. The similarity in their diagnostic classifications does not help us to understand these differences.

A second objection that Bloom and Lahey raised to the categorical system was that children often do not fit neatly into one of these diagnostic classifications. The majority of children with autism, for example, are considered to have mental retardation, as well. So it seems difficult to establish just one cause for the language disorder when more than one categorical label is appropriate.

Naremore (1980) raised another objection: knowing the child's etiological classification may not be much help in deciding what to do for the child. Knowing that a child has mental retardation, for example, does not tell us what kind of language skills the child has, nor does it tell us what intervention goals are appropriate or what approach will succeed best. The etiological category is not terribly useful for guiding clinical practice. Certainly, knowing that a child has a hearing impairment suggests that amplification or cochlear implantation

will be part of the intervention, but this knowledge alone does not answer all the questions about the child's program. Should she be taught to speak, or should an alternative modality, such as sign language, be introduced? This decision is not very different from the decision that must be made in the case of a nonverbal child who is not hearing impaired. So, while it is certainly useful to know that the child has impaired hearing, and we would certainly want to know it, this knowledge in and of itself is not sufficient for clinical management. The categorical model may be helpful for initial placement of children within intervention settings or classrooms, although even for this purpose it will not be completely sufficient. Some other classification schemes will be needed to assess LI thoroughly and to plan intervention.

THE SPECIFIC DISABILITIES MODEL

When we use a categorical model to describe language disorders, we are attempting to describe how the language behaviors of children within one of our categories are similar to each other and different from normal. The specific disabilities model, on the other hand, tries to show us how individuals with language disorders differ in some underlying cognitive abilities relative to other abilities, or how they show within-child variation. In this model, an attempt is made to profile underlying abilities and disabilities and strengths and weaknesses that are believed to influence language development. The idea is to teach to the child's strengths and either remediate or work around the weaknesses (Figure 1-2).

In the 1960s and early 1970s, psychologists and psycholinguists (e.g., Osgood & Miron, 1963; Wepman, Jones, Bock, & Van Pelt, 1960) attempted to devise models to describe how various information-processing capacities interacted to enable the comprehension and production of language. Figure 1-2 gives an example of one of these models. The representation of the interaction of abilities, or capacities, such as perception, discrimination, association, closure, conceptualization, and memory, is demonstrated in this illustration. The models also were used to represent the sequential order in which the processes, or capacities, were thought to be involved in the production and comprehension of language. As Figure 1-2 illustrates, the models were primarily linear, going sequentially in one direction from capacities thought to be lower level, or simpler, to those thought to be higher level, or more complex.

The precise content of the specific disabilities thought to affect language development changes with time and increased experimental investigation. Two "cognitive" theories of LI currently receiving a great deal of research (and clinical) attention are described below.

The Auditory Perceptual Deficit Approach

Because spoken language relies primarily on the processing of auditory information, the specific abilities thought to be most closely associated with oral language disorders are usually identified as auditory processes. This has led many practitioners to the belief that the identification and remediation of specific abilities in the auditory domain will lead to improved language.

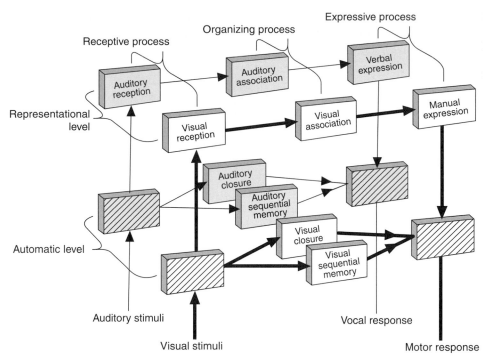

FIGURE 1-2 ✦ Model of the Illinois Test of Psycholinguistic Abilities. (Used with permission from Kirk, S., McCarthy, J., and Kirk, W. [1968]. *Illinois test of psycholinguistic abilities* [revised edition]. Urbana, IL: University of Illinois Press.)

Research examining a variety of auditory skills in children with LIs has shown that these children often perform worse than their peers with normal auditory and language functioning (see Rosen, 2003; Tallal, 2000, for review). In addition, audiometric tests of "auditory processing" are often used to diagnose language and learning disorders, and on these tasks, too, children with difficulty learning language often do poorly (ASHA, 2005). Tallal and Piercy (Tallal, 2000; Tallal & Piercy, 1978) have assembled a large body of evidence demonstrating that children with SLI show difficulty in behavioral tests when asked to identify auditory stimuli that are very brief or are followed quickly by another stimulus. Such a deficit is hypothesized to be detrimental to language development because many phonological and grammatical contrasts are signaled by brief, rapidly occurring sequences in the continuous speech stream (Bishop & McArthur, 2004; Joanisse & Seidenberg, 2003).

Should we therefore accept the "auditory deficit" hypothesis as an explanation for language disorders? There are a number of sources of evidence that suggest this might be a premature conclusion. First, we might predict that if auditory processing deficits played a causal role in language disorder, then the presence of such a deficit should be necessary and sufficient to cause language learning difficulties. In other words, all children with language disorders should exhibit auditory impairments, and all children with auditory impairments should exhibit some degree of language difficulty. This does not appear to be the case. Numerous studies have failed to replicate Tallal's key findings (Bishop, 1999; Rosen, 2003). Although as a group, children with LI score below the average scores of groups of typical children on auditory tasks, some of them do just fine. By the same token, many typically developing children have difficulties on the auditory tasks but have perfectly normal language skills. Even more perplexing, children with known perceptual deficits (children with mild-moderate hearing impairments) outperform children with SLI on syntactic tests (Norbury, Bishop, & Briscoe, 2001, 2002), suggesting there is more to LI than perceptual difficulties.

A second important clinical question concerns whether identifying auditory deficits is necessary to choose specific intervention procedures. Tallal and colleagues (1996) postulated that if poor auditory processing played a causal role in LI, then improving auditory skills should have a beneficial affect on the language system. They have developed an intervention they call Fast ForWord (FFW) (Scientific Learning Corporation, 2003), an Internet- and CD-ROM–based training program. It presents a series of on-screen exercises using synthesized speech sounds that systematically vary in length. The child learns to distinguish sounds of increasingly brief duration. The program consists of 100 minutes per day, 5 days per week for 4 to 8 weeks. The child works on the computer exercises with the guidance of a professional who is certified to deliver the intervention program by its creators. Tallal, Merzenich, Burns, Gelfond, Young, Shipley, and Polow (1997) and Tallal (2000) reported results showing improvements in performance on standardized language tests after this training.

However, it seems very likely that many children would show some change in language function after such intensive intervention. A recent randomized controlled trial (Cohen, Hodson, O'Hare, Boyle, Durrani, McCartney, Mattey, Naftalin, & Watson, 2005) with children who had severe receptive-expressive language disorders contrasted outcomes for children who completed the FFW intervention with children who received a similarly intense intervention program of computer games focusing on language skills. The only difference between the two treatment packages was that the FFW games included modified speech, whereas the other package did not. An encouraging finding from the study is that all children made appreciable gains in language functioning. However, the two groups did not differ from one another, suggesting that the speech modification did not enhance the children's language learning. This finding poses difficulties for the auditory hypothesis.

Should we therefore abandon the auditory deficit hypothesis? Again, this would seem a rash conclusion. Although there is no one-to-one correspondence, there is clearly a strong association between auditory processing deficits and LI that needs explaining. One possibility is that auditory deficits act as one of many possible risk factors for LI. On its own, an auditory deficit may not be sufficient to derail language acquisition, but in conjunction with other risk factors, such as limited processing capacity, it may have more deleterious effects (see the Surface Hypothesis, reviewed in Leonard, 1998). There is some empirical evidence for this. In a twin study, Bishop et al. (1999) found that individuals who had both deficits in auditory processing *and* a deficit in phonological short term memory (see below) had the most severe LI, suggesting that auditory deficits act as an additive risk factor.

A more radical proposal is that although auditory deficits frequently co-occur with LI, they are not causally related to language. Instead, both deficits may be markers of neuro-developmental immaturity (Bishop & McArthur, 2005). The notion of a "maturational lag" has been around for some time (Bishop & Edmundson, 1987) and was first considered in the context of motor deficits that also frequently co-occur with LI (Hill, 2001). In the auditory domain, several researchers noted that whether or not children with LI succeeded on a behavioral auditory task depended crucially on their age, with deficits more likely to be evident in younger participants (Bishop & McArthur, 2004; Wright & Zecker, 2004). This is perhaps not surprising when we consider some of the difficulties in interpreting findings from behavioral tasks. For example, Bishop (1997) pointed out that children with SLI have high rates of attentional problems and that the procedures used to assess auditory deficits in children require a high degree of attention and motivation. She suggests the possibility that the performance deficits seen in children with SLI might reflect generalized attention problems rather than selective impairments in auditory processing. In fact, Leavell et al. (1996) showed that tests purporting to identify auditory processing disorders (APDs) were most consistently related to tests of simple attention, as well as to IQ scores. They conclude that APD tests are, in actuality, sensitive to problems in auditory attention rather than processing difficulties.

However, it is possible to index auditory function using procedures that do not involve attention or overt behavioral responses. Bishop and McArthur (2004) used event-related potentials (ERPs) to measure the brain's physiological response to different tones. Their study is particularly informative because it looked at brain responses as well as behavioral responses in the same children over a period of 18 months. In line with previous studies, Bishop and McArthur found a subset of children with SLI, the youngest ones, who performed poorly on behavioral tests of frequency discrimination (distinguishing between high and low tones). However, the ERP data showed that all children with SLI had immature cortical responses to tones, even the ones who performed well on the behavioral tasks. Bishop and McArthur argue that this pattern of performance would result if we assume a maturational lag of approximately 4 years in the auditory development of children with SLI. Because children reach adult standards of frequency discrimination at about age 9, teenagers with SLI will achieve normal scores on such measures, whereas younger children with SLI will show the predicted deficit. However, neurophysiological responses to sound continue to develop throughout adolescence; thus, ERP responses in SLI continue to look like those of much younger typically developing children throughout the teenage years.

It is theoretically possible that early delays in auditory development will leave lasting "downstream" consequences on language development (Thomas & Karmiloff-Smith, 2003), but there isn't necessarily a causal connection. A second conclusion is that auditory deficits are rarely the only "specific" disability affecting children with LI. Several researchers have noted that language deficits are more severe if they occur in the context of a limited capacity system—in other words, in addition to difficulties in perceiving incoming stimuli, the way children remember and process this information may also go awry. We now consider evidence for the limited processing capacity model of SLI.

Limited Processing Capacity

Spoken language is a transient code; new information is coming in to the system all the time, often before we have completely digested the previous information. Therefore, to some extent, successful comprehension depends on the ability to hold information in temporary memory storage while integrating new, incoming linguistic material. Several investigators have suggested that SLI might result from a specific disability in this aspect of memory (Bishop, 1997; Dollaghan & Campbell, 1998; Montgomery, 2000; Weismer & Evans, 2002), usually referred to as *working memory*.

Two different models of working memory have come under the spotlight in recent years. The model put forward by Just, Carpenter, and Keller (1996) focuses on the tradeoff between storage and processing and is typically assessed using a listening-span task such as the Competing Language Processing Task (Gaulin & Campbell, 1994). In this task, children are asked to make truth judgments about a series of short sentences while at the same time remembering the final word of each sentence (e.g., "pumpkins are purple"; "balls are round"; purple – round). Studies have shown that children with LIs have consistently shorter listening spans than their typically developing peers (Weismer, Evans, & Hesketh, 1999; Weismer & Evans, 2002) and that scores on this span task are associated with deficits in sentence comprehension (Montgomery, 2000). However, it should be noted that all of these listening span tasks involve spoken sentences. By definition, children with LIs are less skilled at comprehending sentences than peers. If the model assumes that increased processing effort results in less efficient storage, then we should not be surprised to find that children with SLI are poor at this task. In this view, their poor performance on listening span measures may be seen as a reflection of their language difficulties, rather than a cause of them.

A slightly different perspective suggests a core deficit in phonological short-term memory (Gathercole & Baddeley, 1990), which is proposed to be a specialized memory system charged with setting-up long-term representations of phonological forms important for learning new vocabulary. The capacity of this system is typically assessed by asking children to repeat non-sense words of increasing syllable length and complexity (e.g., "bannifer" or "trumpetine"; Gathercole & Baddeley, 1996). Numerous studies have now shown that nonword repetition (NWR) is an extremely sensitive test of LI, as children with SLI, and even adults with resolved LI, have difficulty repeating non-sense words of three or more syllables (Bishop, North, & Donlan, 1996; Conti-Ramsden, Botting, & Faragher, 2001; Dollaghan & Campbell, 1998). Twin studies have shown it to be highly heritable, indicating that it is a useful marker for forms of SLI that may have a genetic origin (Bishop et al., 1996; Bishop, Adams, & Norbury, 2005).

But what does the NWR test actually measure? Bloom and Lahey (1978) were among the first to call attention to the limitations of the auditory processing deficit orientation for assessing language and planning language intervention, and a similar argument could be made regarding nonword repetition. They pointed out that auditory processing models generally take a "bottom-up" view of language processing. In a "bottom-up" model, lower-level processes, such as perception and discrimination, provide input necessary to the function of higher-level processes, such as comprehension. But, as Lahey (1988) and Bishop (1997) made clear, these "lower-level" processes do not operate in a vacuum or on a blank slate. Instead, they work in the context of prior knowledge. So prior knowledge, including knowledge of language, always influences how one processes input. For example, suppose that an examiner gave you the two lists of words in Box 1-2 to memorize and repeat.

BOX 1-2	**Hypothetical Word Lists**
List 1	**List 2**
Gigan	Pterodactyl
Gigantis	Giraffe
Angiris	Hippopotamus
Mogra	Triceratops
Megalon	Tyrannosaur
Hedora	Alligator
Mothra	Rhinoceros
Minya	Elephant

From which list do you think you could recall more items? Most people choose List 2. Even though the words in it are long, they are generally more familiar (the names of large animals, living and extinct). List 1, though, would be easier to learn if you had the appropriate background knowledge. You see, List 1 contains the names of characters from several *Godzilla* movies. For *Godzilla* aficionados, this list, too, contains familiar elements and would be readily recalled. In fact, when we began to write out this list for you as an example, we could only recall three or four of the characters' names. We had to put in a quick call to a 6-year-old Godzilla fan we knew, and asked him to name all the monsters in the Godzilla movies he'd seen. He rattled them off without hesitation, producing more than we needed for the list!

Now, let's say you were given List 1 to repeat after one brief presentation without prior knowledge or associations with the words on it. Suppose you scored significantly lower than some other subjects, say, people who were attendees at the Godzilla Fan Club International Convention. Would it follow that you had auditory memory deficit? Of course not! Your familiarity with the stimuli strongly influences how easy they are to remember and recall.

The same might be said of a 5-year-old with an LI who is trying to complete the NWR test. Success on this task is related to the "wordlikeness" of the nonwords or the extent to which they have real words embedded in them (Dollaghan, Biber, & Campbell, 1995; Gathercole, 1995). In other words, the more a nonword resembles a known word in a person's vocabulary (e.g., trumpet – trumpetine), the easier it is to remember. Children with LI who have smaller vocabularies will have fewer words on which to "hook" novel words. So again, this deficit may be seen as more a consequence than a cause of LI. Just as you had trouble remembering "Angiris" because you hadn't heard or used the word before and had no associations with it, our child with LI has the same problem with "trumpetine" because he has very limited experience with the word "trumpet." Ask him to recall several of these relatively unfamiliar terms, and he'll show the same difficulty you had in recalling "Angiris," "Mothra," "Gigan," and "Minya."

Most contemporary views of language and reading (e.g., Bishop, 1997; Treisman, 2001) hold that top-down, or concept-driven, and bottom-up, or data-driven, processes interact when a person is engaged in a task. If this is the case, then prior knowledge, concepts, and expectations always influence the treatment of incoming stimuli. This kind of interaction is illustrated in Figure 1-3.

Another piece of the contemporary understanding of cognitive processing relates to our problem. Information-processing accounts of cognition (see Halford, 2004, for review) suggest that there is a limit to the amount of conscious processing that can go on at any given time. It is possible, however, to overcome some of this limitation by not requiring conscious processing of all aspects of the signal. How? If some part of the signal contains information that is highly redundant, familiar, predictable, or overlearned, it can be handled at an automatic level, thus freeing some of the processing resources for aspects

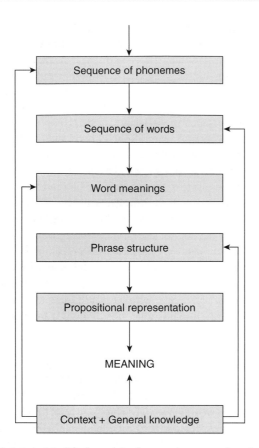

FIGURE 1-3 ✦ Modified model of stages in comprehension from phonological representation to meaning, showing influence of context and general knowledge on earlier stages of processing. (Used with permission from Bishop, D. [1997]. *Uncommon understanding: Development and disorders of language comprehension in children.* East Sussex, UK: Psychology Press Limited.)

of the problem that are new and require conscious attention. Let's take another example to see what this means.

Suppose you're new in town and want to take a drive to the Department of Motor Vehicles (DMV) office to get a new driver's license. You call a colleague on the telephone and ask for directions to the DMV. Your friend tells you to get onto the interstate, take exit 42, turn left at the end of the exit ramp, and follow the road for 3 miles to the DMV building. Now, let's say you arrived in town by plane and have not yet used the interstate highway. So you tell your friend, "Slow down a minute. Tell me how to get to the interstate." Your friend finds out where you're starting from and begins telling you how to get onto the highway, but by the time you've gotten through that, you've forgotten what she said about the exit number. So you ask her to tell you again. Maybe you get a pencil and write it all down. The point is that there was too much new information for you to remember all at once. That's your limited-capacity processor at work. But what if you've taken this section of the interstate to work lots of times? All you really need to get from your friend is what exit to take and how to get to the DMV from the exit. You can get to the interstate on automatic pilot. So you can see how automaticity in one part of a process can make it easier to focus on another part that is

newer and less familiar. The same applies to children with language disorders. Because all their language processing requires effort and attention, they have fewer resources available to take in something new. They are victims of the "Matthew phenomenon": the rich get richer and the poor get poorer. The more automatic, overlearned language you have, the easier it is to pick up something novel. Conversely, the more energy you need to spend on ordinary stimuli, the less you have available to deal with new or difficult input.

In examining the various specific disability models of language disorders, we have seen that, yes, children with LI very often score worse on a variety of processing and auditory perceptual tests than normally developing children. Although performance on such tests does correlate with language ability, we cannot necessarily assume that this correlation implies a causal connection. Nor can we yet conclude that the specific deficits identified need to be remediated for language development to proceed. These difficulties with current versions of the specific disabilities model lead to the consideration of the next model that we will discuss.

THE DESCRIPTIVE-DEVELOPMENTAL MODEL

The last approach to assessing and treating language disorders that will be discussed is the orientation that will be used primarily in this text: the *descriptive-developmental model* (Naremore, 1980). It also is called the *communication-language approach* by some authors (e.g., Lahey, 1988). This model concerns itself with describing in detail the child's current level of language function in terms of the use of vocabulary, meanings expressed, use of syntactic rules and morphological markers, pronunciation of sounds, knowledge of phonological rules, and the appropriate use of language for communication in social contexts. In other words, this model addresses the entire range of language performance, including form, content, and use. Further, the model holds that the normal developmental sequence outlined in research on normal language development (e.g., Haynes & Shulman, 1998b; Miller, 1981; Owens, 2004) provides the best curriculum guide for teaching language to children who have not, for whatever reason, managed to learn it on their own.

The assumptions that this model makes are, first, that it is not always possible to know the cause of a language disorder. As we saw with the examples of Sam and Max and Sharon and Elizabeth, the diagnostic category into which a child is placed may not always either explain or predict language behavior. Although it is important for doing research on language disorders to know as much as we can about etiological conditions, the utility of this information for clinical purposes is really secondary to knowing just what the child does with language.

The second assumption is related to the term *descriptive* in the name of this model. The descriptive-developmental model holds that the most important information for the language clinician to collect is a detailed profile of the child's language skills in each of the relevant areas of language function. It is this information that provides the backbone of the language intervention program. Similarly, the descriptive-developmental approach suggests that it is more important to detail the child's language skills themselves than to have extensive information on auditory perceptual or perceptual-motor abilities, such as those typically tested in the specific disabilities orientation. Instead, the descriptive-developmental approach leads us to focus on detailing the language and communication skills a child demonstrates to assess the child's needs and plan appropriate intervention. So the descriptive-developmental model gets part of its name from its emphasis on in-depth description of language behavior.

The third assumption of the descriptive-developmental approach stems from the other part of its name: developmental. This model holds that the best way to decide what a child should learn next in a language intervention program is to determine where he or she is in the sequence of normal development and what the next phase of normal development for that form or function would be. Going back to the discussion of terminology in language disorders, we said that in general, with some exceptions, most research in disordered language has shown that its course parallels normal development at a slowed down rate with particular, predictable asynchronies. This finding underlies the assumption that leads us to use the normal sequence as a guide to intervention.

What does it mean in practice to use the normal developmental sequence as a guide for intervention? First, it means that we must identify where in the normal sequence a child is currently functioning, as we previously discussed. We also must look at language behaviors relative to the child's overall level of function, as well as comparing linguistic behaviors among the domains of language itself. This is the intralinguistic referencing (Fey, 1986) that we talked about before and will discuss in more detail in Chapter 2. For now, we need to know that a profile of language behaviors can describe a child's level of communicative functioning in several areas. From there, we consult the research on normal language development and find out where in the sequence the client falls for each area of linguistic behavior. We then establish

goals for language intervention by identifying language skills just above the child's current level of functioning. We'll talk more in Chapter 3 about other issues involved in selecting goals for intervention. But, in principle, the descriptive-developmental model suggests that it is the normal sequence of acquisition that serves as the curriculum guide for language instruction.

This suggests that if a 5-year-old is producing primarily two-word utterances, our immediate goal is not to teach him to produce the sentences typical of a 5-year-old but to begin work on expanding the two-word sentences to include the next elements that would appear in normal development, such as three-word agent-action-object constructions or "-ing" marking. The same would be true for a 16-year-old with mental retardation at the same language level. But this is not to say that the two clients would receive the same intervention. The stimuli and materials for intervention for these two clients would differ in that we would attempt to choose props and contexts for intervention that were chronologically age appropriate, even though the words, structure, and meanings being taught were similar in many ways. Let's take an example.

Megan is a kindergartener referred for language evaluation to SLP Ms. Keene by her teacher because she used "short, babyish sentences." Language sampling revealed that most of her utterances were telegraphic, although she used these telegraphic utterances to talk about age-appropriate ideas. After a thorough evaluation, it appeared that semantic, pragmatic, and phonological skills were relatively intact compared with her limited syntactic production, and language comprehension appeared age appropriate. The speech-language clinician decided to target three-word sentences that encoded the same meanings already expressed in the telegraphic utterances. To elicit these sentences, she used a variety of dolls and toys that she manipulated in agent-action-object sequences she expressed verbally for Megan, having Megan imitate some, providing opportunities for her to produce others, and using modeling and expansion of Megan's telegraphic productions.

Ms. Keene also had another client on her caseload by the name of Izzy. Izzy was a teenage boy with Down syndrome placed in a special education class in the high school. Izzy also spoke primarily in telegraphic utterances, although his language comprehension skills were considerably higher than his production level. Although Izzy had some difficulties with phonological production, he could generally make himself understood, and he expressed a wide range of ideas with his simple sentences, engaging often and enthusiastically in social conversation. Ms. Keene decided that Izzy, too, needed help expanding his sentence structures. But rather than using toys and dolls as stimulus materials, she used the tools and equipment that Izzy was learning to use in his vocational education program. She focused on producing sentences that he could use to talk about the work he was learning to do.

These two examples illustrate an important corollary of the descriptive-developmental approach. The normal developmental sequence provides the goals for intervention but other considerations, such as the client's chronological age and the communicative context in which he or she must function,

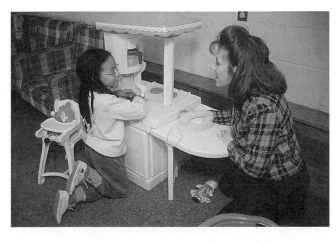

A descriptive-developmental model uses developmentally appropriate intervention methods and materials.

influence the materials and settings the intervention uses. So even if the child's language level is preschool and the goals of intervention target preschool-level structures and functions, the materials and equipment, the particular vocabulary items, the teaching style, and context used are influenced by considerations beyond the language level, such as the child's chronological age or functional needs (Olley, 2005) and the functional communicative demands of the child's environment. Targeting preschool level language structures and functions does not necessarily mean that they must be approached with a preschool style of intervention.

What is the evidence that a descriptive-developmental approach has any efficacy in improving language skills? Extensive reviews (cf. Guralnick, 1997; Law, Garrett, & Nye, 2005) of treatment research done over the past 20 years support the notion that treating language goals directly results in improved language behavior, especially for expressive language behavior. There are still many questions about the best methods for remediating language disorders, the best time to initiate and terminate services, the best candidates for intervention, and other issues. But it does seem clear that language behaviors can be changed for the better when targeted directly and that communication improves as a consequence.

Typologies for the Descriptive-Developmental Model

One disadvantage of the descriptive-developmental model is that it does not provide a convenient form of typology or a general scheme for categorizing children with language disorders. The etiological model categorizes children according to the syndrome that accompanies the language problem, such as hearing impairment or mental retardation. The specific disabilities model uses processing capacities such as auditory disorders, limited

processing capacity, and so on, as a categorization scheme. But how do we classify children within a descriptive-developmental model? There are several alternatives: some (Naremore, 1980) having to do with the amount and type of spoken language present, others (Fey, 1986) with the communicative skills typically used by the client, and yet others with the aspects of the language system that are disturbed (Bishop, 1997; Bloom & Lahey, 1978; Conti-Ramsden, Crutchley, & Botting, 1997; Rapin & Allen, 1987). Table 1-1 gives Rapin and Allen's (1987) scheme, merely to present one example typology.

The most common subtyping scheme uses just two categories: expressive disorders and receptive (or receptive/expressive combined) disorders. Although this scheme is perhaps the easiest to use and has been adopted by both *DSM-IV* and *ICD-10*, there is very little empirical support for its validity or efficacy. While there are a few suggestions in the literature that children with disorders restricted to expressive functions have better outcomes than children whose disorders have both receptive and expressive components (Paul & Cohen, 1984; Whitehurst & Fischel, 1994), this is by no means firmly established (Paul, Spangle-Looney, & Dahm, 1991; Stothard, Snowling, Bishop, Chipchase, & Kaplan, 1998; Young, Beitchman, Johnson, Douglas, Atkinson, Escobar, & Wilson, 2002). Tallal's (1988) review of research on the usefulness of linguistic typologies suggested that there is not a great deal of evidence that subtyping makes a strong contribution to clinical decision-making. Bishop (1997) concludes, likewise, that attempts to classify children with language disorders by statistical methods have been unsuccessful. Part of the problem lies in the fact that the pattern of impairment in language so frequently changes over time (Tomblin, Zhangxy, & Buckwalter, 2004). This means that what might look like two different subgroups may in fact be the same disorder manifesting itself differently at different points in development.

TABLE 1-1   Rapin and Allen's (1987) Clinical Language Subtypes

SUBTYPE	DESCRIPTION
Verbal auditory agnosia	Difficulty in comprehending language, with intact understanding of gestures. Speech is absent or very limited.
Verbal dyspraxia	Comprehension is adequate, but speech is limited with impaired articulation and short utterances. Difficulty cannot be accounted for by dysarthric weakness or incoordination.
Phonological programming deficit syndrome	Speech is fluent with fairly long utterances, but hard to understand. Comprehension is age appropriate.
Phonological-syntactic deficit syndrome	Words are mispronounced, and speech is disfluent. Utterances are short with grammatical errors, omission of function words, and inflections. May appear to affect only expression, but comprehension problems may exist, particularly for abstract or complex language
Lexical-syntactic deficit syndrome	Articulation is normal; word finding problems are present, there is difficulty in formulating connected language in conversation and narration. Expressive syntax is immature. Comprehension of abstract language is worse than for concrete.
Semantic-pragmatic deficit syndrome	Sentences are fluent and well-formed; articulation is adequate. Content is bizarre. Child may use echolalia or unanalyzed "scripts." Comprehension may be overly literal or limited to a few words within each sentence. Language use is odd—the child may be verbose without being communicative. Turn-taking and conversational maintenance are poor.

Subtyping children with language disorders can have important implications. We would like to know whether children with particular profiles have different outcomes, respond differently to different intervention approaches, or have different constellations of concomitant problems that we will need to identify in the assessment. But as things stand as of this writing, there is no well-established subcategorization scheme that has been shown to be useful in addressing any of these issues. Bishop (2000) concludes that a great deal of work still needs to be done to validate and refine classificatory systems in language disorders in order to specify diagnostic criteria and determine whether sharp distinctions exist among subgroups.

For the moment, the use of a descriptive-developmental approach will allow us to gather information about a variety of areas of the child's linguistic and related skills. This descriptive information forms the basis both for careful clinical planning and for research studies that will help to clarify this issue in the future. Although in this book no particular subclassifying system will be advocated for all children with language disorders, the descriptive-developmental model allows clinicians to use any linguistic subtyping scheme that future research shows is clinically useful. Using the descriptive information gathered routinely on each client for every area of language functioning allows us to develop an intralinguistic profile, like the one in Figure 2-2, that can serve as a basis for classifying a language disorder in any subtyping system.

■ CONCLUSIONS

In this chapter we have discussed some of the issues that face language pathologists when engaging in clinical practice with children. We have talked about definitions and terminology, and we have seen some of the difficulties and controversies around these topics. We have given you our views on these questions, but we've tried to make clear, too, that there is not always consensus in the field. Many reasonable people would disagree with the positions we've taken here. Until definitive research allows us to achieve consensus, each clinician must make an independent decision about them. We've tried to give you some of the information needed to make these decisions for yourself.

We've also looked at four different orientations to language disorders in children and have argued that one of them is, in general, better than the others for guiding clinical practice in language pathology. The descriptive-developmental approach makes no assumptions, focusing instead on the manifestations of the language disorder that require intervention. The developmental aspect of this model provides some guidance in determining appropriate targets for this intervention. Does this mean that the other models can be forgotten? Probably not. Each model we discussed provides some information that is useful in developing a fuller picture of the child with an LI. The categorical model is useful for classifying children for research purposes as we attempt to relate causes to the disorders we observe, and it may be essential for procuring services from educational agencies. We'll look at some of these

uses in Chapter 4. The specific disabilities model also has important research implications and may influence the choice of supporting materials, such as visual aids, that we use in conjunction with the language we present. The systems model focuses our attention on the concept of handicap and on the environment in which a child must function. It can lead us to augment our direct services with interventions aimed at making the communicative context more supportive of the child's developing skills. But for the purposes of clinical practice in language pathology—that is, for diagnosing problems in the acquisition of language, detailing the parameters of these problems, and deciding what to do about them—we believe that the descriptive-developmental model serves us best. In the next two chapters, we will discuss how to implement this model in assessment and intervention for children with language disorders.

STUDY GUIDE

I. Definitions of Child Language Disorders
   A. Define "normative" and "neutralist."
   (1) Give an example of each type of criterion as it would be used to identify a child with a language disorder.
   (2) Why are both considered necessary to make the diagnosis?
   B. Give and support your opinion about what constitutes a "significant deficit" in language performance.
   C. Which criterion would result in identifying more children as language disordered: the 10th percentile or more than 1 standard deviation below the mean?
   D. Name and describe the domains of language. Describe an imaginary client who had a deficit in each domain. What would his or her language be like?
   E. Discuss the pros and cons of using chronological age referencing in defining language disorders.
   F. What are two disadvantages of using nonverbal mental age referencing?

II. A Brief History of the Field of Language Pathology
   A. Name the disciplines involved in early studies of language disorders in children.
   B. Discuss changes in the 1950s that influenced the course of clinical practice in language disorders.
   C. How did the study of normal language development influence practice in language pathology?

III. Terminology
   A. What are the implications of calling a child with a language problem delayed? Deviant?
   B. What is the role of the term childhood aphasia in discussing child language disorders?
   C. Discuss synonyms for language impairment, explaining which you would use in your clinical practice and why.

IV. Etiology
   A. What is the evidence for a genetic component in language disorders?
   B. What are some of the brain differences seen in children with language disorders?

V. Models of Child Language Disorders
   A. Where is the communication disorder "located" in a systems model of language disorders?
   B. Define the categorical approach to language disorders. What categories are usually included in this approach?
   C. Explain the difference between "top-down" and "bottom-up" processing.
   D. How does prior knowledge influence performance on tests of processing capacity?
   E. What are the implications for language assessment and intervention of a descriptive-developmental model?

EVALUATION AND ASSESSMENT

CHAPTER OBJECTIVES

Readers of this chapter will be able to do the following:
- Discuss the phases and purposes of each aspect of the diagnostic process.
- List the purposes of assessment.
- Discuss the areas of assessment necessary to evaluate communication.
- Name and define the properties, strengths, and weaknesses of standardized tests.

- Discuss methods of assessment that are alternatives to standardized testing.
- Describe data used and guidelines for making assessment decisions.
- List approaches to dealing with the hard-to-assess child.
- Discuss approaches to integrating and interpreting assessment data.

The approach to language evaluation presented in this chapter derives from the work of Jon Miller, Peg Rosin, Gary Gill, and others at the Waisman Center for Human Development at the University of Wisconsin–Madison. This approach has been developed during the last three decades by these clinicians as a means of implementing a descriptive-developmental model of language disorders in the assessment process. Some of the material discussed in this chapter has been drawn from published sources, such as Miller (1978, 1981, 1996), but much of it derives from the efforts of these gifted clinicians to impart to students like myself some of their considerable experience and thoughtful perspective on the assessment enterprise. Not only the written sources, then, but also the teaching that they did both by precept and example has served as the basis for the approach that I elaborate here.

THE APPRAISAL PROCESS

Many clinicians coming from a medical model, such as Darley (1991) and Peterson and Marquardt (1994), divide the assessment process into two phases: *appraisal* and *diagnosis*. The appraisal portion involves collecting data from existing records and case history, from interviews and questionnaires completed by parents, and from direct examination of the child. The diagnosis is made through the study and interpretation of this information. The diagnosis entails identifying and labeling the problem, often with some inference about its cause. In a

medical model, diagnosis involves classifying the "disease" the client has (see Tomblin, 2000, for discussion). In a descriptive-developmental approach to assessment, these two phases are less distinct. The goal of this approach is to decide whether the child has a significant deficit in communication and to describe that deficit, if identified, in as much detail as possible, relative to the normal sequence of language acquisition. Issues of cause or the identification of a disease category are less central to the language pathologist's mission.

Federal guidelines provided by the Individuals with Disabilities Education Improvement Act of 2004 (PL 108-466), known as IDEA, make a distinction between *evaluation* and *assessment*. For clinicians working under the aegis of IDEA, *evaluation* is used to refer to the initial process of establishing eligibility for educational services. This aspect of the appraisal is focused on determining whether the child meets criteria for educational services. For children under the age of 6, it is not necessary to assign a diagnosis, or label, during this process, only to establish that the child has developmental delays sufficient to qualify for special educational services. Children over 6 will have to meet specific criteria for a disability as defined by IDEA in order to receive special education through the public schools. *Assessment* in this context is used to refer to the rest of the appraisal process, which follows the evaluation. Once a child is deemed eligible for services, clinicians need to describe communicative functioning, determine what the child needs in terms of communication programming, and how best to address those needs.

THE ASSESSMENT TEAM

The processes of evaluation and assessment involve the language pathologist as one member of an assessment team. The team consists of professionals from a variety of disciplines and backgrounds who contribute their expertise to providing a full picture of a client's strengths and needs. Assessment teams can take several approaches to the task of providing diagnostic services. These approaches are summarized in Box 2-1.

Regardless of the team model used, the language specialist participates by focusing on the questions that need to be answered regarding communication and the methods for addressing the questions. Whether the clinician gathers this information independently or through collaborative consultation with others on the team, the information about communicative performance is the "stuff" of the speech-language pathologist's (SLP's) contribution to the overall appraisal process and the basis for developing an intervention program for children in need of speech and language services.

GATHERING CASE HISTORY DATA

The diagnostic process usually begins with a review of historical information about the client. This may include only referral information from a teacher or parent, or it may include data

---

BOX 2-1	**Assessment Team Approaches**

Multidisciplinary—The team is made up of professionals from different disciplines. Each completes an independent evaluation of the client and comes up with a separate set of recommendations, which are reported to the team and the client's family.

Interdisciplinary—The team consists of professionals from different disciplines, but formal communication channels are established between them. A case manager coordinates services among all disciplines. Some professionals may be involved in the assessment on a consultant basis, providing suggestions to those who work directly with the child, but do not interact directly themselves.

Transdisciplinary—Team members are encouraged to share information and skills across disciplines. Assessment is collaborative in that one individual may do all or most of the interaction with the child, whereas others observe or make suggestions for the interactor to use during the assessment process. Team members work together whenever possible. They train and receive training from each other in reciprocal interactions. *Role release* (Woodruff & McGonigel, 1988) is employed; this involves sharing information and having team members help each other perform activities traditionally reserved within disciplines.

---

from previous testing or from intervention that took place at an earlier time. In transdisciplinary team settings, much of the case history data may be gathered collaboratively, with one professional talking with the family and sharing the information with other team members. In other approaches, the language pathologist may need to gather these data independently. When reviewing this information, the clinician needs to determine what information is already in the file and what needs to be learned to plan the appraisal. Basic questions to be answered include the following:

1. What is the problem, or *complaint*, in medical terms? What do people see as this child's area or areas of deficit?
2. When did the problem begin, or has the child always had it? Was the onset sudden or gradual?
3. Does the problem vary in severity, getting worse at some times or with some people and better with others, or is it always about the same?
4. How does the social environment interact with the child's problem? Is the child perceived as failing in school or other important social settings? How does the family see the child and react to the difficulties?

Many agencies use a standard intake questionnaire to collect some of these data before meeting with the family. Appendix 2-1 gives one example of this kind of questionnaire that is filled out by a parent before the child's first meeting with the clinician. McNamara (2007) and Shipley and McAfee (2004) have provided some additional examples. The form in Appendix 2-1 also contains a request for release of information. Such a request must be signed by the parent and must be sent along whenever clinicians attempt to solicit information about a child from another agency. When developing an assessment plan, it is wise to assemble any information available from other agencies where the child may have been a client. Including a form like this one with an intake questionnaire is usually an efficient way to find out whether the child has been seen by other professionals and to get access to the information they collected.

After the history and intake information have been reviewed, additional background information about the client is often helpful in refining the assessment plan. The best way to gather these data is usually to interview the parent or the child, if he or she is old enough. In transdisciplinary teams, one member usually conducts this interview, asking questions developed in collaboration with the team. In other situations, the language pathologist may need to conduct the interview independently. Although techniques for clinical interviewing are beyond the scope of this text, Haynes and Pindzola (1998) have provided helpful information, as have Crowe (1997), McNamara (2007), and Shipley and McAfee (2004). Sensitive interviewing, according to these writers, involves setting a tone of mutual respect; making sure that the person understands the purpose of the interview; listening carefully; asking clear, open-ended questions that are not leading or loaded ("You don't scold him when he makes mistakes, do you?"); and answering questions posed by the parent. The clinician should be prepared for some emotion to surface in these interviews, particularly if the parent has not talked to many people about the child's problem. The purpose of the interview is to gather information, though, not to provide psychotherapy. While a caring and accepting response to the parent's emotion is appropriate, dwelling on the emotion or becoming defensive if it is hostile is not. After expressing sympathy with the parent's feelings, a new, more neutral topic may be introduced.

DEVELOPING AN APPRAISAL PLAN

Once adequate information about the history and context of the problem has been gathered from review of the case history and interview results, the clinician is ready to develop the appraisal plan. The first step in devising this plan is to determine the child's general developmental level; that is, whether the child is functioning at or near age level in terms of day-to-day functioning. If the client is a toddler, does the child walk, feed himself or herself, and so on? As a preschooler, does the child engage in pretend play, drawing, some self-dressing, bathing, toileting, and similar activities? As a school-aged child, is he or she placed in the appropriate grade? As an adolescent or young adult, are daily living skills age-appropriate? This determination of general developmental level, gathered from history and interview data, allows us to determine at what level to begin the communication assessment. As we discussed in Chapter 1, communication skills usually are not more advanced than other areas of functioning, so general developmental level provides a reasonable baseline for beginning to assess communicative performance. If further investigation indicates that communicative skills are above or below this baseline, appropriate adjustments in the plan can be made.

For clinicians working under IDEA guidelines, the first step in the appraisal will be *evaluation*, determining whether the child is eligible for educational services. This will usually involve some testing but will also require gathering information about functioning in home and school from parents and teachers. This information allows us to address the functional criterion for eligibility. We'll talk about ways of gathering this information later on in this chapter. Clinicians will need to know what the specific eligibility guidelines for their work setting are, as these can vary from state to state and district to district. Once it has been determined that the child meets eligibility guidelines, a more detailed assessment can take place.

For this assessment, the clinician needs to decide what areas to evaluate. Even if the complaint is only in one aspect of communication, say articulation, it is usually wise to get as much information about other areas as possible. Although a child may present with only one complaint, such as unintelligible speech, appraisal may reveal that something else is involved. The child may have a hearing loss, a submucosal cleft of the palate, or a syntactic disorder that was masked by the unintelligibility. Whenever possible, the communication appraisal ought to look at aspects of hearing, oral-motor function, and comprehension and production of language. Although history and intake information are important for choosing the areas to be designated as high priorities for assessment, the communication appraisal should always be as comprehensive as we can make it.

We'll also need to decide what methods to use to assess each area. The assessment plan should include a tentative choice of method to be used to address each question about the client's communication. Basic questions about whether a child has a disorder in a particular area can be addressed with standardized tests. More detailed examinations of communicative performance for the purpose of setting remedial goals can be addressed with other approaches, such as language sampling. We'll talk more about the various methods available later in the chapter. In developing an assessment plan, though, the most important thing is to make decisions about the best match between questions and methods, and to be prepared with a "plan B," to make changes in the assessment if some parts of the original plan prove unworkable.

It also is important to think about the order in which the assessments are done so that they provide the client with some variety and maximize his or her potential for success. We might want to start the assessment with a relatively low-structured activity, such as gathering a language sample of parent-child play, to allow the child to warm up to the setting. More structured activities might follow, such as standardized testing. We might want to give the child a break and a snack while we observe oral-motor and feeding skills. A well-thought-out assessment plan often involves alternating high-structure and low-structure activities. We'll want to be careful not to put all the hardest assessments at the very beginning, when the child may feel shy and uncomfortable, or at the very end, when the child is likely to be tired. We'll want to think carefully, too, about how and when to gather information from parents and other adults who are important to the child, as their input is an important part of the information we will need to collect.

The most important thing about an assessment plan, though, is that it be *planned*. We want to get into the habit of reviewing history and intake data carefully and using them to make decisions about the most appropriate goals and methods for the assessment. We should then *write out* a plan that includes the goal and methods decided upon for each area being assessed, keeping in mind that we may have to deviate from the written plan if our interaction with the child suggests this need exists. A sample of a form for such a written plan can be seen in Figure 2-1. Using this approach, we can ensure that we use the client's time well in the appraisal and that we will come out of it with the most comprehensive and valid information possible.

MAKING ASSESSMENT DECISIONS

When developing a plan for evaluating a child, three questions can help structure our thinking about the assessment process: Why shall we assess? What shall we assess? How shall we assess? Let's see how each of these questions might be answered.

Client _____ Age _____
Referral source _____
Probable developmental level _____
Chief complaint _____
Other complaints _____

Areas to assess	Question to be answered	Assessment tool
_____	_____	_____
_____	_____	_____
_____	_____	_____
_____	_____	_____
_____	_____	_____
_____	_____	_____
_____	_____	_____

FIGURE 2-1 ✦ Sample assessment plan.

WHY SHALL WE ASSESS?

Westby, Stevens, Dominguez, and Oetter (1996) identify four basic reasons for evaluating language performance in a child. Each reason involves somewhat different goals and methods. Let's talk about each of the four reasons in turn.

Screening

The first reason we do an appraisal is that we simply want to find out whether the child has a problem using or understanding language. This is a yes-no question, and the assessment ought to provide a clear and definitive answer. Answering the screening question, or determining whether a child has a problem with language, takes us back to our definition of language disorders. To decide whether a child has a problem, we need to know, first, what criterion for language disorder we are using. For clinicians working under IDEA guidelines, these will be defined by the local educational authority (LEA). Screening will be the first step in the evaluation process in these settings. Most screening procedures will make use of screening tests. Here the psychometric properties of the test instrument are especially important, because a test with adequate psychometric properties is essential to provide a fair screening measure. We'll talk more about what makes up these properties in the section on standardized tests. For now, we just need to know that a good screening test is one that meets high psychometric standards.

It is not always necessary to use a test published specifically as a screening instrument to decide whether a child has a problem. Any standardized test that assesses relevant areas of language function and that is adequately constructed can be used. In fact, this is one of the best reasons to use a standardized test: to decide in a fair, norm-referenced manner that a child has a significant language deficit. Deciding *what* standardized test to use has to do with efficiency. When the purpose of assessment is simply screening, all we need to know is whether the child should be considered as having a language

problem and therefore be a candidate for more in-depth evaluation and intervention. In this case, the quickest method of answering the question is the best. It would not, for example, make sense to use a test that has a great number of subtests and items for a screening measure if the same question could be answered as validly by a shorter instrument.

On the other hand, we would not want to use a screening measure that only assessed a narrow range of language behaviors. If, for example, we used the *Peabody Picture Vocabulary Test—IV* (Dunn & Dunn, 2006) as a screening instrument, we might learn that a child does not score below our cutoff (say, the 10th percentile) in terms of receptive vocabulary. Does that mean the client does not have a language problem? Not necessarily. A child could have a normal receptive vocabulary and still have a great deal of difficulty with expressive language skills or even with comprehension of syntax. A test used as an initial screening measure should look at several areas of language function.

In evaluating the results of our screening, we need to ask whether a child who appears to have a language problem is demonstrating a linguistic *difference* or a *disorder*. We need to be aware of this issue for any child who comes from a culturally or linguistically different background, such as the child from a family that speaks Spanish in the home or an African-American child whose family uses a nonstandard dialect of English. For those children, whose experiences with English may be different from those of children from mainstream backgrounds, our first decision will be whether the child has a bona fide impairment or a communication problem that results primarily from a mismatch between the child's experience and the expectations of the social environment. We'll talk in detail about the means for making this decision in Chapter 5.

IDEA Evaluation. If clients fail a screening measure, this does not, of course, mean they definitely have communication problems. Screening is used only to identify children *at risk*. For children who fail screening, a more extensive evaluation will be needed to determine whether they meet eligibility criteria under IDEA. This evaluation will use both testing and other methods, such as interviews, observation, and communication sampling, methods we discuss in more detail later in the chapter.

Establishing Baseline Function

Once the initial screening question has been answered and evaluation has determined that a child is eligible for special services, assessment is used to determine the child's current, or *baseline level* of *functioning*. This purpose is distinct from the screening and evaluation functions and requires the use of different strategies and instruments. To determine baseline function, it is crucial to examine all areas of communicative function, as well as areas related to the child's ability to use language, such as hearing, cognitive skills, and oral-motor abilities. Establishing baseline function involves finding out not only the areas in which the child is experiencing difficulty, but also identifying areas in which the child is functioning relatively well. Miller (1981) suggested that this phase of assessment result in a profile of the child's abilities, like that shown in Figure 2-2, referenced

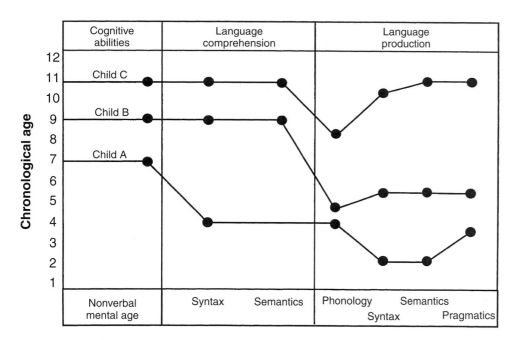

FIGURE 2-2 ✦ Intralinguistic profile. (Adapted from Miller, J. [1981]. *Assessing language production in children.* Needham Heights, MA: Allyn and Bacon.)

intralinguistically and relative to the child's developmental level. Although the practice of using intralinguistic profiling has been criticized on psychometric grounds (Merrell & Plante, 1997), it can be helpful when used to obtain a broad picture of linguistic performance rather than to identify a disorder. Still, the psychometric problems involved mean that we should take these profiles with "a grain of salt" and use ongoing assessment to validate them in the course of the intervention program.

Establishing baseline function may require that we look at the child's communicative behavior in several settings (that is, we may want to know more than how the child uses language in an unfamiliar place, such as the diagnostic clinic, and with an unfamiliar person, such as the language pathologist). Many authors, including Coggins (1991), Losardo and Notari-Syverson (2001), Oetting and MacDonald (2002), Nelson (1998), and Westby, Stevens, Dominguez, and Oetter (1996), have discussed the importance of context in observing communicative behavior. This suggests to language pathologists that we cannot assume that one sample of behavior, gathered in the relatively strange clinical situation, tells us everything we need to know about the child's capacities for communicating. Let's see what this might mean in practice.

Katie was an 8-year-old girl who had been identified as language/learning disabled by her school learning disabilities specialist and SLP. Her teacher noted that she had a great deal of trouble learning to read and write and that her oral language often seemed disorganized and hard to follow. Although the school personnel did an in-depth assessment, her parents felt they wanted to know more about Katie's problem and took her to a diagnostic clinic at the state university's research hospital, about 60 miles from their hometown, for a multidisciplinary assessment. At her first evaluation session, Katie was given a hearing test, some blood was taken for chromosomal testing, and extensive cognitive and psychoeducational testing was done. In the last 2-hour period of the day, Katie went to the communication disorders section for speech and language testing.

Ms. Michaels was the SLP assigned to the case. She offered Katie a large dollhouse with a variety of furniture and characters and invited her to play with her mother and the toys. She turned on a tape recorder and prepared to take notes on Katie's language and communication. Katie played in a desultory way with the toys, then began to whine that she was hungry. When told she could have some crackers in a few minutes, she simply sat quietly and placed all the furniture in the appropriate rooms in the house without further comment.

Should Ms. Michaels conclude that Katie is minimally verbal? Clearly many factors made the day at the diagnostic center a long and difficult one. Would you like being stuck with needles for blood tests? Would you like to answer a lot of hard questions for someone you had never met before? Would you like knowing that your parents brought you all the way to this big, scary place because they think you are not doing well in school?

The point is not that clinic-gathered information is invalid. In some situations with some clients it may be perfectly valid. But we do need to be aware that the context of place, person, materials, and what else has happened to the child that day can all influence performance. Whenever possible, it is to our advantage to sample a child's communicative behavior in more than one setting or with more than one person.

Just as we may want to establish baseline function by getting samples in more than one setting, we may want to get an idea of different aspects of the client's functioning. For example, we may want to know what the child's best performance is under the most ideal conditions, such as interacting with a familiar adult and engaging with novel toys in a free-play situation. But we may also want to know something about how the child performs in more stressful situations, such as a formal testing procedure with an unfamiliar examiner, less appealing materials, and less opportunity for the child to decide how to use them. Both of these environments, the ideal and the more stressful, are "real-life" situations. The ideal situation may be more like the one encountered in the child's home, whereas the stressful one may be like what the child has to cope with at school.

When conducting an assessment, we need to be careful that we don't ignore either aspect of the child's performance—in the ideal situation or in the stressful one—or the difference between the two. Although it is important to look at the child's best performance, the child may not always be at his or her best in all the real-life situations that he or she must confront. Knowing how a child fares under pressure will be a valuable piece of information to gather. Further, it would be important to know whether there is a large gap between the child's best performance and the way he or she behaves under less-than-ideal conditions. So again, assessing the child in more than one situation is an important part of the evaluation process.

This process can be painful for parents to watch. When assessing the child in the formal, stressful context, the clinician may find that the client's parents are anxious and tense, and they may even complain that the testing is unfair. Parents in this situation need reassurance from the clinician that the formal testing procedure is only one piece of the information needed to understand the child's functioning. Explaining that you are trying to see how the child does in this somewhat odd, unnatural situation can help to allay the parents' fears. Seeing the informal aspects of the evaluation can reassure them that their child's best performance also will be taken into account. In any case, it is always wise to explain the purpose of each phase of the evaluation to parents and to make them feel that they are partners in learning as much as can be learned about their child.

Establishing Goals for Intervention

A third purpose for assessment is to identify appropriate targets and procedures for intervention. To do this, when following a descriptive-developmental model, it is necessary first to find at what point in the developmental sequence a child is currently functioning. So establishing baseline function is a crucial prerequisite to this next stage of assessment. Only when the child's level of functioning in each relevant area of language has been described and when all the important collateral areas, such as hearing, cognitive level, and oral-motor functioning, have been assessed, can the clinician make decisions about targets for intervention.

These decisions involve identifying the areas in which the child is functioning below expectations for developmental level. Identified areas—whether they are the comprehension of syntax or vocabulary; the expression of words, sounds, or sentences; or the use of a range of different functions of communication—would then be targeted for intervention. Using the intralinguistic referencing system advocated by Miller (1981), areas that were most delayed relative to other areas of language function would be targeted first (see Fig. 2-2). When these areas of deficit are remediated to the child's highest level of communicative performance, then the target would be to improve overall language functioning so that it more closely approximates nonverbal mental age or chronological age, whichever reference point was being used. Let's see how we might implement this model for a child like the one profiled in Figure 2-3.

Davey is a 6-year-old boy being evaluated for language deficits after failing a kindergarten screening. Comprehensive evaluation indicated that Davey was functioning at age level in terms of performance on cognitive testing. His receptive syntax and vocabulary were found to be below the 10th percentile

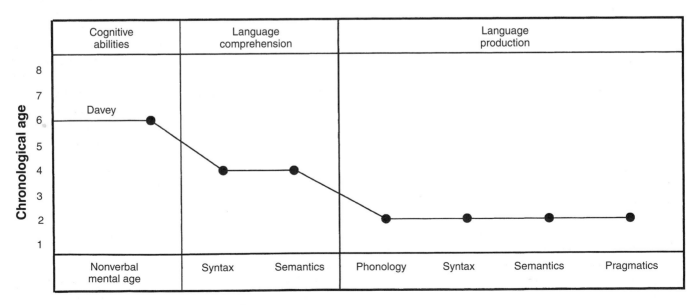

FIGURE 2-3 ✦ Intralinguistic profile for "Davey."

for his age, with age-equivalent scores in the 4-year range. Expressive language was below the second percentile in all areas measured with standardized tests. In addition, language sampling showed infrequent expression of communicative intentions, with only two or three different semantic relations expressed and sentences limited to telegraphic utterances with few grammatical morphemes. Most expressive skills were on the 2-year level.

These data led the speech-language clinician, Mr. Harper, to target expressive skills as the top-priority objective. Goals included increasing sentence length, developing use of grammatical morphemes, improving articulation, and increasing the frequency of expression of communicative intention and the range of semantic relations. After 1 year of intervention, Davey's expressive skills were reassessed and found to approach the 4-year level in terms of semantics and sentence length. Articulation skills were at the 3-year level, but expression of communicative intentions had increased significantly. It was decided to continue working on articulation and to target some receptive skills to move these closer to Davey's chronological age level. Once receptive skills showed improvement, expression would be targeted again, to get it to approximate the receptive level, if expression had not improved spontaneously by that time.

Although there are many other factors to consider when targeting goals for intervention, gathering comprehensive and accurate assessment data is the *sine qua non*. Without these data, the other considerations cannot be adequately addressed. These data also form the basis for the next phase of the assessment process—documenting improvement during the course of intervention.

Measuring Change in Intervention

Assessment is an ongoing process. It does not end when the formal diagnostic evaluation has been completed. The SLP has an obligation to continue to evaluate the client's progress throughout the course of an intervention program.

First, assessment is necessary to determine whether the goals of the program have been met. How will you know when to move on to the next target of intervention without knowing whether the client has yet learned what you've been teaching? If the assessment shows that the client has mastered one of the goals of the program, the next step can be initiated. If not, perhaps the procedures or materials or the therapeutic modality needs to be changed. Programs that are not effective within a reasonable time need to be modified.

Second, ongoing assessment is necessary to decide when to dismiss a client from intervention. Just as we need to decide ahead of time on our criteria for identifying a child with a language disorder, it is important to decide ahead of time what criterion will be used for dismissal (Kemp, 1983). As with so many other issues in the field of language disorders, there are not well-established mandates for determining criteria for dismissal from intervention. Nelson (1998) suggested posing the following questions to determine whether a client is ready to be dismissed from intervention:

▶ Is more change needed?
▶ Is more change possible?

▶ Can more change be achieved without costs that outweigh its benefits?

Fey (1986) suggested that children should be dismissed from therapy for any of the following reasons:

1. They have reached all the goals identified in the diagnostic phases of the program and are no longer viewed as language impaired.
2. They have reached a plateau, and efforts to modify the intervention program do not achieve more progress.
3. They are making progress, but this progress cannot be attributed to the intervention program.

Whatever dismissal criterion we use, ongoing assessment is central in determining when the client meets that criterion.

It is important to remember that although assessment should be ongoing, assessment is not the only activity in which the clinician should be engaged. Most of the time we spend with clients in an intervention program ought to be devoted to teaching them to communicate better, not to testing their current skills. Although the client's progress must be evaluated continually throughout the intervention program, ongoing assessment should involve a minority of the contact time between the client and clinician. In an intervention program, the central aim is to *teach* language or *change* language behavior. Ongoing assessment is an important part of this process but should be confined to a small portion of its time.

One other point needs to be made about assessment for evaluating progress in intervention. When looking for changes in the client's language behavior, we need to know more than whether the child can use or understand a structure or function in the patterned, clinician-controlled exercises that may have formed the basis of the intervention program. We also need to know whether the child can do so in more natural situations, such as less-structured conversations. It would be unwise to dismiss a client from intervention because he or she achieved 80% correct performance on use of "is (verb)-ing" in a delayed imitation format without probing to see whether the child can use the "is (verb)-ing" structure when telling about what he or she is doing during a play situation. To be valid, assessment for any purpose must show how the child functions in naturalistic as well as structured settings. This requirement is especially important when assessing whether a child has learned what we have been attempting to teach in an intervention program. If we only examine how the child performs in a highly structured format, we have not conducted our ongoing assessment adequately. To have learned a form or function, the child must be able to use it in real communicative situations. If the child cannot do this, we have not finished our job.

WHAT SHALL WE ASSESS?

Language Function

The answer to the question "What shall we assess?" may seem simple. We assess language. But there is a bit more to it than that. First, we need to establish the areas of language to be assessed. These consist of the two modalities of communication:

comprehension and *production.* The assessment of these two modalities requires somewhat different approaches. Bloom and Lahey (1978) discussed the differences between language functioning in these two modes and pointed out that it is dangerous to make assumptions about one on the basis of the other. Because comprehension and production capacities function somewhat independently in development, each of these modalities needs to be assessed as a distinct entity.

Comprehension Assessment. Chapman (1978), Miller and Paul (1995), Milosky and Skarakis-Doyle (2006), and Paul (2000*c*) discussed the differences between children's performance on comprehension tasks that are contextualized, in the presence of familiar routines and nonlinguistic cues, and those that are decontextualized. They pointed out that children function quite differently in terms of their comprehension performance in these two settings. When we use standardized tests to measure language reception, we are using a decontextualized instrument to assess comprehension. Such decontextualized information is important to gather and would be part of the assessment of the child's abilities under the less-than-ideal conditions previously discussed. As an adjunct to formal comprehension testing, the clinician may want to assess how the child responds to language in a more familiar, contextualized setting. Lord (1985) and Miller and Paul (1995) suggested pairing traditional comprehension assessment with assessment of the understanding of similar words and language structures in more naturalistic formats that include the presence of familiar situations and nonlinguistic cues such as gestures, gaze, and other contextual support. Comparing the child's performance in these two settings can produce a fuller picture of the child's comprehension skills.

Whether analyzing receptive skills in contextualized or decontextualized formats, it is always important to remember that comprehension is, as Miller and Paul (1995) put it, a private event, something that happens inside the child's mind. What we observe in comprehension assessments is the *product* of the child's comprehension, not comprehension itself. This means that the methods we use to assess comprehension must be chosen very carefully so that these products are valid indications of the underlying process of interest. We talk more about these methods in the "How?" section of assessment.

Production Assessment. Unlike assessment of comprehension, assessment of language production gives us direct access to the thing we are most interested in: how children express themselves with language. But just as children perform differently on comprehension tasks with different contexts, they also perform differently on different types of expressive language tasks. Prutting, Gallagher, and Mulac (1975) have shown, for example, that children make different kinds of grammatical errors when asked to repeat sentences than they do when producing sentences spontaneously. Similarly, Merrell and Plante (1997) showed that a norm-referenced test with high sensitivity and specificity for identifying a language disorder was nonetheless inconsistent in identifying the actual errors children made in spontaneous speech. These studies suggest that to see what kinds of errors a child makes in every-day talk, we need to rely not only on test data but also on spontaneous speech, using language-sample analysis procedures.

That is not to say there is no role for sentence imitation or other standardized approaches to the evaluation of language production. These methods are, in fact, very effective in showing whether children are performing within the normal range of expressive language behavior. In other words, they provide excellent screening information. But to get a realistic picture of baseline level of expressive language function, to see how children actually use language to communicate, to see what errors are typical of a child's speech, and to determine targets for intervention, sampling spontaneous language is the most effective and ecologically valid method.

Domains of Language

Within each of these two modalities—comprehension and production—we would want to evaluate the three domains of language depicted in Figure 1-1:

1. *Form (syntax, morphology, and phonology)*: Inflectional marking of words; sentence components such as the basic noun phrase and verb phrase; and sentence types, such as negative, interrogative, embedded, and conjoined structures. Form also includes the ability to produce sounds, the consistency of sound production, and the use of phonological simplification processes.
2. *Content (semantics)*: Knowledge of vocabulary, the ability to express and understand concepts about objects and events, and the use and comprehension of semantic relations among these objects and events.
3. *Use (pragmatics)*: The range of communicative functions (reasons for talking), the frequency of communication, discourse skills (turn-taking, topic maintenance and change), and the flexibility to modify speech for different listeners and social situations.

Sounds like a tall order? It is. Your first response may be, "It's impossible to do all that!" But don't panic. Remember, not every area needs to be assessed with standardized testing. Standardized testing may be used simply to establish that the child's language is deficient relative to other children's at the same development level. This can easily be done in a 1- or 2-hour testing session, using referral information to decide which areas would be most crucial to evaluate with standardized tests. Standardized testing could start by evaluating receptive vocabulary and syntax. If the client performs significantly below criteria in these areas, then a disorder can be identified and the more comprehensive portion of the appraisal could be devoted to establishing baseline function and determining goals for intervention in production as well as comprehension. If the client's performance in both areas of receptive skill is found to be within the normal range, then some standardized assessment of expression can be used to decide whether the child has a language disorder. This often can be done quickly with a test that measures language production in a standardized format.

Once it has been established that the child functions below criteria on these measures, the evaluation purpose of the assessment has been accomplished. The clinician still needs to know what the child's needs are, to establish baseline function, and to identify goals for intervention from assessment data. But remember, assessment is an ongoing process. It does not have to be completed in the first session, even if that session is the "official" assessment time. Once the child has begun an intervention program, less formal appraisal procedures can be implemented to round out the child's intralinguistic profile. We'll talk about doing that in the "How?" section.

Collateral Areas

As big as the job of assessing language function may seem, it is not the whole task of conducting an appraisal. In addition to analyzing all these aspects of language, a thorough assessment also involves investigating collateral areas that relate to the child's communicative function. The SLP may not gather all this information single-handedly. In an interdisciplinary or transdisciplinary diagnostic evaluation, other professionals may provide some of the necessary data. But even if the evaluation is conceived of as a circumscribed language assessment, it will be necessary to get this information. Upon completing the speech and language portion of the assessment, the language pathologist may need to request additional information from other professionals. This can be done by referring the client for further testing (Appendix 2-2).

Hearing. An obvious but essential piece of collateral data in any evaluation of communicative function involves the child's hearing. No language assessment is complete without an investigation of the child's hearing status. Many speech-language clinicians screen children for hearing impairment, using small, portable audiometers specifically designed for this purpose. The American Speech-Language-Hearing Association (1997) has set guidelines for this screening. More recently, otoacoustic emissions testing has been introduced as a screening method (Hof, van Dijk, Chenault, & Anteunis, 2005). Children who fail either of these screenings need to be referred for comprehensive audiometric assessment.

Speech-Motor Assessment. Another area that needs to be assessed for any child with a language disorder is the integrity of the oral-motor system. Whenever a child presents with difficulty in expression of spoken language, it is imperative to determine whether there are physical barriers to that expression.

Assessing the speech-motor system consists of examining facial symmetry; dentition; the structure and function of the lips, tongue, jaw, and velopharynx; and respiratory, phonatory, and resonance functions as they are used for speech. Shipley and McAfee (2004) and Bukendorf, Gordon, and Goodwyn-Craine (2007) provided some guidance in interpreting the oral-facial examination. Blakely (2000) and St. Louis and Ruscello (2000) provide additional means for assessing oral-motor functions. Figure 2-4 contains a form that can be used to guide this assessment, which is based on information derived from Meitus and Weinberg (1983) and Spriestersbach, Morris, and Darley (1991). The form is used by observing each element outlined on the checklist and marking either *yes* or *no* for each observation on the form. At the end of each section, a judgment of the adequacy of the structures and functions for speech

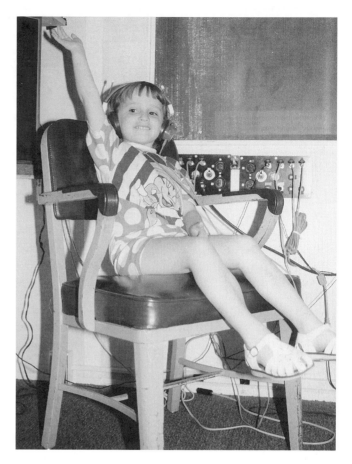

Hearing evaluation is part of every language assessment.

is made, giving an overall impression based on these observations, following Spriestersbach, Morris, and Darley (1991). This overall rating is made as follows:

1. Normal
2. Slight deviation—probably no detrimental effect on speech
3. Moderate deviation—possible effects on speech, especially if other structures also are deviant
4. Extreme deviation—sufficient to prevent normal production of speech; modification of structure required

To prevent the spread of infection, a clinician should always wash the hands thoroughly with soap, then put on surgical gloves for this examination. The hands should be washed again when the gloves are removed.

Examination of the External Face and Head. The face can be examined from a frontal view to determine alignment; spacing of the eyes; proportions of the face; and symmetry of the nares, philtrum, and Cupid's bow. The clinician can observe whether the lips approximate at rest, whether they retract symmetrically when the client smiles or produces /i/, and whether they contract symmetrically when he or she produces /u/. Details for making these observations are provided in Figure 2-4. Normal appearance and terminology for this examination are given in Figure 2-5. Observing the face in lateral or profile view, the clinician examines the alignment of the facial features again, using the guidelines in Figure 2-4. This observation can be conducted on a client of any age, including an infant.

EXTERNAL FEATURES OF FACE AND HEAD

Frontal view

—————— Midline of nose, philtrum, space between central incisors, midline of chin should be aligned at rest when lower jaw is opened and closed.

—————— Eyes should be aligned along horizontal plane, properly spaced (face should be five eyes wide, with one eye width between bony structure that separates eyes).

—————— Lower facial height (base of nose to base of chin) is greater than upper (bridge of nose to base of nose). (Use index finger on bridge of nose, thumb on base. Rotate index finger 180 degrees. Index finger should be on chin with some facial tissue below finger.)

—————— Absence of septal deviations of nose.

—————— Relative size and symmetry of nares, absence of deviations in columella (use inferior view as well).

—————— Deep red color of inferior nasal turbinates.

—————— Nares open, unobstructed breathing (for both one and two nares).

—————— Philtrum.

—————— Cupid's bow.

—————— Lips approximate at rest.

—————— Bilateral symmetry in /i/,/u/, smile.

Lateral view

—————— Bridge of nose, base of nose, point of chin should be in straight or slightly protruded line (class I, normal profile; if upper jaw protrudes relative to lower, class II; if lower protrudes in relation to upper, class III).

Rating: 1 2 3 4 (circle)

FUNCTIONAL INTEGRITY

—————— Raise eyebrows.

—————— Close eyelids against resistance.

—————— Facial expression (smile, frown).

—————— Resting posture of face.

Rating: 1 2 3 4 (circle)

Mandible

—————— Should lower widely without deviation from midline (place index fingers in mandibular condyles; ask client to open mouth widely; fingers should fall in fossa of temporal-mandibular joint when mandible is opened; feel for symmetry).

—————— Ramus should be one third shorter than body. (Place thumbs on angles of mandible, index fingers on top of condyles. Rotate index fingers to planes of mandible. One third of the body of mandible should be in front of index fingers).

Rating: 1 2 3 4 (circle)

INTRAORAL EXAMINATION

Dentition (instructions to client: bite on back teeth and show gums)

—————— Lower molar (or canine for children without molars) is one half tooth ahead of upper (normal, class I occlusion; if lower is one half tooth or more behind upper, class II malocclusion [maxilla is protruded in relation to mandible]; lower more than one half tooth ahead of upper, class III malocclusion [mandible protruded in relation to maxilla]).

—————— One half to one third of crown of lower central incisors should be covered by upper incisor (normal overbite).

—————— Upper incisors should be 1 to 3 mm ahead of lower (normal overjet).

—————— Absence of missing teeth.

—————— Absence of deviant spacing.

—————— Absence of disturbances in axial orientation, rotations.

Rating: 1 2 3 4 (circle)

Pharynx

—————— Absence of blockage of faucial isthmus.

—————— Absence of tonsillary enlargement.

Rating: 1 2 3 4 (circle)

Tongue

—————— Absence of structural abnormalities (lessions, scars, fissures).

—————— Proportional in size in relation to oral cavity.

—————— Nonspeech activities (stick out tongue, lateralize, rapid lateralization, touch nose, touch chin) to evaluate strength, range, symmetry, tone, accuracy of movement.

—————— Absence of resting deviations, fasciculations.

—————— Absence of restrictions by lingual frenum.

—————— Functions normally during swallowing.

Rating: 1 2 3 4 (circle)

Palate

—————— Vault.

—————— Width.

—————— Midline raphe apparent.

—————— Absence of fistulas.

—————— Posterior boundary of hard palate scalloped in appearance.

—————— Boundary continuous.

—————— Pink-white color.

—————— Adequate midline of soft palate.

—————— Single uvula.

Rating: 1 2 3 4 (circle)

Velopharyngeal (VP) port function

—————— Absence of history of VP impairment (nasal regurgitation, family history of clefting, speech disturbance after tonsillectomy or adenoidectomy, history of speech disturbance compatible with VP problems, history of oral-facial myoneural disorder).

—————— Absence of movement during prolongation of /a/.

FIGURE 2-4 ✦ Form for examination of speech mechanism. (Adapted from Meitus, I., and Weinberg, B. [1983]. *Diagnosis in speech-language pathology.* Baltimore, MD: University Park Press; Spriestersbach, D., Morris, H., and Darley, F. [1991]. Examination of the speech mechanism. In F. Darley and D. Spriestersbach [Eds.], *Diagnostic methods in speech pathology* [ed. 2] [pp. 111-132]. Prospect Heights, IL: Waveland Press.)

Velopharyngeal (VP) port function—cont'd

———— Presence of movement during short, repeated phonations of /a/, /a/.
———— Absence of glottal stops.
———— Absence of pharyngeal fricatives.
———— Absence of nasal emissions.
———— Absence of perceived hypernasality on VanDemark sentences.
———— Absence of need for further instrumental evaluation.

Rating: 1   2   3   4   (circle)

Volitional oral movements

———— Stick out your tongue.
———— Blow.
———— Show me your teeth.
———— Pucker your lips.
———— Touch your nose with tip of tongue.
———— Bite your lower lip.
———— Whistle.
———— Lick your lips.
———— Clear your throat.
———— Move your tongue in and out.
———— Click your teeth together once.
———— Smile.
———— Click your tongue.
———— Chatter your teeth as if cold.
———— Touch your chin with tip of tongue.
———— Cough.

———— Puff out your cheeks.
———— Wiggle your tongue from side to side.
———— Show how you kiss someone.
———— Pucker, then smile (demonstrate).

Rating: 1   2   3   4   (circle)

Diadochokinetic function

———— Produces /pa/, /ba/ smoothly, accurately.
———— Produces /ta/, /da/ smoothly, accurately.
———— Produces /ka/, /ga/ smoothly, accurately.
———— Produces /pata/ smoothly, accurately.
———— Produces /pataka/ smoothly, accurately.

Respiratory functions

———— Sustains vowel for 5 seconds.

Rating: 1   2   3   4   (circle)

Phonatory functions

———— Produces soft speech.
———— Produces loud speech.
———— Produces high-pitched sounds.
———— Produces low-pitched sounds.
———— Vocal quality normal. If not, is it:
        ———— Harsh?
        ———— Breathy?
        ———— Hoarse?

Rating: 1   2   3   4   (circle)

Key: 1=Normal   3=Moderate deviation
         2=Slight deviation   4=Extreme deviation

FIGURE 2-4 ✦—cont'd

The functional integrity of the facial musculature can be observed by asking the client to raise the eyebrows, to close the eyelids against the resistance of the clinician's finger holding them open, and to smile and frown. Resting posture of the face can be observed for symmetry. Movement and

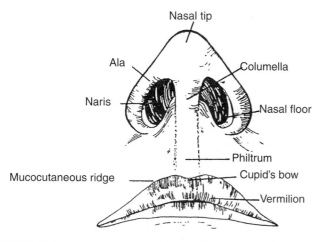

FIGURE 2-5 ✦ Surface view of lips and nose. (Reprinted with permission from Meitus, I., and Weinberg, B. [1983]. *Diagnosis in speech-language pathology* [p. 41]. Baltimore, MD: University Park Press.)

proportions of the mandible also can be evaluated, as outlined in the form in Figure 2-4. A developmental level of 24 months is necessary for the child to perform these assessments. Even a 2- or 3-year-old may have difficulty with some of these activities, though. Young children will probably need to imitate these movements rather than produce them on verbal request. Asking the mother to imitate the clinician first and then have the child do so may be useful. Suggesting that the child pretend to be a clown making funny faces can help; so can using a mirror so that the child can see the funny faces being made. You might even try offering to paint the child's face like a clown for this portion of the assessment. Special paints are available for face painting from many toy stores.

Intraoral Examination. When conducting an intraoral examination, rubber or surgical gloves must be worn for the safety of the clinician as well as the client. Alignment of the teeth (normal appearance and terminology are given in Fig. 2-6) and the occlusion of the mandible can be assessed using the guidelines in Figure 2-4. The eruption, spacing, and orientation of the teeth and the structure and proportion of the tongue also can be observed. Movement of the tongue can be encouraged by using a lollipop and asking the child to lick it as you place it above, below, and on either side of the child's

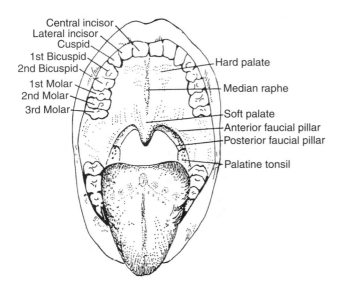

Central incisor
Lateral incisor
Cuspid
1st Bicuspid
2nd Bicuspid
1st Molar
2nd Molar
3rd Molar

Hard palate
Median raphe
Soft palate
Anterior faucial pillar
Posterior faucial pillar
Palatine tonsil

FIGURE 2-6 ✦ View of intraoral structures. (Reprinted with permission from Meitus, I., and Weinberg, B. [1983]. *Diagnosis in speech-language pathology* [p. 43]. Baltimore, MD: University Park Press.)

mouth. Be sure to let the child have the lollipop when you complete the assessment, though!

The structure of the hard palate can be examined using a small penlight, noting the features in Figure 2-4 with reference to the model given in Figure 2-7, *A* and *B*. The clinician should be especially alert for signs of a submucosal cleft of the palate (Fig. 2-8) and the presence of a bifid uvula (Fig. 2-9). These signs include a whitish appearance of the soft palate and a depression in that area that can be felt on palpating the velum. (Stand behind the child with his or her head resting against you as you move a gloved finger along the midline of the palate from the alveolar ridge to the velum.) These findings would indicate the need for further evaluation of the velopharyngeal structures. The function of the velum can be observed by asking the child to sustain /a/ and then to produce short repetitions of /a/-/a/, as indicated in Figure 2-4.

These assessments will be hard to carry out on children younger than 3 years because of their difficulty in tolerating an intraoral examination, as well as their difficulty in imitating sounds on command. To help young children with the intraoral examination, the clinician can let the child use the light to look in the parent's mouth first, then shine the light on his or her own hand to see that it does not hurt. You can ask children to open their mouths so that you can see what they had for breakfast or to see whether there are any elephants (hippos, dinosaurs, or whatever) in there. If the child still refuses to allow the intraoral examination, you might try it again when the child gets to know you better during the course of an intervention program.

Examination of Velopharyngeal Function and Resonance. Even if the velopharyngeal structures appear normal on inspection, it is wise to assess the child's ability to use the velopharyngeal port in speech activities. This can be accomplished quite easily

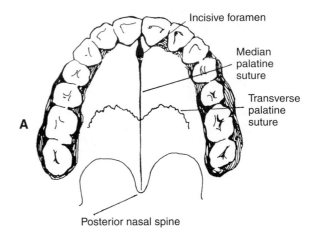

Incisive foramen
Median palatine suture
Transverse palatine suture
A
Posterior nasal spine

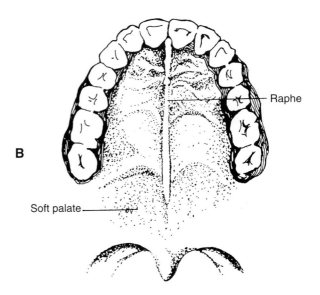

Raphe
B
Soft palate

FIGURE 2-7 ✦ **A,** The hard palate. **B,** Surface view of the soft palate. (Reprinted with permission from Meitus, I., and Weinberg, B. [1983]. *Diagnosis in speech-language pathology* [p. 45]. Baltimore, MD: University Park Press.)

with two quick and efficient instruments. The *Iowa Pressure Articulation Test (IPAT)* (Morris, Spreistersbach, & Darley, 1961) was developed to assess speech errors often associated with velopharyngeal insufficiency. This procedure can be used with children at developmental levels as low as 24 to 30 months. The words used for this test are shown in Figure 2-10; the phonemes within these words that are most important for assessing velopharyngeal function are underlined in the box. The clinician merely asks the client to repeat the words and notes whether the underlined segments are produced correctly. If so, a check is placed on the line for each word. If not, the type of error is recorded, using the key at the bottom of the box. If nasal emissions, glottal stops, pharyngeal fricatives, or nasal snorts are heard, the function of the velopharyngeal port is likely to be compromised. In this case, further investigation as to the cause of this problem should be undertaken with medical consultation. Even if no structural defects can be

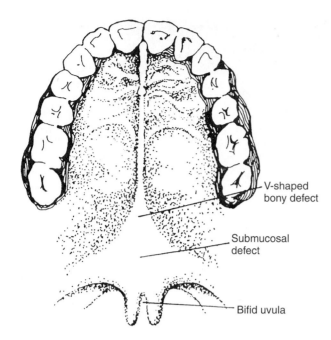

FIGURE 2-8 ✦ Intraoral view of submucous cleft palate. (Reprinted with permission from Meitus, I., and Weinberg, B. [1983]. *Diagnosis in speech-language pathology* [p. 46]. Baltimore, MD: University Park Press.)

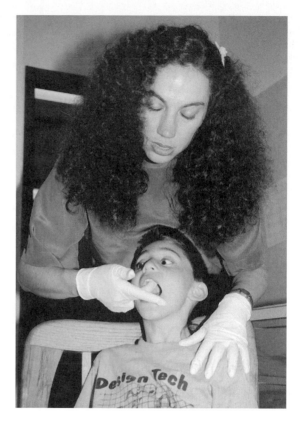

Palpating for a submucosal cleft of the palate.

found, a child producing errors indicating velopharyngeal insufficiency will need treatment for these errors, as well as any necessary language programming.

The degree of perceived hypernasality of speech can be evaluated using procedures developed by VanDemark (1964). The procedure involves asking the child to repeat sentences with a controlled number of nasal sounds. Sentences that can be used for this purpose are given in Box 2-2. The first three sentences contain few nasals. These can serve as a baseline in terms of perceived nasality. The last three have several nasal sounds and can be used to determine whether the nasality of these sounds "spills over" to other words in the sentences. A developmental level of about 36 months is required to perform this task. The child is asked to repeat these sentences after the examiner. The examiner makes a judgment as to whether all sentences sound hypernasal or whether those

containing several nasal sounds have more "spillover" hypernasality than would be normally heard. If either of these conditions pertain, further investigation of the cause is needed. Even if no structural reason can be identified, working on making nasal-oral distinctions in speech should be considered part of the intervention program.

Examination of Volitional Oral Movements. Looking at oral-motor performance in nonspeech activities can be helpful in deciding whether poor speech is related to poor tone or voluntary control of the oral musculature. Some activities to ask children to imitate are listed in Box 2-2. Most children should be able to imitate most of these movements by a developmental level of 36 months.

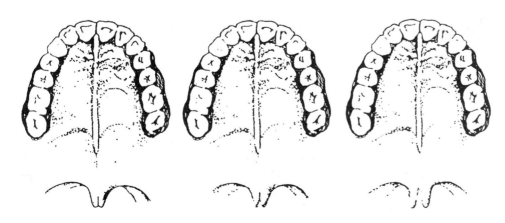

FIGURE 2-9 ✦ Examples of bifid uvula. (Reprinted with permission from Meitus, I., and Weinberg, B. [1983]. *Diagnosis in speech-language pathology* [p. 47]. Baltimore, MD: University Park Press.)

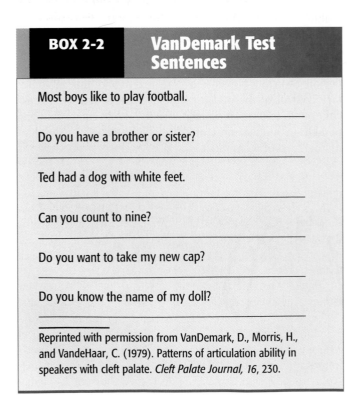

Name: _____	DOB: _____	Age: ____
Date of test: _____		
SCORE: number correct: _____	percentage correct: _____	

tongue _____	sheep _____	fork _____
kiss _____	dishes _____	planting _____
pocket _____	fish _____	clown _____
duck _____	jar _____	glass _____
girl _____	bread _____	block _____
wagon _____	tree _____	wolf _____
dog _____	dress _____	smoke _____
telephone _____	crayons _____	snake _____
knife _____	grass _____	spider _____
soap _____	paper _____	opossum _____
bicycle _____	cracker _____	stairs _____
mouse _____	tiger _____	sky _____
scissors _____	washer _____	books _____
twins _____	stamps _____	stopped _____
		string _____

Key:	√	= OK	G	= Glottal stop substitution
	NS	= Nasal snort	ø	= Omission
	NE	= Nasal emission	D	= Oral distortion
	P	= Pharyngeal fricative		

FIGURE 2-10 ✦ Iowa Pressure Articulation Test (IPAT). (Reprinted with permission from Morris, H., Spriestersbach, D., and Darley, F. [1961]. An articulation test for assessing competency of velopharyngeal closure. *Journal of Speech and Hearing Research, 4*, 48.)

Diadochokinetic Assessment. Diadochokinetic activities can be used to observe the rate, pattern, and consistency of production of syllables. The smoothness and accuracy of the syllables produced during diadochokinetic productions can be noted

BOX 2-2 VanDemark Test Sentences

Most boys like to play football.

_____

Do you have a brother or sister?

_____

Ted had a dog with white feet.

_____

Can you count to nine?

_____

Do you want to take my new cap?

_____

Do you know the name of my doll?

_____

_____
Reprinted with permission from VanDemark, D., Morris, H., and VandeHaar, C. (1979). Patterns of articulation ability in speakers with cleft palate. *Cleft Palate Journal, 16*, 230.

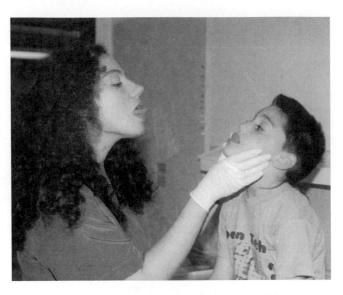

Speech-motor assessment should be done for any child presenting with a speech-language disorder

by the clinician on the form in Figure 2-4. In addition, diadochokinetic rates can be tested in children age 6 years and older using the procedure presented by Fletcher (1978) in Table 2-1. In this procedure the clinician instructs the child to "see how fast you can say these sounds." After a demonstration and practice producing some syllables rapidly, the child is told to "say /pʌ/ as fast as you can a lot of times without stopping or slowing down." The clinician says "Go!" and starts a stopwatch as soon as the child begins. The repetitions of /pʌ/ the child produces are counted silently until the child says it 20 times. The stopwatch is then stopped, and the time to produce 20 repetitions is recorded. The Fletcher test gives average rates per second, with standard deviations, for ages 6 through 13 years. The average number of seconds used to produce 20 repetitions for each age group is given in Table 2-1. If the time used by the client falls within 1 standard deviation of the norm given in Table 2-1, the child's diadochokinetic rate is considered normal. The same procedure is repeated for the syllables /tʌ/, /kʌ/, /fʌ/, and /lʌ/. The child is then asked to produce /pʌtʌ/, /pʌkʌ/, and /tʌkʌ/. The time it takes to produce 15 repetitions of these items is recorded. Finally, the time taken to produce 10 repetitions of /pʌtʌkʌ/ is measured.

This procedure cannot be used with children younger than 6 years. Preschoolers are unlikely to be able to sustain these productions long enough for a stable diadochokinetic rate to be computed. Even though the rate of diadochokinesis cannot be evaluated in preschoolers, diadochokinetic productions can be examined to determine whether the child can make several accurate, smooth, consistent productions of single syllables and to look at the range of consonants for which the child can accomplish this task. The ability to modify tongue position within an utterance to produce syllable sets with two (/pæti/) or three different consonants (e.g., patty-cake) also can be examined. The preschooler who can perform all these tasks would certainly have no diadochokinetic barriers to using speech to communicate.

TABLE 2-1	The Fletcher Time-by-Count Test of Diadochokinetic Syllable Rate

Name: _____   Date: _____

B.D.: _____   Age: _____   Examiner: _____

SYLLABLE	REPETITIONS	#SECONDS	NORMS BY AGE (IN SECONDS)							
			6	7	8	9	10	11	12	13
pʌ	20	_____	4.8	4.8	4.2	4.0	3.7	3.6	3.4	3.3
tʌ	20	_____	4.9	4.9	4.4	4.1	3.8	3.6	3.5	3.3
kʌ	20	_____	5.5	5.3	4.8	4.6	4.3	4.0	3.9	3.7
fʌ	20	_____	5.5	5.4	4.9	4.6	4.2	4.0	3.7	3.6
lʌ	20	_____	5.2	5.3	4.6	4.5	4.2	3.8	3.7	3.5
STANDARD DEVIATIONS ACROSS SYLLABLES			1.0	1.0	0.7	0.7	0.7	0.6	0.6	0.6
pʌtʌ	15	_____	7.3	7.6	6.2	5.9	5.5	4.8	4.7	4.2
pʌkʌ	15	_____	7.9	7.6	6.2	5.9	5.5	4.8	4.7	4.2
tʌkʌ	15	_____	7.8	8.0	7.2	6.6	6.4	5.8	5.5	5.1
STANDARD DEVIATIONS ACROSS SYLLABLES			2.0	2.0	1.6	1.6	1.6	1.3	1.3	1.3
pʌtʌkʌ	10	_____	10.3	10.0	8.3	7.7	7.1	6.5	6.4	5.7
STANDARD DEVIATIONS ACROSS SYLLABLES			2.8	2.8	2.0	2.0	2.0	1.5	1.5	1.5

Reprinted with permission from Fletcher, S. (1978). Fletcher time-by-count test of diadochokinetic syllable rate. *Journal of Speech and Hearing Research, 15,* 763.

Preschoolers who have a great deal of difficulty with these tasks *may* be showing evidence of immaturity or apraxic features, but it is best not to jump to conclusions. With this age group, willingness and motivation can have an especially great effect on performance. To increase this motivation, you can try asking the child to pretend to be a "choo-choo" train by making /pʌpʌpʌpʌ/ sounds, a race car by making /tʌtʌtʌtʌ/ sounds, and so on. If the child's performance on these tasks seems inadequate, ongoing assessment should be conducted as the clinician gets to know the child better. It is well to remember, too, that articulatory and language development are very closely related in young children (Stoel-Gammon, 1991). So it should not be surprising if children who do not talk much show poor performance on these kinds of assessments. Conclusions about a lack of restriction on language production can really only be drawn if the child performs well on oral-motor tasks. If not, it is best to reserve judgment and continue trying these assessments throughout the course of an intervention program to get a valid assessment of their impact.

Evaluating Respiratory and Phonatory Function. In doing this assessment the clinician is again interested in determining simply whether respiratory and phonatory functions are minimally adequate to support basic speech and language. Respiratory function can be evaluated by asking the child to produce any prolonged vowel. Young children may have difficulty persisting in this task for developmental reasons, rather than because they do not have adequate respiratory support for speech. If the child seems unable to sustain vowel production, he or she can be asked to pretend to be a singer and hold a long note in a familiar song or pretend to be the whistle of a train going through a long tunnel. A child who can sustain any phonation for a minimum of 5 seconds can be judged to have adequate respiratory capacity for speech.

Assessment of phonatory function has three components: volume, pitch, and quality. The ability to control volume can be evaluated by asking the child to produce speech that is very soft and then very loud. Having the child pretend to be in a church or library can help for quiet speech. Asking him or her to pretend to yell to a friend across the street or to root for a favorite sports team will elicit loud speech. Children can be asked to demonstrate their range of pitch by imitating the clinician pretending to be a squeaky mouse and a growly bear or by pretending to be a siren with the clinician, who demonstrates the pitch variations in a siren's wail. Vocal quality can be judged in any speech activity, such as the VanDemark sentence task.

Summarizing the Oral-Motor Assessment. For the vast majority of children who are seen for language evaluations, the results of the oral-motor structure and function assessment are "unremarkable," meaning that there is no indication that any aspect of the speech mechanism is interfering with language production. Still, the SLP should be aware that such problems do arise occasionally, and when they do, they must be addressed medically, surgically, or behaviorally for the child to achieve his or her maximum communicative potential.

For some children, oral-motor deficits preclude the development of speech. In these cases, an alternative mode of communication, such as a portable computerized speech synthesizer or a letter, symbol, or picture communication board may be recommended. Most of these children are physically handicapped with conditions such as cerebral palsy or severe dysarthria. For children with milder oral-motor impairments, the speech-motor assessment can help identify oral-motor strengths and needs that can be addressed in an intervention program.

It also is important to remember that the SLP is usually the only professional who will examine the oral mechanism. We cannot assume that the pediatrician, for instance, will have done so before referring a child. Pediatricians and other medical professionals note gross structural defects but may not have looked for signs of a submucosal cleft or for the functional integrity of the mechanism. That examination is the job of the SLP, and unless the child is known to have some orofacial defect or syndrome, it is unlikely that anyone else will have done an examination. Even if only 1 out of every 100 children who present with language deficits is found to have oral-motor problems, it is our responsibility to be the clinician to identify that one child.

Nonverbal Cognition. Another piece of essential information is a measure of nonlinguistic cognition. A model similar to that used to assess hearing also can be followed for evaluating cognition. Although the SLP is not qualified to do IQ testing, there are informal measures of cognitive function based on play assessment, Piagetian tasks, and drawing performance. Table 2-2 lists some of the informal instruments the language pathologist can use as nonverbal cognitive screening measures. In my view, the clinician would be justified in using these informal cognitive screening measures if formal cognitive testing were not available. The clinician could simply assess whether the child is functioning at or near age level on these nonverbal cognitive tasks. If a child does function close to age level on these measures, further information might not be needed. If the child does not, though, the clinician would have a responsibility to make a referral to an appropriate professional for formal developmental testing. An example of a letter of referral for such information is given in Appendix 2-2. Table 2-3 lists formal IQ tests that can be requested to provide this standardized measure of nonverbal cognition for various age groups.

Social Functioning. Since communication is an interactive enterprise, we need to know something about the social environment in which children function to understand their language needs. I want to emphasize strongly that this does *not* mean that we are looking for someone to blame for the child's language disorder. Clinicians are often too quick to conclude that if a family's parent-child interaction patterns are somewhat different from those seen in a typical middle-class family, the child's problems were caused by those interactive patterns. Numerous studies of children with a variety of

disorders (summarized in Caparulo & Cohen, 1983; Leonard, 1989) suggest that the changes in parent interaction styles seen in these families are a result of the parents' functional adaptations to the needs of the child. Except in cases of extreme abuse or neglect, parents are almost never the primary source of their child's communication difficulty.

The real goals of this part of the assessment are as follows:
1. To gather information about how the child uses whatever communicative skills he or she has and to find out how communication problems influence the child's development of daily living skills
2. To assess the child's emotional and behavioral adjustment
3. To find out the family's perceptions of the child's needs and priorities for meeting them
4. To learn about the family's strengths and needs in terms of support from peers and professionals in the difficult task of raising a child with special needs
5. To learn about cultural and language differences present in the home that may affect the child's communication skills or influence the family's perceptions of them

Other aspects of the assessment of social environment may be carried out by a social worker in a multidisciplinary evaluation, either by using published scales or by interviewing. If social-work services are not available, the language pathologist may simply talk with family members about their perceptions, concerns, needs, and hopes for the child. The main purpose of gathering this information is to let the family know that they are crucial members of the team in helping their child achieve the maximum level of functioning possible. It is not only the professionals who decide what the child needs to learn and how to learn it; the family has vital information about these issues that needs to be a part of the management plan. The family also has a right to help determine what goals and methods of intervention most closely meet their needs, as well as the child's, because for the child to function well, the family must be functioning well, too. Recent federal mandates, such those embodied in IDEA (2004) legislation, emphasize the need for family-centered intervention for young children. But all families deserve the same consideration, regardless of the age of their child. The language pathologist has a responsibility to establish an atmosphere in which the family feels that they are partners in the child's progress. Some questionnaire and interview instruments have been developed to assist in the assessment of social environment. These include the *Home and Community Environment Instrument* (Keysor, Jett, & Haley, 2005), the *Homelife Interview* (Leventhal, Selner-O'Hagan, Brookes-Gunn, Bingenheimer, & Earls, 2004), the *Family Strengths Profile* (Trivette, Dunst, & Deal, 1988), the *Measurement of Family Functioning* (Fewell, 1986), and the *Family Environment Scale* (Moos, 1974).

In addition, it may be useful to get some indication of the child's ability to engage in social interaction, apart from language use. Several standardized instruments are available for gathering information about the child's social and daily living skills. The *Vineland Adaptive Behavior Scales-II* (Sparrow, Cicchetti, & Balla, 2005) is a particularly well-constructed

| **TABLE 2-2** | **Informal Assessments Used for Screening Nonverbal Cognition** |

INSTRUMENT	AGE RANGE	AREA ASSESSED	COMMENTS
Cognitive Assessment Battery for Young Children with Physical Impairments (Guerette, Tefft, Furumasu, & Moy, 1999)	18–36 mo	Piagetian skills	Used for children with motor impairments
Cognitive Abilities Scale (ed. 2) (Bradley-Johnson & Johnson, 2001)	3–47 mo	Infant form: exploration, communication, and initiation and imitation. Preschool form: language, reading, mathematics, handwriting, and enabling behaviors	Assess current level of functioning and to identify children who would benefit from special instruction in order to improve their abilities
Developmental Activities Screening Inventory (ed. 2) (DASI-II) (Fewell & Langley, 1984)	Birth–5 yr	Memory, seriation, reasoning, and sensory intactness	Nonverbal format for use with preschool children with disabilities; measures memory, reasoning, sensory intactness
Draw-A-Person Intellectual Ability Test for Children, Adolescents, and Adults (DAP:IQ) (Reynolds & Hickman, 2004)	4–90 yr	Intellectual ability	10 to 12 min. admin. time. Can be administered individually or in groups
Piagetian Concrete Operational Concepts (Goldschmid & Bentler, 1968)	6–12 yr	Concept formation	Used for determining whether child is functioning at school-age level
Piagetian Preoperational Measures (Hohmann, Banet, & Weikart, 1979)	2–5 yr	Classification, drawing	Used for determining whether the child is functioning above a 2-year level
Play Assessment (McCune, 1995)	8–30 mo	Symbolic behavior	Used for establishing level of representational thought
Reynolds Intellectual Screening Test (RIST) (Reynolds & Kamphaus, 2003b)	3–94 yr	Consists of two RIAS subtests: Guess What (a verbal subtest) and Odd-Item Out (a nonverbal subtest)	Helps identify people who need a more comprehensive intellectual assessment or to document the continuing presence of intellectual deficits. 8 to 12 min. admin. time.
Stoelting Brief Intelligence Test (S–BIT) (Roid & Miller, 1999)	6–21 yr	Variety of problem-solving tasks increasing in complexity and difficulty	The examiner pantomimes the instructions and the individual responds by pointing or placing a card in the appropriate position. Provides both norm-referenced and criterion-referenced scores for IQ, Fluid Reasoning, and academically important subtests. 15 min. admin. time
Symbolic Play Test (Lowe & Costello, 1988)	12–36 mo	Play and symbolic ability	Used for establishing level of representational thought
Uzgiris-Hunt Scales of Infant Development (Dunst, 1980)	Birth–24 mo	Sensorimotor skills: object permanence, means-end abilities, imitation, causality, spatial relations, schemes for objects	Used for establishing the presence of basic intentionality and other cognitive skills related to early language

instrument that uses a structured interview format and provides norms for age groups from infants to adults from mainstream as well as handicapped populations. The language pathologist can administer this assessment, with training provided in the test manual. In a multidisciplinary evaluation, a social worker, special educator, or mental health professional may administer it. Some additional scales have been developed recently to assist with assessment of social communicative

TABLE 2-3	Nonverbal Intelligence Assessment	

INSTRUMENT	AGE RANGE	COMMENTS
Comprehensive Test of Nonverbal Intelligence (Hammill, Pearson, & Weiderhold, 1998)	6–90 yr	Has computer-assisted scoring package; designed to reduce bias in intelligence assessment
Hammill Multiability Achievement Test (HAMAT) (Hammill, Hresko, Ammer, Cronin, & Quinby, 1998)	6–17 yr	Uses eight subtests to assess verbal intelligence, overall intelligence, and yields IQ scores
Hiskey-Nebraska Test of Learning Aptitude (Hiskey, 1999)	3–17 yr	Developed for children with hearing impairments
Kaufman Brief Intelligence Test (ed. 2) (Kaufman & Kaufman, 2005)	4–90 yr	Contains vocabulary subtest and matrices subtest; can compare verbal and nonverbal scores
Leiter International Performance Scale–R (Roid & Miller, 1997)	2–18 yr	Uses pantomime for instructions
Merrill-Palmer Scale of Mental Tests (Stutsman, 1948)	18 mo–4 yr	Useful with youngest children
Naglieri Nonverbal Ability Test–Individual Administration (NNAT–Individual Administration) (Naglieri, 2003)	5–17 yr	Assesses general ability in children nonverbally. A companion to the NNAT-Multilevel Form and is the revision of the Matrix Analogies Test-Expanded Form (MAT-Expanded Form). 25 to 30 min. admin. time.
Performance Scale–*Wechsler Preschool & Primary Scale of Intelligence* (ed. 3) (WPPSI-3) (Wechsler, 2002)	2:6–7:3 yr	Part of a full intelligence scale; can compare verbal with performance scores
Performance Scale of *Wechsler Intelligence Scale for Children*–4th ed. (WISC-4) (Wechsler, 2003)	7–16:11 yr	Part of a full intelligence scale; can compare verbal with performance scores
Raven's Progressive Matrices Scale–Colored (Raven, 1977)	5–89 yr (color version)	Requires only pointing response
Reynolds Intellectual Assessment Scales (RIAS) (Reynolds and Kamphaus, 2003a)	3–94 yr	Includes a two subtest Verbal Intelligence Index (VIX) and a two-subtest Nonverbal Intelligence Index (NIX), that taken together form the Composite Intelligence Index (CIX). 20 to 25 min. admin. time.
Swanson Cognitive Abilities Scale (Swanson, 1996)	5 yr–older	Uses high interest materials to engage nonverbal children
Test of Nonverbal Intelligence (TONI-3) (Brown, Sherbenou, & Johnsen, 1997)	5–85 yr	A language-free measure of cognitive ability; requires only a pointing response
Test of Pretend Play (Lewis & Boucher, 1999)	1–6 yr	Assesses level of conceptual development in verbal and nonverbal children
Universal Nonverbal Intelligence Test (UNIT) (Bracken & McCallum, 1998)	K–12th grade	Memory and reasoning abilities

skills, including the *Childhood Communication Checklist—2* (Bishop, 2003), the *Social Responsiveness Scale* (Constantino, 2003), the *Strengths and Difficulties Questionnaire* (Goodman, 1997), and the *Social Communication Questionnaire* (Rutter, Bailey, & Lord, 1999).

Assessment of emotional status may require the involvement of a social worker, psychologist, or psychiatrist. The language pathologist can make a referral to these professionals when the child's behavior and emotional adjustment, as observed during performance on the assessment tasks, appear to be causing problems or standing in the way of successful communication intervention. In making these observations it is always wise to remember that the inability to communicate is a very frustrating condition. The development of maladaptive behaviors often results from being unable to express wants and needs, as we saw in the student with autism we discussed

in Chapter 1. Although evaluating emotional and behavioral aspects of a language disorder is important in planning remedial programming and developing a service plan for the family, we again need to be careful about jumping to conclusions and confusing cause and effect. A child's language disorder may be a result of an emotional disturbance. This is particularly true in cases of selective mutism, when children refuse to speak in certain situations, even though they do speak in others. But it is at least as likely that difficulties in communication caused the behavioral or emotional disturbance observed in a language-impaired child. We'll talk more about this connection in Chapter 4.

Assessing the role of cultural and language differences again involves interviewing the parents about their expectations for communication and their own communicative styles. In some cases, an interpreter who speaks the language of the family may be needed. This issue is discussed further when we talk about culturally and linguistically different children in Chapter 5.

HOW SHALL WE ASSESS?

There are several methods for examining language function: standardized tests, developmental scales, interviews and questionnaires, nonstandardized or criterion-referenced procedures, and behavioral observations, including curriculum-based and dynamic procedures. Each has a place in the assessment process, each fulfills certain functions, but each also has certain limitations. The clinician's aim is to learn to recognize the right instrument to do the job at hand.

Standardized Tests

Standardized or *norm-referenced* tests are the most formal, decontextualized format for assessing language function. They are developed by devising a series of items that are given to (ideally) large groups of children with normal language development and then computing the acceptable range of variation in scores for the age range covered by the test. The advantage of standardized tests, when they are well-constructed, is that they allow a meaningful comparison of performance among children (see Linn & Miller, 2005; Thorndike, 2005, for discussions). They do so because (ideally) they have the following properties:

1. *Clear administration and scoring criteria.* What makes a standardized test "standard" is that it is always given the same way, no matter who administers it, and it is always scored the same way, no matter who scores it or takes it. When evaluating a standardized test, it is wise to read the instructions in the manual and ask yourself whether you understand *exactly* what to do when giving and scoring the test. If questions in your mind cannot be resolved by a careful rereading of the manual, the test procedures may not be stated clearly enough to justify its use.

2. *Validity.* This refers to the extent to which a test measures what it purports to measure. A test is considered valid if its systematic error, or bias, is small. Various types of validity

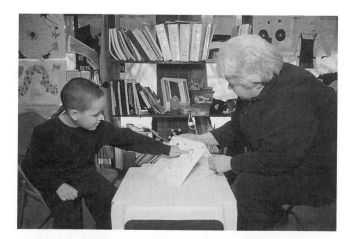

Standardized testing is one method of language assessment.

can be reported. *Face validity* refers to the common-sense match between the test's intended purpose and its actual content. For example, the *Peabody Picture Vocabulary Test—IV* (Dunn & Dunn, 2006) has face validity because it asks subjects to point to pictures that an examiner names, which seems, on the face of it, to be a reasonable way to determine whether a person knows what those words mean. *Content validity* concerns whether the instrument has items that are representative of the content domain sampled by the test (Hutchinson, 1996). This is usually evaluated by having experts in the field judge the instrument as a whole. *Construct validity* has to do with whether the instrument measures the theoretical construct it was designed to measure. This may be evaluated either qualitatively or quantitatively and is, again, generally accomplished by soliciting expert opinion (Thorndike, 2005). *Criterion-related validity* concerns whether the instrument shows strong correlations with other instruments thought to measure the same thing. There are two types of criterion-related validity: *concurrent* and *predictive*. A test has *concurrent validity* when evidence is provided that the test agrees with other valid instruments in categorizing children as normal or disordered. A test has *predictive validity* when there is evidence that this test predicts how the child will perform later on another valid measure of speech or language. These types of validity are generally considered the ones for which mathematical evidence must be presented in the test manual. Tests that do not report some quantitative data on criterion-related validity should not be considered well-constructed instruments (McCauley & Swisher, 1984a; Thorndike, 2005).

3. *Reliability.* An instrument is reliable if its measurements are consistent and accurate or near to the "true" value. Another way to say this is that the amount of random error in the measurement is small. Reliability also can be assessed in several ways. *Test-retest reliability* involves giving the test two different times to the same person and computing the relationship of the two scores. Tests that measure high on this computation are considered *stable*. *Inter-rater reliability* involves having two different examiners either give a test to the same person or score the same person's test. Measuring high on this attribute indicates that a test is not overly influenced by the characteristics of the examiner. Salvia and Ysseldyke (2000) suggested that both these types of validity need to be reported and that for a test to be considered reliable, it must exceed a correlation coefficient of 0.90 with a 95% confidence interval. *Internal consistency reliability* means that the subtests of the instrument rank subjects similarly, or that the parts of the test are measuring something similar to what is measured by the whole. *Split-half reliability,* where scores on the first half of a test are compared with those on the second half, and *odd-even reliability,* where scores on the odd-numbered items are compared with scores on the even-numbered items, are variants of internal consistency measures. *Equivalent forms reliability* means that two

forms of an instrument (such as Form A and Form B of the *Peabody Picture Vocabulary Test—IV* [Dunn & Dunn, 2006]) measure essentially the same thing.

4. *Diagnostic accuracy.* Dollaghan (2003) discussed the requirement that tests demonstrate how accurately they assign clients to diagnostic categories. When a test or other instrument is being used for the purpose of deciding whether or not a child has a particular disorder, measures of diagnostic accuracy are crucial for deciding how confident we can be about the results. This issue is often referred to as *evidence-based assessment practice.* Measures that report these statistics in their manuals provide us with the information we need to make decisions about their accuracy. Dollaghan described several measures of diagnostic accuracy, which are summarized in Table 2-4.

5. *Standardization.* This refers to a set of studies carried out to determine how the instrument works in a known population or norming sample. The characteristics of the norming sample are very important when evaluating a

standardized test. The sample must be big enough, with enough individuals at each age level being tested, to permit statistical conclusions to be drawn. Most authorities on test construction (Salvia & Ysseldyke, 2000) set a minimum of 100 subjects per age group as a lower limit on adequate sample size. The sample also must be representative or contain individuals who are like the subject who will be given the test. This means that the norming sample must (ideally) be drawn from more than one geographic region, both genders, and a range of socioeconomic and ethnic backgrounds. Tests standardized in just one region or on children from a narrow range of economic or racial backgrounds will be less representative. This will mean that they serve as a fair comparison only for children who are like the ones in the norming sample. McFadden and Gillam (1996) discussed the advantages of including not only typical children, but also children with the full range of language abilities in their norming samples. Clinicians should examine standardized tests carefully, looking for

| TABLE 2-4 | **Measures of Diagnostic Accuracy** |

TERM	DEFINITION	FORMULA
Sensitivity	The degree to which a test accurately identifies that a child has the disorder in question; proportion of agreement between a "gold standard" of diagnosis and the test's outcome score	Se = # "true positives" (those testing positive who have the disorder), divided by all those with the disorder.
Specificity	Degree to which a test accurately identifies a child as NOT having the disorder; proportion of agreement between a "gold standard" of normality or absence of the disorder and the test's outcome score	Sp = # of "true negatives" (those testing negative who do not have the disorder), divided by all those without the disorder.
Positive likelihood ratio (LR+)	The degree of confidence that a person who scores in the affected or disordered range on the diagnostic measure truly does have the disorder, or is a true positive. The higher the LR+, the more informative the measure for diagnosing the disorder.	LR+ = sensitivity/(1 − specificity)
Negative likelihood ratio (LR−)	The degree of confidence that a person scoring in the negative (normal) range on the diagnostic measure truly does not have the disorder, or is a true negative. The lower the LR−, the more informative the measure for ruling out the presence of disorder.	LR− = specificity/(1 − sensitivity)
Positive predictive value (PPV)	The probability that the child with a positive test result actually has the disorder. Answers the question, "How likely is it that I will be right when I classify an individual as disordered based on performance on this test?"	PPV = True Positives/(True Positives + False Positives)* *This sum equals all subjects who tested positive.
Negative predictive value (LPV)	The probability that a child with a negative test result actually does not have the disorder. Answers the question, "How likely is it that I will be right when I classify an individual as nondisordered based on performance on this test?"	NPV = True Negatives/(True Negatives + False Negatives)* *This sum equals all subjects who tested negative.

Adapted from Dollaghan, C. (2003). *Evidence-based practice in pediatric communication disorders: What do we know, and when do we know it?* Presentation at the 13th Annual NIDCE-Sponsored Research Symposium, Outcomes Research and Evidence-Based Practice, Chicago, IL; Fleiss, J.L., Levin, B., & Cho Paik, M.C. (2003). *Statistical methods for rates and proportions* (3rd ed.). New York: Wiley.

evidence of adequate size, representativeness, and use of a sample of children with the full range of language abilities when considering the validity of a standardized test.

6. *Measures of central tendency and variability.* If a population taking a test is large enough, the scores of the people taking it will form a normal distribution, or bell-shaped curve like the one in Figure 2-11. This is one reason why it is important for standardized tests to have large norming samples. If they don't, the distribution of scores won't necessarily approximate the normal curve, and they will be more difficult to interpret. When using standardized tests, we usually assume, though, that the scores in the norming population were normally distributed. When they are, most of the scores will fall close to the mean, or arithmetic average of scores for the test. This is the score that is obtained by adding up all the scores and dividing by the number of people who took the test. The further we move away from the mean in either direction, the fewer people in the population will receive that score. That's why the area under the bell curve, representing the percentage of the population who got each score, gets smaller as we move away from the center. The mean is a measure of central tendency, or the tendency of most scores to fall near the middle of the distribution, rather than further out toward its tails, or ends. If we give a test to one

hundred 4-year-olds with normal language function, most of them will score close to the score that is the average for the 100 scores. But how close is close and how far is far? Just knowing the central tendency measure, or mean score, doesn't tell us when a score becomes really different from an average or typical score. That's why we need a measure of normal variability of the test's score, also.

Most standardized tests report, in addition to mean scores for each age group, a *standard deviation.* The standard deviation (SD) represents the average difference of scores from the mean score. It indicates how far from the mean score a typical score fell. In the normal curve, we would expect 68% of scores to fall within 1 SD on either side of the mean for the test. Half of these scores would be higher than the mean, and half would be lower. Ninety-six percent of scores will fall within 2 SDs of the mean. Combining information from the mean and SD of a test allows us to make decisions about when a child's score falls far enough from the mean to warrant deciding that it is really significantly different from normal.

7. *Standard error of measurement.* Any score that we obtain from a client on a test is really only an *estimate* of that client's "true" score. Unfortunately, we can never know the true score with 100% confidence because whenever we measure anything in the real world there is always some

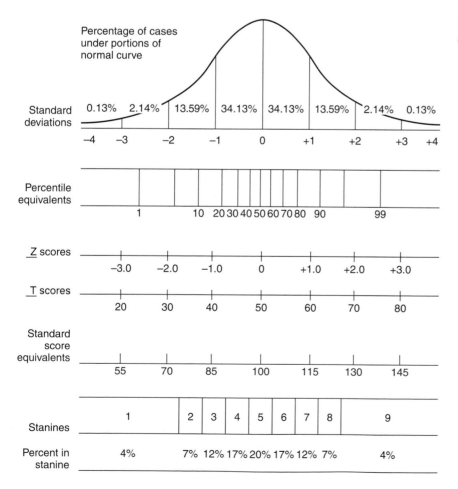

FIGURE 2-11 ✦ Relationships among derived scores and the normal curve.

measurement error involved. For example, if you weigh yourself three times in one day, even on the same scale, the measurements will be slightly different. Which one of them is your "true" weight? If you're like me, you'll say the lowest one! But in fact, none is true. They are all estimates because of the error inherent to the act of measurement.

Measurement error happens because human behavior is never constant. Say you take a typing test. If you did so three times, again, you would get three slightly different scores. None is your true score, but all three are estimates of it. A well-constructed test takes this inevitable human variability into account by reporting a *standard error of measurement,* or SEM. The SEM represents the standard deviation that would be obtained if a person of average ability took the test a large number of times and the distribution of his or her scores were plotted. They would, theoretically, form a normal curve, like the one in Figure 2-11, with the mean being the "true" score. Sixty-eight percent of the time, the subject's observed score would fall within 1 SD or 1 SEM of this theoretical true score. Ninety-five percent of the time the observed score would fall within 2 SDs or 2 SEMs of this true score. In reality, SEM is computed from the reliability coefficients reported for the test. Because we can never, in practice, know a person's true score, we use the SEM to determine a *confidence band* or *confidence interval* around the observed score. We use this band to estimate the location of the true score. The mathematical formula for this estimate is as follows:

Confidence band for true score = Observed score ± SEM

Well-constructed standardized tests provide information about SEM in their manuals and discuss the way to use it to compute a confidence interval for a subject's true score. These tests allow us to say with a certain degree of confidence that, based on the observed score, the subject's "true" score falls within a certain interval. Often, tests that provide SEM information supply a graph on the test form on which this interval can be plotted as a confidence band. Figure 2-12 provides an example of the confidence band computed for a standard score of 86 on the *Peabody Picture Vocabulary Test (PPVT-III)* (Dunn & Dunn, 1997).

SEM and confidence intervals are important because they remind us that a client's score really represents a range of probable performance, rather than a single point. They also are important for comparing performance across time. Suppose a client gets a standard score of 86 on the *PPVT-III.* If the test manual tells us that the SEM around this score is 7 points, then with 90% confidence, or nine times out of 10, we can say that the subject's true score was between 79 and 93. What if we give the test after a course of intervention and find that the client's score increased to 92? Did the intervention provide a true gain? Well, if we take the SEM into account, we cannot truly claim that it did, since the second score fell within the confidence interval for the first. To really believe progress

was made, we would need to see the post-test score move above the confidence interval for the pretest. In general, because of their construction and the inevitability of measurement error, standardized tests are *not* the best way to measure change in an intervention program (McCauley & Swisher, 1984b), although they can be used if SEM information is available. We will discuss some better methods for assessing progress in intervention when we talk about other approaches to assessment.

8. *Norm-referenced scores.* Raw scores, the number of items a client got correct on a standardized test, cannot be interpreted without reference to the *norms* given in the test manual. Only by comparing the client's raw score to scores of other subjects in the norming sample does the test score acquire meaning. Three kinds of comparisons can be made: *standard scores, percentile ranks,* and *equivalent scores.*

   a. *Standard comparisons.* These involve comparing a child's raw score with scores of children in the same population, that is, of the same age, mental age, or grade. The main advantage of these scores is that they represent equal units across the range of scores. A standard score of 85 is just as different from 100 as a standard score of 115 is from 130. This property makes these scores easy to manipulate statistically, so they are best for research purposes. They also are useful for deciding how far apart two scores (such as preintervention and postintervention scores) really are. There are several types of standard comparisons:

      (1). *Z-scores.* Z-scores are simply the number of SD units that a client's score falls from the mean score for that population. Remember that an SD unit reflects the average deviation from the mean in the norming population. In Figure 2-11 you can see that about 34% of children taking a test would, theoretically, earn scores between the mean and 1 SD above it, and 34% would get scores between the mean and 1 SD below it. So about 68% of the population, theoretically, will score within 1 SD on either side of the mean, or average, score for the test. Z-scores have a mean of 0 and an SD of 1, so a Z-score of +1 means a child scores 1 SD above the mean for his or her reference population. A Z-score of –2 means the score falls 2 SDs below the mean.

      (2). *T-scores.* T-scores are very much like Z-scores. The mean is set arbitrarily at 50 and the SD at 10. So a client with a T-score of 35 would be performing 1.5 SDs below the mean, equivalent to a Z-score of -1.5.

      (3). *Scaled scores.* Very often, a test assigns the mean score to a particular value, such as 100, and the SD to a value, such as 15 points. Many IQ tests are constructed this way, with a standard score of 100 representing the mean score and 15 points representing the SD. This form of scaled scoring is sometimes called a *deviation IQ* or *developmental quotient*

Data From Other Tests

Test	Date
PPVT-III (Form IIIA)	

OPTIONAL RELIABILITY CONFIDENCE BANDS

	Level	Standard Score Units
Band of Confidence (Circle one)	68%	± 4
	90%	± 7
	95%	± 8

Standard Score: 79 to 93

Percentile Rank (Norms Table 2): 7 to 30

Normal Curve Equivalent (Norms Table 2): 20 to 38

Age Equivalent (Norms Table 4): 4-6 to 5-3

See manual for complete instructions.

PPVT-III

Peabody Picture Vocabulary Test–Third Edition

by Lloyd M. Dunn & Leota M. Dunn

FORM III B

Performance Record

Name: D.A.

Sex: ☐ F ☑ M

Home Address: 101 Captains Walk   Phone (203) 814-5606

City: Milford   State: CT   ZIP: _____

School: _____   Grade (or education): 1

Language of the Home: ☐ Standard English (or agency)   ☐ Other (specify foreign language, or type of English dialect spoken)

Teacher (or counselor): M.b.   Examiner: _____

Reason for testing: Reported difficulty understanding

Other information on test taker: _____

Date & Age Data

	Year	Month	Day
Date of testing	06	7	28
Date of birth	00	6	24
Chronical age*	6	1	4

*Disregard extra days.

Jan–1 Feb–2 March–3 April–4 May–5 June–6
July–7 Aug–8 Sept–9 Oct–10 Nov–11 Dec–12

RECORD OF SCORES

Raw Score (from oval on page 2): 63

Deviation-type Norms

Standard Score (Norms Table 1): 86

Percentile Rank (Norms Table 2): 18

Normal Curve Equivalent (Norms Table 2): 30

Stanine (Norms Table 2): 3

Developmental-type Norms

Age Equivalent (Norms Table 4): 4-10

Graphic Display of Deviation-type Norm Scores

Mark the obtained standard score on the appropriate line below. Draw a straight vertical line through it and across the other scales. (See manual for more information.)

Optional confidence intervals also may be plotted. To do so, draw two lines vertically across all the scales, one on either side of the obtained standard score line. For the 68 percent band width, use ±4 standard score units. (See manual for other options.)

Standard Score Equivalents	40	50	60	70	80	90	X 100	110	120	130	140	150	160
Percentile Ranks			1	5 10 20 30 40 50 60 70 80 90 95						99	99	99	
Normal Curve Equivalents			1	10 20 30 40 50 60 70 80 90									
Stanines		1	2	3	4	5	6	7	8	9			

Score Range Descriptions	Extremely Low Score	Moderately Low Score	Low Score	Average Score	High Score	Moderately High Score	Extremely High Score

0.13% 2.15% 13.59% 34.13% X 34.13% 13.59% 2.15% 0.13%
−4σ −3σ −2σ −1σ +1σ +2σ +3σ +4σ

FIGURE 2-12 ✦ Confidence band around true score on *PPVT-IIIB*. (With permission from Dunn, L., and Dunn, L. [1997]. *Peabody Picture Vocabulary Test—3rd ed.* Circle Pines, MN: American Guidance Service.)

(DQ). (Recall that IQ stands for "intelligence quotient" and is calculated by dividing mental age by chronological age and multiplying the result by 100.) That's why a child with a mental age the same as his chronological age would have an IQ or DQ of 100: if mental age [MA] and chronological age [CA] are the same, then:

$$MA/CA = 1$$
$$1 \times 100 = 100$$

Many language tests yield DQ scores as well. On a test with this form of standard scoring, a score between 85 and 115 would be within 1 SD of the mean, clearly within the normal range. A standard score between 70 and 84 would fall more than 1 but less than 2 SDs below the mean, and so on.

(4). *Stanines.* Stanines, or standard nines, are normalized standard scores with a mean of 5 and standard deviation of 2. Except for the two extremes (1 and 9), each stanine represents a range of $\frac{1}{2}$ of an SD. Stanines 1 and 9 include all the scores that are $1\frac{3}{4}$ SDs or more from the mean. The fifth stanine comprises the middle 20% of the distribution. The sixth and fourth stanines each contain 17% of the population, and so on out to the first and ninth, which each contain 4% (see Fig. 2-11). Stanine scores are a good way to summarize a child's performance very broadly, but they work best when a child's score falls near the middle of a stanine. Dunn and Dunn (2006) discussed the various uses of these scores further.

(5). *Normal curve equivalents.* These scores are often used by state educational programs as a method of reporting. Normal curve equivalents (NCEs) range from 1 to 99, with a mean of 50 and an SD of 21.06. NCEs of 1, 50, and 99 correspond to percentile ranks of 1, 50, and 99, but other NCE values do not line up directly with percentile ranks (Williams, 2006).

b. *Percentile ranks.* A percentile rank tells what proportion of the norming population scored lower than the subject taking the test. The mean score for a test should be the score at the 50th percentile. A score at the 10th percentile would mean that only 10% of the norming sample population scored below the client's score. Figure 2-11 demonstrates how percentile scores line up with other standard scores, by showing how the percentile scores relate to the theoretical distribution of scores in a normal curve. Percentile rank scores are easy to understand and interpret and are often very useful for discussing a child's performance with parents and teachers. But they do not represent an equal interval scale, as standard scores do. As such, the distance between ranks cannot be assumed to be equal.

c. *Equivalent scores.* The third kind of comparison a standardized test can make is based on equivalent scores. These classify raw scores according to a level, such as age (age-equivalent scores) or grade (grade-equivalent scores). An equivalent score represents the raw score that was the median or middle score earned by subjects in the norming sample who were of a particular age or grade. It is important to note that in equivalent score comparisons, the child is not compared with others in a similar population, that is, to children the same age or in the same grade. Instead, the child's score is assigned to the level representing the age or grade at which the raw score was typical. So a child who got a raw score of 55 on the *PPVT III,* for example, would receive an age-equivalent score of 4 years, 4 months. If this child is actually 7 years old, he is not being compared with other 7-year-olds when the age-equivalent score is reported.

The most important difference between equivalent scores and standard scores is that only standard scores include some measure of normal variation. If we need to decide whether a child's score is *significantly* below expectations for age or nonverbal mental age, we need to know what normal variation around the test mean involves. Otherwise, we don't know how low a score needs to go for it to represent a *significant* deficit. Let's see how this might work in practice.

Suppose a child received a raw score of 29 on the *PPVT–III* (Dunn & Dunn, 1997). This score corresponds to an age-equivalent of 2 years, 4 months. What if our client who took the *PPVT* was 3 years 6 months old? Clearly his score is below age level. Does that mean the child has a deficit in receptive vocabulary? We really can't tell, because the age-equivalent score doesn't give any measure of the normal variability seen in children in the client's population, that is, of the same age. Perhaps that degree of variability is typical of $3\frac{1}{2}$-year-olds taking this test. Only a standard score can tell us if the child's performance is *significantly* different from scores of others that age. In fact, the standard score corresponding to a raw score of 29 for a $3\frac{1}{2}$-year-old is 87, with a percentile rank of 19. This score, then, would fall within the normal range, within 1 SD of the mean for the child's age and above the 10th percentile, and would not justify labeling the child as having a deficit in receptive vocabulary.

Remember, too, that equivalent scores, unlike standard scores, do not represent equal intervals on the scale. A 1-year delay in a 3-year-old is not the same as a 1-year delay in a 9-year-old. Age-equivalent scores are easy to understand but are simply *not appropriate for deciding whether a child has a significant deficit.* Only a standard comparison allows us to make the judgment that a child's performance is significantly below the normal range. Once this significant deficit has been established, we can use the age-equivalent score as an easily understood metric to discuss a child's functioning with parents and teachers and as a means of profiling abilities intralinguistically. But this is acceptable *only* when the child's standard score can be shown to be significantly below normal. If the standard comparison measure falls within the normal range, there is no justification for using or discussing the age-equivalent score. The child is functioning within the normal range of variability on this test, and nothing further ought to be said about it. Reporting an age equivalent in this instance would be misleading.

Standardized tests, as we have seen, need to be evaluated to decide whether they meet accepted criteria to justify their use. If they do not provide clear and unambiguous instructions and information on reliability, validity, standard error of measurement, and standardized comparison scores, we are really not justified in using them since they do not fulfill the role they are purported to serve. Although some years ago it would have been difficult to find tests in our field that met these criteria, the situation is improving as we become more informed consumers of testing materials. Only if clinicians demand well-standardized instruments will the market provide them. It is our responsibility to review the tests available and choose only the best constructed. Hutchinson (1996), Linn and Miller (2005), Sabers (1996), Thorndike (2005), and Salvia and Ysseldyke (2000) provide helpful guidance for clinicians in evaluating standardized tests.

But even if a test is well constructed, can standardized tests ever provide a fair assessment? Much has been written (Duchan, 1982; Dunn, Flax, Sliwinski, & Aram, 1996; Lund & Duchan, 1993; Phelps, 2005; Plante & Vance, 1994) about the inherent dangers of using standardized tests to measure language performance. Should standardized testing be abolished entirely? Anyone who has ever had to qualify a child for services by documenting a deficit will know that standardized testing is essential for this purpose. In fact, standardized testing is the *only* valid, reliable, and fair way to establish that a child is significantly different from other children.

We can do three things to help ensure the fairness of standardized testing with our clients. The first involves choosing tests that meet accepted criteria to be considered psychometrically sound. The second entails interpreting test results properly and judiciously. If we understand the concepts involved in standardized testing outlined in this section, we will be in a position to address both these issues. The third has to do with the uses to which standardized test results are put.

Standardized tests were designed to show whether a child differs significantly from a normal population. To decide whether there is a meaningful discrepancy between the client's score and those of peers, a standardized test is the preferred method. But once that significant discrepancy has been established, other forms of assessment are necessary to establish baseline function, to identify goals for intervention, and to measure progress in an intervention program. Standardized tests were not designed for any of these purposes and they are not valid or efficient approaches for gathering this type of information. Once a significant deficit in communicative performance has been established through use of a limited

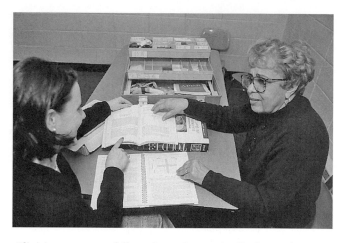

Clinicians must carefully evaluate the standardized tests they use.

number of standardized tests, other tools should be used. We'll talk about some of these other tools now.

Interviews and Questionnaires

Parents, teachers, and other adults who know a child well can provide a wealth of information to supplement our direct clinical assessment. In addition to the clinician-developed interviews and questionnaires we discussed earlier, there are a variety of instruments designed to collect information from adults in a child's life. Many have the same psychometric properties of a well-standardized test, including established reliability, validity, sensitivity and specificity. Instruments with these properties can be very helpful in the evaluation portion of the appraisal, in helping to fill out the picture of the child's level of functioning beyond what can be gathered in a clinical "snapshot." Information obtained from standard interviews and questionnaires can also be helpful in the assessment portion of the appraisal, by giving a more detailed portrait of baseline functioning than we may be able to attain in our limited time with the child. Box 2-3 provides just a few examples of these standard instruments. Additional examples are provided in subsequent chapters, for each developmental level.

Developmental Scales

Developmental scales are interview or observational instruments that sample behaviors from a particular developmental period. Usually they are not fully standardized in that they do not provide standard comparison scores, so they are not appropriate for making the initial decision about whether a child has a significant deficit in communication. But they are formal procedures in the sense that they provide some clearly stated guides for administration and usually provide some sort of equivalent score. Developmental scales such as the *Sequenced Inventory of Communicative Development—Revised* (Hedrick, Prather, & Tobin, 1995), the *Denver II* (Frankenburg, Dodds, & Archer, 1990), and the *Receptive-Expressive Emergent Language Scale-3* (Bzoch, League & Brown, 2003) are often used by language pathologists. It would be a misuse of these instruments to mistake them for standardized tests. Because they only provide

BOX 2-3 **Examples of Standard Interview and Questionnaire Instruments**

Bates-MacArthur Communication Development Inventories (Fensen, Dale, Reznick, Thal, Bates, Hartung, Pethick, & Reilly, 1993)
Child Behavior Checklist (Achenbach & Edelbrook, 2000)
Children's Communication Checklist–2 (Bishop, 2003)
Communication and Symbolic Behavior Scales Infant-Toddler Checklist (Wetherby & Prizant, 2003)
Language Development Survey (Rescorla, 1989)
Social Communication Questionnaire (Rutter, Bailey, & Lord, 1999)
Social Responsiveness Scale (Constantino, 2003)
Vineland Adaptive Behavior Scales–II (Sparrow, Cicchetti, & Balla, 2006)

equivalent score information, they cannot be used to document the existence of a significant deficit. Once that deficit has been identified, however, these scales can be helpful for establishing baseline function by showing the general age-equivalent level at which the child is operating in the areas the scales assess, and they can be used in intralinguistic profiling.

Criterion-Referenced Procedures

Procedures devised to examine a particular form of communicative behavior, not with reference to other children's achievement but only to determine whether the child can attain a certain level of performance, are called *criterion-referenced* assessments. These are not designed to determine whether a child is different from other children. Once it is established that the child has a significant deficit, they are used to establish baseline function and identify targets for intervention by finding out precisely what the child can and cannot do with language. These procedures also are ideal for evaluating whether intervention goals have been met. By using the intervention targets as the criteria for assessment, it can be established whether these criteria are being met in both structured and naturalistic situations. These procedures are often created by the clinician to suit the individual needs of a client, although some criterion-referenced procedures are available in commercial form. Criterion-referenced procedures can be informal and naturalistic because, unlike standardized tests, they do not have to be administered according to rigid rules. But some criterion-referenced procedures are formal and clinician-directed, as well. What distinguishes criterion-referenced approaches to assessment from the other methods we discussed is that the criterion-referenced procedures allow us to look at specific communicative behaviors in depth and to individualize the assessment for a particular child. In this way they lend themselves most effectively to remedial planning and evaluating progress in

intervention. McCauley (1996) discussed in detail the characteristics and uses of criterion-referenced procedures and provided guidelines for their evaluation. Let's look at the kinds of criterion-referenced procedures that might be used for each of the two modalities of language: comprehension and production.

Comprehension. There are several reasons for developing criterion-referenced procedures to assess comprehension. Miller and Paul (1995) and Paul (2000c) discussed these issues in detail. We talked before about the importance of looking at comprehension skills not only in formal, decontextualized settings, but also in more contextualized situations. We also discussed looking at differences in performance between these two conditions. Criterion-referenced procedures are ideally suited to examining contextualized comprehension performance and comparing the response with the same structure in both contextualized and noncontextualized conditions. Let's look at some of the considerations we need to keep in mind when designing criterion-referenced comprehension assessments.

Avoiding Overinterpretation. When we use criterion-referenced procedures to assess comprehension, it is important to remember that we are always inferring something about a private event and we are not observing comprehension directly. That means we must be very careful not to overinterpret what we observe, particularly in the contextualized situation. If a child responds appropriately to an instruction such as, "Put the spoon in the cup," we need to remember that there is a bias toward putting things in containers such as cups. To know whether the child really comprehends the preposition "in," we will need to ask the child to put the spoon "in," for example, a shoe, or something that would be less conventionally expected.

Controlling Linguistic Stimuli. When looking at a child's understanding of language, we need to know exactly what we are testing. If we want to look at comprehension of early developing spatial terms, such as the prepositions "in," "on," and "under," it is important to be certain that any other vocabulary items used in the utterance are well-known to the child. We wouldn't ask a 3-year-old to "Put the spoon in the left-hand drawer," for example. When testing vocabulary comprehension, we need to have established that all the other words in the utterance, besides the one being assessed, are familiar. This can be accomplished either by pretesting or by carefully interviewing the parents about words the child knows.

In the same vein, we need to control the length of sentences used in criterion-referenced comprehension assessment. If we know a child uses only three to four words in his or her own sentences, we had better limit the sentences used in the assessment to that length. Further, we need to be careful to test all structures in sentences of equal length. We shouldn't conclude, for example, that a child has difficulty understanding passive sentences if we give him "The car was pushed by the truck" and "The truck pushes the car." The passive sentence is not only more complex but also longer. If the child does not demonstrate comprehension of it, we don't know whether length or complexity is the problem. The main point is that when devising criterion-referenced comprehension assessments, the linguistic stimuli need to be thought about very carefully to make sure we are assessing what we mean to assess.

Specifying an Appropriate Response. When developing criterion-referenced comprehension assessments, the response is as important as the stimulus. As we've said, we are always inferring comprehension rather than observing it directly, so what we observe needs to be thought about carefully. Criterion-referenced comprehension assessments can use either naturalistic or contrived responses. Either way, though, it is important to specify what response will count as a success so that we clearly understand what we are looking for in the assessment.

Naturalistic responses include behavioral compliance and answers to questions. Behavioral compliance is an appropriate response to observe in children with developmental levels as young as 12 months. It can include touching, moving, picking up, pointing to, or giving objects and can be focused on the assessment of single words ("Give me the *shoe*." "Put it *under* the cup."); morphemes ("This is mommy's cookie."); sentence types ("I *don't* want the spoon."); or speech act intentions ("Can you open the box?"). Specifying a naturalistic response does not have to mean that the assessment involves contextualized language. Both contextualized and decontextualized comprehension can be tested in this format. In fact, it is quite important to distinguish between these two conditions when using a naturalistic response. Remember that a developmentally young child can comply with a request stated as a long, complex sentence such as, "Why don't you open this nice box for me?" (Shatz & Gelman, 1973). But that compliance does not necessarily mean the child comprehends every aspect of the form. Instead, a child might only recognize the words "open" and "box" and comply because the child expects adults to ask children to do things. Unless contextualized and decontextualized variants of a form are contrasted, it will be hard to know whether a child complies with the linguistic stimulus itself or with normal expectations for an interactive situation.

Answers to questions are another naturalistic response that can be used. Usually children will not be reliable in answering questions until they have reached a developmental level of 24 months. Answers to questions can be scored for either semantic or syntactic accuracy. Syntactic accuracy simply involves an answer in the appropriate category. If you ask a child what color an apple is and he says, "Blue," this answer is syntactically appropriate but semantically incorrect. Semantic accuracy involves an answer that would be considered meaningfully accurate by adult standards. Often children can respond with syntactic accuracy before they are entirely semantically correct. Questions, too, can be presented in contextualized conditions, as when picture referents are used or questions concern familiar daily activities. Alternatively, questions can be asked in more decontextualized forms, as with questions about events removed from the immediate situation or about objects and concepts with which the child has only minimal direct experience.

Contrived responses resemble those used in standardized testing. The most common contrived response for a comprehension assessment is picture pointing. Children at develop-

mental levels of 24 months or older can generally respond successfully to picture-pointing tasks. Single-word comprehension ("Point to the shoe."); understanding of sentences ("Point to, 'There are many shoes.'"); or inferential comprehension ("Which picture shows what happened next in the story?") can easily be assessed with this format. Object manipulation is another contrived response, in which children are asked to do something to a set of objects the clinician presents. A developmental level of 20 months or so is generally required for a response in this format. Object manipulation procedures can be used to assess understanding of words ("Find the shoe") and sentences ("Show me, 'The boy is pushed by the girl.'"). They also can be used to assess understanding of connected discourse and inferencing ability by asking children to act out inferred events in a story or what will happen next.

An additional contrived response that can be used in criterion-referenced assessment is a best-fit or judgment response. These types of responses involve some metalinguistic abilities in that they require the child to evaluate language rather than merely use it. As such, they are not appropriate for children younger than 5 years old. But for school-aged children they can be very effective and are easier to construct than picture pointing or object manipulation tasks. Rather than requiring a picture or set of objects to represent each tested item, judgment tasks can involve only two pictures, which the child uses to represent right or wrong, OK or silly, or some other dichotomy. For example, to assess understanding of passive sentences, the child might be given a picture of an "OK" ordinary-looking lady and a "silly" or clownlike lady (Fig. 2-13, *A* and *B*). The child can be told to point to the picture of the lady who would say each sentence. After several demonstrations of what each lady might say (OK lady: "An apple is eaten by a boy." Silly lady: "A boy is eaten by an apple."), the child can be asked to judge subsequent sentences. A similar procedure could be used to assess understanding of connected discourse ("Is it an OK story or a silly story?"), inferencing ("And then he ate the cake. Is that an OK ending or a silly ending?"), speech act intention ("I said, 'Can you pass the salt?' and he said, 'Yes.' Is that an OK answer or a silly answer?"), speech style variation ("He said to the teacher, 'Give me a pencil.' Is that an OK way to ask?"), and other skills.

Whatever type of response we elicit, we need to elicit an adequate number of them. An important advantage of criterion-referenced procedures over standardized tests for establishing remedial goals is that standardized tests usually have only one or two items to test each structure. It can be hard to tell whether the child's performance results from chance, particularly in a picture-pointing format where the child has a chance of being right even if he or she is pointing randomly. Criterion-referenced procedures can include more instances for each form being tested. A good rule of thumb is to include at least four examples for each form and to require the child to get three of the four correct to succeed on that particular form. Another technique is to use contrasting

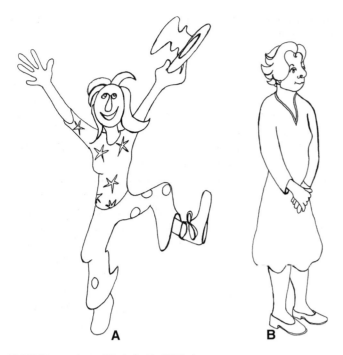

FIGURE 2-13 ♦ A, Silly lady. **B,** OK lady.

sentence pairs ("A boy eats a fish." "A fish eats a boy.") and require that the child perform correctly on both elements in the pair. Both of these approaches can minimize the effects of random guessing.

Production. There are three major approaches to criterion-referenced assessment of productive language: elicited imitation, elicited production, and structural analysis. Because language production does allow us to observe the actual phenomena in which we are interested, issues of inferring information from what the child does are not as crucial as they are in comprehension assessment. Instead, the difficulty in assessing production is to make sure that we get a representative sample of the child's abilities. That's why combining these three techniques, rather than choosing among them, may be the best approach. Let's talk about each one, then see how they might work together.

Elicited Imitation. Asking a child to "say what I say" is probably the easiest way to elicit language. We use this approach in intervention as well as in assessment to provide a model of the speech we want the child to attempt. As we saw earlier, the dangers of elicited imitation are that it tends to result in different kinds of errors than the child would make in spontaneous speech. This is true for both syntactic (Merrell & Plante, 1997; Prutting, Gallagher, & Mulac, 1975) and phonological imitations (Faircloth & Faircloth, 1970; Morrison & Shriberg, 1992; Owens, 2004). Lund and Duchan (1993) also pointed out its pragmatic oddness, since so rarely in real conversations are we asked to repeat what another person says. This might cause children to make changes in the imitated form, not because they could not repeat it but to render it more pragmatically appropriate. If told, for example to repeat, "The red ball is mine," a child might say, "The red

ball (or even "It" since "The red ball" would be redundant in context) is yours." Similarly, a child might be able to repeat a sentence that he or she could not produce spontaneously. For all these reasons, elicited imitation should probably be our last resort as an assessment tool.

Elicited Production. In eliciting production we are tempting the child to say a particular thing by setting up a context in which the target form would be an appropriate remark. Rather than telling the child exactly what to say, as we do in elicited imitation, we give the child a nudge to try to get him or her to say what we would like to hear. There are a variety of ways the child can be nudged into an elicited production.

Patterned Elicitations. Patterned elicitations (Lund & Duchan, 1993) involve modeling a set of similar speech productions, then asking the child to produce a new, analogous production. For example, the clinician might say, "You eat with a fork; you dig with a shovel; you write with a ?" Patterned elicitations also can involve dolls or puppets (Paul, 1992b). For example, the clinician might say, "Here's a grouchy puppet. Whatever we say, he says the opposite. If I say 'It's big,' he'll say 'It's little.' If I say 'It's good,' he'll say, 'It's bad.' Now you be the puppet. If I say, 'It's old,' what does the puppet say?"

Role Playing. Role playing is another way to elicit particular forms from a child. For example, a child can be asked to pretend to be a shy doll's parent. The doll is too shy to answer anyone's questions but the parent's. To elicit question production the client "parent" is told to "Ask him if he likes cookies." The child's ability to produce a variety of question types can then be assessed.

Games. Games of various kinds can be used to elicit specific productions. For example, a game of "I spy" can be played to elicit use of adjectives or relative clauses. In this game, the client and clinician each look at a large, complex picture. The game involves taking turns, with one player (initially, the clinician) describing one element of the picture and the other player pointing to the element described. The clinician models the desired form ("I spy a monkey with a yellow hat." or "I spy a monkey who has a yellow hat.") and notes whether the child can produce it in turn.

Narrative Elicitations. Narrative elicitations have been shown to be a sensitive means of assessing a child's ability to produce connected discourse (Norbury & Bishop, 2003). The child can be told a simple story from a picture book and asked to retell it. Alternatively, a book with vivid pictures that tell a story on their own is given to the child who constructs the story from the pictures (several wordless picture books by Mercer Mayer are ideal for this purpose).

Lund and Duchan (1993) discussed some additional techniques of elicited language production.

Structural Analysis. Structural analysis is the attempt to discover regularities in a spontaneous sample of communicative behavior. In structural analysis, we try to make sense of the communication the child produces spontaneously to find out what structures, forms, and functions a child uses and what contexts influence their use. There are a variety of formats for structural analysis of syntactic production (Crystal, Fletcher,

& Garman, 1976; Hewitta, Hammer, Yont, & Tomblin, 2005; Hubbell, 1988; Lee, 1974; Leadholm & Miller, 1992; Lund & Duchan, 1993; Marinellie, 2004; Owens, 2004; Paul, Tetnowski, & Reuler, 2007; Retherford, 2000; Scarborough, 1990; Tyack & Portnuff Venable, 1998), semantic production (Condouris, Meyer, & Tager-Flusberg, 2003; Lund & Duchan, 1993; Leadholm & Miller, 1992; Miller, 1981; Owens, 2004; Templin, 1957), pragmatics (Bishop & Bishop, 1998; Chapman, 1981; Lund & Duchan, 1993; Owens, 2004; Prutting & Kirchner, 1983; Roth & Spekman, 1984a,b; Tyler & Tolbert, 2002), and phonology (Bleile, 2002; Carson, Klee, Carson, & Hime, 2003; Lund & Duchan, 1993; Ingram, 1976; Paul & Jennings, 1992; Shriberg & Kwiatkowski, 1980; Whissell, 2003). Some of these are discussed in more detail in subsequent chapters.

Structural analysis involves eliciting a representative sample of communicative behavior. Table 2-5 gives some suggestions from Miller (1981) for eliciting a representative speech sample from children of various ages. Miller made some additional suggestions for "good talking" to young children, which include the following:

1. *Listen*: Focus on what the child says, and share his or her focus.
2. *Be patient*: Don't overpower the child with questions or requests. Give space and time for the child to talk. Don't be afraid of pauses.
3. *Follow the child's lead*: Maintain the child's topic and pace. Don't rush on to the next topic or activity.
4. *Don't ask dumb questions*: A good conversational partner has something worthwhile to say. Don't ask questions to which the child knows you already know the answer.
5. *Consider the child's perspective*: Try to see things, such as the assessment situation, as the child does. Take cognitive level and awareness of time, space, and motivation into account. Give the child's comments your undivided atten-

tion and respond positively to them. Be warm and friendly.

Leadholm and Miller (1992), Hewitta et al. (2005), Marinelle (2004), Owens (2004), and Paul, Tetnowski, and Reuler (2007) provided additional discussion of issues of language sampling.

As the sample is being collected, we will want to record it. Recording the sample allows us to examine it in more detail than we could if we had to get all the information from it in real time. Audio recordings are usually used when speech itself is the focus of the assessment and when there is enough intelligible speech present that other information is not needed to figure out to what the client is referring. Video recording can be used when a nonverbal context is necessary to decipher meanings or when nonverbal aspects of communication are of interest. The recorded sample is then transcribed at whatever level is appropriate for the analysis being done. Semantic and syntactic analyses require word-by-word transcriptions of the client's speech, probably with the linguistic context of the other speaker's remarks included. Phonological analysis requires phonemic transcriptions and in some cases phonetic level information, as well. Pragmatic analysis necessitates some information about the nonlinguistic context and perhaps about paralinguistic cues that accompany the speech. The sample is then analyzed not only for errors but also for evidence of patterns or regularities that can be used to identify the child's level of communication and to describe the rules and contexts that influence production. We'll talk in more detail about the methods for analyzing language samples in subsequent chapters on assessment at a variety of developmental levels.

Integrating Approaches. Structural analysis is no doubt the most valid way to look at a child's productive language, since we are observing the very thing we are interested in assessing: spontaneous speech for communicative purposes. One drawback of this approach, though, is that the child may

TABLE 2-5	**Suggestions for Eliciting a Representative Speech Sample from Children**

LANGUAGE LEVEL (BROWN'S [1973] STAGE)	MATERIALS	SAMPLE TYPE
I–III	Familiar and unfamiliar toys; several examples of balls, dolls, eating utensils, cars, etc.	Child-centered conversation on here-and-now topics
III–V	Pretend play materials, such as dollhouse with people, furniture, etc.; introduce some topics about absent objects, people, and events removed from the immediate context in space and time, such as holidays, vacations, etc.	Child-centered conversation on both here-and-now and there-and-then topics
V–on	Picture books, unusual objects to describe	Object description, narration of personal experience, story retelling, or story generation from picture book

Adapted from Miller, J. (1981). *Assessing language production in children: Experimental procedures.* Needham Heights, MA: Allyn and Bacon.

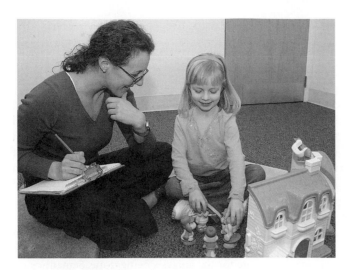

Language sampling ensures validity of expressive language assessment.

not spontaneously produce all the aspects of language that interest us. When talking to an unfamiliar adult, for example, a child may be unlikely to produce questions and negative forms, for pragmatic reasons. If these forms simply do not appear in spontaneous speech, how can we know the child's skills in these areas? The advantage of criterion-referenced assessment is that we can combine approaches as needed to give us access to additional information. One strategy for doing a criterion-referenced production assessment would be to collect a sample of spontaneous communication; record, transcribe, and analyze it; and identify any structures or functions of interest that did not appear in the sample. We could then use an elicited production procedure to try to get some evidence about these forms. If the child still failed to "take the bait," direct elicited imitation might be tried.

Behavioral Observations

Criterion-referenced assessment and structural analysis allow the clinician to examine a child's communicative performance in detail without the restrictions and limitations imposed by standardized testing. With criterion-referenced procedures, however, we are still comparing the child's performance with a predetermined criterion to decide whether the child is meeting this criterion or whether the child needs intervention to accomplish this goal. Behavioral observations differ from this approach in that they are not concerned with comparing a child's performance with a criterion, but only with describing performance in a particular area. Behavioral observations are used to sample whether a particular behavior of interest occurs, the frequency with which it occurs, and the context or antecedents likely to be associated with it. Behavioral observations commonly are designed by clinicians and involve checklists or rating forms that are used to examine or count particular behaviors. Figure 2-14 gives an example of a behavioral observation form that might be used to examine communicative competence in a child suspected of language

disorder. This form was adapted from one developed by Erickson (1987*b*).

The most important aspect of behavioral observation is carefully defining the behavior or behaviors that we want to observe. This means that we must target areas for behavioral observation before we begin the assessment by determining which aspects of the client's communication will be difficult to assess through any of the other methods we've discussed. While standardized and criterion-referenced procedures are useful for looking at language behaviors for which there are well-established norms or comparison data, behavioral observations are suited to those behaviors for which less normative data exist, for which somewhat subjective judgments must be made, or for which standard comparisons are not usually done. For example, computing a mean length of utterance in morphemes in a criterion-referenced structural analysis is a relatively objective, straightforward procedure, one for which some normative data are available. If we want to examine the structural complexity of a child's speech, computing a mean length of utterance in morphemes is a reasonable approach. But what if we want to know how frequently a child responds inappropriately to questions, using either verbal or nonverbal responses, rather than how complex a child's utterances are? The answer to this question might be important if it were part of the initial referral, for example. In this case, a behavioral observation could be done, in which we ask the child questions in a naturalistic format, such as having him or her describe to the examiner illustrations in a picture book and then counting the number of appropriate and inappropriate responses. The observation would give some quantitative information about a communicative behavior and could serve as a baseline for evaluating intervention directed at reducing inappropriate responses.

A second important consideration in devising behavioral observations is to use a recording system designed for the purpose. Performing a behavioral observation does not mean just sitting and watching a client behave. A recording document that contains a way to collect quantitative data about the behavior of interest must be used. The form may allow the clinician to rate the frequency of a particular behavior, as the form in Figure 2-14 does, or it may allow the clinician to rank a behavior on a scale. The rating used in the oral mechanism assessment in Figure 2-4 is an example of this type of observation. The form also could be simply a checklist in which the existence of a particular behavior is noted. For example, the list of articulation errors associated with velopharyngeal insufficiency in Figure 2-4 could serve as a checklist. A child's spontaneous speech also could be rated for these types of errors. The errors could simply be listed on a sheet and a check placed by each if it were heard in the sample. An assessment like this might be important if we need to determine whether the child is using errors in naturalistic conversation that have been eliminated in structured settings by intervention. The main thing to remember about behavioral observations is that we are never justified in doing them unless we know exactly what we will be looking for and have developed a form or document to serve as a record for the observation. Such a

I. Discourse skills

	Frequently Observed	Occasionally Observed	Not Observed	Examples
Starts a conversation	_____	_____	_____	_____
Shows listening behavior	_____	_____	_____	_____
Responds with appropriate content	_____	_____	_____	_____
Interrupts appropriately	_____	_____	_____	_____
Stays on topic	_____	_____	_____	_____
Changes topic	_____	_____	_____	_____
Appropriately ends a conversation	_____	_____	_____	_____
Recognizes listener's viewpoint	_____	_____	_____	_____
Demonstrates topic relevancy	_____	_____	_____	_____
Uses appropriate response length	_____	_____	_____	_____

II. Speech acts and communication functions

	Frequently Observed	Occasionally Observed	Not Observed	Examples
Labels things or actions	_____	_____	_____	_____
Asks for things or actions	_____	_____	_____	_____
Describes things or actions	_____	_____	_____	_____
Asks for information	_____	_____	_____	_____
Gives information	_____	_____	_____	_____
Asks permission	_____	_____	_____	_____
Requests	_____	_____	_____	_____
Promises	_____	_____	_____	_____
Agrees	_____	_____	_____	_____
Threatens or warns	_____	_____	_____	_____
Apologizes	_____	_____	_____	_____
Protests, argues, or disagrees	_____	_____	_____	_____
Shows humor, teases	_____	_____	_____	_____
Uses greetings	_____	_____	_____	_____

FIGURE 2-14 ✦ A worksheet for analyzing communicative skills. (Adapted from Erickson, J. [1987]. Analysis of communicative competence. In L. Cole, V. Deal, and V. Rodriguez [Eds.], *Communication disorders in multicultural populations*. Rockville, MD: American Speech-Language-Hearing Association.)

document is important not only for organizing our observations but for being sure that another clinician could observe the same behavior in the same way. This ensures that progress over the course of an intervention program can be reliably charted. Let's talk about several specific types of behavioral observations that can fill particular "niches" in our overall appraisal.

Dynamic Assessment. All the assessments we have discussed so far fall under the heading of "static" procedures. According to Olswang and Bain (1996), static assessments describe current level of performance by holding contextual support to a minimum. In contrast, dynamic assessment is designed to "systematically manipulate the context to support performance so that a child's optimal level of achievement can be identified" (p. 415). Lidz and Peña (1996) characterize dynamic assessment as a "pretest-intervene-posttest" format (p. 367). In dynamic assessment, the clinician actively engages a child in a learning situation that allows observation of the client's learning process and then attempts to promote change (Elliott, 2000). Clients are encouraged to think out loud throughout the session and to analyze their learning processes. The outcome of a dynamic assessment is not a score. Instead,

it can be described with the following three kinds of information used in assessment planning:

▶ How the child approaches tasks; error patterns, and self-monitoring abilities
▶ The degree to which the client's behavior is modifiable in response to interventions
▶ Intervention styles and methods that will have the greatest potential to promote change

Functional Assessment. Frattali (1998) defines functional assessment as going beyond identifying deficits in specific communicative processes and evaluating their effects on the ability to communicate interpersonally in natural settings. Functional assessment can play a role when a clinician uses a systems approach to communication disorders (that is, we may use functional assessment strategies to analyze communication opportunities and barriers that exist in the client's environment, in addition to assessing the deficits that are "in" the client). Recent studies (e.g., Long, Blackman, Farrell, Smolkin, & Conaway, 2005; Noell, VanDerHeyden, Gatti, & Whitmarsh, 2001) have demonstrated the use of functional assessments for children with communication disorders. Several tools are available for this enterprise, such as the *Communication Supports Checklist* (McCarthy, McLean, Miller, Brown, Romski, Rourk, & Yoder, 1998). These measures are discussed in more detail in subsequent chapters.

A second form of functional assessment is presented by Campbell (1998). He argues that we need to go beyond our traditional assessment of positive change in the specific communication behaviors addressed in the intervention program. *Functional assessment* here refers to the evaluation of the ways in which these newly learned communicative behaviors increase a client's level of autonomy in real-life situations. To accomplish this assessment, he advocates rating a child's use of communication in everyday life on six basic parameters. These parameters were identified by reviewing treatment summaries of children in intervention to identify the most common goals and most frequent parental expectations. Campbell developed a form, similar to the one in Figure 2-15, to be filled out by both the clinician and the parent at the first and last intervention sessions. Using a form like this, it is possible to establish not only that specific communication behaviors have changed as a result of intervention, but also how these changes have an impact on the perceived communicative competence of the child.

Curriculum-Based Assessment. Curriculum-based assessments (CBAs) are frequently used in school settings. They may be constructed by teachers, SLPs, and other professionals to reflect the content of the curriculum. CBAs can be used effectively to assess curriculum-based language use and may be more sensitive to tracking the progress of students from culturally and linguistically diverse backgrounds than traditional standardized testing (Idol, Nevin, & Paolucci-Whitcomb, 1999; Losardo & Notari-Syverson, 2001). You may hear various terms used in reference to these methods, including *authentic assessment* and *performance assessment* (Damico, 1993). Data collected about a client's performance often include various artifacts (examples of written work, projects, language samples, etc.) organized into a portfolio. Scoring rubrics are frequently used to make judgments about the degree to which the performance demonstrates the desired behavior or skill (Kennedy, 2007). We'll talk in more detail about these kinds of assessment in Section III, on school language and learning disabilities.

THE HARD-TO-ASSESS CHILD

Many children can cooperate with a clinician for an extended period so that assessment goes smoothly and quickly, but some cannot. In the course of a diagnostic career, every clinician encounters children who are hard to assess. Some clinicians call these children "untestable." Their clinical report on these youngsters may simply state that the child was unable to cooperate with any testing, so assessment information could not be gathered. My position is that no child is untestable and that, using a variety of clinical tools, it is possible to get at least some useful assessment information about every child, regardless of how hard he or she may be to assess.

When clinicians say a child is untestable, they usually mean that the child does not respond to standardized tests. But remember that standardized tests are only necessary to establish that a child is significantly different from other children. This is usually easy enough to do in a hard-to-assess child. Even if the clinician feels that the standardized test results underestimate the child's true ability, the fact that the child falls below the cutoff is enough to qualify the client for further assessment. From then on, criterion-referenced and behavioral observation procedures can be used. These are less formal and can be adapted to the needs and interests of the child. In addition, if the child refuses to participate in standardized testing at all, standardized interview and questionnaire procedures, such as the *Vineland Adaptive Behavior*

Please answer the following questions about your child's communication. Please check the box of the number that best describes your child's current abilities.

	1 (Never)		2 (Rarely)		3 (Sometimes)		4 (Almost Always)		5 (Always)
Your child attempts to say words									
Your child understands what is said to him/her									
Your child successfully communicates wants and needs to others by speaking									
Your child successfully communicates wants and needs to others without speaking (e.g., using gestures, signs, facial expressions, communication devices)									
Your child communicates successfully with peers									
Your child's speech can be understood by unfamiliar listeners									

FIGURE 2-15 ✦ Functional assessment of children's communication. (Adapted from Campbell, T.F. [1998]. Measurement of functional outcome in preschool children with neurogenic communication disorders. *Seminars in Speech and Language,* 19[3], 223-233.)

Scale-II (Sparrow, Cicchetti, & Balla, 2005), can be used to get a norm-referenced score based on parent report. Again, this can confirm the child's significant difference from peers, and less formal methods can be used to establish baseline function and identify goals for intervention.

Nelson (1991) discussed four kinds of children who may be hard to assess: children who are extremely shy and quiet, those who are noncompliant, those who are hyperactive and impulsive, and those with physical handicaps. For *shy* children, slowing down the pace of the assessment, giving more time to warm up, and starting with comprehension procedures that require little speech on their part can be helpful. A clinician can use misnaming of common objects and playful violations of routine to get these children to engage in criterion-referenced and behavioral observations.

For both *noncompliant and hyperactive* or impulsive children, setting a tone of firm control on the part of the clinician and perhaps asking the parent to wait in an observation room rather than within the child's view may be useful. Nelson (1991) suggested using time-out procedures to gain the cooperation of the noncompliant child. This may require making the assessment longer than planned, but it often results in the ability to get some valid information about the child instead of having to give up in defeat. Avoiding language that gives the child power over the clinician—such as asking the child, "Do you want to do X?" or following a command with "OK?"—can prevent awkward situations in which the child takes the clinician up on the apparent opportunity to reject what the clinician has proposed. Removing extraneous stimulation from the environment can help the hyperactive child focus on the assessment materials. Being flexible about where to do the assessment also can help with this type of child. Instead of insisting that he or she sit at the table, the clinician can do some of the assessment on the floor, in the hall, or under the table. Nelson also suggested taking frequent breaks and doing the assessment in small chunks of time rather than in one extended period.

The child with visual or other *physical disabilities* also presents special problems because of the inability to respond to the usual assessment stimuli in the usual way. Children with physical disabilities who cannot point may be asked to look at the stimulus that best matches what the clinician says. Those with no speech can be given several different alternative communication modes, such as pictures, Blissymbols, signs, or written words, in a dynamic assessment approach to determine what helps them to communicate best. Blind children may be asked to name or describe objects that they feel or to tell about events that they have experienced.

Nelson (1991) provided additional suggestions for working with the hard-to-assess child. The important point is for the clinician to know that something can be learned about every child with a communication problem, even if standardized testing does not seem the most fruitful source of information. In my opinion, we are never justified in writing off a child as "untestable." By making use of our complete repertoire of assessment tools, it is possible to decide for every child whether there is a communication problem, to establish baseline function, and to determine what the child needs to communicate better. This is our mission and, difficult though it may be, it is never impossible.

INTEGRATING AND INTERPRETING ASSESSMENT DATA

Once the interviewing, testing, and observations have been completed, we must interpret the meaning of the assessment data. If a significant deficit is identified by standardized testing, the standard score comparisons may be converted to age equivalents. These can then be combined with information from developmental scales to create an intralinguistic profile of abilities, such as the one in Figure 2-2. The profile can be used to plan what kinds of additional criterion-referenced assessments and behavioral observations may be needed to complete our picture of the child's current level of functioning. This information may be gathered in subsequent assessment sessions or during the early phases of the intervention program. What we do *not* want to decide on the basis of the standardized testing is that we need more standardized testing. Once we have determined that the child has a significant deficit in communicative performance, the important task is to establish baseline functioning in the various areas of language. Interviews, questionnaires, criterion-referenced procedures and behavioral observations, including functional, dynamic, and curriculum-based methods are better suited to this purpose.

When the intralinguistic profile has been established and the baseline level of functioning has been outlined, this information is used to complete the final three parts of the appraisal process: determining the severity of the disorder, making a prognostic statement, and making recommendations for an intervention program.

SEVERITY STATEMENT

Based on the assessment data, a decision is made by the clinician as to the degree of severity of the child's communication disorder. Generally, severity is labeled as *mild, moderate, severe,* or *profound.* The World Health Organization has provided guidelines to the use of each of these terms, which are summarized in Table 2-6.

Severity ratings are important for two reasons. First, they help to establish priorities for intervention. If communicative deficits are severe, whereas deficits in other areas assessed by the multidisciplinary evaluation are less severely affected, then priorities for intervention should include speech and language services. Conversely, if communication is less severely affected than other areas, such as social-emotional development or behavior regulation, these areas might take precedence for intervention resources. The second purpose of the severity rating is to have a benchmark for evaluating the effectiveness of intervention. If communicative skills are initially assessed as severely impaired and after several years of intervention the severity rating improves to moderate, this is one way to

TABLE 2-6	Severity Classifications

CLASSIFICATION	DESCRIPTION
Mild	Some impact on performance but does not preclude participation in age-appropriate activities in school and community Able to function independently with minimal assistance
Moderate	Significant degree of impairment that requires accommodations to function in mainstream settings Able to function in a supervised setting
Severe	Extensive support required to function in mainstream settings May demonstrate some functional skills with supervision
Profound	Few functional skills Requires maximum assistance with basic activities

Adapted from Accardo, P., & Whitman, B. (Eds., 2002). *Dictionary of developmental disabilities terminology* (2nd ed). Baltimore, MD: Paul H. Brookes; Kennedy, M. (2007). Principles of assessment. In R. Paul & P. Cascella (Eds.). *Introduction to clinical methods is communication disorders.* Baltimore: Paul H. Brookes. In press; World Health Organization. (2004). International statistical classification of diseases and related health problems -10th revision (2nd ed.). Geneva: Author.

establish the effectiveness of the intervention, even though fully normal functioning has not been achieved.

PROGNOSIS

The prognostic statement contains the clinician's prediction about what communicative outcome can reasonably be expected at some future time, in light of the current level of functioning. Prognostic statements are similar to severity statements in that they help us to economize intervention resources and aid in accountability. If a clinician states in the prognosis that a child has the potential to achieve normal communicative function, this statement can serve, again, as a benchmark against which to measure progress in intervention. If the child fails to achieve the level of function predicted in the prognostic statement after a reasonable time in intervention, either the prognosis was wrong or the intervention has not been as effective as it should have been. In either case, an accounting of the discrepancy is necessary.

For this reason, we need to be cautious when making prognostic statements, taking all relevant factors into account. Age is usually important in prognosis. The younger a child is when a communication disorder is identified, the less certain the outcome. A teenager with no functional speech has a much clearer and poorer prognosis than a 2- or 3-year-old who has not begun to talk. The social environment can affect prognosis

as well. A client from a well-functioning family that has the resources and energy to work with and advocate for the child has a brighter prognosis than a child from a family in which the parents are ill, addicted to drugs or alcohol, or overwhelmed by a struggle for economic survival. The client's personality and temperament, too, have an effect. A careful, reflective child who has well-developed attentional capacities is in a better position to take advantage of intervention than a hyperactive, impulsive child, who must acquire basic attending behavior before much learning can take place. Similarly, a child who is highly motivated to improve because he or she has a lot to communicate and is willing to take some risks and make some mistakes has a better prognosis than an extremely cautious, shy child who is relatively self-sufficient and does not feel strongly impelled to overcome the communicative deficit. The involvement of other areas of functioning beyond communication also affects prognosis. A 3-year-old with mental retardation and autism who does not talk generally has a worse prognosis than does a sociable nonspeaking 3-year-old with normal cognitive function. Issues of prognosis for various conditions associated with language disorders are discussed in more detail in Chapter 4. Again, the clinician must evaluate each aspect of the prognosis throughout the course of the appraisal, making use of data from interview and observational sources. The clinician's impressions of these elements will be factored into the prognostic statement.

Despite using the best and most extensive data available, though, when we state a prognosis we are always making an educated guess. Whether we make a prognostic statement in writing, in a clinical report, or in conversation with the client's family, this fact has to be respected. It is usually best, then, to make a short-term rather than long-term prognosis and to talk about what it is the child *will* likely be able to do over a specified period, rather than what he or she won't be able to do. For example, a prognosis might contain a statement that with intensive intervention the client will move within 1 year from single-word utterances to the production of some two- and three-word sentences. This prognosis can be evaluated, since it states a specific time period and a measurable outcome. This prognosis also is preferable to one that states that a client will not achieve normal expressive language development, for example. This contains no time period over which an evaluation can be made and states only a negative outcome, not what *can* be expected to happen.

Clinicians who adhere to the rule of making short-term prognoses and stating them in positive terms usually encounter less resistance and hostility from families than those who make blanket long-term projections of which, in truth, no one can really be sure. Even when pressed by a family to predict what the child will be like as an adult, the wise clinician can remind the parents that the important task is to help the child do the best he or she can now and for the next few months or years. An honest admission that human beings are too complicated and unpredictable for us to foretell their future can be coupled with encouragement for the family to work with the child as he or she is now and to advocate for the services he or she needs to achieve the next appropriate developmental step. An assurance that diagnosis and prognosis will be ongoing can help the family to cope with the uncomfortable uncertainties of raising a child with disabilities.

RECOMMENDATIONS

The last, but certainly not the least, task of the assessment process is making recommendations for intervention. These recommendations draw directly on the assessment data. When we talked about the "why" of assessment, we discussed the establishment of goals for intervention as one of the central purposes of the appraisal. In making recommendations, we incorporate the establishment of goals for intervention into a more general statement about the need, directions, and approach to intervention that would be most appropriate for this particular client. The statement of recommendations, then, in either the clinical report or in conference with the family contains three parts:

1. Our recommendation as to whether some intervention by an SLP is appropriate at all. This recommendation is based on whether the child has a significant communication disorder and whether we believe, as a result of the severity and prognostic statements, that intervention would be helpful.
2. The goals we have established for intervention, based on the assessment data and intralinguistic profile.
3. Suggestions for methods, approaches, activities, reinforcers, or any other aspects of the intervention program that the clinician believes would be informed by the data gathered during the assessment. This is the clinician's chance to share the observations and insights gained from working with the child that would help to maximize chances for success in intervention.

PUTTING IT ALL TOGETHER: THE CLINICAL REPORT

A clinical report is simply a summary containing all the information we have been discussed in this chapter. Generally, the clinical report follows a more or less standard format, such as the one given in outline form in Box 2-4. Appendix 2-3 provides a sample of a clinical report. The report starts by stating basic identifying information, such as client name, age, date of birth, address, phone, parents' names, referral agency, and so on. The next section contains a short statement of the presenting problem or complaint. This is followed by a brief review of the historical data. The next section of the report is usually labeled "Assessment" or "Examination Findings" and contains the standardized tests given and the standard score comparisons. Other assessments also are summarized briefly. The next section, entitled "Impressions" or "Behavioral Observations" is where the clinician states some of the insights that come out of working with the child, such as the clinician's opinion about factors in the child's social environment or temperament that may influence current functioning

---

| BOX 2-4 | **Outline for a Clinical Report** |

I. Identifying information
Name:
Sex:
Address:
Date of birth:
Parents:
Date of evaluation:
Phone:
Age:
Referred by:
Examiner:

II. Presenting Problem
III. Historical Information
IV. Examination Findings
Collateral areas
Norm-referenced language measures
Criterion-referenced measures
Behavioral observations

V. Impressions
VI. Summary
Examination findings
Severity statement
Prognosis

VIII. Recommendations
Is intervention needed?
Goals
Suggestions for methods, approaches, activities, and reinforcers

---

or success in an intervention program. In the "Summary" section, the clinician interprets the findings, saying what, in aggregate, the appraisal data mean. This section also generally contains the severity and prognostic statements. The "Recommendations" section should contain the three points we discussed previously.

The language in the clinical report should be clear and simple, but professional. It is not necessary to use every technical term we know or to repeat every confidence expressed in the interview. The purpose of the clinical report is to convey as succinctly as possible the information gleaned from the assessment and to do so in a way that both parents and other professionals will find easy to understand. Toward this end, the use of some personal pronouns (I, we, etc.) is acceptable and would generally be preferred to awkward usages, such as "this clinician found..." In general we want

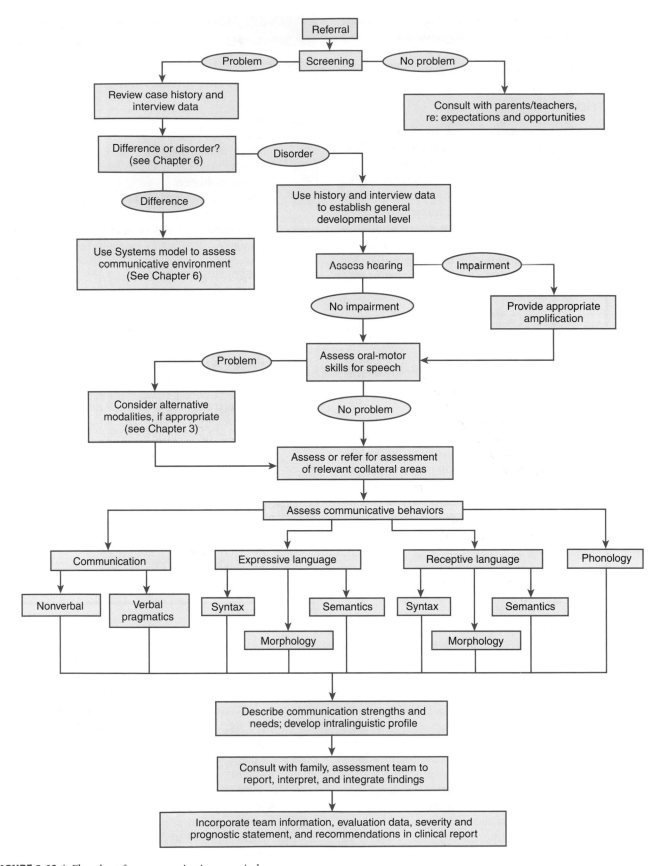

FIGURE 2-16 ✦ Flowchart for communicative appraisal.

to avoid qualifiers, such as "rather" and "very." We need to distinguish between information we gathered or observed ourselves and that reported to us by parents or others, so it is appropriate to use phrases such as, "according to parent report," or "the mother recalls." It's best to avoid judgmental terms such as "good," "poor," "nicely," etc. in describing a child's performance. Usually sentences in active voice are better than passives, although passive sentences can be used occasionally. Short sentences are usually better than long ones. Each new thought should have its own sentence. Keeping the noun and verb in each sentence close together is a good rule. This helps to keep the sentence from getting too strung out and complicated. Jerger (1962, p. 104) provides good advice when he tells us to "write it the way you would say it." We can think of the clinical report as a conversation, in which we try to tell another person who is not an SLP what we saw in this child. This image can help us to choose the words and sentences that work hardest to get our meaning across.

■ CONCLUSIONS

The appraisal process provides the backbone of our intervention program. It tells us whether we need to intervene and what the targets of intervention need to be, and it allows us to decide whether intervention has been effective. The clinician should be familiar with a variety of tools, both formal and informal, for gathering assessment information and must choose these tools carefully to make the most of the time spent assessing the child's skills. The speech-language appraisal is usually part of a larger process that may require the clinician to communicate findings to other professionals and to request further information. The typical sequence of this process is schematized in Figure 2-16. To perform the functions we've been talking about, a clinician needs to develop special writing skills for clinical communication. In writing clinical reports, we are having a sort of conversation with others concerned about the client and want to get across to them not only what we learned from our testing, but what we inferred from our interactions with the child and the family. In acquiring skills as diagnosticians, then, we also are developing some new communication skills of our own.

STUDY GUIDE

I. The Appraisal Process
  A. Discuss the aspects of an assessment that should be included in an assessment plan. What should not be included?
  B. What goes into a case history? From where does the information come?

II. Making Assessment Decisions
  A. What does "screening" mean in a speech-language assessment?
  B. Why do we need to establish baseline function as part of an assessment for a communication disorder?
  C. How do clinicians choose intervention targets?
  D. Give two reasons for doing ongoing assessment as part of an intervention program.
  E. Give the rationale for doing a hearing assessment and a speech-motor assessment for every child suspected of communication disorder.
  F. What is the role of the speech-language clinician in assessing intelligence?
  G. How can the child's social environment be assessed?
  H. Discuss the areas of communication included in a language assessment.
  I. Discuss some of the difficulties of assessing language comprehension.
  J. Discuss the advantages and disadvantages of using speech sampling as an assessment of productive language.
  K. Describe the qualities a clinician should look for in a good standardized test.
  L. Define and give examples of measures of central tendency on standardized tests. Do the same for measures of variability.
  M. Discuss the differences between standard and equivalent scores. What are the uses of each?
  N. Define the standard error of measurement, and tell why it is important.
  O. Discuss the difference between developmental scales and criterion-referenced measures. When would each be used?
  P. Explain how standardized testing and other assessments provide complementary information in the assessment process.
  Q. Explain why behavioral observations are included in an assessment.
  R. Define and discuss *dynamic* and *functional* assessment. What is the purpose of each?
  S. Define the terms associated with measuring a test's diagnostic accuracy.

III. Integrating and Interpreting Assessment Data
  A. State the seven major sections of a clinical report, and describe what would be placed in each.
  B. Give the three components of the recommendations section of a clinical report.
  C. Discuss desirable traits of clinical report writing.

Name: _____

     First   Middle   Last

Birthdate:_____

Age:_____ years _____ months

Parents' names:_____

Address:_____

                 Street

_____

    City   State   Zip Code

Phone:_____

Date:_____

Name of person completing this form

_____

Relationship to child _____

Please answer the following items as completely as you can.

I. REFERRAL SOURCE

Who recommended you to this clinic?

Name _____Phone _____

Address _____Agency _____

II. ACADEMIC INFORMATION

A. School

_____

Name   Phone

_____

Address   Teacher-Grade

B. Briefly indicate how well your child functions in school _____

_____

III. MEDICAL INFORMATION

Indicate the physician who is best acquainted with the client.

_____

Name   Phone

_____

Address

Indicate the physician who has treated the client most recently.

_____

Name   Phone

_____

Address

Is there a physical handicap such as: Cleft palate _____

Paralysis _____ Mouth or teeth deformity _____

Hearing loss _____ Other _____

Comments _____

Has there been a psychological evaluation? _____

When? _____ Where?_____

Is medical treatment being received at the present time?

_____

If so, indicate for what condition treatment is being received.

_____

IV. SPEECH AND LANGUAGE INFORMATION

A. Description

1. Speech

Is child's speech understandable? _____

Are sounds omitted? _____

Is one sound substituted for another? _____

Is the voice unpleasant or different? _____

Explain _____

2. Rhythm

Is there stuttering? _____ Stammering? _____

Rapid speech? _____

Other comments _____

3. Language

Does the child understand more than he or she can say?

_____

Is the language delayed? _____ Immature? _____

Absent?_____ Lost? _____

Are sentences too short? _____

Incomplete? _____ Vocabulary too small? _____

Does the child consistently use specific sounds to designate certain objects, people, or things? _____

_____

_____

4. History

Is the child aware of his or her speech problem? _____

Does it bother him or her? _____

Has the child had speech training? _____

Where, by whom, and how long? _____

_____

Is more than one language spoken in the home? _____

_____

Have others outside the family commented regarding the problem? _____

Please explain _____

V. HEARING INFORMATION

A. Is the hearing problem mild? _____

Moderate? _____ Severe? _____

B. Has there been preschool deaf training? _____

Number of years? _____ Where? _____

_____

C. Describe time spent in other training programs for the acoustically handicapped _____

_____

D. Describe medical assistance for hearing problem, including dates of surgery, etc. _____

_____

E. Is a hearing aid worn? _____ Type _____

Where purchased? _____

Is the aid satisfactory? _____ Left ear _____

Right ear_____ Both ears _____

VI. RELEASE OF INFORMATION

Information that may help us plan a treatment program may be needed from physicians, schools, and other agencies who have assisted in your child's care. Please sign the following release so that we can obtain this information.

REQUEST FOR RELEASE OF CONFIDENTIAL INFORMATION

I hereby authorize you and/or your agency to release any and all information that is available on,

_____

First   Middle   Last

Birth date _____

Month   Day   Year

which may be requested by the staff of the Speech and Hearing Clinic. Additionally, I offer my permission for this "release of information" form to be duplicated and used at the discretion of the administrator of the Clinic. I understand this information will be kept confidential and will be used by professional personnel for the sole purpose of diagnosis and treatment.

Signed _____

Address _____

Date _____

City/State/Zip Code _____

_____

February 17, 2006

Donald McCormack, MS, School Psychologist
Albany Public Schools
Albany, NY

Re: JAMES, Christina
DOB: 11-20-99

Dear Mr. McCormack,

Tina James is a 6-year-old girl being referred to you for a cognitive assessment, following my speech and language evaluation on January 23. Ms. James brought Tina to the diagnostic center on the recommendation of her first-grade teacher, Ms. Taylor. The primary concern was poor articulation and short, immature sentences. Ms. James reports that Tina has always been slow in her development.

The results of my speech and language assessment reveal adequate oral-motor function for speech. Tina makes many substitutions in producing speech sounds and often leaves off the final sounds in words. These processes combine to make her speech difficult to understand. Her comprehension of language is significantly below normal. Receptive vocabulary is at a 3-year level. Understanding of sentence structures is lower, at about a 30-month level. Her production of language is characterized by two- to-three word sentences and frequent omissions of inflectional endings.

As part of my evaluation, I did an informal assessment of cognitive skills, using Piagetian tasks such as copying figures and sorting. It is my impression that Tina's performance on these tasks is below age level. I have recommended that a cognitive assessment be performed to investigate these skills more formally. Because of Tina's problems with language, an assessment of nonlinguistic cognition would be most helpful. Please call me if there is any need to discuss this request further. Thank you for your help.

Yours,

Speech-Language Pathologist

I. Identifying Information

Name: Mark XXXXXX
Sex: Male
Address: 220 Mercer St., NYC
Date of Birth: 11/21/00
Parents: Carol and Jay XXXXXX
Date of Evaluation: 3/3/06

Phone: 673-3788
Age: 6:4
Referred by: Ms. Naughton, kindergarten teacher
Name of Examiner: Ellen Witherson

II. Presenting Problem

Mark's teacher told his parents at the parent-teacher conference that Mark is very hard to understand. When he talks, few of the children know what he means. Ms. Naughton, too, has great difficulty in understanding Mark's speech. The parents were aware that Mark had trouble making himself understood, because they sometimes had difficulty understanding him themselves. Mark also seems to be unhappy about going to school and frequently complains that he is too sick to go.

III. Historical Information

Mark was the product of an unremarkable full-term pregnancy. He weighed 7 pounds 10 ounces at birth and had no newborn difficulties that the parents recall. Mark achieved motor milestones at the normal times, sitting up at 6 months, walking at 14 months, and feeding himself at 1 year. Parents report that speech was late to begin, with few words at 2 and no word combinations until 3. Mark's speech has always been hard to understand, even for members of the family, although by now they can usually figure out what he means. Mother reports that Mark had two or three ear infections before the age of 2, but none after that age. No feeding problems were noted by parents. Medical history is unremarkable. Mark had regular checkups and received all immunizations on schedule.

IV. Examination Findings

Collateral areas: Hearing threshold testing revealed normal hearing in both ears. Examination of the oral mechanism revealed no gross structural abnormalities, but Mark had difficulty producing rapid, smooth repetitions of syllables such as /pʌ/, /tʌ/, and /kʌ/. This difficulty was even more pronounced in utterances with more than one consonant, such as /pʌtʌ/. Cognitive skills were assessed informally with sorting and drawing tasks. Mark appeared to perform at age level on these tasks.

Mark achieved the standardized test scores shown at the bottom of the page.

Nonstandardized assessments of Mark's speech and expressive language skills included an analysis of spontaneous speech and several tasks designed to elicit the production of questions and grammatical morphemes. These analyses revealed that Mark makes numerous changes in his production of speech sounds that are similar to those used by younger children with normal speech patterns. These include leaving off final sounds in words (/da/ for "dog"), making all the sounds in a word more alike (/dadi/ for "doggy"), and substituting earlier-developing sounds for more difficult ones (/top/ for "soap"). When all these changes are put together in connected speech, the speech becomes very difficult to understand. Mark's average sentence length in spontaneous

AREA ASSESSED	TEST USED	SCORE	NORMAL RANGE
Articulation (pronunciation)	Goldman-Fristoe Test of Articulation	5th percentile	Above 10th percentile
Naming	Expressive Vocabulary Test	60th percentile	Above 10th percentile
Producing sentences	Structured Photographic Expressive Language Test	3rd percentile	Above 10th percentile
Understanding words and sentences	Test of Auditory Comprehension of Language —Revised	40th percentile	Above 10th percentile

speech was shorter than would be expected for his age. He used fewer helping verbs and other forms of sentence elaboration than would normally be seen in a 6-year-old. The ideas he expressed were age appropriate, however, in that he talked about past and future events, talked about imaginary topics, and was able to exhibit role-playing. His conversational abilities appeared age appropriate. He attempted to respond to requests for clarification when his speech was not understood, maintained topics for several turns, and changed his speech style when playing a baby and a daddy in the pretend situation.

In the question elicitation task, Mark was unable to change the order of words in a sentence to form a question. In the grammatical morpheme task, Mark consistently left off most morphemes, including ones that are generally easy to pronounce, such as "-ing."

V. Impressions

Mark worked very hard during the assessment and seemed to be trying to do his best. During the expressive test, he was often unable to remember the whole sentence and could only repeat a few words of it. He became frustrated during the free-play session when the examiner was unable to understand him and turned to his mother to provide a "translation."

The parents seem very concerned about Mark's difficulty, but at the same time, they see many positive aspects of his growth. They point out that he is talking more than ever now, that they and his brother can understand him most of the time, and that he tries to imitate them when they correct his speech. They also are pleased that he is very interested in letters and numbers and likes to look at picture books and point out letters he recognizes. They feel he is a bright, capable little boy and think that with some time to mature he will outgrow his speech problems.

VI. Summary

Mark is an apparently bright 6-year-old boy with no significant medical history, but a history of delayed expressive language development. Current assessment reveals normal hearing and language comprehension. His ability to express meanings and engage in conversation appear age appropriate. Mark shows moderate to severe deficits in phonological development and a moderate deficit in expressive language, particularly in the areas of syntax and morphology. His ability to engage with others, his motivation to succeed, and the active support of his family suggest that progress in an intervention program should be significant. Given intensive intervention in phonology and expressive language over the next year, Mark's prognosis for significant improvement in intelligibility and for significant increases in sentence length and complexity is very favorable.

VII. Recommendations

Mark could benefit from speech-language intervention. Individual instruction for working on phonological targets could be combined with group instruction or in-class work with the teacher in consultation with the SLP to improve intelligibility in conversation and increase the complexity of expressive language.

The following specific goals are recommended:
1. Decrease omission of final consonants.
2. Increase production of age-appropriate consonant sounds.
3. Increase self-monitoring of intelligibility in connected speech.
4. Increase use of helping verbs, such as "can," "will," and "be" in sentences.
5. Increase use of grammatical morphemes, at first those that are easy to pronounce, such as "-ing."

Mark enjoys pretend play, and this setting may be useful for working on self-monitoring intelligibility. The parents are very committed to helping him and could be engaged in some homework activities to carry over what is being worked on in the intervention program.

Clinician's Signature

_____

Supervisor's Signature

_____

PRINCIPLES OF INTERVENTION

CHAPTER OBJECTIVES

Readers of this chapter will be able to do the following:
- Discuss the various purposes of intervention.
- List ways in which intervention can change communicative behavior.
- Discuss way of identifying appropriate goals for communication intervention.

- Describe interventions at various points on the continuum of naturalness.
- List and discuss various contexts for providing intervention.
- Describe methods of evaluating treatment outcomes.
- Discuss principles of evidence-based practice.

The result of a successful language intervention program is not simply that a child responds correctly to more items on a test or accurately imitates the language stimuli given by the clinician. Successful intervention results in the child's being able use the forms and functions targeted in the intervention to effect real communication. The goal of our intervention, then, is not only to teach language behaviors but also to make the child a better communicator. To be ethical (American Speech-Language-Hearing Association, 2003b) we also must be able to show that intervention has led to changes in language behavior that would not occur if no intervention were provided. Achieving all these goals is quite a challenge, one that requires us to be more than merely technicians. Effective language intervention involves a great deal of thought and a wide range of decision making.

The developmental-descriptive model of language disorders holds that the best guess at a sequence for teaching language skills is based on what we know about how children learn language normally. In general, a speech-language pathologist (SLP) develops an intervention plan by identifying the child's current level of language use in the various areas documented in the assessment. Looking for semantic, syntactic, phonological, and pragmatic skills that would be next in the typical developmental sequence and targeting these skills will identify the goals of intervention. But many factors go into the process of choosing what, how, and where we will attempt to improve the client's communication. Let's examine these factors in some detail.

▮ THE PURPOSE OF INTERVENTION

The first question we have to ask is, overall, what is the purpose of the intervention we are proposing? Olswang and Bain (1991) discussed three major purposes of intervention. The first is to *change or eliminate the underlying problem*, rendering the child a normal language learner, one who will not need any further intervention. Of course, all of us would like to achieve this with all our clients. Unfortunately, it is not usually possible. Frequently we do not even know what the underlying deficit is, let alone how to alleviate it. In a few instances, though, this might be a realistic goal. For a child with a hearing impairment, for example, if the loss is discovered during early childhood and amplification or cochlear implantation can be used to achieve normal or nearly normal hearing, the language pathologist might need only to provide the child with help in getting language skills to approximate the child's developmental level (ASHA, 2004b; Geers, 2004). Once these developmentally appropriate skills are achieved, normal acquisition could proceed, ideally anyway, without further intervention. Similarly, a young child who suffered a brain injury and developed an acquired aphasia might require intervention to restore language function. Once the brain's normal plasticity is geared up to overcome the damage, further intervention might not be needed and language learning could proceed more or less normally.

In the real world of language intervention, though, cases in which the underlying cause of the impairment is both known and fully remediable are the exception. Most children present with language disorders of unknown origin or associated with incurable conditions, such as mental retardation or autism. In these more common cases, we must settle for something less than changing the child into a normal language learner. Olswang and Bain (1991) identified this second choice as *changing the disorder*. In this case we attempt to improve the child's discrete aspects of language function by teaching specific behaviors. We teach the child, for instance, to expand the number of words and grammatical morphemes in sentences, to produce a broader range of semantic relations, or to use language more flexibly and appropriately. This makes the child a better communicator but does not guarantee that he or she will not need further help at a later time. This purpose is the one most commonly invoked when working with children who have impaired language.

A third option identified by Olswang and Bain is to teach *compensatory strategies*, not specific language behaviors. Rather than, for example, teaching a child with a word-finding problem to produce specific vocabulary items on command, we would attempt to teach the child how to use strategies to aid recall of vocabulary during conversational tasks. We might teach the child to use phonetic features of the target word, as a cue, or to try to think of words that rhyme with the word that the child can't recall. This approach usually requires a good deal of cognitive maturity and is generally used to help older school-aged and adolescent students who have received language intervention for a number of years and will probably always retain some deficits (Wallach, 2005). Rather than trying to make their language normal, the clinician attempts to give them tools to function better with the deficits they have.

There is a fourth option. The goal of language intervention may be focused not on the child at all, but on the child's environment. We discussed this option under the *systems* model of language disorders. In some situations it makes sense to try to influence the context in which a child must function instead of trying to change the individual. Take Justin, for example.

Justin was born with severe cerebral palsy. After years of intervention he was still not able to produce much intelligible speech. In middle school, his language comprehension and literacy skills were near age level, though, and he had been given an augmentative communication device that included a communication board and a computerized speech synthesis system. But his parents commonly forgot to bring the device along when they went out, and often forgot to send it to school with him, so he was forced to revert to vocal attempts to communication, which were usually not very successful. Without an easy way to communicate with him, his classmates usually left him alone with his aide, so he had few peer interactions. His teacher interacted mostly with the aide, rather than Justin, giving her assignments to have Justin complete. His parents requested additional therapy for the oral language since they felt he was trying so hard to communicate that way. Instead, his clinician set up sessions with the family to teach them to use the system, to find out what was getting in the way of using it, and to give Justin a signal to use as a request for the device. In addition, the clinician showed Justin's classmates how to use the device, so that they could talk to HIM by using it, as well as allowing him to talk to them. The classmates thought the computerized device was pretty cool and started spending more time interacting with Justin. The clinician encouraged the teacher, too, to use the device to give Justin his assignments directly, rather than talking to the aide. Now Justin can usually get someone to set up his device when he wants to say something. He also spends more time interacting with peers and participating, through his device, in class discussions.

Often this fourth option is combined with one of the other three to maximize the child's communicative potential. On occasion, though, modifying the environment alone will be the purpose of the clinician's activities.

Choosing which of these options to pursue as an overarching purpose is an important first step in an intervention plan. This choice enables the clinician to talk realistically with the family about the long-term goals and prognosis for the client. If alleviating the basic deficit is the purpose, the clinician can tell the family how long it will take for this to happen and how much intervention should be needed to achieve it. Since the long-term purpose is normal acquisition, only the short-term goals for intervention need to be specified. If modifying the disorder is the goal, both short- and long-term objectives need to be identified. If teaching compensatory strategies is the purpose of the intervention, then short- and long-term goals are formulated very differently than they would be for modifying language behavior itself. So the first decision to be made in developing an intervention plan is the basic purpose of the intervention.

This decision is based on the age and intervention history of the client, the nature of the disorder, and the way the environment interacts with the child's communicative function, as well as on the data collected from the communication appraisal. Young children with treatable or transient conditions may be restored to normal language learning with limited intervention. Older children with long histories of intervention who are likely to have lifelong deficits may benefit most from a compensatory-strategies approach. Modifying the environment may be the primary purpose for some clients and a secondary purpose with others. Most commonly, though, the purpose of intervention is to modify the language disorder. Given this purpose, how is the change accomplished?

How Can Intervention Change Language Behavior?

According to Olswang and Bain (1991), when the purpose of intervention is to modify the disorder, language behavior can be changed in several ways. These alternatives are depicted in Figure 3-1.

Facilitation

The first role intervention can play is that of *facilitation*. With facilitation, the rate of growth or learning is accelerated, but the final outcome is not changed. In other words, facilitative language intervention helps children to achieve language mile-

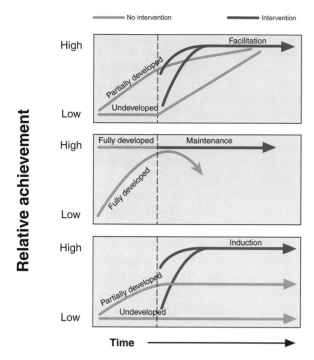

High

Low

High

Low

High

Low

Relative achievement

Time

— No intervention   — Intervention

Facilitation

Partially developed

Undeveloped

Fully developed   Maintenance

Fully developed

Induction

Partially developed

Undeveloped

FIGURE 3-1 ✦ Purposes of intervention. (Reprinted with permission from Gottlieb, G. [1976]. Roles of early experience in species-specific perceptual development. In R. Aslin, J. Alberts, and M. Peterson [Eds.], *Development of Perception.* Vol. I. Orlando, Fl: Academic Press.)

stones sooner than they would have if left to their own devices, but it does not mean that they ultimately achieve higher levels of language function than they would have without intervention.

If all facilitation does is increase the rate of acquisition of a particular behavior without altering the child's eventual language status, why bother to intervene? Gottlieb (1976) argued that facilitation could help a child increase his or her ability to differentiate among perceptions. In other words, facilitation can bring language to a higher level of awareness. This awareness can influence other aspects of development. For example, perhaps a child with a phonological disorder would outgrow his multiple articulation errors without intervention by age 8 or 9. But if intervention to overcome these errors is provided earlier, this intervention may not only improve articulation but also may focus the child's attention on the sound structure of words. This increased awareness may contribute to the child's phonological analysis skills, which, as we shall see later, are important for the development of literacy. Some writers (e.g., Whitehurst, Fischel, Lonigan, Valdez-Menchaca, Arnold, & Smith, 1991) suggest that if therapy is merely facilitative and the child would eventually outgrow the disorder anyway, there is no justification for intervening. But many clinicians (Olswang & Bain, 1991; Paul, 1991a; Robertson & Weismer, 1999) have argued that facilitative intervention is justified because of the other systems in development that accelerating language skills may affect. Take a child like Sammy.

Sammy is a cute, apparently bright 3-year-old who has trouble communicating. His speech is hard to understand, his sentences are limited to two or three words, and he tends to push first and talk later. An appraisal by the local education agency (LEA) revealed that his problems were pretty much limited to expressive language; his cognitive and receptive language skills were at age level. He was having some difficulty with social skills and was showing some behavior problems, though, and seemed to be very frustrated about not getting his ideas across. His parents were quite anxious and concerned, particularly about his difficulties in getting along with other children. The LEA reported that he did not qualify for intervention because his deficits were limited to expression and were in the mild-to-moderate range. His parents were told that he would probably outgrow these deficiencies by the time he got to school. But they didn't want to wait. They were able to arrange for him to see a clinician through a private charitable agency. After 6 months his intelligibility, although still not normal for a child nearly 4 years old, had improved so that at least half of his utterances were comprehensible to peers. Sammy seemed a happier little boy; his aggressive behavior had decreased, neighbors were inviting him over to play more often, and his parents were feeling much more at ease.

This example illustrates how improving communication can affect a child's social skills, behavioral repertoire, self-esteem, and family relations. These outcomes also are considerations in deciding whether to initiate intervention. Communication influences many aspects of a child's life, and increasing its maturity, even if a problem would eventually be outgrown, can often result in changes that go beyond the language behavior itself.

MAINTENANCE

A second way that intervention can change behavior is through *maintenance.* Olswang and Bain (1991) explained that intervention for the purpose of maintenance preserves a behavior that would otherwise decrease or disappear. Gottlieb (1976) argued that maintaining behaviors is important to "keep an immature system intact, going, and functional so that it is able to reach its full development at a later stage" (p. 28). A toddler with a cleft palate, for example, for whom surgery was delayed for medical reasons, might need intervention to maintain babbling and early vocal behaviors. These behaviors would then be functioning and available for building intelligible language once the palatal vault was closed by surgery.

INDUCTION

Finally, intervention can serve the role of induction. *Induction* of a behavior means that the intervention completely determines whether some endpoint will be reached. Without the intervention, the outcome is not achieved. For example, a hearing-impaired 4-year-old who uses very little spoken language, who comes from a hearing family, and who has no access to the deaf community will not learn sign language as a form of communication unless intervention takes place. The use of intervention to teach the child sign language as a form of communication would be an example of induction.

Induction is the most dramatic form of intervention and the one for which we would most like to take credit. Unfortunately, in most real-life situations we do not know ahead of time whether our intervention is accomplishing facilitation or induction. Induction, of course, is the most cost-effective purpose of intervention, and when deciding whether to intervene, we feel more at ease if we can convince ourselves that the effect of the intervention will be induction rather than facilitation. In truth, though, we often do not have enough information to know. In these cases, I would argue that we be familiar with the role of facilitation in language learning and be prepared to assert the importance of facilitation as a valid outcome of intervention.

◼ DEVELOPING INTERVENTION PLANS

Once a decision to establish an overall purpose for intervention has been made and we specify, or at least think about, how we expect our intervention to change client behavior, the next step is to develop a specific plan. Like assessment, intervention should be carefully considered and planned in detail before it is implemented. One aspect of this planning involves making use of the available scientific evidence in choosing our intervention methods. This aspect of planning is referred to as using *evidence-based practice*. Let's talk about some of the ways we as clinicians can use evidence to decide on what constitutes our best practice for our clients.

EVIDENCE-BASED PRACTICE

Let's imagine you are a clinician working with a preverbal 3-year-old named Brendan. One day, Brendan's parents come to you with a newspaper article, which says that exposing children who don't talk to a certain kind of auditory stimulation (through a special set of earphones) leads to speech. There's a Web address in the article, and the parents have looked it up; the program is available for $2000; all they have to do is send for it and have the child wear the earphones for 20 minutes three times a day. They ask you whether you think they should purchase the program, and whether you would include 20 minutes of this treatment within each of Brendan's sessions with you. How will you answer them? These kinds of questions lead us to the need for evidence-based practice (EBP).

Ochsner (2003) defined evidence-based practice as "the conscientious, explicit, and unbiased use of current best research results in making decisions about the care of individual clients" by integrating clinical expertise with the best available external clinical evidence from systematic research (Sackett, Strauss, Richardson, Rosenberg, & Haynes, 2000). Dollaghan (2004) discusses these issues and reminds us that EBP does not *only* mean solving clinical problems by going to the external evidence, defined primarily as published literature, to find the best available scientific support for the use of specific intervention approaches,

although it does mean that, too. Fey and Justice (2007) tell us that EBP includes evaluating internal evidence as well. Internal evidence comes from characteristics of the client and family, their willingness to participate in a treatment approach, and their preference; as well as our own clinician preferences, professional competencies, and values; and the values, policies, and culture of the institutions in which we work. Let's talk about how we can evaluate external evidence first, then we'll consider how internal evidence is included in this decision-making process.

Dollaghan (2004) suggested we approach external evidence using three principles:

1. The opinions of expert authorities (including expert panels and consensus groups) should be viewed with skepticism.
2. All research is not created equal. Everything that gets published is not necessarily true (or to paraphrase your grandmother, you can't believe everything you read). Some studies are better, and therefore better suited to inform clinical decisions, than others.
3. Clinicians must be critical about the quality of evidence they use to guide clinical decision-making.

Let's see what these principles might mean to us in practice. First, they tell us that we can't take "experts" at their word. If you go to a workshop and a famous clinician tells you about a new approach that can't fail, you have to ask yourself, "How does she know?" If the answer is not based on data presented, but rather on her confidence and experience, we have to consider her endorsement with a few grains of salt. Why? Well, maybe the approach does work for her, but it works because she is an especially talented clinician and another person doing the same thing may not get the same results. Or maybe she works with certain kinds of clients, who are not like the clients in your practice. There could be lots of reasons. The point is, her saying it works is not enough. If you decide to try the approach, you should carefully monitor its effects on your clients, and perhaps compare it to other approaches you are using before deciding that it is really right for your practice and your clients.

Dollaghan's second and third principles tell us that not only must we view experts with skepticism, we must read published research with the same critical attitude. When we say "critical" in this context, though, we don't just mean finding fault. We have a very specific set of criteria in mind that we want to measure the studies we read against. Fey and Justice (2007) outlined a series of questions we can ask ourselves to help determine the type and quality of a study. These are summarized in Figure 3-2. The answers to these questions allow us to classify a report we read in the literature according to the levels of evidence it provides. These levels are summarized in Table 3-1. The higher the level of evidence we can find for a particular approach, the more confident we can be that the approach has strong scientific support. Finn, Bothe, and Bramlett (2005) provide additional guidance for evaluating claims about evidence.

But suppose we find strong scientific support for a particular practice. Is that the end of our decision-making process? Perhaps, but perhaps not. I'll give you an example. As we'll see in Chapter 4, the strongest support available for any approach to eliciting initial speech from young children with autism

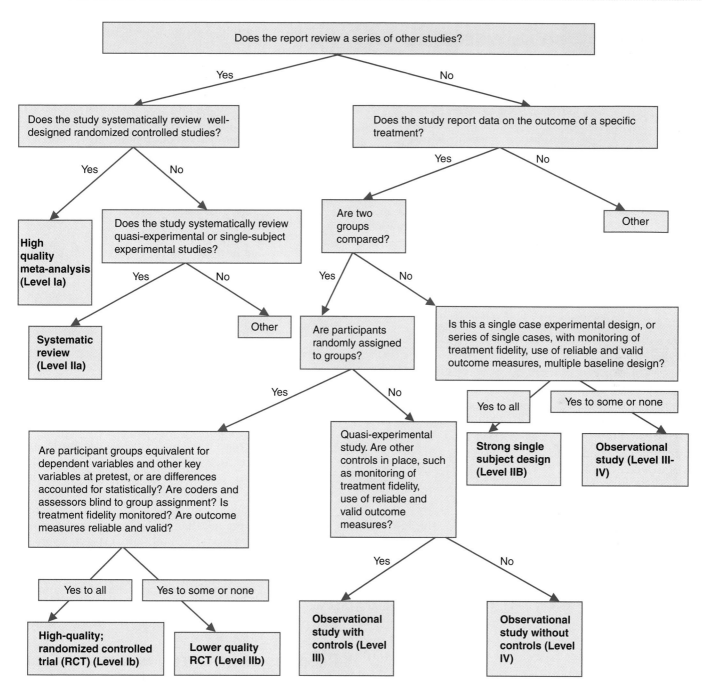

FIGURE 3-2 ✦ Flowchart for evaluation of published reports. (Adapted from Fey and Justice, 2007.)

spectrum disorders (ASD) is for behavioral, or operant, methods. These methods have been carefully investigated for many years, and have the greatest number of studies as well as the highest quality of research evidence behind them. Does this strong scientific evidence mean to us that every preverbal child with ASD must be given operant training? You've probably already thought of some reasons why the answer is "not necessarily." Perhaps the clinician is not well trained or experienced in this approach, or perhaps it conflicts with her values. Maybe the parents don't like it, and think it would make their child too passive. All these are examples of the

internal evidence that also needs to go into deciding about an approach to intervention.

What does EPB require of us, then? Do we have to read every published study in order to be EBP practitioners? Of course not—that would be impossible! Should we disregard scientific evidence if our own or a family's values or experiences don't match it? That would not be very responsible, either, since research does provide some helpful guidance in making clinical decisions. Fey and Justice (2007) and Sackett et al. (2000) outlined a reasonable approach to incorporating EBP that includes the following steps:

TABLE 3-1	Levels of Evidence

LEVEL	TYPE(S) OF EVIDENCE
Ia	A systematic meta-analysis of multiple well-designed randomized controlled studies
Ib	A well-conducted single randomized controlled trial (RCT) with a narrow confidence interval
IIa	A systematic review of nonrandomized quasi-experimental trials *or* a systematic review of single subject experiments that documents consistent study outcomes
IIb	A high quality quasi-experimental trial *or* a lower quality RCT *or* a single subject experiment with consistent outcomes across replications
III	Observational studies with controls (retrospective studies, interrupted time-series studies, case-control studies, cohort studies with controls)
IV	Observational studies without controls
V	Expert opinions without critical appraisal *or* theoretical knowledge *or* basic research

Adapted from Fey and Justice, 2007; Robey, 2004.

1. Formulate your clinical question, including the four "PICO" elements:
   P—Patient or Problem
   I—Intervention being considered
   C—Comparison treatment (such as the prevailing approach or no treatment)
   O—desired Outcome
   Example: Would Brendan, a 3-year-old with ASD and no speech (P) show greater improvement with an intervention that targets speech through an operant approach (I), or one that uses an alternative modality, such as a Picture Exchange Communication System (PECS; Bondy & Frost, 1998) as shown by increases in verbal communicative acts (O)?
2. Use internal evidence (such as clinical experience and family preferences) to determine what your typical, "first stab" approach would be.
   Example: Brendan's parents saw a newspaper article about PECS use in a nearby town. The child in the paper started saying a few words after working with PECS for several months. The parents think it makes sense and want to try it. You attended a PECS workshop several months ago, have used it with a few clients, and feel more confident using this technique than an operant approach with which you have little experience. You would opt for trying PECS first, other things being equal.
3. Find the external research evidence base. Use the ASHA database (www.asha.org) or other databases (such as MEDLINE or PsychInfo) available from libraries to search for information on your question. Start by reading review articles to find out what has been written recently; read abstracts of papers to decide if reading the whole paper will

be worth your time. Choose just a few articles that come closest to answering your question to read in their entirety. If you have to choose just one or two, choose the most recent, since these will review earlier papers on the topic.
4. Grade the studies for (a) relevance to the clinical question (b) the level of evidence provided by the study based on its design and quality, and (c) the direction, strength, and consistency of the observed outcomes, using the criteria in Table 3-1 and Figure 3-2.
5. Integrate internal and external evidence.
   Example: After reading several reviews and recent papers on behaviorist approaches, you are impressed with their high level of scientific support. You have read a few studies supporting PECS, but their quality is not very high. Still, the internal evidence for PECS seems strong, and besides Brendan has started doing more vocalizing, so he may be ready to use speech, once he learns some communication skills through PECS.
6. Evaluate the decision by documenting outcomes.
   Example: You take a baseline sample of play between Brendan and his mother for communicative acts using verbal and nonverbal means before starting PECS. Brendan is producing fewer than one communicative act/minute; most are vocal but not verbal. After six weeks of PECS, you take another sample of communication; Brendan now produces two acts/minute spontaneously, using both PECS and vocal behavior. He produces a one word approximation, with prompting from Mom: /mʌ/, for *more*, using it three times to request repetition of a tickle game. You conclude that PECS is doing its job, and decide to continue with the program, but to re-evaluate in another six weeks to be sure verbal communication continues to emerge. If it does not, you will consider a more direct speech approach, perhaps using more operant methods, at that time.

As you can see from this brief introduction to EBP, it offers a framework to help us make the crucial clinical decisions that go into the planning of an intervention program. Let's look at some of the other elements that go into this planning process.

PRODUCTS OF INTERVENTION: SETTING GOALS

McCauley and Fey (2006) and McLean (1989) suggested that there are three aspects of the intervention plan: the intended *products*, or objectives, of the intervention; the *processes* used to achieve these objectives; and the *contexts*, or environments, in which the intervention takes place. Let's see what each of these aspects entails.

A major source of information for goal setting is the assessment data. The appraisal tells us about the child's current level of functioning in the various language areas. McCauley and Fey (2006) describe intervention goals at three levels. These include the following:

Basic goals: Identify areas selected because of their importance for functionality or because of the severity of the deficit; these are general goals and usually correspond to long-term objectives in an educational plan (e.g., new grammatical forms).

Intermediate goals: Provide greater specification within a basic goal; usually there are several levels of intermediate goals associated with each basic goal (e.g., auxiliaries, articles, pronouns).

Specific goals: Specific instances of language form, content, or use are identified as intermediate goals. These are considered steps along the way to the broader and more functional basic goals, and should be based on the child's functional readiness, those which the child uses correctly on occasion or for which the child produces obligatory contexts without producing the target form (e.g., is, are, a, the, he, she).

Because many children with language impairments have multiple linguistic deficits, it is helpful to have some criteria for setting priorities among the deficits identified in the baseline assessment. Nelson, Camarata, Welsh, Butkovsky, and Camarata (1996) found that both forms that did not appear in the child's speech at all and forms that were used correctly some of the time were equally amenable to improvement with intervention. This research suggests that both these types of forms make suitable intervention targets. Fey (1986) and Fey, Long, and Finestack (2003) suggested, though, that forms that the child is already using a majority of the time correctly, even if some errors are still being made, should not be targeted for intervention. These forms are well on their way to mastery and will probably improve without direct teaching. Their suggestions are summarized in Box 3-1.

This strategy for goal setting can be thought of as targeting the child's *zone of proximal development* (Schneider & Watkins, 1996; Shepard, 2005; Vygotsky, 1978). The zone of proximal development (ZPD) is the distance between a child's current level of independent functioning and potential level of performance. In other words, the ZPD defines what the child is ready to learn with some help from a competent adult. Figure 3-3 gives a schematic representation of the ZPD. Choosing a goal within the child's current knowledge base is wasting the child's time, teaching something that is already known. Unfortunately, this error is sometimes made in intervention out of a misguided desire to ensure that the child succeeds on an intervention task. If a goal, such as production of a plural morpheme, is identified, and a child is found to perform at 80% correct on the first activity involving this morpheme, this indicates that the child does not need to be taught it. To persist in providing intervention on such an objective is to work short of the child's ZPD. The client is not being challenged to assimilate new knowledge and is simply demonstrating what he or she has already learned. This may make the clinician feel good, but it does not help the child acquire new forms and functions of language.

If the child is only 40% correct in the first sessions on a certain morpheme, however, the clinician can feel relatively confident that the form is within the child's ZPD. If continued intervention eventually produces 80% correct responses, the clinician would be justified in continuing to provide opportunities for the child to use this form, to stabilize and generalize its use. After several sessions in which the form is used correctly

---

BOX 3-1 | **Suggestion for Setting Priorities among Intervention Goals**

Highest Priority

Forms and functions client uses in 10% to 50% of required contexts.

High Priority

Forms and functions used in 1% to 10% of required contexts, but understood in receptive task formats.

Lower Priority

Forms and functions used in 50% to 90% of required contexts. Forms the client does not use at all and does not demonstrate understanding of in receptive task formats.

Adapted from Fey, M. (1986). *Language intervention with young children.* San Diego, CA: College-Hill Press; Fey, M., Long, S., and Finestack, L. (2003). Ten principles of grammar facilitation for children with specific language impairments. *American Journal of Speech Language Pathology, 12*, 3-15.

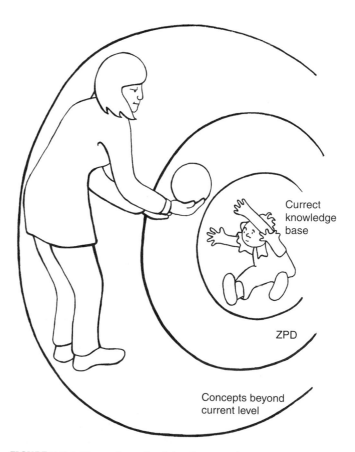

Currect knowledge base

ZPD

Concepts beyond current level

FIGURE 3-3 ✦ Zone of proximal development (ZPD).

almost all the time, though, the notion of ZPD suggests that it is best to move on to another target, checking back on plural morphemes occasionally to be sure that they are maintained in the child's repertoire. Focusing on targets for longer than necessary to get them stabilized into the child's knowledge base and generalized into conversational use does not make the most of intervention resources.

Similarly, it is important to choose objectives that are not beyond the client's ZPD. If a goal is too far above the current knowledge base, the child will be unable to acquire it efficiently and may not learn it at all. For a child in the two-word stage of language production, for example, using comparative "-er" forms, which are normally acquired at a developmental level of 5 to 7 years (Carrow-Woolfolk, 1999), is in most circumstances too far from the child's current level of functioning to be an appropriate goal. Again, the probable range of the ZPD is based on detailed assessment data, which pinpoints where the child is already functioning, and on knowledge of normal development, which allows us to determine the next few pieces of language development to fall into place. Lidz and Gindis (2003) and Schneider and Watkins (1996) point out that using dynamic assessment techniques to establish the ZPD also is helpful. This would mean identifying a particular form that is used infrequently or not at all in the client's spontaneous speech. Diagnostic teaching could be used to determine whether adult scaffolding makes it possible for the child to produce the form more accurately or often. If so, the form is within the child's ZPD and makes an appropriate therapy target.

Even in a descriptive-developmental model, though, we need to take some other considerations—besides the child's current level of functioning and the ZPD—into account when setting long- and short-term goals. Let's examine what some of these considerations might be.

Communicative Effectiveness

Fey (1986), Lahey (1988), and McCauley and Fey (2006) all emphasized the importance of choosing objectives not only on developmental grounds, but also on the grounds of how efficient the targeted behaviors will be in increasing a child's ability to communicate. This suggests that when a variety of aspects of semantic and syntactic skill emerges in a child's repertoire, it makes sense to choose skills that most readily accomplish social goals as highest-priority targets.

For example, suppose a 6-year-old is using primarily four- and five-word utterances. Let's say the child is producing all grammatical morphemes correctly, except appropriate forms of the verb "to be" and is expressing a range of age-appropriate meanings and communicative functions in simple, unelaborated sentences. What should be targeted first? Developmentally appropriate goals could include both forms of "to be" and elaborated sentence types such as passive sentences, sentences with embeddings, and conjoined sentence forms. But which might be most efficient for increasing communicative ability? Although the "be" forms might appear earlier developmentally than elaborated sentence types, use of "be" forms is usually redundant in context. In other words, no new meaning is added

by saying, "They are going away," instead of "They is going away." The former is correct by adult grammatical standards but not really much more efficient in terms of communication. So it may make sense to target sentence elaboration objectives as a higher priority. Passive sentences, although developmentally appropriate, would again not add much to the child's communicative repertoire, since the same ideas can usually be expressed in active form. Embedded sentences, such as relative clauses, might help the child encode more than one proposition within a sentence, making expression more compact, efficient, and sophisticated. Conjoined sentences also could be used to combine propositions within sentences. A decision as to which of these two forms to target first might be made by looking at what meanings the child is already attempting to combine in his discourse. If the child is producing sentence pairs that attempt to specify objects ("I like that gum. It has stripes."), relative clauses could be targeted to allow the production of more sophisticated versions of what he's already saying ("I like the gum that has stripes."). If temporal or causal meanings are being juxtaposed ("He went home. He got tired."), conjoinings with appropriate conjunctions to specify these relations could be targeted ("He went home because he got tired.").

Decisions about communicative effectiveness of language objectives are particularly important for children who are not likely ever to achieve adult communicative levels, such as those with severe autism or mental retardation. For these children especially, goals that may come next in the developmental sequence but do not allow the child to function as a more effective communicator take lower priority. These decisions are also important for children who are producing a very limited range of meanings or communicative functions. For these clients, expanding the range of ideas and intentions that can be expressed may be more important than syntactic accuracy, even when syntactic goals would appear to be suggested by the developmental sequence. The key is to remember that the overarching goal of intervention is not only to improve language but also to improve communication. With this goal in mind, developmental considerations can be kept in perspective.

New Forms Express Old Functions; New Functions Are Expressed by Old Forms

This dictum, articulated by Slobin (1973), tells us that when choosing targets for intervention, we must be careful to require that the child do only one new thing at a time. In targeting a new form, such as color vocabulary, we need to ask the child to use this form to serve a communicative function that has already been expressed with other forms. For example, if a child has used "big" and "little" to express attribution relations in two-word sentences, we could ask him or her to produce color words in these two-word attribution utterances. But if the child is not yet producing any utterances encoding the semantic relation of attribution, color vocabulary might not be a wise choice, or it ought to be taught in a simple labeling context using one-word utterances rather than two-word phrases.

Similarly, if a new communicative function, such as requesting information, is the target, the form used to express this function needs to be within the client's current repertoire. If the child is producing two-word phrases to express a meaning of location, such as, "Sit chair," the first information requests could be about locations. The clinician might play a sort of "musical chairs" game, bringing several different chairs into the clinic room and saying, "Where do I sit?" The child then can be given a turn to ask. "Where sit?" would be an acceptable phrase for the client to use. Thus the new function of requesting information would make use of a semantic relation and sentence form that the child is already using. In these cases, the clinician would have observed the rule of requiring only one new thing at a time in the intervention program.

Client Phonological Abilities

Another consideration in choosing intervention targets was pointed out by Fey (1986) and Schwartz and Leonard (1982). This concerns the phonological abilities of the client. Schwartz and Leonard showed that children are less likely to acquire the production (but not necessarily the comprehension) of new words if the new words contain phonological segments or syllable shapes that the children are not already producing in their other words. So "shoe" would not be a good word to choose as one of the vocabulary goals for a child who was not using any words containing the /ʃ/ sound, even though "shoe" might be a good choice from other perspectives. Similarly, plural morphemes might not be a high-priority goal for clients who did not produce any /s/ sounds in their current vocabulary. Phonological considerations are especially important for children in the first stages of language development, when mean utterance lengths are less than three morphemes, and less important for more developmentally advanced clients. Still, for developmentally young children, phonological constraints can be quite powerful and should be factored into decisions about targets for language production.

Teachability

Fey (1986) also pointed out that the ease with which a form or function can be taught should be considered in choosing objectives for intervention. He suggested that forms that are more teachable are (1) easily demonstrated or pictured; (2) taught through stimulus materials that are easily accessed and organized; and (3) used frequently in naturally occurring, everyday activities in which the child is engaged.

These certainly are reasonable criteria to add to the list to be used for selecting intervention goals. Objectives that are teachable by these standards will make the intervention process more efficient by minimizing the clinician's preparation time and maximizing the chances that the client will grasp the concepts and have the opportunity to use them in real communicative situations. However, Fey warned of a danger here. Teachability should only be used in conjunction with the other criteria we have discussed, never as the primary criterion. In other words, goals should not be chosen primarily on the basis of the materials the clinician has available or whether it is easy to obtain pictures for the target. Developmental and communicative considerations should take priority, and teachability

considerations should be invoked only after these other standards have been considered.

PROCESSES OF INTERVENTION

Once the specific objectives of the intervention have been determined, it is time to decide on a general approach or combination of approaches to use in the program and to choose or design particular intervention activities. Let's look at the options available to SLPs in these areas.

Intervention Approaches

Fey (1986) discussed a continuum of naturalness in intervention approaches. This continuum represents the extent to which the settings and activities in intervention resemble "real life" or the world outside the clinic room (Fig. 3-4). We can vary intervention activities along this continuum of naturalness. Activities in language intervention can be a lot like the activities a child engages in during the rest of his or her life, or they can be very different. We can go from very naturalistic settings and activities such as play in the child's home to very contrived activities, such as drill, in a setting such as a clinic room, or we can choose settings and activities somewhere midway along this continuum. Three basic approaches to intervention identified by Fey (1986) will be outlined here. I don't mean to suggest that a clinician has to choose just one of them. Our aim should be to make the best match among a particular client, a particular objective, and an intervention approach. Some clients may do better with one approach than another. Other clients may do well with one approach for one objective and a different approach for another. One objective may be well suited to a highly structured approach; another may be better served by a more open-ended approach. Often, several activities are designed to address a particular objective—some highly structured, some with a low level of structure, and others a compromise between the two. The important thing is to be aware of the range of approaches available for planning intervention activities and to be able to take advantage of this range of approaches in setting up a comprehensive, economical, efficient intervention program that meets each client's individual needs. We should also, as we saw earlier in the chapter, evaluate the available evidence in the

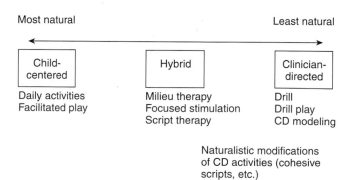

FIGURE 3-4 ✦ The continuum of naturalness. (Adapted from Fey, M. [1986]. *Language intervention with young children.* San Diego, CA: College-Hill Press.)

research literature for the effectiveness of particular approaches with particular goals for particular kinds of clients.

The Clinician-Directed Approach. In these approaches, the clinician specifies materials to be used, how the client will use them, the type and frequency of reinforcement, the form of the responses to be accepted as correct, and the order of activities—in short, all aspects of the intervention. Clinician-directed (CD) approaches, also referred to as discrete trial intervention (DTI), attempt to make the relevant linguistic stimuli highly salient, to reduce or eliminate irrelevant stimuli, to provide clear reinforcement to increase the frequency of desired language behaviors, and to control the clinical environment so that intervention is optimally efficient in changing language behavior. CD approaches tend to be less naturalistic than other approaches we will discuss, since they involve so much control on the part of the clinician and since they purposely eliminate many of the natural contexts and contingencies of the use of language for communication. Peterson (2004) defined these approaches as ones in which the clinician selects the stimulus items, divides the target language skill into a series of steps, presents each step in a series of massed trials until the client meets a criterion level of performance, and then provides an arbitrary reinforcement. Roth and Worthington (2005) provide an excellent introduction to this approach. Their summary of this basic training protocol appears in Box 3-2.

An advantage of CD approaches is that they allow the clinician to maximize the opportunities for a child to produce a new form, producing a higher number of target responses per unit time than other approaches allow. This provides excellent opportunities for the child to get extended practice using a new form or function.

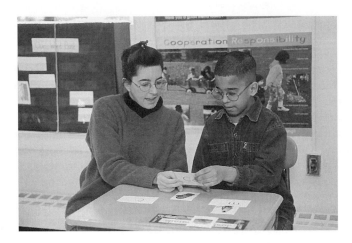

Clinician-directed intervention provides a high level of structure.

Proponents of this approach (e.g., Connell, 1987; Fey & Proctor-Williams, 2000) also point out that its unnaturalness is itself an advantage. They argue that if clients were going to learn language the "natural" way, by listening and interacting with others, they would not need intervention. The fact that the child has, for whatever reason, failed to learn language through natural interactions suggests that something else is needed. The something else, in this view, is the highly structured, clinician-controlled, tangibly reinforced context of the behaviorist's intervention.

There is something to be said for this position. CD approaches have been shown in a large literature of research studies to be consistently effective in eliciting a wide variety of new language forms from children with language disabilities of many types (see Abbeduto & Boudreau, 2004; Fey, 1986; Goldstein, 2002; Paul & Sutherland, 2005; Peterson, 2004; Rogers, 2006, for reviews). The proponents of the CD approach appear to be justified in arguing that children who have not learned language the "old-fashioned way," by interacting naturally with their parents, benefit from formal behavior modification procedures. Further, some research (Friedman & Friedman, 1980) suggests that while children with higher IQs learn better in a more interactive intervention program, those with lower IQs or more severe disabilities perform better when a CD approach is used. Connell (1987) showed, using an invented morpheme, that children with normal language acquisition learned more efficiently when the form was merely modeled for them, whereas children with impaired language learned the form better when they were required to imitate the instructor's production of it. These studies tend to support the behaviorist position that CD approaches to language intervention work better than more naturalistic ones for children with language impairments.

But, of course, that's not the whole story. Cole and Dale (1986), for example, were not able to replicate the Friedman and Friedman results and found no differences between interactive and CD approaches. Nelson et al. (1996) showed more rapid acquisition of grammatical targets and increased generalization with a conversational intervention treatment than an imitative one. Camarata, Nelson, and Camarata (1994) reported that children with language impairments learned

---

BOX 3-2 **Training Protocol for Clinician-Directed Intervention**

- Clinician gives instructions in declarative form ("Say the name for the picture after me.").
- Clinician presents stimulus or antecedent event ("Big ball.").
- Clinician waits for client to respond, allowing sufficient time for client to formulate response.
- Clinician presents consequent event or reinforcement (primary, such as food, or secondary, such as social praise ["Good talking!"], tokens to accumulate for a prize, or feedback regarding the acceptability of the response).
- Feedback might include biofeedback instrumentation or information on performance ("You said four of the five correctly!").

Adapted from Roth, F. & Worthington, C. (2005). *Treatment resource manual for speech-language pathology* (3rd ed.). Clifton Park, NY: Delmar.

syntactic targets more quickly under naturalistic conditions than with a CD approach, and a meta-analysis by Delprato (2001) suggested that naturalistic interventions showed a consistent advantage over CD methods. More fundamentally, perhaps, numerous studies (e.g., Hughes & Carpenter, 1983; Mulac & Tomlinson, 1977; Zwitman & Sonderman, 1979; see Peterson, 2004, for review) show difficulties in generalization to natural contexts of forms taught with a CD approach, even when use reaches high levels of accuracy within the CD framework. Gillum et al. (2003), while generally favoring more naturalistic approaches, argue that clinicians and researchers need to determine which developmental profiles in clients are best matched to particular intervention methods.

It seems, then, that while CD approaches can be highly efficient in getting children to produce new language forms, they are not so effective in getting them to incorporate these forms into real communication outside the structured clinic setting, and that more naturalistic methods can also provide an efficient means of addressing language targets. What shall we make of these findings? Some writers, including Hubbell (1981), Norris and Hoffman (1993), and Owens (2004), have argued that the lack of generalization seen in CD approaches renders them useless and that the only approaches that are right for language intervention are more natural and interactive. This view, in my opinion, involves "throwing the baby out with the bath water." Since CD approaches have proven efficacy in eliciting new language forms, why not take advantage of this efficacy? CD approaches can be used in initial phases of treatment to elicit forms that the child is not using very much spontaneously. Fey, Long, and Finestack (2003) argue that drill formats that emphasize contrasts between two forms (such as past/present or singular/plural) are the most effective use of CD approaches. Either simultaneously, or later, once the form or function has been stabilized with a CD approach, some of the more naturalistic approaches we will discuss can be used to help bring the form into the child's conversational repertoire. Let's look at three major varieties of CD activities: drill, drill play, and modeling.

Drill. Shriberg and Kwiatkowski (1982a) defined several types of clinical activities in terms of their degree of structure. The most highly structured in their framework is drill, which makes use of the classic DTI format. In a drill activity, the clinician instructs the client concerning what response is expected and provides a training stimulus, such as a word or phrase to be repeated. These training stimuli are carefully planned and controlled by the clinician. Often they contain *prompts* or instructional stimuli that tell the child how to respond correctly, for example by imitating the clinician. If prompts are used, they are gradually eliminated or *faded* on a schedule predetermined by the clinician. When prompts are used, the client provides a response to the clinician's stimulus. If this response is the one the clinician intended, the child is *reinforced* with verbal praise or some tangible reinforcer, such as food or a token. A *motivating event* also may be provided. For example, if the child is to label clothing items, he or she may be asked to place a sticker of the item in a sticker album after it has been named appropriately and the response has been reinforced. If the client's response is not the intended target, the clinician attempts to *shape* the response by reinforcing the production of parts of the complete target and gradually increasing the number of components that must appear correctly to obtain the reinforcement. Drill is the most efficient intervention approach in that it provides the highest rate of stimulus presentations and client responses per unit time.

One problem with drill in Shriberg and Kwiatkowski's study was that neither the clients nor the clinicians liked it very much. The clients did not find it very motivating, and the clinicians were uncomfortable with its high degree of structure and low level of motivation. It is interesting to note that the clinicians in the study did not like drill even though it was obvious that it got the job done and provided an efficient and effective form of intervention.

Drill Play. Drill play is another CD approach, which differs from drill only in that it attempts to provide some motivation into the drill structure. It does this by adding an *antecedent* motivating event, that is, one that occurs not only after the target response is reinforced but also before it is even elicited. Thus there are two motivating events in drill play, one that goes along with the original training stimulus the (*antecedent* motivating event) and one that follows the reinforcement (the *subsequent* motivating event). For example, take the activity mentioned before—using stickers to motivate naming clothing items. As an antecedent motivating event, the client may be allowed to choose any sticker from a sheet of clothing stickers that he or she would like to put in the album. The training stimulus would elicit the name of clothing item represented by the sticker. After reinforcement for correct labeling, the client would be allowed to put the sticker in the album, as a subsequent motivating event.

Shriberg and Kwiatkowski (1982a) found drill and drill play to be equally efficient and effective in eliciting responses in phonological intervention. Further, clinicians in the study liked drill play a lot better than they did drill and believed that their clients did, too. Do these findings about phonological intervention transfer to language? We don't really know, since this question has not been addressed in language intervention research in as clear a manner as Shriberg and Kwiatkowski have addressed it. But it seems reasonable to expect the two modes of intervention to produce similar outcomes with semantic, syntactic, pragmatic, and phonological goals. These findings suggest that many of the advantages of highly structured CD approaches can be retained while client motivation and clinician comfort are increased, by small but well-thought-out modifications of the basic DTI approach.

Does this mean that we should never drill, if drill play is just as effective and more fun? Not necessarily. Some children, in fact, may enjoy the predictability and simplicity of drill. Many computer language-teaching programs are, in fact, drill formats that use their own graphic displays as subsequent motivating events, and many children find these to be quite a treat. The bottom line, in my opinion, is that if drill works for a certain client, we should by all means use it initially to elicit new forms and functions. If it doesn't work, we should use whatever works better. The important thing is to have a range of techniques and approaches on our clinical palate from which to draw, mix, and match to suit the needs of clients.

Modeling. Fey (1986) presented a second CD alternative to straight drill procedures. This arises from social learning theory and involves the use of a third-person model—thus the name, *modeling* approaches. Like drill, modeling uses a highly structured format, extrinsic reinforcement, and a formal interactive context. But here, instead of imitating, the child's job is to listen. The client listens as the model provides numerous examples of the structure being taught. Through listening, the child is expected to induce and later produce the target structure. The child never has to imitate a structure immediately after the model. Instead this procedure implicitly requires the child to find a pattern in the model's talk that is similar across all the stimuli presented. In Leonard's (1975a) modeling procedure, a "confederate," such as a parent, is used by the clinician as a model. The clinician, after pretesting the client on the target structure, gives the model a set of pictures not used in the pretest and asks, "What's happening here?" The confederate provides, for example, a *be + (verb) + -ing* utterance that describes each picture presented by the clinician (e.g., "the boy is drinking," "the girl is eating," "the cat is walking"). After 10 or 20 of these descriptions, the client is asked to "talk like" the model and to describe a similar but not identical set of pictures. In this phase the model and client alternate their productions until the child produces three consecutive correct versions. Then, the child is asked to continue until a criterion (say, of 10 consecutive correct responses) is reached. At this point, the client would be tested on the pretest stimuli without models. This method can easily be adapted when a confederate is not available by using a doll or puppet (with the clinician's voice) as a model.

All three variations we've discussed—drill, drill play, and modeling—share the tightly structured, formal, clinician-controlled features that characterize operant approaches to intervention. They share the advantages these approaches provide: specification of linguistic stimuli, clear instructions and criteria for appropriate responses, reinforcement designed to increase the frequency of correct responding, high levels of efficiency in evoking maximal numbers of responses per unit time, and proven effectiveness in eliciting new language behaviors. They all share certain disadvantages, too. They are relatively "unnatural" and are dissimilar to the pragmatic contexts in which language is used in everyday conversation. Perhaps as a result, their targets are not spontaneously incorporated into everyday language use, even when they reach criterion levels in the structured intervention situation. I've argued that these facts imply that CD approaches ought to be considered in initial phases of intervention to evoke use of forms the child is not using very often in spontaneous conversation, because of their great efficiency for this purpose. Because of their drawbacks, though, I've suggested that CD approaches be combined with other modalities to effect the transition from use in formal intervention contexts to use in everyday interactions. Let's see what some of these alternative approaches might be.

Child-Centered Approaches. You can lead a horse to water, but you can't make it drink. That's the problem with CD approaches. Some children simply refuse to engage in CD activities, no matter how good it is for them. Some clinicians might call these children "behavior problems" and would spend long stretches of intervention time trying to train them to participate in CD formats. These "hard-to-treat" children rebuff any attempt to get them to say what the clinician tells them to say, no matter how tempting the reinforcement.

For these children, an alternative intervention approach seems warranted. That is, even if we believe that CD approaches are the most efficient means of language change, we may need to have another weapon at our command for children who refuse to engage in them, at least until we can establish a better relationship with the client and get him or her to want to cooperate with us. Sometimes we need to win a child's trust.

For another kind of client, too, the CD approach may not be the best first step. This is the child that Fey (1986) called "unassertive." An unassertive child responds to speech, but rarely initiates communication. These children are passive communicators who let others control interactions. In a sense, a CD approach panders to these clients' propensity to sit back and let others do the interactive work. Having these clients respond when and how they are told to is essentially reinforcing them to continue the old, maladaptive communication pattern.

For both these children—the obstinate child and the unassertive communicator—CD approaches may not be the most appropriate first step in an intervention program. That is not to say that other approaches never work for these clients, only that we may need to do something else first before we ask them to work with us. For the obstinate and unassertive child particularly, the child-centered (CC) approach (Fey, 1986; Girolametto & Weitzman, 2006; Sheldon & Rush, 2001) may be a good introduction to intervention. CC approaches can be appropriate adjuncts to the program for many children with language disorders. CC approaches go by several names, including *indirect language stimulation* (ILS; Fey, 1986), *facilitative play* (Hubbell, 1981), *pragmaticism* (Arwood, 1983), and *developmental* or *developmental/pragmatic approaches* (Prizant & Wetherby, 2005). In using a CC approach, a clinician arranges an activity so that opportunities for the client to provide target responses occur as a natural part of play and interaction. From the child's point of view, the activity is "just" play. A clinician may use a variety of linguistic models as instructional language when they seem appropriate in the context of the child's activity. There are no tangible reinforcers, no requirements that the child provide a response to the clinician's language, and no prompts or shaping of incorrect responses when they do occur, although the clinician does *consequate*, or follow up, any child remarks in specific ways, as we'll see.

CC intervention puts the child in the driver's seat. Apart from choosing the materials with which the child will play, the clinician does not direct the activity. Rather, we follow the child's lead, doing what he or she is doing and talking about what he or she is talking about or doing. This has a great many advantages for both obstinate and unassertive clients. Rather than

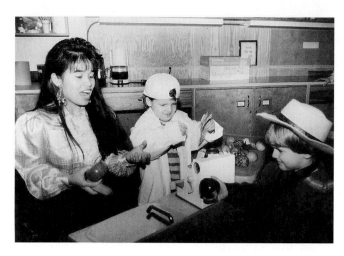

Child-centered intervention.

spending all their energy resisting, in the case of the obstinate child, or passively complying, as the unassertive one will do, clients engaged in a CC activity spend their time in natural, enjoyable play with a very accepting and responsive adult who makes a consistent and salient match between what they are doing and the language used to talk about it. And all clients can benefit from opportunities to see how actions and objects are mapped onto words in the context of fun, familiar activities.

When we use CC intervention, the first (and perhaps hardest) thing we must learn to do is *wait*. The key to this approach is to *respond* to the client. To do this, we have to wait for the client to do something. Ideally, that something will be to talk. If it is, we can respond to the child's language with one of several specific verbal techniques. Sometimes, though, we must interpret some action of the child's and act as if it were intended to communicate, even though the client may not truly have had such an intention. Once the child has said or done something that we can interpret as communicative, we then respond to the behavior in a way that models communicative language use. Unlike in the CD approach, we are not trying to elicit specific structures from the client. Instead, we react to the child's behavior, placing it in a communicative context and giving it a linguistic mapping.

The clinician does this mapping by using a variety of techniques that constitute the indirect language stimulation approach. These techniques can be summarized as follows:

1. *Self-talk and parallel talk.* In *self-talk* we describe our own actions as we engage in parallel play with the child. If the child is building a block tower, we copy the tower with our own blocks, saying as we do, "I'm building. I'm building with blocks. See my blocks? I'm building." Self-talk provides a clear and simple match between actions and words. By using the child's actions and matching our own words and actions to them, we model how to comment on our actions with language.

   In a sense, in *parallel talk* we provide self-talk for the child. Instead of talking about our own actions, we talk about the client's, providing a running commentary, something like the play-by-play at a sporting event. To take the

same block-building example we used before, parallel talk might sound like, "You're building. You put on a block. You did it again. You put on another block. Now it's big! You're building a big one!" Parallel talk also can help us make connections to children with severe disorders whose choice of actions may not be typical. For example, children with autism, if given a set of toys, may use them in unconventional ways. Instead of building a tower with blocks, an autistic child may smell them or focus on the texture of the rug underneath the blocks. Parallel talk allows us to share this child's focus. Again, we talk about the child's focus of attention; for example, "You see the rug. It's green. It's a green rug. It's soft. Can you feel it? It's soft. The blocks are on the rug. They're on the soft, green rug."

Self-talk and parallel talk are helpful for children who are not talking at all in the clinical setting. The clinician's use of these techniques maximizes the chances that the child will use the model in producing a spontaneous utterance. Once the child does, the clinician can respond with other techniques included in the indirect language stimulation approach. These techniques are designed to provide a verbal response that is highly contingent on the child's own utterance. Let's look at these contingent response possibilities, too.

2. *Imitations.* We often ask children to *imitate* what we say in intervention. But instead, we can turn the tables and imitate what the child says. Folger and Chapman (1978) showed that adults often repeat what normal toddlers say, and that when they do, there is a substantial probability that the child will imitate the imitation. Research suggests that children who imitate show advances in language development (Carpenter, Tomasello, & Striano, 2005). Moreover, we know that anything that increases the amount of child talk is associated with acceleration of language development (Gallagher, 1993; Hoff-Ginsberg, 1987; Sachs, 1983). The more the child says, the more the opportunities exist for practice of phonological, lexical, and syntactic forms and the more opportunities there are for feedback. If the child repeats our imitation, we can go on to use some of the other forms of contingent responses available in indirect language stimulation to provide more focused and extensive feedback. Or, alternatively, we can use the child's imitation to initiate a repeated back-and-forth exchange that will help the child develop this basic turn-taking structure for conversation.

3. *Expansions.* In *expanding* the child's utterance we take what the child said and add the grammatical markers and semantic details that would make it an acceptable adult utterance. For example, if the child puts a toy dog in a dollhouse and says "doggy," or "doggy house," this could be expanded as "The doggy is in the house." Expansions have been shown to increase the probability that a child will spontaneously imitate at least part of the expansion (Scherer & Olswang, 1984). Again, any talk is good talk in our book. It's practice, and it gives us yet another opportunity to provide additional contingent feedback. Moreover, Saxton

(2005) reviewed literature to suggest that expansions specifically have been associated with grammatical development for a number of structures in a number of diagnostic groups. In more current literature, these are sometimes called *recasts* (Camarata & Nelson, 2006).

4. *Extensions.* Some writers call these responses *expatiations* (Fey, 1986). They are comments that add some semantic information to a remark made by the child. In our "doggy house" example, saying "He went inside" or "Yes, he got cold" could extend this remark. Cazden (1965) and Barnes, Gutfreund, Satterly, and Wells (1983) showed that adults' extensions are associated with significant increases in children's sentence length.

Owens (2004) called the latter three kinds of responses—imitation, expansions, and extensions—*consequating behaviors* on the part of the adult. They decrease the amount of information in the adult utterance that the child has to process (Proctor-Williams, Fey, & Loeb, 2001). They do this by taking the form and meaning the child has already expressed and pushing it a small step further, into the ZPD, we might say. All three behaviors increase the likelihood that the child will imitate some part of the consequating utterance. This is important because anything that increases the rate of child talk has positive consequences for language development, in general, as we've seen. In particular, these consequating remarks provide the child with information about how to encode in a more mature linguistic form the ideas they are already expressing.

5. *Buildups and breakdowns.* Weir (1962) studied the before-sleep monologues of a 2-year-old child. She found that the monologues commonly contained sequences in which the child took her own utterance, broke it down into smaller, phrase-sized pieces, and then built them back up into sentences. We can do this *breaking down* and *building up* for the client, in an attempt to demonstrate how sentences get put together. We start by expanding the child's utterance to a fully grammatical form. Then we break it down into several phrase-sized pieces in a series of sequential utterances that overlap in content. Let's take the "doggy house" example again. To do a buildup and breakdown on this utterance, we might respond, "Yes, the doggy is in the house. The house. He's in the house. In the house. The doggy is in the house. The doggy. The doggie's in the house." Cross (1978) found that these types of responses, too, are associated with language growth in normally developing children.

6. *Recast sentences. Recast sentences* are similar to expansions. Expansions, you'll remember, elaborate the child's utterance into a grammatically correct version of the intended sentence type. In recasting we expand the child's remark into a different type or more elaborated sentence. If the child makes the statement "doggy house," we can recast it as a question, "Is the doggy in the house?" or a negative sentence (used as a playful denial of the child's utterance), "The doggy is *not* in the house!" or even a negative question, "Isn't the doggy in the house?" Camarata et al. (1994), Nelson et al. (1996), and Proctor-Williams, Fey, and Loeb

(2001) showed that recast treatment was effective in teaching grammatical forms to children with specific language impairment, but only when the recasts were presented at rates that are much greater than those available in typical conversations with young children. This finding reminds us that one of the ways therapeutic conversation differs from ordinary talk is in its conscious attempt to greatly increase the "dose" of helpful input it provides. When engaging in any CC language activity, it is essential to focus attention on using our linguistic input to maximize the intensity of our client's exposure to helpful examples of language.

One particular type of recast sentence has been found in research (Hoff-Ginsberg, 1990) to be particularly helpful to normal children in learning the verb structure of English, a system that gives children with language impairments a particularly hard time. This is the *verbal reflective question.* Verbal reflective questions are recasts that repeat part of the child's utterance but pass the conversational turn to the child by turning the partial repetition into a question. So if the child says, "doggy house," a verbal reflective question response would be "The doggy is in the house, isn't he?" Again, these responses seem to be useful, like the other consequating behaviors we've discussed, because they provide a scaffold to elicit talk from the child that is contingent on the child's own topic. However, Fey and Loeb (2002) found that it was important to provide these recasts only to children for whom the targeted form was within the ZPD. Providing them to children whose language levels were too low did not result in increased learning for the new form. This is one reason that careful assessment of language level is so important; it helps us identify the appropriate "next step" in the child's language development, so we can provide just the right input to make that step possible.

Indirect language stimulation, then, attempts to provide a simple, accessible model of the mapping between the child's actions and the language that can be used to describe them. Its purpose is to "tempt" the child to talk by following the child's choice of activities and topics, providing an attentive and responsive person with whom the client can interact and supplying models of more mature language that are within the child's ZPD. Research on both children with typical acquisition and those with language disorders suggests that these techniques are indeed helpful in accelerating language growth (see Camarata & Nelson, 2006; Girolametto & Weitzman, 2006; Peterson, 2004; Saxton, 2005, for reviews), particularly at Brown's stages IV and V of language development (Gillum et al., 2003). It's interesting to note, though, that Shriberg and Kwiatkowski (1982a) found that clinicians did not like the ILS approach, even though the clients did. This finding probably reflects the discomfort many of us feel in leaving the child in some sense in charge of the intervention, relinquishing the control that CD approaches afford us.

Despite this discomfort, in my view, there is a place for indirect language stimulation in our clinical arsenal. For obstinate and unassertive clients it may be the best bet for establishing a relationship that allows them to take some responsibility for communication. For any client who is functioning at a mean length of utterance (MLU) level below three morphemes (where these techniques have been shown to be effective for normally developing children), ILS can be an especially useful adjunct to more structured intervention activities. Augmenting more structured approaches with ILS gives the child a chance to see how the forms being trained are used for real communication and gives the client an opportunity to try for spontaneous usage in a safe and responsive environment with a good deal of scaffolding and support. ILS, then, is an ideal first step for certain developmentally young clients and can be a useful adjunct to the intervention program for any client in the early stages of language acquisition. It is important to remember, however, that to be effective, ILS techniques must provide high levels of intensity of input. Proctor-Williams, Fey and Loeb (2001) estimated that it is necessary to provide about one consequating remark per minute in order to make this method work.

We can summarize our discussion of the CC approach to language intervention by saying that it is at the opposite end of the continuum from CD approaches in terms of naturalness, degree of adult control, use of external reinforcement, and adherence to pragmatic principles. Is there anything in between? Fey (1986) suggested that there are approaches that fall midway on this continuum. He referred to these as *hybrid* approaches.

Hybrid Approaches. According to Fey (1986), hybrid intervention approaches have three major characteristics. First, unlike CC approaches, which focus on general communication, hybrid approaches target one or a small set of specific language goals that are identified through the processes we discussed earlier. Second, the clinician maintains a good deal of control in selecting activities and materials but does so in a way that consciously tempts the child to make spontaneous use of utterances of the types being targeted. Finally, the clinician uses linguistic stimuli not just to respond to the child's communication but to model and highlight the forms being targeted. We'll discuss several forms of hybrid intervention: focused stimulation, vertical structuring, milieu teaching, and script therapy.

Focused Stimulation. In this approach the clinician carefully arranges the context of interaction so that the child is tempted to produce utterances with obligatory contexts for the forms being targeted. The clinician helps the child succeed in this by providing a very high density of models of the target forms in a meaningful communicative context, usually play. The child is not required to produce the target forms, however—only tempted. Because the clinician provides many models of the target form in a meaningful context, this approach is very effective for improving comprehension of a form, as well as production (Weismer & Robertson, 2006). Box 3-3 gives an example of a focused stimulation approach to teaching use of "is" as a copula.

The example demonstrates how the clinician provides multiple exemplars of the target form in a structured but interactive play context. Note how the clinician first provides opportunities for the client to use the form, but when the child

---

BOX 3-3	A Focused Stimulation Approach to Teaching Copula "Is"

Materials: Toy barn, farmer, farm animals, toy truck that can hold animals.

Clinician: Let's pretend we're farmers. We're taking our animals to the fair. We want to be sure we don't forget any. Here they are in the barn. I'll put some in the truck. OK, now the cow *is* in the truck. The horse *is* in the truck. The sheep *is* in the truck. What about the dog?

Client: Bark.

Clinician: Yes, the dog can bark. He says, "Ruff, ruff." Let's put the dog in the truck. Now he *is* in the truck. Good! Let's see. The cat *is* in the barn. Let's put her in the truck. Good, now she *is* in the truck. The goat *is* in the truck. How about the chicken?

Client: Chick in truck.

Clinician: Yes, she *is*. The chicken *is* in the truck. That's good. *Is* the pig in the truck? He *is*. He *is* in the truck. Tell the farmer. Tell him, "The pig *is* in the truck."

Client: Pig is in truck.

Clinician: Good, now everyone *is* in the truck. Now we can go to the fair.

---

responds with something other than the target, the clinician responds contingently anyway, then goes on to give further models. The clinician gives feedback similar to an expansion when the child makes an unsuccessful attempt. She asks the child to attempt the form, but if the child declines to do so, the clinician simply goes on giving additional models. Weismer and Robertson (2006) provide an extensive review of the evidence supporting the use of focused stimulation to teach language form, content, and use for both monolingual and bilingual children (e.g., Cleave & Fey, 1997; Leonard, Camarata, Rowan, & Chapman, 1982; Robertson & Weismer, 1999; Skarakis-Doyle & Murphy, 1995), when implemented by both clinicians and parents (e.g., Girolametto & Weitzman, 2006; Lederer, 2001; Robertson & Weismer, 1999) for improving both functional comprehension and use of the target structures.

Vertical Structuring. Vertical structuring is a particular form of expansion used like focused stimulation to highlight target structures. Box 3-4 provides an example dialogue that uses vertical structuring. There we see that the clinician responds to a child's incomplete utterance with a contingent question. The child responds to the question with another fragmentary remark. The clinician then takes the two pieces produced by the child and expands them into a more complete utterance. The child is not required to imitate this expansion. The fact that children often imitate adult expansions of their own utterances in normal development is the basis for the hope that children with language impairments will take these expanded

---

BOX 3-4 **Example of Vertical Structuring**

Materials: A picture of children visiting a zoo.
Clinician: Look at this. What do you see? (If the child does not respond or makes a remark unrelated to the picture, the clinician directs the child's attention to a specific referent in the picture and asks again, "What do you see here?")
Client: Lion.
Clinician: Yes, and what is the lion doing?
Client: Roar.
Clinician: Yes, he's roaring. The lion is roaring.

---

models of their own intended utterances as a cue for spontaneous imitation. If they don't, the clinician simply goes on to elicit another set of related utterances from the child and offers the vertically structured expansion again.

Vertical structuring is obviously less naturalistic than standard ILS techniques in that the clinician provides a specific nonlinguistic stimulus, such as a picture; targets a particular form; and attempts to elicit particular language behavior from the child. But it does use a naturalistic response on the part of the clinician and takes the child's spontaneous utterance as the basis for the clinician response, rather than requiring an imitation. Vertical structuring has been used primarily to target early developing language forms and has been shown to be effective when used for this purpose (Schwartz, Chapman, Terrell, Prelock, & Rowan, 1985). Skarakis-Doyle and Murphy (1995) used the technique to target more advanced language structures *(should, must)*. They demonstrated that vertical structuring used after focused stimulation enhanced the effectiveness of the intervention. Box 3-5 gives an example of a dialogue that uses vertical structuring to elicit sentences with relative clauses.

BOX 3-5 **Example of Vertical Structuring Used to Elicit Sentences with Relative Clauses**

Materials: A picture of children visiting a zoo.
Clinician: Tell me about one of the children in this picture.
Client: This boy sees the lion.
Clinician: Uh-huh. Tell me something else about him.
Client: He's wearing a baseball cap.
Clinician: Yeah, the boy who is wearing a cap sees the lion.

Milieu Teaching. Milieu teaching includes several different techniques that apply operant principles to quasi-naturalistic settings. Hancock and Kaiser (2006) discuss three major components that characterize this approach: (1) environmental arrangement (2) responsive interaction, and (3) conversation-based contexts that use child interest and initiation as opportunities for modeling and prompting communication in everyday settings. These methods make use of imitative cues and extrinsic reinforcement but do so during interactive activities that have been carefully arranged by the clinician to elicit child initiations, necessitate social communication on the part of the client, and provide natural consequences for the communication.

Hart and Risley (1975) introduced the *incidental teaching* method, as one example of this approach. Here the clinician arranges the setting so that things the client wants or needs to complete a project are visible but out of reach. The child selects the topic of conversation by making some kind of request, such as gesturing or looking toward the desired item. The clinician responds first with *focused attention*. This involves moving toward the child, making eye contact, and waiting expectantly to see whether the child will offer a more elaborated request. If not, the clinician asks a question. The question form varies, depending on the clinician's goal. "What?" may be used if the target is simply for the client to produce verbal requests. "Which one do you want?" could attempt to elicit sentences with adjectives. "Why do you want it?" might be used if the goal is sentences with "because" clauses. If this question produces the target response, the clinician provides a confirmation, which includes a model of the target form (Client: "Want red marker." Clinician: "Oh, you want the red marker. Here it is."). If the question fails to produce the target response, a prompt is provided. Prompts can be general requests for the target, such as "You need to tell me." Or they can be requests for partial imitations, such as, "Say, 'I need a marker because... .'" They can also be requests for complete imitations, such as, "Say, 'I want a red marker.'" If the child responds appropriately to the prompt, a confirmation is provided and the communicative goal is achieved (the child gets the marker). If not, one more attempt to prompt is made. If this also fails, the child still gets what he or she wants. The clinician tries again to elicit more elaborated language on the child's next attempt at communication.

A similar method is the *mand-model* approach of Rogers-Warren and Warren (1980). There are two major differences between this and incidental teaching. The first is that the clinician does not need to wait for the child to initiate communication. The clinician carefully observes the child, and when the child seems to show some interest in some aspect of the environment, the clinician "mands" (requests) an utterance with a stimulus, such as "What's that?" or "Tell me what you need." The second difference is that the goals are stated very generally. Rather than specific form or meaning targets, the clinician is merely trying to elicit one-word utterances from some clients, two-word sentences from others, or complete grammatical sentences from more advanced clients. In this way the mand-model approach can be easily adapted to work with groups of clients, where each might have his or her own set of goals, and prompts are individualized to the goals of each client. If the child provides the target response, he or she is verbally reinforced *and* given the desired item ("Good talking! You asked for the marker, so here it is!"). If the child does not, prompts similar to those used in incidental teaching are used.

Warren et al. (2006) and Yoder and Warren (2001, 2002) discuss an additional variation: *Prelinguistic Milieu Teaching* (PMT). This method is designed for children not yet using spoken language, at developmental levels of 9 to 15 months, although they may be of chronological ages up to six years. The goal of PMT is to develop the basic intentional communication skills necessary for early language development by increasing the frequency, maturity, and complexity of nonverbal communicative acts. Table 3-2 lists the five essential goals of this approach. We'll discuss PMT in more detail in Chapter 7.

Finally, Hancock and Kaiser (2006) discuss *Enhanced Milieu Teaching* (EMT). This method has been shown to be especially effective for children who meet the following criteria: (1) produce some verbal imitation, (2) have at least 10 productive words, and (3) are in the early stages of language development, with MLUs from 1 to 3.5. The approach has been used with clinicians, parents, and teachers as agents of intervention, but most of the research on EMT has focused on parent-delivered therapy. It incorporates methods from both incidental teaching and the mand/model approach, using activities like those in Box 3-6.

A large literature base exists on the effectiveness of various examples of milieu teaching. Hancock and Kaiser (2006), Peterson (2004), and Warren et al. (2006) review over 50 studies that provide evidence for the usefulness of these approaches with preschool children with intellectual and language disorders, autism spectrum disorders, as well as children from high-risk and low-income families. Delprato (2001), as we saw, used meta-analysis to argue that these techniques lead to better generalization than strict CD approaches. Milieu teaching has been shown to increase children's frequency of talking both to

TABLE 3-2	**Goals and Activities for Prelinguistic Milieu Teaching**
GOAL	**ACTIVITIES**
Establish interactive routines to serve as contexts for communication	Imitate child's actions Imitate child's vocalizations Interrupt patterns of action with an adult turn; wait for child to take a turn Perform an action child finds silly, pause for child reaction, repeat When a child performs one part of a routine, perform the act needed to complete it

Increase frequency of vocalizations	Recast the child's vocalization with a word if s/he is focused on a referent
	Imitate vocalizations in varying ways:
	    Precisely as child produces them
	    With different sounds and syllables within the child's repertoire
	    With sounds and syllables outside the child's repertoire

Increase frequency and spontaneity of coordinated gaze	Create a need for communication within a routine in which the child looks at an object, then:
	    Give the child the object or action only if s/he looks at it
	    Verbally prompt for gaze
	    Move the object to your face to get the child to look at you
	    Intersect the child's gaze by moving your face into the child's line of sight
	    When the child looks, acknowledge the look with a pleased facial expression

Increase use of nonconventional and conventional gestures	Create a need for communication within a routine in which the child looks at an object, then:
	    Give the child the object or action only if s/he uses a gesture, such as pointing
	    Pretend not to understand if child fails to gesture; ask "What do you want?"
	    If needed, give a more specific cue ("Show me which one")
	    Give an explicit cue ("Show me!")
	    Model an appropriate gesture
	    Verbally acknowledge when the child complies by producing a gesture

Encourage combinations of gaze, vocalization, and gesture	If the child produces two of the three elements, wait expectantly for the third
	If the child does not supply it:
	    Ask, "What do you want?"
	    Intersect the child's gaze
	    Model the gesture
	    Model the word
	    Provide feedback and praise

Adapted from Warren, S., Bredin-Oja, S., Fairchild, M., Finestack, L., Fey, M., & Brady, N. (2006). Responsivity education/prelinguistic milieu teaching. In R., McCarthy & M. Fey (Eds.). *Treatment of language disorders in children* (pp. 47-75). Baltimore: Paul H, Brookes. In press.

BOX 3-6	**Activities Used in Enhanced Milieu Teaching**

- Choose materials of interest to child; arrange environment to support engagement and requesting.
- Use environmental arrangement to elicit child initiations.
- Mirror child actions to take a nonverbal turn; pause and wait expectantly following an adult remark to give child a chance to take a turn.
- Recognize and respond to what child communicates verbally or nonverbally.
- Expand child utterances to those at child's current ZPD.
- Use models following child requests to elaborate child form.
- Use requests or questions that give child a limited choice for responses.
- Use time delay/expectant waiting to elicit child speech.

Adapted from Hancock, T.B., Kaiser, A.P. (2006). Enhanced milieu teaching. In R. McCauley and M. Fey (Eds.) *Treatment of language disorders in children*. Baltimore: Paul H. Brookes. In press.

the teacher and to each other (Hart & Risley, 1980; Warren, McQuarter, & Rogers-Warren, 1984) and to be helpful for addressing a broad range of expressive communication targets (Camarata & Nelson, 2006). These approaches are particularly useful in small-group or classroom settings in which clinicians want to retain some of the positive aspects of clinician-directed language intervention but to expand their effects to a broader communicative context. They allow the clinician to use imitation, prompting, and cueing during the course of naturalistic activities, thus showing the child how the language being trained works to accomplish real communicative ends.

Script Therapy. Olswang and Bain (1991) discussed script therapy as a way to reduce the cognitive load of language training by embedding it in the context of a familiar routine. Here the clinician develops some routines or scripts with the child in the intervention context. For example, a clinician may institute a routine of placing a nametag on a peg when the client enters the room or always passing out supplies for snacks in the same sequence. Alternatively, the clinician re-enacts scripts the child already knows. These already known scripts could include eating at a fast-food restaurant, for example. In the intervention activity the known script is disrupted in some way, challenging the child to communicate to call attention to or repair the disruption. Disruptions can be accomplished by violating the routine. For example, the teacher can begin to give out cookies before the napkins have been distributed. The clinician can withhold turns, passing over one child when she is distributing drawing supplies. The clinician can violate the normal uses of objects in routines. For example, she can wear

the clients' nametags on her head one day, or she can hide objects needed to complete routines. If she locks the classroom each day as the class leaves for recess, she can hide the key and pretend to leave without locking up.

Verbal scripts or routines also can be used in this kind of activity. If the group always begins a session by singing a good-morning song, the clinician can start one day by singing, "Good-night." If the clinician has read the clients a book several times so that the children know it by heart, she can misread various portions. If a finger play such as "Where is Thumbkin?" is part of the group's routine, the clinician can purposely hold up an incorrect finger for one part of the rhyme. If the class has been learning nursery rhymes, the clinician can substitute words that rhyme but are inaccurate ("Humpty Dumpty sat on a wall; Humpty Dumpty had a great *doll*") or that don't rhyme ("Tom, Tom, the piper's son/Stole a pig and away he *walked*.").

Violations of verbal scripts also can be encouraged in clients, as a way to provide a scaffold from a known form to a slightly different or more complex variant. For example, a particular book, song, finger play, or poem can be included as part of every intervention session. The clients can be encouraged to "play with" this script once it has been overlearned. These violations can be pegged to specific intervention goals. For example, clients can be asked to change some words in the script to their opposites, if opposites are a target concept in the intervention. They can be asked to recast a present-tense text in past tense or vice versa. ("Let's read *The House that Jack Built* as if it is just happening now. I'll do the first page. 'This is the house that Jack *builds*' [or '*is building*']. 'This is the malt that lies in the house that Jack builds.' Now you try the next page.")

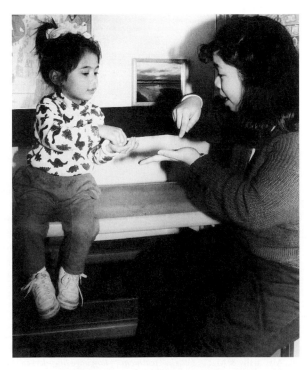

Finger plays can be used in script therapy.

Literature-Based Scripts and Interactive Book Reading. One variant of script therapy that has been subject to a good deal of research involves scripts based on picture and story books. This approach capitalizes on the familiarity and naturalness of interacting with young children around story book reading. Cole, Maddox, and Lim (2006) argue that book-sharing contexts are particularly effective because the book provides parents with greater opportunities for asking questions, making comments, and taking turns than do unsupported conversational settings. But they emphasize that simply reading to children is not enough, the reading must be accompanied by specific interactive techniques if it is to be effective as a language therapeutic tool. They review studies (e.g., Crain-Thoreson & Dale, 1999; Dale, Crain-Thoreson, Notari-Syverson, & Cole, 1996; Hargrave & Senechal, 2000) showing that children with language disorders associated with a variety of disabilities, as well as children with limited English proficiency (Lim & Cole, 2002), benefit from interacting with adults who use specific picture book interaction methods. They also cite studies demonstrating that clinicians can teach parents, teachers, and librarians to use and disseminate these techniques (Crain-Thoreson & Dale, 1999; Dale, Crain-Thoreson, Notari-Syverson, & Cole, 1996; Huebner, 2000). The critical pieces of this method include the following:

Commenting: The adult notices what the child is interested in on the page, makes a comment, and waits for a child response (e.g., Child points to picture of dog; adult says, "Our dog looks like that one!")

Asking questions: The adult asks a question at the child's language level about what the child has shown an interest in on the page (e.g., Child looks at picture of dog and says, "Dog;" adult says, "What shall we call that dog?")

Responding by adding a little more: After the child talks, the adult expands, extends or recasts the child's remark, then waits for the child to take a turn. (e.g., Child says, "Go on bus;" adult says, "Yes, they're getting on the bus. They're ready for school.")

Giving time to respond: Adults consistently use expectant waiting before giving another remark, allowing the child an opportunity to take a turn.

Using the Continuum of Naturalness

Are naturalistic activities always better than "unnatural" ones? Fey (1986) argued that highly naturalistic activities are best only if they improve the child's language. If two activities are equally effective in getting a child to produce a form or function he or she has not used before, then the naturalistic activity would be preferred, since it will presumably be more helpful to the child in moving the new form into everyday usage. But if the less naturalistic activity is more efficient in eliciting usage of the new form or function, the unnatural activity is the better choice.

Remember the argument the behaviorists use? They remind us that children with language impairments have been engaging in natural language activities since they were born and have not been able to take advantage of them the way normally speaking children have. Children with language impairments have particular difficulty abstracting conventional

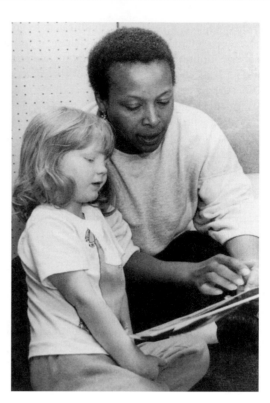

Interactive storybook reading builds language and preliteracy skills.

language structures from natural interactions. Some children with language impairments are excellent communicators. They get messages across with gestures and vocalizations very effectively and in a natural communicative environment can continue to do so indefinitely. Their communication will not necessarily change in an intervention program that merely provides more of the natural opportunities and consequences that they have been exposed to throughout their history.

So the point to be made about naturalness is that, all things being equal, a natural activity is better than an unnatural one, but only if all things are equal. If it can be shown that the child gives a greater number of correct responses in an unnatural activity, then the unnatural activity is better for eliciting the form, at least initially.

When thinking about naturalness in intervention, it is important to recall, too, that as Craig (1983) pointed out, communication can look natural to the child but does not have to be natural to the clinician. It is possible to design intervention contexts that appear to be natural but actually require a good deal of contrivance on the part of the clinician. For example, a clinician could set up a situation in which a child is supposed to build a block structure, a naturalistic activity. The clinician could give the child all the materials, then ask for each piece he or she needed to build a duplicate of what the child was building. Each request could be framed in an exactly parallel way, "Can you pass me the [X] please, [client]?" Clearly, this is not a natural way to talk. In real conversation we would vary our request forms, make a request for several items at once, just take some things that were in reach, and so on. But this stilted, unnatural style provides a clear and consistent model of how the client is to phrase a polite request. Suppose the tables are then turned and for the next building project the clinician has all the materials. The child has been exposed to an intensive dose of the forms he or she needs to request the desired materials.

So, in dealing with the continuum of naturalness in intervention, we have several options. We can complement CD activities with more naturalistic hybrid or CC activities throughout the intervention program. Or we can engineer the environment, carefully designing settings and activities that appear natural from the child's point of view. A third option was also presented by Fey (1986). We can use highly structured, clinician-directed activities and modify their format to increase the extent to which they resemble real-life communication. Fey gave the following guidelines for increasing the naturalness of CD activities.

Make the Language Informative. For example, instead of having the client simply imitate the clinician's "is (verb)-ing" description of a picture ("The boy is jumping."), we can display two similar action pictures and describe one, asking the client to point to the one we're talking about. Then we can give the client the same two pictures and ask him or her to describe one so the clinician can point to the picture being talked about. If the client chooses to imitate the same description as the clinician ("The boy is jumping."), well and good; a drill-like response has been given, and the clinician can point to the matching picture. If the client chooses to describe the other picture and uses a correct "is (verb)-ing" form, well and good again. If the client describes either picture with an incorrect form, the clinician can feign confusion, present the correct form as a model, and ask the client to give him or her another chance ("I'm not sure I heard you right. Did you say, 'The girl is running?' This picture shows 'The girl is running.' Tell me again which picture you want me to point to, so I can be sure to get it right.").

Increase the Motivation to Communicate Within the Task. This principle concentrates on getting the client to initiate communication within the CD format. One way to do this is to use a barrier or have the clinician and client sit back-to-back and talk to each other on toy telephones. In this format, the clinician can make a comment designed to pique the curiosity of the client to find out more about the clinician's topic, which is hidden from the client's view. In an activity designed to elicit questions, for example, the clinician can say, "WOW!" The client will presumably want to know what the excitement is about and initiate further communication by asking a question. Or, if the clinician wants to elicit negative statements, grossly false assertions can be made and the client can be allowed to correct the clinician by pointing out the error. The clinician might show the child a set of pictures and describe each one with an incorrect verb (for a picture of a boy jumping, the clinician might say, "He's sleeping. Uh-oh, I think I made a mistake. Can you straighten me out?").

Use Cohesive Texts. Many CD intervention activities have the child respond with a series of utterances that are syntactically related, in that they have the same form, but are semantically unrelated. In real conversation, though, there is usually a topic about which several related remarks are made. We don't usually say, "A boy is jumping. A girl is running. A dog is sitting." We usually establish a topic of conversation and then elaborate on it; for example, "A girl is running. She's going very fast. She's going over the finish line now. She wins the gold medal!"

Lee, Koenigsknecht, and Mulhern (1975) dealt with this problem in their *Interactive Language Development Teaching*. This CD program comprises a series of stories, each of which targets several syntactic forms. The clinician reads a story that is illustrated with simple flannelboard figures and contains examples of the target form. A question is then asked that is, essentially, a request for the client to imitate one of the statements heard in the narrative. The "exchange techniques" given in Box 3-7 are used to consequate the child's response so that the intended target is produced fully and accurately. Box 3-8 gives an example of an *Interactive Language Development Teaching* lesson.

Clinicians also can develop their own materials to serve the same purpose. For example, in eliciting use of auxiliary "can," the clinician could use a picture book about dressing. The clinician can show each page of the book to the child, while saying, "Here are some things my friend Sam can do. Sam can put on his shoes. Sam can put on his socks. Sam can put on his shirt," and so on. "Now let's talk about what you can do. Look at each page. Tell me what you can do to dress yourself. Here is a boy. He can put on his shoe. What about you?"

Move From Here and Now to There and Then. When first attempting to teach language use to developmentally young children, parents and clinicians both use language to talk about objects and events in the immediate environment. This helps the child to see how language is used to map, or refer to, things in the world. But eventually children begin to use language to convey new information about things that are not present in

---

| **BOX 3-7** | **Interchange Techniques** |

(In response to client's utterance, "There one more.")
1. Complete model: a prompt to imitate ("There's one more.")
2. Reduced model: a prompt to imitate that contains only a portion of the target response ("There's . . .")
3. Expansion request: the clinician asks for an expansion but does not present a model ("Tell me some more. Say the whole thing.")
4. Repetition request: the clinician asks the client to repeat his or her utterance but does not present a model ("What did you say? Tell me again.")
5. Self-correction request: the clinician asks the child to monitor his or her response ("Did you say that right?")

Adapted from Lee, L., Koenigsknecht, R., and Mulhern, S. (1975). *Interactive language development teaching.* Evanston, IL: Northwestern University Press.

| **BOX 3-8** | **Sample Lesson from Interactive Language Development Teaching** |

Concepts: baiting a hook, camping, fishing, hurrying
Vocabulary: bait, campfire
Flannel-board materials: figures of Mommy, Daddy, Timmy, Bobby; cutout of tent, table, four fishing poles with strings and hooks, worms, pond, boat

Elicited Structures

Primary Emphasis

Personal pronouns: he, she, his, her, him, we, us, our, them, their, they
Main verbs: *-s, -ed, am, are, can* + verb, *will* + verb, *do* + verb, *could* + verb, *should* + verb, *does* + verb, *did* + verb
Secondary verb: gerund
Negative: *couldn't*, uncontracted negative

Secondary Emphasis

Secondary verbs: later-developing infinitives
Interrogative: Reversal of modal and obligatory *do*

Narrative	**Target Response**
This is Mommy. Who is this?	This is Mommy.
This is Daddy. Who is this?	This is Daddy.
Mommy and Daddy are on a camping trip.	
Mommy and Daddy are fixing breakfast on their camping trip.	
They are fixing breakfast.	
They are hungry. What are they doing?	They are fixing breakfast.
Where are Bobby and Timmy?	
I do not see them. Where are they? Do you see them?	I do not see them.
Here are Timmy and Bobby!	
They were playing in the woods.	
They smelled the bacon so they came back.	
Why did they come back?	They came back because they smelled the bacon.
Timmy and Bobby say: We're hungry.	
Mommy and Daddy say: We're hungry.	
Mommy says: Breakfast is not ready yet. We will have to wait because breakfast is not ready.	
What does Mommy say?	We will have to wait because breakfast is not ready.
Now breakfast is ready.	
Mommy says: Breakfast is ready. Come and eat. Come and eat, because breakfast is ready.	
What does Mommy say?	Come and eat because breakfast is ready.
Everyone is sitting around the campfire.	
Timmy says: I wish we could stay longer. This is fun. I wish we could stay longer.	
What does Timmy say?	I wish we could stay longer.
Bobby says: Couldn't we stay. Daddy? Couldn't we? Couldn't we stay?	
What does Bobby say?	Couldn't we stay?
(Lesson continues to address other goals listed above.)	

From Level II, Lesson 26.
Reprinted with permission from Lee, L., Koenigsknecht, R., and Mulhern, S. (1975). *Interactive language development teaching.* Evanston, IL: Northwestern University Press.

the here and now. This shift is important. It shows that the child realizes that language is primarily used, not to tell people things they can see with their own eyes, but to impart information that is not present in the immediate environment. This ability to use language to talk about events removed in time and space is what frees the child from dependence on the immediate context. Eventually, this shift allows the child to use the kinds of decontextualized language that are important for literacy development and school success (Nelson, 2005; Wallach & Miller, 1988; Westby, 2005).

Spradlin and Siegel (1982) discussed the importance of teaching children to use language to accomplish things that cannot be accomplished in other ways. One basic function of language is to tell people about things they do not already know, about places they have never been, or about things they have never seen. So it seems important to give children with language impairments the opportunity to practice using language for this informative purpose. One way to increase the naturalness of CD intervention is to contrive contexts for children to drill forms in such a way as to use them in reference to "there and then" rather than "here and now."

But for many children with language impairments, this is no easy task. Fey (1986) suggested that one way to scaffold this kind of activity is to talk about events outside the immediate context and to rely on familiar activities or "scripts" for doing so. For example, a child working on basic subject-verb-object (S-V-O) sentence structures might make popcorn with the clinician. Each step in the process can be labeled by the clinician and, using a CD format, repeated by the child. ("We get the popcorn. We fill the popper. We plug in the popper. . . .") After completing the activity, the clinician can invite a parent, peer, aide, or puppet to join the client in eating the popcorn. The client can then be asked to retell the steps in making popcorn to the confederate ("You get popcorn. . . ."). This activity requires the client to talk about a nonpresent set of actions without using props, but provides the strong scaffold of recent personal experience.

Using these techniques to increase the naturalness of CD activities can be another means toward our end of helping the child not only to produce target forms, but also to use them to communicate. Whether we use a mix of approaches, engineer the environment to make intervention appear natural from the child's point of view, modify CD approaches to increase their naturalness, or do all of these, our overriding objective is to make the language we teach to children a meaningful tool for accomplishing social goals.

Intervention Activities

Once a general approach to intervention for a specific set of goals has been established and a mix of approaches for the entire intervention program has been set out, we need to plan the individual activities that will comprise the "meat" of the intervention. Although it is impossible in a textbook to outline all the activities that can be part of an intervention program, we can talk about some features of these activities so that the clinician will have a menu of choices for putting activities together. Let's see how we can structure specific activities to achieve changes in clients' language skills.

Modifying the Linguistic Signal. When we deliver language intervention, one of our most important tools is our own linguistic input to the client. Linguistic input is one of the major means of structuring what the child has to deal with in the intervention. Because it is such an important tool, we need to think very carefully about the input we present to the child, in terms of both its meaning and its formal properties.

Linguistic input can be manipulated in many ways to make it a more effective, efficient vehicle for encouraging change in the client's language use. As language pathologists, our linguistic signal is our richest and most flexible device for accomplishing this change. That's why we have to use it wisely. Let's look at some of the ways we can modify our input.

Rate. Reducing the rate of speech is a fundamental means of modifying input. In speech to normally developing young children, adults produce fewer words per minute and take longer pauses between words and utterances than they do in speaking to adults (Sheng, McGregor, & Xu, 2005). Talking more slowly may help the child by reducing the number of units that need to be processed per unit time, by providing somewhat more stable auditory models, and by encouraging increased clarity of articulation on the clinician's part, thus supplying a higher-quality model for the child. Further, in activities involving choral speech or song, the clients' speech-motor capacities may preclude their participation at normal speech rates. Slower delivery gives them more time to formulate and execute their speech-motor capacities. Montgomery (2005) and Weismer and Heskith (1993) have shown that slowing the rate of speech improves both comprehension and production of new words by children with language impairments. Weismer (1996) showed that reducing speaking rates also aids in the acquisition of grammatical morphemes in children with language disorders.

Slowing down the rate of speech is often easier said than done, particularly when working with a group of children or with very active clients, whose behavior tends to influence our own sense of pacing. Consciously trying to speak slowly and distinctly, conveying a sense of calm control, is a good habit for a clinician to cultivate. When working in a script therapy format using songs, rhymes, or finger plays, slowed rate is especially important. If the goal of these activities is to allow the client to internalize a verbal script, it is vital that the script be easily accessible. Singing may be more fun when it is "up tempo," but it will do the client less good. In my own work in supervising student clinicians, I have often seen students leading a group of young children in a song, the students themselves merrily singing away at normal tempo while the clients sit silent, unable to keep up the pace. When the clinicians are encouraged to slow the song down, the clients often begin to join in. Again, a slower-than-natural rate of speech, song, and rhyme often helps the language-learning child.

Repetition. "If I've said it once, I've said it a hundred times." This should be the language clinician's motto. Research has shown that children with language disorders need many more exposures before acquiring language forms and concepts than typically developing children do (Camarata & Nelson, 2006; Proctor-Williams, Fey, & Loeb, 2001). In normal development, clear examples of the match between a particular linguistic form and its nonlinguistic referent are often few and far between. For children with normal development, these few widely spaced exemplars may be enough. But children with language disorders are, by definition, less efficient language learners. They may need many more experiences of this match concentrated in relatively short periods of time to assimilate them. Intervention that exposes clients to multiple examples of target forms and their nonlinguistic mapping may be a key to their learning.

This implies that intervention can sometimes entail providing clients with what they would normally get from natural interactions, but simply increasing the frequency of both these focused interactions and the particular forms used within them. It could be taken to suggest a rationale for ILS and other naturalistic forms of intervention. It also could be seen as a rationale for drill forms of intervention or for focused stimulation, which also supply numerous examples in concentrated formats. The point is that there are a variety of ways, both naturalistic and contrived, to provide a client with intensive experience with form-meaning matches. What matters is providing the repetition.

One additional way to supply the child with useful, repetitive information about how language works is to provide contrasting forms from which the child can induce linguistic rules. This approach is sometimes called "inductive teaching" (Connell, 1989) or "contrastive drill" (Fey, Long, & Finestack, 2003) and is frequently used in both phonological and language intervention. This approach provides the client with a large number of examples of the operation of a linguistic rule, presented in a concentrated manner. If the goal were use of plural forms, the client might be shown a set of picture pairs. Each pair would contain one card with a picture of a single item and one card with a picture of more than one (not always the same number) of the same item. The clinician would then go through the sets, naming each picture with an appropriate singular or plural label for the client ("cat/cats," "dog/dogs," "bike/bikes," "car/cars," and so on). The clinician might then, after the multiple exemplars, explain the rule in simple terms for the child ("When we see more than one, we put an /s/ sound at the end."). The client could then be asked, with help from the clinician, to label the same sets of pictures. When success on this task is achieved, a new set of pictures that the child has not heard labeled could be tried.

Although adults see repetition as redundant and boring, it may not be so for the child, as you know if you have ever heard a child ask to watch a video he or she has already seen a dozen times. It is not necessary, as it is in adult conversation, to come up with a new and different way to say the same thing each time. In intervention the opposite may be true. We should strive to say the same thing the same way in the same context over and over and over. In this way we can maximize clients' opportunity to add it to their repertoire.

Increasing Perceptual Saliency through Prosody and Word Order.
In speech to normally developing young children, adults typically stress more than one word per utterance and use exaggerated intonation contours. This style of speech does not sound natural in other contexts, but it may help the very young listener direct attention to the auditory signal and highlight the segments containing the most salient information. These prosodic changes are available for talk in intervention, too. Weismer and Hesketh (1993) showed that children with

language impairments produced new words that had received emphatic stress during an intervention program more often than they produced words that had been trained with neutral stress. Weismer (1998) showed that this effect was specific to the production modality. These findings suggest that intonational highlighting helps get children to produce new structures. Sheng et al. (2005) called this complex of changes clinicians make in their speech to highlight language forms for clients a *therapeutic register*. Their research suggests that this register takes time and experience to acquire, so beginning clinicians will need to consciously practice and cultivate it.

Fey (1986) and Weismer and Robertson (2006) discussed a second means of increasing the perceptual saliency of language forms: by varying word order. Some forms that are particularly difficult for children with language-learning problems, such as auxiliary verbs and forms of the verb "to be," are usually found in the middle of sentences where they receive very little stress or intonational highlighting. One way to make these forms more perceptually salient is to present them in sentence variants that naturally place stress on them, such as questions that put them in the initial sentence position ("*Will* he ride the bike?" "*Is* he here?") or elliptical responses to questions that put them in final position ("Who will ride the bike? He *will*." "Where is Thumbkin? Here he *is*."). Using these forms as initial instructional contexts for auxiliaries and copulas avoids unnatural stress conditions in declarative sentences. When usage reaches criterion in these more perceptually salient contexts, efforts could be made to generalize the forms to their less marked variants in declarative sentences.

Complexity. When talking to very young children, adults generally produce sentences about two morphemes longer than the child's MLU (Paul & Elwood, 1991). The sentences parents produce when talking to normal language learners are shorter than those they use when talking to adults (Sheng et al., 2005). They also are semantically simple in that they generally use a limited vocabulary to refer to concrete objects and perceptions in the child's immediate environment (Chapman, 1981). But they are not simplified syntactically. Parents produce many questions when talking to young children, rather than more straightforward declaratives. And their sentences are fully grammatical and well formed—in fact, more so than sentences spoken to adults, which often contain garbles and false starts (Owens, 2005). So it would seem that normally developing children learn language from a semantically restricted but syntactically well-formed database.

What does this imply for the complexity of language used in intervention? My answer would be that we should adhere to the same principles. Our sentences should be slightly longer than those the child is using, they should refer to concepts that are semantically accessible to the child, and they should be well formed. Some clinicians "simplify" their input by leaving out function words and grammatical details, producing instructions such as "Get ball." They believe that these utterances are easier for children to process, so they model exactly the kinds of sentences the children are likely to produce.

My own belief, shared by Chapman (1981), Fey, Long, and Finestack (2003), and Hubbell (1981), is that the sentences children hear should, like those heard by normally developing children, be slightly longer and more advanced than those the child currently can produce and include only grammatically correct forms. For children whose comprehension skills are ahead of their current levels of production, the inclusion of grammatical markers in the linguistic input, even if the child cannot reproduce them in his or her own speech, helps to build an accurate auditory image of what well-formed sentences are supposed to sound like. Incorporating grammatical markers in the utterance gives it a rhythmic frame that may eventually help the child fill in the slots created by the rhythm. It also gives children additional exposure to these forms and, as we've seen, children with language impairments need higher levels of exposure before forms are learned. Furthermore, there is no evidence that simplifying sentences to telegraphic forms helps children to understand them (Fey, Long, & Finestack, 2003). Semantically constrained, well-formed, grammatically correct input does not hinder, but may help, language development.

Obligating Pragmatically Appropriate Responses. When using linguistic stimuli to elicit talk from a client, we should try to elicit language that is not only semantically and syntactically correct, but pragmatically appropriate. This suggests that if we want a client to produce a whole sentence as a response, our linguistic stimulus should obligate that form and not provide a context for an elliptical sentence. For example, if we want a client to produce, "He is running," we should not use the linguistic stimulus, "What is the boy doing?" The pragmatically appropriate response to this question is, "running." To have the client give this response, and then to tell him or her, "No, say the whole thing," in effect teaches a pragmatic error. If we want "He is running," as the response, we had better choose a stimulus that properly evokes this form. For example, we might say, "Let's look at these pictures. Here, the girl is running. Here the dog is running. Now you tell me about the boy."

There are times when the elliptical response may be the one we want. For example, we may decide to elicit elliptical responses to questions containing inverted auxiliaries to highlight these forms perceptually. In this case a question such as *Will he run?* will elicit the ellipted auxiliary form, "He will," if we make it a rule of the game that the child cannot say "yes" or "no" but must use some other words as an answer. This format supplies linguistic input that elicits the target form in a pragmatically appropriate context.

Careful selection of linguistic stimuli is one of the most important aspects of our clinical work. It is one thing that allows a trained clinician to provide a more efficient and effective form of linguistic input to a client than an untrained conversationalist. We have an obligation to show the child not only how to produce a syntactically correct sentence but also how to choose which of many possible forms of the sentence is pragmatically appropriate in a given linguistic context. That is, part of our job is not only to teach the child what to say but also when to say it. To tell a client to "say the whole thing" when we have given a stimulus that normally elicits less than the whole sentence violates this obligation. We fulfill our mission to teach language as real communication when we create the linguistic context that obligates a target sentence form in a pragmatically appropriate way.

Determining the Intervention Modality. Besides deciding how to manage the input to the child in the intervention program, we must decide how we will require the child to respond. This decision involves choosing the modality of the child's communication, and again we have a range of choices available. Let's explore what some of these choices are.

Comprehension versus Production. One fundamental decision we make in intervention is whether we work toward the child's ability to show that a target was understood or whether we require that the child use the target in his or her own speech. In normal development, children sometimes use forms, such as correct word order, before they show the ability to comprehend the same forms (Chapman & Miller, 1975; Paul, 2000c). So it is not necessarily true that comprehension precedes production. It follows that it is not always necessary to train comprehension before having a child produce a target form.

For forms and functions that assessment indicates are comprehended but not produced, production training is clearly indicated. Fey (1986) argued that such targets should be high priorities for production training, since they are clearly within the child's ZPD and the child is "ready" to learn to use them. But what about structures and meanings that assessment indicates are neither comprehended nor produced? Should they be targeted for production training, for comprehension, or not at all? Behaviorists (e.g., Guess, Rutherford, & Twichell, 1969; Lovaas, Berberich, Perloff, & Schaeffer, 1966; Sundberg & Michael, 2001) have stressed production, in imitation, as a first step in language learning. They believe that to be learned, behavior must be reinforced, and to be reinforced, it must be produced.

Lahey (1988), on the other hand, emphasized the fact that equivalent comprehension and production responses are often not present in normal language learners. She argued that a child should be exposed through multiple meaningful exemplars in the input language to forms that the child does not have in the comprehension repertoire. But she concluded from her review of research on comprehension versus production training that comprehension responses, such as pointing to contrastive stimuli, do *not* need to be trained before production of the forms is targeted. Guided production activities appear to facilitate both comprehension and production of new forms in children.

In light of this discussion, I would suggest that for forms the child comprehends, production training should be a high priority. For forms and functions that the child does not yet appear to comprehend, but that are chosen as intervention targets on the basis of other considerations we've discussed, an input component should be part of the intervention plan. This might include focused stimulation activities or CC activities that provide multiple opportunities for the clinician to demonstrate use of the structure in context. These approaches should be presented along with activities that elicit production of the target. It is not necessary to wait until the child demonstrates comprehension in pointing activities before trying to elicit the use of target forms.

Augmentative and Alternative Modalities. Speech is the most universal form of human communication. A child who can speak will have the most direct access to the greatest number of communication partners. For some children, though, speech is simply not a realistic option. These children have severe deficits in hearing or oral-motor structure or function that prevent them from using vocal communication. It might seem, on the surface, that these children should be easy to identify. But this is not always the case. Remember when we talked about etiological models of language disorders? We said that the etiology doesn't always explain the language level that a child attains. For example, you might have two children with the same level of hearing, one with very intelligible speech and one with almost none. One may need to use signs as a form of communication, whereas the other does quite well with spoken language. Moreover, some children do not have any obvious barriers in sensory or motor domains, but simply do not begin speaking; children with moderate to severe levels of mental retardation sometimes present this picture, as do some children with autism spectrum disorders. For clients who present these profiles, Beukelman and Mirenda (2005) advocate a "communication needs" model for delivery of AAC services. In this model, any child who needs a means to communicate because of a lack of speech is provided with some communication system, regardless of whether they have identifiable barriers to vocal expression.

Once the decision to adopt an alternative form of communication is made, a variety of communication systems are available to us. The process of choosing an AAC system has two components: *choice of the symbols* to be used and *choice of the interface* between communicator and the system, or how the child will access the symbols.

Symbols can be either aided or unaided. Unaided symbols include gestures, vocalizations, and body language. Aided symbols include productions that require some tool outside the client's own body. Examples of aided systems include objects, pictures, graphic symbols (such as Blissymbols [Fig. 3-5]), and alphabet letters. Both types of symbols can differ in their degree of *iconicity*, or the degree to which the symbol visually resembles its referent (Millikin, 1997; Romski, Sevcik, Cheslock, & Barton, 2006). In general, it is thought that iconic systems are easier to learn and easier for communication partners who have not been taught the system to understand (Hetzroni, Quist, & Lloyd, 2002). However, Romski and Sevcik (1996) and Romski, Sevcik, Cheslock and Barton (2006) discuss their System for Augmenting Language (SAL), an approach developed for use with school-aged clients with severe cognitive disabilities who had fewer than 10 spoken words, some intentional communication, and a history of many years of unsuccessful communication experiences. SAL differs from other AAC systems in that it uses abstract visual symbols, rather than pictures, to stand for words, and it employs a speech-generating device that "speaks" the word for each symbol selected by the client.

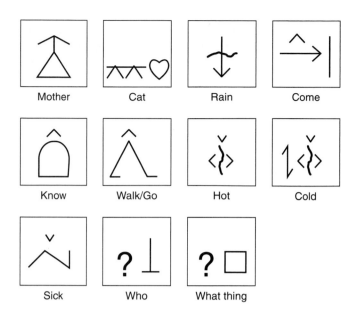

FIGURE 3-5 ✦ Blissymbols. (Reprinted with permission from Millikin, C. [1997]. Symbol systems and vocabulary selection strategies. In S. Glennen and D. DeCoste [Eds.], *Handbook of AAC* [p. 120]. San Diego, CA: Singular.)

Their research has shown that this computer-based form of alternative communication that employs visual symbols and voice output can increase not only communication but vocal production and intelligibility, as well, in older clients without spoken language. Still, children just introduced to an AAC system are commonly given a highly iconic one to start with. The disadvantage of iconic systems, though, is that they are somewhat limited in generativity, or the degree to which they can support the user in producing a full range of novel, original communicative messages. For this reason, we want, whenever we can, to move clients toward less iconicity in their AAC systems as their development and skill with the system proceed, with a written system as the ultimate goal. Daniel (2004) discussed additional considerations in moving students along a continuum of AAC devices. Figure 3-6 presents an outline of the varying levels of iconicity seen in several aided and unaided AAC symbol systems.

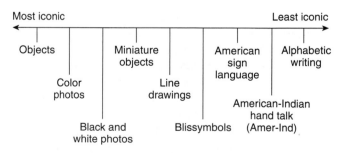

FIGURE 3-6 ✦ Symbol iconicity. Hierarchy of AAC symbols. (Adapted from Millikin, C. [1997]. Symbol systems and vocabulary selection strategies. In S. Glennen and D. DeCoste [Eds.], *Handbook of AAC* [p. 120]. San Diego, CA: Singular.)

The second issue in choosing an AAC system concerns *interface*. Communication boards containing words, letters, pictures, or symbols are sometimes used. Clients can indicate what they want to point out with a finger, head stick, headlight, or other device. Portable computers that either type out or produce synthesized speech versions of client messages also are available. These can be activated in a variety of ways: with a finger; stick; headlight; or a switch operated by sucking and puffing, head tap, eye movements, or whatever motor abilities the client can muster. These devices allow the client to select the letter, word, symbol, or picture he or she wants from an array presented on the computer screen, either by direct selection or by scanning through a series from which the client chooses when a cursor gets to the desired item. (See Beukelman and Mirenda [1998, 2005] and Glennen and DeCoste [1997] for a more complete discussion.)

The choice of a particular augmentative or alternative system is always a matter of experimentation to see what works best for a particular individual. The clinician working with a client who needs an augmentative or alternative system should give the client the opportunity to try the full range of devices that his or her abilities allow. Choice of a system should depend on the ease, accuracy, and efficiency with which the client can use the system, and these won't be obvious until the client gives several systems an extended try. Electronic systems with speech synthesis devices are available and often very useful, especially since it is known that voice output capacity not only increases vocalization and intelligibility, as Romski and Sevcik (1996) and Romski et al. (2006) showed, but also improves phonological awareness skills, which may help in the development of literacy (Foley, 1993; Millar, Light, & McNaughton, 2004). So use of a voice output communication aid (VOCA) may serve as an ultimate goal. However, some clients may need to start with a simpler system.

Bondy and Frost (1998) and Charlop-Christy and Jones (2006) discuss the Picture Exchange Communication System (PECS), one method that may serve as this first step for some children. PECS is an AAC method for eliciting initial communication from nonspeaking children without known sensory or motor disabilities. This approach begins by teaching children to exchange pictures for desired objects, and goes through a progression of steps to train higher levels of communicative behavior. These are summarized in Table 3-3. Charlop-Christy and Jones (2006) reviewed reports on this approach that suggest it can lead to increases in communicative behavior, decreases in maladaptive behavior, and increased use of vocalization and speech in some children; however they caution that the evidence is not strong. It is as yet unclear which children make the best candidates for PECS or whether it is superior to other AAC approaches. They and Rogers (2006) also note that it is not yet clear whether PECS is a better choice than direct speech training for nonspeaking young children without known sensory or motor impairments.

Another important consideration in choosing an AAC system should be the client's communication partners. Parents, siblings, teachers, and whoever else interacts regularly with the child should be involved in this decision from the beginning and should also be part of the process of training for using the system. Remember that communication is a two-way street. The client won't be able to use the system effectively if the people in the environment are not able to comprehend the messages (if, for example, the child is signing to people who don't know sign), or are uncomfortable with the particular system, or don't know how to enable the client to use it (Calculator, 1997b). Kent-Walsh and McNaughton (2005) discussed the importance of including training for communication partners (family, teachers, aides, peers) when implementing an AAC system for a client. They identified four interactive skills that research has supported as leading to increases in conversation participation, turn-taking skills, and the range of communicative functions expressed by the AAC user. These functions are listed in Box 3-9. They emphasized the importance of systematically describing, demonstrating, practicing, and providing feedback to partners in a structured, direct instructional program in order to achieve positive changes in the partners' interactive use of the AAC system. When implementing an AAC system for a client, it will be important to include a carefully designed program for helping communication partners participate in the client's new communication modality.

Consequating Client Language. Once we have succeeded in getting the client to produce some language, whether in the form of speech, sign, or some other modality, our responsibility as clinicians—rather than ordinary interlocutors—is to provide the client with a consequence for the production. One type of consequence is what behaviorists call *reinforcement*. The intent of reinforcement is to increase the frequency of the behavior being reinforced. Reinforcement can be tangible, such as a raisin or a sticker given for correct imitation of a sentence, or it can be a token, such as plastic chips or hash marks on paper, that are accumulated to "buy" an object or activity the client likes. Reinforcement also can be social. Social reinforcement takes the form of praise or approbation (such as the dreaded "Good talking!"). These kinds of reinforcement that are outside of the interactive frame and do not contribute to the interaction itself are called *extrinsic reinforcements*.

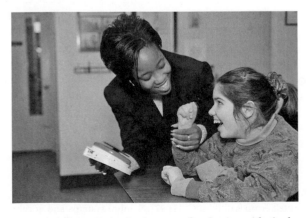

Augmentative communication use often begins with single message switch devices.

TABLE 3-3	Phases of the Picture Exchange Communication System

PHASE	GOAL	ACTIVITIES
1	Physical exchange	Client is taught to hand a picture card to a communicative partner in exchange for a desired item.
2	Expanding spontaneity	Client is taught to go to the communication board, get a picture, seek a partner, place the card in the partner's hand to receive a reinforcer. Distances between child and partner and child and board are gradually expanded. Response is trained in new settings.
3	Picture discrimination	Child is taught to choose among several pictures on their board.
4	Sentence structure	Child is taught to find their board, create a "sentence" on a strip by combining the *I want* card with the card for the desired object, find a partner to give the strip to. Partner reads the strip, leaving a time period after reading "I want" for the child to supply the name of the item. If the child does, s/he receives praise and the item; otherwise just the reinforcer is given.
5	Answer question	Child is taught to respond to "What do you want?"
6	Comment	Child is taught to respond to the question "What do you see?" by choosing a card and combining it with the *I see* card to gain a reinforcer that is NOT the pictured item.

Adapted from Charlop-Christy, M., & Jones, C. (2006). The picture exchange communication system. In R. McCauley & M. Fey (Eds.). *Treatment of language disorders in children* (pp. 105-122). Baltimore: Paul H. Brookes; Frost, L., & Bondy, A. (1994). *The Picture Exchange Communication System training manual.* Cherry Hill, NJ: Pyramid Educational Consultants.

BOX 3-9	**Interactive Functions of Communication Partners that Increase Communication Opportunities for Clients Using AAC Systems**

- Use extended pause time and expectant waiting to increase opportunity for client to take a conversational turn.
- Respond to all user attempts to communicate, whether with the device, or by means of vocalization, gesture, or gaze; treat behaviors with the AAC device as if they were communicative and respond even when user's intent is not entirely clear.
- Use open-ended questions to encourage more elaborated response from user.
- Model using the AAC system to communicate; accompany speech with indicating symbols on the user's device to show that the device is a means anyone can use for communication.

Adapted from Kent-Walsh, J., & McNaughton, D. (2005). Communication partner instruction in AAC: Present practice and future directions. *Augmentative and Alternative Communication, 21,* 195-204.

Reinforcement also can be more *intrinsic* to the communication process. It can be a naturalistic social reward, such as the achievement of the intended goal of a child's request (the child says, "Want crayon" and is given one) or the control of the clinician's attention or actions through the client's language (the child says, "See!" and the clinician looks at what the child points out). All these consequences are reinforcement, though some are clearly more natural reinforcers than others. A behaviorist would accept any of these forms of reinforcement as a valid way to increase the frequency of the desired behaviors. A pragmatically oriented clinician, on the other hand, would only accept natural communicative consequences as an acceptable form of reinforcement.

A second kind of consequence we can provide is somewhat different from reinforcement. This kind of consequence is *feedback.* Unlike reinforcement, feedback is not intended to increase the frequency of the client's behavior. Instead, its intent is to give the client information about the communicative value or linguistic accuracy of an utterance. In addition, it often provides the child with a scaffold to a more acceptable production. We talked about many forms of feedback under the CC approaches. CC approaches generally consequate client language behavior with feedback rather than reinforcement, except when they use natural communicative consequences as reinforcement, as we saw earlier.

It is possible to use feedback in CD approaches also, though. Lee, Koenigsknecht, and Mulhern (1975), for example, provided a set of "interchange techniques" in their CD program, *Interactive Language Development Teaching.* A clinician can use these, too, as feedback to consequate an incorrect production. Some of these feedback techniques are given in Box 3-7.

Should we reinforce or provide feedback in intervention? If we reinforce, should we use natural or extrinsic reinforcement? You've probably already guessed my answer. It depends. Extrinsic reinforcement is usually used in CD approaches. When CD approaches are the best way to intervene for a particular client, these forms of reinforcement are appropriate. Lahey (1988) argued that natural reinforcers are more effective than extrinsic ones in facilitating language development. She believes that language can only be learned in social interactions, so any reinforcement should be the natural consequence of these interactions. Even Lahey conceded, though, that there are some children for whom natural communicative consequences are simply not that rewarding. Children with autism can serve as examples. My approach would be to attempt to use natural consequences as reinforcement in any activity in which it is possible. When an activity does not allow for natural reinforcement, or when a client does not find natural reinforcement rewarding, I would suggest using food or tokens for a limited time. We would begin fading them out as soon as we could, moving first to a more and more intermittent schedule for the tangible reinforcement, then to direct praise, and finally to natural consequences.

Feedback, on the other hand, is always appropriate. It can be combined with reinforcement or used apart from it in a variety of activities from CD to CC. There is one form of feedback that we should be careful to avoid, though. Feedback that focuses on and repeats the child's error, rather than providing an appropriate alternative, is an extremely ineffective form of language consequation (Muma, 1971). If a child makes an error, we should never imitate it. We can either ignore it, in a CC approach, or provide a correct model or a scaffolding form of feedback, like those in Box 3-7, that helps the child correct the error. To allow the client to hear us make the same error he or she did can only be confusing. The client should hear only appropriate language as feedback from the clinician.

Generalizing Language Gains. The goal of language intervention is not only to get the client to produce appropriate forms in response to our stimuli but also to get the child to use these forms in real conversations. Moving from use of communication in structured, formal situations to using the same forms and functions in real life is the process we call *generalization*. Traditionally, generalization is thought of as the last step in the intervention process, something we work toward after all other objectives have been met. I would argue, though, that generalization ought to be incorporated into every intervention session, though not every activity, just as I advocated using more naturalistic activities for every goal, but not for every activity.

Although our hope is that generalization will just happen as a result of our intervention, we know that this is often not the case. As we saw when we talked about CD approaches to intervention, years of research have shown that children do not always generalize the forms learned in this manner to spontaneous conversations, even when high levels of accuracy are achieved in the structured setting. An argument that is commonly used for more naturalistic clinical approaches is that they are more likely to lead to generalization, since they are more similar to the other settings in which the targets will be used. But even when we use naturalistic approaches we cannot assume that the client will spontaneously generalize the language behaviors we train to people, places, and purposes outside the clinic.

So what do we do? If even a careful mix of structured CD and less formal hybrid and CC approaches does not guarantee that the client will spontaneously transfer learning, how can we achieve generalization? Costello (1983) argued that this could only be done by carefully planning generalization training within the context of the intervention program. She provided guidelines for achieving this transfer of training, and I will summarize some of them for you here.

First, Costello suggested that we use *many exemplars* of target forms and functions. This means that we should not stop training when the client is responding with high degrees of accuracy to a limited set of exemplars, such as a set of pictures. Nothing is wrong with using a limited set of stimuli in a repetitive CD format to elicit new forms from clients who use them very infrequently. Once this has been done, though, we cannot assume that the client will generalize the form's use. We need to work toward that generalization by providing many different examples of how the form can be used, when it can be used, and who can use it in real conversations. And one or two real situations may not be enough. We may need to provide quite a few. If we are teaching a client to use "is (verb)ing" to describe ongoing action, it may not be enough to have the child use it to tell about making pudding. The child may have to tell about making a collage, a pizza, and a birthday card, too.

Another aspect of the multiple exemplars idea is the notion of *sequential modification*. Sequential modification happens when the intervention environment is extended from one place to another until spontaneous generalization to new environments occurs. For us it means that in addition to providing multiple exemplars of target forms, we should do so in multiple settings. These could include the client's home, the classroom, outdoors, or in the cafeteria. How many different settings? Costello suggested that two or three are enough. This does not have to be an overly arduous or expensive process. One or two sessions in one or two alternate environments every few months of intervention may be adequate. For school-aged and adolescent clients this may suggest the "pull-out/sit in" model of service delivery, in which some sessions take place in the clinician's office and some in the child's classroom. For preschoolers, it may mean that now and then the clinician travels to the child's home, day-care center, or preschool. This form of generalization training involves doing what the clinician normally does with the client in a different place.

Costello also suggested that we *make the treatment material similar to things used in the natural environment*. This may mean, for example, using classroom textbooks rather than specially designed materials in intervention for school-age children or using the storybooks read in the preschool class instead of commercial "speech therapy" materials.

Intermittent or delayed reinforcement is another important generalization tool. Costello warned that these schedules would probably not be effective in the early stages of training, when more consistent reinforcement is necessary to stabilize target productions. Once stabilization is achieved, though, extrinsic reinforcement should, as discussed earlier, be less and less frequent, and the use of natural contingencies should be increased. In this way the contingencies of training become more similar to those found in the natural environment.

Another one of Costello's ideas for promoting generalization involves introducing *distracter items* into the intervention stimuli. The theory is that we should use some stimuli that are semantically relevant but not direct targets of intervention because this more closely resembles what happens in natural conversation. In other words, occasionally within a training sequence used to elicit particular language targets, the clinician should inject a relevant comment that will elicit a nontargeted response from the child.

These suggestions are important because children's language use cannot be maintained in the natural environment if they cannot withstand the inconsistent, delayed, and indirect reinforcement contingencies that the natural environment provides. An additional way to guard against this danger is to attempt to increase the frequency of the child's communication by targeting high rates of response within the initial phases of training and to provide multiple opportunities for the child to produce the same responses in hybrid and CC settings. Focused stimulation and script activities may be particularly useful in this regard. Increasing rates of production also may help the child to automatize production processes, freeing resources to be devoted to more complex levels of language formulation. In other words, practice makes perfect. Providing extended practice with new forms and functions may increase generalization and provide a scaffold to higher levels of language complexity.

Another strategy that may be useful in helping children to transfer learning is the use of *self-monitoring*. This requires encouraging the child to become the internal "teacher" who constantly judges performance. If we can get clients into the habit of evaluating their own communicative effectiveness in the clinic setting, they are more likely to do so in other situations. Self-monitoring is particularly effective for clients at advanced language levels who have higher degrees of metalinguistic and meta-cognitive ability than preschoolers. A client learning a particular communicative function, such as using questions to elicit information, can engage in a conversation with the clinician that is recorded via audiotape. The client can listen to the tape. The clinician can stop it after each client remark and ask, "Was that a good way to find out?" Roles can be switched and the client can make the same requests for self-monitoring to the clinician. During a third round of listening, clients can be prompted to ask the same question for each of their own utterances.

Even young children can do simple self-monitoring. They can begin by monitoring the clinician. Almost all children enjoy the opportunity to correct an adult's "mistakes." They can then be asked to make intentional mistakes themselves and let the clinician "guess" if they produced the target right or not, earning a point each time the clinician "discovers" an "error." They also can be given self-monitoring prompts, like those suggested by Lee, Koenigsknecht, and Mulhern (1975), "Did you say that right?"

Another way we can increase children's tendency to generalize language training is by encouraging them to take advantage of models in the environment. We can do this, first, by making imitation or use of a model in the intervention setting very rewarding. We accomplish this by praising and reinforcing clients for their efforts to imitate as well as for their production of specific forms. Second, we can provide the client with some very salient and appealing models. Hart (1981) suggested using *peer models*. Putting the client in a structured communication situation with a peer with the clinician available as a "troubleshooter" may be a helpful way to attain this end and effect generalization.

We've discussed a wide variety of techniques for encouraging clients to generalize the results of our intervention to real communication. The most important point to take away from this discussion is that generalization needs to be built consciously into our intervention programs. Using CD approaches will not ensure it. Using naturalistic approaches cannot guarantee it, either. The only way to be sure that our teaching generalizes to real conversation is to make a concerted effort to see that it does and then to evaluate the use of targets in natural settings, as we discussed in the assessment section. Hoping for generalization, or assuming it will happen, will not make it so.

THE CONTEXT OF INTERVENTION

The context of intervention, according to McLean (1989), involves the physical and social settings in which the intervention takes place. Let's look at some of the ways we can manipulate the context of intervention to achieve our objectives for the client.

Choosing the Nonlinguistic Stimuli

We've talked already about the importance of controlling the linguistic stimuli in intervention. In addition, though, we need to choose the nonlinguistic context of objects and events in which the intervention takes place. Let's examine some of the choices we have available.

Types of Stimuli. Clinicians often use pictures, toys, and real objects as nonlinguistic stimuli in intervention. Pictures are popular choices because they are convenient and easy to obtain. For young children, though, pictures may not be a best first choice. They may contain too few central aspects of the referent. For example, an important thing to know about the meaning of the word "ball" is that balls roll. A picture of a ball may not convey this notion. Leonard (1975b) showed that children acquired certain syntactic forms more readily when given demonstrations of event referents for the sentences than when shown pictures. This is not to say that we should not use pictures, only that we should not use pictures exclusively. Further, the younger the client, the more advantageous the use of objects and real events is going to be. Lahey (1988) pointed out that young children also seem to be more interested in moving objects than static ones and are most likely to talk about objects they act on themselves. For example, a toy with a button that a client pushes may be more interesting than one with a key that the clinician must operate for him. This suggests that successful intervention for young children includes allowing them to manipulate real objects and providing objects that do

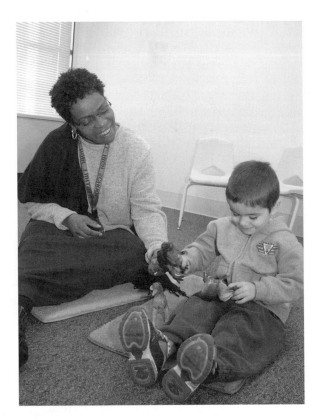

Real objects are more compelling than pictures for language stimulation activities.

something interesting when they are manipulated, such as make a noise, move, fit onto something, light up, or play music.

For older clients, though, pictures, particularly in the form of photographs, can be very engaging. Tarulli (1998) discussed a variety of uses of photography in intervention for school-aged children, most of which focus on linking the client's personal experiences, as recorded in the photos, with language use. Examples include using photographs from class events as a basis for labeling, describing, and writing about the events or to compare and contrast experiences in which the child participated, such as a field trip to an aquarium, with those described in a nonfiction text, such as a book on marine life. The advent of digital photography makes collecting and printing pictures to use in intervention a real possibility for most clinicians and families.

What about pictures on a computer screen? Many software programs designed to provide computer-assisted language intervention use amusing pictures or moving images as either stimuli or reinforcement for child language behavior. These are often very entertaining for children. Most enjoy pushing the buttons on the computer and being involved with such a "grown-up" piece of apparatus. Steiner and Larson (1991) pointed out that using a computer often can be very exciting for children because it allows them to "command the machine." The danger in this is that the human-machine interaction may overshadow the interpersonal communication that is the goal of our intervention. When children enjoy computers and when programs are available that target goals identified in the client's

assessment, there is every reason to include them as part of the intervention program, so long as the clinician interacts with the child as he or she uses the machine. Cochran and Masterson (1995) report on several research studies that show clinician-mediated computer-based activities to be comparable in efficacy with more traditional approaches. They find no evidence, though, that children with speech and language problems show improvements in interactive communication as a result of *independent* computer use. This is true even of Fast ForWord (Scientific Learning Corporation, 2000), perhaps the most popular computer-assisted language development program as of this writing. Cohen, Hodson, O'Hare, Boyle, Durrani, McCartney, Mattey, Naftalin, and Watson (2005) compared results of Fast ForWord intervention with other computer-assisted intervention activities, as well as with traditional intervention. They found that children receiving all three kinds of intervention made gains, although there was no advantage for either computer method over regular speech-language therapy. Troia and Whitney (2003), in studying Fast ForWord, found that positive changes were seen in tested expressive language, but not in academic or social skills. Loeb, Stoke, and Fey (2001) also saw changes on expressive test scores following Fast ForWord training, but did not find that these translated to functional language use. A small study of children with autism, however (Hetzroni & Tannous, 2004), suggests that these children do show some improvement as a result of exposure to an interactive video game focused on social communication.

Cochran and Masterson (1995) discussed several uses to which computers can be put into clinical practice. One is as a context for treatment. In this use, the computer program or game functions as the topic of conversation. For example, an activity might involve using a graphics program, such as *Walt Disney Comic Strip Maker* (The Walt Disney Co., 1983), to create a greeting card, or a creative writing program, such as *Mystery at Pinecrest Manor* (Klug, 1983) or *Tiger's Tales* (Hermann, 1986), to generate a story. Here the computer serves as the shared context for structured conversation, much as a board game or craft activity can in more traditional activi-

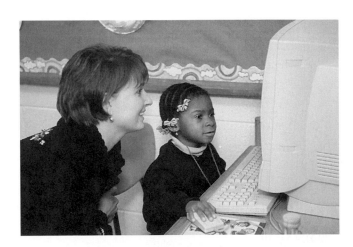

Computer-assisted language therapy is often popular with young clients.

ties. For school-age children and adolescents with language learning disorders there is a wealth of educational software designed to teach mathematics, history, geography, and other topics. *Where in the World Is Carmen Sandiego?* (Bigham, Portwood, & Elliott, 1986) provides just one example. Since many students with language-learning disabilities have low levels of general information because they have difficulty acquiring new knowledge from language and print, these programs can often help to fill in the gaps in their knowledge base. These programs generally require reading skill, so the clinician can either read the text to the client or choose programs carefully to match the client's reading ability. Adolescents with language-learning disorders, for example, may benefit from educational software designed for elementary students. Content-related educational software also can give the clinician a base of information to be used to help clients work on, for example, discourse comprehension skills such as summarizing, getting the main idea, and paraphrasing. Lots of other materials can serve the same function, including classroom texts, Internet sites, library books, newspapers and magazines, carefully chosen children's literature, and commercial instructional materials. The point is that computer software is useful if it motivates clients, but a skilled clinician can find many ways to motivate clients. Commercially available multimedia programs also can be adapted for use with children with language disorders, and numerous resources are available on the Internet, at sites such as www.communicationdisorders.com, to give just one example. But as Steiner and Larson (1991) pointed out, good clinical practice always integrates computer-based instruction with other activities. The computer is just one tool, which always needs to be supplemented with other kinds of communicative activities.

A second important use for computers for school-aged clients is word processing as a way to facilitate the development of written language skills. Cochran and Masterson (1995) emphasize the advantages of "talking" word processors, not only for motorically impaired students who use them as an alternative communication mode, but for speaking students as well. They argue that the auditory feedback provided by these programs helps writers develop a better sense of audience as well as identify grammatical errors. They cite research demonstrating that students given word processing opportunities improved in written language skills.

Some software (e.g., *Micro-LADS* [Wilson & Fox, 1983] and *Language Carnival* [Ertmer, 1986]) is specifically designed to teach language to children with disabilities. It often contains fixed vocabulary, uses too heavy a reinforcement schedule, or is very expensive when it is applicable to only a few children in the caseload. Programs designed for more general use, such as *Stickybear ABC* (Hefter, Worthington, Worthington, & Howe, 1982) or *The Factory* (Kosel & Fish, 1984), may be just as useful as more expensive software designed for children with language disorders and can be adapted for a variety of intervention goals. Coufal (2002) and Westby and Atencio (2002) provide additional discussion of these issues.

Timing. Besides deciding what the client needs as a referent for the linguistic signal, we also need to decide when the referent will appear. This simply means that we need to be careful about the timing of our nonlinguistic stimuli to be sure that they correspond appropriately to what is being said. This is sometimes not as simple as it sounds. Take past-tense forms, for example. To demonstrate an action referred to with a past-tense form, it is important to be sure that the action is completed before the speech act begins. We might throw a paper airplane across the room, then say to the client, "Tell me what I did." "You threw (or flew) the airplane," would be an appropriate response. But if we asked the question *while* throwing the paper airplane, our question would be inappropriate. We must plan our linguistic stimuli carefully to be sure that they elicit the target response appropriately, and the same is true of the timing of the stimuli in reference to the nonlinguistic context.

Service Delivery Models

There is one final aspect of the context of intervention. This refers to where, when, and with whom the intervention takes place. Traditionally we think of language intervention as taking place in a clinic room with a clinician providing therapy to a client or a small group for several 30- to 60-minute sessions each week. This model is often referred to as a *pull-out*, or *clinical*, form of service delivery. But language intervention can be delivered in a variety of ways. We'll discuss the options briefly here and return to them in later chapters when we talk about which service delivery models are most appropriate for clients at different ages and developmental levels.

The Consultant Model. The traditional answer to the question, "Who delivers language intervention?" is "the language pathologist." But an additional role for the SLP has evolved—that of consultant. In a consultant role, the language pathologist still determines the intervention targets, procedures, and contexts. But instead of relating directly to the client, the SLP relates to another agent of intervention, giving that person information and a rationale for the intervention targets and more or less detailed instructions for the intervention procedures. The SLP also meets regularly with this individual to provide feedback on the intervention process, discuss problems that arise, and plan further intervention targets and activities. When acting in a consultant role, the SLP remains responsible for evaluating the client's progress in the intervention program, for deciding when targets have been met, and for troubleshooting the intervention procedures and contexts to ensure that they are effective.

The alternative agents of intervention may be parents, classroom teachers, speech-language aides, or peers. Girolametto and Weitzman (2006) review research showing that parents can be trained to use focused stimulation techniques that will result in positive changes in language form and content. Cole, Maddox, and Lim (2006) showed that interactive story book sharing techniques could be effectively implemented by parents and teachers to improve children's language skills. Law, Garrett, and Nye (2004) reported few differences in the outcomes of language therapy for preschoolers when the intervention was delivered by clinicians or trained parents. Given these findings, it is likely that clinicians will find themselves frequently playing the role of consultant to parents or educators who will work directly to improve language skills in children with communication problems. It will be important for clinicians not only to know how to deliver effective intervention themselves, but to have effective means of teaching these techniques to others. Girolametto and Weitzman (2006) provide some guidelines, and more will be discussed in Chapters 6, 7, and 9.

Peers of the client also can be important agents of intervention. Paul (2003a) reviewed literature that suggests peers may be the most effective agents for teaching social communication skills to children with primary deficits in the area of pragmatics. When training peers it will, again, be important to have effective ways of teaching them how to support and expand clients' communication attempts. Several programs for peer training are discussed in Chapters 9 and 14.

The Language-Based Classroom Model. Here the clinician is the classroom teacher for a group of students with language disorders. Mainstream students also may be members of the class, although the focus is on intervention for the group with disorders. Language-based classrooms at the preschool level resemble traditional nursery-school programs. Many of the themes and activities resemble those used in mainstream preschools. The main difference is that SLPs in these settings use their expertise in language development and intervention to maximize the students' opportunities to attend to and practice oral language. What distinguishes them from the clinical model is that the SLP provides a continuous form of intervention embedded within a context of day-to-day activities.

For school-age clients, language-based classroom instruction may comprise either the entire school day or part of the day, depending on the severity of the student's needs. This organization places children identified as having special needs in a "resource room" with the SLP as the classroom teacher. The SLP provides instruction for each client, according to his or her Individual Educational Plan (IEP), and also organizes activities that focus on oral language skills for the group. Many students in this setting also spend part of their school day with a regular teacher in a mainstream classroom.

For adolescents with language disorders, the language-based classroom model often takes the form of one of the student's classes. When the mainstream students go to English for a 50-minute period, for example, the student with a language-learning disorder may go instead to a language classroom taught by an SLP. The organization of this classroom is similar to that of the resource room at the elementary level. But because the students usually spend less time there, perhaps one period a day for one or two marking periods of the school year, instruction is more concentrated. Theme-based and curriculum-based approaches are often used to help the students develop not only oral language abilities, but also study skills, thinking skills, and the ability to deal more proficiently with written forms of language.

Collaborative Models. Midway between the consultant model and the language-based classroom model, in terms of intensity of client contact, is the collaborative model. The SLP works with one or more students who have been identified as having a language disorder, but does so in the mainstream classroom in collaboration with the regular teacher. Instead of seeing the client in a clinic or pull-out setting, the clinician delivers the intervention mandated in the IEP in the context of the regular classroom. This model, too, can be implemented at any developmental level, from preschool through adolescence.

The collaborative model requires consultation and cooperation with the classroom teacher. The SLP and teacher must meet together to decide what classroom material will fit in with the goals identified on the client's IEP and how the SLP can either develop activities in line with those themes or use the regular teacher's normal classroom activities to work toward IEP goals. The SLP then plans the specific activities to be used and works within the classroom alongside the regular teacher. The SLP focuses primarily on the children identified as having a language disorder, whereas the regular teacher focuses on the other students. Ehren (2000a,b) and Prelock (2000) provide some additional guidelines in implementing collaborative practice. Here's an example of how a collaborative activity might work.

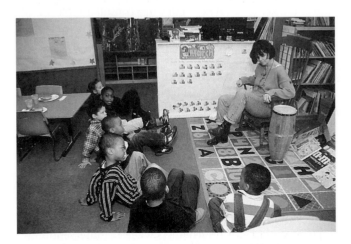

Language-based classroom intervention provides opportunities for functional language use.

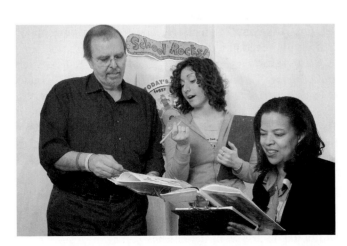

Collaborative planning is needed for clients in integrated settings.

Suppose George and Martha are students identified as having a language disorder. Both are in Ms. Marshal's fourth-grade class. One of the goals identified on George's IEP is producing complex sentences. Martha has production and understanding of narratives as an IEP goal. Mr. Taylor, the SLP, consults with Ms. Marshal about doing some in-class activities to work toward these goals. They decide together that Ms. Marshal's literature unit on fantasy novels might be a good context for the intervention activity. The class has been reading children's books that tell fantasy stories. So Mr. Taylor decides to have the class write a fantasy story of their own in small, cooperative learning groups. He puts George and Martha in separate groups and arranges with Ms. Marshal that he will supervise these two groups while she supervises the other three.

Mr. Taylor introduces the lesson and has the class talk about the differences between fantasy and reality, give examples of fantasy books they've read, and generate some ideas for fantasy stories about magical animals. He then tells the students that each group is to work together to write a fantasy story, but first he wants to talk about what makes a good story. He writes two short choppy sentences on the board (such as, "The dragon was fierce. The dragon breathed fire.") and asks students to judge whether these tell a story well. Then he asks for suggestions from the class about how to better convey these thoughts, by combining them into one sentence. After letting several mainstream students model this process, he asks George to do one. Then he asks the class to think about what parts their story should have. He can ask them to recall some of the fantasy stories they've read and identify parts, such as main character, setting, a problem that gets the story going, and so on. He can have several mainstream students identify these parts in books they have read. Then he can ask Martha to do so.

Next he tells the class that each group is to write a short fantasy story about a magical animal. He reminds them to make their sentences more informative by sometimes combining two ideas into one. He reminds them about the parts that a good story should have. Then he and Ms. Marshal work with their cooperative learning groups. Mr. Taylor is careful to be sure that George and Martha are fully involved in their respective groups and have opportunities to contribute. He reminds them about complex sentences and narrative structure as he "troubleshoots" for them within the activity. This project may take more than one collaborative classroom session to complete. When the project is finished, the groups may illustrate, display, and share their stories.

Collaborative intervention does not need to be an all-or-nothing affair. Some clinicians use a "pull-out/sit-in" version. In this approach, some intervention is provided in a pull-out or clinical format, perhaps once or twice a week. Additional intervention, perhaps once a week, is delivered collaboratively in the student's classroom.

All the service delivery models we've discussed—clinical, consultative, language-based classroom, and collaborative—are valid contexts for language intervention. The choice depends on the needs of our clients and the clinician's relations with other professionals who work with them. We'll talk more about criteria for making these choices when discussing intervention for different developmental levels. The important thing for now is to be aware of the range of service delivery options that are available and not think of ourselves as being limited to one option to the exclusion of others.

EVALUATING INTERVENTION OUTCOMES

We've talked about the importance of planning each aspect of language intervention: the selection of objectives, the choice of procedures, and determination of contexts. But we have an additional responsibility: to demonstrate that we have not wasted the client's time; that we have, in fact, achieved the goals that we set for the intervention. This responsibility is known as *accountability*. We are accountable to the client, and to whoever paid for our services, for making a significant change in language behavior. Further, we should be able to show that the changes we made would not have happened if our intervention had not taken place. Let's talk about how we can fulfill these responsibilities.

TERMINATION CRITERIA

One way to demonstrate that intervention objectives have been met is to specify ahead of time what criterion we will use to decide that a goal has been achieved. This specification is called the *termination criterion*. ASHA (2004e) has proposed a list of criteria for terminating services. These are summarized in Box 3-10.

The termination criterion for individual objectives, as opposed to termination from an intervention program, is simply the

---

BOX 3-10 **Discharge Criteria**

Intervention may be terminated if one or more of the following conditions are met:
1. Communication is now within normal limits.
2. All goals and objectives of intervention have been met.
3. The client's communication is comparable to those of others of the same age, sex, and ethnic and cultural backgrounds.
4. The individual's speech or language skills no longer adversely affect social, emotional, or educational status.
5. The individual uses an AAC system and has achieved optimal communication across partners and settings.
6. The client has attained the desired level of communication skills.

Adapted from American Speech-Language-Hearing Association (2004e). Admission/discharge criteria in speech-language pathology. *ASHA Supplement, 24,* 65-70.

level of use of a targeted structure that the client must achieve for the structure to be considered learned. In behaviorist intervention formats, this criterion is usually set quite high, at 80% to 90% correct usages. However, usage is measured within the structured intervention context. Lee, Koenigsknecht, and Mulhern (1975) have argued that termination criteria should be set lower, at 50%, but be measured in natural contexts such as spontaneous conversation. It seems to me that to claim we have truly changed language behavior, we have an obligation to show that the client does use the targeted forms in natural, spontaneous speech. Further, we know that once children use forms a majority of the time in spontaneous speech, they are very likely to progress toward consistent correct usage on their own without intervention. So a criterion of 50% correct usage in spontaneous speech seems to me to be a responsible terminal objective for any particular intervention goal.

But how will we know when to take that spontaneous speech sample to determine whether 50% correct usage is achieved? Here it seems to me that we would want to see high (80% to 90% correct) levels of usage in the structured intervention setting before we would expect the child to use the forms spontaneously. Therefore, some charting of progress in structured intervention formats is an important part of the intervention program. A simple form such as the one in Figure 3-7 can be used to track performance in structured activities. As we discussed in Chapter 2, it is not necessary to chart every activity, but only to take samples periodically throughout the structured portion of the intervention program. Further, we know that high degrees of accuracy in CD formats will not guarantee that usage will generalize to spontaneous speech. So once we get those high levels of use in structured activities, we should use the generalization techniques we discussed if we have not done so already. We also would be wise to give the client some opportunities to use the forms in hybrid and other more naturalistic intervention formats. When all these have been accomplished—high levels of accuracy in structured formats; provision of activities designed to promote generalization; and use of hybrid, CC, or naturalistically modified CD intervention activities—then we should monitor the use of target forms in unstructured conversation, using speech sampling or other criterion-referenced techniques.

If correct use of the forms in this context exceeds 50%, I suggest discontinuing direct intervention for that target. The target form should be monitored every few months in spontaneous speech, though, to see that its correct usage is increasing. If not, it can be returned to the intervention program. If the target form or function is not used correctly a majority of the time in spontaneous speech, even if the client is very successful in producing it in the structured context, more generalization training and naturalistic activities are needed to help the client make the transition to spontaneous usage. By using a termination criterion that requires use of intervention targets in real communication, we can be sure of fulfilling our obligation to demonstrate meaningful change in language behavior.

EVALUATING THE EFFECTIVENESS OF INTERVENTION

The second aspect of accountability concerns our obligation to make changes that would not happen without our intervention, as ethical practice requires (American Speech-Language-Hearing Association, 2003b). There are a variety of ways to evaluate the efficacy of intervention (see Dollaghan, 2003, 2004; Fey & Justice, 2007; McReynolds & Kearns, 1982; Ochsner, 2003, for discussions including using single-subject research designs, in which each client serves as his or her own control). Fey (1986) argued that the most appropriate of these, for clinical purposes, is the *multiple-baseline* design. Multiple-baseline designs give us the opportunity to show that the behaviors we targeted in intervention improved more than other language behaviors that were not subjected to intervention. By demonstrating this facilitative effect of intervention, we can ensure that the time and money spent on intervention were worthwhile.

The procedures for conducting a multiple-baseline single-subject research design are schematized in Figure 3-8. The first step in implementing a multiple-baseline design to study the effects of intervention is to identify several intervention objectives, based on assessment data. Using some of the other criteria we discussed earlier, certain of these objectives will be chosen as targets of the intervention program. Others will not be chosen, perhaps because they are not considered high in communicative effectiveness, because they require phonological skills the client does not yet have, or because we feel they are low in teachability. The goals that were not chosen could be considered *control goals*.

When choosing control goals, we need to be careful to choose language behaviors different enough from the targeted goals so that response generalization is unlikely. Goals that are similar in form to the target goals can be chosen as *generalization goals*. These would be tracked along with the target and control goals to determine whether training is generalizing, as expected, to these similar behaviors. If, for example, "is (verb)ing" were the target, we would probably not want to choose copula "be" as the control goal, since it is quite likely that some learning from the "is (verb)ing" intervention program might generalize to copula use. Instead, we would designate copula "be" as a generalization goal. We might choose to use the auxiliary "will" as a control goal.

The second step in the multiple-baseline procedure is to gather baseline data on the target, generalization, and control goals. Elicited production procedures, such as the ones we discussed in Chapter 2, can be used to compute a percentage of usage in obligatory contexts for both target and control forms. It is important to establish a stable baseline for each form so we know that the baseline is a reliable reflection of the child's ordinary use of the form. Baseline measures may be taken two to three times during the course of a few sessions, and percentage of usage may be averaged to achieve this stability.

The next step is to institute intervention for the target, but not the control or generalization goals, using all the principles of intervention that we have discussed. Although multiple-

RESPONSE DATA FORM

Name of client: _____ Name of clinician: _____ Date: _____

Bahavioral objective: _____

Therapy materials: _____

Reinforcement type and schedule: _____

Trials

Stimulus presented	1	2	3	4	5	6	7	8	9	10	Comments
1.											
2.											
3.											
4.											
5.											
6.											
7.											
8.											
9.											
10.											
11.											
12.											
13.											
14.											
15.											
16.											
17.											
18.											
19.											
20.											
Total Number of Responses: Total Correct Responses: Total Incorrect Responses: Percent Correct:											Key:

FIGURE 3-7 ✦ Response data form. (Reprinted with permission from Roth, R., and Worthington, C. [2005]. *Treatment resource manual for speech language pathology*, ed 3. Clifton Park, NY: Delmar.)

baseline designs are often used in applied behavior analysis, Fey (1986) pointed out that this fact in no way restricts us to CD intervention programs. We can make use of all the intervention approaches we have talked about when we implement multiple-baseline studies. Intervention is continued until our termination criterion for the target goal is met, including both high levels of correct use in structured formats and use of the targets in spontaneous conversation.

We would then evaluate the child's use of the target and control goals. We can use the same elicited production tasks we used in the baseline studies, as long as they are not exactly the same as what we did in the intervention program. If use of

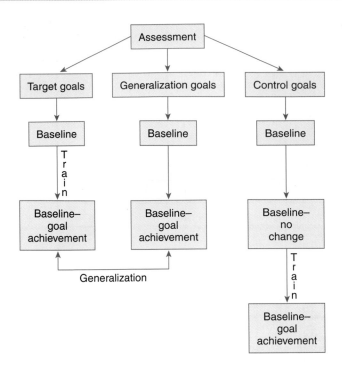

FIGURE 3-8 ✦ The proposed steps in a multiple-baseline intervention design. (Redrawn with permission from Fey, M. [1986]. *Language intervention with young children* [p. 110]. San Diego, CA: College-Hill.)

the target and generalization goals shows a significant increase over the baseline, whereas use of the control goal remains unchanged, then we have demonstrated that our intervention was what made the difference in the client's use of the target form. If we graphed the data from such a study, it could resemble the graph displayed in Figure 3-9. We might then choose to go on and target the control goal for intervention as well.

Finally, we need to remember that meeting goals in a structured setting is not our ultimate aim. Our real objective is improved functional communication, what Kovarsky, Culatta, Franklin, and Theodore (2001) called "communicative participation." Before deciding that a goal has been reached, we need to demonstrate that the goal has been incorporated into the child's functional communicative repertoire. ASHA has developed functional communication measures for children, which are listed in Appendix 3-1. Jacoby, Lee, Kummer, Levin, and Creaghead (2002) showed that it was possible to document improvement in intervention using these FCMs, such that a majority of children (76.5%) improved by at least one FCM level following 20 hours or more of therapy. So we can identify a child's pretreatment FCM and use this as a baseline for determining whether and to what extent functional changes have occurred in children's communication following intervention. To determine these kinds of functional changes, Olswang, Coggins, and Timler (2001) suggested that communicative behaviors be assessed in a core set of salient contexts. These contexts include role-playing tasks, narrative tasks, structured peer interactions, and natural observation in real settings. Although we may not always sample every goal in

every one of these contexts to establish its level of functional use, we do need to demonstrate that each communicative behavior we teach has become functional for the child in real social situations before claiming "effectiveness." Table 3-4 provides some examples of Olswang et al.'s advice.

DETERMINING RESPONSIVENESS TO INTERVENTION

One additional concept that has recently become of interest in the evaluation of treatment outcomes is the idea of measuring responsiveness to intervention (RTI) as an assessment technique. Graner, Faggella-Luby, and Fritschmann (2005) discussed this concept as an emerging method of determining whether children qualify for special educational services. RTI approaches are designed to overcome the problem of identifying children with language and learning disorders based on a discrepancy, for example, between verbal and nonverbal test scores. We've already discussed the issues with this kind of identification for children with language disorders in Chapter 1, and the same problem occurs in identifying school children with learning disabilities (Graner et al., 2005), as well as preschoolers at risk for reading failure (Justice, 2005). In addition, children from poor and minority backgrounds often under-achieve in school and are frequently placed inappropriately in special education (Moore-Brown, Montgomery, Bielinski, & Shubin, 2005). RTI provides one possible solution to these problems. Using RTI, children are exposed to a series of levels of instruction, which Troia (2005) and Ehren and Nelson (2005) defined as follows:

Tier I: classroom instruction for all children that is evidence-based, with frequent progress monitoring implemented by classroom teachers with adaptations provided by the SLP for children at risk. Progress is monitored by regular in-class evaluation. Children who show difficulties in learning at this level are given Tier II instruction.

Tier II: targeted, short-term research-based instruction designed to address weaknesses in children who struggle with language and literacy, as identified through progress monitoring; this intervention supplements regular instruction, is delivered in small groups by paraprofessionals or volunteers in consultation with the SLP and special educators; monitoring continues. Children who continue to struggle with language and learning at this level are given Tier III instruction.

Tier III: students who continue to struggle in Tier II instruction are considered in need of intensive, therapeutic intervention; SLP collaborates to determine this eligibility by evaluating response to Tier I and II instruction, and provides specialized language and literacy intervention in collaboration with others using an individualized instructional plan once identification of special educational need is made.

The SLP has several roles to play in the RTI process. SLPs can consult with teachers and educate staff about how language influences all aspects of school performance, the identification of evidence-based practices in reading, writing, and spelling

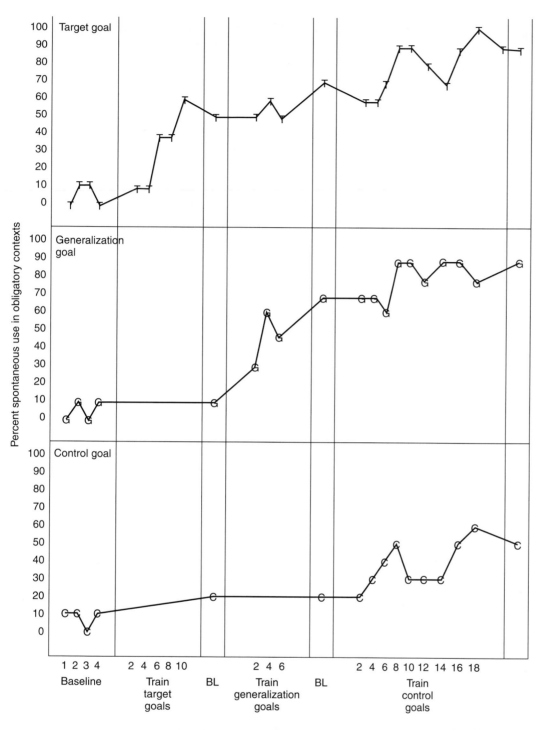

FIGURE 3-9 ✦ Multiple-baseline study data. (Reprinted with permission from Fey, M. [1986]. *Language intervention with young children* [p. 110]. San Diego, CA: College-Hill.)

instruction, and the need for language-facilitating approaches in all areas of the curriculum. For Tier II instruction, SLPs can help to select or design the procedures to be implemented in small group instruction, such as the provision of phonological awareness training for young children or the use of morphological and "word study" approaches to spelling for older children (see Chapters 9, 12, and 14), and can train paraprofessionals and volunteers to deliver them. SLPs may provide, or collaborate in providing, Tier III instruction for children identified through the RTI process as having special educational needs. But perhaps the most important role that SLPs play in this process is through our knowledge and experience in evaluating treatment outcomes, since ongoing monitoring is a central element of RTI. Just as we've talked about evaluating the outcomes of our own intervention, we can use the same techniques—including determining termination or outcome criteria, tracking individual behaviors, developing nonstandard assessments including functional, dynamic, and curriculum-based methods, and using single subject design procedures—to determine whether the Tier I and II instruction has accomplished its goals. In this way, our expertise not only in language and literacy, but in evaluation methods can

TABLE 3-4	Tasks for Documenting Functional Use of Communicative Goal Behaviors	

CONTEXTS	EXAMPLE GOAL	EXAMPLE ACTIVITY
Role-playing	Negative sentence forms	"Let's imagine you're shopping for a pair of shoes, and the clerk is trying to sell you a pair you don't like. I'm the clerk. Act out what you would say to tell him why you don't want these shoes."
Narrative	Use of articles (*a, an, the*)	"Tell me about your class trip to the fast food restaurant. Tell me about the equipment you saw that they use when they make food there."
Structured peer interaction	Use of polite forms	"I'm going to give you and Aisha some toys to play with. Some are for you and some are for Aisha. If you want to use each other's toys, you have to ask nicely."
Natural setting observation	Use of quantity terms (*more, less, all,* etc.)	Observe student during math lesson in which teacher gives instructions using quantity terms ("What's one more than two?")

Adapted from Olswang, L., Coggins, T., & Timler, G. (2001). Outcome measures for school-age children with social communication problems. *Topics in Language Disorders, 22(1)*, 50-73.

contribute to the team's ability to use RTI to identify children at risk and work toward preventing school failure.

You might be feeling that, with all the thought and work involved in planning an intervention program, maybe trying to evaluate it, too, is just too much to expect. While I can understand that feeling, I must caution against giving in to it. The respect that we can command as professionals and as a profession rests to a large degree on our ability to prove that we make a difference. Because we don't usually cure our clients, but rather facilitate their language development, the fruits of our labor are not always easy to see. The client's continuing deficits may overshadow them, or they may not seem very different from maturational change. Because our results can sometimes seem invisible and because it really is important to document that we are making ethical use of time and resources, it is incumbent upon our profession to fulfill our obligation to be accountable. Only by doing so can we earn the respect we deserve and be in a strong position to advocate for the importance of the services we provide to our clients.

PREVENTION OF LANGUAGE DISORDERS IN CHILDREN

We've talked for a long while now about ways to change communication disorders. But any humane and responsible person would like to work toward preventing the devastating effects of these disorders by eliminating their root causes and thereby inhibiting the disorders from ever occurring. Why should prevention be our concern? Are we not language *pathologists*, people who diagnose and treat disorders of language learning? Isn't remediation our business? Certainly it is. In all areas of health care, though, including our own (ASHA, 2004d; Marge, 1993), there is a national trend away from exclusive attention to rehabilitation and toward prevention efforts. This trend arises partly from our knowledge of the enormous cost of rehabilitation and the burden it places on all levels of the economy. In 1984, the American Speech-Language and Hearing Association (ASHA) estimated that preventing even one case of mental retardation can result in long-term savings of more than $1 million, and that figure would be even higher today. The U.S. Public Health Service (PHS), in its *Healthy People 2010: National Health Promotion and Disease Prevention Objectives* (Department of Health and Human Services, 2005; http://www.cdc.gov/ncbddd/dh/hp2010.htm), has established national goals for improving health, reducing risk factors, providing screening and early identification resources, and increasing public awareness and information about health and the prevention of disease; disability is one of their focus areas. ASHA has worked with the PHS to develop objectives for reducing the incidence of communication disorders. As responsible health professionals, we have an obligation to contribute to these efforts.

There is another reason, too, why SLPs would be concerned about preventing communication disorders. As the professionals who deal day to day with these problems, we know the suffering they bring to our clients and their families. We know how a parent of a preschooler with little speech feels when she sees her child made fun of or left out by other children because the child cannot talk. We know how a language-impaired fourth grader who has trouble understanding the teacher feels when he fails yet another spelling test, even after he studied hard for it. We know how a teenager with a language-learning disability feels when he can't get a date for a school dance because his pragmatic skills are so poor. We know how a high-functioning adolescent with autism feels when he sees his classmates "rapping" and using slang that he cannot master or understand and when they giggle at his attempts to join them. We know because we try every day to help our clients overcome these problems. But how much better it would be, from a purely human standpoint, if they never happened in the first place! Although our job is the remediation of language disorders, our concern is for the welfare of our children and their families. It is this concern and our knowledge of the central role of communication in human development that urges us to work toward not only treating but also preventing disorders of language learning. This has, in fact, happened in some cases. The last major epidemic of rubella was in 1965. Since the introduction of inoculation against this disease, new cases of profound hearing impairment caused by rubella are very rare, despite the fact that rubella was one of the most common causes of acquired deafness in children before the availability of the vaccine. But this ideal situation, in which we eliminate the cause of a disorder, is not always achievable. Sometimes prevention has to occur in a more modest way. Epidemiologists look at prevention as happening at three levels. Definitions of each of these levels of prevention, as discussed by the Committee on Prevention of Speech, Language, and Hearing Problems of the American Speech-Language-Hearing Association (ASHA, 1991, 2004d), are found in Table 3-5.

PRIMARY PREVENTION AND THE SPEECH-LANGUAGE PATHOLOGIST

ASHA (2005d) and Marge (1993) identified several primary prevention strategies that can be applied to disabilities that lead to communicative disorders. They include proper health and medical care, including immunizations and prenatal care; public education; genetic counseling; mass screening and early identification; environmental quality control; governmental action; and the elimination of poverty. Donahue-Kilburg (1993) argued that wellness promotion is another primary prevention tactic in which SLPs can engage. This approach involves optimizing psychological, physical, and behavioral well-being to increase resistance to disease or disorder. Donahue-Kilburg suggested that family-centered early intervention programs are ideal settings in which to promote wellness as a means of preventing communication disorders. Wellness promotion in these settings might involve encouraging good maternal nutrition and prenatal care to promote optimal fetal growth, helping parents of premature babies to become aware of infant states and receptive capacities so that they can maximize interaction, and working to help pregnant women avoid drug and alcohol use during pregnancy. Table 3-6 lists some suggestions

for primary prevention activities that SLPs employed in a variety of settings can initiate. "May Is Better Hearing and Speech Month," sponsored by ASHA, is always a good opportunity to introduce efforts like these.

When primary prevention is accomplished, the incidence of a disorder is reduced. *Incidence* is defined as "the rate of new occurrences of a condition in a population free of the disorder within a specified time period" (ASHA, 2005d). In other words, incidence refers to the number of new cases of a disorder that appear. For example, Down syndrome has an incidence of 1 in every 800 live births. This means that for every 800 babies born, 1, on average, has Down syndrome. This one baby out of 800 who is born with Down syndrome contributes to the total number of individuals in the population who have this condition. Epidemiologists have another term for this total: prevalence. *Prevalence* is defined as "the total rate or proportion of cases in a population at, or during, a specified period of time" (ASHA, 2005d). For example, the prevalence of learning disabilities is thought to be 5% to 10% of school-aged children. This means that at any given time, about 10% of a population of school-aged children will be affected by this disorder. Primary prevention is aimed at reducing the incidence, and thereby decreasing the prevalence, of disorders.

THE SPEECH-LANGUAGE PATHOLOGIST'S ROLE IN SECONDARY AND TERTIARY PREVENTION

Unfortunately we will never be able to prevent all disorders. In some cases, such as specific language disorders, we do not know the cause and so cannot ward off its effect. In other cases, in this imperfect world, primary prevention efforts will fall short of their goals. When this happens, we must fall back on secondary and tertiary prevention to minimize handicapping effects. SLPs can and should be active participants in early identification and treatment efforts, as well as in research programs to identify risk factors and preventive intervention methods. The advent of mandatory newborn hearing screening, as well as preschool and kindergarten speech/language screening programs are good examples of secondary prevention.

TABLE 3-5	**Levels of Prevention as Defined by ASHA**	
LEVEL	**DESCRIPTION**	**EXAMPLE**
Primary prevention	The elimination or inhibition of the onset and development of a disorder by altering susceptibility or reducing exposure for susceptible persons.	Inoculation to prevent rubella.
Secondary prevention	Early detection and treatment are used to eliminate the disorder or retard its progress, thereby preventing further complications.	Newborn hearing screening to detect hearing loss and provide early amplification or cochlear implantation.
Tertiary prevention	Intervention is used to reduce a disability by attempting to restore effective functioning.	Providing rehabilitation and special educational services to a child with Down syndrome.

Reprinted with permission from American Speech-Language-Hearing Association Committee on Prevention of Speech, Language, and Hearing Problems. (1991). The prevention of communication disorders tutorial. *American Speech-Language-Hearing Association*, 33(9, suppl. 6).

TABLE 3-6	Primary Prevention Activities in Various Employment Settings

SETTING	SUGGESTED ACTIVITY
Preschool or early intervention program	Work with health officials to set up a low-cost on-site inoculation clinic. Set up a "parenting" class to help parents deal with issues of discipline and prevent child abuse. Provide contraceptive and family-planning services to teens who have had one child, to prevent a subsequent pregnancy before the mother finishes school. Display posters, hold short education sessions to discuss dangers to fetuses of drugs, alcohol, and smoking for mothers who may become or are already pregnant again. Make arrangements with local health-care agencies to refer mothers for free or low-cost prenatal care if they become pregnant again. Set up a "health education" class, using a curriculum such as "Smooth Sailing into Next Generation" (Plumridge & Hylton, 1987) to educate parents about family planning and preventing birth defects in future children.
Elementary school	Work with health officials to set up a low-cost on-site inoculation clinic. Set up a "parenting" class to help parents deal with issues of discipline and prevent child abuse. Make arrangements with local health care agencies to refer mothers for free or low-cost prenatal care if they become pregnant again. Set up assembly programs with local police agencies to talk to students about seat-belt and helmet use. Send home a calendar on which each student is to mark the days on which everyone in the family used a seat belt in the car or on which every child in the family wore a bike helmet. Students who achieve a given number of days of use win a prize or have names posted on a bulletin board. Collaborate with drug and alcohol education programs by "guest lecturing" to students about the dangers these substances pose. Hold an essay or drawing contest, "How I Will Get My Family to Use Seat Belts and Helmets." Display winning entries in the school newspaper with an interview with winners about how they convinced others to take these precautions.
Middle and high school	Hold an essay contest on "How I Will Get My Family to Use Seat Belts and Helmets." Display winning entries in the school newspaper with an interview with winners about how they convinced others to take these precautions. Set up assembly programs with local police agencies to talk to students about seat belt and helmet use. Collaborate with drug and alcohol education programs by "guest lecturing" to students about the dangers these substances pose for unborn children. Work with health teachers to initiate a curriculum module such as "Smooth Sailing into Next Generation" (Plumridge & Hylton, 1987), to educate students about family planning, contraception, avoiding early sexual activity, and preventing birth defects in future children. Work with health teachers to initiate a curriculum module on parenting, discipline, and preventing child abuse. Set up a language stimulation class for teen mothers to help them learn techniques for encouraging language development.
Hospital or clinic	Arrange with obstetrics section for low-cost prenatal care for mothers of children on caseload, if they should become pregnant again. Develop referral network for getting families in touch with parenting classes, family-planning programs. Work with health educator and public relations office to offer classes in language development and preventing birth defects to families in the community. Encourage agency to mount public information campaigns to address drug abuse, child abuse, and seat-belt use.
Private practice	Offer parenting classes as part of your practice; include family planning and prevention of birth defects, using a curriculum such as "Smooth Sailing into the Next Generation" (Plumridge & Hylton, 1987), as well as methods of discipline and language stimulation techniques. Work with local pediatric practices to provide inoculations for clients who are lacking them. Offer to contract with local high schools to work with teen parents on a language-stimulation module within an existing parenting class, or on preventing pregnancy and birth defects in an existing health class. Offer low-cost speech and hearing screenings at community events that focus on children, such as toy "expos," etc. Involve practice in local public education campaigns regarding drug abuse, child abuse, seatbelt and helmet use, and similar issues.

Then, too, old-fashioned tertiary prevention, or rehabilitation, will always be needed. Some children will "fall through the cracks" of even the most aggressive screening program and will turn up with problems in communication that need to be addressed by attempting to reduce the already-present disability. Some will need ongoing support as their disability persists throughout development. But this traditional role of the SLP, regardless of its clear importance and centrality to our mission, is no longer sufficient. To be the kind of professionals we all strive to be, who serve not only our individual clients but their families and communities, we need to expand our conception of what being an SLP means. It means not only picking up the pieces after disabilities strike but also working toward preventing them.

■ CONCLUSIONS

Planning and evaluating language intervention requires us to make a series of decisions. We need to decide on the overall purpose of the program, the specific long-term and short-term goals, the procedures we will use to achieve these goals, the evidence available to support the use of these procedures, the context in which the intervention will take place, and how we will demonstrate that we have made a real difference in the client's communication. What I have tried to do in this chapter is give you a broad overview of the range of options we have for making these decisions. I have tried to suggest that as clinicians we do not need to pick just one approach, orientation, or style of intervention. We do not have to identify ourselves as behaviorists, milieu therapists, or pragmaticists; or as classroom teachers, consultants, or parent trainers. What we can strive for, instead, is access to the fullest possible set of tools for improving communication. We can then choose the right tool for the job of improving the communication skills of each individual client in our charge. We can work, too, toward preventing communication disorders by engaging in activities to promote communicative wellness and community education. We who know the high cost of these disorders, in both fiscal and human terms, should be among those most motivated to work for their prevention.

STUDY GUIDE

I. The Purpose of Intervention
   A. What are the three basic purposes of intervention? Give an example of a client for whom each would be used.
   B. What are three ways that intervention can change language behavior?

II. Developing Intervention Plans
   A. Discuss the difference between short- and long-term goals.
   B. Define and give examples of the *zone of proximal development*.
   C. What criteria are used to decide which goals identified in the assessment will be targeted in the intervention program?
   D. Name the three basic approaches to intervention discussed in this chapter. Give an example activity for teaching "is (verb)ing" as it might be done in each approach.
   E. Why is it suggested that intervention focus on selecting production as a target response rather than comprehension?
   F. Discuss the role of perceptual salience and pragmatic appropriateness in determining the linguistic stimuli to be used in intervention.
   G. What is meant by the *continuum of naturalness* in intervention? Give examples of three activities and settings at different points along this continuum.
   H. Discuss the considerations involved in determining the modality of language for the client to use.
   I. Describe and give examples of both extrinsic and intrinsic reinforcement.
   J. Describe five activities for promoting generalization of plural forms.
   K. Discuss the uses of computers in language intervention.
   L. Name and define the four models of contexts for language intervention. Give situations in which each one would be the best choice for teaching use of the conjunctions "because," "unless," and "although."
   M. Discuss the criteria you would use for evaluating a new technique to decide whether it is evidence-based.

III. Evaluating Intervention Outcomes
   A. Define *termination criteria*, and discuss the guidelines suggested in the text.
   B. Describe how to implement a multiple-baseline study of language intervention.
   C. Why is it important to evaluate the effectiveness of intervention?
   D. How can functional use of communication be evaluated?

IV. Prevention of Language Disorders in Children
   A. Define and discuss levels of prevention identified by ASHA.
   B. Compare and contrast the meaning of the terms *incidence* and *prevalence*.
   C. What kinds of primary prevention efforts are appropriate for SLPs?
   D. What is the role of the SLP in secondary prevention of communicative disorders?

FUNCTIONAL COMMUNICATION MEASURES FOR CHILD LANGUAGE

Spoken Language Production

Level 1: Child attempts to communicate, but attempts are not meaningful to familiar or unfamiliar individuals at any time.

Level 2: Child attempts to communicate, but even with consistent maximal cuing, child rarely produces meaningful communication with familiar people in routine situations.

Level 3: With moderate cueing the child usually produces meaningful communication in routine events of daily living with persons familiar to the child. This communication is much simpler than expected for chronological age.

Level 4: With minimal cues, child can communicate in routine events of daily living. When moderate cues are given, child occasionally communicates in familiar and novel settings, using simpler sentences than are appropriate for his chronological age.

Level 5: With minimal cues, child usually communicates in familiar and novel settings, using simpler sentences than are appropriate for his chronological age. With maximal cueing, child occasionally uses age-appropriate sentences in familiar settings.

Level 6: Child usually communicates using age-appropriate sentences in most adult-child, peer, and directed group activities but some limitations are still apparent. Minimal cueing is occasionally required from the communication partner.

Level 7: Child's ability to participate in adult-child, peer, and directed group activities is not limited by language production. Cueing is rarely required.

Spoken Language Comprehension

Level 1: Child understands a limited number of common object and action labels and simple directions only in highly structured, repetitive daily routines, with consistent maximal cueing.

Level 2: Child understands a limited number of common objects and action labels and simple directions only in highly structured repetitive daily routines.

Level 3: Child understands a limited number of common objects and action labels and simple directions in novel situations.

Level 4: Child understands simple word combinations/sentences. Child usually requires rephrasing and repetition to ensure understanding of brief conversations.

Level 5: Child understands brief conversations. Child usually requires rephrasing and repetition to ensure understanding of the type and length of sentence typically understood by chronologically age-matched peers.

Level 6: Child understands communication of the type and length typically understood by chronologically age-matched peers but occasionally requires rephrasing and repetition. Child's ability to participate in adult-child, peer, and group activities is sometimes limited by language comprehension.

Level 7: Child's ability to participate in adult-child, peer, and group activities is not limited by language comprehension. Repetition and rephrasing are rarely required.

Adapted from American Speech-Language-Hearing Association (1999). *National outcomes measurement system (NOMS): Pre-kindergarten speech-language pathology training manual.* Rockville, MD: Author; Jacoby, G., Lee, L., Kummer, A., Levin, L, & Creaghead, N. (2002). The number of individual treatment units necessary to facilitate functional communication improvements in the speech and language of young children. *American Journal of Speech-Language Pathology, 11,* 370-380.

SPECIAL CONSIDERATIONS FOR SPECIAL POPULATIONS

CHAPTER OBJECTIVES

Readers of this chapter will be able to do the following:
- Discuss the role of a developmental-descriptive approach to language disorders in understanding these disorders as they appear in a range of conditions.
- Describe the way in which several syndromes of mental retardation, as well as nonspecific retardation, affect communication development.
- Discuss language disorders associated with sensory deficits.

- Describe the effects of abuse, neglect, and maternal substance abuse on language development.
- Discuss the interactions of social, emotional, and language development.
- Outline the communicative characteristics and needs seen in autism spectrum disorders.
- Describe the effects of acquired disorders on communicative function.
- Discuss several syndromes of specific speech and language disorders.

According to the descriptive-developmental model of language disorders advocated in this book, it is more important in clinical practice to describe the nature of a child's language disorder than to identify its cause or associate it with an etiological category. We talked earlier about how the diagnostic category that a child is placed in may not always either explain or predict language behavior. We discussed some examples of children in the same diagnostic group who had very different types of language problems. We also talked about the fact that children often don't fit neatly into one diagnostic classification. Children with mental retardation (MR) also can have autism spectrum disorders (ASD), for example. So it seems difficult to establish just one cause for a language disorder when more than one categorical label is appropriate. Finally, we've said that knowing a child's diagnostic label often doesn't precisely indicate the child's needs in terms of assessment or intervention. Knowing that a nonverbal child has ASD, for example, does not automatically prescribe the program. Should he or she be given intervention in the speech modality, or should an alternative modality such as Sign language be introduced? This decision is not very different from the decision that must be made in the case of a non-speaking child who has a hearing impairment or MR.

Is there any other reason, then, to include etiological categories in the clinical decision-making process, given our descriptive-developmental orientation? Although etiological category may not be the primary determiner of clinical decisions about children with language disorders, knowledge of etiological categories associated with language disorders can come in handy in several ways. First, as we discussed in Chapter 1, the assignment of a child to one of these categories is often needed to qualify a child for special services, especially at school age. The speech-language pathologist (SLP) is not necessarily the person who diagnoses these etiological conditions. Usually a medical professional or psychologist is required at least to consult in the diagnosis, and information from several sources must often be gathered before the diagnosis can be made. In the case of MR, for example, both IQ and adaptive behavior must be significantly below the normal range for the diagnosis to be conferred. Accordingly, professionals who evaluate both these aspects of development need to be involved in the diagnostic process. Although the SLP does not make the diagnosis, we are often asked to supply information that leads to it. In the case of a child with ASD, for example, the SLP may be required to document the social communication difficulties the child displays, which are part of the core symptoms of these conditions. To fulfill this role, it is important to know the standard definitions of each etiological category. These definitions are discussed in this chapter.

Second, although the etiological classification associated with a language disorder does not dictate the assessment and intervention strategies appropriate for each child, knowing the classification often provides hints about what areas to look at in the assessment or what areas might receive priority in intervention. For example, if we know that a child has ASD, we can make an informed guess that pragmatic aspects of language will be impaired, among other things. This could suggest that we include a detailed pragmatic evaluation procedure in the assessment. It also might lead us to be especially careful to provide pragmatic contexts in the intervention. That's because knowing a child has ASD implies, as we'll see, that he or she will not spontaneously generalize language learned to appropriate use in context. Again, decisions of this sort are not unique to this population. But knowing something about the typical characteristics of a diagnostic category can be helpful when making some preliminary decisions about practice with a particular child, as long as we remember that these decisions must be tentative, to be borne out by the careful observation and description of the language the child exhibits. Remember, too, that although characteristics may be *typical* of a particular diagnostic category, they are neither inevitable nor universal and cannot be assumed to exist on the basis of diagnostic category alone. Not all children with ASD echo, for example, although echolalia is a typical symptom in this disorder. The diagnostic classification can, as we've said, provide *hints* about assessment and intervention. These hints must be followed up, though, by a detailed description of the individual's actual language performance.

Third, the clinical reports and medical histories of clients often contain information about these diagnostic categories. To read these documents intelligently, we need to understand what the labels mean. Let's look at some of the major categories of disorders often associated with language-learning problems, outline standard definitions of each of these conditions, then talk about typical (not universal) characteristics of each and the hints they might provide for clinical practice in language pathology.

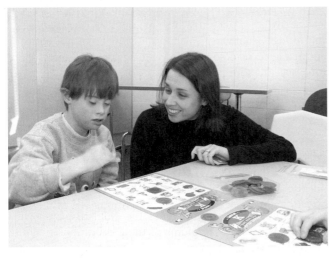

Language disorders can be associated with a variety of congenital conditions.

MENTAL RETARDATION

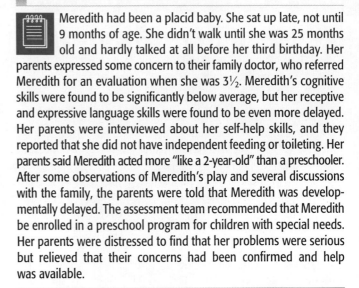

Meredith had been a placid baby. She sat up late, not until 9 months of age. She didn't walk until she was 25 months old and hardly talked at all before her third birthday. Her parents expressed some concern to their family doctor, who referred Meredith for an evaluation when she was 3½. Meredith's cognitive skills were found to be significantly below average, but her receptive and expressive language skills were found to be even more delayed. Her parents were interviewed about her self-help skills, and they reported that she did not have independent feeding or toileting. Her parents said Meredith acted more "like a 2-year-old" than a preschooler. After some observations of Meredith's play and several discussions with the family, the parents were told that Meredith was developmentally delayed. The assessment team recommended that Meredith be enrolled in a preschool program for children with special needs. Her parents were distressed to find that her problems were serious but relieved that their concerns had been confirmed and help was available.

Meredith is just one example of the kind of child who can receive the diagnosis of *mental retardation (MR)* and has just one of several possible types of communicative disorders associated with her condition. In Meredith's case, as in a significant proportion of cases of children with MR, the cause of the retardation is unknown. The diagnosis of MR is based on behavioral, not medical, characteristics, and the diagnosis can be conferred regardless of whether the etiology of MR for a particular child is known. Let's look at the standard definition of MR and its various levels. Then we'll discuss some of the typical (not universal, remember) relations we may see between language disorders and retardation in general. Finally, we'll talk about language characteristics associated with some specific syndromes of MR.

DEFINITION AND CLASSIFICATION IN MENTAL RETARDATION

The American Association on Mental Retardation (AAMR; Luckasson, Borthwick-Duffy, Buntinx, Coulter, Craig, Reeve, Schalock, Snell, Spitalnik, Spreat, & Tasse, 2002) provides the following definition of MR:

> Mental retardation is a disability characterized by significant limitations both in intellectual functioning and in adaptive behavior as expressed in conceptual, social, and practical adaptive skills. This disability originates before age 18.

In addition, AAMR's (2002) definition makes the following assumptions:

> Limitations in present functioning must be considered within the context of community environments typical of the individual's age peers and culture.

> Valid assessment considers cultural and linguistic diversity as well as differences in communication, sensory, motor, and behavioral factors.

Within an individual, limitations often coexist with strengths.

An important purpose of describing limitations is to develop a profile of needed supports.

With appropriate personalized supports over a sustained period, the life functioning of the person with mental retardation generally will improve.

This definition emphasizes the role of adaptive skills both in the definition of retardation and in the ability of the individual to achieve optimal functioning. "Significant limitations in intellectual functioning" is defined as an IQ of approximately 70 to 75 or less, based on assessment that includes an individually administered standardized test developed to assess intellectual function. This range of scores translates to a criterion of at least 2 (or so) standard deviations (SDs) below the mean; that is, below the second percentile on a well-standardized IQ test. Fewer than 2% of a normally distributed population will score more than 2 SDs below the mean (see Fig. 2-11). You'll note that the IQ criterion is not absolute, though. This definition has some "wiggle room" that allows a person to receive a diagnosis of MR, even when IQ is slightly more than 70, *if there are related, significant limitations in adaptive skills.*

The definition also holds that an individual must show significant deficits in adaptive behavior *relative to his or her own cultural group.* This criterion is necessary because people from non-mainstream backgrounds may have different expectations of individuals at different ages. In our culture, we expect children to be able to separate from their mothers easily at age 5 to attend school, for example; other cultures tolerate much longer-term dependency on mothers. Too many children have in the past been placed in classes for the retarded because their experiences were different from those of middle-class children, which resulted in their scoring low on IQ tests that contained culturally biased items. Similarly, it is important to rule out linguistic differences as a source of "failure to adapt." In the "old days," it sometimes happened that children were labeled retarded simply because they did not speak English and could not respond to testing or questions in the school language. The emphasis on an adaptive behavior standard is a safeguard against such misdiagnoses.

Although adaptive behavior is often evaluated subjectively, standardized measures exist for various aspects of adaptive performance. Some examples include the *Adaptive Behavior Assessment System—2nd Edition* (Harrison & Oakland, 2003), the *Comprehensive Test of Adaptive Behavior* (Adams, 1984), the *Scales of Independent Behavior* (Bruininks, Woodcock, Weatherman, & Hill, 1996), and the *Vineland Adaptive Behavior Scales—II (VABS)* (Sparrow, Cicchetti, & Balla, 2005). Ecological inventories and environmental assessments (see Chapter 8) also can be used to assess various aspects of adaptive performance.

The definition of MR also includes the requirement that onset occur before 18 years of age, or during the developmental period. This criterion is used to differentiate MR, which is considered a *developmental disorder,* from forms of dementia that result in mental deterioration during adulthood. Of course, there can be muddy cases. Suppose an apparently normal child is in a serious accident at age 10 that results in brain damage so that the child scores within the retarded range afterward. By the AAMR definition, this child would be considered to have MR, although the onset is clearly traumatic rather than developmental. Still, the child would probably benefit from intervention that is in some ways similar to that we would design for a child who had MR from birth, so perhaps the fence-straddling nature of these cases is not of such great consequence. Again, for the purposes of clinical practice, we will always look at the child, not the name of the disorder, to determine our program.

Before the current AAMR definition, the degree of MR an individual displayed was described according to four levels of severity, which were defined in terms of the number of SDs below the mean that an individual's score on an IQ test fell. Table 4-1 gives an overview of these levels as they have traditionally been defined. The newer definition, however, focuses on an individual's adaptive strengths and weaknesses and on the level of intensity of support needed to maximize the person's ability to function in daily life. In this system, diagnosis is a three-step process:

Step 1. Use the definition (previously described) to determine whether a person is eligible for supports because of a diagnosis of mental retardation (Intellectual Functioning and Adaptive Skills criteria).

Step 2. Identify strengths and weaknesses and areas of need for supports (Psychological/Emotional considerations, Physical/Health/Etiological considerations, Environmental considerations); identify optimal environments that will facilitate the individual's continued growth and development.

Step 3. Identify level of support and specific types of supports needed to maximize performance in each of the four areas considered (Intellectual Functioning and Adaptive Skills, Psychological/Emotional, Physical/Health/Etiological, Environmental). Levels of support are as follows:

Intermittent: "As needed;" supports are episodic or short term; may be needed during transitions such as school-to-work or a job loss; intermittent supports may be of high or low intensity when given

Limited: May be consistent over time, or time limited, but not intermittent; require fewer staff and less cost than higher levels of support

Extensive: Regular (e.g., daily) involvement in at least some of the client's living environments (e.g., employment, residential), long term, not time limited

Pervasive: Constant, high-intensity support provided in all environments; potentially life sustaining

The AAMR has developed an instrument, the *Supports Intensity Scale* (Thompson, Bryant, Campbell, Craig, Hughes, Rotholz, Schalock, Silverman, Tassé, & Wehmeyer, 2005), to assist in identifying supports for these clients.

Many children identified with MR today may carry a diagnosis of a specific syndrome of retardation, some of which will be discussed later in this section. For some children with MR,

TABLE 4-1	Levels of Retardation as Defined before 1992			
LEVEL	PERCENT OF PEOPLE WITH MR IN THIS CATEGORY	STANDARD IQ SCORE RANGE	STANDARD DEVIATION RANGE ON AN IQ TEST	SUPPORTS NEEDED
Mild ("educable")	89	55–69	−2 to −3	May require some special education, can function in mainstream classrooms with support. May eventually achieve up to early secondary school level. As adults, many are capable of holding jobs and living independently, although they may need some supervision and support.
Moderate ("trainable")	6	40–54	−3 to −4	Usually require special education, but can develop academic skills commensurate with intermediate elementary grades. In adulthood, can work independently at unskilled or semiskilled occupations, but often require some support and supervision in their living situation.
Severe	3.5	25–39	−4 to −5	With special education can develop self-care skills and improve their communicative abilities, but rarely attain functional literacy or computational skills.
Profound	1.5	<25	More than 5	With special education, some motor and communication skills (often through AAC) may be developed. Self-care skills, such as feeding and toileting, can be learned. Many have serious physical anomalies and neurological damage, and there is a high childhood mortality rate. As adults, need care and supervision and generally cannot live independently.

Adapted from Owens, R. (2004). Language impairments. In R. Owens (Ed.), *Language disorders* (ed. 4) (p. 23). Columbus, OH: Merrill/Macmillan.

however, no specific syndrome or cause can be identified; these children are said to have nonspecific MR (NSMR). We'll talk briefly about some of the general characteristics of children with NSMR before looking at several of the more well-known syndromes of retardation.

COGNITIVE CHARACTERISTICS AND NONSPECIFIC MENTAL RETARDATION

Owens (2004) discussed the cognitive skills of individuals with MR. He reported that in general, cognitive development is not tremendously dissimilar from that seen in normal children, although it is slower. Still, researchers have found cognitive differences in this population that cannot be entirely attributed to low IQ. Individuals with MR can attend to tasks as well as mental-age mates but have trouble directing their attention to the most relevant aspects of the situation without guidance. They have trouble with discrimination tasks, primarily because they attend to fewer dimensions of stimuli than they need to distinguish among them. Discrimination skills can be improved by direct instruction, though. People with MR have more problems in organization and recall than their mental age would predict, for the most part because they use fewer strategies spontaneously to aid storage and recall. Retrieval processes are slower in this population, and short-

term memory appears to be an area of weakness. Generalization is a particular difficulty for people with MR (Owens, Metz, & Haas, 2003). Cognitive skills do continue to grow through adulthood, though, and special educational services continue to be warranted to abet this growth (Edwards, 2002).

LANGUAGE DISORDERS AND NONSPECIFIC MENTAL RETARDATION

Limitation in communicative skill is often one of the first signs of MR. Weiss, Weisz, and Bromfield (1986) indicated that until a mental age of 10 years, children with MR follow a slowed-down sequence of language acquisition similar to that seen in normal development, except that sentences are somewhat shorter and less language is produced. For many children with MR, though, communicative skills are less mature than would be expected, based on their nonverbal mental age (Chapman, 2003; Owens, 2004), as seen in Meredith's case. Miller and Chapman (1984) reported that about half of individuals with various kinds of retardation have language skills commensurate with cognitive level. In the rest of the population with MR, two patterns of language disorder were identified: 25% diagnosed with MR had comprehension skills that were on par with mental age, but production skills were poorer; the other 25% had deficits in both production and comprehension relative to mental age, as Meredith did. Abbeduto and Boudreau (2004) report that this variation is often related to a particular cognitive skill, such as auditory memory. As we've discussed, simply knowing that a child has MR will not tell us which of these patterns of language skill the individual displays or what specific gaps occur within the receptive and expressive modalities. As usual, in-depth assessment and description of communicative skill are needed to answer these questions. Let's look at some of the typical findings of research on language skills in the general MR population. Remember, though, that not every individual with MR will follow these patterns, and we will look more specifically at several distinct syndromes of MR a bit later.

Syntax and Morphology

Children with MR display few differences in the sequence of learning grammatical rules when compared with mental-age mates, particularly when mean length of utterance (MLU) in morphemes is less than 3 (Abbeduto & Boudreau, 2004; Owens, 2004). When MLU is above this level, children with MR tend to use shorter, less-complex sentences with fewer elaborations and relative clauses than do their mental-age peers. Children with MR learn grammatical morphemes in about the same order as normally developing preschoolers. They do appear, though, to reach each MLU level at later mental ages than do children with normal development.

Phonology

Shriberg and Widder (1990) reported that articulation errors were more common in children with MR than in nonretarded children, and errors were likely to be inconsistent. They found consonant deletions to be the most common type of error. The phonological processes used by children with MR were similar to those used by young children with normal development, although children with MR used the processes more often and for a longer time period (Klink, Gerstman, Raphael, Schlanger, & Newsome, 1986; Moran, Money, & Leonard, 1983).

Semantics

Vocabulary appears to be learned more easily than syntax by children with MR, particularly children with Down syndrome (DS) (Layton, 2001). Children with MR produce utterances encoding semantic relations similar to those used by mental-age mates (Coggins, 1979; Kamhi & Johnston, 1982). Word meanings are more concrete and literal than those of typical peers (Semmel & Herzog, 1966). Adjectives and adverbs are used less frequently, whereas words with concrete meanings are used more often (Owens, 2004).

Pragmatics

As in the other areas of language development, the pattern of acquisition of pragmatic skills is similar between children with and without retardation, although Abbeduto and Boudreau (2004) report that children with MR sometimes have difficulty using language forms in the socially appropriate contexts. Communication development, like that of language forms, is closely tied to cognitive level in youngsters with and without

retardation (Owens, 2004). Mundy, Seibert, and Hogan (1985) pointed out that the cognitive deficits of children with MR, particularly in the first 2 years of life, may affect the quality of the prelinguistic input they receive. This may, in turn, influence their later communicative development. Still, children with retardation do use gestures to convey early communicative intentions in much the same way as children of similar mental ages (Owens, 2004). When word use begins, they show mental-age appropriate presuppositional skills (Leonard, Cole, & Steckol, 1979). In conversations they display turn-taking, topic maintenance, and speech act choice commensurate with mental age and can adjust their speech style, to some extent, to the needs of the listener (Guralnick & Paul-Brown, 1986; Hoy & McKnight, 1977). They do have difficulty with referential communication tasks and with seeking clarification in conversation (Owens, 2004). Mundy, Seibert, and Hogan (1985) also reported that children with MR do not use questions as efficiently as mental-age peers to gather new information. People with MR also tend to be less assertive in conversation (Bedrosian & Prutting, 1978). Boudreau and Chapman (2000) report that narrative production in children with MR is mental-age appropriate, but shows poorer use of linguistic cohesive devices.

Summary

The sequence of language acquisition in children with NSMR follows, in general, the sequence of normal acquisition, although some differences can be identified. More than one half of retarded individuals display less advanced language skills than would be expected for mental age. Productive deficits are common, with some children with NSMR showing deficits relative to mental age only in this area and others having both receptive and expressive limitations relative to mental age. Although we have talked about some "typical" patterns of language development in the MR population, these patterns do not tell us conclusively about the language of any individual child or what to do about it. A thorough description of each client's language performance is always necessary.

COMMON SYNDROMES OF MENTAL RETARDATION

Down Syndrome

Down syndrome (DS), named for the 19th-century English physician who first published a description of a group of clients with the syndrome, results most commonly from a chromosomal abnormality called trisomy 21, or an extra (third) copy of the 21st chromosome. Symptoms include mild to moderate MR; hypotonia (low muscle tone); a characteristic face with a shortening of the front-to-back dimension (brachycephaly); hyperflexibility of joints; heart and respiratory problems; ear anomalies; oral-motor difficulties; and deficits in speech, language, and hearing (Chapman & Hesketh, 2000). Articulation and intelligibility problems, as well as delayed language development, are almost universal in this population. Anomalies of the ear and upper respiratory tract lead to recurrent otitis media, which has effects on both speech and language development.

DS appears in about 1 of every 800 live births, making it the most common form of organic retardation. Its occurrence increases with advancing maternal age.

Because DS is a relatively common and diagnosable form of MR and because speech and language deficits are a prominent aspect of the syndrome, a great deal of research has been carried out on the communicative characteristics of this population. Layton (2001) reported that early linguistic environments appear to be facilitative for most children with DS and not a primary factor in causing their language delays. Mundy, Kasari, Sigman, and Ruskin (1995) found that preverbal requesting in young children with DS was disturbed and that this difference was associated with later expressive language development. They argue that some of the language problems seen in children in DS stem from these early deficits in nonverbal communication.

Layton (2001) also reported that symbolic play skills in children with DS are similar to those of mental-age–matched peers, although children with DS retain more immature behaviors in their play for longer periods. Casselli and Casadio (1995) found that children with DS produced a greater percentage of symbolic gestures than did typically developing children, suggesting a strength in gestural expression that can be built upon by using an augmentative and alternative communication (AAC) approach with these children. Layton (2001) reported that studies show the use of manual communication can facilitate early expression and support the development of spoken words in this population.

Although language development in DS follows the normal sequence in general, some specific asynchronies in acquisition among language domains have been found. Craniofacial anomalies associated with the syndrome have multiple effects on speech and hearing development. Because of the tendency to recurrent otitis media, Dahle and Baldwin (1992) recommend that children with DS be monitored continuously for middle-ear disease, even after early childhood, when the risk decreases for non-DS children. Layton (2001) reported that speech problems typically seen include a rough, breathy, and low-pitched voice and poor speech intelligibility. Unintelligibility is very common in this group (Abbeduto & Murphy, 2004), and includes a high incidence of speech-sound omissions and vowel distortions. Sound changes also are more inconsistent in DS than in other forms of retardation, even after intensive intervention. However, children with DS are more accurate in articulatory imitation tasks than in spontaneous production. These findings are thought to reflect a specific speech-motor control deficit. For this reason, intensive evaluation of oral-motor skills is especially important in this population. When the deficit is severe, an AAC method may be considered, and there is some evidence that strengthened gestural development facilitates the use of Sign or other visual AAC methods.

Lexical development in DS has been a topic of intense research interest recently. A large body of research, summarized by Rice, Warren, and Betz (2005), suggests that vocabulary is less impaired than grammar. Early vocabulary comprehension often lags behind cognitive development, but typically "catches up" to be on par with nonverbal cognitive ability. Children

with DS use words and multiword meanings very similar to those used by mental-age mates with typical development, though acquisition is at a slower pace. Semantic development is generally thought to be an area of strength in DS.

In terms of syntax, Layton (2001) reports that children with DS have been found to show production skills that lag behind comprehension, and this gap appears to increase with age. Even so, their scores on tests of syntactic comprehension are lower than those of other groups with MR (Abbetduto & Murphy, 2004). Syntactic skills also have been shown to be less advanced than cognitive and vocabulary abilities in children with DS, and these children show more expressive difficulties than children with other types of retardation. Rate of syntactic growth appears variable, with spurts of rapid acquisition and long plateaus not seen in typical development. Layton concludes that children with DS exhibit a specific deficit in language production, which is most pronounced in the area of morphosyntax and widens as the child gets older. Chapman, Seung, Schwartz, and Kay-Raining Bird (1998) found that children with DS omitted more grammatical function words and morphemes than did controls matched for mental age and that expressive vocabulary acquisition was more rapid than was syntax. They point out, however, that these deficits are not associated with a reduced amount of talk, and that although plateaus occur, they do not represent ceilings on development. Their research showed that even adolescents with DS can continue to show growth in sentence length and complexity and argue that this finding indicates a need for continued language intervention, even for adolescents with DS. Pragmatic skills have traditionally been thought to be a relative strength in DS, but more detailed studies (e.g., Abbeduto & Murphy, 2004) showed that although children with DS did have strengths in describing objects in a referential communication task, they had more difficulty in inferring others' informational state (theory of mind), and using linguistic markers to signal cohesion (Chapman & Hesketh, 2000).

A new area of research in DS concerns literacy development. Until recently, it has been thought that reading cannot be achieved until mental age reaches 6 years. Since many individuals with DS never reach this milestone, it was assumed that learning to read was not possible for them. However, in the past decade more literacy-related goals have become of interest for children with a variety of disabilities, and some studies of reading development in DS have appeared (e.g., Byrne, Buckley, MacDonald, & Bird, 1995; Fowler, Doherty, & Boynton, 1995). These studies report that children with DS appear to have reading levels in advance of their language and cognitive abilities. The studies of children with DS suggest that they approach reading with a different strategy than is typical in normal acquisition. They tend to rely more on whole word recognition, rather than phonological analysis. Regardless of the path they take to reading, these studies suggest that literacy is an appropriate and attainable goal for children with DS and should be part of the communication intervention program.

In summary, children with DS have physiological characteristics that can affect communication and need to be investi-

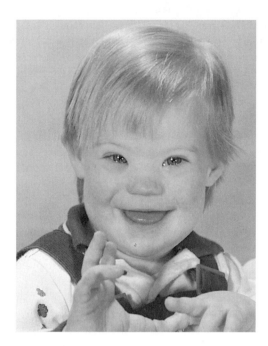

FIGURE 4-1 ✦ Children with Down syndrome have characteristic features. (Reprinted with permission from Zitelli, B.J., and Davis, H.W. [2002]. *Atlas of pediatric physical diagnosis* [ed. 4]. St. Louis, MO: Mosby.)

gated in any assessment process (Fig. 4-1). Their language development shows uneven patterns that make it impossible to generalize from one aspect of their communication to another. Each area will need to be evaluated carefully. These uneven patterns also give some hints about where intervention should be focused. Without intervention, for example, syntax is likely to develop more slowly than vocabulary size. This might suggest that syntactic goals receive priority in an intervention program for children with this disorder. The deficits found in prelinguistic communication emphasize the need for early intervention, whereas the slow rate of acquisition, coupled with the knowledge that development occurs even in adolescence, indicates a need for continued language intervention throughout the developmental period. Early communication appears to be fostered through the use of manual AAC. Once expressive communication has been established, literacy development should be targeted.

Fragile X Syndrome

It has been known since the 19th century that there are many more males with MR than females and that some families show an X-linked pattern of inheritance of MR. But it was not until 1969 that Lubs noticed that the X chromosomes cultured in the laboratory from retarded members of these families showed fragility, or breakages, under certain conditions. The gene associated with this fragility has been isolated (Brown, 2002), leading to the discovery of the source of the gene's instability: the size of a particular DNA fragment that acts as a "switch" controlling the gene. This fragment can exist in either a smaller "premutation" form, which can be passed on to future generations without

affecting its carrier, or in a larger "full mutation" form, which leads to expression of the fragile X syndrome. When the full mutation is present, the gene (known as *FMR1*, or *Fragile X Mental Retardation-1*) is shut off so that it no longer produces the specific protein it is intended to make. The gene appears to be involved in the maturation of synapses and the pruning of synaptic connections in the developing brain (Churchill, Beckel-Mitchener, Weiler, & Greenough, 2002).

Fragile X syndrome is second only to DS as a known genetic cause of MR. Since DS is not passed down from one generation to another, fragile X is considered the most common inherited form of MR. The syndrome is seen in about 1 in 4000 males and 1 in 8000 females (Abbeduto & Murphy, 2004). About half of these females with the full mutation have MR; the rest have learning disabilities. One in 250 females and 1 in 700 males are unaffected carriers for this condition (Dykens, Hodapp, & Leckman, 1994). Boys with fragile X syndrome are typically moderately retarded, with an IQ range similar to that seen in DS; IQ can range from low normal to the severely impaired range. These boys do not have clearly dysmorphic features and during early childhood are often difficult to identify, unlike children with DS, whose physical features mark them from birth. With increasing age, though, certain physical features tend to appear (Fig. 4-2). These include an elongated face, highly arched palate, larger-than-average head size, enlarged ears, flat feet, large hands with hyperextensible finger joints, hypotonia, and large testes in boys (macroorchidism) after age 8 (Hockey & Crowhurst, 1988). Increased frequency of strabismus and seizure disorders also has been noted.

The physical differences found in boys with fragile X have little direct effect on speech, although low muscle tone is thought to affect speech production and may lead to vulnerability to ear infections (Schopmeyer & Lowe, 1992). Otitis media is common in this population and may affect communicative development (Hagerman, Altshul-Stark, & McBogg, 1987).

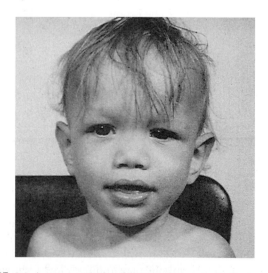

FIGURE 4-2 ✦ Boys with fragile X syndrome typically have long, narrow faces and large ears. (Reprinted with permission from Simko, A., Hornstein, L., Soukup, S., and Bagamery, N. [1989]. Fragile X syndrome: Recognition in young children. *Pediatrics* 83, 547-552.)

Again, aggressive monitoring for middle-ear disease is important for these children. Increased latencies of auditory brain stem response also have been reported in this population (Spiridigliozzi, Lachiewicz, Mirrett, & McConkie-Rosell, 2001).

Behavioral problems also are common. Hyperactivity, impulsivity, poor interactive skills, anxiety, social withdrawal, and short attention spans are more common in boys with fragile X than in other children with MR (Abbeduto & Murphy, 2004). About 16% of males with ASD also have been found to have fragile X, and 35% of boys with a primary diagnosis of fragile X exhibit some autistic behaviors, such as unusual hand movements and poor eye contact (Scharfenaker, 1990; Rice, Warren, & Betz, 2005). Sensorimotor disturbances—such as hypersensitivities, tactile defensiveness, and poor balance—as well as poor fine-motor skills are often seen (Spiridigliozzi, Lachiewicz, Mirrett, & McConkie-Rosell, 2001). Gross motor milestones, however, are within the normal range.

Boys with fragile X exhibit an uneven profile of cognitive skills. They do better on "gestalt" or "simultaneous processing" tasks, such as identifying a picture of an object with a part missing, than on "sequential processing" tasks, such as recalling a series of digits in correct order. Long-term memory appears to be a relative strength, as are visual memory skills (Merritt, Roberts, & Price, 2003). These allow boys with fragile X to learn to read and spell words by memorizing their visual configuration (Spiridigliozzi, Lachiewicz, Mirrett, & McConkie-Rosell, 2001). Imitation of both visual and verbal material also is a strength. This finding leads to the suggestion that good language and behavioral models, such as those found in mainstream classroom environments, are particularly important for boys with fragile X, in order to make use of their tendency to imitate what they see and hear and to prevent their propensity for imitating maladaptive behaviors.

Spiridigliozzi, Lachiewicz, Mirrett, and McConkie-Rosell (2001) described several weaknesses in the cognitive profiles of boys with fragile X. Abstract reasoning, problem-solving, and calculation appear to be problematic. Boys with fragile X also are reported to have trouble initiating and completing tasks, although they can be prompted to do so. Longitudinal studies suggest that IQ in this population declines over time, not because the boys lose skills but because their rate of development, relative to typical peers, slows down as they get older.

Communication problems are universally seen in boys with fragile X. In fact, language delays are often the first sign of difficulty in this population, so the SLP may be the first professional who encounters these children. SLPs who see young children with early language delays should consider fragile X as a possible explanation for some of these problems. Roberts, Mirrett, Anderson, Burchinall, and Neebe (2002) provided an outline of early communicative development in this syndrome. They found that boys with fragile X showed relative strengths in verbal and vocal production, with relative weaknesses in the use of gestures and symbolic play. Young children who present with this pattern, as well as the physical features just described, and/or a family history of learning disorders or MR, should be considered for referral for genetic testing.

Although a pattern of language characteristics has been associated with fragile X in boys, this pattern is by no means universal and many of the characteristics of the disorder are seen in children who do not have this syndrome. Communication skills are, to some extent, related to the degree of retardation, which varies widely in these boys. Boys with fragile X do, however, show a relative strength in verbal performance, relative to visual/spatial cognition (Rice, 2004). The "typical" pattern of language performance has been summarized by Spiridigliozzi, Lachiewicz, Mirrett, and McConkie-Rosell (2001). Early markers of the syndrome include oral hypotonicity and sensory defensiveness, poor sucking and chewing, and drooling. Delayed onset and development of expressive language is very characteristic, particularly in syntax, with receptive skills and vocabulary a relative strength (Rice, 2004). Speech is characterized by phonological errors similar to those used by young normal children; reduced intelligibility; a fast, uneven rate; poor juncture; and disturbed rhythm, with a hoarse and breathy vocal quality and uneven loudness (Rice, 2004; Scharfenaker, 1990). Some dyspraxic qualities, such as impaired planning, sequencing, and execution of fluent speech, as well as poor intelligibility, are present (Paul, Cohen, Brag, Watson, & Herman, 1984). Language sequencing and organization are often poor with a staccato-like rhythm, giving the speech a cluttered quality, with increasing impairment as sentences get longer (Hanson, Jackson, & Hagerman, 1986). Formulating verbal responses on demand and answering direct questions, even when they know the answer, also has been shown to be difficult for boys with fragile X. Word-finding problems also may be seen. Syntax is usually delayed but, unlike in DS, is consistent with the individual's mental age. Pragmatic deficits are often noted, including gaze avoidance, perseveration, frequent use of "canned" phrases ("Oh my, oh my!"), lack of communicative gestures, and poor topic maintenance and turn-taking (Schopmeyer & Lowe, 1992). Verbal imitation skills may be a relative strength (Scharfenaker, 1990).

Unlike most X-linked disorders, in which females are unaffected carriers, fragile X syndrome has been demonstrated to produce some affected females as well. Affected girls are usually more mildly impaired and may function in the learning disabled range. Their physical appearance may be normal or share some of the features seen in boys, such as a long face; prominent ears; and high, arched palate. Low muscle tone and hyperextensible finger joints also are sometimes seen (Spiridigliozzi, Lachiewicz, Mirrett, & McConkie-Rosell, 2001). Sensory and motor deficits are seen in girls with less magnitude and frequency than in boys with the syndrome, but Spiridigliozzi, Lachiewicz, Mirrett, and McConkie-Rosell (2001) emphasize the need for comprehensive occupational therapy evaluation to define strengths and needs in girls with fragile X. Social deficits of girls with fragile X also are milder than those seen in males. They may be shy or anxious, or they may show attention problems that affect learning, but they are less likely than boys with the syndrome to have hyperactivity. Cognitive skills in girls with fragile X are generally less limited than those of boys, but one-third to one-half of this group has been found to have MR. Performance on the Arithmetic, Digit Span, and Block Design subtests of the Wechsler scales (Wechsler, 1990, 1991) tends to be lower than performance on other subtests, with mathematics a particular weakness (Spiridigliozzi, Lachiewicz, Mirrett, & McConkie-Rosell, 2001). Girls with fragile X often do not often demonstrate any specific communication deficits (Scharfenaker, 1990). When they do, their most common problems include difficulties with abstract thinking, use of tangential language, poor topic maintenance (Schopmeyer & Lowe, 1992), and narrative skills (Madison, George, & Moeschler, 1986). Wolff, Gardner, Lappen, Paccia, and Meryash (1988), however, reported that girls with this syndrome did more poorly than control subjects in expressive language and auditory memory, whereas their receptive skills, vocabulary, and visual memory were on par with those of peers.

In summary, boys with fragile X syndrome display language difficulties beyond what would be expected on the basis of their level of retardation. The "typical" characteristics cited suggest that thorough language assessment should be conducted for any boy diagnosed with the syndrome. Conversely, if a boy with mild to moderate retardation shows some of these language characteristics, DNA testing for fragile X might be suggested to the family. Intervention strategies for these boys should keep their frequent attentional and behavioral problems in mind. Addressing their prosodic, dyspraxic, and cluttering difficulties will most likely be the focus of an intervention program. Poor eye contact is often a problem, but insisting on more direct eye contact has not been shown to be helpful (Spiridigliozzi, Lachiewicz, Mirrett, & McConkie-Rosell, 2001). Because of their declining rates of development in later childhood, early intervention is particularly crucial in this population. More research is needed to define the communication characteristics of girls affected by fragile X.

Williams Syndrome

This syndrome has only been recognized as a genetic entity since 1961. It is relatively rare (estimated to occur in 1 in 20,000 births). We now know that Williams syndrome (WS) results from a small deletion on Chromosome 7. Children with WS have dysmorphic facial features, hoarse vocal quality, heart and kidney problems, joint abnormalities, some hypersensitivity to sound, the appearance of an overly-friendly personality, and mild to moderate MR (Rice, 2004). Facial features include a small upturned nose, long philtrum (upper lip length), wide mouth, full lips, small chin, and puffiness around the eyes (Fig. 4-3). Blue- and green-eyed children with WS can have a prominent "starburst" or white lacy pattern on their iris. WS is found in about equal numbers in boys and girls. Although it has been thought for some time that children with WS show a sparing or even special ability in language, more recent research has suggested that this is not the case. While they may show relative strength in verbal ability, WS children do have delays in language development. They show late acquisition of first words and word combinations and have slow acquisition of grammatical forms. However, morphological development occurs at a more normal pace after onset. Rice (2004) describes language development in WS as being delayed in onset but eventually reaching expected

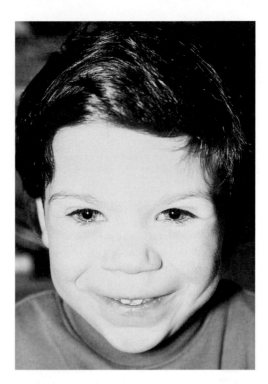

FIGURE 4-3 ✦ Children with Williams syndrome have upturned nose and small chin. (Reprinted with permission from Zitelli, B.J., and Davis, H.W. [2002]. *Atlas of pediatric physical diagnosis* [ed. 4]. St. Louis, MO: Mosby; courtesy R.A. Mathews, MD, Philadelphia.)

or higher levels of growth, relative to their nonverbal cognitive skills. Children with WS are unique in showing a pattern of language acquisition that, while not precocious or completely typical, is generally higher than their performance in nonverbal cognitive areas. Social communication tends to be a relative strength, although Laws and Bishop (2004) do identify some pragmatic difficulties in these children.

Prader-Willi Syndrome

Prader-Willi syndrome (PWS) results from the loss of function of genes on Chromosome 15. Children with the syndrome are hypotonic in the early years and show developmental delays, characteristic facial appearance, short stature, and obesity (Fig. 4-4). The syndrome is rare, occurring once in 10,000 to 15,000 live births, with boys and girls equally affected (Cassidy, 1997). Lewis, Freebairn, Heeger, and Cassidy (2002) studied communication performance in a relatively large group of children with PWS. They reported that communication is generally below mental-age expectations. Speech sound development tends to be delayed, and poor oral motor and articulations skills are a hallmark of the PWS. A variety of voice disorders, including hypernasality and hyponasality and high and low pitch, were observed. Receptive skills tended to be somewhat better than expressive, although both are impaired. A particular weakness in narrative abilities was noted. Pragmatic problems include maintaining a topic, taking turns appropriately in conversation, and maintaining appropriate physical distance. Areas of strength were seen in vocabulary, reading decoding and comprehension, and visual/spatial skills.

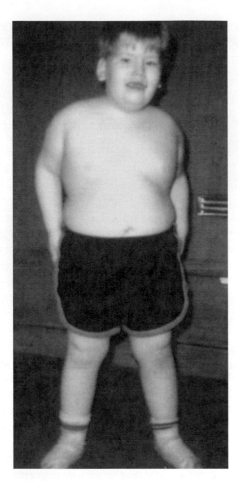

FIGURE 4-4 ✦ Children with Prader-Willi syndrome have small hands, short stature, and truncal obesity. (Reprinted with permission from Zitelli, B.J., and Davis, H.W. [2002]. *Atlas of pediatric physical diagnosis* [ed. 4]. St. Louis, MO: Mosby; courtesy Jeanne M. Hanchett, MD, The Children's Institute, Pittsburgh.)

ASSESSMENT AND INTERVENTION ISSUES IN MENTAL RETARDATION

Evaluation

Most states no longer require a discrepancy between cognitive and language level in order for a child to qualify for speech-language services. Instead, eligibility is decided on the basis of functional use of communication and informed clinical opinion. Many children with MR will benefit from SLP services, even if there is no gap between mental age and language level. Children with WS, for example, may have higher verbal than nonverbal scores, but if they have functional difficulties using the language they have in order to interact in the classroom or with peers, these difficulties can be addressed by the SLP.

Assessment

One thing that emerges very clearly from the descriptions above is that there is a great deal of variation within the population of children with MR in terms of communicative ability. This suggests that, following the developmental-descriptive model, an in-depth assessment of a range of relevant areas of communication is

warranted for every child in this category. We can't assume that, because we know the particular syndrome a child has, we will have the information we need to plan an appropriate program; we will need to carefully investigate each child's development.

Intervention

Children with MR, like other children with communication impairments, can benefit from a range of approaches. Studies have suggested that children with MR benefit from clinician-directed, behavioral methods (Yoder, Warren, & Hull, 1995) as well as more hybrid and naturalistic approaches (Vilaseca, 2004; Yoder & Warren, 2002). In addition, the characteristics of the child predict (to some degree) what intervention will work best. Abbeduto and Boudreau (2004), for example, review literature suggesting that indirect language stimulation is effective with children with MR who have MLUs above 2.0; for those with MLUs below 2.0, more clinician-directed approaches have a better track record. Gillum and Camarata (2004) argue that language comprehension in MR is often resistant to intervention, but report that milieu teaching has been shown to be associated with receptive language gains.

LANGUAGE DISORDERS ASSOCIATED WITH SENSORY DEFICITS

Helen was a very bright toddler. At age 2 she was already saying sentences, prattling on to anyone who would listen. She liked to draw and had great fun playing 'family' with her dolls. When she was 2½, she suffered a serious bout of meningitis, resulting in hospitalization. Her hearing was tested during her hospital stay, and she was found to have a severe loss in both ears. She was fitted with hearing aids before she returned home. Her parents were distraught that she had suffered permanent damage from her disease, but they were determined to minimize it. They made sure she wore her aids at all times and were careful to speak clearly and directly to her and to be sure she was watching them when they spoke to her. When she turned 3, they enrolled her in a preschool program that combined hearing-impaired and mainstream children in an intensive language stimulation program. When their physician saw Helen for follow-up, she discussed the possibility of a cochlear implant to improve Helen's hearing. Her parents spent a great deal of time carefully considering the risks versus the benefits of this treatment option.

Helen has one kind of sensory disability that has a profound effect on communicative development. Her story illustrates that, even today, common childhood diseases can have devastating consequences. Her case also points out the powerful role that families play in the outcome of a disorder. If her family had reacted differently to her loss, by becoming overwhelmed and unable to cope, for example, Helen's prognosis would change dramatically. Finally, Helen's experiences show us the tough choices families and clinicians often face in selecting the best intervention strategies for a particular child with a sensory deficit. Let's look at some of the characteristics associated with the two major forms of sensory loss: hearing impairment and blindness.

HEARING IMPAIRMENT

Hearing loss can be classified by both degree and type. The degree of hearing loss is defined by the audiometric classification of Bess and McConnell (1981). Their system is given in Table 4-2. It is based on the *pure tone average*, or the average threshold a client displays in pure tone testing at the "speech" frequencies 500, 1000, and 2000 Hz. People with losses in the 35- to 69-dB range are called *hard of hearing* in some classification systems, whereas those with losses of more than 70 dB are called *deaf* (Northern & Downs, 2002). Helen's audiogram appears in Figure 4-5.

TABLE 4-2	Degrees of Hearing Loss

HEARING THRESHOLD LEVEL	DEGREE OF HEARING LOSS CLASSIFICATION
26–40 dB	Mild
41–55 dB	Moderate
56–70 dB	Moderately severe
71–95 dB	Severe
96+ dB	Profound

Adapted from Bess, F., and McConnell, F. (1981). *Audiology, education and the learning-impaired child.* St. Louis, MO: Mosby.

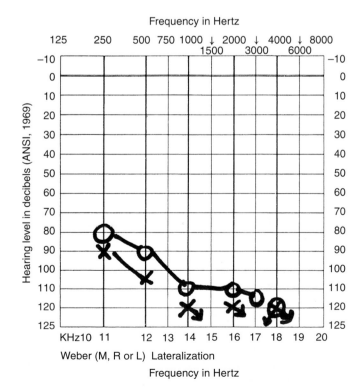

FIGURE 4-5 ✦ Helen's audiogram.

Of course, these designations of degree of loss say nothing about the language of a child with hearing impairment (HI). As we saw in Chapter 1, two children with very similar audiograms can have very different communication skills. Also, as Boothroyd (1982) pointed out, a child's unaided audiogram is not his or her fate. With amplification, children can be moved from one classification to another. Cochlear implants and tactile aids also are used to provide auditory information to children who would otherwise be considered deaf (Roeser, 1988). Again, the bottom line is that diagnostic classification itself is not enough to tell us what a child with hearing impairment needs. Individualized assessment of language skills and careful consideration of individual needs are necessary to plan the intervention program.

Three types of hearing loss are usually discussed: conductive, sensorineural, and mixed. *Conductive* losses result from interference in the transmission of sound from the auditory canal to the inner ear, while the inner ear itself functions normally (Northern & Downs, 2002). Conductive losses are usually medically treatable and reversible. The most common conductive losses in children are associated with *otitis media*, the inflammation or infection of the middle ear. These losses are usually fluctuating and intermittent. *Sensorineural* losses result from damage to the inner ear. They can be congenital or result from injury, infection, ototoxicity, or the degenerative effects of aging. They are usually not directly treatable or reversible, although cochlear implants are used to provide one form of surgical intervention. *Mixed* losses are caused by problems in both the conductive and sensorineural mechanisms. Let's look at the communicative characteristics associated with sensorineural and mixed losses first. Then we'll talk about conductive losses.

Communication in Sensorineural and Mixed Hearing Impairment

Quigley and Kretschmer (1982) found that a variety of factors influence communication development in children with hearing losses. These factors include not only the degree of loss but also (1) the age of onset (children who lose their hearing later do better than those who lose it earlier since the later the loss, the greater the language experience on which development can build), (2) the audiometric slope of the loss, (3) the age of identification and amplification (early identification and amplification have strong positive effects on language outcomes), and (4) the amount and type of habilitation. These factors would suggest, for example, that Helen's chances for a good outcome are excellent since she had learned some language before her loss occurred; she was amplified immediately; and her parents provided early, intensive habilitation.

Multiple handicaps are common in the HI population, with 13% to 33% of children with HI suffering from some other handicap (Levitt, McGarr, & Geffner, 1988; Shepard, Davis, Gorga, & Stelmachowicz, 1981). Despite the high incidence of multiple handicaps and the auditory deprivation these children experience as a result of their hearing losses, Levitt, McGarr, and Geffner (1988) reported that with intensive special education, children with HI do make slow-but-steady progress in communicative skills. Recent changes in treatment options, though, including the use of cochlear implantation (CI) to restore auditory signals, have resulted in dramatic changes for this population. Let's look at some of the ways in which children with HI have developed, without CI. Then we'll talk about how CI is changing this picture.

Infant Communication. Infant vocalization in the first half of the first year of life is similar in infants with and without normal hearing (Oller, Levine, Cobo-Lewis, Eilers, & Pearson, 1998). Oller and colleagues report that normally developing infants begin to display reduplicated, or *canonical*, babbling by 10 months of age. Their research suggests that children who do not begin babbling by this age should be referred for hearing testing.

Studies of mother-infant communication have shown that deaf mothers interacting with their deaf babies use heightened physical touch and facial expression and support their communication with contextual cues, whereas hearing parents of deaf babies use fewer of these strategies spontaneously (Kretschmer & Kretschmer, 2001). The deaf babies, however, emit signals of interest in interaction that are similar to those seen in hearing infants.

Phonology. Children with HI have been found to use at least partially rule-governed phonological systems (Dodd, 1976). They use phonological processes as do young children with normal hearing, although more processes are used. Consonant deletions are especially common in both initial and final position. One difference from normal development is that vowels are often distorted or neutralized. Prosodic features also are affected, including reduced speech rate, slow articulatory transitions with frequent pauses, poor respiratory control, poor coordination of breathing with syntactic phrasing, inappropriate use of duration to create stress patterns, and distorted resonance (Dunn & Newton, 1986). Speech often shows decreased intelligibility, particularly as utterances become more linguistically complex (Radziewicz & Antonellis, 1997; Schauwers, Gillis, & Govaerts, 2005), but with early identification and intervention, including hearing aids, the number of children with severe HI and intelligible speech has increased (Uchanski & Geers, 2003).

Cognition and Language. The cognitive development of children with hearing losses has been studied since the early 20th century. For a time it was thought that children with HI were retarded or developed qualitatively different forms of cognition, but later 20th-century research demonstrated that language mediates cognitive development in this population, as it does in children with normal development. As a result, it must be expected that if language development is seriously delayed by the hearing impairment, cognition will be affected as a result (Quigley & Paul, 1984). Meadow (1980) showed that on IQ tests, deaf children scored within the normal range but significantly lower than normal-hearing peers. This difference is thought to be attributable to the effects of language deprivation and the influence of the delays in language development experienced by children with HI. Kretschmer and Kretschmer (2001) argued that these language deficits are the explanation for any social or cognitive differences found in children who

are deaf. Some writers go further and see deaf children not as deficient but as culturally different (Kannapell, 1980; Padden, 1980). Advocates of Deaf culture argue that deafness does not have to be seen as a disability, but simply as one of many differences among people. They view Deaf culture as providing a rich and fulfilling social world for its members, complete with a fully developed language, set of beliefs, and social mores. Advocates of Deaf culture interpret findings such as Meadow's to reflect the cultural bias of IQ tests rather than real deficits on the part of children with HI. Tests specifically designed to assess intelligence in children with HI attempt to address this problem. The *Hiskey-Nebraska Test of Learning Aptitude* (Hiskey, 1966) was normed on children with HIs, for example.

Syntax. Grammatical acquisition in children with HI follows the same general order as it does in normal development, although it is greatly delayed, and the delays affect all modalities: receptive and expressive, oral and written (Kretschmer & Kretschmer, 2001; Quigley, Power, & Steinkamp, 1977). Inflectional morphemes, adverbs, prepositions, quantifiers, and indefinite pronouns seem to be especially difficult for children with HI. Nelson (1998) reported that relative clauses, complex sentences, verb marking, and pronominalization also are particularly troublesome for this population. Quigley, Smith, and Wilbur (1974) found some syntactic structures not seen in normal development in the HI population. It appeared that the children with HI were generating their own syntactic rules that were a combination of those in English and the approximations of English grammar that they were attempting. Wilbur, Goodhart, and Montandon (1983) suggested that many syntactic structures seemed to be learned as separate lexical items, rather than as generative structures.

Semantics. Children with hearing impairments who are learning speech express a range of semantic relations from an early age, as normal children do, although at a slower rate (Curtiss, Prutting, & Lowell, 1979; Schauwers, Gillis, & Govaerts, 2005). Children learning Sign as a first language encode the same semantic relations in the same order as hearing children (Launer, 1982). Children with HI who are learning speech generally show delays in verbal semantic ability throughout the developmental period (Radziewicz & Antonellis, 1997). They show difficulty in using concept words and figurative and multiple meanings (Nelson, 1998), although children learning Sign use figurative expressions in signed communications (Marschark & West, 1985). In addition, children with HI have trouble understanding connected discourse in both spoken and written modes, and these problems persist throughout adolescence (Moeller, Osberger, & Eccarius, 1986).

Pragmatics. Unlike the other areas we've outlined, pragmatic abilities in children with HI are on par with those of normal-hearing peers (Curtiss, Prutting, & Lowell, 1979). Young children with HI use a wide range of means, including gestures, vocalizations, and invented signs (Goldin-Meadow & Feldman, 1977), to get their messages across, although they do so with less frequency than normal-hearing peers. Still, their ability to communicate tends to be ahead of their ability to encode semantic concepts at this level (Curtiss, Prutting, & Lowell, 1979).

Kretschmer and Kretschmer (2001) report that preschoolers who are deaf, whether learning speech or Sign, show adequate turn-taking abilities, are socially sensitive, and are able to maintain conversational exchanges, although they had some difficulty with topic management. Nohara, MacKay, and Trehub (1995) looked at conversations between preteens, who were deaf and consistently had amplification, and their parents. These dialogues were found to be no different from those between dyads of mothers and normally hearing preteens. In general, children with HI show a rate and pattern of pragmatic development similar to that seen in normal-hearing children. Some gaps have been identified, though. These include poor conversational initiation and ability to respond to partners' initiations, especially comments (McKirdy & Blank, 1982), and difficulty in using rules for entering and continuing conversation, particularly in classroom settings (Weiss, 1986). Other problems seen in preschoolers included difficulty in use of deixis and in using linguistic means of marking cohesion. Ciocci and Baran (1998) reported that deaf children make adequate attempts at conversational repair but use different strategies from hearing children. Children who are deaf tended to revise utterances when asked for repair, whereas hearing children tended to repeat. Some aspects of narrative skills also appear to be impaired (Yoshinaga-Itano & Snyder, 1985), although deaf adolescents make inferences in stories as well as normal-hearing peers (Sarachan-Deily, 1985). Kretschmer (1997) emphasized that children with HI have reduced access to hearing and overhearing the everyday narratives used to convey ordinary experience in the family and stressed the need to develop a variety of discourse structures, including narration, description, explanation, and persuasion, in the communicative program for children with HI.

Written Language. Reading and writing present particular problems for children with HI, primarily because of the language basis necessary for acquiring these skills. Average reading comprehension level for adolescents with HI is third to fourth grade (Allen, 1994; King & Quigley, 1985; Trybus & Karchmer, 1977). Geers and Moog (1989) studied profoundly hearing-impaired high school seniors who had been enrolled in either oral or mainstream high school programs. They found that three things were related to literacy development in this population: hearing level, early intervention, and spoken language skills. This group of orally educated deaf youngsters, unlike most other people with HI, were able to achieve reading levels commensurate with those of age mates. The authors concluded that the reasons for this level of achievement were that these students had at least average nonverbal IQs; good use of residual hearing; early amplification; and strong oral English language ability, including vocabulary, syntax, and discourse skills.

Prinz and Strong (1998) found a positive relationship between American Sign Language (ASL) and English literacy in students attending a school in which ASL was used for face-to-face communication and English for reading and writing. Padden and Ramsey (1998) attribute this relationship to the use of finger spelling and initialized signs (those that use the handshape of the first letter in the English spelling of the word as part of the Sign), which help the Signer to use the alphabetic cues inherent in the English writing system (see Chapter 10). Prinz and Strong suggest the importance of specialized instruction and practice with these aspects of ASL to bridge the gap between ASL and written English for Signing students.

Another factor that may contribute to literacy development in this population is early exposure to print. Because parents and educators are often so focused on developing a primary language in these children, less attention is paid to the establishment of important preliteracy skills. Kretschmer and Kretschmer (2001) pointed out that children with HI exhibit more emergent literacy behaviors when they are provided with engaging, print-rich environments at home and at school and when their early attempts at writing in these environments are similar in form and content to those of children with normal hearing. Clearly, exposing children with HI to books, reading them stories, demonstrating the uses of writing in everyday activities, and providing attractive writing materials and opportunities will be useful in this population, as in others, in fostering the acquisition of literacy.

Language Development in Children with CI

Since the 1990s, the rate of cochlear implantation in children with HI has increased rapidly, the age at which children receive implants has decreased (Mellon, 2005), and several research groups have been following the progress of the communication development of these children. Schauwers, Gillis, and Govaerts (2005) summarized the early studies, in which children received implants at ages 2 to 5 years. They report that when implantation occurs during the preschool period, the rates of speech and expressive and receptive language development, which are significantly delayed in children without CI, accelerate to match those of normal children, although gaps may remain, since the children did not start hearing until after the first three critical years. Intelligibility, vocabulary, and syntax all benefit from implantation, although children appear to dwell at the two-word stage for a longer than normal period of time. Age at implantation seems to have a significant effect on outcome in these studies, with children implanted earlier achieving higher outcome levels.

More recently, children have received implants earlier. Children identified as hearing impaired at birth (due to mandatory newborn hearing screening in most states) can now be implanted by their first birthday, and many are implanted even earlier (Shafer, 2005). Research is currently being carried out to determine the optimal age for implantation.

Geers (2004), Geers, Nicholas, and Sedley (2003), and Tomblin, Shriberg, Nishimura, Zhang, and Murray (1999) summarized research on the effects of early implantation by reporting that children who received implants early in life, followed by a period of appropriate rehabilitation, were able to speak intelligibly, converse fluently, and read at close to age-appropriate levels (ASHA, 2004). For these children with CI, Geers (2004) found that an oral education program was more effective than total communication in producing speech and oral language outcomes. Oral language and literacy in these children exceeded those observed in deaf children with hearing aids. Geers (2004) reported that use of a cochlear implant resulted in a majority of children who produced and understood English language at a level comparable with that of their hearing-age mates.

This research suggests that implantation outcomes are improved by auditory training and the use of classroom assistive listening devices (Ertmer, 2002; Teagle & Moore, 2002). However, Ertmer, Strong, and Sadagopan (2003) and Tye-Murray (2003) emphasize that although early milestones are typically attained easily by these children, progress toward more advanced language, such as consistent use of word order, intelligible speech, and fluent conversation, was slower. They argue that these findings suggest the continued need for auditory training and speech-language intervention for children with CI to ensure that they achieve their communicative potential.

Implications for Clinical Practice

Choosing a Communication Modality. There have been long and heated debates within the field of deaf education about the efficacy of oral versus manual language instruction. This debate is in some ways less urgent with the advent of CI, because many families who wish to have their child educated orally can opt for CI and, with early identification, implantation, and education, see their child achieve oral language skills that are similar to those of hearing peers. However, deaf parents of deaf children may feel it is more important for their child to be fluent in Sign and comfortable in Deaf culture, and so wish to allow their child to participate in it through the acquisition of Signed communication. For these families, instruction in Sign may make more sense. When embarking on a Sign program, the clinician needs to determine whether to use strictly signs or total communication (TC), which is the use of speech and Sign simultaneously. TC is viable if one of the several forms of signed English is being taught. Signed forms of English combine signs from ASL with inflectional markers and grammatical morphemes represented as gestures to produce a direct translation from English to a manual language form. Signed forms of English are thought to help children with hearing impairments learn not only to communicate but also to read and write, because they mimic the structure of English. But speakers of ASL disdain them as a "pidgin" language that distorts the very different syntactic structure of ASL. ASL is the living language of the Deaf community and uses different forms of morphology and word order than English. If ASL is taught, rather than a signed form of English, it is not possible to use a TC approach because one could not directly translate the English being spoken into the Sign being produced simultaneously (Coryell & Holcomb, 1997).

Kretschmer and Kretschmer (2001) suggest that if some manually coded form is the mode of choice, the family members must either have proficiency in the system or develop it as quickly as possible. It is crucial that the manual system, whatever it is, be used consistently with the child and even between parents if the child is present so that learning through "overhearing" can take place. Language interactions in ASL must, of course, be as authentic, interactive, and meaningful as is parent-child communication in spoken language.

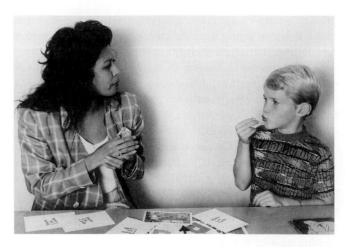

Sign language is often used as a communication modality for children with HI.

Even children who go the ASL route will need to develop literacy skills in English to participate in the mainstream culture. Radziewicz and Antonellis (1997) suggested using an English as a Second Language (ESL) or bilingual approach to this problem, teaching spoken and written English to students who use Sign as a first language, just as we would for hearing children who come to school with a mother tongue other than English. Strong (1988) proposed a story-based method for this type of instruction. Hanson and Padden (1989) have developed a computer and video instructional method. CD-ROM and Internet technology may offer additional approaches to ESL instruction for users of Sign in the future. Other writers, though (e.g., Nover, Christensen, & Cheng, 1998; Singleton, Supalla, Litchfield, & Schley, 1998) emphasize the inherent differences between ASL and English and stress the unique aspects of learning a *spoken* language when the first language is in the visual modality. They suggest that written English may be an important link between the two modalities. This emphasis again focuses our attention on the central role of literacy in English in providing communication programming to children using Sign as a first language.

Deaf children of hearing parents may have families who believe that spoken language achievement is their most important goal. Not every child is a good candidate for CI (ASHA, 2004b). Kretschmer and Kretschmer (2001) emphasize that when speech is the chosen modality for a child who does not receive CI, parents and professionals must ensure that the child receives appropriate amplification and that all amplification systems are consistently monitored and maintained. Here, too, the importance of natural interactive communication cannot be overemphasized.

Regardless of what the family wants, though, some children may do better in one modality than the other. It would be wise to offer trial instruction in each modality to see how well the child adjusts. If the child shows no clear preference, the family's wishes can prevail. If the child seems to do much better in the modality not preferred by the family, some consultation may be in order to try to find the best educational approach for all concerned. A resource such as *Choices in Deafness* (Schwartz, 1996) may help parents to make this difficult decision.

Intervention and the SLP. Brackett (1997) reported that hearing impairment is the most common disability of school-age children in mainstream settings. SLPs in school-based practice are very likely to have children with HI, with and without CI, in their caseload. Brackett suggests that SLPs advocate for sound-treating classrooms in which these children are placed, using sound absorbing materials such as carpet, acoustic ceiling tiles, curtains, and corkboards. FM listening systems should also be requested for these clients. Brackett urges SLPs, in our consulting role, to suggest that teachers use visual enhancements such as outlines, writing on the board, and visual demonstrations to support oral presentation of information. Box 4-1 gives Brackett's suggestions for the responsibilities of the SLP with regard to the client with HI.

Communication in Children with Mild, Fluctuating Conductive Hearing Losses Caused by Otitis Media

According to the U.S. Department of Health and Human Services, otitis media (OM) is one of the most common diseases of young children. Three quarters of all children experience at least one episode during the preschool years (Roland & Brown, 1990). Children who experience OM, particularly when it is accompanied by effusion (OME), often suffer some degree of conductive hearing loss during the episode. It has long been thought that such mild, fluctuating hearing losses, when experienced over and over during the sensitive language development period, can have a negative effect on language learning. Shriberg and Kwiatkowski (1982*b*), for example, found that one-third of children enrolled in speech or language intervention had histories of recurrent middle-ear disease.

The degree of increased risk for speech and language disorder in children with a history of OM has been a matter of intense debate, though. Many studies have reported adverse effects on various aspects of speech and language associated with chronic OM (Downs, Walker, & Northern, 1988; Friel-Patti & Finitzo, 1990; Friel-Patti, Finitzo-Hieber, Conti, & Brown, 1982; Holm & Kunze, 1969; Hubbard, Paradise, McWilliams, Elster, & Taylor, 1985; Lehmann, Charron, Kummer, & Keith, 1979; Menyuk, 1986; Needleman, 1977; Paden, Novak, & Beiter, 1987; Roberts, Burchinal, Koch, Footo, & Henderson, 1988; Schlieper, Kisilevsky, Mattingly, & Yorke, 1985; Shriberg & Smith, 1983; Silva, Kirkland, Simpson, Stewart, & Williams, 1982; Teele, Klein, Rosner, & the Greater Boston Otitis Media Study Group, 1984; Wallace, Gravel, McCarton, & Ruben, 1988; Yont, Snow, & Vernon-Feagans, 2001). Often, though, these studies looked only at effects in the first 2 years of life (e.g., Friel-Patti & Finitzo, 1990; Wallace, Gravel, McCarton, & Ruben, 1988). In longer-term follow-up studies, effects do not always persist (Gravel & Wallace, 1992; Teele, Klein, Rosner, & The Greater Boston Otitis Media Study Group, 1984). Effects are often statistically significant but of questionable clinical significance (Friel-Patti & Finitzo, 1990; Paul, Lynn, & Lohr-Flanders, 1993; Roberts et al., 1988). Some researchers find no important differences between the verbal skills of children who do and do not have histories of OM (Bishop & Edmundson, 1986; Fischler, Todd, & Feldman, 1985; Greville, Keith, & Laven, 1985; Roberts, Burchinal, Davis, Collier, & Henderson, 1991; Roberts, Sanyni, Burchinal, Collier, Ranney, & Henderson, 1986). Casby (2001) reported on a meta-analysis of earlier studies that suggests that the detrimental effect of OME on language learning in young children is small, but potentially significant. Roberts (2004) also used meta-analysis to argue that, on average, OME does not appear to constitute substantial risk in typically developing children for later speech/language development or academic achievement. Bishop

---

| **BOX 4-1** | **Brackett's (1997) Suggestions for the SLP's Role with Children with HI** |

1. Assume responsibility for amplification: select, monitor, and maintain classroom amplification; train school staff to troubleshoot the equipment.
2. Establish an auditory learning program: using assessment data, identify areas of need. Use programmed approaches (such as Ling, 1989; Stout & Windle, 1992). Teach client to maximize the use of available auditory information, using words and phrases from the classroom setting.
3. Interpret performance relative to hearing impairment: analyze errors to determine which are caused by auditory perception problems and by lack of linguistic knowledge or inability to place articulators. Concentrate on these latter errors in intervention.
4. Be familiar with typical patterns of performance: be aware of likely areas of deficits in children with HI.
5. Select targets from multiple deficit areas: include speech, language, listening, and social-interactive goals. Use curriculum-based materials and activities.
6. Recognize subtle areas of difficulty in milder impairments: assist the classroom teacher in understanding the impact of mild hearing losses on classroom performance, and plan objectives collaboratively for students with mild HI.
7. Act as consultant to the classroom teacher: sample classroom lessons and analyze them for communication requirements, then plan with the teacher to optimize access to this instruction for the client with HI. Help the teacher develop methods for checking clients' comprehension in classroom situations.

and Edmundson (1986) and Roberts and Schuele (1990) suggest that OM alone may not constitute an increased risk for language disorder. Klein and Rapin (1992) argue that chronic otitis media may interact with other risk factors in vulnerable children.

What does this mean for a clinician who sees a young child with delayed communicative skills and a history of chronic OM? Since the research is equivocal about whether that history will have a strong influence on this child's outcome, what are we to do? In general, we will probably want to take a "better-safe-than-sorry" stance. Children with chronic OM and otherwise normal development who are not having communication problems are probably at low risk for later difficulties. We can counsel their families to be sure to have each ear infection treated and to discuss with their physician preventive measures such as prophylactic antibiotics and myringotomy tube placement. In addition, Lahey (1988) suggested advising these families to provide extra language stimulation. They also can be encouraged to have their child's language development monitored periodically during the preschool years. For children with a history of ear infections who are demonstrating some delays in communication, we might suggest that families be especially careful to read to the child every day, to talk slowly and directly to the child, and to match language to ongoing activities. Additional suggestions for families of these children appear in Box 4-2. They may be helpful in reducing whatever risk there is of long-term effects of middle ear disease. In talking with families of these children, though, it is important to emphasize that the OM is only one aspect of the child's language-learning problem. Eliminating the recurrent otitis, through antibiotics or myringotomy tubes, will probably not entirely eliminate the language delay.

Children with craniofacial syndromes or DS are particularly vulnerable to OME. These children should be monitored especially closely for middle ear disease. Roland and Brown (1990) asserted that these children almost always require myringotomy tubes.

BLINDNESS

Visual impairments do not have as negative an effect on language development as hearing impairments (Pérez-Pereira & Conti-Ramsden, 1999). Children who are blind learn spoken language and also can learn to read with the help of specially adapted writing systems such as Braille and computers that scan print and convert it to speech. For many years it was believed that blindness had no effect at all on language development (cf. Chomsky, 1980). There was even a folk myth, now discredited (Erin, 1990), that blind people have superefficient auditory systems that automatically compensate for the loss of visual information. Despite the apparent normality of language in children who are blind, though, some risks for language development have been identified in this population (Andersen, Dunlea,

---

| **BOX 4-2** | **Suggestions for Parents of Children with Chronic OM and Language Disorders** |

- Be aware of signs of ear infection (pulling on the ear, fever and congestion related to a cold, decreased attentiveness).
- Secure the child's attention before speaking to make sure he or she is listening, and give reminders to pay attention.
- Provide focused language input by presenting language forms with high frequency in contexts in which meaning is clear and language is matched to ongoing events.
- Be sure that the child is close to the person speaking.
- Face the child and talk at the child's eye level to provide clearer visual and auditory information.
- Speak slowly and clearly and repeat important words, but in a natural tone of voice. Build redundancy into input and limit its complexity.
- Increase opportunities to be close by reading to the child and playing word games and other communicative activities.
- Use intonation and stress to highlight important information.
- Use visual support whenever possible, such as pictures, photographs, or objects.
- Be responsive to the child's attempts to talk.
- Provide a quiet environment for conversation by moving to an area with carpeting and draperies and by closing doors.
- Reduce distractions during conversations by turning off TV, radio, or music.
- If the child has recurrent OME, consider personal amplification on a temporary basis until the problem resolves.
- Have the child seen by an audiologist for routine hearing tests.
- Be aware that children with OM may have fluctuating hearing losses and will appear to have trouble hearing or paying attention.
- Provide opportunities for small-group interaction.

Adapted from Kretschmer, L., & Kretschmer, R. (2001). Deafness and hearing impairment in young children. In T. Layton, E. Crais, & L. Watson (Eds.), *Handbook of early language impairment in children: Nature* (pp. 541-626). Albany, NY: Delmar Publishers; Roberts, J., & Schuele, C. (1990). Otitis media and later academic performance: The linkage and implications for intervention. *Topics in Language Disorders, 11*(1), 43-62; Watkins, R. (1990). Processing problems and language impairment in children. *Topics in Language Disorders, 11*(1), 63-72.

& Kekelis, 1993; Erin, 1990; Fraiberg, 1977; Mills, 1983; Warren, 1984). I'll briefly summarize some of the findings on language development in blind children.

Semantics

Blind children are often late in acquiring vocabulary (Lahey, 1988). Early words used by blind children are similar to those used by sighted peers, even "sighted" verbs such as *look* (Andersen, Dunlea, & Kekelis, 1984; Landau & Gleitman, 1985). But the meanings attached to these words are more limited and often are not extended beyond the original context in the one-word period. Dunlea (1984), Landau and Gleitman (1985), and Urwin (1978) all found that blind children begin to combine words and express a range of semantic relations similar to those used by sighted children. But blind children were more likely to talk about their own actions than those of others and less likely to describe than sighted children were. The blind children were more likely to talk about past events, whereas the sighted children tended to talk about the here-and-now during the two-word stage.

Syntax

Syntactic development may be slow in the third year of life, but blind children generally have age-appropriate MLUs by their third birthday. They show lags, though, in acquisition of auxiliary verbs (Landau & Gleitman, 1985). Unlike sighted children, blind children use past tense as one of their earliest grammatical markers (Dunlea, 1989; Dunlea & Andersen, 1992), but they use locative prepositions later than sighted peers. Andersen, Dunlea, and Kekelis (1993) concluded that blind children seem to deal with concepts of time before space, whereas the opposite is true for sighted children.

Pragmatics

Blind children produce fewer spontaneous vocalizations than sighted peers and initiate communication less often (Fraiberg, 1977). Andersen, Dunlea, and Kekelis (1993) reported that blind children have more trouble than sighted peers in establishing and maintaining topics, in producing cohesive discourse, and in using deictic markers. They may display use of routine phrases, echolalia, pronoun reversals, flat intonation, and a lack of creativity in their utterances in the early phases of development (Fraiberg, 1977; Urwin, 1984). According to Urwin, blind children use language first in solitary play and only later in communication. These findings reinforce the suggestion of Andersen, Dunlea, and Kekelis (1993) that blind children have more trouble than sighted peers in figuring out the purpose of language.

Implications for Clinical Practice

Despite differences in early acquisition, most blind people eventually develop language that is not different from that of sighted people, although they may get there via a slightly different route (Mills, 1992). But, because we know some of these children will experience delays of various kinds, direct intervention may be considered. Some blind children may benefit from intensive language stimulation by a language pathologist. Junefelt (2004) pointed out that congenitally blind children rely more than do others on language for understanding the external world and for creating their inner world. In this sense, it would be wise to provide as rich a linguistic input as possible, to provide the child with the largest array of tools for constructing these worlds. For many blind children, though, parent education may be sufficient to provide this enriched input. It is probably wise to monitor the language development of children who are blind. Those who have delays after age 3 are most likely to be in need of direct services.

For blind children younger than 3, the best approach may be consultative intervention that focuses on helping parents understand how the child's blindness affects interaction and identifies alternative ways for parents to engage with their children. Fraiberg (1979) identified a set of behaviors that parents of blind infants can be taught to look for as substitutes for visual interaction patterns. These include smiling in response to parents' voices, seeking comfort from and being calmed when embraced by parents, vocalizing in response to parent vocalizations, manual and tactile seeking behaviors, stranger avoidance, and anxiety at separation from parents and comfort at reunion. When parents learn to recognize and elicit these signs of social interaction, they can begin to normalize some of the interaction patterns that are problematic with blind infants.

In addition to teaching parents to "read" these cues in the child's first year of life, we can encourage them to provide some more enriching linguistic stimulation during the second and third years. Some suggestions we can glean from the literature on parent input to blind children might include advising parents to do the following:

1. Provide both labels and descriptions of objects the child handles.
2. Ask both open-ended and more directive questions.
3. Provide more variety in the topics that they discuss with their children, talking about both the child's own actions and other things going on in the environment.
4. Model and encourage the child to engage in pretend play.

Counseling parents of blind children to take advantage of these techniques can help to minimize the effects of the child's visual impairment on communicative development.

DEAF-BLINDNESS

Children with significant deficits in both hearing and vision are considered *deaf-blind*, even though some may have useful residual vision and/or hearing. There are two major causes of deaf-blindness. One is *Rubella syndrome*, a congenital condition that arises when the mother contracts rubella, or German measles, during the first months of pregnancy. Thanks to widespread immunization for Rubella, deaf-blindness attributable to this syndrome has been greatly reduced. The second major cause is *Usher's syndrome* (Shprintzen, 1997), a disease transmitted genetically.

Because of the multisensory deprivation that children with deaf-blindness experience, Nelson (1998) recommends using contextualized and dynamic assessment techniques to evaluate skills and identify communicative needs in this population. It is well to remember, too, that although these children have complex and severe disabilities, they may have normal cognition. When accurate cognitive assessment is not available or feasible, it is best to set aside questions of basic intelligence and work to expand conceptual, social, and communicative skill as far as possible. Some form of AAC is almost always useful in these cases. Communication devices that emulate the receiving and transmitting modes of tactile finger spelling have been shown to be useful with this population (van Kraayenoord & Schonell, 2003). Box 4-3 presents some additional types of AAC interventions to try with these clients.

DISORDERS WITH ENVIRONMENTAL COMPONENTS

Communication disorders that result from maternal abuse of toxins, such as alcohol, or from parental behavior disorders, such as abuse and neglect, are some of the most tragic aspects of our clinical practice because these kinds of disorders could have been prevented. As Joseph's story indicates, these factors often operate in concert to produce a range of long-term developmental problems. Let's look at some of the communication patterns we may see in children exposed to these hazards to understand how they might influence clinical decision making. We'll talk about two major types of environmental stressors: maternal substance abuse and maltreatment.

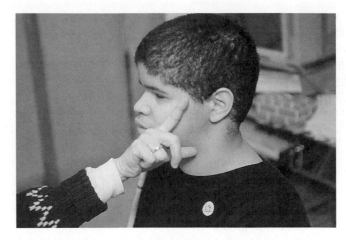

Finger spelling is one means of communication used with students who are deaf-blind.

Joseph was born in 1990 to a mother who had been severely alcoholic during her pregnancy. During his stay in the hospital, it was noted that he had some dysmorphic facial features, including microcephaly (small head size), micrognathia (small jaw size), a thin upper lip with an indistinct philtrum, and a flat midface. He was extremely irritable in the newborn nursery.

| **BOX 4-3** | **Recommended AAC Intervention for Children with Deaf-Blindness** |

Unaided Techniques

Signaling—Simple body signals such as coordinated rocking with reciprocal cues to start and stop.

Gestures—Conventional gestures such as *hi, bye-bye,* or head nods.

Anticipatory cues—Cues used to signal an upcoming action so the child may anticipate events, such as rubbing the child's cheek with a washcloth to signal bath time.

Adapted signs—The child's hand can be shaped to produce Signs, and the child can be encouraged to feel the clinician's hand shape to perceive Signs. At first, gross approximations can be accepted and then gradually shaped to more conventional Signing.

Finger spelling—Finger spelling can be introduced by first manipulating the fingers in playful interactive games. Eventually, familiar objects and actions within routines can be labeled with finger-spelled words.

Speech—Children with residual hearing may be taught speech, but other modes of communication can coexist with speech instruction.

Print/Braille—Children with significant residual vision can be introduced to print when level of functioning appears appropriate. Braille may be appropriate for those who can make fine tactile discriminations.

Aided Techniques

Opticon—This device changes print to a tactile representation and may assist higher functioning deaf-blind students who rely on Braille for academic information.

Teletouch—This device allows sighted people to type messages on a standard keyboard, so that each letter is reproduced as Braille.

Communication boards—Pictures or symbols can be labeled with Braille or more concrete tactile cues and used for both receptive and expressive communication.

Typing and writing—Computers and dedicated electronic augmentation devices can be used and can be coupled with speech synthesis software to allow an individual's message to be written out and spoken.

Adapted from McInnes, J.M., & Treffry, J.A. (1982). *Deaf-blind infants and children: A developmental guide*. Toronto, Canada: University of Toronto Press; Nelson, N. (1998). *Childhood language disorders in context: Infancy through adolescence* (ed. 2). Columbus, OH: Merrill.

During his preschool years, Joseph's mother continued to drink, and she also began using cocaine. She was often absent, leaving Joseph with whatever neighbor would take him, while she earned money by prostitution to buy drugs. Joseph grew slowly in size. He experienced many developmental delays, including late motor milestones and slow language development. When his mother enrolled herself in a drug treatment program when Joseph was 3, he was assessed and found to function in the low to borderline normal range on an IQ test. At that time, he was diagnosed as having fetal alcohol syndrome (FAS). He was enrolled in early intervention while his mother was involved in the drug rehabilitation program. Both made significant progress. At age 5 he was able to function in a regular classroom, but he required special education periodically throughout his school career. He often charmed his teachers with his chatty manner, but he had difficulty understanding classroom directions and comprehending reading assignments. Arithmetic was his worst area. In high school his poor judgment often got him into trouble. He was easily convinced by friends to buy them cigarettes or skip school. He didn't seem to have any "common sense." At 16, he dropped out of school.

MATERNAL SUBSTANCE ABUSE

Maternal substance abuse can affect a child's development in the following two ways, which interact with each other:

1. Substances such as alcohol and cocaine can have negative effects during prenatal development. These substances can cross the placental barrier and affect the intrauterine environment. In the case of alcohol, the fetus is unable to metabolize the alcohol as an adult does. Alcohol acts as a teratogenic agent and interferes with chemical processes in fetal cells. Abuse of street drugs, such as cocaine, can lead to increased chances for prematurity, which carries its own set of risks.
2. Communication development also is influenced through the effects of substance abuse on the caregiving environment. A mother who is frequently drunk, high on drugs, or driven to get drugs by any means necessary is not a person who can devote much energy to child rearing. These mothers often have difficulty understanding their children's communications and interpret the children's communicative bids as demands, often rejecting or criticizing their efforts (Sparks, 2001). If other parent figures are not present in the child's life to mitigate the mother's neglect, the child's development will suffer.

Sometimes it is hard, as in Joseph's case, to separate the effects of prenatal toxicity from those of neglect during childhood. Moreover, people who abuse one drug tend to drink, smoke, and abuse other drugs. This issue becomes even more complicated when the mother's substance abuse leads to HIV infection, which can be passed on to the fetus. Then the caregiving environment is affected not only by the mother's drug use but also by her illness and its consequent debilitation. The child, too, may become ill, and then development is affected by the child's own vulnerability to infection. We'll look at the effects that the abuse of two broad classes of substances—alcohol and street drugs—have on communicative development and touch briefly on the way in which HIV infection interacts with these stressors.

Alcohol-Related Disorders

Sparks (1993) pointed out that alcohol has been suspected of causing birth defects from ancient times and cites the biblical passage in *Judges 13:7* that warns women who would bear children to "drink no wine or strong drink." The syndrome was not recognized scientifically until 1974, however (Jones, Smith, Streissguth, & Myrianthopoulos, 1974), and it was not until 1981 that the U.S. surgeon general recommended that pregnant women abstain from alcohol. As recently as the 1960s, physicians often told expectant mothers to have a cocktail before bedtime to help them relax and sleep well!

The syndrome of birth anomalies associated with excessive alcohol intake during pregnancy, referred to as FAS, has three diagnostic criteria (O'Leary, 2004; Sparks, 1993, 2001):

1. Growth deficiency
2. A specific pattern of minor anomalies of the facial features, including short eye slits (palpebral fissures), a flat midface, a short upturned nose, a long philtrum, and a thin upper lip
3. Neurobehavioral effects, including reduced head circumference (microcephaly), tremors, hyperactivity, fine or gross motor problems, attentional deficits, learning disabilities, cognitive impairments, or seizures

Because prenatal alcohol exposure is not the only potential cause of this constellation of problems, the diagnosis of FAS also must include information that the mother did, in fact, abuse alcohol during pregnancy. Fetal alcohol effects (FAE) are a milder version of FAS. Here, a child whose mother had a known history of alcohol abuse during pregnancy displays some but not all three of the characteristics that warrant a diagnosis of FAS. FAS and FAE last throughout the lifespan, and there is a predictable progression of maladaptive behaviors and communication problems (Box 4-4).

Sparks (1993) and Streissguth (1997) provided a set of characteristics typically seen in children and adolescents with FAS or FAE. These are summarized in Box 4-4. Communication disabilities are almost universal in this population (Cone-Wesson, 2005) and are related to the level of intellectual impairment. In children with more severe impairments, perseveration and echolalia are often present. Cone-Wesson (2005) also points out that the facial anomalies often seen in these children predispose them to OME, so that careful monitoring of hearing and health is especially important.

Disorders Related to Drug Abuse

As we've said, many women who abuse street drugs during pregnancy take more than one drug and may abuse both drugs and alcohol. Attributing effects on development to just one drug may be a mistake. The effects of the mother's drug abuse on her care-taking ability are just as important as any biological effects the abuse may have caused before birth. As far as

| BOX 4-4 | **Common Characteristics of Children and Adolescents with FAS and FAE** |

Infancy and Early Childhood

- Sleep disturbances
- Poor sucking response
- Failure to thrive
- Proneness to middle-ear disease
- Poor habituation
- Delays in walking and talking
- Delays in toilet training
- Difficulty following directions
- Temper tantrums

School Years

- Hyperactivity, distractibility
- Poor attention
- Delayed motor, cognitive, and speech development
- Difficulties in understanding consequences of actions
- Temper tantrums and conduct problems
- Fine-motor difficulties
- Learning and memory problems
- Lack of inhibition
- Interest in social engagement, but poor social skills
- Indiscriminate attachment to adults
- Withdrawal, depression
- Poor judgment, difficulty matching aspirations to ability, failure to learn from past experience
- Good verbal facility, giving appearance of strong verbal skills, but poor receptive vocabulary and comprehension
- Better performance in reading, writing, and spelling than in mathematics
- Better performance on word recognition than reading comprehension
- Good performance on concrete tasks, but poor abstract reasoning

Adolescence

- Reach academic ceiling
- Depression, social isolation
- Naïve, childlike manner
- Sexual difficulties (inappropriate behavior, easily exploited)
- Poor impulse control
- Difficulty seeing cause-effect relationships
- Memory, learning, attention, activity, and judgment problems persist
- Pragmatic difficulties
- Truancy and school dropout problems

Adapted from Sparks, S. (1993). *Children of prenatal substance abuse*. San Diego, CA: Singular Publishing Group; Streissguth, A., LaDue, R., & Randels, S. (1988). *A manual on adolescents and adults with fetal alcohol syndrome with special reference to American Indians*. Seattle, WA: University of Washington; Streissguth, A., Aase, J., Clarren, S., Randels, S., LaDue, R., & Smith, D. (1991). Fetal alcohol syndrome in adolescents and adults. *Journal of the American Medical Association*, 265, 1961-1967; Streissguth, A. (1997). *Fetal alcohol syndrome: A guide for families and communities*. Baltimore, MD: Paul H. Brookes.

biological effects are concerned, Sparks (1993, 2001) pointed out that less than one-half of children exposed to drugs prenatally experience low birth weight, prematurity, intrauterine growth retardation, or small head circumference. Sparks (1993) and Chiriboga (2003) reported that drug-exposed newborns are often irritable and stiff and show arousal and attention problems, but these traits do not appear to last past the first year. In general, cognition is not impaired, except when reduced head size is seen. Still, catch-up head growth is a marker of good prognosis for long-term development (Sparks, 2001). Several studies (Bandstra, Vogel, Morrow, Anthony, & Lihua Xue, 2004; Cone-Wesson, 2005; Lewis, Singer, Short, Minnes, Arendt, Weishampel, Klein, & Min, 2004; Morrow, Vogel, Anthony, Ofir, Dausa, & Bandstra, 2004) have found that children with a history of cocaine exposure show delays in language acquisition, particularly in the area of expressive language, with exposure to higher doses prenatally resulting in higher levels of impairment. However, these studies also find that effects are modified by an enriched environment; children placed in foster or adoptive homes show higher levels of communicative skill than those who remain with biological mothers. Box 4-5 lists some of the risks posed by drug exposure for both physical and communicative development. Remember, though, that only a minority of children exposed to drugs prenatally experience these problems. In general, the developmental problems these children exhibit are not much different from those of other children who live in chaotic homes but who did not have prenatal drug exposure. Still, there do appear to be some problems specifically associated with drug exposure. Deficits in representational play (Lundgren, 1998) and difficulty in forming secure attachments have been noted (Sparks, 2001). Timler, Olswang, and Coggins (2005a) report that children with FAS show pragmatic difficulties including difficulty in providing sufficient information and failure to take listener perspectives into account in conversation. Nonetheless, not all drug-exposed children show these effects, and even those who do respond well to traditional early intervention procedures. In fact, early intervention is even more promising for children exposed to cocaine than it is for children with FAS (Sparks, 1993).

BOX 4-5 — Risks of Prenatal Drug Exposure for Physical and Communicative Development

Physical Risks

- Small head circumference
- Low birth weight as a result of prematurity or intrauterine growth retardation
- Small strokes or heart attacks (intrauterine cerebral and cardiac infarctions) before birth
- Congenital malformations of the heart, genitourinary tract, and limbs
- AIDS and other infections

Behavioral Risks

Infancy
- Irritability
- Hypertonicity or hypotonicity
- Hyperactivity
- Tremulousness
- Deficiencies in organization of state and interactive abilities
- Seizures

Childhood
- Reduced self-regulation
- Distractibility
- Reduced pretend play
- Flat affect
- Attachment problems

Adapted from Sparks, S. (1993). *Children of prenatal substance abuse.* San Diego, CA: Singular Publishing Group; Sparks, S. (2001). Prenatal substance use and its impact on young children. In T. Layton, E. Crais, & L. Watson, (Eds.), *Handbook of early language impairment in children: Nature* (pp. 451-487). Albany, NY: Delmar Publishers.

HIV INFECTION

Children can acquire HIV—the infection that leads to AIDS—after birth, but 80% of children with HIV acquired the infection through maternal-infant transmission before or during the birth process (Scott & Layton, 2001). Because most mothers acquire HIV themselves through exposure to contaminated needles, HIV infection in children is to some extent a byproduct of maternal drug abuse.

Because of advances in pharmacological treatments, many of these children will remain healthy. However, because of their vulnerability to infection, they also experience frequent ear infections, which require careful monitoring and management. The medications that prolong their health, too, may have effects on feeding and swallowing, which need to be monitored (McNeilly, 2005). Blanchette, Smith, King, Fernandez-Penney, and Read (2002) followed a group of these children to age 7 and found normal cognitive development with only modest motor deficits.

MALTREATMENT

Nelson (1998) distinguished four types of maltreatment that children may experience. These include physical abuse (e.g., shaking, beating, or burning), sexual abuse, emotional abuse (excessive belittling or verbal attack or overt verbal rejection), and neglect (abandonment, inadequate supervision, or failure to provide food, clothing, and shelter). Children with communicative and other developmental disorders are, as Knutson and Sullivan (1993) pointed out, more likely than normally developing children to experience abuse. Fox, Long, and Anglois (1988) suggested that a child with a communication disorder may be less satisfying for a parent to care for and provide less-rewarding interactions. These difficulties might predispose a child to abuse. This suggests that SLPs should be alert to signs that parents may not be coping well with a child's disorder and provide referrals and counseling before abuse takes place. In the event that clear signs of abuse—such as repeated scars, bruises, or burns—are seen in a client, these, of course, must be reported to appropriate authorities.

Maltreatment itself also constitutes a risk for language disorder. Culp, Watkins, Lawrence, Letts, Kelly, and Rice (1991) argued that language development is particularly vulnerable in the maltreatment situation, because of the disruption in social interaction it entails. Coster, Gersten, Beeghly, and Cicchetti (1989) showed that maltreated toddlers had shorter MLUs and more limited expressive (not receptive) vocabularies during play with their mothers than peers from nonabusing homes. Both Allen and Oliver (1982) and Eigsti and Cicchetti (2004) found that preschoolers with a history of maltreatment had significantly lower language scores than peers of similar socioeconomic level, with impairments in both vocabulary and syntactic production. Lynch and Roberts (1982) showed that children with a history of maltreatment scored significantly lower on verbal IQ relative to nonverbal scores. Fox, Long, and Anglois (1988) found that maltreated children had receptive language deficits, with neglected children suffering greater lags than those shown by children who were abused.

In general, severe neglect seems to be a greater risk factor than abuse for communicative handicap (Allen & Oliver, 1982; Culp, Watkins, Lawrence, Letts, Kelly, & Rice, 1991; Pears, 2005). The few cases we know of in which children were raised in isolation, such as the famous case of "Genie," who was discovered at age 13 after years of being tied to a potty seat in a dark room with no language spoken to her (Curtiss, 1977), confirm the dire consequences of neglect. Although both language and cognition are severely impaired in such grossly neglected children, gains are made in both areas after rescue. Still, if severe neglect persists past early childhood, the prognosis for normal language development is very limited, even with intensive intervention.

The sources of risk for language and cognitive development in maltreated children can be found in several places. Abusing and neglecting mothers have been found to be less responsive to their infants (Crittenden, 1988). Babies of these mothers show insecure, avoidant, or disorganized patterns of attachment (Coster & Cicchetti, 1993), and attachment has been shown to be significantly related to language development (Gersten, Coster, Scheider-Rosen, Carlson, & Cicchetti, 1986). Crittenden (1981), Eigsti and Cicchetti (2004), and Wasserman, Green, and Allen (1983) also showed that maltreated children received more negative and rejecting communications from their mothers and less complex and stimulating language input. Few of these children's utterances exchanged information about their own internal states, and they made fewer references to events removed from the here-and-now. Coster and Cicchetti (1993) concluded that maltreated toddlers and their mothers have a language interaction style that gets things done but is not used to exchange social and affective messages. This style can cause a child problems in learning to use language (instead of hitting or pushing) to express feelings and solve problems and in sustaining cohesive narratives and dialogue over an extended round of conversational turns.

As in the case of substance abuse, sorting out the effects of maltreatment is difficult. As a result of being maltreated, children may suffer psychosocial harm that affects their communication. The maltreatment also can result in physical injury—brain damage as a result of shaking or blows to the head or malnutrition as a result of neglect—that will likewise affect communicative potential (Oates, Peacock, & Forrest, 1984). The social services initiated to stop the maltreatment, which often include removal from the family and placement in a series of foster homes, can sometimes result in poor attachment and interactive opportunities for children with a history of abuse and neglect.

Clinical Implications

Like any child with a language disorder, a client whose problem has an environmental component must qualify for services, and standardized tests of language performance will be part of the assessment to document this need. And, as in the case of any child with a language disorder, standardized tests will not tell the whole story and will need to be supplemented with structured observations and criterion-referenced procedures, as we discussed in Chapter 2. Family assessment, using some of the scales we talked about there, may be especially pertinent for children with these kinds of problems.

Intervention for communication disorders in children experiencing parental substance abuse or maltreatment must, as Sparks (1993) argued, be comprehensive and family centered. Just treating the language deficits will not address the underlying problems that these children face. Without changing parental behavior, we cannot have a significant impact on the child. Skuse (1993) pointed out that the factor most related to improvement in cases of severe abuse, like that of Genie, is not the specific type of intervention but the quality of the interactions the child develops with caregivers. It is these interactions that must be ameliorated in children who are experiencing maladaptive caretaking. We'll talk in more detail about family-centered assessment and intervention in Section II; the principles and procedures outlined there will be very useful for working with children who have language problems of environmental origin. In general, it will involve a two-pronged approach: addressing the needs of the parent and working with the parent to help improve interaction with the child.

When thinking about addressing parents' needs, we need to remember that not all children with addicted or abusive parents come from poor families and not all have the same needs. Sparks (1993) suggested starting by asking the mother what she needs and attempting to get it for her through referrals to social service agencies or model comprehensive programs. This can help the mother to feel that the clinician is on her side.

Despite the fact that parental substance abuse and maltreatment can occur at any socioeconomic level, there is an increased incidence of these problems in families who live in poverty (Trickett, Aber, Carlson, & Cicchetti, 1991). In cases in which poverty is a factor, intervention must address at least some underlying issues such as the parent's need for medical care and treatment for addiction, education, housing, a job, child care, and so on. Of course, not every program can address all these areas, but this should, at least, be the ideal. Sparks suggested that clinicians help improve the mother's literacy as part of the intervention program, since better reading and writing give the mother more opportunities for rehabilitation and employment. If a comprehensive program is not available, parental needs related to poverty must be referred to social service agencies, but the SLP can help to coordinate the requests, help the mother follow up when the response is not immediate, and generally advocate for the family.

The second prong of the intervention program entails working with parents to improve their interactions with the child. Sparks (1993) provided guidelines for this aspect of the intervention, which are outlined in Box 4-6.

You'll find additional approaches and resources for training parents to maximize their interactions with their children in the chapters on early assessment and intervention (see Chapters 6 and 7). These resources will be useful supplements to Sparks' guidelines for working with families of children experiencing parental substance abuse or maltreatment. For children from birth through 5 years, these approaches are generally the primary form of intervention, since research has shown that ameliorating the interactive environment generally leads to rapid gains in language skills in children whose disorders have an environmental component (Blager, 1979; Lewis et al., 2004).

For children of school age with a history of these experiences or who are continuing to suffer from them, problems in language and reading comprehension and in pragmatic skills appear to be the greatest risks (Blager, 1979; Fox, Long, & Anglois, 1988; Oates, Peacock, & Forrest, 1984). And, as we saw, some long-term consequences of FAS and FAE may be present in children at this age level. Both of these aspects of a child's communication disorder may be addressed directly in an intervention program by following the principles we discussed in Chapter 3 and paying particular attention to pragmatic and interactive abilities. Sparks (1993, 2001) gave some suggestions for the direct aspect of the intervention program, which are summarized in Box 4-7. Still, a family-centered, multidisci-plinary approach including parental involvement will continue to be important even at school age for children with language problems that have an environmental component.

COMMUNICATION IN PSYCHIATRIC DISORDERS

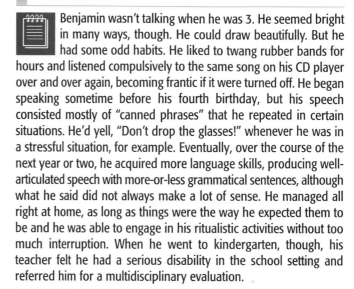

Benjamin wasn't talking when he was 3. He seemed bright in many ways, though. He could draw beautifully. But he had some odd habits. He liked to twang rubber bands for hours and listened compulsively to the same song on his CD player over and over again, becoming frantic if it were turned off. He began speaking sometime before his fourth birthday, but his speech consisted mostly of "canned phrases" that he repeated in certain situations. He'd yell, "Don't drop the glasses!" whenever he was in a stressful situation, for example. Eventually, over the course of the next year or two, he acquired more language skills, producing well-articulated speech with more-or-less grammatical sentences, although what he said did not always make a lot of sense. He managed all right at home, as long as things were the way he expected them to be and he was able to engage in his ritualistic activities without too much interruption. When he went to kindergarten, though, his teacher felt he had a serious disability in the school setting and referred him for a multidisciplinary evaluation.

Benjamin has a disorder that influences the meaning and appropriateness of his communication more strongly than it affects the form of language. Problems such as his come under the category of psychiatric disorders because the major handicap involves social and emotional aspects of communication rather than ability to use sounds, words, and sentences in and of themselves. Let's look at two types of psychiatric disorders and their impact on communication: behavioral-socioemotional disorders and pervasive developmental disorders, or ASD.

| **BOX 4-6** | **Guidelines for Intervention in Caregiver-Child Interaction for Children with a History of Parental Substance Abuse or Maltreatment** |

- Listen to parents about their needs and goals for the child.
- Provide education about child development and the physical and psychological needs of children.
- Attempt to get as much togetherness between mother and child as the mother's rehabilitation will allow. Attachment can only evolve when the mother is with the child.
- Observe some good points of the mother-child interaction, and point them out to the mother and to others. Make her feel good about her parenting skills.
- Organize play groups in which mothers' positive behaviors are pointed out as good examples. Attribute positive intentions even when they may not be there; for example, tell a mother who shifted the child on her lap into a face-to-face position just to get more comfortable, "Look, Maria moved Max so she could see his face. See how happy Max looks now!"
- Use videotaping to point out positive mother-child interactions, and show them repeatedly to the parent or group.
- Provide model strategies for play and talking with children, such as reciting nursery rhymes, finger plays, and songs.
- Set up respite child care so parents can get a break from caretaking.
- Work with parents to maximize child attendance at preschool or intervention.

Adapted from Sparks, S. (1993). *Children of prenatal substance abuse.* San Diego, CA: Singular Publishing Group.

| **BOX 4-7** | **Suggestions for Direct Intervention with Children with a History of Maternal Substance Abuse or Maltreatment** |

Infants

- Be sure interactions take place when the child is in a quiet, alert state (see Chapter 6). Help parents learn to recognize this state.
- Use swaddling and pacifier to help quiet the baby.
- Help parents understand that the child may have digestive difficulties as a result of their exposure to drugs. Explain that this may make the baby irritable to prevent the parent from displaying negative reactions to the child's difficulties.
- Infants with prenatal drug exposure may sleep for long periods. Be sure the child is wakened for feedings, if necessary, to ensure adequate nutrition.

Children

- Monitor child's health and development carefully.
- Organize the learning environment to minimize distractions.
- Make routines predictable and repetitive.
- Help children develop self-regulation and attention skills; teach them to use language to regulate their own actions.
- Keep groups small, work collaboratively with others.
- Include structured play activities to encourage interaction and pragmatic development (see guidelines in Chapter 9).
- Use language instead of punishment to control problem behaviors; provide clear and immediate consequences for inappropriate behavior.
- Emphasize functional communication skills.
- Establish a small number of clearly stated rules.
- Use approaches that focus on narrative skills (see Chapters 9 and 12) and pragmatic abilities (see Chapters 9, 12, and 14), and develop receptive abilities in both oral and written language (see Chapters 12 and 14).
- Build caregiver confidence, trust, and attachment.

Adapted from Sparks, S. (2001). Prenatal substance use and its impact on young children. In T. Layton, E. Crais, & L. Watson, (Eds.), *Handbook of early language impairment in children: Nature* (pp. 451-487). Albany, NY: Delmar Publishers; Sparks, S. (1993). *Children of prenatal substance abuse.* San Diego, CA: Singular Publishing Group.

BEHAVIORAL-SOCIOEMOTIONAL DISORDERS

Disorders of behavioral and emotional development fall on that fuzzy boundary line between problems that have a clear environmental origin (such as those resulting from parental neglect) and those that have a biological basis. Andreasen (1984) suggested that most psychiatric disorders serious enough to be diagnosed have some form of neurological component. As we learn more about the relationships between the brain and behavior we may be in a better position to tease out the effects of biology and environment in behavioral and socioemotional disorders.

One thing that is known about these disorders is that there is a very high coincidence with communicative problems. Benner, Nelson, and Epstein (2002) found, in a meta-analysis, that over 70% of children diagnosed with emotional-behavioral disorders (EBD) had clinically significant language deficits. The deficits were broad-based and included expressive, receptive, and pragmatic aspects of language. This finding has been confirmed in studies of bilingual children, as well (Toppelberg, Medrano, Pena Morgens, & Nieto-Castanon, 2002). In addition, over 50% of children diagnosed with language deficits also had diagnosable EBD. Further, the number of children who

have both communicative and behavioral-socioemotional disorders increases as children with language disorders get older (Baltaxe, 2001; Benner et al., 2002). These findings shouldn't really be a surprise, because everything we know about communication development emphasizes the interrelationships among language, communication, and social and emotional development. Brinton and Fujiki (2005) discuss the issues involved in providing for the needs of these children. Sadly, children with these overlapping disorders often do not receive the comprehensive services they need (Benner et al., 2002; Gallagher, 1999). As SLPs we need to become familiar with what these comprehensive needs are and how we might begin to meet them. Let's look at the major categories of behavioral-socioemotional disorders and see how each might affect communication. Then we'll talk about how socioemotional and behavioral considerations can be included in the program for children with primary communication disorders who are, as we've seen, at risk for behavioral-socioemotional involvement.

Conduct and Oppositional Disorders

Conduct and oppositional disorders involve aggressive and sociopathic behavior, such as fighting; defiance of adults; persistent negative, hostile behavior patterns; truancy; stealing; vandalism; cruelty to people and animals; and so on. Baltaxe (2001), Giddan (1991), and Gilmour, Hill, Place, and Skuse (2004) showed that between one and two thirds of children referred for conduct disorders had concomitant speech and language difficulties. Cohen, Barwick, Horodezky, and Isaacson (1996) and Gilmour et al. (2004) found these disorders to be particularly related to receptive language and pragmatic difficulties. As Prizant, Audet, Burke, Hummel, Maher, and Theadore (1990) showed, many youngsters with these disorders have speech and language problems that may have gone unidentified for some time. Children with these disorders should be screened for communicative skills. If deficits are identified, a focused program that addresses both language and social and emotional communication skills should be part of the intervention program.

Attention Deficit/Hyperactivity Disorders

The most common and fastest-growing disability category in school-age children is attention deficit/hyperactivity disorder (ADHD; Damico, Tetnowski, & Nettleton, 2004). According to the *Diagnostic and Statistical Manual, Fourth Edition* of the American Psychiatric Association (APA; 1994), this disorder involves three components: excessive inattention, overactivity, and impulsivity. More recent research (Giddan & Milling, 2001) suggests, though, that there are really only two, rather than three, primary dimensions of the disorder: inattention and overactivity/impulsivity. When ADHD is primarily of the inattentive type, problems with poor attention and concentration, distractibility, poor organizational skills, and difficulty in completing tasks without close supervision occur. Barkley (1995) uses the concept of "behavioral disinhibition" to characterize the second dimension of overactivity/impulsivity. He argued that this aspect consists primarily of deficiencies in the regulation and inhibition of behavior. Put another way, we can say that children with this type of ADHD are deficient in the ability to "stop and think" before acting. These children tend to be restless and fidgety, to run, climb, and talk excessively, although they often convey little information, despite their verbiage. Westby and Watson (2004) report that ADHD is now viewed as a condition with primary deficits in *executive functions* (the ability to regulate feelings and behaviors necessary to select and guide actions in the context of rules and goals) and *working memory*, which is necessary for holding information in mind long enough to construct, maintain, and update mental representations so they can be used to recall facts, draw inferences, and plan responses.

These disorders appear to be present very commonly in conjunction with a variety of other developmental disabilities, including fragile X syndrome, ASD, learning disabilities, and specific language impairment (Tetnowski, 2004). In fact, comorbidity of ADHD with certain developmental disabilities is so high that some researchers have argued that the conditions are not really distinct but part of the same syndrome. Shaywitz, Fletcher, and Shaywitz (1995), for example, suggested that there is a specific subtype of ADHD, which they call "cognitive inattentive," that is characterized by significant academic underachievement with linguistic skill deficits. They believe this subtype coexists or is perhaps synonymous with language-learning disorders.

Diagnosing ADHD is a difficult business because of a lack of objective criteria for establishing either poor attention or excessive activity/impulsivity, especially in young children. Rapoport and Ismond (1984) reported that a large proportion of children with ADHD show "soft neurological signs," such as difficulty moving the fingers of one hand while keeping those on the other still or being unable to stand on one foot without falling. These signs are neither specific to ADHD nor diagnostic of it, though. Another diagnostic problem is that the condition can be so context dependent. Many children with ADHD can show normal attention in highly motivating situations, such as playing a video game. Barkley (1990) speculated that these children have lower levels of internal motivation than normal and are less able to derive reinforcement from routine activities. Sometimes children are considered to have attention and activity problems in school, whereas at home, their behavior (whether it is similar or different from their behavior in school) is considered acceptable. Often, attention and activity problems are not diagnosed until the child reaches school age. Does that mean the child has a problem that wasn't recognized before, or that it is the child's interface with the school context that is creating a problem that did not previously exist? Some researchers (e.g., Damico, Augustine, & Hayes, 1996; Damico, Damico, & Armstrong, 1999; Damico, Muller, & Ball, 2004; Nelson & Hawley, 2004; Weaver, 1993) suggest that ADHD is really part of a system of the child within the environment. In this model, similar to the systems model we discussed in Chapter 1, the problem is not so much "in" the child as it is in the interaction of the child's level of attention and activity with the specific home and school environments in which he or she must function.

Chan, Hopkins, Perrin, Herrerias, and Homer (2005) report in a survey of primary care physicians that diagnostic practices for school-aged children with ADHD varied widely, especially with respect to use of *Diagnostic and Statistical Manual of Mental Disorders* diagnostic criteria and whether or not ADHD-specific diagnostic instruments were used. Physicians reported using a range of tools including teacher or school information such as report cards and rating scales, ADHD-specific rating scales, and global behavior scales. The *Child Behavior Checklist* (Achenbach, 1991) is perhaps the most commonly used behavior scale and provides a particularly well-constructed and well-normed measure of ADHD symptoms. Standardized measures of cognitive functioning may be used to establish a discrepancy between achievement and intelligence, but they do not make or rule out a diagnosis of ADHD. Instead, neuropsychological tests are usually used to assess specific cognitive and attentional functions. The most helpful type of neuropsychological measure appears to be the Continuous Performance measure, which examines vigilance by having the child press a button each time a particular stimulus appears. The *Gordon Diagnostic System* (Gordon, 1983) has adequate psychometric and normative properties for this purpose. Both these tests require specific computerized equipment for administration and are usually only available in specialized diagnostic/research centers.

Medical evaluation is always important in the diagnostic process to rule out other conditions that mimic the symptoms of ADHD, such as high blood pressure, cardiac disorders, or tic syndromes (Chan et al., 2005; Giddan & Milling, 2001). Attempts are being made to find more physiological methods of diagnosing ADHD. Smith, Johnstone, and Barry (2003), for example, report that evoked potentials provided some help in assigning the diagnosis in children aged 8 to 12, but were less useful for younger and older children. Even in this age range, overall classification accuracy was only 70%. For the present, it appears that behavioral observations, ratings, and neuropsychological assessment will remain necessary for making this diagnosis. Of course, thorough communication assessment also is crucial to understanding the child with ADHD. This is because so many of the manifestations of this disorder are in the social/communicative domain and because it is easy to overlook linguistic deficits that might underlie the more obvious learning and behavior problems of these children. Damico, Tetnowski, and Nettleton (2004) point out that much of the self-regulation and inhibition that are absent in ADHD normally take place through the medium of internalized language. Given this insight, it would appear that SLPs have much to contribute in assisting these children to develop the executive functions they lack by working on guiding their internalization of language with prompts first provided externally.

Voeller (2004), in reviewing treatment of ADHD, reports that optimal treatment requires both medical and behavioral intervention. According to Blum and Mercugliano (2002), Fabiano and Pelham (2002), and Pelham (2002), behavior management combined with carefully monitored pharmacological treatment provides the most effective approach to improving behavior in children with ADHD. Behavioral techniques include positive reinforcement, such as tokens to collect for tangible rewards; response cost, such as loss of accumulated tokens for undesirable behaviors; and time-out, or removing access to social interactions as a punishment for inappropriate behavior (Barkley, 1995). Alternatives to the behavioral approach can include cognitive-behavioral strategies such as self-monitoring, self-reinforcement, and self-instruction, as well as other meta-linguistic and meta-cognitive activities, such as Think-alouds, and Directed Reading-Thinking Activities (Damico & Armstrong, 1996; Damico, Damico, & Armstrong, 1999) (see also Chapters 12 and 14). However, Giddan and Milling (2001) point out that although both behavioral and cognitive-behavioral approaches are effective, they do not usually generalize to spontaneous use, and the student with ADHD may continue to need guidance in using them.

The most common classes of medication used to treat children with ADHD are stimulants such as methylphenidate (Ritalin), dextroamphetamine (Dexedrine), Adderall, and pemoline (Cylert). Antidepressants, clonidine, and phenothiazines also are occasionally used, but these have been found to be less effective and to have more common and more worrisome side effects than the stimulants. Newer medications, including selective serotonin reuptake inhibitors (SSRIs) such as fluoxetine (Prozac), also may have a role in the treatment of ADHD

(Batshaw, 2002). Stimulant medications have very beneficial effects for some, though not all, children with ADHD (Lahey, Carlson, & Frick, 1992). They mainly increase attention and decrease motor activity and impulsiveness, although they do not affect learning disorders or self-image directly. Despite their demonstrated safety and effectiveness, many are concerned about the wide-spread use of medication to treat so common a childhood disorder, particularly as its diagnosis, and therefore its treatment with medication, increasingly extends into the preschool period (Damico, Tetnowski, & Nettleton, 2004). There are also newer, nonstimulant drugs emerging for the treatment of ADHD. One example is atomoxetine (Strattera), which has also been shown to be safe and effective in children (Weiss, Tannock, Kratochvil, Dunn, Velez-Borras, Thomason, Tamura, Kelsey, Stevens, & Allen, 2005). Although there is some concern that medication is overused, particularly with young children, these treatments are clearly helpful in overcoming attention and activity problems and in improving school performance. Their use must be carefully monitored, though, to ensure that they are providing significant benefits. The SLP may be involved in monitoring the behavior and attention of children using these medications, as well as assessing their effect on language and communication skills. These observations can be helpful in making the best choice of medication and dosage (Giddan & Milling, 1999). As we've seen, however, the most effective intervention programs combine behavioral, educational, and pharmacological treatments (Batshaw, 2002; Voeller, 2004).

Children receiving language intervention who also have attention and activity disorders need to have these behavioral and educational interventions built into the communication program. Damico and Armstrong (1996), Damico, Damico, and Armstrong (1999), Dunaway (2004), Giddan (1991), Heyer (1995), and Maag and Reid (1996) have suggested intervention strategies for SLPs to use in providing communication intervention for children with ADHD. These are summarized in Box 4-8.

Anxiety and Affective Disorders

These problems involve depression; inordinate difficulties in separation; and avoidant disorders, such as excessive fear in social settings, or excessive anxiety about performance in social settings, school, or sports, or about appearance or health. Many children with primary diagnoses of ASD and selective mutism also exhibit anxiety and affect disorders. Communication in primary affect and anxiety disorders may be affected in a variety of ways, and some children with these disorders fail speech and language screenings, as Benner, Nelson, and Epstein (2002) and Prizant et al. (1990) reported. Intervention for children with these problems who have documented speech or language deficits should incorporate socioemotional contexts. Giddan (1991) suggested encouraging and reinforcing these clients for the smallest approximation of participation. It is especially important to make sure that these children see themselves as "succeeding" within the intervention setting.

An SLP also may be asked to consult on the social-communicative aspects of psychotherapy for some of these youngsters. When this occurs, we can make several helpful

| **BOX 4-8** | **Suggestions for Communication Intervention for Children with ADHD** |

In Language Intervention Sessions

1. Begin intervention only after medication, if used, has taken effect.
2. Schedule frequent, short sessions.
3. Give personalized individual attention.
4. Remain calm, steady, and consistent, avoiding matching the frenzied pace of the client with ADHD.
5. Use highly structured tasks with lots of physical involvement in holding, placing, or moving things.
6. Reinforcement should be rapid, and there should be frequent shifts in activities.
7. Encourage making choices within the intervention program, eventually allowing the client to choose and arrange the sequence of four or five activities within a session.
8. Use sessions to develop self-talk, analyze classroom discourse rules, role-play difficult situations, encourage use of graphic organizers.
9. Target social-pragmatic and more traditional speech and language goals, such as the following:
   • Good listening skills; i.e., looking at the speaker, repeating what was heard to check comprehension
   • Waiting until an entire question is asked before answering
   • Looking for cues as to when it is appropriate to take a conversational turn
   • Learning not to interrupt or intrude in conversations
   • Complimenting others rather than criticizing or complaining
   • Learning strategies for persuasion
   • Practicing empathy and "putting oneself in another's shoes"

In Classroom Consultation and Collaboration

1. Teach self-talk for modulating activity. For example, have the clients tell themselves, "I need to stay here until I finish my work."
2. Have the child keep a journal or planner to organize time, predict a schedule, and record assignments.
3. Encourage students to tape record class sessions for later study. Help teachers break down information into smaller units.
4. Provide classroom materials modified for the client with fewer examples per page, fewer repetitions.
5. Help teacher identify environmental triggers for inappropriate behavior; find ways to modify the environment to eliminate triggers.
6. Encourage teachers to remove time limits to allow students to perform optimally in testing situations.
7. Use cooperative learning and peer tutoring to induce and reinforce learning.
8. Create a structured, predictable environment in the classroom with picture schedules, redundant instructions, opportunities for peer group re-teaching.

Adapted from Damico, S., & Armstrong, M. (1996). Intervention strategies for students with ADHD: Creating a holistic approach. *Seminars in Speech and Language, 17,* 21-36; Damico, J., Damico, S., & Armstrong, M. (1999). Attention-deficit hyperactivity disorder and communication disorders: Issues and clinical practices. In R. Paul (Ed.), *Child and adolescent psychiatric clinics of North America* (pp. 37-60). Philadelphia, PA: W.B. Saunders; Dunaway, C. (2004). Attention deficit hyperactivity disorder: An authentic story in the schools and its implications. *Seminars in Speech and Language, 25,* 271-285; Giddan, J., & Milling, L. (1999). Comorbidity of psychiatric and communication disorders in children. In. R. Paul (Ed.), *Child and adolescent psychiatric clinics of North America* (pp. 19-36). Philadelphia, PA: W.B. Saunders; Heyer, J. (1995). The responsibilities of speech-language pathologists toward children with ADHD. *Seminars in Speech and Language, 16,* 275-288; Maag, J., & Reid, R. (1996). Treatment of attention deficit hyperactivity disorder: A multi-modal model for schools. *Seminars in Speech and Language, 17,* 37-58.

contributions. We can encourage therapists to develop emotional and empathic vocabulary; to provide opportunities for the children to engage in extended discourse in the therapy setting; and to role-play difficult communication situations, such as asking a teacher a question or asking a peer to play. Empathic development also can be encouraged in psychotherapy through pretend play, with dolls as the objects of empathic communication at first. We also can suggest that therapists provide simple, formulaic verbal means of expressing fears and anxiety and encourage children to learn to regulate their own and others' behavior with language rather than maladaptive actions.

Selective Mutism

The SLP is often the first professional consulted when a child is not speaking in school. A refusal to talk in certain situations, when the child is known to understand and use language in others, is known as *selective mutism*. *DSM-IV* (APA, 1994) defines selective mutism as a persistent refusal to talk in one or more major social situations, including school, despite the ability to comprehend and use spoken language. Selective mutism often occurs in conjunction with anxiety disorders and is usually seen as a psychiatric or emotional disorder, rather than a developmental disability (Black & Uhde, 1995; McInnes & Manassis, 2005). The problem has been recognized for at least a century (Kussmaul, 1877) and is relatively rare, with prevalence rates of 0.3 to 0.8 per 1000 (*DSM-IV*, APA, 1994). Selective mutism is most often seen in school settings, where the child refuses to speak despite being verbal at home. Cultural and linguistic differences (CLDs) can exacerbate the problem, especially when the child has limited English proficiency (LEP) and feels uncomfortable using the language of the classroom (Elizur & Perednik, 2003; Giddan, Ross, Sechler, & Becker, 1997). Although most CLD children eventually overcome their reluctance to talk in school, some, as well as up to 50% of monolingual English speakers who experience selective mutism along with other kinds of school-related anxiety, remain selectively mute for extended periods of time (McInnes, Fung, Manassis, Fiksenbaum, & Tannock, 2004).

To qualify for this diagnosis, the disturbance must last for at least 1 month other than the first month of school and must not be better explained by some other communication disorder, such as hearing impairment, stuttering, or ASD. The condition shows a 2:1 ratio in favor of girls (McInnes et al., 2004). Despite the fact that children with this diagnosis must be known to have the ability to use language in some situations, a high incidence of speech and language difficulties has been reported in this population. Seventy-five percent of selectively mute children have been found to have articulation disorders and expressive language problems; 60% show significant deficits in receptive language (Giddan et al., 1997; Kolvin & Fundudis, 1981). Although nonverbal cognition and receptive language can be assessed using nonspoken modalities, assessing expressive language skills in these children is a special challenge. McInnes et al. (2004) suggest asking parents to collect a narrative sample on audiotape in order to assess spontaneous speech.

Although selective mutism is seen primarily as an anxiety disorder, the SLP often is called upon to develop a treatment program. This is due to the disorder's frequent co-occurrence with other speech and language problems (McInnes & Manassis, 2005) and the fact that the SLP is considered to be the member of the team of school professionals who deals with problems in talking. The team usually includes a psychologist, pediatrician, or child psychiatrist; classroom teacher; parents; and the SLP (Giddan et al., 1997). Several recent reports have given examples of effective intervention strategies implemented by SLPs to deal with selective mutism. Thompson (quoted in Banotai, 2005) cautions that we should not try to force the child to talk; instead the child should be provided with inviting, tempting opportunities to interact with familiar peers, first in small, safe environments within the school setting before attempting speech in classroom or other public environments. McInnes and Manassis (2005) argued that intervention should take into account the child's social anxiety and begin

by encouraging children to answer simple, factual questions (What color is this?) and avoiding questions that require any self-disclosure (What is your favorite color?). They also suggest starting with private interactions, at first including a parent or someone the child does talk to, before attempting public speech. Techniques that have been used successfully with this population are summarized in Box 4-9. In addition to implementing these techniques to address the child's silence, the SLP also should address any receptive language problems identified in the assessment. Once speech has been established, any articulation and expressive language difficulties that are present should be added to the intervention program. Drug treatment with antidepressant medication is sometimes considered when behavioral interventions prove ineffective (Harris, 1996).

AUTISM SPECTRUM DISORDERS

Previously called pervasive developmental disorders (PPDs), autism spectrum disorders (ASD) are psychiatric conditions that have a more clearly established neurological base than do the behavioral and socioemotional disorders we were just discussing. ASD represent a spectrum of difficulties in socialization, communication, and behavior. Box 4-10 gives a brief description of each of the disorders identified within this spectrum.

Like many other developmental disabilities, ASD, which involves more than language disorders alone, require a multidisciplinary team for its identification. In addition to documenting communicative disorders, the team needs to document a significant deficit in social skills, imaginative behavior, and stereotypical or ritualistic behaviors. Research teams often use a structured observational format called the *Autism Diagnostic Observation Schedule (ADOS)* (Lord, Risi, Lambrecht, Cook, Leventhal, DiLavore, Pickles, & Rutter, 2000) that provides opportunities for the client to demonstrate social overtures, play, joint attention, imitation, requesting, reciprocity, and nonverbal communicative behavior. The *Autism Diagnostic Interview (ADI)* (Lord, Rutter, & LeCouteur, 1994) looks at similar behaviors through a parent interview. In clinical settings, the most widely used instrument is the *Childhood Autism Rating Scale (CARS)* (Schopler, Reichler, & Renner, 1993), which contains just 15 items (on social relations, communication, sensory functioning, emotional reactions, and resistance to change), each of which is rated on a scale from 1 to 4. This instrument, though brief, has been shown to have high reliability and validity as a diagnostic tool (Schopler et al., 1993).

Although you may have heard the term *infantile ASD*, we now know that ASD is a lifelong disability in more than 95% of people diagnosed with the syndrome (Grandin, 1997; Howlin, 2005). Kanner (1943), who first described the autistic syndrome, suggested it was associated with cold parents, but a wealth of recent research has established that parents of children with ASD are not different than parents of other children with disabilities and that this disorder clearly has biological roots (Anderson & Hoshino, 2005; Volkmar, Carter, Grossman, &

| **BOX 4-9** | **Strategies for Intervening with Selective Mutism** |

Step 1: Elicit responses in a one-to-one setting with the SLP. Accept nonverbal means, such as writing, gestures, head nods, drawing, and pantomime.

Step 2: Discuss with the client how hard he or she finds it to talk. Let the client listen as the clinician discusses that talking is sometimes easy and sometimes harder. Let the child use nonverbal means to participate in this discussion.

Step 3: Give communication "homework assignment" cards that the child must complete and return with signatures to the SLP. At first, these can include tasks that the client already can do easily, such as talking to Mother at home. Later, they can include progressively more difficult tasks, such as talking to a relative on the telephone.

Step 4: Have the client make audiotapes to play for the clinician. At first the child can sing a song with a parent on the tape. Later the client can read or tell a story or convey a message. At first the clinician listens to these when the child is not present and comments on them in the session. Later, the clinician can ask permission to play them in the child's presence.

Step 5: Encourage the child to whisper, mouth, or use a puppet to communicate with the clinician. At first have the child produce rote language, such as counting to 10 or naming colors. Encourage increased eye contact during these activities.

Step 6: Encourage other kinds of vocalization, such as playing a kazoo, making animal sounds, or coughing. The clinician and client can sit back-to-back. The clinician can ask the child to whisper or vocalize more loudly so the response can be heard.

Step 7: Use barrier games in which the client and clinician take turns creating patterns with shapes that the other must reproduce without seeing. Have the child whisper an instruction, and encourage louder speech so the clinician can clearly understand what needs to be done.

Set 8: Have the child choose a favorite game and teach the rules to the clinician. Have the child reiterate the rules throughout the game, telling the client that the clinician has forgotten and needs to be reminded for the game to continue. BE SURE TO LET THE CLIENT WIN.

Step 9: Repeat steps 5, 6, 7, and 8 with the child's psychotherapist, peer, or teacher in a private setting.

Step 10: Encourage the child to speak in a soft voice in group or classroom situations. Provide rewards for raising the hand, participating nonverbally, and writing notes at first. Gradually shape these responses to whispering, soft speech, and full voice.

Adapted from Furst, A.L. (1989). Elective mutism: Report of a case successfully treated by a family doctor. *Israel Journal of Psychiatry and Related Science, 26,* 96-102; Giddan, J., Ross, G., Sechler, L., & Becker, B. (1997). Selective mutism in elementary school: Multidisciplinary interventions. *Language, Speech, and Hearing Services in Schools, 28,* 127-133; Harris, F. (1996). Elective mutism: A tutorial. *Language, Speech, and Hearing Services in Schools, 27,* 10-15; Weise, M. (June, 1998). A case study in the treatment of elective mutism. Poster presented at the Symposium of Research in Child Language Disorders. Madison, WI.

| **BOX 4-10** | **Autism Spectrum Disorders** |

1. Autism

 A. Qualitative impairment in social interaction (at least two of the following):

  1. Markedly impaired nonverbal behaviors, such as gaze, postures, and gestures to regulate communication.

  2. Lack of social or emotional reciprocity.

  3. Failure to engage others in enjoyments and interests.

  4. Failure to develop appropriate peer relationships.

  5. Lack of social or emotional reciprocity.

 B. Qualitative impairment in communication (at least 1 of the following):

  1. Delay or absence of spoken language not accompanied by an attempt to compensate with other forms of communication.

  2. Marked impairment in the ability to initiate and sustain conversation when speech is present.

  3. Stereotyped and repetitive use of language or idiosyncratic language.

  4. Lack of varied and appropriate imitative or pretend play.

 C. Restricted patterns of behavior, interest, and activities (at least 1 of the following):

  1. Insistence on sameness; inflexible adherence to nonfunctional routines or rituals.

  2. Persistent preoccupations, especially with parts of objects, such as the wheels of a toy car.

  3. Stereotyped or repetitive motor mannerisms, such as rocking or hand-flapping.

  4. Preoccupation with stereotyped or ritual patterns of interest.

 D. Delays or abnormal functioning before age 3 in social development, language used for social communication, or play; not better accounted for by Rett's disorder or childhood disintegrative disorder.

BOX 4-10   Autism Spectrum Disorders—cont'd

2. Asperger's Syndrome

A. Qualitative impairment in social interaction (at least one of the following):
  1. Markedly impaired nonverbal behaviors, such as gaze, postures, and gestures to regulate communication.
  2. Lack of social or emotional reciprocity.
  3. Failure to engage others in enjoyments and interests.
  4. Failure to develop appropriate peer relationships.
  5. Lack of social or emotional reciprocity.
B. No clinically significant delay in language or cognitive development.
C. Restricted patterns of behavior, interest, and activities (at least one of the following):
  1. Insistence on sameness; inflexible adherence to nonfunctional routines or rituals.
  2. Persistent preoccupations, especially with parts of objects, such as the wheels of a toy car.
  3. Stereotyped or repetitive motor mannerisms, such as rocking or hand-flapping.
  4. Preoccupation with stereotyped or ritual patterns of interest.

3. Rett's Disorder

A. Apparently normal development and head circumference during the first 5 months of life.
B. Onset of all of the following after at least 5 months of normal development:
  1. Deceleration of head growth
  2. Loss of purposeful hand movements and development of stereotyped movements
  3. Loss of social engagement
  4. Poorly coordinated gait and trunk movements
  5. Severely impaired language and cognitive development

4. Childhood Disintegrative Disorder

A. Apparently normal development for the first 2 years, with age-appropriate communication and social, adaptive, and play behavior.
B. Significant loss of previously acquired skills before 10 years of age in the following areas:
  1. Communication
  2. Social or adaptive skills
  3. Bowel or bladder control
  4. Play
  5. Motor skills
C. Abnormal functioning in the following areas (at least two):
  1. Qualitative impairment in social interaction
  2. Qualitative impairment in communication
  3. Restricted, repetitive and stereotyped patterns of behavior, interests, and activities, including motor stereotypes

5. PDD-NOS

A. Severe and pervasive impairment in social interaction and communication or stereotyped behavior, interests, and activities are present, but criteria for other specified PDDs are not met.
B. May include late onset, atypical symptoms, or subthreshold symptoms.

Adapted from American Psychiatric Association (1994). *Diagnostic and statistical manual of mental disorders* (ed. 4). Washington, DC: American Psychiatric Association.

Klin, 1997). A variety of neurophysiological correlates have been observed in children with ASD, including abnormal cellular organization in the limbic system and cerebellar areas of the brain, elevated levels of the neurotransmitter serotonin, and larger-than-normal head circumference and brain size (Minshew, Sweeney, Bauman, & Webb, 2005). Recent imaging studies (Minshew, Sweeney, Bauman, & Webb, 2005; Schultz & Robins, 2005) suggest increased volume in several areas of the cortex—but not the frontal lobes, corpus callosum, or hippocampus—as well as altered activations of brain regions during tasks such as looking at faces, listening to speech, and watching social scenes. Reduced connectivity of brain regions that are related in people with typical development has also been reported (Just, Cherkassky, Keller, & Minshew, 2004). Genetic factors also have been shown to play a major role in the causation of ASD, although genetic mechanisms are not yet clear (Rutter, 2005).

Social, Affective, and Cognitive Development in ASD

It is important to recognize that the majority of children with ASD also have MR. Tager-Flusberg, Paul, and Lord (2005) reported that 80% of children with ASD function in the MR range on intelligence and adaptive behavior measures. Although people with ASD sometimes have "splinter skills" (unusually high levels of ability in one or two areas, such as drawing, mathematics, or music), these skills do not decrease the validity of IQ scores (DeMyer, Hingten, & Jackson, 1981), and children with low IQs tend to have less favorable outcomes in adulthood than children who score higher on these tests (Howlin, 2005).

Although children with ASD are often described as "untestable," DeMyer, Barton, and Norton (1972) have shown convincingly that every autistic child can be tested and a mental age profile constructed, when easy items are presented first and tangible reinforcement is given. We talked about the issue of the "hard-to-test" child in Chapter 2, and everything discussed there applies to clients with ASD. No child should be denied an in-depth assessment of communicative skills simply because of a presumed diagnosis.

Some of the most interesting findings in studies of cognition in ASD concern what people with ASD *can* do, rather than what they cannot do. Sigman, Dissanayake, Arbelle, and Ruskin (1997) report that ASD is not associated with deficits in discrimination or short-term memory; in fact, subjects with ASD often perform better on these tasks than do matched controls. People with ASD often perform above normal, too, on tasks involving identifying small differences between stimuli. However, children with ASD do show differences in sensory processing abilities. They are overly responsive to some stimuli, becoming excessively excited or upset in response to a noise or bright light (Ritvo, 1976; Tsatsanis, 2005). They can, at the same time, be undersensitive to other stimuli, failing to respond when spoken to, for example. Neuropsychological studies (Tsatsanis, 2005) show intact memory, visuospatial, and sensoriperceptual abilities, as well as single-modality problem solving. Difficulties are seen in the ability to transfer information across sensory modalities and to solve complex tasks involving multiple domains of information processing. Dawson (1996) reported difficulties in selective attention, orienting, and shifting attention that may be related to some of these differences.

Another important piece of this picture, though, is the contribution of social skills to the ability to solve cognitive problems. Hobson (2005) reported that children with ASD show deficits in the ability to recognize facial expressions and imitate others' actions, particularly others' expression of emotions. These children do themselves express emotions and form attachments, but the quality of their attachment is often unusual and their emotional expression somewhat impoverished.

Lack of eye contact is often imputed to people with ASD, but Watson and Ozanoff (2001) report that these children do not differ from peers in terms of frequency of duration of gaze. They are, though, less likely to combine eye contact with a smile and do not use gaze to regulate joint attention.

"Social cognition" entails understanding how other people think and feel, as opposed to what they look like and do. Conceiving of other people's mental states, or having a "theory of mind" as Baron-Cohen (1995) called it, is another deficit in ASD (Carter, Davis, Klin, & Volkmar, 2005). It leads to problems in guessing what other people know; in inferring other people's beliefs; and in understanding psychological causality, or what makes people act as they do (Negri, 1992). These deficits contribute to making social interactions incomprehensible to people with ASD. When they cannot figure out other people's motivations and intentions, others' actions make little sense or seem unpredictable.

Social deficits form the core of the autistic syndrome. As young children, these clients tend to spend much of their time in solitary activity and often fail to respond to others. Some may avoid social contact; others may passively accept interaction but rarely initiate it. Older children with ASD may be interested in social interactions but have difficulty participating successfully; they may be socially "active but odd" (Wing & Gould, 1979).

ASD and Communication

Like the other psychiatric disorders we've been talking about in this section, ASD is a disorder primarily of communication rather than of language. We see this clearly in the major criteria for the disorder, which refer to impaired social functioning, communication, and delay or deviance in early engagement in social communication and play. Even the obsessive behaviors seen in the syndrome relate to communication. For example, obsessive interests are often expressed through compulsive talk about preoccupying topics and an inability to switch topics from these areas in conversation. Although certain language characteristics are associated with ASD, what distinguishes it from more specific language disabilities is its impact on communicative competence, over and above more specific linguistic deficits. Let's look at the language and communication characteristics that are "typical" of ASD, remembering that every child with ASD is different, just as every normally developing child is.

From early in development, children with ASD show differences in intentional communication. Chawarska and Volkmar (2005) note that two major differences are seen in 1-year-olds later diagnosed with ASD: a lack of joint attentional behavior and an abnormal response to human faces and voices. These babies use gestures to show and point less often than language-matched controls, although they do use gestures to request, protest, and regulate others' behavior (Tager-Flusberg, 1995). In general, they do not communicate in order to share focus as normal infants do but only to express wants and needs (Wetherby, Woods, Allen, Cleary, Dickinson, & Lord, 2004). Some children with ASD do not develop speech, although the proportion who do not is declining as earlier identification and intervention is being implemented (Paul, Chawarska,

Klin, & Volkmar, 2006; Rogers, 2006). When speech is absent, it is not spontaneously replaced by communicative gestures, as it is in children with HI, for example. Furthermore, children with ASD may develop maladaptive means for expressing requests and protests. They may begin head-banging, for example, to express rejection of an activity. In children with ASD who do develop speech, some expansion of communicative intentions occurs, along with an elaboration of more socially acceptable means of communicating (Tager-Flusberg et al., 2005).

Children with ASD begin speaking late and develop speech at a significantly slower rate than other children (Tager-Flusberg et al., 2005). About 25% of children with ASD appear to acquire a few words by 12 or 18 months, and then lose them or fail to acquire more (Lord, Shulman, & DiLavore, 2004). When children with ASD begin talking, aspects of language form, including phonology, syntax, and morphology, are relatively spared. These children generally show skills in language form that are at or close to those of mental-age mates (Tager-Flusberg et al., 2005), although a subgroup of children with ASD show deficits in language form that are similar to those of children with specific language impairment (Tager-Flusberg & Joseph, 2003). Vocabulary skills also are usually on par with developmental level. Meaning and pragmatic aspects are disproportionately impaired, though (Tager-Flusberg, 1995). When they talk, children with ASD show sparse verbal expression and a lack of spontaneity. They have trouble adapting what they say to the needs and status of the listener, distinguishing given from new information, following politeness rules, making relevant comments, maintaining topics outside their own obsessive interests, and giving listeners their fair share of conversational turns (Tager-Flusberg et al., 2005).

Children with ASD may use nonreciprocal speech—that is, speech not directed or responsive to others (Dewey & Everard, 1974). The classic example is from Kanner (1943). He told the story of his autistic client who would scream, "Don't throw the dog off the balcony" at odd times. The remark was incomprehensible until the boy's parents explained that he had once been told not to throw a toy dog off the balcony of a hotel in which the family was staying. Ever after this event, he used the statement as an admonition to himself when he had an impulse to do something he shouldn't do. This use of language that is "stuck" in its original context and cannot be interpreted with only the knowledge that is normally shared among conversational partners is a classic characteristic of autistic communication. Similarly, speaking children with ASD show extreme literalness in their use of language (Tager-Flusberg et al., 2005). They have trouble accepting that words can have synonyms or multiple meanings or that there can be different interpretations of the same utterance in contexts such as jokes (e.g., What do you call an overheated puppy? A *hot dog*.)

Another classic characteristic of autistic language is echolalia, either immediate or delayed (Kanner, 1943; Tager-Flusberg, 1995). Although echolalia was long thought to be a dysfunctional language behavior, investigators such as Fay (1969) and Prizant and Duchan (1981) have shown that children with ASD often use echolalia for communicative purposes. Echolalia in ASD is selective, as it is in normal development (Carr, Schriebman, & Lovaas, 1975). Children with ASD who echo tend to do so when they do not understand what has been said to them or when they lack the language skills to generate an original reply (Prizant, 1996). Although echolalia is a "classic" symptom of autistic disorders, not all verbal children with ASD use it. Fay (1992) estimated that it appears, at least briefly, in about 75% of autistic children who speak. Also, echolalia is used by children with other syndromes, such as blindness and fragile X syndrome. As language skill in children with ASD improves, echolalia decreases, as it does in normal development. These findings suggest that echolalia is not a language behavior we want to extinguish in intervention. Instead, we want to work with it, using it as an index of the child's level of comprehension and as a springboard to more appropriate responses.

Kanner (1943) also identified pronoun reversals as characteristic of autistic language. Fay (1971) pointed out, though, that what children with ASD are doing is not reversing pronouns, but *failing* to reverse them: saying the same "you" as the speaker used, rather than changing it to "I." The problem is likely to be related to the autistic child's tendency to echo and to the deictic nature of pronoun reference: the referent shifts, depending on the point of view of the speaker. This shifting reference is particularly difficult for children with ASD because of their literalness and lack of flexibility.

These characteristics of meaning and pragmatic aspects of language in verbal children with ASD suggest that these clients do intend to communicate, but they have limited skills in acquiring and applying the conventional rules for communication. The strategies they use to maintain interaction, such as echolalia, are often interpreted as rejecting communication, when in fact they are the best the child can do. As clinicians, we need to learn to work with these behaviors instead of against them.

Paralinguistic aspects of communication also are affected in verbal children with ASD. Intonation is often monotonous and machinelike, and stress, vocal quality, rate, rhythm, and loudness deviances also have been reported for approximately half of higher functioning speakers with ASD (Shriberg, Paul, McSweeney, Klin, Cohen, & Volkmar, 2001). The reasons for these paralinguistic differences are not known. Paralinguistic aspects of communication do, though, carry some of the pragmatic and emotional information in the message. The deficits in affective development seen in children with ASD may, then, form some part of the explanation.

Prognosis

The outcome for children with ASD is related primarily to two factors: performance on IQ tests and language ability, although neither predictor is perfect (Howlin, 2005). Children who score within or close to the normal range on IQ measures have a better chance for some degree of independence in adulthood. Children who develop functional speech by age 6 also have a better prognosis. Watson and Ozonoff (2001) also reported that poorer prognosis is associated with a history of normal development followed by a regression. Even for those with good outcomes, whose high IQs allow them to attend college, obtain employment and live independently, ASD remains a lifelong disability with residual deficits in social skills, empathy, and pragmatic communication (Howlin, 2005; Schroeder, LeBlanc, & Mayo, 1996).

Clinical Implications

Assessment. As the criteria for diagnosing ASD demonstrate, impaired communication is always a part of the syndrome, and communicative intervention of some kind is virtually always appropriate for children with this syndrome. For this reason, SLPs should always be part of the multidisciplinary assessment and planning team for children with ASD (ASHA, 2006). Although SLPs will not generally have the responsibility to make a diagnosis of ASD independently, information on communication skill will play a large role in the diagnostic process. Paul (2005) and Prizant et al. (2006) provide guidelines for assessment of children with ASD. Some of these are summarized in Table 4-3.

Early Identification and Intervention. One of the most important recent findings about ASD is that early intervention works (Lord & McGee, 2001). Children with ASD derive most benefit from intervention when it is begun between 2 and 4 years of age and when the intervention is intensive—15 or more hours per week for more than 2 years. When this level of early intervention is provided, children with ASD make gains more rapidly than children with other kinds of disability (Rogers, 1996; 2006). Much of the current emphasis in research on ASD is on finding ways of making earlier diagnoses that will allow treatment to begin in the crucial first years of life. Early screening measures, which attempt to accurately identify children at risk for ASD in the first or second year of life (see ASHA, 2006 for review), are in rapid development. When it is possible to identify infants with ASD, the next challenge will be to develop effective programs to remediate their early deficits in communication.

Intervention. There has been a great deal of debate over the years about the modalities and targets of intervention for this population. Goldstein (2002), Paul and Sutherland (2005), and Rogers (2006) provide resources that describe various treatment approaches.

One particularly "hot" debate concerns the advantages of highly structured behavioral programs versus those of more naturalistic approaches. Intensive, individualized intervention using discrete trial training methods stands at one end of this continuum. A large body of research has demonstrated that these approaches are an effective means of initially developing attention to and understanding of language, as well as initiating speech production in preverbal children with ASD (Goldstein, 2002; Rogers, 2006). Discrete trial instruction (DTI) involves dividing the chosen skill into components and training each component individually, using highly structured drill-like procedures, until the goal is successfully accomplished. Intensive training utilizes shaping, prompting, prompt fading, and reinforcement strategies. A discrete trial is one cycle of a DTI teaching sequence. The program first teaches attending behavior, then following directions, imitation, and prompted verbal responses (Lovaas, 1987). Early proponents claimed to "cure"

close to half the children with ASD who are treated, provided that 40 hours per week of this type of intervention was given. More recent reanalyses of these data and other studies using the same approach (Shea, 2005), however, conclude that although this approach is beneficial, early results were greatly overstated. Follow-ups of children originally seen by Lovaas, who were selected for their IQs within the normal range and their ability to imitate verbal production, show them to continue to evidence social difficulties despite their relatively high IQs. Further, research has demonstrated that benefits similar to those shown in the Lovaas studies can be derived from 12 to 20 hours per week of DTI (Sheinkopf & Siegel, 1998).

Moreover, just like the CD approaches we have discussed for other disorders, DTI is limited in its generalization. Other approaches have also been developed to address the communicative deficits in ASD. More broadly based behavioral approaches, generally known under the rubric of applied behavioral analysis (ABA), have also been used with a wide range of autistic behaviors over the past 20 years. ABA frequently involves using the information acquired through functional analysis of antecedents and consequences to interpret the relationship between behavior and the circumstances in which it appears (Jensen & Sinclair, 2002). The primary emphasis in ABA is the use of intensive, direct instructional methods that alter particular behaviors in systematic and measurable ways (Anderson, Taras, & O'Malley-Cannon, 1996). While DTI is one method used within an ABA framework, it is not the only method included within this broader approach. Generally, these methods are an attempt to apply operant principles to more functional communicative situations, and would come under the heading of what we have called *incidental* or *milieu teaching* approaches. Their major insight concerns the importance of making access to the object of the child's interest contingent on the child's initiating some communicative exchange about it. Goldstein (2002) and Rogers (2006) reviewed studies showing that more naturalistic ABA approaches are as effective as DTI and may show increased generalizablity. Approaches we would call *child centered* have also been advocated for children with ASD. Usually referred to as *developmental* or *pragmatic* approaches when used with this population (Prizant & Wetherby, 2005), these methods do the following:

▶ Use the normal sequence of communicative development to serve as the best guidelines for determining intervention goals.

▶ Provide intensified opportunities for children with ASD to engage in activities that are similar to those in which typically developing peers engage, in the belief that these are the most effective contexts for learning social and communication skills.

▶ Exploit learning opportunities ("teachable moments") that naturally arise in the course of interactions, rather than relying on a predetermined curriculum.

▶ Facilitate interactions, including symbolic play, rather than addressing teacher-chosen goals.

Research is beginning to emerge on these approaches, as well. Currently, the literature (reviewed by Paul & Sutherland, 2005; Rogers, 2006) suggests that developmental methods can be effective in eliciting early communicative behaviors in

TABLE 4-3	Guidelines for Assessment of Children with ASD

STEPS IN ASSESSMENT	QUESTION TO BE ANSWERED	INSTRUMENTS	EXAMPLES
1: Screening	Is the child at risk for ASD?	Autism-specific screeners	*Infant-Toddler Checklist* (Wetherby & Prizant, 2003) *Pervasive Developmental Disorders Screening Test—II* (Siegel, 2005) *Social Communication Questionnaire* (Rutter, Bailey, & Lord, 2003)
2: Evaluation	Does the child meet criteria for ASD?	Autism-specific instruments	*Communication and Symbolic Behavior Scales Caregiver Questionnaire* (Wetherby & Prizant, 2003) *Childhood Autism Rating Scale* (Schopler, Reichler, & Renner, 1993). *Autism Diagnostic Observation Scale* (Lord et al., 2000). *Autism Diagnostic Interview* (Lord, Rutter, & Le Conture, 2002)
3a: Assessment of strengths and needs: Preverbal	What are the child's communication skills? Ability to respond to and initiate joint attention; Frequency, range, and means of communicative acts; Symbolic behaviors (e.g., play); Ability to imitate sounds and gestures; Ability to respond to words.	Observation in interactive context using: communication temptations, play assessment, assessment of language comprehension; Interactive vocal and gestural play; (See Chapter 6), parent report.	*Communication and Symbolic Behavior Scales—Behavioral Sample* (Prizant & Wetherby, 2003) *Communication Checklist* (see Chapter 7) *Play Scale* (Carpenter, 1987) *McCune Play Scale* (see Chapter 7) *Communication Development Inventory* (Fensen et al., 1993)
3b: Assessment of strengths and needs: Speakers	What are the child's strengths and needs in terms of language and social communication? Use of echolalia; Level of grammatical development; Appropriate word use; Understanding of discourse; Ability to engage in conversation, especially with peers; Ability to understand and produce narrative.	Language sampling; Observation in peer interactions; Standardized testing; Parent and teacher report.	*Comprehensive Assessment of Spoken Language* (Carrow-Woolfolk, 1999b) *Test of Pragmatic Language* (Phelps-Terasaki & Phelps-Gunn, 1992) *Test of Problem Solving-Elementary* (Bowers, Barrett, Huisingh, Orman, & LoGiudice, 1994) *Test of Problem Solving-Adolescent* (Bowers, Barrett, Huisingh, Orman, & LoGiudice, 1991) *Vineland Adaptive Behavior Scales-II* (Sparrow, Cicchetti, & Balla, 2005) *Children's Communication Checklist—2* (Bishop, 2003) *The Strengths and Difficulties Questionnaire* (Goodman, 1997)
4: Dynamic Assessment	What facilitates or interferes with the child's successful communication? Use of stereotypies; Maladaptive behaviors; Unconventional, labile emotional expression; Sensory sensitivities; Modality preferences.	Functional behavior analysis (see Chapter 12); Diagnostic teaching (see Chapter 2).	Systematically manipulate the context to identify optimal supports (visual, written, tactile, etc.) SCERTS Assessment (Prizant et al., 2006) Use think-aloud protocols for speakers (see Chapters 13 and 14)

preverbal children, such as increasing rates of communication and joint attention. Fewer data are available on their effectiveness for eliciting speech from preverbal children or social communication in older children with ASD who speak.

Many clinicians (e.g., Lord & McGee, 2001; Prizant & Wetherby, 2005) also point out, though, that it is not necessary to choose one approach or the other. Many highly regarded programs (such as the TEACCH [Treatment and Education of Autistic and related Communication-handicapped Children] Program at University of North Carolina, the Denver program developed by Sally Rogers, the Douglass [New Jersey] Developmental Disabilities Center, the SCERTS program [Social Communication, Emotional Regulations, and Transactional Support developed by Prizant et al., 2006], and the LEAP Program [Lifeskills and Education for Students with Autism and other Pervasive Behavioral Challenges] at the Kennedy Krieger Institute in Baltimore) borrow from both the more clinician-directed DTI and ABA methods and more child-centered and hybrid procedures. Still, programs that are eclectic in the sense of mixing a variety of methods are not necessarily the most effective (Eikeseth, Smith, Jahr, & Eldevik, 2002; Howard, Sparkman, Cohen, Green, & Stanislaw, 2005); programs work best when each clinician is an "expert" in one approach and uses it consistently, so that the child experiences a variety of approaches, each presented by a highly trained and experienced practitioner of that method.

Nonverbal Children with ASD. For children with ASD who do not speak, establishing some means of functional communication will be our goal, as it is with all nonspeaking clients. The first objective for these clients is to assess whether any intentional communication is taking place, and if so, for what purposes and by what means. In Chapter 7 we'll discuss in detail some assessment techniques that can be used to answer these questions. In developing assessment protocols for non-speaking children, we'll want to look not only at the means they use to express their intentions, but also at comprehension abilities. The criterion-referenced methods for assessing comprehension that we'll discuss in Chapter 6 will be useful here. Knowing how much the child understands will help both to structure our own input and to select among goals in production, as we discussed in Chapter 3. We'll also want to examine clients' use of comprehension strategies, using the procedures detailed in Chapter 6. Research on language comprehension in ASD (see Tager-Flusberg, Paul, & Lord, 2005, for review) indicates that these children use strategies for comprehending that are in many ways similar to those seen in normally developing children. Knowing about how the child takes advantage of nonlinguistic information in attempting to process language can be useful both for structuring input and for developing contexts for language activities.

As we saw, a likely finding for this population will be that some requests and protests are expressed, but joint attention or social interactional intentions are not. When this is the case, we'll want to do two things. First, we'll want to provide some conventional means—gestures, signs, vocalizations, words, or some form of augmentative communication such as a picture board—for expressing the intents the child is already producing. Second, we'll want to provide extensive support for eliciting joint attentional and social interactive behaviors. When these emerge in presymbolic form, we'll then try to find more conventional means of expression for them. Bono, Daley, and Sigman (2004), for example, showed that joint attentional behaviors predict the amount of growth in a language intervention program, and Kasari (2005) demonstrated that activities aimed at increasing joint attention also had positive effects on language production. Koegel and Koegel (2006), Quill (1998), Paul and Sutherland (2005), and Prizant et al. (2006) have provided some guidelines for intervention programs for nonspeaking children with ASD. Some drawn from Koegel and Koegel (1998) and Paul and Sutherland (2005) are outlined in Box 4-11.

Augmentative Communication in ASD. The issue of alternative modes of communication is often raised for nonverbal children with ASD. Although these children have no known motoric impediments to speech, advocates of AAC, using a "communication needs" model, recommend providing AAC to any non-speaking child, regardless of the reason, because everyone needs some way to communicate (Beukeleman & Mirenda, 2005). Sign is one alternative often used. Some studies (e.g., Carr, Binkoff, Kologinsky, & Eddy, 1978) have reported communicative gains from the use of signs, and there have been reports indicating that the introduction of signs is sometimes followed by the onset of vocalization or speech (Tincani, 2004). Layton and Watson (1995), though, found that few children used the signs functionally, and Grove and Dockrell (2000) report no evidence of language development beyond Brown's stage I with the use of signs. In current practice, AAC systems for people with ASD often begin with object or picture exchanges (Bondy & Frost, 1998; Watson & Ozonoff, 2001). Here the child is given an object (such as a spoon to represent a bowl of cereal to eat) or picture that represents the desired goal, and is taught to give it to the clinician to obtain the goal. One popular example of this approach is the picture exchange communication system (PECS; Bondy & Frost, 1998). Several studies (e.g., Charlop-Christy, Carpenter, Le, Leblanc, & Kellet, 2002; Ganz & Simpson, 2004) show that children with ASD who are taught PECS have increased communication and speech, but no direct comparisons between PECS and more explicit speech instruction have been done. Other forms of AAC, such as communication boards have also been studied (e.g., Garrison-Harrell, Kamps, & Kravits, 1997), as have the use of voice output communication aids (VOCAs; Mirenda, 2003). Like Sign and PECS, these methods appear to be helpful, but studies are few and small. In general, nonverbal children with ASD who are taught signs or other alternative modes of communication show gains, but not dramatic transformations in communicative skills. Overall, we can say that AAC methods have been shown to be compatible with the development of speech, although efficiency relative to straightforward speech treatment has not yet been established. For children with autism, though, we know that the acquisition of speech by school age is one of the most powerful predictors of outcome (Howlin, 2005), so it would seem impor-

BOX 4-11	Guidelines for Enhancing Communication for Nonspeaking Children with Autism

Establish receptive joint attention. Use loud, exaggerated cues and intense reinforcement to encourage child to look at what the clinician points out or looks at.

Establish initiation of joint attention. Whenever the child looks at or attends to an object or event, follow the child's lead AS IF the child intended to establish joint attention. Look at, touch, and interact with the object or event the child is engaged with. Intrude so that the child's attention shifts to the clinician, then provide exaggerated praise for looking at and sharing with the clinician.

Encourage the development of social interactive routines. Using enjoyable social routines, such as "If you're happy and you know it," or tickling routines, require the child to say or do something and look at the adult before proceeding with the game.

Encourage imitation. Play "copy cat" games in which reinforcement is provided for vocal or gestural imitation. Start by imitating the child; then reward the child's imitation of the adult.

Use sounds the child is already producing to encourage first word use. At first, associate sounds the child already makes as babble with a meaningful object or outcome. If the child says "oo" spontaneously, show him a train each time he says it, and say, "Choo-choo! Yes, this is a choo-choo." Encourage and reinforce imitation/approximation of the adult's rendition of the child utterance.

Replace unconventional communicative means. Teach gestures (such as nodding), vocalizations, or actions (such as walking toward the door) to replace maladaptive behaviors.

Establish multiple means of communication. Model using simple words and phrases, ritualized utterances, songs, rhymes, etc. to express intents; model and accept gestures, vocalizations, gaze and other behaviors as communications.

Expand the range of communicative functions. Use communication temptations to encourage socially oriented intents.

Develop strategies to maintain communication and repair breakdowns. Use highly motivating activities to keep the client focused. At first respond to behavior as if it were communicative; later up the ante to requiring more conventional signals. Create opportunities for repair by delaying responses or feigning misunderstanding.

Provide environmental supports to enhance social communication. Use visually cued instruction (such as PECS, visual schedules and calendars, pictographic symbols) and modified linguistic input (exaggerated intonation and facial expression; simple, routine, repetitive language).

Adapted from Koegel, R., & Koegel, L. (2006). *Pivotal response treatments for autism: Communication, social and academic development.* Baltimore: Paul H. Brookes Publishers: Paul, R., & Sutherland, D. (2005). Enhancing early language in children with autism spectrum disorders. In F. Volkmar, R. Paul, A. Klin, & D. Cohen (Eds.). *Handbook of autism and pervasive developmental disorders–vol.2* (pp. 946-976). New York: Wiley; Prizant, B., Schuler, A., Wetherby, A., & Rydell, P. (1997). Enhancing language and communication development: Language approaches. In D. Cohen & F. Volkmar (Eds.). *Handbook of autism and pervasive developmental disorders* (pp. 572-605). New York: John Wiley & Sons.

tant to make every attempt to elicit speech during the crucial preschool period. Direct speech instruction, using DTI methods (such as those described by Partington & Sundberg [1998] or Tsiouri & Greer [2003]) or other methods focused on verbal imitation and speech production (such as Koegel, Sze, Mossman, Koegel, & Brookman-Frazee, 2006) can be combined with AAC as well as approaches that foster preverbal communication skills such as joint attention. However, we know very little about the relative efficiency of these approaches, and more research is needed to guide clinicians as to what mix of approaches will yield the most direct route to spoken language. For nonverbal preschoolers with ASD, though, it would seem important to include direct attempts to elicit and develop speech in order to give them the maximum opportunities to reach their potential.

Verbal Children with ASD. Children with autism who speak are typically referred to as "high functioning" (Tager-Flusberg et al., 2005). For these children, it will be necessary to devote some assessment time to learning how echolalia or other unusual

forms of language are used. We can analyze the communicative functions of autistic language patterns and then teach more adaptive patterns, starting with formulaic phrases such as "I don't understand" to replace them. Again, assessing comprehension, using both standardized and more contextualized methods, is an important part of the evaluation process (Miller & Paul, 1995). Prizant et al. (2006) emphasized the importance of providing simple-input language to children with ASD to minimize their comprehension difficulties. In general, formal aspects of language are more advanced than pragmatic skills in these children, but there is a subgroup of children with ASD whose language resembles that of children with specific language impairment (Tager-Flusberg & Joseph, 2003). For children with non-pragmatic language deficits, form and content deficiencies can be addressed as we would for a child with SLI. The focus of intervention for most verbal children with ASD, however, will be making the language forms they already possess more effective for communication. Myles and Simpson (1998), Paul and Sutherland (2005), Prizant et al. (2006) and Prizant, Schuler, Wetherby, and Rydell (1997) provided guidelines for intervention procedures with verbal children with ASD.

Paul (2003a) emphasized the importance of social skills training for children with ASD. Role playing and giving these children practice with social situations in which they can try out communicative strategies, following a clinician's model, can help develop skills for expressing emotion, empathy, and social participation, even though these may never become completely "natural" for these clients. Visual cues, including both graphics and writing, can be useful in helping them to structure their interactions. Posting a series of steps to go through in greeting a friend, for example, can help children with ASD internalize these skills (Quill, 1998; Timler et al., 2005a; see Fig. 4-8). Video modeling, using a videotaped interaction of peers engaging in a social script being taught to the child has been shown to be an effective method of improving social behaviors (Charlop-Christy, Le, & Freeman, 2000; Nikopoulos

& Keenan, 2004). Gray (1995b, 2000a) has developed a method using "social stories" to promote appropriate social behavior. These stories are written to give clients an explanation of social situations at their level of comprehension. The stories use descriptive statements to help the child understand situations and provide scripted verbal models for the child to use when he or she has difficulty. An example social story appears in Figure 4-6. Preliminary research, summarized by Sansosti, Powell-Smith, and Kincaid (2004), provides some degree of evidence of the usefulness of this approach for decreasing problem behaviors in children with ASD, although evidence for their efficacy in improving social skills is more limited. Gray (2000a) also suggests using comic strips, like those in Figure 4-7, to help students understand the distinction between what people say (in word bubbles) and what they think (in thought bubbles).

In addition, many of the meta-cognitive approaches discussed in Chapters 12 and 14 may also be useful for school-

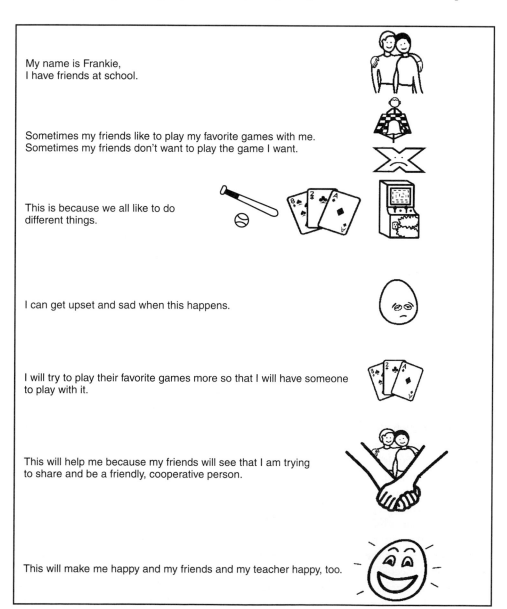

FIGURE 4-6 ✦ Sample social story. (The Picture Communication Symbols, 1981-2006 by Mayer-Johnson, LLC.)

My name is Frankie, I have friends at school.

Sometimes my friends like to play my favorite games with me. Sometimes my friends don't want to play the game I want.

This is because we all like to do different things.

I can get upset and sad when this happens.

I will try to play their favorite games more so that I will have someone to play with it.

This will help me because my friends will see that I am trying to share and be a friendly, cooperative person.

This will make me happy and my friends and my teacher happy, too.

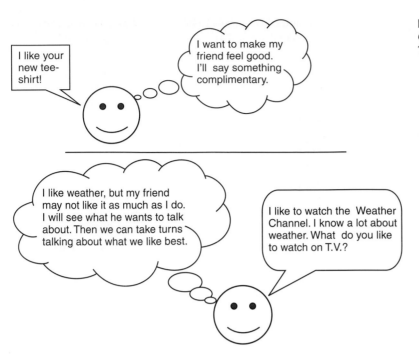

FIGURE 4-7 ✦ Comic strip conversations. (Adapted from Gray, C. [1994]. *Comic Strip Conversations*. Arlington, TX: Future Horizons.)

age verbal clients with ASD, as will the use of graphic and written supports (such as in Timler et al. [2005a] and Fig. 4-8). The strong rote memory abilities often seen in this population can be invoked to memorize communicative procedures. Again, their responses to others may be less than spontaneous but can at least be made to more closely approximate conventional acceptability. An important element in social skills training is the inclusion of peers as models and trainers (Paul, 2003a). English, Goldstein, Shafer, and Kaczmarek (1997), Paul (2003c), Terpstra (2002), Timler, Olswang, and Coggins (2005b), and Werner, Vismara, Koegel, and Koegel (2006) provide guidelines for teaching peers to model and train social skills in peers with ASD. In addition, Koegel, Klein, Koegel, Boettcher, Brookman-Frazee, and Openden (2006) provide information on training paraprofessionals, who are often the primary agents of intervention for these children in inclusive settings, to improve socialization and social skills instruction.

Borderlands of the Autism Spectrum

As a spectrum disorder, autism can be difficult to distinguish from conditions that share some of its features. Because there is no laboratory test to determine whether a child's condition falls within the autism spectrum, it can be hard to decide whether a given constellation of symptoms fall on or off of this continuum. Bishop and Norbury (2002) talked about the "borderlands" of the autism spectrum; generally three additional conditions would be considered to reside in these borderlands: Asperger syndrome (AS), nonverbal learning disability (NLD), and pragmatic language impairment (PLI). Much controversy surrounds these classifications: whether there is any real distinction among them; whether they should all be considered to be part of the autism spectrum; whether some are more closely connected to specific language impairment than ASD; whether they have different genetic and biological roots that provide a justifi-

cation for keeping them as separate categories even when the behavioral presentation is similar. One clinician seeing a child called AS by another may feel NLD or PLI is the more appropriate label. Only AS is listed as an "official" diagnosis in the *DSM-IV*; whether NLD and PLI are categories that can be used for educational services varies from district to district. We'll outline these three disorders as they have been described in the literature, but remember that these distinctions are still in flux and may have changed by the time you read this section!

Asperger Syndrome. In 1944, the Viennese psychiatrist Hans Asperger published a paper describing a group of children with marked social deficits in the presence of normal intelligence. The disorder came to be known by his name in Europe but was virtually unrecognized in the United States until his paper was translated into English over 20 years later. During the past few years there has been a dramatic increase in the number of children receiving a diagnosis of AS, which is made on the basis of autistic-like deficits in social and pragmatic skills in the presence of a history of normal cognitive and language development (see Box 4-10). Controversy still exists as to whether AS is a disorder separate from other high-functioning forms of autism, with some researchers arguing that the two are distinguishable (Klin & Volkmar, 2003; Klin, Volkmar, & Sparrow, 2000; Rourke, Ahmad, Collins, Hayman-Abello, Satyman-Abello, & Warriner, 2002) and others (Adams, Green, Gilchrist, & Cox, 2002; Lord & McGee, 2001) suggesting that few differences between high-functioning children with autism and those diagnosed with AS can be found. Klin et al. (2000) provide an in-depth resource on this disorder.

Whatever the final resolution of this issue, children with AS-like presentation have clear needs for identification and intervention (Winner, 2003). Bishop's (2003) *Children's Communication Checklist-2* (CCC-2), a parent report measure, may be a helpful part of the evaluation process for providing

Card 1
STOP, LOOK AND LISTEN

FIGURE 4-8 ✦ Checklist for social skills training.

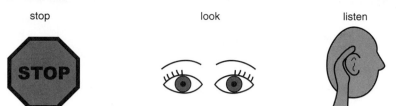

stop   look   listen

1. Did I pay attention to the conversation?

    _____ YES! _____ NO, I need help!

2. What do I know?

3. How do I know this?

think

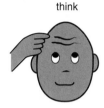

Card 2
SEEING AND HEARING LEADS TO
THINKING AND KNOWING!

look listen   I see I hear   think   know

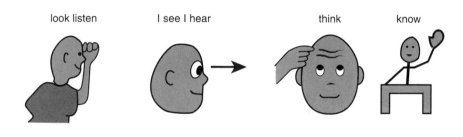

1. Did I pay attention to what others saw
   and heard?

    _____ YES! _____ NO, I need help!

2. What does everyone else think or know?

3. How do they know this?

friend

documentation of pragmatic skills that are significantly different from normal. Assessment will need to focus on documenting social communication and pragmatic language deficits, following guidelines like those in Box 4-12 for speaking children with ASD and discussed in Paul (2005), Wetherby and Prizant (2005), and ASHA (2006). Intervention for these children will focus on social cognition and social communication and include strategies similar to those appropriate for other speakers with ASD, such as using visual cueing, social skills training, and script-based and meta-cognitive strategies. Tsatsanis, Foley, and Donehower (2004) discussed programming guidelines for

students with AS and suggest focusing on peer-mediated interventions, working with teachers to provide supports within the classroom, and planning for transition to postschool settings. Winner (2003) argues for the need to develop social thinking skills, which focus, using meta-cognitive and meta-linguistic strategies (see Chapter 14), on helping students learn why we use certain social behaviors, such as looking at others, before modeling and practicing these skills. For example, she suggests encouraging students to be detectives, using their eyes to watch people and learn about how they use their faces to express thoughts and feelings and to use that information to increase

---

BOX 4-12 | **Guidelines for Enhancing Communication in Verbal Children with Autism**

Emerging Language

Expand vocabulary—Teach words for social control (stop, help) and for expressing emotions and labels.

Reward efforts for communication and speech—Focus on encouraging clients to produce communicative acts rather than stressing proper form.

Expand communicative functions—Use communication temptations to elicit social interactional and joint attentional expressions, such as greetings and comments.

Teach clients to direct attention—Use adult and peer modeling to demonstrate conventional ways of drawing attention to their efforts to communicate (such as touching someone on the shoulder, or saying, "Listen.")

Encourage multiword utterances—Use vertical structuring and naturalistic procedures (such as creating a need for more specific information than one word can provide) to encourage clients to combine words.

Expand sentence types—When sentences emerge, create opportunities for use of negatives, questions, and comments in real communication situations (see Paul, 1992, for suggestions).

Develop emergent literacy—Use procedures such as those in Chapter 9 to develop reading and writing.

Teach functional use of imitation—Use the client's tendency to imitate to introduce forms that are useful in real communication.

Capitalize on memorized forms—Talk multiword utterances that the child produces in delayed imitation, and use build-up/break down strategies to demonstrate how they can be segmented.

Developing and Advanced Language

Talk about there-and-then—Provide practice in reviewing and discussing routine events first, then events more removed from the here-and-now. Use visual organization and support for these activities.

Address conversational skills—Teach verbal conventions for initiating conversations, exchanging turns, and ending conversations; model and discuss use of paralinguistic behaviors to support conversation; provide strategies for recognizing and repairing conversational breakdowns.

Provide scripts for specific events—Use meta-cognitive planning, with visual/written support, to prepare clients for common experiences, such as ordering in a restaurant or buying a bus pass.

Use reading and writing for communicative purposes—Encourage the use of letters, thank you notes, memos, etc., to augment face-to-face communication.

Use meta-linguistic strategies—Help students learn to monitor their own communication. Encourage students to be aware of what they and others say and look for clues as to how others respond.

Adapted from Paul, R., & Sutherland, D. (2005). Enhancing early language in children with autism spectrum disorders. In F. Volkmar, R. Paul, A. Klin, & D. Cohen (Eds.). *Handbook of autism and pervasive developmental disorders–vol. 2* (pp. 946-976). New York: Wiley; Prizant, B., Schuler, A., Wetherby, A., & Rydell, P. (1997). Enhancing language and communication development: Language approaches. In D. Cohen & F. Volkmar (Eds.). *Handbook of autism and pervasive developmental disorders* (pp. 572-605). New York: John Wiley & Sons.

---

their understanding of communication, rather than simply telling students to "look at me." Adams (2005), Brinton, Robinson, and Fujiki (2004), Myles and Simpson (1998), Rubin (2004), and Timler et al. (2005a) provide additional information on developing interventions for these students.

Nonverbal Learning Disability. Byron Rourke and colleagues (Rourke, 1995; Rourke et al., 2002) have advanced the idea that one subtype of learning disability is a syndrome in which children show a profile of skills that is opposite of the one seen in language-learning disabilities like the ones we discuss in Chapter 10. Children with nonverbal learning disabilities (NLD) have normal verbal IQs, but nonverbal IQs that are significantly lower. They show preserved single word reading and talk fluently, but have difficulty with nonverbal problem solving, visual-spatial skills, tactile perception, psychomotor coordination,

and, despite superficially normal language form, show deficits in pragmatic use of language (Volden, 2002; 2004). Their discourse is described as verbose, rambling, disorganized, incoherent, tangential, repetitive, monotonous, and loose (Volden, 2002). Some writers (Klin, Volkmar, Sparrow, Cicchetti, & Rourke, 1995) have seen a connection between Asperger's syndrome (AS) and NLD, and hypothesize that both reside in deficits in right hemisphere brain functions (Rourke, 1989). And like children thought to have AS, those with NLD are also often difficult to qualify for SLP services because of their relatively strong skills in language form. The same strategies we discussed for evaluating students with AS can be applied to those with NLD: the *CCC-2* can be helpful in establishing eligibility, assessment will focus on observation, parent and teacher report, and tests that provide some description of pragmatic abilities.

Interventions like those prescribed for high functioning children with autism or AS will also be appropriate.

Pragmatic Language Impairment. Rapin and Allen (1983) were the first to propose a subgroup of children with developmental language disorders whose primary deficits were not in language form, but in semantic and pragmatic aspects of communication. They called this subgroup semantic-pragmatic disorder. Bishop and Rosenbloom (1987) also identified a similar subtype of SLI, which was distinguishable from other SLI children only on the basis of pragmatic skills, and more recent research by this group (Bishop, 2000) has shown that these children do not have semantic deficits per se. Bishop argues that they can be seen as distinct from children with ASD because of their lack of difficulties with peer relations or special interests, but with symptoms that overlap both SLI and ASD. Most researchers interested in this group of children now call their disorder Pragmatic Language Impairment (PLI). Like those with NLD, these children are described as verbose, having poor turn-taking and topic management skills and having difficulty with nonliteral language and drawing inferences (Adams, 2001). Again, many writers would see these children as having disorders on the autism spectrum.

Adams (2001) suggests using the *CCC-2* as a way to identify these children. Narrative and conversational assessments are also recommended to assist in program planning. Children with PLI have been shown to produce less information in a retelling task than children with SLI (Conti-Ramsden, Crutchley, & Botting, 1997).

Conversational analysis focusing on initiation and responsiveness to topics may also be helpful in distinguishing PLI from SLI. Adams (2005) provided elements of a social communication intervention program (SCI) to address the needs of students with PLI and similar difficulties. Adams, Baxendale, Lloyd and Aldren (2005) documented the usefulness of this approach in a series of case studies. Its elements are summarized in Table 4-4.

TABLE 4-4 Elements of the Social Communication Intervention (SCI) Program

SCI ELEMENT	EXAMPLES
Adaptation and compensation	Establish a highly adapted environment by training parents, teacher and peers to provide positive social experiences
	Adapt the school curriculum; use trained paraprofessionals to implement individualized instruction and support generalization in classroom
	Train adults to monitor their responses to the child so that they provide elaborations using language within the child's level to extend the child's topic
Flexibility	Use social stories, cartoons, scenarios and real experiences to discuss and become aware of own and others' feelings; encourage talking and thinking about empathy
	Regularly add small changes to routines to increase flexibility; warn child about changes, and encourage anticipation and understanding of change
	Use picture and cartoon stories to increase understanding of verbal and nonverbal cues and use these cues to infer thoughts and feelings
	Introduce and discuss figurative language; provide direct instruction in using the social context to derive meaning from figurative forms
	Build sequences in narratives and goal-directed events; focus on coherence as a basis for understanding
Meta-pragmatics	Talk about rules for conversation (turn-taking, staying on topic, using the right style for the situation) and practice them
	Discuss why these rules help people communicate

Materials used to support these elements:

Black Sheep Press. *Activities for pragmatics and problem solving*. Keighley, England: Author.

Brinton, B., & Fujiki, M. (2005). Social competence in children with language impairment: Making connections. *Seminars in Speech and Language*, 26, 151-159.

Gray, C. (1995). *New social story book*. Arlington, VA: Future Horizons.

Gray, C. (2000). *Comic strip conversations*. Arlington, VA: Future Horizons.

Silver Lining Multimedia (2004). *Mindreading*. Peterborough, NH.

Paul, R. (1992). *Pragmatic activities for language intervention*. San Antonio, TX: Communication Skillbuilders.

Rinaldi, W. (2001). *Social use of language programme-Revised*. Windsor, England: NFER-Nelson.

Silver Lining Multimedia. *My community*. Author: Peterborough, NH.

Silver Lining Multimedia. *My school day*. Author: Peterborough, NH.

Silver Lining Multimedia. *School rules*. Author: Peterborough, NH.

Thinking Publications. (2004). *Nickel takes on anger*. Eau Claire, WI: Thinking Publications.

Thinking Publications. (2004). *Nickel takes on teasing*. Eau Claire, WI: Thinking Publications.

Adapted from Adams, C. (2005). Social communication intervention for school-age children. *Journal of Child Psychology, Psychiatry, & Allied Disciplines*, 43, 973-988.

ACQUIRED DISORDERS OF COMMUNICATIVE FUNCTION

Freddie had been a very bright preschooler. In fact, he was so bright that his parents had him tested to determine whether he could enter school at 4 instead of waiting until he was 5. The results of this testing, of which the parents kept copies and showed to every clinician who saw Freddie later, indicated an IQ in the superior range and very advanced verbal skills. When Freddie was 7, he experienced a series of seizures for no apparent reason. After Freddie was hospitalized several times and underwent much experimentation with drugs and dosage, the seizures were partially but not fully controlled. His parents began to notice, though, that Freddie's speech was beginning to deteriorate. His sentences got shorter. He couldn't think of words he wanted to use. His concentration was poor. He became extremely impulsive, so that they had to lock cabinets and keep dangerous substances away from him, as you would with a toddler. Even when the seizures were fairly well controlled, the language and cognitive problems did not go away. His parents struggled for years to find a way to release the bright Freddie they had known as a little child from the tyranny of the seizures' after-effects. They took him to numerous specialists, showing each one his early test results, trying to impress on them that somewhere inside, Freddie must still be as smart as he was when he was 4. But he had a terrible time in school. Although his nonverbal skills were age appropriate, his oral communications was telegraphic and he had severe comprehension deficits. Eventually his parents reluctantly agreed to place him in a special education resource class so that his needs could be addressed.

As Freddie's case illustrates, acquired brain damage can have severe and long-lasting effects on communication and school performance. In this section, we'll discuss some of the implications of these facts for clinical practice with children who acquire communication disorders. Let's look at four kinds of injury that can result in acquired language disorders and see what they might suggest to us for clinical practice.

FOCAL LESIONS

Lesions that are focal, or localized to a specific area of the brain, are usually caused by cerebrovascular accidents (CVAs) such as strokes and are relatively rare in children; however, children with congenital heart problems are particularly vulnerable to CVAs, and premature babies may suffer focal damage as a result of intracranial bleeding during their first weeks of life outside the womb. Recent research (Booth et al., 2000; Chilosi, Cipriani, Bertuccelli, Pfanner, & Cioni, 2001; Chilosi, Pecini, Cipriani, Brovedani, Brizzolara, Ferretti, Pfanner, & Cioni, 2005; Dick, Wulfeck, Krupa-Kwiatkowski, & Bates, 2004; Levin, Song, Ewing-Cobbs, Chapman, & Mendelsohn, 2001; Reilly, Losh, Bellugi, & Wulfeck, 2004; Vicari, Albertoni, Chilosi, Cipriani, Cioni, & Bates, 2000; Weckerly, Wulfeck, & Reillly, 2004; Wulfeck, Bates, Krupa-Kwiatkowski, & Saltzman, 2004) suggests that children with very early focal lesions show delays in the acquisition of language, particularly if the lesion is on the left side of the brain, and some atypical lateralization of language functions in the brain. Delays continue to be shown through early development in children with early-acquired lesions, particularly for those with left-lateralized damage, although in general delays are mild. Children who acquire damage before age 10 usually go through a mute period immediately following the injury, but generally regain most functional language use, with mild deficits in efficiency of language processes. For children with right hemisphere damage, development may appear normal after initial recovery, but there may be difficulty with some higher-level language abilities for those over 10 years. Thus, most children who suffer focal lesions make more or less complete recovery in terms of communication, although when seizures persist after the injury, prognosis is more guarded.

ACQUIRED APHASIA SECONDARY TO SEIZURE DISORDERS

Some children, like Freddie, go through a period of normal development, then suddenly or gradually lose language skills in association with a seizure disorder. The affected child usually stops paying attention to speech, although audiological testing shows normal hearing; the child may stop talking, or regress in language ability, although nonverbal skills are preserved. The seizure disorder itself is often of unknown origin. This condition is known as *Landau-Kleffner syndrome (LKS)*, named after a paper by Landau and Kleffner (1957) that first described it. LKS usually has its onset between 3 and 6 years of age, although it can occur any time between 2 and 13 years (Miller, Campbell, Chapman, & Weismer, 1984). In general, prognosis is worse the earlier the onset of the syndrome, which is more common in boys than in girls. Cognitive functioning is usually impaired as well. Unlike aphasias associated with focal lesions, LKS may result in a permanent aphasia. Another difference between LKS and aphasias arising from focal lesions is that comprehension is more severely affected in LKS, and reading and writing may be relatively spared (Aram, 1988; Glos, Jariabkova, & Szabova, 2001). Some children can successfully use Sign language as a form of communication (Sieratzki, Calvert, Brammer, David, & Woll, 2001). Clinical seizures are not always apparent (Harrison, 2001; Robinson, 2003), but abnormal EEG activity is one of the two diagnostic criteria for the syndrome; the other being a loss of previously acquired language function. Communication deficits persist in many subjects with LKS (Miller et al., 1984), although recently developed treatments have shown some potential to limit chronic effects. Both surgical and pharmacological management have been used. Drug therapy is used to treat the seizures, which can usually be controlled by anticonvulsant medication. These drugs do not, unfortunately, affect the language disorders associated with the syndrome. Treatment with corticosteroids, usually prednisone, has been shown to lead to improvement in communication and EEG abnormalities in some cases if given within 3 years of the onset of the condition (Harrison, 2001; Robinson, 2003). For children not helped by these medications, surgical intervention is also an option. A procedure known as multiple subpial transection (MST), which severs horizontal fibers in the cortex while preserving vertical fiber connections (Robinson, 2003), is used. Although it is only useful in a minority of cases, Robinson (2003) reports dramatic changes when surgery is effective. Robinson, Baird, Robinson, and Simonoff (2001) emphasize that full recovery has only been seen in children who had the condition for less than 3 years. Van Slyke (2002) reminds us that even when treatments are effective, recovery is not immediate; that it can take months or years for a child to regain functional communication skills, and delays in some areas may persist. Long-term outcomes are generally unknown, due to the relatively recent application of new medical and surgical approaches.

Van Slyke (2002) suggests the following guidelines for working with children with LKS:

▶ A small, language-based instructional setting for at least part of the day
▶ A high level of individual support and one-to-one instruction
▶ Intensive language intervention focusing on using residual skills functionally and re-teaching the typical developmental sequence of acquisition
▶ Use of Sign as an augmentative modality
▶ Use of visual supports, such as picture schedules, color coding, cue cards, etc.
▶ Use of written channels, whenever developmental level allows, to bypass auditory deficits
▶ Use of computer programs to provide multimodal, individualized input

Brain Damage after Tumors, Infection, or Radiation

The mortality due to acute lymphocytic leukemia in children has been greatly reduced by the advent of brain radiation treatment, but this "cure" sometimes has the unfortunate consequence of causing learning problems, loss of developmental skills previously acquired, or seizures (Riddle, Anderson, Cicchetti, McIntosh, & Cohen, 1991). Brain tumors also can affect cognitive and communicative functioning. In addition, brain damage that can affect language development may also result from infectious diseases, such as meningitis. As in the case of the other acquired language disorders that we have been talking about, the long-term sequelae of these kinds of insults can be subtle and variable, depending on timing, location, size, and area of the brain affected by the damage. Children with these injuries, again, may retain a great deal of language function but have deficits that only surface during complex tasks, such as those required for school. They may have expressive skills that are relatively intact, but poor comprehension. This can result in adults' being fooled into thinking comprehension is on par with production and being frustrated when the child "refuses" to follow instructions. The range of severity of these effects can extend from almost nonexistent to severe enough to result in a diagnosis of MR.

Traumatic Brain Injury

Traumatic brain injuries (TBIs) can be focal in nature. These are usually *open-head injuries*, such as bullet wounds, and their course is similar to that described for focal lesions. *Closed-head injuries*, such as those resulting from blows or collisions, tend to involve diffuse damage, affecting large areas of the brain and are the more common type in children. Falls and car accidents cause most of these childhood TBIs, although Blosser and DePompei (2001) report that 10% to 15% can be attributed to child abuse. Boys are twice as likely to suffer TBIs as girls. Like children with acquired aphasias associated with focal lesions, children with TBIs of both types show a great deal of spontaneous recovery. Recent research (Anderson et al., 2005; Catroppa & Anderson, 2004; Hanten, Zhang, Barnes, Roberson, Archibald, Song, & Levin, 2004; Russell, 1993; Yeates, Swift, Taylor, Wade, Drotar, Stancin, & Minich, 2004) suggests that outcome is generally predicted by the degree of coma, the length of time a child spends in an impaired state of consciousness after the injury, and by the length of the post-traumatic amnesia (PTA) period; that is, the period of time between the injury and the time the child regains a continuous memory for ongoing events. PTAs longer than 24 hours are considered signs of severe injury, and children with more severe injuries are also at higher risk for long-term consequences. In addition, the research suggests that children with lower pre-injury adaptive skills and low socioeconomic status and family functioning have highest risk levels. Again prognosis appears to be better the later in childhood the injury occurs, contrary to previous belief (Wolcott, Lash, & Pearson, 1995). The onset of deficits may be delayed for long periods after the injury has taken place. Although some children retain physical disabilities from TBIs, many do not show obvious physiological damage. Still, a substantial minority of these apparently recovered children suffer long-term deficits in cognitive and communicative function (Blosser & DePompei, 2002; Satz & Bullard-Bates, 1981; Yeates et al., 2004). When the damage caused by the injury has been severe, swallowing and speech motor control deficits also may be long-term consequences (Murdoch & Theodoros, 2001).

Gerring and Carney (1992) and Murdoch and Theodoros (2001) described the language recovery process in TBI. Children tend at first, during the phase of post-traumatic amnesia, to be mute. They may comprehend only simple commands. Early language productions often reflect the confused state that the child is in and are often dysarthric or nonfluent. Speech may be slow, and prosody may be affected so that the speech sounds monotonic and "flat." Swallowing disorders also are common during this phase of recovery. Gerring and Carney distinguished the following two types of language patterns that can emerge during this period:

1. Sparse language production, in which the child is not spontaneous and will only answer questions with single words or short phrases, often lacking in affective prosody.
2. Excess speech production, in which the child talks too much; makes tangential statements; wanders from the conversational topic; and makes irrelevant, inappropriate remarks.

Once the post-traumatic amnesia period has passed, language functions begin to show improvement even in severe cases (Catroppa & Anderson, 2004), but language impairment sometimes remains as a chronic deficit. The following two types of language deficits can persist (Hagen, 1986; Murdoch & Theodoros, 2001):

1. Specific language problems with minimal cognitive involvement, similar to an acquired aphasia in adults. Problems that tend to persist in this type are word-finding problems, auditory and reading comprehension deficits, and paraphasic errors (substitutions of inappropriate sounds, words, or phrases). Schwartz-Cowley and Stepanik (1989) suggested that this outcome is relatively rare in children with head injuries.

2. Disorganized language secondary to a primary cognitive impairment resulting in difficulties in using language. This type of residual handicap is the more common of the two. The cognitive functions often impaired in TBI include attention and concentration, short- and/or long-term memory, speed of processing information, organization, and reasoning (Russell, 1993). Many of these have to do with "executive functions," those by which the brain orients and organizes itself to accomplish activities. These processes support and enable the understanding and use of language. When they are disrupted, the result is language that can sound inappropriate, irrelevant, fragmented, illogical, tangential, concrete, and confused, even though basic syntax, morphology, and phonology are spared. Russell (1993) referred to this complex as a *cognitive-communication disorder* and outlined the linguistic characteristics that tend to be associated with it. These are listed in Box 4-13. Chapman, McKinnon, Levin, Song, Neier, and Chiu (2001) reported that discourse abilities, such as narrative skills, were also a common long-lasting effect, particularly in children with the most severe injuries.

Clinical Implications

Nelson (1998) put her finger on the hardest thing for teachers and families to accept in a child with acquired brain injury: they are, in many ways, dealing with a different person than the one who inhabited the child's body before the neurological damage took place. Both the child and the adults may feel confused, frustrated, and angry that things that came easily before seem impossible now. The child may seem to be less compliant, to be "lazy" or unmotivated, to be scattered and inattentive, to have a different personality entirely. Freddie's family's response exemplifies this problem. They keep trying to find the "old" Freddie, trying to convince clinicians and teachers that he's in there, looking for a way to get out. They may, in fact, be right. But in clinical practice, we need to deal with the Freddies as we

---

BOX 4-13 **Linguistic Characteristics in Cognitive-Communication Disorders After TBI**

- Intact syntax, morphology
- Age-appropriate basic comprehension and production of words and sentences
- Intact story grammar in short narratives
- Intact cohesive skills at sentence level
- Islands of preserved premorbid abilities
- Limited disruption of overlearned abilities, such as counting
- Comprehension affected by decreased attention and speed of processing
- Difficulty with verbal abstractions, drawing conclusions
- Dysarthria, apraxia, or both
- Disruption of recently acquired linguistic skills resulting from recent memory deficits
- Difficulty expressing complex thoughts, identifying main ideas, organizing information in oral or verbal form
- Difficulties in word fluency, confrontational naming, and word finding
- Ineffective, tangential, or inappropriate social discourse
- Impaired cohesion at discourse level, resulting in long, fragmented, or irrelevant utterances in discourse
- Inappropriate social and pragmatic behavior; poor social problem solving
- Inflexibility and impulsivity in language and behavior
- Difficulty in detecting semantic anomalies
- Deficits in pragmatic language use

Adapted from Russell, N. (1993). Educational considerations in traumatic brain injury: The role of the speech-language pathologist. *Language, Speech, and Hearing Services in Schools, 24,* 67-75; Blosser, J.L., & De Pompei, R. (2002). *Pediatric traumatic brain injury: Proactive intervention* (2nd ed.). San Diego: Singular; Hanten G., Zhang, D., Barnes, M., Roberson, G., Archibald, J., Song, J., & Levin, H. (2004). Childhood head injury and metacognitive processed in language and memory. *Developmental Neuropsychology, 25,* 85-106; Yeates, K., Swift, E., Taylor, H., Wade, S., Drotar, D., Stancin, T., & Minich, N. (2004). Short- and long-term social outcomes following pediatric traumatic brain injury. *Journal of International Neuropsychological Society, 10(3),* 412-426.

find them today, working with them to establish as great a degree of functional skill and independence as we can.

Assessment Issues. Identifying a child's stage of recovery from brain injury can be important for assessing needs and planning programs. Gerring and Carney (1992) suggested that the Ranchos Los Amigos Cognitive Function Scale (Hagen, 1986), which was developed to identify stages in the course of recovery from head trauma for adults, can be adapted for use with younger clients to guide rehabilitative planning. A summary of the stages in this scale appears in Box 4-14.

Blosser and DePompei (2001) suggested that there are three stages to the assessment process in this population:

Phase I: the child is recovering medically, usually in an acute-care facility

Phase II: the child is medically stable and ready to begin rehabilitation

Phase III: ongoing assessment in the child's educational and daily living settings takes place

During phase I, assessment focuses on the physical care needs that affect treatment, such as respiratory, swallowing, or motor control problems. This also is a time to collect case history data from the family about premorbid functioning—the level at which the child performed before the TBI—and to help families understand the child's condition. In phase II, assessment focuses on determining the child's functional strengths and needs in behavioral, cognitive, and communicative domains. Phase III entails using formal and informal methods, as we discussed in Chapter 2, to establish baseline function, identify goals for intervention, and evaluate change in the therapy program. Phase III also may entail environmental assessment (Blosser & DePompei, 2001), in order to identify the demands and expectations of the child's daily living situations. This assessment can be used to develop a profile of the most important environmental requirements that should serve as the focus for treatment. It should also include assessing areas of higher level language function known to be residual

---

BOX 4-14 | **Stages of Cognitive and Communicative Functioning from the Rancho Los Amigos Level of Cognitive Functioning Scale**

I. No Response—Client appears to be in a deep sleep and is completely unresponsive to any stimuli.

II. Generalized Response—Client reacts inconsistently and nonpurposefully to stimuli in a nonspecific manner. Responses are limited and often the same, regardless of stimulus presented. Responses may be physiological changes, gross body movements, and/or vocalization.

III. Localized Response—Client reacts specifically, but inconsistently, to stimuli. Responses are directly related to the type of stimulus presented. May follow simple commands such as "Close your eyes" or "Squeeze my hand" in an inconsistent, delayed manner.

IV. Confused-Agitated—Behavior is bizarre and nonpurposeful relative to immediate environment. Does not discriminate among persons or objects, is unable to cooperate directly with treatment efforts, verbalizations are frequently incoherent and/or inappropriate to the environment, confabulation may be present. Gross attention to environment is very short, and selective attention is often nonexistent. Client lacks short-term recall.

V. Confused, Inappropriate, Nonagitated—Client is able to respond to simple commands fairly consistently. However, with increased complexity of commands, or lack of any external structure, responses are nonpurposeful, random, or fragmented. Has gross attention to the environment, but is highly distractible and lacks ability to focus attention on a specific task; with structure, may be able to converse on a social or automatic level for short periods of time; verbalization is often inappropriate and confabulatory; memory is severely impaired; often shows inappropriate use of subjects; may perform previously learned tasks with structure, but is unable to learn new information.

VI. Confused-Appropriate—Client shows goal-directed behavior, but is dependent on external input for direction; follows simple directions consistently and shows carry-over for relearned tasks with little or no carry-over for new tasks; responses may be incorrect because of memory problems, but appropriate to the situation; past memories show more depth and detail than recent memory.

VII. Automatic-Appropriate—Client appears appropriate and oriented within hospital and home settings, goes through daily routine automatically, but is frequently robot-like, with minimal to absent confusion; has shallow recall of activities; shows carry-over for new learning, but at a decreased rate; with structure, is able to initiate social or recreational activities; judgment remains impaired.

VIII. Purposeful and Appropriate—Client is able to recall and integrate past and recent events, and is aware of and responsive to the environment; shows carry-over for new learning and needs no supervision once activities are learned; may continue to show a decreased ability, relative to premorbid abilities in language, abstract reasoning, tolerance for stress, and judgment in emergencies or unusual circumstances.

Reprinted with permission from Hagen, C. (1986). Language disorders in head trauma. In J.M. Costello & A.L. Holland (Eds.), *Handbook of speech and language disorders*. San Diego, CA: College-Hill Press.

deficits in children with TBI (Chapman et al., 2001; Savage, DePompei, Tyler, & Lash, 2005; Schoenbrodt, 2001b; Semrud-Clikeman, 2001). This assessment also can involve helping to sensitize communication partners to the child's needs and eliminating barriers in the environment to successful communication and interaction. Gerring and Carney (1992) explained that performance on formal tests may look quite good for children who are recovering from acquired brain damage because these structured procedures provide support that helps the child compensate for the impairments in executive functions that frequently disrupt performance in less-structured settings. They pointed out the importance of contrasting performance on formal tests with informal assessment in naturalistic situations, as we discussed in Chapter 2. Looking at performance in both optimal and stressful settings gives us a broader picture of the client's abilities. Blosser and DePompei (2002), Sohlberg and Mateer (1989), and Russell (1993) provided guidelines for conducting this two-pronged assessment for children with acquired brain damage. Many of them are recognizable from the general discussion of assessment principles in Chapter 2. They are summarized in Box 4-15.

Another important contrast to make in assessment, which is unique to the population of children with acquired brain damage, is a comparison of premorbid and present levels of performance. Assessment in the rehabilitation setting should include obtaining school records and discussing the child's academic status with teachers and parents. Skills in which the child was very proficient before the injury would be good targets for retraining, because overlearning may have helped to preserve these areas. Inconsistent performance is one of the hallmarks of acquired brain injury, though. We can't assume that because a child can, for example, do long division, he or she will necessarily be able to do simpler addition and subtraction. Each area needs to be probed. Hotz, Helm-Estabrooks, and Nelson (2001) have developed an assessment designed specifically for children with TBI that can also be useful in this endeavor. Additional resources on assessment of this population can be found in Savage et al. (2005), Schoenbrodt (2001b), and Semrud-Clikeman (2001).

Intervention Issues. Schwartz-Cowley and Stepanik (1989) suggested that there are three distinct phases of the intervention process in acquired brain injury, each of which requires a somewhat different approach. In the early phase of recovery from a focal lesion or TBI, when a client is still in a hospital or rehabilitation setting and spontaneous recovery is taking place, the goal of multidisciplinary intervention is to improve residual functions beyond levels they would reach without intervention. Sessions should be short and aimed at stimulating one modality at a time, with tactile and motor stimulation coming before visual and auditory. Once a response to stimuli has been established and is reliable, more functional activities can be introduced. These might include nodding answers to questions, basic self-care, and simple visual motor activities (copying shapes).

In the middle phase of recovery from focal lesions or TBI, intervention should emphasize structured tasks, such as those we discussed under clinician-directed and hybrid approaches in Chapter 3. Because of the frequent difficulties with attention, concentration, and impulsivity in children with acquired brain damage, the context of these activities should be free of distractions and be repetitive and predictable. Their goal would be to develop functional and adaptive behaviors. These would include work on language comprehension, simple verbal problem solving, and the use of self-monitoring to detect and self-correct errors.

In the late phase of recovery, the child with a focal lesion or TBI will be moving out of a rehabilitation setting and back to the home and school environments. Children with brain damage resulting from tumors, infections, irradiation, or seizure disorders also require programming appropriate for this phase. Blosser and DePompei (2002), McKerns and Motchkavitz (1993), Murdoch and Theodoros (2001), and Semrud-Clikeman (2001) provided some suggestions for working with children in this stage. Additionally, Russell (1993) and Blosser and DePompei (2002) emphasized that intervention in this stage should be collaborative and classroom based, to help the client adjust to the demands of the crucial school setting. Here the clinician may serve in a consulting role, helping the classroom teacher reintegrate the student into the mainstream program, as well as providing collaborative lessons that focus on integrating communication skills within the classroom program. Suggestions for collaborative intervention appear in Chapter 12. For children with severe disabilities related to TBI and who have deficits in basic language skills, the SLP may provide some individual treatment, as well as consulting with the classroom or resource room teacher to infuse these retrained skills into the academic program. Blosser and DePompei (2002) also provided some suggestions for helping reintegrate students with acquired brain damage into the school setting. These guidelines, summarized in Box 4-16, are appropriate for both direct intervention and for consulting with classroom teachers.

In addition to these strategies to help the student succeed in the classroom, additional intervention goals are suggested by Savage et al. (2005) and Ylvisaker and Szekeres (1989). These focus primarily on meta-cognitive functioning, or retraining clients to use executive functions to monitor their own cognitive processes and regulate their learning behavior. We'll talk a lot more in the chapters on language-learning disabilities about developing meta-cognitive skills in our students. Meta-cognitive goals, using cognitive behavior modification (Meichenbaum, 1977); reciprocal teaching (Brown & Palinscar, 1987, see Chapters 12 and 14 for detailed description); and a variety of other techniques discussed in the chapters on language-learning disorders, are appropriate for students with acquired brain damage.

Another area of intervention we often need to address with these students is pragmatics. As we saw, specific disorders of language form are not always present in students with acquired brain injuries, but language use is often disrupted. Malkmus (1989) discussed using videotapes to teach gaze, paralinguistic, and other pragmatic behaviors to students with acquired brain damage, by having students observe and rate the behaviors they viewed in the videotape. Students then make their own

BOX 4-15	**Guidelines for Formal and Informal Assessment in Acquired Brain Damage**

Formal Assessment

1. Use standardized tests to examine all major areas of cognitive and communicative functioning:
   - Intelligence (e.g., Bayley Scales of Infant Development–ed. 3. [Bayley, 2005]; Leiter International Performance Scale–Revised [Royd & Miller, 1997])
   - Executive function (e.g., *Wisconsin Cart Sorting Test* [Berg & Grant, 1980])
   - Judgment and reasoning (e.g., *Ross Test of Higher Cognitive Processes* [Ross & Ross, 1976])
   - Problem solving (e.g., *Test of Problem Solving–Adolescent* [Bowers, Barrett, Huisingh, Orman, & LoGiudice, 1991])
   - Attention and concentration (e.g., *Child Behavior Checklist* [Achenbach, 1991]; *Attention Deficit Disorder Evaluation Scale* [McCarney, 1986])
   - Memory (e.g. Denman Neuropsychology Memory Scale [Denman, 1984])
   - Perceptual and perceptual-motor (e.g., Beery-Buktenica Developmental Test of Visual-Motor Integration, 5th Ed. [Beery, Buktenica, & Beery, 2003]; Test of Visual Motor Skills [Gardner, 1986]; Test of Visual Motor Skills-Upper Extension [Gardner, 1992])
   - Academics and achievement (e.g., *Portage Guide to Early Education* [Bluma, Shearer, Frohmam, & Hilliard, 1976]; *Peabody Individual Achievement Test* [Dunn & Markwardt, 1970]; *Woodcock-Johnson Psycho-Educational Test Battery–Revised* [Woodcock & Johnson, 1990])
   - Social-emotional (e.g., *Vineland Adaptive Behavior Scales* [Sparrow, Cicchetti, & Balla, 1984])
   - Receptive and expressive language (e.g., Communication and Social Behavior Scales [Wetherby & Prizant, 1993]; MacArthur-Bates Communicative Development Inventories [Fenson et al., 1993]; Test of Language Development: P-3 [Newcomer & Hammill, 1997]; Test of Adolescent and Adult Language-3 [Hammill, Brown, Larsen & Wiederholt, 1994])
   - Speech (e.g., *Comprehensive Apraxia Test* [DiSimoni, 1989]; *Frenchay Dysarthria Assessment* [Enderby & Roworth, 1984])
   - Pragmatic skills, including narrative and conversational skills (e.g., *Test of Pragmatic Language* [Phelps-Terasaki & Phelps-Gunn, 1992])
2. Use multiple measures of each function to look at inconsistencies of performance.
3. Modify tests by giving items that are below the suggested basals and above suggested ceilings to look for areas of preserved function. Extend time limits on tests. Use both normative and observational information from these modifications to interpret test results.
4. Provide additional modifications of testing to gather additional information, such as infusing auditory and visual distractors, allowing the student to respond by pointing or underlining instead of talking, enlarging print and decreasing the amount of print per page, giving multiple examples to clarify instructions, giving breaks to offset fatigue and attention drift.

Functional Assessment

1. Use an observational protocol with a comprehensive breakdown of task components and areas of potential disruption.
2. Use multiple observations in different natural environments.
3. Use both quantitative and qualitative methods.
4. Use curriculum-based assessment methods (see Chapter 11).
5. Identify relevant environmental and contextual factors that can be provided to optimize performance.
6. Assess responses to cueing and use of compensatory strategies.

Adapted from Blosser, J., & DePompei, R. (1994). *Pediatric traumatic brain injury*. San-Diego, CA: Singular Publishing Group; Savage, R.C., DePompei, R., Tyler, J., & Lash, M. (2005). Pediatric traumatic brain injury: A review of pertinent issues. *Pediatric Rehabilitation, 8(2),* 92-103; Semrud-Clikeman, M. (2001). *Traumatic brain injury in children and adolescents: Assessment and intervention*. New York: Guilford Press; Sohlberg, M., & Mateer, C. (1989). The assessment of cognitive-communicative functions in head injury. *Topics in Language Disorders, 9(2),* 15-33; Russell, N. (1993). Educational considerations in traumatic brain injury: The role of the speech-language pathologist. *Language, Speech, and Hearing Services in Schools, 24,* 67-75.

tapes and observe and rate their own behaviors. Structured discourse sessions also can be useful. Here the clinician begins with ritual speech acts, such as greetings, introductions, requests for repetition and clarification, modeling, and having students practice these acts. Later, less routine speech acts (e.g., requesting, describing, suggesting, negotiating) and expressing and responding to feelings are monitored and practiced in the controlled setting. Students are then encouraged to try their skills in the context of family or peer interactions, to report back, discuss, and monitor their effectiveness. Other pragmatic

| BOX 4-16 | Guidelines for Reintegrating Students with Acquired Brain Damage |

1. Plan small-group activities to help develop interaction skills.
2. Clarify verbal and written instructions by reading written instructions out loud and accompanying verbal instructions with written ones. All instructions should be repeated, with unfamiliar terms defined or paraphrased.
3. Explain core vocabulary and concepts, or "pre-teach" this material in individual sessions.
4. Pause when giving instructions to allow extra processing time.
5. Give the student extra time to respond, since processing speed may be slow.
6. Avoid figurative language or paraphrase it.
7. Give the student a classroom "buddy" to help him or her keep on top of instructions, assignments, and classroom transition times (see Chapter 14).
8. Let the student use assistive devices, such as a typewriter, computer, or calculator.
9. Help the student "get organized" by having him or her keep a written log of classes, assignments, due dates, and so on. Monitor the log frequently.
10. Set aside time for the student to talk to a trusted adult about feelings and frustrations in readjusting (see Chapter 14).
11. Plan extracurricular activities based on interests before the injury as well as on current abilities.
12. Avoid direct, confrontational questions in class. Ask leading or indirect questions (e.g., "Tell me about . . .") to encourage responsiveness. Let the student answer questions privately with the teacher or clinician or in a small group to check comprehension.
13. Decrease distractions in the classroom, perhaps using an individual carrel on the student's desk. If mobility problems are present, carefully arrange classroom furniture to permit easy movement.
14. Modify assignments by reducing the number of questions to be answered or the amount of material to be read. Let the student tape lectures, give test answers verbally, or otherwise change the format of testing to accommodate the student's abilities. Go over tests and explain errors (see Chapters 12 and 14).
15. Augment textbooks with pictures and vocabulary lists, or highlight key information in the student's book. Provide a tape-recorded summary of textbook material. Assign the student to answer review questions on material. Use reciprocal teaching techniques (see Chapters 12 and 14).
16. Teach compensatory strategies (see Chapter 14).
17. Announce and clarify conversational/lesson topics.
18. Support many forms of communication through gestures, pictures, written forms, etc.
19. Require and expect communication; reinforce all communicative attempts; construct opportunities to communicate (lunch buddies, paired classroom activities, etc.).
20. Practice higher level reasoning skills in small groups with peers engaged in problem-solving activities.
21. Encourage memory skills by teaching strategies such as categorizing, association, rehearsing, visualizing, and chunking.

Adapted from DePompei, R., & Blosser, J. (1987). Strategies for helping head-injured children successfully return to school. *Language, Speech, and Hearing in Schools, 18,* 292-300; Blosser, J., & DePompei, R. (2002) *Pediatric traumatic brain injury* (ed. 2). San Diego, CA: Singular Publishing Group.

training programs, including Kilman and Negri-Schoultz's (1987) as well as social-skills training programs, are discussed in Paul (2003a,b). These, too, are appropriate for students with acquired brain damage.

Many of the techniques used in intervention for the client with an acquired language disorder are similar to the ones used for students with language-learning disorders. The cognitive and communication patterns in children with acquired brain damage are in many ways similar to the ones we see in specific learning disabilities. There is a scattering of abilities, with some areas of relatively unimpaired function and others with deficits of varying degrees of severity. Attention, memory, and impulsivity problems also are common in both conditions. Despite these similarities and the fact that similar intervention methods are often appropriate, it is wise to be aware of some of the ways in which these two conditions differ. Blosser and DePompei

(2002) summarized these differences, which are listed in Table 4-5. When working with students who have acquired language disorders, special consideration needs to be given to these differences and their effects on communication and learning. Several books have appeared recently that aim to help parents of children with TBI with adjusting to, coping with, and understanding their children's difficulties. These include Schoenbrodt (2001a) and Cera, Vulanich, Brady, and Blosser (2003). Semrud-Clikeman (2001) is a useful resource for school personnel.

SPECIFIC LANGUAGE DISORDERS

SPECIFIC LANGUAGE IMPAIRMENT

As we discussed in Chapter 1, some kinds of language disorders have no known concomitants. These disorders have been

TABLE 4-5	**Differences between Language-Learning Disabilities and Acquired Language Disorders**

LANGUAGE-LEARNING DISABILITY	ACQUIRED LANGUAGE DISORDER
1. Mild memory problems	1. Severe recent memory problems, with difficulty carrying over new learning
2. Early onset	2. Later onset
3. Central damage can only be assumed from "soft neurological signs"	3. Direct evidence of neurological impairment
4. No pre/post contrast	4. Marked pre/post contrast of abilities, self-perception, and perception of self by others
5. Skills and knowledge show uneven development	5. Some old skills and knowledge remain, but there are inconsistencies of performance
6. Physical problems usually include only mild motor incoordination	6. Physical disabilities may include paresis (weakness) or spasticity
7. Basic cognitive skills may be intact	7. Basic cognition is commonly disrupted
8. Acquisition of new skills is slow, but what is learned is usually retained	8. What is learned may not be retained; much repetition and practice using compensatory strategies are needed
9. Status changes slowly	9. Status may change rapidly during recovery
10. Visual perceptual problems often unaccompanied by visual impairment	10. Visual problems often include double vision, poor depth perception, inability to adjust from near (book) to far (blackboard) vision, partial loss of vision
11. Client is distracted by external events	11. Client is distracted by both external and internal events, with internal events related to the brain damage
12. Normal or high activity level	12. Recovery from coma may include slowness or lethargy
13. Seizure medication, which can cause dulling of cognitive function, used only if frank seizures are present	13. Seizure medication may be used to prevent seizures, even if they have never occurred, and their cognitive dulling effects may influence learning
14. Usually aware of own learning problems	14. Injury may cause lack of awareness of learning problems in some cases
15. Behavior modification strategies are often effective	15. Organic dysfunction and memory losses may decrease the success of behavior modification
16. New learning can often be linked to past learning, although memory problems are present	16. Loss of some long-term memory may make linking new learning to old more difficult
17. Emotional reactions connected with present situation	17. Emotions can be labile and unpredictable and may not be linked to immediate situation

Adapted from Blosser, J., and DePompei, R. (Nov., 1992). *Serving youth with TBI: Circumventing the obstacles to school integration.* Mini-seminar presented at the annual convention of the American Speech-Language-Hearing Association, San Antonio, TX; Blosser, J., and DePompei, R. (2002) *Pediatric traumatic brain injury* (ed. 2). San Diego, CA: Singular Publishing Group.

traditionally defined by exclusion, that is, by the absence of the other factors we've discussed in this chapter—MR, sensory disorders, neurological damage, emotional problems, or environmental deprivation. We've talked about the change in terminology, from *childhood aphasia* to *specific language disorder* or *specific language impairment (SLI)*, that has taken place in labeling these disorders. We have also discussed the reasons for this change: the lack of clear evidence of specific neurological structural or functional differences to define the disorder.

Rescorla and Lee (2001) have argued on the basis of recent evidence regarding the development of very young children with delayed speech (e.g., Paul, 2000; Rescorla, Roberts, & Dahlsgaard, 1997) that it is not appropriate to make the diagnosis of SLI until age 4. Research suggests that younger children with delayed language have a good chance of "out-

growing" their slow start, although their language functioning may seem very similar to children with SLI at earlier ages (Dale, Price, Bishop, & Plomin, 2003) and they frequently retain subtle weaknesses when compared to socio-economic peers (Rescorla, 2002, 2005; Snowling, Adams, Bishop, & Stothard, 2001; Weismer & Evans, 2002). We'll restrict our use of the term SLI to mean children who retain significant deficits in language acquisition after age 4, but we will talk about what this condition can look like in younger children, as well.

We've talked before about the issue of subtyping language disorders syndromes. As you know, the *DSM-IV* of the APA (1994) recognizes only two types of SLI: Expressive Disorders, restricted to deficits in the production modality, and Mixed Receptive/Expressive Disorders, in which difficulties are seen in both modes. Not all writers in the field accept this limitation, however. Bishop (1997), for example, has argued that detailed assessment reveals that most children with SLI have some impairment in comprehension, even though the productive disorder may be more salient. Curtiss and Tallal (1985) reported that patterns of performance on language testing over time in a longitudinal study were the same for children with SLI regardless of the subgroup in which they had been placed (Expressive versus Mixed). Bishop contends that the differences among children with SLI may be more a matter of degree than a sharp distinction between subgroups. She suggests that instead of identifying subtypes, we may do better to try to characterize the dimensions of communicative functioning that are impaired in this population at different points in time. Let's try to understand the SLI population better by looking at some of the linguistic, psychological, social, and behavioral characteristics typical of this disorder.

Linguistic Characteristics

We mentioned earlier that, in general, language acquisition in SLI follows the normal sequence. Communication patterns of children with SLI are similar to those of children at comparable levels of language development, as indexed by MLU. While this pattern holds true when looking at one specific feature of development at a time, Leonard (1991) pointed out that children may be 1 year below age level in one set of features, 1½ years below in another, 6 months below in a third, and so on. The result will be that the overall profile of language skills in a child with SLI may not resemble that of a child with normal language function at any point in development. This does not mean that language development is deviant, but rather that it is in some ways asynchronous, just as the language profiles of children with Down syndrome typically are (Rice, Warren, & Betz, 2005).

Early lexical usage in children with SLI is very much like that of normally developing children at similar language levels but is acquired at a slower pace. Vocabulary sizes of normally developing 2-year-olds are more than 200 words, whereas those of children with SLI are in the range of 20 words (Paul, 1996; Rescorla & Alley, 2001; Rescorla, Mirak, & Singh, 2000; Rescorla et al., 1997). Moreover, children with SLI talk and communicate less often than same-age peers (Rescorla & Lee, 2001). While these children acquire sounds and use phonological simplification processes that are similar to those of peers, their repertoires of consonant sounds are smaller, and they take longer to acquire CVC syllables and multisyllabic productions (Paul & Jennings, 1992; Rescorla & Ratner, 1996; Roberts, Rescorla, Giroux, & Stevens, 1998). The development of sounds and words is closely related in this population (Stoel-Gammon, 2002).

Although vocabulary deficits are the first sign of language delay, these typically resolve by age 3 to 4 (Paul, 1996; Rescorla, Mirak, & Singh, 2000). Studies of the ability of children with SLI to acquire new words in "fast mapping" or "quick incidental learning" studies, in which they receive brief exposure to new words, show impairments in both production and in comprehension, although production impairments are more pronounced (Alt, Plante, & Creusere, 2004; Dollaghan, 1987; Kiernan & Gray, 1998; Rice, Buhr, & Oetting, 1992; Weismer &

Evans, 2002). Use of early semantic relations appears similar to that of language-matched peers (Leonard, 1989). Vocabulary in school-aged children with SLI lags behind that of peers (Rice, Warren, & Betz, 2005), perhaps because of reduced experience through reading (which is often problematic for these children).

The first delay to be seen in the syntax of children with SLI is a failure to combine words spontaneously at 18 to 24 months (Paul, 1996; Rescorla et al., 1997; Rescorla, Dahlsgaard, & Roberts, 2000; Rescorla & Roberts, 2002). Follow-up studies indicate that these children continue to lag behind in syntactic development (Rescorla, Dahlsgaard, & Roberts, 2000; Rescorla & Mirren, 1998). They appear to acquire syntactic structures in roughly the same order as do normally speaking children, although they make more errors for longer periods and use higher rates of ungrammatical sentences (Rescorla & Lee, 2001; Rescorla & Roberts, 2002). Children with SLI do have particular difficulty with learning grammatical morphemes, however. These include certain bound morphemes (plural s, possessive 's, -ed, copula be verbs); auxiliary verbs (e.g., is, do, can); and small, closed-class morphemes (such as articles a and the). Morphemes that complicate the phonological structure of the output word (such as plural s that turns cat into a word with a final cluster, cats) seem to pose some special difficulties (Cleave & Rice, 1997; Leonard, 1989), even relative to younger children at the same language level. However, the question of whether these differences are the result of a specific grammatical disability (Gopnik & Crago, 1991; Rice & Wexler, 1996), deficits in phonological and working memory (Gathercole & Baddeley, 1990), particular aspects of auditory processing (Tallal, Miller, Bedi, Byman, Wang, Nagarajan, Schreiner, Jenkins, & Merzenich, 1996), or more general processing difficulties (Bishop, 1997; Leonard, 1998) is still a matter of debate (see Botting & Conti-Ramsden, 2001; Eadie, Fey, Douglas, & Parsons, 2002; Evans, 2000; Weismer & Evans, 2002; also see Chapter 1).

Pragmatic skills are generally better than skills in language form, and this is one of the characteristics that differentiates SLI from ASD (Caparulo & Cohen, 1983). While children with SLI have been reported to be less interactive than age-matched peers, they are often similar to younger language-matched children (Rescorla & Lee, 2001), and pragmatic deficits seen are usually in the mild range (Rice, Warren, & Betz, 2005). Rice, Warren, and Betz (2005) suggest that apparent pragmatic differences in children with SLI are secondary to their primary difficulties in morphosyntax. Lahey (1988) argued that pragmatic deficits were more closely related to comprehension than expressive level; when normal and SLI groups are matched for comprehension level, most areas of language use appear to be similar. Still, Marton, Abramoff, and Rosenzweig (2005) report finding significant deficits in social knowledge in children with SLI. As we've seen, though, there are some children with SLI whose deficits extend into the pragmatic realm. Whether these children should be thought of as SLI or ASD is often a matter of disagreement. One other area in which children with SLI may have deficits is in prosody. Wells and Peppe (2003) reported that, as a group, children with SLI scored lower on a prosodic measure than age mates, and more like younger children with normal language.

Cognitive Skills

How specific are specific language disorders? Children with SLI are at greatly increased risk for attention and activity problems (Cantwell, Baker, & Mattison, 1979; Tallal, 1988; Tetnowski, 2004), as we've seen. Other "soft" neurological signs also are commonly present in children with SLI (Benton, 1964; Eisenson, 1972). The involvement of nonverbal cognitive skills in SLI also has been investigated and is still a matter of intense interest and debate. Several researchers (Bavin, Wilson, Maruff, & Sleeman, 2005; Johnston & Ramstad, 1978; Johnston & Weismer, 1983; Kamhi, 1981; Kamhi, Catts, Koenig, & Lewis, 1984; Rescorla & Goossens, 1992; van der Lely, 2005) have demonstrated that children with SLI do have problems with certain kinds of nonverbal cognition, including symbolic play, classification, figurative thinking, mental rotation, haptic perception, and hypothesis formation. Botting (2005) showed that children with SLI lost 20 nonverbal IQ points between the ages of 7 and 14. These findings have led to the hypothesis that children with SLI may have not just a language problem but a general representational deficit, affecting a variety of kinds of symbolic functioning. Casby (1997) argued, however, that these findings are not definitive. The differences found between groups in these studies were usually frequency differences, not qualitative ones. He also pointed out that it is hard to separate language difficulties from these performances, since children with SLI may not understand directions or explain their behaviors in words so that the examiner can appreciate the complexity of their mental representations. Leonard (1987) reported that although some children with SLI fall below age mates on such tasks, they still do better than younger children with comparable language skills.

Auditory and Information Processing

Another area in which deficits have been explored is the rate of information processing and responding, particularly in the auditory modality. We talked in Chapter 1 about Tallal's contention that SLI can be traced back to difficulties in discriminating rapidly presented tones and in sequencing tones presented in rapid sequence. Tallal et al. (1996) has argued that children with SLI are specifically impaired in the ability to process rapidly presented information. Other investigators, including Weismer and Hesketh (1996) and Kail (1994), have provided corroborating evidence on this account. Although these studies show that length and complexity of the tasks used have a large effect on performance, in general it appears that children with SLI process information somewhat more slowly than typically developing children. This suggests that interventions that involve slowing the rate of input may help these children to improve their processing of language. We must remember Bishop's (1997) arguments, though, about the possibility that slow auditory processing could be a *result* rather than a cause of language disorder. Some evidence is accumulating to call Tallal's assertion into question (Rosen, 2003; Rosen & Adlard, 2004; van der Lely, 2005), and Bishop's group has been active in advancing the suggestion

that auditory processing is immature, rather than disordered in these children (Bishop, 2005; Bishop & McArthur, 2004; Mengler, Hogben, Michie, & Bishop, 2005). (For a further discussion of auditory and information processing in SLI, as well as theories of its etiology, see Chapter 1.)

Neuromotor Skills

Since specific language disorders have been recognized, it has been known that children with SLI typically display "soft" neurological signs such as clumsiness, poor attention, mild motor difficulties, and poor visual-motor integration (Rescorla & Lee, 2001). These findings have led to speculation about a neuromaturational lag as one root of SLI. Several investigators (e.g., Beitchman, Hood, Rochon, Peterson, Mantini, & Majumdar, 1989; Powell & Bishop, 1992) have demonstrated correlations between language disorders and neuromotor deficits.

Social and Behavioral Functioning

We talked earlier about the common associations between socioemotional and behavioral disorders and SLI. Young children with delayed language tend to have social skill deficits that go beyond their verbal difficulties (Paul, 1991a). Older preschoolers with SLI have been shown to be less likely to initiate interactions with peers and this, in turn, limits their opportunities to learn and practice communication and social skills (Redmond & Rice, 1998), although these difficulties tend to decrease as the children grow (Redmond & Rice, 2003). Behavior problems, such as overactivity, aggressiveness, and moodiness, are often perceived by parents of children with delayed language, but these, too, tend to resolve as linguistic skills improve (Paul & Kellogg, 1997). As we saw earlier, ADHD commonly co-occurs with SLI. Rescorla and Lee (2001) and Tetnowski (2004) reported that ADHD is the most commonly co-occurring disorder in children with SLI, particularly in those whose disorder has a receptive component. Conti-Ramsden and Botting (2004) found that over one-third of children with SLI had poor social adjustment at age 11. Redmond (2002), though, suggests that many of the rating scales used to identify social and behavioral disorders contain items that are verbal in nature and could be biased toward overidentifying children with SLI, and suggests augmenting such forms with more direct observation and assessment.

SLI and Learning Disabilities

Estimates of the co-occurrence of SLI and school learning problems run as high as 60% (Schoenbrodt, Kumin, & Sloan, 1997). Tallal (1988) has suggested that many children with mild to moderate forms of SLI "change diagnoses" when they get to school age, not because the underlying nature of their problem changes, but simply because the demands of the school situation put stress on their "wobbly" (Nelson, 1998) language skills. Children with SLI, particularly those with mild to moderate impairment, often outgrow the most obvious aspects of their linguistic deficits by the end of the preschool period (Paul, 1996, 2000; Rescorla, 2002, 2005; Scarborough & Dobrich, 1990; Tallal, 1988). The deficits that remain often surface only in situations requiring complex language skills, such as phonological awareness, meta-linguistic, and narrative tasks. These situations are just the ones, though, that are required for success in learning to read, write, spell, and do mathematical problems. Although not all children with learning disabilities have a history of SLI, a very high proportion of children with SLI also have trouble in school, particularly in learning to read (Eisenmajer, Ross, & Pratt, 2005; Mackie & Dockrell, 2004). For this reason, children who "outgrow" SLI often seem to "grow into" learning disabilities. Leonard (1991) argued that this progression may reflect language skills that are simply limited relative to those in the general population, rather than reflecting a specific pathology. Tallal (1988) has suggested that language disorders and language-learning disabilities should not be considered separate, but simply different manifestations of the same problem at different ages. Bishop and Snowling (2004), on the other hand, argue that there are two components of reading disorders that relate to different aspects of language: decoding deficits, which relate to phonological awareness problems, and comprehension deficits, which relate to semantic and syntactic difficulties. Whether we consider the two disorders as separate or unitary, the knowledge of their likely co-occurrence has clinical implications. It tells us that building emergent literacy skills in young children with language disorders is especially important, and that we need to address not only the phonological awareness skills that will impact decoding, but also the development of more sophisticated semantics and syntax that will affect reading comprehension. Chapter 9 gives detailed methods for accomplishing this goal. It also suggests that when we work on oral language in school-aged children with language-learning disorders, we need to use targeted procedures to provide them with specific skills that help them make the transition to literacy. These approaches are presented in Chapters 12 and 14.

Prognosis

As we've said, one aspect of the natural history of SLI is that it tends to change shape with age. In children with mild to moderate disorders, oral language problems predominate in early childhood, whereas learning difficulties are more obvious during the school years. For children with this degree of severity, several factors appear to affect prognosis. Range of areas affected is one. Children with deficits limited to articulation have the best prognosis (Hall & Tomblin, 1978), whereas those with expressive language disorders but intact comprehension skills fare better than those with deficits in both language modalities (Thal, Reilly, Seibert, Jeffries, & Fenson, 2004; Whitehurst & Fischel, 1994). The degree of the impairment also is a factor (Bishop & Edmundson, 1987), with more severely delayed preschoolers showing less favorable outcomes at school age. Nelson (1998) reported that better prognosis in SLI is associated with few perinatal problems, higher nonverbal IQ, and willingness on the child's part to participate in groups. Paul and Fountain (1999) suggest that the ability to communicate for adaptive purposes, even when language is limited, is related to outcome in young children with delayed language. Certain measures have been shown to be good predictors of school-age outcome in preschoolers with mild to moderate SLI. These include

measures of nonword repetition (Botting & Conti-Ramsden, 2001), the ability to learn words through "fast mapping" (Weismer & Evans, 2002), narrative skills (Bishop & Edmundson, 1987), certain motor abilities (Paul & Fountain, 1999), and performance on sentence repetition tasks (Lee, 1971; Aram, Ekelman, & Nation, 1984).

The proportion of children who show persistent problems in language varies from study to study. Both Bishop and Edmundson (1987) and Shriberg and Kwiatkowski (1988) reported that about 20% of children with disorders restricted to phonology required special services by the time they reached school age. Whitehurst and Fischel (1994) and Paul (1996) reported that a similar proportion of children with specific expressive language delays as preschoolers had deficits in oral language skills by kindergarten age. For children with both expressive and receptive deficits, risk estimates for persistent problems in oral language and academic skills range from 40% to 80% (Nelson, 1998). For children whose problems do persist, deficits tend to narrow in their focus and to be concentrated in subtle difficulties of language organization and efficiency, rather than frank errors. Academic problems tend to involve primarily reading and writing. Some mild social deficits also may be seen. Despite their persistent problems, though, most of these children finish high school, some go on to college, and most live independent lives (Hall & Tomblin, 1978; Rescorla, 2005; Snowling, Adams, Bishop, & Stothard, 2001).

For children with severe SLI, the prognosis is more guarded. Paul and Cohen (1984) studied long-term outcomes in children diagnosed with SLI as preschoolers who were not speaking in full sentences by the time they were 6. By the time they were adolescents, these subjects were likely to score in the retarded range on IQ tests, even if they had scored in the normal range at the preschool level. These children, all receiving intensive language intervention, made steady progress in receptive language skills throughout their school years, and progress in expressive ability was at a rate that exceeded their growth in age. Still, 90% of these subjects were significantly below the normal range in both areas by adolescence, and all required intensive special education, with most in special classrooms, schools, or residential facilities.

SEVERE SPEECH PRODUCTION IMPAIRMENTS AND LANGUAGE DISORDERS

Many disorders can affect the orofacial structures or neuromotor functions that serve speech production. Some of these can leave the understanding and formulation of language, as well as general cognitive skill, more or less intact, resulting in circumscribed speech impairments. Cerebral palsy, certain congenital facial anomalies, and brain injuries specifically affecting neuromotor tracts are some examples. In Chapter 3 we discussed some principles to use in making decisions about augmentative communication for children with severe speech and physical impairment (SSPI). We'll want to apply those principles when choosing an augmentative or alternative system for these clients. Many such disorders also affect feeding and swallowing. These problems require an intervention program beyond the scope of this text, but clinicians should be aware of the need for assessing and planning treatment (perhaps in collaboration with physical and occupational therapists) for these aspects of the disability in children with SSPI.

Sturm and Clendon (2004) discuss some of the reasons why children with SSPI may have trouble learning language. Some have to do with the external barriers they face. They cannot learn through the usual sensorimotor interactions with people and objects because of their physical disabilities. They don't have constant access to their mode of communication as speakers do; if they use a board or device, someone has to get it and set it up for them before they can communicate. Their limited mobility gives them fewer opportunities to interact with other people. They aren't able to develop from babble to speech by playing with sound and using sound as an interaction tool; devices and outputs are chosen for them and may not be the best match for their abilities and intentions. Gerber and Kraat (1992) and Sturm and Clendon (2004) discussed the issues involved in designing language-learning programs for children who use AAC systems. They argued that although the developmental model certainly has limitations in working with these clients, it still provides the best working position to guide us in determining the content of language programs for AAC users. One necessary modification involves the issue of modalities of language. When we invoke a developmental model, we usually assess comprehension and production independently, use an index of productive capacity such as MLU to summarize the child's overall level, and focus primarily on production targets. This approach may not work best for children using AAC systems, though. Instead, Gerber and Kraat suggested focusing on comprehension skills in the assessment. Miller and Paul (1995) provided a variety of techniques for comprehension assessment that can be used with this population. It also is important to assess pragmatic and cognitive skills in these clients, since these assessments give some idea of the concepts and social interactions the client is using spontaneously. Intervention can follow the developmental model in terms of targeting words and word combinations that would be expected given the child's cognitive, comprehension, and communicative profile.

One finding of research on language development in children who use AAC is that a communication device that provides voice output, so that the machine "speaks" what the child selects to communicate, is very facilitative in stimulating both speech and language growth (Foley, 1993; Romski & Sevcik, 1996). These voice output communication aids (VOCAs) should, whenever possible, be part of the AAC system for clients with SSPI. Dowden and Marriner (1995) review the features of various VOCAs available.

In building a first lexicon for prelinguistic AAC users, Gerber and Kraat suggested following the normal sequence in introducing words that are typical of normal children's early vocabularies. They emphasized, however, the importance of offering a range of types of lexical items, using both single words that refer to objects and some fixed language chunks that the child can use as speech acts (e.g., "Don't do that," "Lemme see"). This diversity would allow AAC users to choose

from the range of language-learning styles seen in normal development (Nelson, 1973), rather than restricting them to a referential, one-noun-at-a-time style. Such choice might expand the child's possibilities for development.

Gerber and Kraat proposed that when teaching word combinations and sentence structures, our knowledge of normal development should guide the choice of semantic relations the child can be encouraged to express. But normal development may not be the best guide to choosing the syntactic forms to include on the AAC device. It may be more important to provide AAC users with opportunities to express some more complex ideas, on par with their cognitive or communicative level, than to learn all the appropriate grammatical morphemes for expressing these ideas. We may, then, want to provide the child with opportunities to produce sentences of the form "I play outside yesterday." If a child's productions are limited by the number of words that can be placed on a communication board, increasing the number of content words may be more important in providing communicative flexibility than using a full complement of grammatical markers. On the other hand, since speech synthesis devices can be programmed with whole sentences, children using these devices might be given ways to produce sentences such as "I drank all my milk." These sentences might be possible through the device before the point at which irregular past forms would normally be acquired in the developmental sequence. Paul (1997b) has suggested that programming the communication device with some "giant phrases" (See you later, alligator!), often used as gestalt forms by young children, can help the child using AAC to develop the analytical skills these forms facilitate in typical speakers.

Gerber and Kraat suggested including talk about "then and there" in the intervention program. The focus on a communication device may bias the intervention toward talk about the "here and now" for a longer period than would be typical in normal development. Bedrosian (1997) and Wood and Hood (2004) suggest that interactive storybook reading is an especially natural format in which such talk can take place. It will be important for clinicians who work on teaching first language skills to AAC users to begin to introduce some talk about past time, predictions about future events, discussions of pretend, and so on. Following some of the guidelines given in Chapter 9 for incorporating play contexts in language intervention can be helpful in achieving this goal. Finally, Sturm and Clendon (2004) emphasize the importance of having people who communicate with the AAC user use AAC themselves. Because children learn language partially through the desire to emulate others, it is important that others use AAC as a means of interacting with the client.

Although for many years children with SSPI were given little access to literacy, much has changed in the last 20 years (Koppenhaver, Coleman, Kalman, & Yoder, 1991). Considerable research and clinical effort has been devoted to developing literacy skills in these children and to providing a variety of AAC devices, from letter boards to computer-assisted devices, to transmit their written messages. This change has literally revolutionized the communicative capacity of many children with SSPI. Written output, which is understandable by most adults and older children in our culture, allows the child with SSPI to express the full range of meanings available in language to the broadest possible audience. Koppenhaver et al. (1991), Paul (1997b), and Sturm and Clendon (2004) have argued that to complete this revolution, it will be important in the coming years to make a variety of literacy experiences available to children with severe speech impairments to maximize their ability to use written communication. Although Sandberg (2001) and Smith (2001) reported that children with SSPI performed below developmental expectations on literacy measures despite instruction, there are methods that can be used to improve their chances for access to the written word. Improving basic language development is an important part of this picture (Sturm & Clendon, 2004), as is the provision of early, intensive exposure to storybook reading (Wood & Hood, 2004), opportunities for adapted writing (Sturm, 2003), and carefully scaffolded phonemic awareness and letter-sound association (Blischak, Shah, Lombardino, & Chiarella, 2004). Fallon, Light, McNaughton, Drager, and Hammer (2004) described a successful program for teaching beginning reading to students with AAC. This program is summarized in Table 4-6.

Additions suggestions for helping to develop literacy skills in these clients are summarized in Box 4-17.

CHILDHOOD APRAXIA OF SPEECH

Children with severe, persistent speech disorders accompanied by certain language and behavioral features are often said to have a *childhood apraxia of speech (CAS)* (Hall, 2000; Rosenbek & Wertz, 1972; Yoss & Darley, 1974). Alternative terms for this problem include *developmental verbal apraxia* or *dyspraxia*.

Davis (1998) discussed some of the controversies surrounding this disorder. Like "developmental dysphasia," CAS was originally defined as an analogue to an adult acquired neurological disorder: apraxia of speech, or a neurologically based

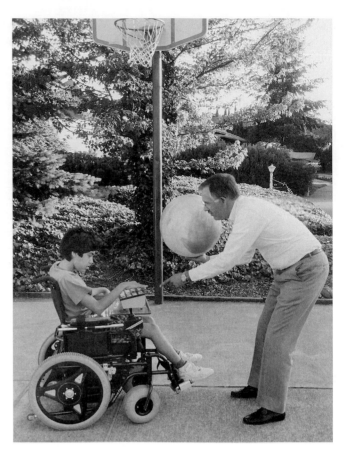

AAC systems increase communicative opportunities for children with severe speech production impairments.

difficulty in programming speech movements, thought to take place at a prearticulatory motor planning level. Intensive investigation, however, has not been able to document any consistent neuropathology in children who show this speech

---

TABLE 4-6	Methods for Teaching Early Literacy to Students with AAC

METHOD	ACTIVITY
Phonological awareness: Matching phonemes to initial sounds in words	Teacher labels each of four picture choices (*mop, cup, net, sun*). Teacher produces a phoneme. Client selects picture that started with the target sound.
Phonological awareness: Blending sounds into words	Clinician slowly produces the series of individual sounds that make up each target word (/m/, /a/, /n/). Client chooses the word from a set of four pictures (*man, pan, met, mat*).
Single word reading	Clinician models saying the sound for each letter of a word written on a card, blending the sounds, then saying the target word and matching it to a corresponding picture from a group of four. Clinician tracks letters with her finger, encourages child to say each sound "in his head," then choose the picture the word represents. Client tracks letters on the card and chooses the appropriate picture independently.

Adapted from Fallon, K., Light, J., McNaughton, D., Drager, K., and Hammer, C. (2004). The effects of direct instruction on the single-word reading skills of children who require augmentative and alternative communication. *Journal of Speech, Language, and Hearing Research, 47,* 1424-1439.

BOX 4-17	**Suggestions for Developing Literacy Skills in Children with Severe Speech Production Impairments**

- Use story-reading activities in intervention.
- Provide opportunities for clients to interact with normal children during story-reading activities to expose them to models for questions, comments, and retellings.
- Create "story boards" with reproductions of a series of individual pictures from a storybook that clients can use during story-reading activities to allow them to interact with the adult.
- Use repeated readings to facilitate development of story grammar.
- Read a variety of types of stories and nonfiction to clients to expose them to different literary *genres*.
- Provide independent access to text, writing, and drawing materials, using adaptive equipment such as computers.
- Get print into the environment within the client's line of vision. Show shopping lists, open mail and comment on it, point out product labels and signs, and label classroom objects with word cards.
- Encourage families to read to clients and display the print in the books to them. Encourage families to have clients watch literacy-related televisions shows such as *Sesame Street, Reading Rainbow,* and *Ghost Writer.*
- Pair pictures with printed words on communication boards and devices.
- Provide voice output communication devices early in the AAC program, as these are known to promote phonological awareness (Foley, 1993), which is highly related to success in reading (Swank & Larrivee, 1999).
- Include opportunities for student to "write" with adapted devices.
- Provide structured experience with sound awareness and analysis activities to build phonological awareness skills:
  a. Provide experience with hearing rhymes in rhyming stories, songs, and poems.
  b. Program communication devices to allow children to select a rhyme to complete poems in cloze activities.
  c. Have children identify how many syllables a word has by hitting a switch for each syllable.
  d. Have children identify which words begin with the same sound from an array on the communication device; later look for words with the same last sound.
  e. Go on "treasure hunts" for the child to identify by eye-pointing words that begin with their "special sound" for the day.
  f. Use commercial phonological awareness computer programs to give children practice with sound segmentation.

Adapted from Koppenhaver, D., Coleman, P., Kalman, S., & Yoder, D. (1991). The implications of emergent literacy research for children with developmental disabilities. *American Journal of Speech-Language Pathology: A Journal of Clinical Practice, 1,* 38-44; Paul, R. (1997). Facilitating transitions in language development for children who use AAC. *AAC, 13,* 141-148; Sturm, J.M., & Clendon, S.A. (2004). Augmentative and alternative communication, language, and literacy. *Topics in Language Disorders, 24(1),* 76-91.

pattern, even with sophisticated new techniques. Partly as a result of this failure to identify a neurological lesion similar to the one that causes apraxia in adults, some authors (Guyette & Diedrich, 1981) have suggested that CAS is not a clinically definable entity. The fact that the behavioral symptomatology associated with CAS overlaps so much with other conditions, such as developmental phonological disorders and expressive language delays, contributes to this view, and makes the diagnostic process difficult. Hall (2000) provides an in-depth discussion of the disorder that is helpful for educating parents.

Although traditionally, checklists of symptoms have been used to identify CAS, Shriberg, Campbell, Karlsson, Brown, McSweeny, and Nadler (2003a) and Shriberg, Green, Campbell, McSweeny, and Scheer (2003b) argued that this approach casts too wide a net, and results in overidentification. Shriberg, Aram, and Kwiatkowski (1997) and Shriberg et al. (2003a,b) contrasted linguistic behaviors in children with suspected CAS and those of children with developmental speech disorders (functional articulation problems) to find out whether the two groups could be differentiated on the basis of behaviors directly related to speech praxis, the generation of volitional

movement patterns for the purpose of performing an action. They, along with Munson, Bjorum, and Windsor (2003), concluded that two linguistic behaviors distinguished the two groups: inconsistent production of stress in tasks involving the naming of two-syllable words, and the degree of variation in the timing of speech. These results led Shriberg et al. to develop automated speech recognition methods for distinguishing speech samples of children with and without CAS (Hosom, Shriberg, & Green, 2004). These methods are likely to lead to more accurate diagnosis of this condition in the near future. Sample activities for addressing CAS are presented in Box 4-18.

Dowden and Marriner (1995) stressed that supplementation with AAC also should be considered for any child whose speech problem makes communication difficult. It will be important for these children to receive appropriate, intensive speech therapy, following guidelines like those in Box 4-18, as well as augmentative communication, and remedial activities with a broader focus on language and communication. Research (Lewis et al., 2004) suggests that speech disorders tend to improve in these children as they reach school age, while language and learning problems persist. The danger of the overuse of

---

BOX 4-18	Motor and Prosodic Approaches to Intervention for Children with Suspected CAS

Motor Approaches

- Massed practice: Schedule frequent, short sessions; use a small set of stimuli (5-7 words or phrases) practiced over and over before moving on to another small set.
- Use block practice schedules early on: Practice each utterance or stimulus many times in a row in the early stages of learning, as these facilitate retention.
- Use random practice schedules later: When production is stabilized, use random practice, where items are interspersed in random order, to facilitate generalization.
- Provide feedback: Provide feedback after a small number, but not every, response. Provide the feedback quickly, within less than a second of the production. Fade the amount of feedback as the intervention proceeds, and encourage client self-monitoring.
- Provide slowed-down models: Provide extra time for the client to process and program the target movement. As accuracy of movement increases, increase rate of presentation of stimuli gradually.
- Practice, practice, practice: The fundamental tenet of a motor approach is that learning takes place as a result of repeated successful trials that lead to habituation and automatization of processing. Develop strategies for imitation and practice that go beyond basic sit-and-drill to maintain interest and motivation.

Prosodic Approaches

- Practice analyzing words into syllables: Have clients clap out the syllables in a word, or have them use large blocks to represent stressed syllables in a word and small blocks to represent unstressed syllables. Be careful *not* to produce unnatural stress in word productions.
- Identify stressed syllables in words (Which part of rhiNOSceros is the loudest?), and imitate multisyllabic words with appropriate stress. If necessary, use backward chaining to achieve this (e.g., have the child say *y, city, tricity, lectricity, electricity*).
- Match phrases with meaning according to stress patterns: Have clients match *BLACKboard* to a picture of a chalk-board, and *BLACK BOARD* to a picture of a painted one, for example.
- Have children identify stressed words in sentences: Initially use exaggerated stress, then gradually fade the exaggeration.
- Use "wh-" questions: Have children use stress to contrast between answers to "wh-" questions, such as: Who ate the cheese? The *mouse* ate the cheese. What did the mouse eat? The mouse ate the *cheese*. What did the mouse do to the cheese? The mouse *ate* the cheese.

Adapted from Strand, E. (1995). Treatment of motor speech disorders in children. *Seminars in Speech and Language, 16,* 126-139; Velleman, S. (October, 1998). Lexical stress errors in developmental verbal dyspraxia: The problem and some possible solutions. *ASHA special interest division, Language Learning and Education* (newsletter).

CAS as a category lies in its tendency to lead clinicians to ignore the language needs of these children to focus on speech production or alternative modes of communication exclusively. If children who present with speech problems that resemble CAS receive careful assessment in both speech and language production skills, and if both areas are carefully attended to in intervention, this danger can be avoided.

■ CONCLUSIONS

For a book that takes a descriptive-developmental approach to assessment and intervention of child language disorders, this has been a long discussion of etiological factors and clinical categories. How come? Again, we want to use these factors to give us hints about assessment and intervention procedures. We also need information about these categories to interpret

the medical records we read in case histories and to aid in making placement decisions when etiological categories are used for this purpose by the educational and social service agencies with which we work. It's important to remember, as we emphasized in Chapter 1, that these categories are the beginning, not the end, of the process of planning assessment and intervention for children with language problems. There is a great deal of overlap in the communicative characteristics associated with these clinical categories, so knowing the etiological category alone doesn't indicate a unique pattern of language problems. Communication profiles in FAS, TBI, and language-learning disabilities in children with a history of specific language impairment are similar in many ways, for example. The categories are not mutually exclusive; children whose parents abuse drugs also can have hearing impairments, be mentally retarded, or acquire brain damage. So can

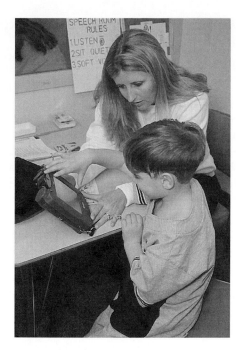

Aided AAC devices are sometimes used with children with severe CAS.

children with ASD, and so on. Finally and most importantly, knowing the clinical category tells us only a small amount of what we will need to know about a child's communicative function. To learn the rest we need to do thorough, comprehensive assessment of a broad range of language and related functions using the guidelines presented in Chapter 2. Then we need to develop intervention goals and methods based on the assessment data, choosing among a repertoire of procedures and contexts that we discussed in Chapter 3. That's the real work of designing a language program. While it is influenced by the clinical category associated with the child's disorder, it cannot be fully determined by it.

STUDY GUIDE

I. Mental Retardation
   A. Define *mental retardation*, and describe the diagnosis of retardation as mandated by the American Association of Mental Retardation.
   B. Describe the cognitive and linguistic characteristics typical of children with MR.
   C. Discuss syntax, morphology, phonology, semantics, and pragmatics in NSMR.
   D. Describe the most common syndromes of mental retardation, and discuss how they relate to communication assessment and intervention planning.

II. Language Disorders Associated with Sensory Deficits
   A. Discuss the types and degrees of hearing loss.
   B. Describe the cognitive and linguistic characteristics, including written language skills, of children with sensorineural hearing losses.
   C. Discuss the issues involved in manual Sign versus oral

language intervention for children with sensorineural hearing losses.
   D. Discuss the effects of otitis media on communication development.
   E. What clinical implications can be drawn from the research on otitis media and language disorders?
   F. How does blindness affect language development in terms of syntax, semantics, and pragmatics?
   G. What kinds of advice can be given to parents of young blind children to promote language growth?

III. Disorders with Environmental Components
   A. Describe the physical and cognitive characteristics associated with fetal alcohol syndrome. How do these affect communicative development?
   B. Discuss the definition of fetal alcohol effects. How does it differ from fetal alcohol syndrome?
   C. How does FAS interact with other environmental risks for communication disorders?
   D. What are some of the risks to communication development associated with maternal drug abuse? Why are these considered *risks* for language disorders rather than causes?
   E. Why are children with language disorders at increased risk for maltreatment?
   F. How does maltreatment affect communicative development?
   G. Describe the aspects that will be important in a parent training program for children who have experienced parental substance abuse or maltreatment.
   H. What are some implications for direct intervention with children who have a history of parental drug abuse or maltreatment?

IV. Communication in Psychiatric Disorders
   A. Discuss the co-incidence of communication disorders and socioemotional and behavioral problems.
   B. List and describe the kinds of socioemotional and behavioral problems that can be associated with language disorders.
   C. What can an SLP contribute to a consultation with the psychotherapist of a child with socioemotional and behavioral problems?
   D. Give some ideas for incorporating socioemotional and behavioral dimensions in the assessment and intervention program for children with language disorders.
   E. Discuss the behavioral features of ASD and other pervasive developmental disorders.
   F. Describe the cognitive, communicative, social, and sensory characteristics of children with ASD.
   G. Discuss considerations that should be kept in mind when developing an assessment and intervention program for a verbal child with ASD.
   H. What goals and methods can be considered in developing a communication program for nonspeaking children with ASD?
   I. Discuss the issue of alternative modes of communi-

cation in children with ASD.

J. Describe Asperger's syndrome, and give some clinical implications of this diagnosis.

V. Acquired Disorders of Communicative Function

A. Describe the four types of acquired brain damage that can affect communicative function. What kinds of communication problems are most typically associated with each type?

B. What concerns must be kept in mind when assessing children with acquired language disorders?

C. Describe the three phases of recovery from acquired brain damage and the intervention approaches appropriate for each.

D. Discuss reintegration in the classroom of children with acquired brain damage. What can the SLP contribute?

E. Describe the differences between language-learning disorders and acquired language disorders. What are their implications for clinical practice?

VI. Specific Language Disorders

A. Discuss the course of language development in children with SLI. Is it delayed or deviant? What other characteristics does it have?

B. How specific are specific language impairments? What other kinds of problems tend to accompany them?

C. Discuss what is known about auditory processing in SLI.

D. Discuss the relationship between SLI and language-learning disorders.

E. Describe the debate about the issue of subtyping in SLI.

F. Discuss the role of literacy in working with children who have severe speech production impairments.

G. How can SSPI affect language development?

H. Discuss the application of the developmental model in designing a language program for a child with SSPI.

I. Define and describe childhood apraxia of speech. Why is it a controversial category?

J. What concerns should be addressed in assessment and intervention for children suspected of having childhood apraxia of speech?

CHILD LANGUAGE DISORDERS IN A PLURALISTIC SOCIETY

CHAPTER OBJECTIVES

Readers of this chapter will be able to do the following:
- Describe the distinction between language disorders and language differences.
- Discuss the role of communication in culture.
- List a range of assessment procedures for evaluating communication in children with cultural and linguistic differences.

- Describe intervention issues and strategies for clients with cultural and language differences.
- Discuss the role of the speech-language pathologist in addressing communicative competence in bilingual and bidialectical clients.

In his book on the Civil War, James McPherson (1988) recounted an episode that occurred during General Lee's surrender to General Grant at the Appomattox Courthouse. General Grant's staff included a Native American of the Seneca tribe, by the name of Ely Parker. General Lee, upon being introduced to Parker, noticed Parker's Native American features and remarked, "Well, it's nice to see a real American here." And Parker replied, "We are all Americans."

Unless you've been stranded on the space shuttle for the past decade, it must be obvious that the cultural composition of American society is changing. Sources of this change include an increase in immigration from Africa, Central and South American countries, the Caribbean Islands, and many parts of Asia and the Pacific Rim, as well as an increase in internal migration of Native Americans away from reservations toward metropolitan areas. Robinson-Zanartu (1996) reported that, whereas 90% of Native Americans lived on reservations in 1940, only 20% do today. In fact, the U.S. Census Bureau (Hobbs & Stoops, 2002) reports that the percentage of Native Americans living in a metropolitan area increased more in the last 35 years than in any other group. A second source of the change is seen in the fact that although the overall percentage of children in the United States is declining, the proportion of children from nonwhite, non–Western European, non–English-speaking backgrounds is increasing (Children's Defense Fund, 1990; Hobbs & Stoops, 2002). This is a result both of higher birth rates in non-European and non-American populations (National Center for Health Statistics, 1985) and of the higher

number of females of child-bearing age in these groups, relative to the European and American populations (Hanson, 1998; Hobbs & Stoops, 2002). The result of these trends is that one in every four people in the United States is now of a race other than white, and the Hispanic population in the United States has doubled in the last 20 years (Hobbs & Stoops, 2002). In some states, such as California and Texas, a majority of residents are of a non-European background. By the year 2050, it is predicted that the percentage of individuals from non-European backgrounds will increase, as the percentage of whites declines to slightly over half of the population (Goldstein & Iglesias, 2006). In some cities, such as Miami, Philadelphia, and Baltimore, "minority" children are a majority in the public schools (Adler, 1993; Brice, 2002). But as Goldstein and Iglesias (2006) point out, there is a misperception that individuals from culturally and linguistically diverse populations exist mainly in large, urban areas. Children from culturally and linguistically diverse populations are well-represented across the nation's school systems. In 2001, 40% of children in U.S. schools were from culturally and linguistically diverse backgrounds; over 6% of all students were learning English as a second language, and it is predicted that this proportion will rise to 20% by 2010 (U.S. Department of Education, 2003). And, unfortunately, a disproportionate number of these children will be from poor, single-parent (usually single-mother) families and at risk for a variety of disabilities (Battle, 2002b; Brice, 2002; Hanson, 2004; Iglesias, 2001).

And yet, as Ely Parker so aptly observed, we are all Americans. This is the challenge that speech-language pathologists (SLPs) face as we progress through the new century: to appreciate the vibrant possibilities of the diversity that makes up our multi-faceted American civilization and to contribute to our clients' ability to participate in it. Appreciation entails understanding, sensitivity, and respect for the many ways people look at the world and use communication, given their differences in culture and experience. Contributing means that we use every tool available to ensure that all clients—regardless of cultural background—get the most informed, most effective assessment of their difficulties and the most efficient, sensitive support in maximizing their potential for successful communication.

The term *culture* refers to the ways of thinking, talking, understanding, and relating to others that are characteristic of groups of people with a shared history. Cultures evolve to serve a purpose: to make groups coherent and to preserve their values and beliefs over time. In general, people come to America because they want a better life for themselves and for their children. Some come to escape repressive or intolerant societies in their homelands. Others want a chance to participate in our prosperity and engage in our pursuit of happiness. However, the opportunity to participate in the economic and political freedom that America affords should not have to entail giving up all that was unique about the cultures from which each American came. For all of us, the achievement of participation in mainstream American life is a tug-of-war between opposing aspirations—the desire, on one hand, to enjoy the benefits of engagement in the wider society and the need, on the other hand, to maintain our cultural heritages and links to our past and our roots.

As clinicians, we help balance these desires by trying to provide access, through effective communication, to the opportunities of American society without depriving clients of the communication styles and strategies of their home cultures. This approach is often called "bicultural" education. Bicultural education simply means that a person can learn to take part in two (or more) sets of cultural styles and can switch back and forth when appropriate to maximize effectiveness in each. The foundation of bicultural education is understanding and sincere respect on the part of teachers and clinicians for cultures that contrast with those of the mainstream and that influence clients' communication.

DEFINING LANGUAGE DIFFERENCES

We should focus here for a moment on the distinction between a language difference and a language disorder. A *disorder* is what we defined in Chapter 1: a significant discrepancy in language skills relative to what would be expected for a client's age or developmental level. A language *difference*, on the other hand, is a rule-governed language style that deviates in some way from the standard usage of the mainstream culture. Some children from culturally different backgrounds have language disorders. When they do, the SLP's job is to provide reme-diation in a culturally sensitive way. But many children from

culturally different backgrounds who are referred for language assessment do not have disorders, only language differences. One of the primary jobs of the SLP in dealing with children from culturally and linguistically different (CLD) backgrounds is to diagnose language disorders accurately and to distinguish them from language differences.

When careful assessment, such as the kind described later in this chapter, reveals a difference rather than a disorder, we have two choices. One is to do nothing about it and simply inform the parents and teachers of the difference and distinguish it from a disorder. The other is to address the difference, as such, in an educational program. The clinician may deliver that program or consult on its development with a classroom or English as a Second Language (ESL) teacher. Because of the importance of communication to success both in school and in vocational settings, there is good reason for SLPs to collaborate in working with children who have language differences to improve their ability to communicate in the mainstream culture. We'll talk about developing Standard English proficiency in bicultural programs in the intervention section of this chapter.

First, though, let's look at few of the larger cultural groups likely to be encountered in language pathology practice with children. We'll talk first about some information useful in understanding the communication patterns of children from some of these minority groups. Additional information is available in Goldstein (2000). Then we'll look at some of the tools we can use to provide the most effective assessment and intervention services to these children.

LARGER MINORITY GROUPS IN AMERICA'S CULTURES

AFRICAN-AMERICAN CULTURE AND COMMUNICATION

As Terrell and Jackson (2002) pointed out, African-Americans, currently the largest single minority group in the country, are

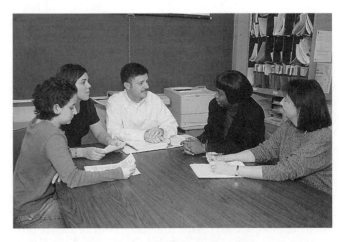

Cultural sensitivity is needed when working with families whose backgrounds differ from the clinician's.

not all alike. Some are wealthy, some are poor, and some are middle class. Socioeconomic class makes a good deal of difference in the attitudes and experiences of African-Americans, as it does in all Americans. However, one set of cultural experiences is common to many African-Americans: the history of forced abduction from their homelands, of slavery, and the tradition of racism and discrimination that has existed in the United States. Terrell and Terrell (1996) argued that the reaction to this set of experiences has formed many of the elements of contemporary African-American culture, including its music, religion, attitudes, and communication styles. Moreover, these experiences, according to Terrell and Terrell (1996), have led many African-Americans to develop a sense of cultural mistrust that can affect their performance on evaluations administered by white clinicians. Willis (2004) provides additional information on cultural features that were shaped by these experiences and are shared by families with African-American roots.

The communication style shared by many, though not all African-Americans, is often called African American Vernacular English, or AAVE. AAVE is considered a *dialect* of American English. Dialects are regional or cultural variations within a language that are used by a particular group of speakers. Dialects use a set of rules that are similar in many ways to those of the standard form of the language but differ in the frequency or circumstances of use of certain structures, lexical items, and other elements. All dialects of a language are mutually intelligible—any speaker of the language can understand them—and all are equally complex and legitimate. But some dialects have a higher status than others. The relative value or status of dialects is not inherent, though. It is said that a *language* can be defined as "a dialect with an army and a navy." In other words, the choice of which dialect has the role of the "standard" form of the language has more to do with power relations within the society than with anything intrinsic to the linguistic structure of any of the dialects involved.

Speaking a nonstandard dialect does not, in itself, constitute a disorder, but merely a difference in language use (Seymour, 2004). Still, the use of a nonstandard dialect such as AAVE can in some situations be a handicap to the user, if speakers of the standard dialect view the nonstandard form as inferior or deviant (Fitts, 2001). Terrell and Terrell (1983), for example, found that when two groups of equally qualified African-American women applied for secretarial jobs advertised in newspapers, applicants who spoke AAVE were less likely to be offered jobs. When they were, significantly lower salaries were offered to AAVE speakers than to speakers of Standard American English (SAE). Prejudice against speakers of AAVE, then, can have important economic implications.

Not all African-Americans use AAVE, and many who do are bidialectical. Some speakers use AAVE, for example, at home and with friends and switch to SAE, or whatever the predominant regional dialect of the mainstream is, when operating in the academic or employment setting. Use of AAVE varies, to some extent, with geographical region. Washington and Craig (1992), for example, found that AAVE speakers living in the urban Midwest did not use as many AAVE changes in their phonology as did children from the South. The use of AAVE changes over a person's lifetime, as well. Issacs (1996) and Craig, Thompson, Washington, and Potter (2003) found that use of nonstandard dialect decreased through the elementary school grades, with the biggest dip occurring between kindergarten and first grade (Craig & Washington, 2004). AAVE use also differs across contexts: Thomson, Craig, and Washington (2004) found that African-American third graders used less AAVE in more literate contexts, such as writing, than in picture description, while Curenton and Justice (2004) found that African-American preschool AAVE speakers used literate language forms as often as Caucasian peers in a story-telling task from a wordless picture book. However, some African-Americans live in relatively isolated settings and may have little exposure to Standard English (Willis, 2004; Wolfram, Hazen, & Tamburro, 1997). Despite the great variability in its use, some characteristic differences between AAVE and SAE are useful for clinicians to know. These differences are summarized in Box 5-1. For more detailed information on the linguistic structure of AAVE, Green (2002), Mufwene, Rickford, Baugh, and Bailey (1998), and Rickford (1999) are excellent resources.

Understanding these characteristics can help the clinician to communicate more effectively with African-American clients, to distinguish between a difference and a disorder, and to identify points of interference when developing a bidialectical educational program. It also is helpful in this enterprise to understand the normal sequence of acquisition in AAVE, which is described in Craig and Washington (2002, 2005), Jackson and Roberts (2001), and Kamhi, Pollack, and Harris (1996).

As we'll often see in this chapter, developing bidialectical programs does not mean that the home dialect, in this case AAVE, is defective in any way or that the AAVE speaker has a disorder. It only means that we want to give access to SAE to those normally developing speakers of AAVE who *elect* or whose families want them to learn the mainstream dialect to avoid encountering bias in the mainstream culture. Of course, we never want to "extinguish" use of AAVE; rather, our goal is to develop bidialectical individuals who can *code switch*, or move back and forth between AAVE and SAE, as appropriate to the situation.

HISPANIC-AMERICAN CULTURE AND COMMUNICATION

Americans of Hispanic heritage come from a variety of cultures and races. What they share is a background of Spanish-speaking ancestry, although they may not actually speak Spanish themselves. Hispanic-Americans (or *Latinos*) come from Mexico, Cuba, Puerto Rico, Spain, the Caribbean Islands, Central and South American countries, and even Asia or Africa, and account for close to 10% of the U.S. population (Goldstein, 2001). This diverse group speaks many dialects of Spanish; the major six spoken in the United States are Mexican, Central American, Caribbean, Chilean, and Puerto Rican. Some Hispanics are

| BOX 5-1 | Some Differences between AAVE and SAE |

Phonological Differences

Changes in Medial and Final Consonants
1. Voiced and voiceless *th* replaced (*toof* for *tooth*; *nofin* for *nothing*).
2. /r/ and /l/ deleted (/fo/ for *four*; *potect* for *protect*).
3. Voiced stops; (/b/, /d/, and /g/) devoiced with vowel lengthened in consonant-vowel-consonant words (/pIk/ with lengthened vowel for *pig*).
4. /m/ and /n/ deleted and replaced by a nasalized vowel (/pĬ/ with nasalized vowel for /pIn/).
5. /ŋ/ changed to /n/ in -ing forms.
6. Change in order of consonants in cluster (/ɛksep/ for *escape*).

Changes in Initial Phonemes, Syllables, and Initial Consonant Blends
1. Liquids often dropped from initial consonant blends (/p/ for /pr/; /b/ for /br/, etc.)
2. Certain consonants (particularly /w/ and /d/) omitted in specific words (*was, one,* and *don't*); final /r/ deleted.
3. Unstressed initial syllables dropped (*mato* for *tomato, cause* for *because*).
4. Word initial interdental fricatives; (*th*) replaced by stops.
5. *Thr* clusters pronounced as *th* (*tho* for *throw*).

Deletion of Final Consonants and Clusters
1. Final consonant is dropped in final clusters such as /nd/, /sk/, /sp/, /ft/, /ld/, /st/, /sd/, /nt/.
2. Variable deletion of certain consonants, including /l/, /b/, /p/, /d/, /t/, /g/, /k/.

Syntactic and Morphological Differences

Verb Marking
1. Regular past tense marking (*-ed*) is not obligatory and is sometimes omitted.
2. Irregular past tense is marked on some verbs and not on others (*see* is not changed to *saw*).
3. Regular and irregular third-person marking is not obligatory.
4. Future tense is often marked by *gonna* rather than *will*. When *will* is contracted, its pronunciation may be reduced. When *will* is required before *be* in SAE, it may be deleted in AAVE ("I be home later" instead of "I will be home later"); or *bouta* (He *bouta* fall).
5. Contractible forms of copula and auxiliary *be* verbs are not obligatory ("He here"), though contractible forms are obligatory ("Is he here?").
6. Perfect tense in AAVE is expressed by *been* to denote action completed in the distant past ("*She been gone*"); SAE uses adverbs to express this idea ("*She left long ago*").
7. Habitual state of verbs is marked with uninflected *be* in AAVE ("She be workin' two jobs"), whereas SAE uses adverbs and inflected forms of *be* ("She's working two jobs now").
8. Double modals are allowed in AAVE ("We might could go"), but not in SAE.

Noun Inflections

1. Plurals are not obligatory when quantifiers are present (*two dollar*).
2. Possessives are not obligatory when word order expresses possession ("Get mother coat"; "It be mother's").

Pronouns and Demonstratives

1. Pronominal apposition (noun followed by pronoun) is used in AAVE ("My mother she home").
2. Reflexive pronoun forms are regularized in AAVE so that all reflexive forms are produced by adding *–self* to a possessive pronoun (his-*hisself* in AAVE, but *himself* in SAE; their-*theirself* in AAVE, but *themselves* in SAE).
3. Relative pronouns are not obligatory in most cases, although in SAE only the *that* form is optional (AAVE: "He the one made it"; SAE: "He's the one *who* made it"; but SAE: "He's the one [that] you like").
4. *These here* and *them there* combinations used in AAVE, but not in SAE.
5. *Them* substituted in AAVE for forms used in SAE (*these, those*).

Comparative and Superlative Markers

1. Endings *–er* and *–est* can be added to most adjectives in AAVE (*baddest, worser*), unlike in SAE in which only certain forms can take these endings.
2. *More* and *most* can be combined with superlative comparative markers in AAVE (*most stupidest*).

BOX 5-1 **Some Differences between AAVE and SAE—cont'd**

Negation

1. Double- and triple-negative markers may be used in AAVE ("Nobody didn't never write to me"), but not in SAE ("Nobody ever wrote to me").
2. *Ain't* is used as a negative marker in AAVE.

Questions

1. Indirect questions are produced with the same form as direct questions in AAVE ("What is it?" "Do you know what is it?").
2. A clause beginning with *if* in SAE is produced with *do* in an indirect question in AAVE ("I want to know *do* you want to play ball with us?").

Semantic Differences

Many lexical items are used in AAVE that are not used in SAE or that come into SAE from their use in AAVE. Some examples include *funky* and *rap*. Other words are used to denote meanings in AAVE that are not part of their meaning in SAE, although often these meanings migrate into mainstream use as well. Some examples are *hog* (expensive car), *all that* (excellent), and *dude* (man or person).

Pragmatic Differences

1. Silence is used in AAVE when the speaker is in unfamiliar situations, when a speaker means to refute an accusation, or when a question considered intrusive is asked. The silence is often misinterpreted by mainstream listeners as a lack of innocence of an accusation or lack of knowledge, rather than as a communication strategy.
2. Direct eye contact is used in AAVE in the speaker's role, but indirect eye contact is considered proper listening behavior. Making direct eye contact with speakers by children and by speakers with lower status is considered disrespectful in AAVE. SAE speakers may misinterpret the indirect eye contact as "not listening" or "not making appropriate eye contact."
3. Wit and sarcasm are important elements in AAVE language interactions. These often involve ritualized insults and retorts. Skill at parrying in these interactions is highly valued. Such interactions, often perceived as hostile by SAE speakers, may in fact be friendly and playful.
4. Asking personal questions of a new acquaintance about his or her job, family, and similar matters is considered rude and intrusive in AAVE, although an SAE speaker may intend such inquiries to be friendly.
5. Conversations are considered private; butting in is seen as rude in AAVE, although SAE speakers may intend this behavior to be a helpful addition to the discussion.
6. Interruption is tolerated and access to the conversational floor is given to the most aggressive speaker in AAVE, whereas in SAE turn-taking rules attempt to give most participants at least some time to hold the floor, and interruption is considered rude.
7. Dynamic, intense behavior in public conversations in AAVE is acceptable, including intense verbal arguing; SAE requires more restraint, less emotion, and less intensity in verbal argument.
8. Narrative style in AAVE is more associational than topic-centered, as SAE narratives are. AAVE narratives flow from comments made in association with the last statement, rather than from a central theme.
9. Touching a child's hair during conversation is considered an insult in AAVE, whereas in SAE it is meant as a sign of affection.

Adapted from Adler, S. (1993). *Multicultural communication skills in the classroom*. Needham Heights, MA: Allyn & Bacon; Iglesias, A., and Goldstein, B. (2004). Language and dialectical variations. In J. Bernthal and N. Bankson (Eds.) (2004). *Articulation and phonological disorders*, ed. 5 (pp. 348-375). Boston, MA: Allyn & Bacon; Craig, H., Thompson, C., Washington, J., and Potter, S. (2003). Phonological features of child African American English. *Journal of Speech, Language and Hearing Research, 46,* 623-635; Haynes, W., and Shulman B. (1998). Ethnic and cultural differences in communication development. In W. Haynes and B. Shulman (Eds.), *Communication development: Foundations, processes, and clinical applications* (pp. 363-386). Boston, MA: Allyn & Bacon; Labou, W. (1998). Co-existent systems in AAE. In S. Mufwene, J. Rickford, J. Baugh, and G. Bailey (Eds.), *African-American English: Structure, history, and use* (pp. 110-153). London: Routledge; Owens, R. (1998). *Language development: An introduction* (ed. 4). New York: Macmillan; Rickford, J. (1999). *African-American Vernacular English*. Oxford: Blackwell Publishing. Stockman, I. (1996). Phonolgical development and disorders in African American children. In A. Kamhi, K. Pollack, and J. Harris (Eds.), *Communication development and disorders in African American children* (pp. 117-153). Baltimore, MD: Paul H. Brookes; Goldstein, B. (2000). *Cultural and linguistic diversity resource guide for speech-language pathology*. San Diego: Singular Publishing Group; Reid, D.K. (2000). Ebonics and Hispanic, Asian, and Native American dialects of English. In K. Fahey & D.K. Reid (Eds.). *Language development, differences, and disorders* (pp. 219-246). Austin, TX: Pro-Ed; Blond-Steward, L. (2005). Difference or deficit in speakers of African American English? *ASHA Leader, 10*(6), 6-30.

monolingual Spanish speakers; others are bilingual, to one degree or another, in English and Spanish. Brice (2002), Goldstein (2001, 2004), Roseberry-McKibben (2002a), and Zuniga (2004) provide detailed information about many aspects of the Latino culture of these diverse peoples.

Many children of Hispanic heritage come to school with *limited English proficiency (LEP)*; that is, they know a little English but are not fluent communicators in English and have trouble functioning in a monolingual English classroom, at least for a while. Again, LEP is not a disorder, nor is it a permanent condition. Most normally developing LEP children, with help and opportunities to interact with peers, eventually master English and become bilingual, able to communicate effectively in two languages.

Brice (2002), Haynes and Shulman (1998a), Kayser (2002), Scheffner Hammer, Miccio, and Rodriguez (2004), and Tabors, Paez, and Lopez (2002) provide a detailed discussion of what is known about normal development of Spanish in children learning it as a first language. This information can be useful to clinicians attempting to differentiate between a language difference and a disorder in a child whose dominant language is Spanish. When looking at the Spanish language development of these children, comparing production to available information on normal acquisition of Spanish can help to establish the stage of development a child is demonstrating in the first language. We'll talk in more detail later in the assessment section about some methods of looking at level of first language acquisition in children with LEP.

In working with Hispanic children with LEP, some characteristic difficulties or interference points come up between English and Spanish in what we might call Spanish-influenced English (SpIE). These characteristics are summarized in Box 5-2. Hispanic children with LEP who make changes such as those listed in Box 5-2 in their use of English would not be considered as having a disorder. To determine whether a Hispanic child with LEP were having inordinate problems in learning English, we would need to look for other types of errors that would not be typical of SpIE. We'll talk in more detail in the assessment section about methods of looking for these atypical kinds of errors.

NATIVE AMERICAN CULTURE AND COMMUNICATION

Joe and Malach (2004) reported that at the time of Christopher Columbus, there were at least 1000 Native American tribal entities, each with a distinct language, culture, set of beliefs, and governance structure. Even though many Native Americans have moved away from reservations to more urban areas, more than 1 million people still live on hundreds of reservations located in remote rural areas where medical, educational, and rehabilitative services are not readily available. Even Native Americans in cities share many of the cultural and child-rearing practices of their relatives on reservations (Joe & Malach, 2004; Westby & Vining, 2002). Like the other cultural groups being discussed, the Native American population encompasses great diversity. However, Joe and Malach (2004) and Robinson-Zanartu (1996) have pointed out some of the common themes among communication styles of the many first American peoples.

Native American children from a variety of tribal groups have been found to score higher on motor, social, and self-help skills than their mainstream peers, although they score lower on language areas (Westby, 1986). These differences are thought to reflect the experience of the Native American children, whose cultures rely much more heavily on visual than on vocal channels of information exchange. Native American children are taught to learn by watching—being quiet, passive observers of cultural practices. Demonstration of skills to Native American children does not usually involve verbal accompaniment nor are children expected to show their knowledge by verbal performance. Instead, they are required to display their physical mastery of a task, such as dancing or weaving, by just doing it.

Basso (1979) reported that Apache children were scolded for "acting like a white man" if they talked too much. Native American children are taught that important questions deserve thoughtful answers and are encouraged to take time to consider a question carefully before answering. The long pauses they use before responding to questions are often misinterpreted as a processing problem or lack of knowledge of the correct answer. Similarly, Joe and Malach (2004) report that it is considered rude in many Native American cultures to ask too direct a question or to make direct eye contact with one in authority. Westby (1986) emphasized that a Native American child's reluctance to speak, to look at the teacher, to ask questions, or a tendency to have long latency of response should not be misinterpreted as a lack of communicative competence. Instead, it should be understood as an appropriate expression of cultural patterns of communication.

Robinson-Zanartu (1996) noted that many Native American languages do not have words for concepts such as *hearing loss, retardation,* or *disability*. Children so labeled by the mainstream culture may be considered as simply part of the traditional community by its members. This can have profound effects on the ways professionals need to communicate with families about assessment and intervention services.

Westby and Vining (2002) and Reid (2000) identified several general differences that are commonly seen between English and Native American languages, and give some examples, primarily based on the Navajo language, as reported by Young (1967). These are summarized in Box 5-3. For more detailed and specific comparisons, clinicians will need to consult native speakers of the languages with which they come in contact, or resources such as Mithun (1999) and Patrick (2002). Again, in analyzing the language skills of a Native American child with LEP and attempting to decide whether a language difference or disorder exists, it will be necessary to determine whether the errors made in the child's use of English are different or more pervasive than those of peers at similar stages of exposure to English. It also will be important to keep pragmatic differences in mind. Being sensitive to these differences will

BOX 5-2 Characteristics of Spanish-Influenced English

Phonology

1. Some phonemes of English are not used in Spanish and will typically be changed in SpIE:
   - /θ/ in English is changed to /t/ in SpIE.
   - /ð/ in English is changed to /d/ in SpIE.
   - /z/ in English is changed to /s/ in SpIE.
   - /ʃ/ in English is changed to /tʃ/ in SpIE.
   - /v/ in English is changed to /b/ in SpIE.
   - /ʤ/ in English is changed to /j/ in SpIE.
2. Final consonants are usually devoiced in SpIE.
3. Addition of schwa vowel before /s/ initial consonant clusters in SpIE (*estudy* for *study*, *eschool* for *school*).
4. Spanish has fewer vowels than English. The vowels /ɪ/, /æ/, and /ə/ are absent from Spanish and will be substituted for when they appear in SpIE. /ɪ/ in SAE is usually pronounced as /i/ in SpIE, for example.

Syntax and Morphology

Verb Marking

1. Regular past -*ed* is not obligatory in SpIE.
2. Regular third-person–singular marking is not obligatory in SpIE.
3. Copula will sometimes be produced as *have* in certain constructions ("I *have* eight years").
4. Future tense can be expressed by "go + to" in SpIE (for example, SpIE: "I go to have lunch." SAE: "I am going to have lunch").

Noun Inflections

1. Possessive markers used in SAE will be substituted by prepositional phrases ("the book *of my sister*"), or, in the case of body parts, by articles ("I cut *the* finger").
2. Plural /s/ marker is not obligatory in SpIE.
3. Articles are often omitted in SpIE ("I go to store").
4. Subject pronouns may be omitted in SpIE when the subject has been given in the previous sentence ("Jose is sick. Got chicken pox").
5. *More* is used as a comparative marker in SpIE instead of the -*er* ending ("He is more short").
6. Articles are optional ("That is big dog").

Negatives

1. *No* may be used in SpIE as a negative marker in place of *not* ("She no go to work today").
2. No may be used instead of *don't* in negative imperatives ("No go too fast!").

Questions

1. "*Do* insertion" is not obligatory in questions in SpIE (SpIE: "You want some?" SAE: "Do you want *some?*").
2. Intonation is used more frequently in SpIE to mark questions than it is in SAE ("Carmen will be here?").

Semantics

1. Number, color, and letter words often receive less emphasis in parent-child interactions in Hispanic households.
2. Names and labels for objects, donors of objects, and particularly for relatives are emphasized in Hispanic parent-child interactions.

Pragmatics

1. Speakers of SpIE tolerate closer personal distance during conversation than speakers of SAE.
2. Direct eye contact is avoided in SpIE; lack of eye contact can signal attentiveness in SpIE, although it can mean just the opposite in SAE.
3. There is a greater incidence of touching between conversational partners.

Adapted from Kayser, H. (2002). Bilingual language development and language disorders. In D. E. Battle (Ed.), *Communication disorders in multicultural populations*, 3rd ed. (pp. 205-232). Boston: Butterworth-Heinemann; Goldstein, B. (2001). Transcription of Spanish and Spanish-Influenced English. *Communication Disorders Quarterly, 23,* 511-560; Haynes, W., and Shulman, B. (1998). Ethnic and cultural differences in communication development. In W. Haynes and B. Shulman (Eds.), *Communication development: Foundations, processes, and clinical applications* (pp. 363-386). Englewood Cliffs, NJ: Prentice-Hall; Owens R. (2005). *Language development: An introduction,* 6th ed. Boston: Allyn & Bacon; Reid, D. K. (2000). Ebonics and Hispanic, Asian, and Native American dialects of English. In K. Fahey & D.K. Reid (Eds.), *Language development, differences, and disorders* (pp. 219-246). Austin, TX: Pro-Ed.

BOX 5-3 | **Features of Native American Dialects of English**

Phonology

1. Native American dialects retain the phonemic patterns, phonological rules, and stress patterns of the tribal language. For example, the Navajo language does not use consonant clusters in syllable final position. Navajo dialects of English simplify these clusters.
2. Native American dialects retain intonation patterns of the tribal language. For example, Navajo uses particles rather than intonational contours to express questions, exclamations, and other forms. Navajo dialects of English may not include intonational changes to mark emotional overtones in speech.

Syntax and Morphology

1. Native American dialects carry over syntactic forms from the tribal language. For example, in Navajo, possession is expressed by personal pronouns prefixed to the possessed noun (*man his-boots*). Navajo dialects may include these rather than standard ('s) possessive markers.
2. Native American dialects carry over morphological rules from the tribal language. For example, in Navajo, opposites are not expressed morphologically, but rather with a standard negating or opposite marker:
   Navajo dialect: agree-not agree; SAE: agree-disagree
   Navajo dialect: tie-not tie; SAE: tie-untie
3. Constructions found in other nonstandard forms of English also can be found in Native American dialects (e.g., *ain't*, uninflected forms of *be*).
4. Specialized meanings of negative markers may be used; e.g., "The man does not do anything like this" (implies women may do it) and "The man does not do nothing like this" (implies he does something else).

Pragmatics

1. Cultural norms dictate who may be addressed by whom and what is appropriate to discuss at what season of the year.
2. Silence is more than absence of speech. It is a rule-governed practice used to express respect, thoughtfulness, that the question is worthy of serious consideration, or that the situation is unfamiliar.
3. It is rude to tell someone something he or she already knows. For example, if a teacher asks a question to which the answer is obvious, she must already know the answer (e.g., the teacher holds up a picture of a dog and says, "What is this?"), and therefore the child may not answer.
4. Greetings are not always used when entering or leaving, out of a desire not to intrude or interrupt.
5. Tempo of speech is slower and more fluid than in SAE.
6. Native Americans show a preference for "hearing out" a whole story or discourse before any questions or discussion takes place.
7. It is rude to correct or interrupt a peer.
8. Narratives are discursive, circling around a central point, rather than proceeding directly to it.

Adapted from Reid, D.K. (2000). Ebonics and Hispanic, Asian and Native American dialects of English. In K. Fahey & D.K. Reid (Eds.), *Language development, differences, and disorders* (pp. 219-246). Austin, TX: Pro-Ed; Young, R. (1967). *English as a second language for Navajos: An overview of certain cultural and linguistic factors.* Washington, DC: Navajo Area Office, Division of Education, Bureau of Indian Affairs; Westby, C. & Vining, C. (2002). Living in harmony: Providing services to native American children and families. In D.E. Battle (Ed.), *Communication disorders in multicultural populations,* 3rd ed. (pp. 135-178). Boston: Butterworth-Heinemann.

---

optimize the chances of obtaining information that is truly representative of the child's communicative competence.

ASIAN-AMERICAN CULTURE AND COMMUNICATION

Although Asians have been coming to America for more than two centuries, their numbers have increased greatly in the past three decades. Chan and Lee (2004) and Cheng (2001,2002a) discussed the diversity of peoples included in the "Asian-American" category and provided valuable information on many linguistic, social, religious, educational, and historical characteristics of the major cultural groups subsumed under the "Asian-American" umbrella. They come from China; Japan; Korea; India; Vietnam; Thailand; Cambodia (Kampuchea); Laos; and various Pacific Islands, including Guam, Samoa, and the Philippines. They speak hundreds of different languages—more than 80 languages are spoken in China alone. Asian-Americans come out of both rural and urban backgrounds and adhere to a variety of religions, including Buddhism,

Christianity, Confucianism, Hinduism, Islam, Shinto, Taoism, and various local animistic belief systems. Like many cultures, those from Asia have specific cultural practices and beliefs relating to child development and language learning that need to be addressed when working with these families (Johnston & Wong, 2002). Clinicians who find children from these groups on their caseload will benefit from reviewing Chan's, Cheng's, and Johnston and Wong's detailed descriptions.

Like the Native American languages discussed earlier, the Asian languages that can influence the speech of Asian-Americans are so many and diverse that it would be impossible to outline all the points of interference. Cheng (2001), Goldstein (2000), Owens (2005), and Reid (2000) provided some characteristics that Asian language speakers in America have in common. These are outlined in Box 5-4. Cheng (2002b) provides specific guidelines for assessing Asian-language

---

BOX 5-4 **Features of Asian Dialects of English**

Phonology

1. Most Asian languages have open (consonant-vowel) rather than closed (consonant-vowel-consonant) syllables. Many Asian dialects of English omit final consonants.
2. In many Asian languages, /r/ and /l/ occur in the same phonemic category and will be confused in Asian dialects of English.
3. Consonant blends are common in English but rare in many Asian languages. Some Asian-Americans may simplify them.
4. Many Asian languages are monosyllabic. Asian dialects of English may involve truncated or telegraphic-sounding forms, and stress may be misplaced.
5. Many Asian languages are tonal; prosodic changes carry semantic information rather than defining sentence types or conveying communicative intent, as they do in English. These intonational patterns may be difficult for Asian-Americans to learn, and they may be misinterpreted.

Syntax and Morphology

Verb Marking

1. *Be* verbs may be omitted or improperly inflected ("I going." "I is going").
2. Auxiliary *do* may be omitted or uninflected ("He not going." "He do not go").
3. Past *-ed* may be omitted ("He want ice cream yesterday"), overgeneralized ("He eated the cake"), or doubly marked ("She didn't saw me").
4. Past participle may be unmarked ("I have eat") or overgeneralized ("He has wented"); *have* auxiliary may be omitted ("He been there").
5. Noun-verb agreement may be in error ("He have." "You goes").

Nouns and Pronouns

1. Plurals may be omitted with quantifiers (*two shoe*) or overgeneralized (*the sheeps*).
2. Subject-object confusion ("Him here").
3. Errors of possessive marking (*him book*).
4. Errors on demonstrative pronouns (*those horse*).
5. Errors on comparatives (*gooder, more gooder*).
6. Gender is not marked ("He and his husband go").

Negatives

1. Double marking ("I didn't hear nothing").
2. Simplified marker ("He no want").

Questions

1. No reversal of auxiliary verb ("You are going?").
2. Auxiliary omitted ("You like football?").

Other

1. Omission or misuse of prepositions ("She is at room." "We go car").
2. Omission of conjunctions ("You I leave now").
3. Omission or overinclusion of articles ("I go to store." "You go to the home").
4. Word-order errors including adjectives following nouns (*shoe new*), possessives following nouns (*hat mine*), subject-verb-object order ("He gave out them").

Semantics

1. Literal translations from native language (*open-light*|=|turn on light).
2. Difficulties with idioms and colloquialisms.

| BOX 5-4 | Features of Asian Dialects of English—cont'd |

Pragmatics

1. Giggling may be used to indicate shyness rather than humor.
2. Praise is responded to with embarrassment; praise is not usually given outside the family.
3. Feelings are not openly expressed; Asians may retain composed facial expression even when agitated. Reprimands may be responded to by lowering the eyes and maintaining silence.
4. Kinship terms may be used to address elders as sign of respect, even when they are not actually related.
5. Professionals have high status and command respect. They are regarded as authorities.
6. Social status is important and must be established early in an interaction. Formal introductions by a third party are preferred to self-introductions, particularly for introductions of high-status professionals (such as SLPs).
7. Social status is established on the basis of age, marital status, and employment. Questions on these facts are deemed appropriate to ask directly of new acquaintances to establish proper social order among conversationalists.
8. Children are expected to be seen and not heard; children are not expected to talk during meals. In school, children are discouraged from interrupting teachers and may appear passive to Western adults.
9. Direct eye contact is avoided.
10. Repeated head nodding is used.
11. It is rude to say "no." It is hard for Asians to disagree directly, especially with a high-status professional.

Adapted from Owens, R. (2005). *Language development: An introduction* (ed. 6). New York: Macmillan; Cheng, L. (1987). Cross-cultural and linguistic considerations in working with Asian populations. *American Speech-Language-Hearing Association, 29(6),* 33-41; Cheng, L. (2001). Transcription of English influenced by certain Asian languages. *Communication Disorders Quarterly, 23,* 40-46; Reid, D.K. (2000). Ebonics and Hispanic, Asian, and Native American dialects of English. In K. Fahey & D.K. Reid (Eds.), *Language development, differences, and disorders* (pp. 219-246). Austin, TX: Pro-Ed.

---

speakers. Again, though, a clinician working with an Asian-American child with LEP will need to get more specific information about the child's first language to determine the extent to which a child's communication problem represents a language difference, or a disorder in need of intervention. Hwa-Froelich, Hodson, and Edward (2002), for example, discuss this issue for Vietnamese.

HIGH- AND LOW-CONTEXT COMMUNICATION

As we've seen from this brief review of some of the communicative characteristics of several of the larger minority groups in America today, there is nearly as much diversity within each group as there is between each and the mainstream. Knowing a little about communicative characteristics typical of particular minorities can be useful in sensitizing ourselves to differences we might expect, so long as we are careful not to stereotype anyone on the basis of cultural background. In addition to the commonalities that exist within each cultural group, some general tendencies in communicative style are common across traditional cultures. Awareness of the possibility of these differences, too, can help us to be cognizant of the cultural factors that operate when we assess and remediate communication skills in children whose cultural backgrounds and perspectives diverge from our own.

Westby and Rouse (1985) and Lynch (2004a) discussed these general tendencies under the rubric of high-context versus low-context cultures, as defined by the anthropologist

Hall (1983). Hall suggested that there is a continuum of contextualization of communication along which cultures can vary. Mainstream North American culture, particularly the culture of the classroom, tends toward the lowest end of this continuum, with communication being highly *decontextualized.* Many traditional cultures, however, locate their communication at the higher end of the contextualization continuum. Table 5-1 presents some of the contrasts between high- and low-context communicative styles. Understanding these differences in communicative styles can help to head off problems with clients

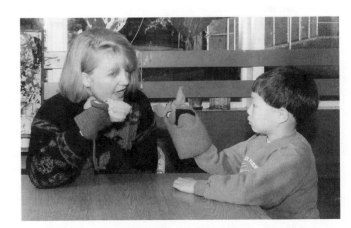

SLPs will often have clients from cultural backgrounds different from their own.

| **TABLE 5-1** | **Contrasts between High- and Low-Context Communicative Styles** |

LOW-CONTEXT STYLES USED IN MAINSTREAM CULTURE	HIGH-CONTEXT STYLES USED IN TRADITIONAL CULTURES
Most information is transmitted verbally.	Most information is in the physical context or is in shared knowledge among participants.
Learning takes place through words.	Routines and behaviors are taught through observation.
Society undergoes rapid change; there is great opportunity but life is less predictable. Planning of the future and delaying gratification for future rewards are encouraged.	Change is slow, life is predictable. As a result, little planning is needed. Talk about the future may be discouraged.
The role of the individual is to achieve and excel.	The role of the individual is as a member of the cultural group; most activities are controlled by the group rather than by an individual; individuals should not stand out from peers.
Monochronic concept of time: single events happen one at a time. Planning and scheduling are critical. Actions are tightly scheduled. What matters is sticking to the timetable.	Polychronic concept of time: time is flexible; timelines and schedules may not exist. What matters is the completion of transactions, not time.

Adapted from Westby, C., & Rouse, G. (1985). Culture in education and the instruction of language learning disabled students. *Topics in Language Disorders, 5(4)*, 15-28; Hall, E. (1983). *The dance of life*. New York: Anchor Press/Doubleday.

who come from relatively high-context cultures. We might, for example, talk about the objectives and procedures for the immediate present, perhaps one session at a time, in our discussions with these families and focus less on planning intervention strategies and goals for the longer-term future.

Westby and Rouse (1985) pointed out that children from more traditional, high-context cultures may have particular difficulty adjusting to the demands of low-context communicative situations, particularly those of the classroom. They suggested that SLPs, in a consulting role, can encourage teachers to incorporate some higher-context activities in programs designed for such children. These might include substituting a more high-context activity for the usual "sharing time" monologue required in typical classrooms. Instead of being asked to relate an experience without contextual support, children can be asked to respond as a group to a question about personal experiences, such as, "What happens when you have a guest in your home?" Rather than singling out a child, teachers can invite children to make a contribution when they have one and use the support provided by others' contributions as a scaffold. Westby and Rouse (1985) also suggested supplying parents with a few low-context activities that they can do with the child at home. One idea might be to send home books at the child's level for the parents to read to their children (or if they are unable to read English, to talk about the pictures with their children). Parents can be given a list of specific questions to ask the children about the books, such as, "What is the story about?" "How did the character feel?" and "Why did she do that?" Increasing the contextualization of some activities at school while providing some experience with decontextualized talk at home can help to ease the transition for children from more traditional cultures, especially children with language and learning difficulties.

Narratives

Another place in which high- and low-context cultural styles affect communication is the area of narrative development. Narratives differ from conversation in that they are monologues that are tied into cohesive units by linguistic markers and thematic unity. Like conversation, narratives are important communicative structures used by all cultures to accomplish specific communicative purposes. High- and low-context cultures differ in narrative style, though. They contrast in the degree to which the various narrative genres are used, in the way in which narratives are organized, and the extent to which children are expected to produce each genre. Heath (1986) and Goldstein (2000) described four basic narrative genres: recasts/recounts, event casts, accounts, and stories. Descriptions of each type are summarized in Box 5-5.

These genres are used for different purposes and to different degrees in high- and low-context cultures. High-context, traditional cultures expect children to use *recast/recounts* to retell events with extensive verbal imitation, role-playing, and use of present tense. Low-context cultures, such as those of the classroom, use them to summarize succinctly, using past tense. *Event casts* are used frequently in low-context cultures to explain activities or series of events that are being planned or will take place in the future. They are very prone to metalinguistic or metacognitive commentaries, in which the speaker talks about the language being used or thinks out loud about how best to convey the ideas. These types of narratives are used often in classroom communication but are rarely expected of children in high-context, traditional cultures. *Accounts* are used in both high- and low-context cultures to share experiences. Low-context cultures require that they have a predictable progression of events so that the listener can anticipate what is coming. In low-context situations in which these narratives are used, such

---

| BOX 5-5 | **Narrative Genre Descriptions** |

Recast/Recount—Retells events and experiences from the past, with sequential chronology and consistent point of view. Example: summarizing a section of a textbook.

Event cast—Verbal replies or explications of activities or procedures that are currently being done or are planned. Example: telling how to bake a pie, explaining what will happen on a field trip.

Account—Shares an experience. Example: telling about your vacation.

Story—Fictional account of people (or animals or inanimate objects that take on human characteristics) who must overcome some problem that has social or moral significance to the culture. Example: *The Three Little Pigs*.

Adapted from Goldstein, B. (2000). *Cultural and linguistic diversity resource guide for speech-language pathology*. San Diego: Singular Publishing Group; Heath, S. (1986). Taking a cross-cultural look at narratives. *Topics in Language Disorders, 7(1)*, 84-94; Kayser, H. (2002). Bilingual language development and language disorders. In D.E. Battle (Ed.), *Communication disorders in multicultural populations*, 3rd ed. (pp. 114-157). Boston: Butterworth-Heinemann.

---

as the show-and-tell situation in school, accounts are judged by not only their truth value but also by their degree of organization. In high-context cultures, less stress is on organization. *Stories* are used by both high- and low-context cultures, but they differ across cultures in terms of their internal organization and focus. Although most cultures expect children to listen to stories, cultures differ in the degree to which children are expected to tell stories. In some traditional high-context cultures, only elders or others with high status are expected to be storytellers.

Goldstein (2000) and Hester (1996) discussed the different structures that stories can have in high- and low-context cultures. Low-context cultures tend to have a storytelling style that Gee (1985), Michaels and Collins (1984), and Tannen (1982) referred to as "topic-centered." These stories have a linear progression that follows the story-grammar model (Stein & Glenn, 1979), in which an initiating event or problem motivates a character to develop a plan and carry out an attempt to solve the problem. The problem is resolved one way or another, and some form of external evaluation of the resolution ("and they lived happily ever after") takes place. (Story grammars are discussed in more detail in Chapters 10 to 14.) High-context cultures tend to use a more topic-associated style of narrative organization. This style is more anecdotal than linear. Westby and Vining (2002) reported that topic-associated stories consist of segments in which the overall theme may be implicit but never stated. Focus of person, place, and time often shifts and relationships must be inferred by the listener. These stories are longer than topic-centered narratives and may appear to the naive listener to have no beginning, middle, end, or central point. Westby (1989a) cited Kaplan's (1966) diagrammatic representation of the different forms that topic-associated narrative can take. These appear in Figure 5-1. However, Goldstein (2000) pointed out that this difference in structure may be more related to task demands than to underlying narrative ability. In fact, Fiestas and Peña (2004) found that bilingual children did include elements of story grammar in their stories in both English and Spanish, although there were differences in the particular elements included in each language.

Skill in producing and understanding topic-centered narratives has been shown to be closely related to literacy development and to success in school (Bishop & Edmundson, 1987; Boudreau, 2006; Boudreau & Hedberg, 1999). Children from high-context cultures with little experience of this narrative style may encounter difficulties in the many academic tasks that require processing and producing these narratives. As Westby (2005) pointed out, topic-centered narratives form a bridge between high-context, oral language styles and the low-context, literate language style of the classroom for mainstream as well as for culturally different children. Moreover, Fiestes and Peña (2004) argue that narrative production requires children to manage cognitive load in planning extended discourse, and thus is a good way to assess higher-level cognitive-linguistic skills. They report data indicating that

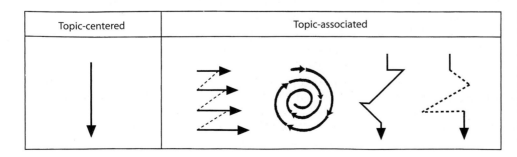

FIGURE 5-1 ✦ Narrative structures across cultures. (Adapted from Westby, C. [November, 1989a]. Cultural variations in storytelling. Paper presented at the National Convention of the American Speech-Language-Hearing Association. St. Louis, MO; Kaplan, R. [1966]. Cultural thought patterns in intercultural education. *Language Learning, 16,* 1-2.)

narrative is a valid and relevant task for assessing higher-level language skills in bilingual children. When assessing narrative development in clients, it is important to be aware of the possible problems children from traditional cultures can have with the topic-centered narratives. In thinking about narrative intervention for children from culturally different backgrounds, again, we will want to take a *bicultural* approach. That means being careful not to imply that the topic-associated narrative styles with which the client is familiar are wrong. Rather, we will want to encourage students to learn an additional style to be used when telling stories in the classroom or mainstream setting.

Working with Families from Culturally Different Backgrounds

As we'll see when we talk in the following chapters about working with young children, best practice in child language disorders is *family-centered*. This practice involves helping families to identify concerns, priorities, and resources for their child and including them as integral members of the intervention team (Donahue-Kilburg, 1993). Family-centered practice with families whose cultural background differs from our own operates on exactly the same principles. We must respect the concerns and priorities of families whose experiences and values diverge from ours, just as we do those of families whose beliefs are more familiar to us. As Hwa-Foerlich and Westby (2003) pointed out, differences in beliefs and values about learning, parenting, and disabilities can lead to confusion and misunderstanding. Therefore, we need to be aware of how our own assumptions and expectations affect our interactions with CLD families. Goldstein and Iglesias (2006) suggested the following strategies for culturally sensitive family-centered practice:

▶ Be sure family members (and in many CLD families, family members other than parents will be involved) understand the purpose of each assessment or intervention session.
▶ Attempt to involve family members in making decisions about assessment methods and interpretation, intervention targets and procedures, etc.
▶ Match assessment and intervention goals to family priorities.
▶ Allow ample time for questions after each session, and be prepared to answer the same question different ways for different family members, if necessary.
▶ Research the language and culture of each client (using sources like those cited in this chapter) to make use of culturally appropriate practices.

Cheng, Battle, Murdoch, and Martin (2001), Coleman and McCabe-Smith (2000), Goldstein (2000), Johnston and Wong (2002), Lynch (2004b), and McNeilly and Coleman (2000) discuss issues related to developing cultural competence for working with families of CLD children. Clinicians would benefit from reading and studying these texts to develop culturally sensitive practices.

We'll talk in more detail about family-centered practice in the next few chapters. The important point to remember here is that the principles and communication strategies we'll discuss apply to families that come from diverse cultures as well as to families in the mainstream.

ASSESSING CULTURALLY AND LINGUISTICALLY DIFFERENT CHILDREN

LANGUAGE DISORDER OR LANGUAGE DIFFERENCE?

The first problem in assessing a culturally or linguistically different child is determining whether a real disorder exists or whether there is merely the perception (usually on the part of teachers or other professionals) of a disorder that is based on a language difference. Laing and Kamhi (2003) point out that overdiagnosis and underdiagnosis of language and literacy problems are common in CLD children, and that standardized tests are often plagued by biases that reduce their validity for assessing these children fairly. Taylor (1986) suggested that a language disorder exists in a culturally or linguistically different (CLD) child when the child's language skills deviate significantly from the norms and expectations of the child's home community. Wilson, Wilson, and Coleman (2000) outlined the criteria for identifying language disorders in CLD clients. A language disorder is likely to exist if the client's communication:

▶ Is considered defective by the individual's cultural community
▶ Operates outside the norms of acceptability for that community
▶ Calls attention to itself or interferes with communication within that community
▶ Results in difficulties in adjustment for the client

So the initial step in the assessment process for any CLD child is to determine whether language is disordered or simply different. This decision involves invoking the Systems model of communication problems as discussed in Chapter 1—that is, we need to find out whether a problem is perceived because of a difference in cultural expectations for communication or because the child has a genuine disability, even in the home culture. Let's take an example.

Harry was a Native American child recently arrived from the reservation to an urban Head Start program. He seemed to the teachers to be inordinately quiet. When asked a question, he took an exceedingly long time to answer, causing the teachers to question his comprehension skills. He had a great deal of difficulty presenting information during sharing time and did not seem to process teachers' verbal directions. He was referred for speech and language assessment. Ms. Lopez, the SLP, observed his classroom behavior and saw the same problems that the teachers had indicated.

Before deciding Harry had a disorder, however, she interviewed Harry's parents. She found that they spoke both English and Navajo in the home. Both were fluent in English and had jobs in which they conversed with English speakers regularly. They believed that Harry was proficient in English; he watched English-language TV and played with English-speaking children in the neighborhood and seemed to get along with them all right. They didn't really understand why he should be having so much trouble in school.

Ms. Lopez decided to collect a language sample from Harry during a play period with a peer. She analyzed the sample and found that

Harry's use of syntax and semantics was generally age-appropriate. Receptive language testing, using a standardized picture-pointing test, showed that Harry's receptive vocabulary score was somewhat below the normal range. Ms. Lopez asked the parents about the items Harry failed to identify on the test, and they explained that he was unlikely to have encountered those words in their home or on the reservation. Ms. Lopez assessed Harry's comprehension of classroom directions with some criterion-referenced measures. She found that Harry could follow most directions, but was very slow and careful about doing so. When she asked his parents why this might be the case, they explained that he had been taught at home to think carefully before acting. They commented that Harry had once said that the teachers seemed to want him to act like a "show off" in school.

Ms. Lopez concluded that there was a mismatch between the teachers' expectations and Harry's communication style. While Harry would need some help in developing some of the vocabulary items with which he'd had no previous experience, consulting with teachers about some concepts to emphasize in the course of their regular program could do this. Ms. Lopez also shared her nonstandardized assessment results with the teachers and talked with them about Harry's need to consider before answering and his unwillingness to stand out from the group in sharing time. She suggested some ways they could modify their interactions with Harry that could bring their communicative expectations more in line with his. She also suggested that they talk with him about some of the different ways people can be expected to act at school and at home, so that some of the school rules might seem less foreign to him.

In Harry's case, the assessment suggests a difference rather than a disorder of communication. The remedy for this situation is two-pronged. Some work must be done to help Harry adjust to the communicative demands of the classroom. This work, however, should be culturally sensitive; care should be taken not to invalidate the styles of communicating that are appropriate at home. The second prong involves making some adjustments in the classroom's communication requirements. This would include consultation with teachers to make them aware of Harry's communication style, assuring them that it is a difference rather than a disorder and that Harry has the potential to communicate effectively. It also would involve finding ways to accommodate his communication in the classroom setting. As discussed in Chapter 1, using a Systems model to evaluate communication suggests that when a mismatch is found, the remedy lies in ameliorating both sides of the communicative team, not just in changing the client's communication.

Recently, at least one assessment method has been developed to address this issue directly in children who speak AAVE. *The Diagnostic Evaluation of Language Variation* (DELV) (Seymour, Roeper, & deVilliers, 2005) was developed as a valid and reliable assessment that allows the clinician to identify AAVE speakers with language impairments regardless of the dialect of the child. The DELV is available in both screening and full diagnostic forms, and also provides items that identify speech delays in AAVE speakers. Based on extensive research of both typical and delayed development in AAVE (Pearson, 2004),

the DELV provides clinicians with at least one psychometrically sound tool for diagnosing language disorders in AAVE speakers. We'll talk in the following sections about some more specific techniques we can use to help us determine whether a language difference or disorder is present in clients from various CLD backgrounds.

Another approach is suggested by Laing and Kamhi (2003). They report on the use of processing-dependent tasks, which require minimal use of prior knowledge or experience. Examples of processing-dependent tasks include various memory tasks, such as digit span (repeating a series of numbers in random order), working memory (children hear a sentence, are asked to tell whether it is true, and then recall the last word in the sentence), and nonword repetition (repeating nonsense words varying in length from one to four syllables that have no resemblance to familiar English words). These tasks are thought to be less biased because they do not depend on knowledge of culturally determined information, such as vocabulary (which children learn from hearing their parents talk). Instead they tap directly the processes that go into learning language. Laing and Kamhi, Hwa-Froelich and Matsuo (2005), and Weismer et al. (2000) reported that when children perform poorly on processing-dependent measures, there is a high likelihood that they will have some type of language learning difficulty. The use of processing-dependent measures with CLD populations makes sense because they are not biased toward life experience, socialization practices, or literacy knowledge, and they are quick and easy to administer. Moreover, many nonword repetition and working memory measures are included in currently existing standardized measures, including the *Comprehensive Test of Phonological Processing*, or in clinical literature, such as *the Non-word Repetition Test* (Campbell, Dollaghan, Needleman, & Janosky, 1997), as just two examples.

A third approach to this question is the use of dynamic assessment procedures. We talked about dynamic assessment in Chapter 2. From there, you will remember that one approach to dynamic assessment is to test, teach, and then retest. This method of dynamic assessment has been shown to differentiate stronger and weaker language learners in Puerto Rican, African-American, and Native American preschool and kindergarten children (Laing & Kamhi, 2003; Ukrainetz, Harpell, Walsh, & Coyle, 2000). Another method of dynamic assessment was examined by Peña, Iglesias, and Lidz (2001). They used Mediated Learning Experiences (MLE), designed to teach children principles or strategies for learning a task, to determine whether these supports would distinguish language difference from language disorder in preschool African-Americans and Latino American children with low levels of language performance. All children received pretest standard language measures. Children were then taught new vocabulary items; some received MLEs organized around theme-based play and book-sharing activities, others received no mediation. All were post-tested on the same tests. Findings revealed that changes in the post-test scores on knowledge of the new vocabulary were associated more closely with the presence of mediation than with pretest standard scores. Miller, Gilliam, and Peña

(2001) reported similar findings for a dynamic narrative assessment task.

Dynamic assessment also allows us to learn, for those children who do not improve in quantitative test scores after an intervention, whether their responses are qualitatively improved; for example, whether they provide longer responses, or responses closer to the target than they did before. These changes, too, are indicative of a benefit from the intervention and can be used to help distinguish a language difference from a disorder. Gutierrez-Clellen and Peña (2001) provide information on various dynamic assessment techniques, which are summarized in Table 5-2.

TABLE 5-2	**Dynamic Methods for the Assessment of CLD Children**		
METHOD	**DESCRIPTION**	**PURPOSE**	**EXAMPLE**
Test the limits	Traditional test procedures are modified by providing feedback about the correctness of the answer, why it was correct or incorrect, and an explanation of the principle in the task; or by asking the child to describe the test question and tell why they gave the answer they did.	To get a more accurate assessment of the child's knowledge of items on the test; modified responses cannot be included in standard scoring, but supply deeper information about the child's knowledge.	When child is incorrect on expressive vocabulary test, point to the stimulus and say, "Yes, we do eat that. Do you know a special name for this thing?"
Interview on responses	Generate questions to help children understand how they are thinking about test problems and help them become aware of target skills.	To understand how the task appears from the child's point of view.	When child is incorrect on expressive vocabulary test, ask questions such as, "How did you know that?" or "What would happen if you wanted one of these from the store? What would you say?"
Graduated prompting	Identify Zone of Proximal Development (ZPD) by providing a hierarchy of prompts to vary the level of contextual support.	Child responses to the prompts are used to make predictions about response to intervention. Number of prompts needed to elicit targets can predict gains after intervention.	To predict readiness for production of 2-word utterances, provide a hierarchy of prompts for single words; such as: modeling (It's a baby), modeling with elicitation (It's a baby; what is it?), and modeling with obstacle (withhold object until child says word). Fewer cues needed for word production predicts readiness for multiword speech.
Test-teach-retest	Identify deficient or emerging skill; provide intervention by teaching principles of the task; post-test to find out how modifiable the child's performance is.	To equalize students' experiences that can affect test performance.	If a child performs poorly on a language test, provide instruction on items similar to those in the test by giving verbal explanation, models, examples, and prompts. Post-test on an alternate form of the pretest.
Measure modifiability	Likert scales developed by the clinician used to rate the child at the beginning and end of the intervention phase of dynamic assessment.	To document change in child behaviors not measured by pre- or post-tests.	Amount of support provided: 1 2 3 Maximal Minimal Child responsiveness to tasks: 1 2 3 Maximal Minimal

Adapted from Gutierrez-Clellen, V., & Peña, E. (2001). Dynamic assessment of diverse children: A tutorial. *Language, Speech, and Hearing Services in Schools, 32*, 212-224.

Establishing Language Dominance

As a first step toward determining whether there is a language difference or disorder, we need to identify the child's dominant language. That is, we need to determine whether the child's primary language is English or some other language. The reason that establishing language dominance is important concerns our responsibility to do least-biased assessment. The Individuals with Disabilities Education Act (Part B)—the federal law that guarantees a free, appropriate public education in the least restrictive setting to every child regardless of handicapping condition—requires that testing be provided in the language or other mode of communication in which a child is most proficient. If we test a child with LEP in English, of course, all we will find out is that he or she has limited English skills. We won't know whether the child really has a language disorder or simply hasn't yet had the opportunity to develop fluency in English. For this reason, when we meet a CLD child suspected of having a language disorder, we need to determine in what language(s) testing should take place.

Kayser (1995) provided some suggestions for establishing language dominance in CLD children. Observation is one method. Here the clinician would observe the child in the classroom and in less formal settings, such as the lunchroom or playground, and chart communicative behaviors in each. Heavy reliance on gestures in situations requiring English or a preponderance of the home language in informal situations would suggest that English is not dominant for this child. A second method is the use of structured questionnaires to assess language dominance. Some examples include the *Assessment Instrument for Multicultural Clients* (Adler, 1991), the *Basic Inventory of Natural Language* (Herbert, 1977), the *Bilingual Language Proficiency Questionnaire* (Mattes & Santiago, 1985), the *Bilingual Syntax Measure* (Burt, Dulay, & Hernandez-Chavez, 1975), the *Home Bilingual Usage Estimate* (American Speech-Language-Hearing Association, 1982a), the *Oral Language Evaluation* (Silvaroli & Maynes, 1975), *PAL Oral Language Dominance Measure* (Apodaca, 1987), and the *Teacher Language Observation Report* (American Speech-Language-Hearing Association, 1982b).

If English is found to be the dominant language, testing in English can proceed. With a CLD child, however, testing in English requires sensitivity to pragmatic, experiential, and dialectical differences that must be evaluated before deciding whether a disorder is present. As we saw in Harry's case, a child can be English-dominant and still have a culturally different communication style. As discussed in Chapter 2, standardized tests do not provide all the information we need to answer these questions in a CLD child, just as they do not for any other child. Particularly for the CLD child, however, standardized measures should be supplemented with criterion-referenced and other nonstandardized information to obtain a full picture of the child's communication skills. When working with a CLD child, it is wise to keep the Systems model of communication problems in mind. In this way, we can be alert to communication difficulties that might be coming from *both* sides of the communicative dyad.

If English is not the CLD child's dominant language, Kayser (1995) suggested testing further in both English and the dominant language. Naturally, scores in English will be lower than those in the dominant language, but comparing performance in the two gives the clinician an idea of whether the child is progressing adequately for age in the home language and where gaps in English proficiency are found. Owens (2004) suggested testing in the dominant language first, then following up with testing in English. As Appendix 5-1 shows, there are a variety of tests available in a range of languages for children with CLD. If the clinician has a child who is dominant in one of these languages on the caseload, testing may be carried out by a trained native-speaking paraprofessional or speech assistant who can report results to the SLP for interpretation.

Obtaining Interview Data

Just as we need to gather data on hearing, speech-motor, and nonverbal skills for every client suspected of a language disorder, we need to gather these data on children with CLD: obtaining information about a child's medical, language, feeding, and developmental history; interviewing parents about current skills in communication and related areas; and finding out about family concerns and priorities are important parts of the assessment for each child we see. For the CLD child, however, these tasks become more complicated, because the SLP and the client's parents may not speak the same language. One solution to this problem is to employ interpreters.

Bilingual individuals can often interpret between clinicians and parents, giving the clinician access to crucial information about clients. Not everyone who is bilingual can be an interpreter, though. Interpreting for clinical purposes requires special skills. Kayser (1991) suggested that interpreters need to have at least a high school education, an ability to relate to people with disabilities, and strong linguistic and literacy skills in both languages. They should be able to say things in different ways and retain chunks of information while interpreting. Lynch and Hanson (2004b) point out that the interpreter needs to be able not only to translate from one language to another, but also to interpret cultural cues and convey the nonverbal aspects of the message as well as its words. Interpreters also need to have good command of medical and educational vocabulary and be able to rephrase terms for parents. They must be trained to maintain confidentiality and neutrality. Langdon (2002) advocates following a three-step process that includes briefing, interaction, and debriefing (BID) in preparing interpreters for a session. This process is summarized in Box 5-6. Derr (2003) emphasized that, for these reasons, it is usually better for the interpreter not to be a member of the client's family or close personal friend. The American Speech-Language-Hearing Association (ASHA, 1988) recommended using professional interpreters from language banks, bilingual professional staff from other disciplines, or bilingual teachers' aides or paraprofessionals as interpreters. Langdon (2002) and Langdon and Chen (2002) provide detailed guidance for SLPs on working with interpreters.

BOX 5-6	Langdon's (2002) BID Process for Working with Interpreters

Briefing: Clinician and interpreter review client's background information and outline the purpose of the session.

Interaction: Each team member addresses the client or family when speaking, even when through the interpreter ("Are you..." rather than, "Ask Ms. X if she..."). The clinician must always be present with the interpreter, to monitor task presentation and client/family reactions.

Debriefing: Clinician and interpreter review the session and develop a follow-up plan. Clinician should give interpreter feedback on performance and seek interpreter's impressions of client/family responses.

Interpreters function essentially as paraprofessionals under the direction of the SLP, with the clinician maintaining responsibility for decisions in assessment and intervention. It is important, however, that they understand the rationale and procedures being used in the interview and that time is spent with them before the parent conference discussing the information the clinician hopes to obtain. They can be asked to review the clinician's questions for cultural appropriateness and to help find alternative ways to get information that families may be uncomfortable giving. Bernstein (1989) suggested that one way to evaluate whether an interpreter has been trained adequately is to borrow a technique from anthropology. Here two interpreters are used. One translates the clinician's questions into the second language and the other translates the questions back into English. In this way the clinician can assess whether the interpreter will correctly convey the sense of the interview to the family.

Westby (1986) suggested that a good interview question to begin with in obtaining history information on CLD clients is, "Is this child like your other children or different in some way?" Interpreters translating parents' answer to such a question should understand and have discussed with the clinician the kinds of differences that will contribute to a decision about a language disorder, so that these can be reliably conveyed to the clinician.

USING STANDARDIZED TESTS WITH CLD CHILDREN

When assessing CLD children's communication in the dominant language and in English, we have basically the same methods available as discussed in Chapter 2: standardized tests, developmental scales, criterion-referenced procedures, dynamic assessment, and behavioral observation. As we saw in Chapter 2, the primary purpose of standardized tests is to find out whether a child is significantly different from other children in the area assessed by the test. However, there are dangers in using tests standardized for monolingual English speakers with CLD children (Paradis, 2005). In recent years, a variety of standardized tests have been developed in languages other than English for just this purpose. Spanish language tests are the most common, although some tests have been normed in other languages, as well. Appendix 5-1 presents a sample of standardized tests that can be used to assess CLD children. These tests also can be given along with standardized tests that assess English versions of similar areas. Results can then be compared not only to help determine whether the child is progressing normally in the home language (L_1) but also to identify areas of English (L_2) that are less developed than the dominant language. However, as we would when using any standardized test, we need to be cautious about understanding the properties, strengths, and weaknesses of these measures. Restrepo and Silverman (2001), for example, reviewed the psychometric properties of the *Spanish Preschool Language Scale–3*, a widely used instrument. They found that there were problems in the test's norming sample, reliability, and validity data. This suggests that we need to carefully review the manuals for any test we select for use with our clients, and attempt to find those that meet high psychometric standards.

Brice (2002), Goldstein (2000), Kayser (1995), Roseberry-McKibben (2002a), and Wyatt (2002) have made suggestions for modifying standardized tests to gain information about language proficiency in CLD children. They suggest that adapting tests should be a group effort, since a monolingual SLP making the modifications in isolation might not make adaptations that are optimal for speakers of a different language. The SLP can enlist bilingual ESL teachers, psychologists, special educators, and community members to make the modifications. Suggestions for adaptations of tests are given in Box 5-7. Adler (1993) and van Keulen, Weddinton, and DeBose (1998) also presented some modifications of standardized tests that can be applied when testing speakers of nonstandard dialects.

For many CLD children, however, standardized tests of the home language will not be available. In this situation we have some alternatives. An obvious alternative is to have an interpreter translate a standardized test into the child's home language. Cheng (2002a), Goldstein (2000) and Wilson, Wilson, and Coleman (2000), however, cautioned against this practice. Words and concepts common in mainstream culture may be unfamiliar to the CLD child, so failure to use or recognize them in the home language would not necessarily indicate a deficit. Translating also invalidates the standardization of the test, defeating the purpose of using it in the first place. Goldstein (2000) and Kayser (1995) suggested that it is wiser to modify or adapt test items than to translate them directly. When these modifications are made, of course, the adapted instrument is no longer a standardized test. We are, in effect, using the standardized test as a criterion-referenced measure. Although this method will not tell us if a child is significantly different from other children, it can tell us what forms and functions a child uses and understands in the language being tested.

| **BOX 5-7** | **Suggestions for Modifying Standardized Tests for Assessment of CLD Children** |

1. Review test content for items that tap knowledge or experiences CLD children are unlikely to have. Determine whether modification can reduce bias.
2. Have members of the team perform the tasks on the test and make suggestions about how to make them less culturally biased.
3. Consider administering the test to an adult from the community to get information on the appropriateness of the test items.
4. Review past testing of CLD children to look for items or subtests that were problematic for many of these children. Modify or eliminate these items.
5. Make an effort to identify tests that include substantial numbers of individuals from CLD backgrounds in the norming sample.
6. Determine appropriateness of vocabulary for community; poll team for most appropriate vocabulary to use for local children.
7. Review pictures for familiarity. Substitute other pictures or objects for those likely to be unfamiliar.
8. Reword instructions to make them more comprehensible for CLD children.
9. Give additional practice items to teach children how to take the test.
10. Provide additional response time; repeat items and instructions if needed.
11. Continue testing beyond ceiling.
12. Record children's comments, explanations, and changes of response for qualitative analysis.
13. Observe *code switching* (alternations between languages within an utterance) and *language interference* (the influence of one language on another, such as mispronunciations due to accent), and interpret how these affect performance and results.
14. Compare children's answers not only to "right" answer according to test norms, but also to dialect, home language, or second-language learning features. Rescore articulation and expressive language results, giving credit for these kinds of variations.
15. On picture-pointing tests, have children name the items as well as point to those named by the tester, to examine the appropriateness of the children's label.
16. Have children explain why they answered as they did, if answer is incorrect according to test norms.
17. Report all modifications when writing up assessment information; use norm-referenced scores with caution, and only if they are valid for the population to which the client belongs.

Adapted from Goldstein, B., & Iglesias, A. (2006). Issues of cultural and linguistic diversity. In R. Paul & P. Cascella (Eds.) *Introduction to clinical methods in communication disorders*, 2nd Ed. (pp. 261-280.) Baltimore: Paul H. Brookes; Erickson, J., & Iglesias, A. (1986). Assessment of communication disorders in non–English-proficient children. In O. Taylor (Ed.), *Nature of communication disorders in culturally and linguistically diverse populations*. San Diego, CA: College-Hill Press; Kayser, H. (1995). Speech and language assessment of Spanish-English speaking children. *Language, Speech, and Hearing Services in Schools, 20,* 226-244; Wyatt, T. (2002). Assessing the communicative abilities of clients from diverse cultural and language backgrounds. In D.E. Battle (Ed.), *Communication disorders in multicultural populations* (pp. 415-459). Stoneham, MA: Andover Medical Publishers; Weddington, G. (1987). Guidelines for use of standardized tests with minority children. In L. Cole & V. Deal (Eds.), *Communication disorders in multicultural populations* (pp. 21-22). Rockville, MD: American Speech-Language-Hearing Association.

Wyatt (2002) cautioned that when we do adapt standardized tests for use with CLD children, we need to be especially careful to note the adaptations in clinical reports on the client. She recommended that any changes made in standardized administration or scoring procedures be fully documented in the report. The report should also state whether an interpreter was used and how the interpreter was trained to administer and score the test. When testing takes place in two languages, the languages used and the order of use of the languages (English first, Spanish second, for example) should be given.

Norm-referenced scores should be reported only when they are appropriate for the way the test was administered. If the test was adapted in any way, norm-referenced scores cannot be used without reservations. If published developmental data are used for comparison to the child's performance, full bibliographical reference to the published data should be made.

Another alternative for assessing a CLD child's language proficiency is to develop local norms for standardized tests (Goldstein & Iglesias, 2006). This option only makes sense when a large number of CLD children from similar backgrounds reside in an SLP's district. Kayser (1995) warned that developing local norms is not as easy as it sounds. Groups of CLD individuals are heterogeneous in terms of socioeconomic status, length of time in this country, and degree of acculturation. All these differences can affect their performance on a test. Adler (1990) suggested that developing local norms may not really help identify CLD children with genuine language disorders, because the "culture fair" data represented in the local norms may not be relevant to the realities of classroom expectations. Harris (1993) advised that if local norms are to be developed, they should have at least 50 individuals at each age or grade level who are randomly selected from the community to provide the norms. Both means and standard deviations should be computed. Children falling 1, 1.5, or 2 standard deviations below the mean for their community group might be identified as language disordered, depending on the criterion for language disorder being used by the clinician. However, Carter et al. (2005) remind us that these local norms should show a normal distribution, or bell-shaped curve. If they do not, the assessment should be modified so that a normal distribution is achieved. Bayles and Harris (1982) found that using local norms in this way decreased the percentage of children from CLD families identified as having language impairments.

Whether we adapt tests or develop local norms, several guidelines should be followed. These are outlined by Carter et al. (2005), and include the following:

▶ Include native speakers of the home language in the development of the instrument, including paraprofessionals, teachers from the community and other local informants.

▶ Pilot-test the assessment on a representative sample of typically developing children from the home community.

▶ Pilot-test pictures to be used in the assessment by asking young, typically developing children from the community to identify them. Any pictures not recognized by the pilot sample should be redrawn or discarded.

▶ Pilot-test instructions, practice items, etc. as well before using the test to identify deficits in the home language.

▶ Whenever possible, have the assessment administered by native speakers of the home language.

▶ Use materials familiar to children from this community; for example, types of trees and flowers in pictures should be those with which the children will be familiar.

▶ For children who are unfamiliar with the testing situation, consider giving extra practice items.

Terrell, Arensberg, and Rosa (1992) suggested an additional alternative use for standardized tests with CLD children: Parent-Child Comparative Analysis (PCCA). This is a method of assessing children who come from cultural groups too small for development of local norms. Here an identical battery of tests is given to both parent and child. The child's performance is compared not to test norms but to the parent's responses. Any patterns that match patterns produced by the parent are considered dialectical variations rather than errors. If the child's patterns do not match the parent's, the child's responses are compared to age expectations, using developmental charts and normal language data, such as those found in Owens (2005)

or Haynes and Shulman (1998b). Deviations from Standard English patterns that do not match the parent's and are not typical of normally developing children of the client's age are considered aspects of a language disorder.

Developmental scales that look at nonlinguistic areas can be a useful adjunct to assessment of the CLD child. As discussed in Chapter 2, developmental scales and collateral, nonverbal assessments can provide information about motor, self-help, nonverbal cognitive, problem-solving, and play skills that can help to identify gaps between linguistic and nonlinguistic development in CLD children, as they can in clients from mainstream backgrounds. Many of the instruments we talked about in Chapter 2, particularly those that are nonverbal or minimally verbal in format, are appropriate for rounding out our picture of the skills of the CLD child. Ortiz (2001) also suggests determining the degree of "cultural loading" on these assessments; that is, the degree to which a test requires specific knowledge and experience with mainstream culture. His article provides a list of tests of cognitive and collateral areas classified by their degree of cultural loading.

CRITERION-REFERENCED ASSESSMENT OF CLD CHILDREN

Criterion-referenced assessment is used with CLD children in much the same way as for a mainstream child (that is, we use criterion-referenced measures once standardized testing has established that the child is significantly different from peers—in the CLD child's case, peers from the home culture—in linguistic development). The criterion-referenced assessments are then used to establish baseline function, identify goals for intervention, and document progress in the remedial program. Interpreters can be especially helpful in carrying out criterion-referenced assessments. When testing a child who is not English dominant, we may want to assess forms of interest in both the first language and English, to identify gaps between the two as well as establish level of functioning in the dominant language.

Since standardization is not an issue for criterion-referenced assessments, many of the criterion-referenced procedures in the following chapters can be translated directly by an interpreter into a CLD child's first language. The only thing we will need to be careful about is that the forms and procedures used in the assessment are culturally appropriate. For example, if a child's home culture's communication style dictates that you don't tell people something they already know, asking a child to tell what color a picture is may be inappropriate, even if the question is asked in the native language. Perhaps the situation would have to be modified so that the question concerns a picture that the examiner cannot see, to make the question pragmatically appropriate for the CLD client. Here, too, consulting ahead of time with the interpreter about culturally appropriate procedures can help prevent problems.

We talked in Chapter 2 about the importance of structural analysis of spontaneous speech samples as one aspect of criterion-referenced assessment and about some guidelines for collecting speech samples that truly represent a child's productive language skills. Language sample analysis can be a part of the assessment of communication in the CLD child, too, but certain cautions need to be kept in mind. Stockman (1996) points out a central concern to us: language sampling is not used to identify a disorder in mainstream children. Instead, it is used when a disorder has been identified with standardized testing and we want to investigate baseline function and target expressive language goals for intervention. Because language sampling procedures do not meet psychometric standards of reliability, validity, sensitivity, and specificity, they cannot properly be used to decide that a child is significantly different from other children. We can use language sampling with CLD children just as we use it for children from mainstream backgrounds: to describe current functioning in the dominant language and in English, to identify goals for intervention by establishing the next steps in the normal sequence of acquisition of either language, and to target these goals in an intervention program.

When collecting a language sample for these purposes from a CLD child, it is important to remember that conversational rules are culturally determined. To get a valid sample of a CLD child's language, then, we need to attend to the cultural rules that govern conversation for that child. Perhaps children are not expected to speak extensively to adults in a certain culture. In this case, a more valid sample might be collected from a peer interaction. Leonard and Weiss (1983) emphasized the importance of incorporating culturally appropriate materials and topics into the evaluation. These all help to obtain a more representative picture of the child's linguistic skills. To monitor the representativeness of a speech sample collected from a CLD child, we will want to learn some details of the cultural conversational practices from interviews with community members. Ethnographic methods such as those given in Table 5-3 can be useful, as can asking community members about conversational rules in their culture. In addition, we may want to observe the client in several conversational situations to select the most representative one to use as the basis for our

TABLE 5-3	Dimensions of Communicative Competence to Assess Using Ethnographic Methods

DIMENSIONS	CHARACTERISTICS
Conversational partners	How often does the child interact with adults, peers, older or younger siblings, others?
	How many people are usually involved in a conversation?
Mode of communication	How much of the interaction is verbal? Nonverbal?
	How is silence used?
	Can people be comfortable together without talking?
	Are children supposed to be seen and not heard?
	How is gaze used?
	Where do people look when they are talking, listening, asking, scolding, being scolded, joking, and so on?
Conversational duration	How long do conversations usually last? Adult-adult? Adult-child?
Amount of talking	Do children talk more or less in conversations with particular people?
	Do children talk more or less in conversations in particular settings?
Conversational structure	Who starts, continues, ends conversations?
	How may a child request a conversational turn?
	Are children's bids treated differently than adults'?
Topics	What are acceptable topics for conversations with children?
	What topics are considered rude?
Adult talk to children	Does it have "motherese" features?
	Do adults use minimal or expanded talk to children?
	Is adult talk contingent on child remarks?
Speech acts	Are certain types (questions, stories) used only by certain speakers?
	Who can joke, tease, or threaten?
	Is labeling used in looking at picture books?
	Who may give orders or make requests of whom?
Social beliefs	How do people think children learn language?
	What kinds of language play are allowed?
	How does the culture view disabilities?

Adapted from Crago, M., & Cole, E. (1991). Using ethnography to bring children's communicative and cultural worlds into focus. In T.M. Gallagher (Ed.), *Pragmatics of language: Clinical practice issues* (pp. 99-132). San Diego, CA: Singular Publishing.

speech sample analysis. It also is a good idea to check with a parent or familiar adult to ask whether the sample we plan to analyze sounds like the way the child usually talks.

Language samples can be collected in the home language from children who are not English dominant. In this case, the child may interact with a parent or another fluent speaker of the language. The sample can be collected on audiotape and transcribed by an interpreter. Again, the interpreter will need to be carefully trained by the clinician so that the transcription accurately represents the child's pronunciation, use of grammatical morphemes, word order, and any other aspects of speech that the clinician wants to examine. Without training, the interpreter may be tempted to "normalize" the child's speech, correcting the child's errors in the transcription and removing an important source of information about the child's linguistic patterns. A translation of the sample will need to retain some indication of these errors to be analyzed by the clinician in collaboration with the interpreter.

The language sample from the home language will be especially useful for determining whether the child is learning normally in the first language. Norms for Spanish acquisition are available (see Haynes and Shulman, 1998b, for example), and a Spanish-speaking child's spontaneous speech can be compared with these normative data. Linares (1981) and Goldstein (2001) provided rules for computing mean length of utterance in morphemes in Spanish. For languages for which normative data are not available, the interpreter and the clinician can consult with the parent and other bilingual individuals in the community.

Collecting a sample of the child's speech in English also can be helpful. Here we would compare the child's errors in English to those made in the home language to look for similar difficulties in the two languages. The child might be substituting a /t/ for an /s/ in both languages, for example, or leaving plural morphemes out of both, even where they are required in the home language. These kinds of similarities could indicate that the child is having trouble acquiring language in general, not just in using English. Second, this comparison can identify structures that the child uses correctly in the home language but makes errors on in English. These errors can be examined to determine whether they arise from interference from the home language. If so, they are likely to resolve on their own as the child develops English proficiency, if no other language disorders are present.

Stockman (1996) has made an additional suggestion for the use of spontaneous speech data as a way to establish whether, in fact, a child is demonstrating a language difference or disorder. The Minimal Competency Core (MCC) is a criterion-referenced measure that represents the least amount of linguistic knowledge needed to be judged normal at a given age within a speech community. Although most speakers will know more than this core, the MCC is designed to identify the linguistic features that the least competent normal child could demonstrate. Because this core includes common obligatory features, it is less affected by contextual and vocabulary differences among situations and speakers. The use of this metric requires,

of course, a detailed and well-researched set of MCC features for each age and dialect. Stockman (1996) has presented one such set for 3-year-old speakers of AAVE. This is presented in Table 5-4.

Craig and Washington (1995) looked at the production of complex sentence types (those containing more than one main verb) in the speech of a representative sample of low income African-American boys aged 4 to 5.5 years old who were living in the urban Midwest. Like Stockman, they found that complex sentence production of at least 3% of a speech sample represented typical performance. They suggest that the appearance of complex sentences within spontaneous speech samples of AAVE speakers as they enter school can serve as a screening criterion for determining presence of language disorder within this population. Craig and Washington (2000) explored this idea further and showed that a combination of MLU, % complex sentences, and number of different words derived from free speech samples provided a sensitive and culturally fair method of identifying expressive language impairment in school-aged AAVE speakers. When combined with receptive measures of responses to *wh*-questions and passive sentences, sensitivity and specificity of this informal measure were excellent for identifying language impairments in this population. Craig and Washington (2002) provide norm-referenced information on these measures from typically developing AAVE speakers. Further, Craig and Washington (2004b) show that adding a measure of non-word repetition (imitating nonsense syllables) and a measure of nonverbal cognition to this battery produced a valid, relatively unbiased screening for language impairment in young African-American children.

Leonard and Weiss (1983) suggested another approach. They advocate looking for features with surface realizations that differ from those expected in Standard American English. For example, several features of SAE are not obligatory in AAVE. If a child who speaks AAVE omits a plural marker, we will not be able to tell whether the omission represents an error or a rule-governed feature of AAVE. Instead, we can look for features that are not omitted but are realized differently in AAVE (or whatever the child's linguistic variation is) than in SAE. Leonard and Weiss provided some examples for AAVE, which are listed in Box 5-8. Coles-White (2004) added a related suggestion. She found that typically developing African-American children were similar to Caucasian peers in understanding various negative forms, even when their production of these forms was influenced by AAVE. She suggests that testing understanding of forms like the one in Figure 5-2 will be helpful in distinguishing children with dialect usage from those with language disorders.

Another approach to analyzing language samples from children who speak AAVE dialect was proposed by Nelson (1998). She presented a modification of the criteria for the *Developmental Sentence Score* (Lee, 1974), called the Black English Sentence Scoring (BESS). This procedure uses a set of criteria based on those developed by Lee (see Chapter 8 for details of these criteria) with changes based on patterns typical of AAVE dialect. For example, under the first stage of personal pronoun

TABLE 5-4	Minimal Competence Core Features for 3-Year-Old AAVE Speakers

Language sampling context: Two-hour speech sample gathered while subject played with race track and cars, then looked at pictures in books.
Productivity criteria: Four correct productions observed anywhere in the 2-hour sample.

LANGUAGE DOMAIN	CORE FEATURES
Phonological	• Correct production of the following word-initial consonants: /m/, /n/, /p/, /b/, /t/, /d/, /k/, /g/, /f/, /s/, /h/, /w/, /j/, /l/
Pragmatic functions	• Comment on objects by labeling or describing
	• Regulate interaction by requesting information or requesting objects or actions
	• Initiate conversational repairs with general query ("Huh?") or spontaneously repeating or revising utterances
	• Respond to speech by answering questions, acknowledging or imitating prior utterances
Semantic relations	• Existence
	• State
	• Locative state
	• Action
	• Locative action
	• Specification
	• Possession
	• Time
	• Negation
Morphosyntax	• Simple sentences with two to three constituents (subject-verb: I eat; subject-verb-object: I eat candy.)
	• Simple, elaborated two to three constituent sentences with lexical or inflectional modifiers (He eats; I am eat*ing the* candy.)
	• MLU 2.7
	• Use of two or more different grammatical morphemes
	• 3%–10% complex sentences in sample

Adapted from Stockman, I. (1996). The promises and pitfalls of language sample analysis as an assessment tool for linguistic minority children. *Language, Speech, and Hearing Services in Schools, 27,* 355-372.

development, Lee places *I, me, mine, you,* and *yours.* The BESS includes *mine's* in this category, since it is used in AAVE. Similarly, in the main verb category, absent copulas would be given an "attempt mark" or a score of zero in Lee's procedure. The BESS awards these constructions 1 point, since they are typical of AAVE. Using the BESS to analyze a speech sample from a child known to be an AAVE speaker is another way to reduce the bias of our structural analysis of the speech of CLD children. Toronto (1976) developed a similar adaptation of the *Developmental Sentence Score,* the *Developmental Assessment of Spanish Grammar,* for evaluating the syntactic skills of Spanish-speaking children using spontaneous speech samples. Gutierrez-Clellen, Restrepo, Bedore, Peña, and Anderson (2000) discuss the issues involved in conducting language sample analyses on Spanish transcripts. They advocate using a measure of number of syntactic/morphological errors/T-unit. This measure has been shown to have a cut-off of 10 errors in 50 utterances for identifying language disorders in Spanish-speaking five year-olds. However, its use for children of younger ages, or those with bilingual development, has not yet been established. Gutierrez-Clellen et al., also warn against counting episodes of code-switching (going from Spanish to English forms within an utterance, or vice versa) as errors.

As we discussed in Chapter 2, language samples can be used for a variety of purposes. Cheng (1987) suggested collecting language samples from several tasks to look at pragmatic skills in a CLD child. These tasks included relating a past experience, describing an object, and describing a picture. Samples collected can be used to look at language function as well as form and content, as Stockman (1996) demonstrates. Bernstein (1989) found this approach to be particularly helpful in getting a broad picture of the communicative skills of CLD children from a variety of backgrounds.

Terrell et al.'s PCCA (1992) also can be applied to language sample analysis. Here a speech sample using a similar sampling context, such as relating a personal experience or narrating a story, would be collected from both parent and child. Again, the child's linguistic patterns—in terms of syntax, semantics, phonology, or pragmatics, depending on the presenting complaint—would be compared with those of the parent. Any child language characteristics that match those produced by the parent are considered dialectical variations rather than errors. If the child's patterns do not match the parent's, the child's responses are compared with age expectations, using developmental charts and normal language data, such as that found in Miller (1981), Haynes and Shulman (1998b), or Owens

BOX 5-8	Features Realized in AAVE but Not in SAE

Distributive *be:*
AAE: "I be good."
SAE: "I am good sometimes."

Remote time *been:*
AAE: "I been walked."
SAE: "I already walked."

Complete aspect *done:*
AAE: "I done went fishing."
SAE: "I already went fishing."

Inflectional marking after consonant cluster reduction:
AAE: *desses, tessing*
SAE: *desks, testing*

Embedded *do* inversion:
AAE: "He wants to know did she get here."
SAE: "He wants to know if she got there."

Preposed negative auxiliary:
AAE: "Couldn't nobody do it."
SAE: "Nobody could do it."

Existential *it:*
AAE: "It's a new kid in the building."
SAE: "There's a new kid in the building."

Pronoun apposition:
AAE: "My mother she did it."
SAE: "My mother did it."

Adapted from Leonard, L., & Weiss, A. (1983). Application of nonstandardized assessment procedures to diverse linguistic populations. *Topics in Language Disorders, 3,* 35-45.

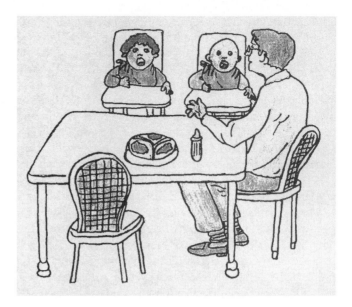

FIGURE 5-2 ✦ A true double negative item from the grammatical judgment task. In the item depicted, a man is sitting at a table and preparing to feed one of two hungry babies; the baby with hair or the baby without hair. A correct response to the verbal prompt, "He didn't feed the baby with no hair, which one did he feed?" would be to point to the baby with the hair.
(Reprinted with permission from Coles-White, D. [2004]. Negative concord in child African American English: Implications for Specific Language Impairment. *Journal of Speech, Language, and Hearing Research, 47,* 212-222.)

1993), the *Basic Inventory of Natural Language* (Herbert, 1977), the *Bilingual Syntax Measure* (Burt, Dulay, & Hernandez-Chavez, 1975), and the *Oral Language Evaluation* (Silvaroli & Maynes, 1975). These procedures provide a somewhat structured method of analyzing natural conversational data. Each requires the child to produce a short language sample using a picture description or picture sequence task. Criteria for evaluating the language produced in both English and the home language are provided in the manuals for these procedures.

Other Assessment Procedures

Recently, a variety of alternative approaches to making the distinction between language difference and disorder have been presented in the literature. Roseberry and Connell (1991) found that teaching an invented morpheme to children with LEP reliably differentiated normal bilingual children from those with specific language deficits. The children with LEP who were language impaired were much poorer at learning the invented rule and failed to use the morpheme in naming pictures given during post-teaching probes. Lidz and Peña (1996) and Owens (2004) advocated a similar approach, using mediated learning experiences in a pretest-intervention–post-test format to teach vocabulary items on the *Expressive One-Word Picture Vocabulary Test–2000 Edition* (Brownell, 2000). Both these approaches use dynamic assessment procedures, as we defined them in Chapter 2. Dynamic assessment, you'll remember, attempts to determine the degree to which mediation in the learning processes assists

(2005). Deviations from Standard English patterns that do not match the parent's and are not typical of normally developing children of the client's age are considered aspects of a language disorder. The PCCA is especially useful for analyzing speech that is influenced by languages or dialects with which the clinician has little experience and for which there are no published data on typical variations from SAE or interference points with English. Comparative analyses can also be done by comparing a child's speech to that of another, typically developing child from the same language/cultural group (Goldstein, 2000).

Some of the measures we discussed as indices of language dominance also can be used to elicit and analyze samples of spontaneous speech from CLD children. These include the *Assessment Instrument for Multicultural Clients* (Adler, 1991;

a child in grasping new material. For children who can benefit from this mediation, normal language learning capacity can be inferred. For those who do not find the mediation helpful, underlying deficits in language learning ability may be present. Approaches such as mediated learning, dynamic assessment, and language processing evaluations like the ones we discussed earlier are especially promising because they can be used no matter what first language the client speaks and regardless of the clinician's familiarity with or access to normative developmental data regarding the first language.

Restrepo (1998) identified a set of measures that discriminate language difference from disorder in Spanish-speaking 5- to 7-year-olds. Her analysis showed that high sensitivity and specificity could be achieved with only two of the measures: parental report of the child's speech and language skills and the number of errors per T-unit (see Chapter 11) in a speech sample derived from three contexts (picture description, interview, and story retelling). The speech samples were collected

in Spanish and analyzed by a native Spanish speaker for morphosyntactic errors. Findings suggest that more than 10 errors per 50 T-units and more than 10 speech or language problems reported by parents on a form such as the one in Figure 5-3 are sufficient to identify a child as having a language disorder in Spanish. Similarly, Patterson (2000) reported that using parent reports of vocabulary size and ability to combine words provided valid information about whether bilingual Latino two-year-olds were acquiring language normally.

Of course, these methods will only help to decide whether a child with CLD really has a language problem—the screening aspect of our assessment. If, with the help of these procedures, we decide that a CLD child would benefit from intervention, we will still need to do additional assessment to establish baseline function and document progress in intervention, just as we would for any client. For these purposes, both the criterion-referenced procedures we've discussed and observational methods will be helpful.

*(More than 10 "yes" responses indicate significant language problems in 5- to 7-year-olds)**		
In comparison with other children of the same age, do you think that your child has problems expressing himself/herself or being understood?	Yes	No
In comparison with children of the same age, do you think that your child has speech problems?	Yes	No
Do your family or friends think that your child is delayed in language?	Yes	No
For his/her age or in comparison with other children, does your child have difficulty producing correct phrases?	Yes	No
Do your family or friends think that your child is difficult to understand?	Yes	No
For his/her age, does your child produce very short phrases?	Yes	No
Do you think that your child has problems with grammar?	Yes	No
When your child talks about the same person, does he/she have difficulty using the correct pronoun such as *he, she, they?*	Yes	No
When your child talks about something that happened, does he/she have difficulty explaining when this happened or use words in different times; for example, talking about yesterday, does the child say "fall" instead of "fell"?	Yes	No
Does your child make mistakes in sentences more than a little of the time?	Yes	No
When your child talks, does he/she have difficulty expressing whether he/she is talking about a man or a woman?	Yes	No
In comparison with other children of the same age, does your child use many words that are too general and not descriptive or exact, such as *this, that,* or *thing?*	Yes	No
Does your child have difficulty finding the exact words to express himself/herself?	Yes	No
Does your child have difficulty explaining or describing things?	Yes	No
Is it difficult for your child to tell you what he/she did during the day?	Yes	No
Is your child frustrated because he/she cannot talk well?	Yes	No
Do you or your child's brothers and sisters have to repeat what you say to him/her more often than when talking to other children?	Yes	No
Do you have to repeat questions or directions to your child more often than to other children?	Yes	No
Does your child have trouble understanding more than a little of what he/she is told?	Yes	No
Do you think that your child has trouble learning new words?	Yes	No
In comparison with children the same age, is it difficult for your child to learn new ideas?	Yes	No
In comparison with children the same age, does your child have a very low or limited vocabulary?	Yes	No
Do you think that your child has a learning problem?	Yes	No
Does your child have dyslexia?	Yes	No
For his/her age, does your child have difficulty paying attention for a long period?	Yes	No
Is your child hyperactive?	Yes	No
Does your child have difficulty attending to an activity or game?	Yes	No
For his/her age, does your child have difficulty pronouncing words?	Yes	No
Is your child's pronunciation easy to understand?	Yes	No
*In conjunction with more than 10 errors/50 T-units in a language sample.		

FIGURE 5-3 ✦ Parental report of child speech or language problems.
(Reprinted with permission from Restrepo, M. [1998]. Identifiers of predominantly Spanish-speaking children with language impairment. *Journal of Speech, Language, and Hearing Research, 41,* 1398-1411.)

USING BEHAVIORAL OBSERVATION WITH THE CLD CHILD

In Chapter 2, we talked about using behavioral observation to describe aspects of a child's communication when our concern is not to compare the child to some standard but simply to get a picture of current communicative skills. Figure 2-14 gives an example of a form that we might use to look at communicative competence, and this form is appropriate for CLD as well as for mainstream clients (Erickson, 1987). Clinicians can devise other forms to look at behaviors of interest as well.

Cheng (2002a) and Crago and Cole (1991) have argued for the importance of ethnographic assessment with CLD children. Ethnographic assessment differs from other forms of naturalistic behavioral observation in that it makes a greater attempt to look at the larger, sociocultural context in which communication takes place and to look at how language is used to share knowledge and establish social order within a particular culture. Ethnographic observation also differs from the kinds of structured behavioral observations discussed in Chapter 2 in that we may not know ahead of time exactly what categories and attributes of behavior we wish to examine. We are using the ethnographic method because of our unfamiliarity with the cultural norms of the child being observed and will use the observation itself to discover the relevant parameters.

Crago and Cole discussed several methods of ethnographic assessment. These include participant observation, audio and video recorded data, and open-ended interviews. Participant observation is described as "hanging around and taking notes" (p. 114). The clinician watches and may participate in a natural interaction, taking brief notes to be expanded later, to get a rounded and unencumbered view of a set of events. Although participant observation is usually easier to accomplish than, say, videotaping a child in a classroom or on the playground, notes of the participant observation are usually less inclusive than transcripts of a recording. The relative advantages of each method need to be weighed before deciding what method to use in observing a particular child.

Open-ended interviews with families of CLD children are another method of gathering ethnographic information about the communicative competence of the CLD child. McCracken (1988) suggested that interviewers develop a series of skeletal questions, without preconceived categories of response, and proceed by a series of indirect prompts for further information while listening carefully for signals that topics are inappropriate or that miscommunication has occurred. When interviewing speakers of a different language through an interpreter, all the cautions in using interpreters that we talked about earlier need to be considered especially carefully. Crago and Cole suggested some dimensions of communication that can be explored through the ethnographic methods we've just been talking about. These are summarized in Table 5-3.

LANGUAGE INTERVENTION WITH THE CLD CHILD

Once a language disorder has been identified and baseline function in the dominant language has been established, intervention for the CLD child generally follows the guidelines we discussed in Chapter 3. We need to address a few problems particular to CLD children when we plan their intervention programs, though. The first type of problem arises when we find that a child who is not SAE dominant has a language disorder. If an SLP who is fluent in the child's dominant language or dialect is not available, how should intervention be managed? A second problem concerns the child who is progressing adequately in the dominant language or dialect but has limited proficiency in SAE or uses a nonstandard dialect. What is the SLP's role with this client? Thirdly, we have a problem in making our intervention culturally appropriate. How can we be sure of not creating just another setting in which cultural differences get in the way of communication and learning? Let's take these questions one at a time.

THE MONOLINGUAL SLP AND THE CLIENT DOMINANT IN A DIFFERENT LANGUAGE OR DIALECT

Because SAE proficiency is so important for access to mainstream culture and its economic opportunities, children with language disorders who speak a language or dialect other than SAE should, at some point, be given the opportunity to learn to communicate in Standard English. In early stages of intervention, however, research (Cobo-Lewis, Eilers, Pearson, & Umbel, 2002; Lopez & Greenfield, 2004; Perozzi, 1985; Perozzi & Chavez-Sanchez, 1992) suggests that instruction in a client's native language facilitates the development of both the first language and English. These findings indicate that early stages of intervention for CLD children with language disorders should be given in the native language, whenever possible, with gradual transition to intervention and instruction in English. When a clinician fluent in a client's native language is available, this approach is clearly preferable.

Too often, however, in a diverse society such as ours, clinicians who speak the language or dialect of every client on the caseload are not to be had. Take Lilly's case, for example.

Ms. Engle was an experienced SLP who had worked for 10 years in a pediatric hospital. But she had never been confronted with a problem such as the one she faced when Lilly found her way onto her caseload. Lilly's family had recently emigrated to the United States from China, and no one in the family, including Lilly, spoke much English. Lilly had recently, at age 4, suffered a series of seizures, and her language use in her native dialect of Mandarin Chinese appeared to be deteriorating. Distraught, her parents brought her to see doctors at the hospital, using friends in the neighborhood as interpreters. Ms. Engle used parent interviews, a speech sample carefully translated in collaboration with the neighborhood interpreters, and some developmental scales and modifications of standardized tests to establish that Lilly's language had been normal when she was younger but had indeed gotten worse since the seizures. Lilly appeared to be communicating at a telegraphic level, to have difficulty understanding anything beyond simple one-step commands, and to rarely initiate communication. In addition to medication to control the seizures, the diagnostic team at the hospital recommended language intervention. Since Mandarin Chinese was Lilly's first, and at this point, only language, Ms. Engle believed it was important to deliver the intervention in that language. Ms. Engle, however, did not speak this dialect.

Juarez (1983) suggested that direct therapy with a mono-lingual SLP is not the optimal approach for clients with language disorders who are dominant in a different language or dialect. However, as Goldstein and Iglesias (2006) point out, there are important services the monolingual SLP can provide, including in-service training, consultation, diagnostic service, and paraprofessional training.

In-Service Training

The SLP can train ESL and classroom teachers who work with these clients. Training can focus on topics such as normal language acquisition processes, the relation of communication to language development, the importance of interaction in language acquisition, appropriate and inappropriate uses of standardized tests, informal and criterion-referenced assessment procedures, techniques for eliciting and evaluating language samples, and methods of designing language intervention programs. The SLP also can provide answers to some of the most commonly asked questions about CLD children with language disorders. These questions include the following:

1. Did the child's bilingual background cause the language disorder?

   The answer to this question is a definitive *no*. Cheng's (1996) and Owens' (2005) reviews of a broad range of literature on this topic concluded that normally developing bilingual children acquire both languages at a comparable rate, with no deficits in either language. Kay-Raining Bird (2006) and Restrepo (2005) showed that children with mental retardation growing up in bilingual home environments found learning two languages no more difficult than learning one. Even children with significant developmental disorders were able to acquire two languages with no greater delays than their counterparts learning just one. The key to development is the opportunity to hear and use both languages in familiar, interactive environments. This, of course, may not be the case for many CLD children who hear the minority language exclusively at home and do not encounter the dominant language until they get to school. Still, a child exposed to two languages simultaneously will learn both with no trouble. A normally developing child exposed to one language at home and another at school will go through a period of limited English proficiency but will communicate normally in the home language and will eventually master the dominant language, given adequate opportunity. Juarez (1983) suggested that it may take 5 to 7 years to achieve English skills sufficient to succeed in English-only academic programs (cognitive academic linguistic proficiency, or CALP). Most normally developing bilingual children learn enough English to engage in ordinary social interactions (basic interpersonal communication skills, or BICS) in 2 to 3 years, though. So if a child is having trouble in the first language, exposure to the second is not what caused it.

2. Should CLD parents speak to their children only in English?

   Again the answer is a resounding *no*. Parents should never feel guilty about using the native language in the home. They should not speak to the CLD child with a language disorder in English, if English is not their own first language. Research (Cummins, 1981; Ramirez & Politzer, 1978) has shown that it is the quality of the language input that makes a difference in development, not the particular language spoken. Parents should be encouraged to engage in many kinds of communicative interactions with their children, including reading books to them, telling them stories, engaging in pretend play, and hearing and telling personal experiences. The language in these interactions should be the one in which the parent is most comfortable and fluent. In this way, the child can receive an optimal model of language structure and function that serves as a strong foundation for development in both languages.

3. Can a language disorder exist in one language and not the other?

   Once more, the answer is *no* (Cummins, 1981; Juarez, 1983; Kay-Raining Bird, 2006). If a child has a deficit in the first language, that deficit will affect the acquisition of English as well. If a child is developing normally in the first language, on the other hand, but has limited English, the problem is most likely to be lack of adequate opportunity to develop English language skills. This lack of opportunity may be a result of recent arrival in the United States, in which case time and understanding teachers may be all that are needed to solve the problem. The lack of opportunity could also stem from social isolation, though. A CLD child may be exposed to English only in limited, formal contexts in school and interact exclusively with people who speak the minority language at all other times. The monolingual SLP can make this clear by observing the child in school. The SLP can document who the CLD child spends informal time with during recess and lunch and what language is spoken.

   If it turns out that the CLD child is socially isolated from English speakers, the SLP can use the in-service training setting to encourage teachers to foster some social interaction. This might include helping teachers to arrange an English-speaking "buddy" to pair off with the child during some informal parts of the day; organizing sports, craft activities, or games between mixed groups of CLD children and English-speaking classmates during recesses; or developing a lunchtime club with invited members from both linguistic groups who get to eat in a special place (such as the teachers' room) and talk together in English.

For normally developing children with limited English skills, such social interactive opportunities go a long way toward building English proficiency.

Damico and Damico (1993) discussed the process of acculturation in students from linguistically and culturally different backgrounds. They emphasized that a crucial factor in acculturation is the degree to which a person feels affiliated with the mainstream culture. An attitude of acceptance and respect on the part of mainstream professionals is certainly an important factor in creating this feeling of affiliation. In addition, however, teachers and clinicians who work with children from culturally different backgrounds would perform a service by setting up opportunities for playground or extracurricular interactions with mainstream peers. These interactions will go a long way toward developing feelings of solidarity with the dominant culture that provide children with LEP the motivation to improve their English language skills.

Consultation

In addition to training teachers in general techniques for developing language skills in children, monolingual SLPs can consult on the interventions for particular CLD children with language disorders. Clinicians can work with teachers to increase their use of culturally sensitive teaching strategies, such as those discussed in the "Multicultural Teaching Techniques" section. We also can encourage the use of script-based interventions, literature-based scripts, and many of the other intervention strategies we discussed in Chapter 3. Clinicians can demonstrate in English how to use such approaches, so the bilingual staff can adapt them to the minority language.

SLPs also can, in collaboration with other staff, develop child-centered or curriculum-based language activities that can be translated by the bilingual staff. These would involve consulting with bilingual staff about the language status and goals for particular clients and about the current classroom themes and curriculum. The SLP can then design a set of activities to address these goals in the context of classroom themes and can consult with staff about translating this program into the child's first language.

In addition, SLPs can fulfill their consultation role by becoming familiar with new tests and materials that address particular language groups. As we see in Appendix 5-1, a variety of tests are available in several languages. As time goes on, more materials in more languages will come onto the market. The SLP can serve as a resource for bilingual staff by watching for and alerting them to new materials in the languages of their clients.

SLPs consulting to classroom programs with CLD children also are important in helping decide when to introduce or focus more sharply on instruction in English. Since CLD children with language disorders should have the opportunity to develop English-language skills, the monolingual SLP needs to observe their progress to determine when some intensive intervention in English is warranted. This involves careful monitoring of both English and first language skills. Using the techniques for assessing first language and SAE skills in CLD children that we talked about earlier, the clinician can use both standardized and informal procedures to track growth in each language. Criteria we might use to make the decision to introduce English-language intervention include the following:

1. The client's English skills have progressed to about the same level as first language skills. English-language intervention can "shadow" forms and functions being acquired in the first language.
2. The client has reached a plateau in first language learning and is not making rapid progress. English skills commensurate with those in the first language can be targeted. Miller (1984) suggested that language intervention in English should begin with features the child already knows in the first language.
3. The client has been in a bilingual program for a considerable time. English intervention can be introduced to begin the transition to more participation in the mainstream program.

Diagnostic Services

Monolingual SLPs have the obligation to determine whether a CLD child is different or disordered in communication skills. This diagnostic responsibility can be fulfilled by using all the techniques we talked about before, including establishing language dominance, training interviewers and obtaining interview data, using and modifying standardized tests, doing speech sample analyses and other criterion-referenced assessment, gathering information from behavioral observation of the child, doing dynamic assessments, and getting ethnographic information about cultural styles of communication from bilingual members of the community.

Training Paraprofessionals to Deliver Services in the First Language

When professional staff such as ESL teachers or bilingual clinicians fluent in a client's language are not available, we may be able to draw on bilingual paraprofessionals, aides, or community volunteers to deliver first-language services. SLPs may sometimes need to recruit such people to assist with their programs for

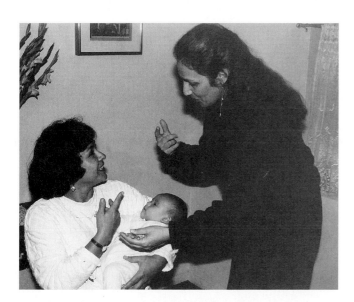

Bilingual SLPs can deliver services in clients' first language.

CLD children with language disorders. Community agencies, churches, and local colleges and community colleges can be contacted to locate bilinguals willing to work as aides or volunteers to teach language skills to children in their cultural group.

The monolingual SLP has the responsibility to plan out the client's program and train the paraprofessional to deliver it. Again, the SLP will need to complete the diagnostic process and arrive at goals for first language learning. Commercially available materials in the first language can be selected and assembled to address some of the goals. The SLP can carefully review the procedures for use of these materials with the paraprofessional.

The SLP can train the paraprofessional to use the child-centered language approaches we talked about in Chapter 3 when working with clients in early stages of first language acquisition. These include, you'll remember, indirect language stimulation or facilitative play. The clinician can train the paraprofessional to engage in child-centered activities and provide enriched input in the form of self-talk, parallel talk, recasts, expansions, and extensions in the client's first language. Literature-based script activities also can be taught to the paraprofessional, with an emphasis on clear and repetitive input paired with engaging activities and materials selected to highlight vocabulary and language forms and functions that the child needs to develop. Focused stimulation and clinician-directed activities also can be designed by the clinician and translated in collaboration with the paraprofessional.

When working with a paraprofessional, of course, the SLP maintains the responsibility to monitor progress in the intervention program, by reviewing assessment data gathered by the paraprofessional in the course of the program. The SLP will be the one to decide when to introduce new goals, when to modify procedures, when to terminate intervention, and when to switch to English language instruction or to pair intervention in the two languages.

ASHA (1998, 2004c) has provided guidelines for monolingual SLPs working with clients who speak another language. These are summarized in Box 5-9.

The Worst-Case Scenario

Suppose you have a certain CLD child with a language disorder on your caseload. You don't speak her language and neither does anyone else in your facility; there is no ESL program in your area; the client's parents do not speak English; and you've been unable, after some effort, to recruit a community member to work with her. What can you do? In this worst-case scenario, we have no choice but to deliver intervention in English. We would want to assess, as well as we can, where the child is functioning in the first language to get some sense of baseline function. Then we would begin using indirect language stimulation with age-appropriate materials. When the child has begun to use English in this setting, some script-based or focused stimulation activities can be introduced. We would proceed essentially as we would with a child in the emerging language stage (see Chapter 7). Vocabulary and themes can be related to classroom work if the client is in school. Again, this will be our least-favored approach to working with the CLD child, and we will only adopt it when we have no other resources available.

| **BOX 5-9** | **ASHA Guidelines for Monolingual SLPs Working with Clients Who Speak Another Language** |

Monolingual SLPs may do the following:
- Test in English
- Perform oral-peripheral exams
- Conduct hearing screening
- Complete nonverbal assessments
- Conduct family interviews with appropriate support personnel
- Research client's language and culture
- Advocate and refer

Monolingual SLPs should seek help with CLD clients by doing the following:
- Establishing contacts and hiring bilingual SLP as consultants
- Establishing cooperative groups among several school systems to hire bilingual SLPs
- Establish networks and links between universities and clinical setting to recruit and train bilingual SLPs
- Establish Clinical Fellowship Year and graduate student practicum sites for bilingual SLPs in training
- Establish interdisciplinary teams in which monolingual SLPs collaborate with and cross-train bilingual professionals from other fields
- Recruit and train support personnel from the community to serve as bilingual aides and paraprofessionals
- Follow ASHA guidelines for supervising bilingual support personnel

Adapted from American Speech-Language-Hearing Association (1998). Provision of English as a second language instruction by speech-language pathologists in school settings; position statement and technical report. *ASHA Supplement, 18*; American Speech-Language-Hearing Association. (2004c). *Preferred practice patterns for the profession of speech-language pathology*. Retrieved from http://www.asha.org/members/deskref-journal/deskref/default

THE SLP AND NORMALLY DEVELOPING CHILDREN WITH LIMITED PROFICIENCY IN STANDARD ENGLISH

Several court cases (*Lau v. Nichols*, 1974; *Martin Luther King Junior Elementary School Children et al. v. Ann Arbor Michigan School District Board*, 1979) have ruled that it is unconstitutional for schools to fail to take into account the languages with which children come to the classroom. These decisions do *not* mean that students' home languages must be the language of instruction. They do mean, however, that public institutions have the obligation to educate teachers about students' native languages or dialects and to attempt to eliminate negative attitudes and diminished expectations on the part of teachers based on their perceptions of their students' language differences. Ms. Salford's story shows how such attitudes can affect adults' perceptions of CLD children.

> Ms. Salford was a new SLP in an inner city school with about 90% African-American and Hispanic-American students. When she arrived, she noticed that the students rarely talked to adults unless they were directly asked a question. On the playground students did lots of talking, yelling, and arguing, but inside they were mostly sullenly silent. Teachers complained that the students had "poor verbal skills" and were "language delayed" and wanted large numbers of students included on Ms. Salford's caseload for language intervention. Ms. Salford sat in on a few classroom sessions to learn more about the students' communication skills. She noticed that the teachers frequently corrected their students, insisting that they use "proper" English when they talked. Students were often told that the teacher couldn't understand them, that their speech was "sloppy." Yet in her playground observations, Ms. Salford heard sophisticated verbal negotiations and a lot of creative use of language for ritualized, playful put-downs. She even heard students getting together in small groups in corners of the playground to add verses and make up new lyrics to their favorite raps. She began to suspect that there was a serious discrepancy between what she heard on the playground and what the teachers were reporting about the children's language skills.

When a normally developing CLD child has LEP, the SLP needs to decide, based on thorough assessment in both languages or dialects, that the child is indeed developing normally in the first one and is limited in SAE only. For these children who do not have a disorder, but rather have a limitation in the use of Standard English, direct services by the SLP are usually not indicated. Still, as Fitts (2001) reminded us, even though LEP or use of nonstandard dialect may not be a disorder, it can constitute a social and educational handicap. Blake and van Sickle (2001) and Mehan (1984) emphasized the importance of being able to master the code of classroom language to succeed in school and thereby obtain wider opportunities for economic advancement and security. In light of the importance of using and understanding SAE to "make it" in the mainstream, a legitimate aspect of our scope of practice can be to offer our expertise to professionals who deal with normally developing LEP children, even when we don't provide services

to these children directly. ASHA (2002) provides guidelines for these kinds of services, and considers them *elective*, rather than required. The main roles we will generally play in this enterprise will be in terms of in-service training and consultation.

In in-service presentations to other professionals and in consultation activities, we will want to emphasize the importance of creating social opportunities for LEP children to interact with SAE speakers. Taylor (1986) gave some suggestions for encouraging the development of a second language or dialect through interaction. These are summarized in Box 5-10. In addition, many of the recommendations that we talked about earlier for creating social opportunities for CLD children also are applicable here.

Another aspect of our responsibility for educating other professionals about CLD concerns the need to convey the importance of language skills for success in the classroom. We need to help our colleagues see how language skills pervade the curriculum at all levels, from preschool through secondary grades. Some of the suggestions for in-service training given in Chapter 12 can be used to make this point. To take it one step further for the CLD child, Adler (1990) emphasized that we need to make colleagues aware of how negative attitudes about language differences can affect children's performance. We also need to help minimize the handicap conferred by a language difference by increasing colleagues' awareness of the problem.

Blake and van Sickle (2001) stressed that improving SAE does not mean eliminating the nonstandard dialect or use of the minority language. On the contrary, programs aimed at improving SAE in culturally different children should have the aim of helping children become bilingual or bidialectical *code-switchers* (that is, speakers able to move back and forth between language styles, choosing the one most appropriate for the situation). This goal requires not only instruction in SAE forms, but also discussion of the functions of a variety of

---

BOX 5-10 | **Principles for Developing Second Language or Dialect Skills**

1. Give children opportunities to engage in genuine, spontaneous conversations with peers.
2. Create situations in which some information is missing, so the child must identify the gap and request more information.
3. Set up goal-oriented conversations with peers, such as assigning children to cooperative learning groups in which they must complete a class project. Be sure that the CLD child has opportunities to negotiate verbally with the other members of the group.

Adapted from Taylor, O. (1986). A cultural and communicative approach to teaching Standard English as a second dialect. In O. Taylor (Ed.), *Treatment of communication disorders in culturally and linguistically diverse populations.* Austin, TX: Pro-Ed.

communicative styles. As a metalinguistic approach, this sort of intervention is ideally adapted to classroom situations. Talking about language use is a metalinguistic activity that will benefit all students, not just those who are CLD. Let's look at some specific techniques we can present to colleagues as consultative suggestions for classroom programming in this area.

Cole (1985) suggested a variety of activities that can be used to teach SAE as a second dialect to AAVE speakers, many of which are applicable for children with LEP as well. These are outlined in Box 5-11.

Taylor (1986) presented a detailed program for developing skills in SAE for children who speak a nonstandard dialect. This program is referred to as *A Cultural and Communication Program for Teaching Standard English as a Second Dialect* (*ACCPT*, pronounced as "accept," for short). These procedures also can be adapted for bilingual children with LEP. The sequence of instruction in this program is schematized in Figure 5-4.

The first and perhaps most crucial step in this program is developing positive attitudes toward the children's own language or dialect. This requires, of course, that the teacher

---

| **BOX 5-11** | **Methods for Teaching English as a Second Dialect or Language** |

1. Modeling and expansion. The instructor models the SAE version of a child's utterance, making no direct attempt to change the child's production. The SLP works with the teacher to identify a small set of forms to be especially careful to notice and model whenever they appear in the child's speech. When use of these forms moves closer to SAE usage, new forms can be targeted.

　　Example: If an AAVE- or Spanish-speaking student in the class has difficulty using SAE negative marking, a child who remarks, "He no like beans" can be told, "You're right. He doesn't like beans."

2. Script-based approaches. Specific forms are targeted by teaching the group a script based on a song, story, poem, finger play, or chant.

　　Example: If a Hispanic child in a class has difficulty using comparative endings, the group might be taught the song "I Am Bigger" to the tune of "Where Is Thumbkin?" Each student adds a verse to the song, after several models by the instructor. Each verse has the following form:

　　"You are big, but I am bigger. I am bigger, I am bigger" (You are X, but I am X-er).

3. Call and response. This is a type of interaction between a speaker and group of listeners in which calls from the speaker elicit responses from the group. Responses can be either scripted or spontaneous. For scripted responses, the teacher establishes a classroom routine, to which students are expected to respond when they hear a particular call. For example, when a child uses a "school talk" form spontaneously, the teacher might ask the group, "What do we say to that?" who respond, "Smooth talking; give your back a pat!" Spontaneous responses use the teacher's call as a guide; usually these include requests for repetition. Foster (2000) provides the following example.

　　Example: When teaching a new word such as *paleontologist*, the teacher (T) might say to the class (C):

T: Here's a new word we need to learn for our dinosaur study. The scientist who studies dinosaurs is a paleontologist. How many parts to that?

　C: Six.

T: OK, let's say the first three together: pay lee on

　C: pay lee on

T: Yes, just like when you owe your friend, you'll say I'm gonna Pay Leon!

　C: Pay Leon

T: (whispers) Pay Leon

　C: (whispers) Pay Leon

T: (louder) PAY LEON

　C: (louder) PAY LEON

T: OK! PAY LEE ON to lo gist

　C: to lo gist

T: Let's say the whole word, FAST: pay lee on to lo gist!

　C: Pay Leon tologist

4. Literature-based scripts. The group reads or listens to a story selected to give numerous examples of a target form (see Appendix 9-1 for an extensive list of examples of such stories). After the first reading, children participate in telling the story by acting it out, using flannel board figures or similar means. Students fill in parts of the script of the story as the instructor rereads it.

　　Example: If a CLD child has trouble with subjective pronoun use, *The Very Busy Spider* (Carle, 1984) can be read to the group and acted out. The CLD child can be asked to narrate some sections of the acting-out, so that opportunities for using the subject pronoun ("*She* was very busy . . .") are provided.

| **BOX 5-11** | **Methods for Teaching English as a Second Dialect or Language—cont'd** |

5. Dialect stories. Stories are read to the group that contain characters from the same cultural group as the CLD child. The speech of the characters is read in dialect, whereas the rest of the text is read in SAE. The instructor has the children contrast the two styles, talk about how they differ, and explain why different styles are used in different parts of the story. The dialect sections can be "translated" into SAE and the SAE sections into dialect or into the CLD child's first language by the CLD child. Again, the group can discuss the differences.

Example: The group can read *Liza Lou* (Meyer, 1976), *We Be Warm Til Springtime Comes* (Chaffin, 1980), or *Cornrows* (Yarbrough, 1981). The characters can be given dialogue in AAVE by AAVE speakers in the group. These forms can be contrasted with the way the rest of the story is written.

6. Situational contrastive drills. Children act out a variety of everyday situations, using both SAE and the home language or dialect. They are encouraged to talk about which is appropriate for each situation, to list situations in which they might use one or the other. They can brainstorm about why "home talk" is appropriate at home, but a different "school talk" form is needed at school or in more formal situations.

Example: Suppose Marta's dad runs out of gas on his way to work. He walks to a gas station near his factory. What do he and the gas station attendant say to each other? What if he ran out of gas right near his apartment, where nearly everyone speaks Spanish and walked to the station right on his corner. What would he and the attendant say to each other then? How do we decide which way to talk?

7. Linguistic contrastive analysis. The instructor gives the children examples of specific contrasts of standard and nonstandard forms. The students contrast the two versions of each form to find out about the rules that differentiate the two types.

Example: Here are two ways to say the same thing:
"I look for him last week." "I looked for him last week."
"I walk to school yesterday." "I walked to school yesterday."
"I help the teacher a lot last year." "I helped the teacher a lot last year."

How are the two ways of saying the same thing different? Can you say what the rule for the first speaker is when talking about things that happened in the past? What about for the second speaker? Which speaker is using "school talk?" "Home talk?"

8. Paraphrasing and retelling. Students listen to or read a story in SAE and retell it in the home language or dialect.

Example: The students read a story, such as a chapter of *Stuart Little* (White, 1974). In cooperative learning groups, they "translate" it into the home language or dialect.

9. Role projection. Students take on a role and respond to realistic situations within their role.

Example: Willy isn't feeling well, so his mom takes him to the doctor. What do Willy's mother and the doctor say to each other as the doctor examines Willy?

Adapted from L. Cole (1985). *Nonstandard English: Handbook for assessment and instruction.* Silver Spring, MD: Author; Foster, M. (2002). Using call-and-response to facilitate language mastery and literacy acquisition among African American students. *ERIC/CLL Digest*, July, EDO-FL-02-04.

---

have such attitudes as well. The SLP can be very important in this process by using in-service training opportunities to talk about the legitimacy and importance of having a strong base in the home language or dialect on which SAE proficiency can be built. At the same time, the SLP can encourage teachers to convey an accepting and positive attitude about the home language or dialect to students. Taylor (1986) suggested that students be introduced to the idea that each culture has its own language and to see language as a tool for communication that can be looked at and be of interest for its own sake. Activities such as learning a simple song, rhyme, or finger play in each of several languages can be a first step. The teacher can convey acceptance of the students' own language or dialect through activities such as asking students to bring in songs or games that they play at home and teach them to the group or

asking the students to "teach" how they greet someone in the home language or dialect.

The next step in this program involves developing an awareness of language differences, first in general and later in contrasting the home language or dialect with SAE. Adler (1993) suggested that students be taught to recognize two different language styles, designated "everyday talk" and "school talk." Two puppets might be introduced, one who talks everyday talk and one who talks school talk. Children can be encouraged to listen to how the puppets talk differently and decide which puppet uses which style. Next, pictures of different settings, such as classroom, playground, doctors' office, and kitchen, might be shown. Children can be asked to say whether everyday talk or school talk would be most appropriate for each setting.

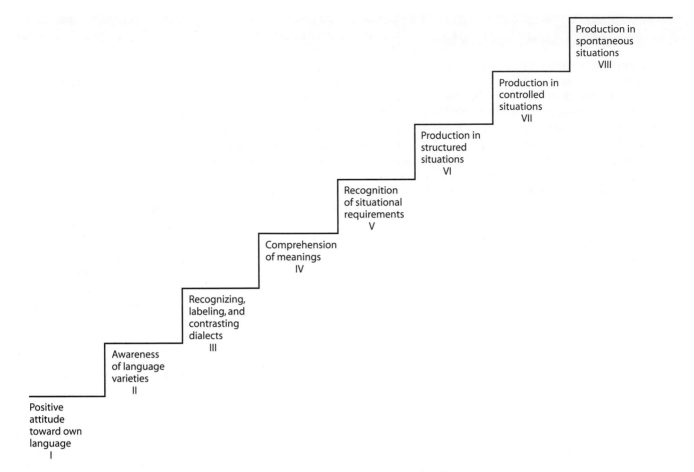

FIGURE 5-4 ✦ A sequence of oral communication training for bilingual or bidialectal children. (Reprinted with permission from Taylor, O. [1986]. *Treatment of communication disorders in culturally and linguistically diverse populations* [p. 168]. Austin, TX: Pro-Ed.)

Additional activities can include reading poems and stories in "old" or more archaic forms of English. Classic poems such as Mary Howitt's "The Spider and the Fly" or Henry Wadsworth Longfellow's "The Midnight Ride of Paul Revere" might be used. Children can retell each in their own language, the teacher can retell them in contemporary SAE, and the retellings might be taped for later contrastive analysis. Children also can listen to different regional dialects, taped by the instructor from popular television shows, and "translate" these scripts into the home dialect.

Steps III and IV of Taylor's scheme involve recognizing and labeling differences in the form and meaning of messages sent in standard and nonstandard styles. For children beyond the primary grade levels, analysis of form could include contrastive linguistic analyses and attempts to characterize the rules for use of the different languages or dialects. Work on comprehending meanings of various forms of the same message can involve talking about the different meanings words can have in different dialects (When does /fæt/ mean "overweight" and when does it mean "cool" or "hip"?). Wheeler (2005) has shown that contrastive analysis and encouraging code-switching through awareness of differences between dialects works better than merely correcting dialectical usage. She argues that correcting

children's dialect use is ineffective (Wheeler & Swords, 2004), and leads to increasing gaps between SAE and AAVE speakers as they progress through school. Wheeler shows that contrastive analysis with an emphasis on conscious code-switching results in significant decrease in the use of AAVE features in writing, and in consequent narrowing of the achievement gap.

Looking at the situational requirements for different language styles (Step V) can involve role-playing and metalinguistic discussions of the needs of speakers and listeners in different communicative settings. Activities such as those suggested in Box 5-11 can be used in these contexts. In Step VI of Taylor's sequence, children are given practice and support to produce forms in SAE in structured situations. One kind of structure that can be employed is the call-and-response form. This form has a long history in African-Americans traditional discourse (Cazden, 1999) and may be familiar to students for this reason. Foster (2002) reported that primary classrooms whose teachers used call-and-response improved reading and code-switching to SAE more than classrooms that did not use the technique. A description of call-and-response discourse appears in Box 5-11. Taylor also suggested activities such as choral reading and Readers' Theater, in which students read short poems or stories of their own choosing to an audience.

The poems and stories in this exercise are in SAE style. Step VII involves similar activities with somewhat less structure and support. Students use role-playing and story-telling contexts to produce SAE forms. In these activities, the content of the message is familiar and predictable. Familiar situations, such as visiting a doctor, ordering a hamburger, or buying stamps at the post office, would be appropriate for role play in SAE style. Retelling an often-heard story, such as the plot of a popular movie or TV episode or a folktale well-known in the community, is another vehicle for this level of instruction. Although the students must produce their own spontaneous language in SAE style, the task is somewhat more constrained than normal conversation, providing the students with a better chance to focus on the SAE forms, since the function and content of the message have already been determined for them.

Blake and van Sickle (2001) suggest using a Writers' Workshop approach to address this step for older students. Here, students are encouraged to write about their own experiences in their own dialect. Brief mini-lessons are presented to address writing mechanics and text structures. Students get feedback on their work through dialogue journals, in which teachers comment not only on content, but on dialect features of the writing and make suggestions for changes to SAE. Students then share their writing with the class, and discuss when/how/why they did or did not choose to use dialect features within their compositions.

The final step in Taylor's program involves spontaneous production of SAE forms in the appropriate context. Here instruction would remind children what they have learned about the different communicative demands of different contexts. Role-playing would be used for less-constrained production activities to allow students to practice emerging SAE skills. Situations appropriate for this level might include asking a teacher about a homework assignment, giving a formal talk on bike safety to a group of younger students, or telling the student's life story to a reporter writing an article for the school newspaper.

Adler (1993) also presented a comprehensive program for developing SAE proficiency in normal children with LEP or dialect differences. It included detailed lesson plans for children at both preschool and elementary school levels. Like Taylor's approach, this one emphasizes acceptance of children's home language styles, contrastive analysis and awareness of language differences, and practice in structured communication situations. Adler's method also included an incidental learning component. That is, teachers are encouraged to label "everyday" or "home talk" as such when it comes up in the classroom. In this situation, the teacher reminds the child about the different settings in which home talk is appropriate and states in a positive way that "school talk" is the style that should be used in school. The teacher can then translate the child's remark into SAE or ask the child to do so. Either way, an atmosphere of understanding of language differences rather than of judging language deficiencies is maintained on the teacher's part.

Brice and Roseberry-McKibbin (2001) made suggestions for working with children who come from non—English-speaking backgrounds. They emphasized the importance of using the native language as a medium for improving students'

communication in the second language, and outlined a series of strategies for implementing this suggestion in the bilingual or monolingual classroom. These strategies are summarized in Table 5-5, and can serve as helpful consultation suggestions for SLPs working with classroom teachers of children learning English as a second language.

Any of the programs we've been discussing, or ideas from them, are appropriate information to share with classroom and ESL teachers in our consulting role. For SLPs who work in schools with large numbers of CLD children, these also are ideal opportunities to do some collaborative teaching, coming into the classroom of a CLD child who does have a disorder and doing activities such as the ones we just discussed to help the whole class improve their proficiency in SAE. When we offer these activities as consultative suggestions, however, we'll need to remember that it won't be enough just to do the activities, if the teacher doesn't convey a genuine sense of acceptance of language difference. Using the collaborative teaching situation may be one of the best ways for us to provide a model of this kind of attitude to teachers who work in classroom settings with CLD children.

MULTICULTURAL TEACHING TECHNIQUES

How can we make intervention more culturally appropriate and therefore more accessible to CLD children? Tharp (1989) showed that when similarities between the school and home culture are increased, the performance of CLD children improves. In both our consulting role with teachers and in our own direct interactions with CLD children, we can incorporate some procedures and activities that will help reduce cultural conflicts. Remember, however, that different cultures will have different expectations. As we saw earlier, Asian-Americans may expect teachers to talk and children to listen, speaking only when spoken to first. Native Americans, on the other hand, may not find speaking in a teacher-directed group a familiar or comfortable experience. The suggestions we'll talk about here may be helpful for some children from some cultural groups, but no one suggestion will be appropriate for everyone. We'll always need to use judgment and rely on advice from community members about what techniques will work best for particular children and cultural groups.

One issue that faces us when we work with children with CLD concerns their view of themselves and their potential. Smyer and Westby (2005) recount what happened when they invited students in a low-income, all-minority school to enter an essay contest for scholarships to a summer science camp. They were surprised when, after a long silence, one of the students replied, "That's for smart white kids, not us." (p. 23). Smyer and Westby conjecture that the persistent achievement gap between CLD children and mainstream students has roots in this feeling that only "smart white kids" succeed in school and academic pursuits. They argue that an important aspect of multicultural teaching includes an explicit refusal to accept this assumption, and a concerted attempt to convince the children themselves of their potential as learners. Danzak and

TABLE 5-5	Consulting Suggestions for Teachers Working with Bilingual Children in Classroom Settings	

STRATEGY—ENCOURAGE TEACHERS TO DO THE FOLLOWING:	DESCRIPTION	EXAMPLE
Reiterate	Repeat what the other speaker said for emphasis and clarification.	Student: He take it? Teacher: Did he take it? I think he did.
Check and expand vocabulary	Checks vocabulary understanding and use. Introduce new words in English, talk about Spanish equivalents and discuss vocabulary items explicitly.	Student: I need a …. Teacher: You need an eraser? You need to erase your answer, to change it? You need an eraser, then. We use an eraser to erase, or get rid of what we want to change. How do you say that in Spanish?
Maintain flexible language environment	Allow students multiple forms of participation in classroom discourse, including flexible turn-taking, increasing wait time for responses, accepting answers in either language, rewards for participation.	The teacher may occasionally respond to a student with "*si*" rather than "*yes*," or prompt with "*y que mas*" sometimes, instead of "*and what else.*"
Value native languages	Convey acceptance and appreciation of multiple languages by recognizing appropriate uses of each language, asking students how to say things in their native languages, including material from native languages within the curriculum.	Teacher reads students a Mexican folktale in English, then asks students, "What's the word for this bowl in Spanish? How would you ask the girl in the story's name in Spanish?"
Encourage code-switching	Allow code-switching in student contributions to encourage spontaneous language use.	Encourage students to help others master classroom concepts by presenting what the teacher said in English to peers in Spanish.
Ask questions	Encourage bilingual students to answer teacher questions, in the native language if necessary, to increase class participation and provide opportunities to hear English versions of their Spanish responses.	Teacher: There's a grandmother in this story. What do you call your grandmother? Student: Abuelita. Teacher: Abuelita, that's what you call your grandmother? I call mine "Gran." Abuelita, Gran, two names for grandmother.

Adapted from Brice, A., & Roseberry-McKibben, C. (2001). Choice of language in instruction: One language or two. *Teaching Exceptional Children, 33,* 10-16.

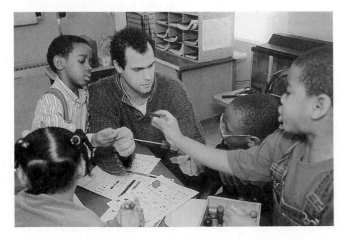

Working with culturally different clients may involve teaching SAE as a second dialect.

Silliman (2005) echo this notion, and argue that becoming a competent English language speaker involves building a new aspect of identity; that of a "smart kid" who communicates in English at least some of the time. To accomplish this end, Smyer and Westby describe a literature-based program in which they encouraged students to read (or listen to) and discuss stories of individuals, particularly those from nontraditional backgrounds, who had overcome obstacles, defied others' expectations, and used courage and determination to achieve great things. A list of some of the literature they used in this program appears in Box 5-12. Smyer and Westby also report that, following this literature program, several of their students successfully applied for the summer scholarships. In our consultant and collaborative roles, we can encourage teachers to adopt similar approaches to raising students' expectations of themselves.

BOX 5-12 Books Used to Overcome Low Expectations

Adler, D. (1996). *A picture book of Thomas Alva Edison*. New York: Holiday House.

Bridges, R. (1999). *Through my eyes*. New York: Scholastic.

Coleman, E. (1999). *White socks only*. Morton Grove, IL: Albert Whitman.

Cooper, R. (1996). *Mandela: From the life of the South African statesman*. New York: Philomel.

Farris, C. (2003). *My brother Martin: A sister remembers*. New York: Simon and Schuster.

Demi (2001). *Gandhi*. New York: Margaret K. McElderry.

Krull, K. (2003). *Harvesting hope: The story of Cesar Chavez*. San Diego: Harcourt.

Lasky, K. (2003). *The man who made time travel*. New York: Farrar, Straus, & Girouz.

Pinkney, A. (1994). *Dear Benjamin Banneker*. San Diego: Harcourt Brace.

Ringgold, F. (1999). *If a bus could talk: The Rosa Parks story*. New York: Aladdin.

Wiles, D. (2001). *Freedom summer*. New York: Atheneum.

Wishinsky, F. (2002). *What's the matter with Albert? A story of Albert Einstein*. Toronto: Maple Leaf Press.

Wishingsky, F. (2003). *Manya's dream: A story of Marie Curie*. Toronto: Maple Leaf Press.

Woodson, J. (2001). *The other side*. New York: Penguin Putnam.

Yin, C. (2003). *Coolies*. New York: Puffin.

Adapted from Smyer, K., & Westby, C. (2005). Using children's literature to promote self-identity in CLD students. *Perspectives in Language Learning and Education, 12,* 87-96.

One important aspect of multicultural teaching concerns the role of literacy for the CLD child. Kayser (2004) reported that the International Reading Association advocates encouraging CLD students to become biliterate as well as bilingual, and suggests beginning literacy instruction in the child's first language. While this may not be possible for children from smaller language groups, many programs working with Spanish first-language users do adopt this approach. Even if first-language literacy instruction is not possible, however, Kayser suggests SLPs work with teachers of CLD children to improve their literacy development by providing parents with books to read to their children in their native language, and building bridges between home literacy and school. Parents can be encouraged to participate in the classroom and share stories from their own culture with students. Literacy training, both in the form of basic literacy instruction and on ways to share written materials with children can also help parents feel more a part of their child's school culture and education.

We talked earlier about some of Westby and Rouse's (1985) suggestions for working with CLD children with language and learning disorders in classrooms. They suggested adding some high-context activities in the classroom to increase the child's chances for success there. In addition, they advocated providing parents with structured, lower-context activities to do at home to build these skills in a nurturing atmosphere. Westby and Rouse also suggested using cooking, crafts, and pretend play activities to provide high-context opportunities for language learning. In these activities, the clinician or teacher first introduces the tools or props to be used, names them, and discusses their function. The adult outlines the sequence of activities to be carried out. For cooking or craft activities, this would involve telling the students the steps to follow to complete the project. For pretend play, the adult can set the scene and outline the script ("We'll pretend to have a birthday party for Maria. First we'll have to bake her a cake. Someone will have to go to the store to buy ...") Children are invited to contribute, but are not singled out or required to give a particular response. The purpose of the interactions is to provide rich, contextualized language input with models of the kinds of discourse appropriate for the situation and to give children opportunities to talk in a nonthreatening setting. Children are encouraged to comment and relate personal experiences, rather than to display knowledge as they are in traditional classroom activities.

Westby and Rouse stressed the importance of teaching planning and metacognitive skills to CLD children, since many high-context communicative styles do not place strong emphasis on planning future activities. They suggested that book reports, particularly reports developed by a group rather than an individual, offer an especially helpful context for learning these skills. Harris (1995) emphasized the importance of allowing CLD children to read or hear the whole story before asking any questions, since this holistic approach more closely mirrors a high-context communicative style.

Having a group of children develop an oral or written book report on a book they have read or listened to is valuable for several reasons. First, the book sets the topic and can be used by the teacher to get a child back on topic if an associative remark is made. Having the group negotiate the best way to retell or interpret the story provides valuable experience in applying metacognitive and metalinguistic processing to a text, such as a remembered story, for which there is little contextual support. Looking for characters' strategies, motives, and attempts to carry out intentions, then evaluating the results of characters' attempts, all help focus attention on the planning aspect of human behavior. Westby and Rouse emphasized that the purpose of all these activities is to help CLD children learn how to learn in a low-context culture such as the classroom and to allow them to use the high-context learning styles with which they came to school to acquire that knowledge.

Harris (1995) suggested modifying the timing and rhythm of presentation of material. Teachers and clinicians are encouraged to give CLD children more time to answer questions and to pause after a child's answer before giving an evaluation. These changes are particularly relevant for Native American children who feel speech needs to be considered carefully before a response is given. When these wait times were increased, Winterton (1976) found that Native American children were twice as likely to participate in classroom interactions as when shorter wait times and fewer pauses were used. Modifying rhythm of presentation means talking more slowly and fluidly, with fewer self-interruptions and digressions. Decreasing the rate of presentation of material will probably benefit many students, as well as improving the participation of CLD children.

Cheng (1996) argued that the key to success in working with CLD clients is both to support the students' transition to the classroom culture and to encourage children to make conscious comparisons and contrasts between home and school cultures. This can best be done, according to Cheng, by encouraging CLD students to bring their experiences with the home culture into the classroom conversation. There are several ways to structure these experiential activities.

One suggestion is to use a *multicultural calendar*. Here the clinician or teacher would use the typical classroom theme of holidays and special days to incorporate the experience of the CLD child. Each month, mainstream holidays and holidays from the cultures of the CLD children would be marked on the calendar. Weekly or monthly themes for language activities would revolve around these special days. For example, Thanksgiving might be a theme for November. Here, activities around the traditional American celebration would be combined with discussion of harvest festivals of other cultures. CLD children could be asked to find out how the harvest is celebrated in their culture; to share artifacts, pictures, songs, or dances with the class; and to compare how these holidays are observed. Depending on the developmental level of the class, projects might include making group picture books with labels for objects used in American Thanksgiving and other harvest festival celebrations; making greeting cards to send to family members with pictures, ideas, and phrases typically associated with the mainstream and other holidays; writing recipes and cooking foods associated with each festival; writing descriptions of how to celebrate each holiday; and so on.

Cheng (2002a) pointed out that *map study* provides another opportunity for incorporating the experience of CLD children in the classroom. Maps can be studied to identify the place of birth of each class member or to follow routes of trips that class members have taken (for CLD children, this can include the route to their country of origin). Students can work in groups to make maps of various places associated with their personal experience, such as their house, home town or village, or home country. Life stories can be written and illustrated with maps relevant to each student's story.

Hyter and Westby (1996) suggested the comparative study of *folktales* as another method to bring the CLD child's experience into school. Here, again depending on the developmental level of the group, age-appropriate folktales from mainstream culture can be read. CLD children can be asked whether they know any similar stories. The clinician or teacher may consult in advance with a librarian about parallel stories from different cultures and obtain books that tell parallel tales. *Little Red Riding Hood* and its Chinese version, *Lon Po Po* (Young, 1989), for example, may be read and compared. Paul Galdone's (1970) traditional retelling of *The Three Little Pigs* can be contrasted with *The Three Little Hawaiian Pigs and the Magic Shark* (Laird, 1981) or *The Three Javelinas* (Lowell, 1992). Various culture's renditions of the Cinderella story, such as *Mufaro's Beautiful Daughters* (Steptoe, 1987), *The Talking Eggs* (San Souci, 1989), *Turkey Girl* (in Verlarde, 1989), and *Yeh-Shen* (Louie, 1982), also can be compared. Folktales from Asia have been compiled by the Children's Book Press (1461 Ninth Ave., San Francisco, CA 94122). Many West African folktales (Appiah, 1989; McDermott, 1972), too, have parallels in folktales familiar to mainstream students.

Comparative folklore studies have many advantages. They not only bring students' experience into the classroom, but they also allow metalinguistic focus on different ways of telling stories and support narrative development. Cheng suggested doing activities such as having parents tell stories in the native language, having them translated, and having the CLD child retell the story to the class. Collective stories, in which each member of a group retells a part of a story, also can be used. These group stories can be "published" in class books, with the mainstream and CLD child's version side by side. Discussions of similarities and differences can follow. Related activities might have groups generate yet another version of the same story to write, illustrate, and publish.

Hyter and Westby (1996) also encouraged the use of stories as a way to help children learn to take multiple perspectives. For both mainstream and CLD students these activities help us to learn to try to "walk a mile in another's moccasins," or see how things might look from another's point of view.

Multiple perspective activities include the following:

▶ Discussing versions of stories told through different characters' eyes, such as *The True Story of the Three Little Pigs by A. Wolf* (told from the wolf's point of view; Scieszka, 1989) or *The Untold Story of Cinderella* (told from the point of view of the stepsisters; Shorto, 1990).

▶ Discussing controversial topics, such as racial prejudice, through books such as *Roll of Thunder, Hear My Cry* (Taylor, 1975), or *Maniac Magee* (Spinelli, 1990).

▶ Talking about books that give a first person perspective, such as *Hatchet* (Paulsen, 1987) or *Toning the Sweep* (Johnson, 1993).

▶ Reading and talking about "trickster tales," stories that involve deception and the need to distinguish between what is intended and what is said; many cultures have tales of traditional tricksters, including Brer Rabbit (Appalachian; Lester, 1990), Anansi the Spider (West African; McDermott, 1972), Raven (Northwest Native American; McDermott, 1993), Iktomi (Plains Native American; Goble, 1990), and Coyote (Southwest Native American; McDermott, 1994).

Cheng (2002a) also suggested the use of cultural "capsules" or "clusters." These are elements, activities, and events that are unique to a culture. They might include the African-American

Kwanza celebration or the Mexican-American use of piñatas. Items related to cultural clusters or capsules can be displayed and discussed, used for vocabulary development, and incorporated into role-playing activities in which children use language forms appropriate for the objects and events. Scripts can be developed ahead of time and rehearsed, so that students can demonstrate their cultural capsules to an audience such as parents or another group of students. Such scripts also will support the students' development of communicative competence about their own culture.

Mainstream culture capsules also can be included in the intervention program. Here objects and events that may be unfamiliar to the CLD child (such as erasers, rulers, or "lining up") can be introduced and studied as other culture capsules are. This approach brings home the point that there's nothing more "right" or "natural" about the school culture than the home culture. What is important is to know the language and behavior that is expected in each. Again, role playing and previously developed scripts can be useful to help CLD students interact with the culturally specific materials. Teacher-student, storekeeper-customer, doctor-patient, and other familiar roles can be played out to give CLD students additional experience with the language and organization of commonly occurring activities in the mainstream culture.

Cheng (1989) also suggested using the *"personal weather report"* (Fig. 5-5) to help develop vocabulary for emotional expression. Since this is an area in which traditional cultures often differ from our American style of "letting it all hang out," CLD students may need extra help developing a precise and differentiated lexicon of feelings, beyond *happy, sad,* and *mad.* Clinicians can start each session by giving their own personal weather report and asking the students to identify their emotional state on a chart such as the one in Figure 5-5. The label for the chosen emotion can be given, and discussion of the various emotions expressed can be used to compare and contrast the various words and the feelings they represent. Later, figurative uses of words such as "cold" and "warm" to discuss feelings can be added to the activity. Other figurative uses of such words ("That's a hot car!") also might come up.

Scott and Rogers (1996) discussed ways of helping the older CLD student improve writing abilities in the classroom. They emphasized that the writings of CLD students often sacrifice self-expression for the sake of using SAE features. They suggest that students be encouraged to write first for voice and meaning by giving a verbatim transcription of the way the student would convey the message in speech. Through successive editing passes, each attending to only one feature of SAE at a time, the students bridge the gap between their oral speech style and an SAE version. Goldstein (2000) made additional suggestions for SLPs to use in consultation or collaboration with teachers in classrooms with CLD children. These are summarized in Box 5-13.

■ CONCLUSIONS

We started our discussion of multicultural issues in child language disorders with the reminder that, despite our differences, we are all Americans. Most of us who are SLPs now have ancestors who, at some point, were newcomers to this country and spoke little English, too. Most of us have lost the languages with which our families came to these shores. That has some advantages, like the fact that we can all talk to each other in a rich common tongue that has borrowed elements from many of the languages our families brought here. But the loss of the old languages is sad, too. So many of us are now monolingual, which limits our communication in some ways in this ever-smaller world. As we think about our role in helping new arrivals and those who have been excluded from the mainstream to find their place in the bubbling multicultural mixture that is America, we might do well to remember the pluses and minuses of this historical pattern. We certainly want to help and encourage CLD children and their families to develop proficiency in Standard American English, which will give them the broadest opportunities for scholastic and economic success. But at the same time, we might recall the advantages that being bilingual or bicultural can confer. In working with CLD clients, our challenge is to strike a delicate balance. We must provide the tools of SAE communication that will allow participation in the mainstream culture, but we must do so without confiscating the tools of communication that make the life of the individual rich and integrated and the mosaic of our country increasingly vibrant as new elements continue to be added to its texture.

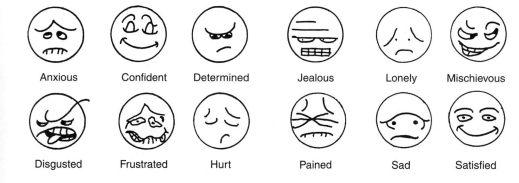

FIGURE 5-5 ✦ Personal weather report.
(Reprinted with permission from Cheng, L. [1989]. Intervention strategies: A multicultural approach. *Topics in Language Disorders, 9*[3], 91.)

Anxious	Confident	Determined	Jealous	Lonely	Mischievous
Disgusted	Frustrated	Hurt	Pained	Sad	Satisfied

BOX 5-13	Suggestions for Multicultural Teaching

Adapt classroom materials

Build on prior knowledge

Provide context and background information

Control new vocabulary

Use social and pragmatic activities

Modify curricular material

Use a variety of narrative styles (recounts, event casts, etc.)

Use culturally appropriate materials

Use a variety of social organizations for classroom activities

Use role playing

Use cooperative learning groups

Use peer tutoring

Focus on communication in reading and writing

Use dialogue journals in which teacher/clinician responds to, rather than corrects, student writing

Use language experience stories, in which the teacher writes down students' oral narratives

Provide written materials in both English and the first language

Read aloud to students throughout the elementary grades

Use visual supports

Use semantic webs

Use word maps

Use scripts

Use "What I know" charts

Develop a bicultural approach

Talk about differences between "home talk" and "school talk"

Encourage extracurricular activities that come from the home culture and that expose children to mainstream culture activities

Encourage high levels of interaction between CLD and mainstream students, or students with different non-mainstream backgrounds

Adapted from Goldstein, B. (2000). *Cultural and linguistic diversity resource guide for speech-language pathology*. San Diego: Singular Publishing Group.

STUDY GUIDE

I. An Introduction to Cultural Diversity
   A. Define bicultural education.
   B. Distinguish a language difference from a language disorder.
   C. Describe some of the factors that contribute to the unique style of communication used by African-Americans.
   D. List and discuss differences between AAVE and Standard American English.
   E. Define bidialectical.
   F. Discuss the meaning and importance of code switching.
   G. What is meant by limited English proficiency?
   H. Describe some characteristics of Spanish-influenced English.
   I. Discuss some features of Native American dialects of English.
   J. List some features of Asian dialects of English.
   K. Describe the contrasts between high-context and low-context communication. How are these styles associated with CLD children? How do they affect narrative skill?

II. Assessing Culturally and Linguistically Different Children
   A. How can language dominance be established? Why is it important to establish it?
   B. How can interview data be obtained from families of CLD children if the clinician does not speak their language?
   C. Discuss the appropriate uses of standardized tests with CLD children.
   D. What are some appropriate modifications to make if standardized tests are not available in the client's dominant language? What are inappropriate modifications? How can the results of these modifications of tests be interpreted properly?
   E. Describe the Parent-Child Comparative Analysis procedure. Under what circumstances would it be used?
   F. Discuss the use of speech sample analysis with the CLD child. How can it be done if the clinician does not speak the child's dominant language? How can it be used to differentiate limited English proficiency from a language disorder?
   G. Explain what the Minimal Competency Core means. Give elements of this core for preschool speakers of AAVE.
   H. How can dynamic assessment be used with CLD children?
   I. What are the uses of behavioral observation with the CLD child?
   J. What is ethnographic assessment, and how can it be used in the evaluation of a CLD child?

III. Language Intervention and the CLD Child
   A. What are the service delivery options for a CLD child whose dominant language is not English when the clinician is monolingual in English?
   B. What is the SLP's role with the normally developing child who has LEP or a nonstandard dialect of English?
   C. Describe a general approach to improving proficiency in SAE for children with LEP or nonstandard dialects. Give several specific examples of activities that might be used in such a program.
   D. Describe several approaches and activities for making instruction culturally appropriate for CLD children.

A SAMPLE OF MULTICULTURAL
TESTS AND ASSESSMENT MATERIALS

Name	Description	Available from
African American English: Structure and Clinical Implications (C. Temple Adger, N. Schilling-Estes, N.W. Wolfram)	Assesses phonological, grammatical, and pragmatic characteristics of AAE in school-age children. Includes an interactive CD-ROM and manual. Helps you understand more about the structure, features, and rules of AAE, in order to work more effectively with children who speak vernacular dialects.	American Speech-Language-Hearing Association 10801 Rockville Pike Rockville, MD 20852
All India Institute of Medical Sciences Test for Auditory Comprehension of Language; All India Institute of Medical Sciences Test of Articulation (S. Bhatnager)	Instrument for diagnosing speech and language disorders in Hindi.	Subhash Bhatnagar Dept. of Communicative Disorders College of Liberal Arts University of Mississippi University, MS 38677
Ann Arbor Learning Inventory-Revised (AALI-R) (B. Vitale and W. Bullock) (Available in Spanish)	Assesses central processing skills important to learning, such as visual discrimination, visual memory, auditory discrimination, and auditory memory. Valuable for determining the best form of instruction for a child with disabilities. Offers comprehensive and detailed examination of skills that underlie reading, writing, speaking, listening and spelling. Grades K-8.	Academic Therapy Publications 20 Commercial Blvd. Novato, CA 94949
Assessment Instrument for Multicultural Clients (S. Adler)	A criterion-referenced instrument for examining a broad range of 22 communication behaviors in children with LEP.	In Adler, S. (1991). Assessment of language proficiency in LEP speakers. *Language, Speech, and Hearing Services in Schools,* 22(2), 12-18.
Assessment of Phonological Processes (B. Hodson) (Available in Spanish)	Identifies error patterns while deemphasizing differences related to dialect variations.	Los Amigos Research Associates 7035 Galewood, Suite D San Diego, CA 97120
Basic Inventory of Natural Language (C. Herbert) (Available in Spanish and 31 other languages)	Used for grades K-12. A language sample is scored for fluency, complexity, and average sentence length.	CHECpoint System, INC. 1520 N. Waterman Ave. San Bernardino, CA 92404
Ber-sil Spanish Test (M. Beringer) (Available in Philippine, Tagalog, Ilokano)	Also available in Cantonese, Mandarin, Korean, Persian. Assessment of receptive vocabulary for ages 5-12 years (elementary) and 13-17 years (secondary).	Ber-Sil Co. 3412 Seaglen Dr. Rancho Paols Verdes, CA 90274
Bilingual Classroom Communication Profile (C. Roseberry-McKibbin)	Observational screening tool to help classroom teachers distinguish communication differences from communication disorders.	Academic Communication Associates PO Box 566249 Oceanside, CA 92056
Bilingual Language Proficiency Questionnaire (L. Mattes and G. Santiago)	Parent interview questionnaire regarding bilingual children's development and use of speech and language. Items listed in both English and Spanish.	Academic Communication Associates, Publications Divisions, Dept. 2C PO Box 6044 Oceanside, CA 92056

Name	Description	Available from
Bilingual Syntax Measures I and II (M. Burt and H. Dulay)	Identifies students' mastery of oral syntactic structures in English and/or Spanish. Pre-K to 12th grade.	Harcourt Assessment 19500 Bulverde Rd. San Antonio, TX 78259
Bilingual Syntax Measures— Chinese and Tagalog (C. Tsang)	Test of language dominance in Chinese/Tagalog speakers.	Asian-American Bilingual Center 2134 Martin Luther King Jr. Way Berkeley, CA 94709
The Bilingual Verbal Ability Tests (BVAT) (A.F. Moñoz-Sandoval, J. Cummins, C.G. Alvarado, and M.L. Ruef)	Assesses the following in 5 year olds to adults: Cognitive Ability; Picture Vocabulary, Oral Vocabulary, and Verbal Analogies. Comprised of three subtests from the Woodcock-Johnson-Revised Tests of Cognitive Ability; Picture Vocabulary, Oral Vocabulary, and Verbal Analogies. These three subtests have been translated from English into eighteen languages. The languages available in BVAT are Arabic, Chinese Simplified, Chinese, Traditional, French, German, Haitian-Creole, Hindi, Hmong, Italian, Japanese, Korean, Navajo, Polish, Portuguese, Russian, Spanish, Turkish, Vietnamese	Riverside Publishing Company 425 Spring Lake Dr. Itasca, IL 60143
Bilingual Vocabulary Assessment Measure (L. Mattes) (Available in Spanish, French, Italian, Chinese, Vietnamese)	Initial screening for expressive vocabulary.	Academic Communication Associates PO Box 566249 Oceanside, CA 92056
Black English Scoring System (N. Nelson)	Speech sample analysis for AAVE speakers; an adaptation of the Developmental Sentence Scoring procedure.	Nelson, N. (1998). In Appendix C of *Child language disorders in context.* Columbus, OH: Merrill Publishers
Boehm Test of Basic Concepts-3 (A. Boehm)	Designed to measure children's mastery of basic concept vocabulary. The test manual and instruments are available in Spanish.	Harcourt Assessment 19500 Bulverde Rd. San Antonio, TX 78259
Bracken Basic Concept Scale-Revised (B. Bracken) (Available in Spanish)	Assess 258 basic concepts including color, quantity, shapes. Spanish version for criterion-referenced use only.	Harcourt Assessment 19500 Bulverde Rd. San Antonio, TX 78259
Bracken School Readiness Assessment (B. Bracken)	Assesses the following concepts in children 2; 6-7; 11 years: Colors, Letters, Numbers/Counting, Sizes, Comparisons, and Shapes. National norms are provided for English only, but Spanish norms can be developed for local Spanish-speaking population. Includes information on how to develop local norms based on your school or area population to be more reflective of your clients.	Harcourt Assessment 19500 Bulverde Rd. San Antonio, TX 78259
Brigance Diagnostic Assessment of Basic Skills, Spanish Edition (Brigance)	Constructed using the comprehensive *Inventory of Basic Skills* (not a direct translation).	Curriculum Associates 153 Rangeway Rd. North Billerica, MA 01862
Brigance Diagnostic Assessment of Basic Skills, Portuguese Edition (H. Groomsman)	Adaptation of the Brigance Test.	Dr. Herbert Groomsman, Director of the Bilingual/ Multicultural Special Education Programs Division of Special Education and Rehabilitation Services San Jose State University San Jose, CA 95192

Name	**Description**	**Available from**
Chinese Oral Proficiency Test	Test of oral comprehension and word association in Chinese and English for children in grades K-6.	The National Hispanic University 255 East 14th St. Oakland, CA 94606
Chinese Test, Chinese Literature and Cultural Test, Chinese Bilingual Test (A. Metcalf)	Test and materials for use with speakers of Chinese.	Chinese Bilingual Project San Francisco Unified School District San Francisco, CA 94102
Clinical Evaluation of Language Fundamentals-4 (E. Semel, E. Wiig, and W. Secord) (Available in Spanish)	Uses a range of subtests to assess school-related academic skills.	Harcourt Assessment 19500 Bulverde Rd. San Antonio, TX 78259
Compton Speech and Language Screening Evaluation: Spanish Adaptation of Revised Edition (A. Compton and M. Kline)	Measure of speech and language in Spanish-speaking children, ages 3-6 years.	Carousel House PO Box 4480 San Francisco, CA 94101
Denver Developmental Screening Test II-Spanish (W. Frankenburg et al.)	Determines whether a child's development is within normal range. Identifies children ages 1 mo to 6 years likely to have motor, social, and/or language delays.	Denver Developmental Materials PO Box 371075 Denver, CO 80237
Developing Skills Checklist (DSC) (C.K. Tanner) (Available in Spanish)	Comprehensive checklist that evaluates a wide range of skills in children in pre-K and kindergarten. Measures language, mathematical concepts and operations, fine- and gross-motor skills, visual memory, auditory skills, printing, and writing.	CTB/McGraw-Hill PO Box 150 Monterey, CA 93942
Developmental Assessment of Spanish Grammar (A. Toronto)	A language-analysis procedure for Spanish-speaking children; an adaptation from the Developmental Sentence Scoring procedure in English.	In Toronto, A.S. (1976). Developmental assessment of Spanish grammar. *Journal of Speech and Hearing Disorders, 41,* 150-171.
Developmental Indicators for the Assessment of Learning-3 (DIAL-3) (C. Mardell-Czudnowski and D. Goldenberg) (Available in Spanish)	Screens development in motor, concept, language, self-help, and social function areas. Identifies children ages 3-7 years who are likely to need special services.	American Guidance Service 4201 Woodland Rd. Circle Pines, MN 55014
Developmental Programming for Infants and Young Children (D. Schafer, M. Moersch, and D. D'Eugenio) (Available in Spanish)	Assesses function and facilitates development of children, ages birth to 6 years, in six areas: perceptual/fine motor, cognition, language, social/emotional, self-care, and gross motor.	University of Michigan Press PO Box 1104 Ann Arbor, MI 48106
Diagnostic Evaluation of Language Variation (DELV-Criterion Referenced) (H.N. Seymour, T.W. Roeper, and J. de Villiers)	Assesses comprehensive speech and language, including pragmatics, syntax, semantics, and phonology in 4- to 9-year-olds. Helps distinguish language differences from language disorders. Criterion referenced scoring.	Harcourt Assessment 19500 Bulverde Rd. San Antonio, TX 78259
Dos Amigos Verbal Language Scale (D. Critchlow)	Assesses language functioning in English and Spanish students between the ages of 5-13 years.	United Educational Service Box 605 East Aurora, NY 14052

Name	Description	Available from
El CIRCO Assessment Series	Assesses comprehension of mathematical concepts and basic linguistic structures in Spanish and English. Also screens facility in Spanish before administration. Developed for Spanish-speaking children from Mexican-American, Puerto Rican, and Cuban backgrounds.	CTB/McGraw-Hill Del Monte Research Park Monterey, CA 93940
Evaluating Communicative Competence (C. Simon) (Available in French-Canadian)	Ages 10 years and older. Uses a series of 21 receptive and expressive language tasks to document a profile of functional communication proficiency.	Thinking Publications 424 Galloway St. Eau Claire, WI 54703
Expressive One-Word Picture Vocabulary Test—Spanish-Bilingual Edition (R. Brownell, Ed.)	Offers an assessment of expressive vocabularies of individuals who are bilingual in Spanish and English. By permitting examinees to respond in both languages, this test assesses total acquired vocabulary. The test is co-normed on a national sample of Spanish-bilingual individuals ages 4-0 through 12-11. Record forms include acceptable responses and stimulus words in both languages.	Academic Therapy Publications 20 Commercial Blvd. Novato, CA 94949
IPT 2004 Language Proficiency Tests	Grades pre-K through 12, available in English and Spanish. Assesses oral, reading, and writing proficiency. Scoring software available.	Ballard and Tighe, Publishers PO Box 219 Brea, CA 92821-0219
Language Assessment Scales-Oral (LASA-O) (S. Duncan and E. deAvila)	Assesses oral language proficiency in English and Spanish. Available at three levels: Pre-LAS for preschoolers, LAS I for grades K-5, and LAS II for grades 6-12.	CTB/McGraw-Hill Del Monte Research Park Monterey, CA 93940
Lindamood Auditory Conceptualization Test-Spanish Version (C. Lindamood and P.C. Lindamood)	Criterion-referenced test that measures phonological awareness and segmentation skills. Examiner's cue sheet for testing Spanish-speaking subjects.	DLM Teaching Resources 1 DLM Park Allen, TX 75002
Logramos (Riverside Publishing)	Assesses reading, language, and math in K through 12th grades. Standardized test designed to measure the academic progress of Spanish–speaking students. Depending on grade level, can require up to 8 subtests to be administered.	Riverside Publishing Company 425 Spring Lake Dr. Itasca, IL 60143
Look Listen and Tell: A Language Screening Instrument for Indian Children	Language screening device for Native American children ages 3-7 years. Can be used by child-care workers without training in speech-language pathology. It is not standardized.	Southwest Communication Resources, Inc. PO Box 788 Bernalillo, NM 87004
MacArthur Inventarios del Desarrollo de Habilidades Comunicativas (Inventarios) (Translated and adapted by D. Jackson-Maldonado, E. Bates, and D. Thal)	Assesses expressive and receptive vocabulary sizes and early grammatical production in infants 8 to 30 months. Parent-report instrument. Reports good validity when compared with direct observation measures. The CDIs (English version of instrument) were normed on approximately 1,800 children in three locations, and the Inventarios were normed on more than 2,000 children.	Brookes Publishing PO Box 10624 Baltimore, MD 21285
Medida de Sintaxis Bilingue, I and II (Bilingual Syntax Measure, I and II) (M. Burt, H. Dulay, and E. Chavez)	Uses pictures and questions to elicit language samples to be analyzed for proficiency levels in English and Spanish. BSM is available at two levels: BSM I for grades K-2, BSM II for grades 3-12.	Harcourt Assessment 19500 Bulverde Rd. San Antonio, TX 78259

Name	Description	Available from
Medida Espanola de Articulacion (Spanish Articulation Measure) (M. Aldrich-Mason, B. Figueroa-Smith, and M. Martinez-Hinshaw)	Assesses early development of phonemes in Spanish.	Martha Lerma San Ysidro School District 4350 Otay Mesa Rd. San Ysidro, CA 92073
Multicultural Vocabulary Test (G. Trudeau)	Tests expressive vocabulary of body parts in any language. Yields age equivalents 3-13 years.	Los Amigos Research Associates 7035 Galewood, Suite D San Diego, CA 92120
PAL Oral Language Dominance Measure (R. Apodaca)	Picture descriptions yield information for determining oral language proficiency in English or Spanish.	Susie Snyder El Paso Public Schools PO Box 2100 El Paso, TX 79998
Preschool Language Assessment Instrument: The Language of Learning in Practice-Spanish Language Edition (M. Blank, S. Rose, and L. Berlin)	Assesses 3- to 6-year-olds' ability to name, imitate, sequence, match, define, predict, remember, and describe. Provides information on how children handle language demands of the classroom and how to effect appropriate programming.	The Speech Bin 213 Clarksville Rd. PO Box 218 Princeton Junction, NJ 08550-0218
Preschool Language Scale (PLS-3) (I. Zimmerman, V. Steiner, and R. Pond) (Available in Spanish)	Diagnostic measure of receptive and expressive language. Subtests measure grammar, vocabulary, memory, attention span, temporal and spatial relations, and self-image. Record forms are available in English and Spanish (Mexican-American).	Order Service Center The Psychological Corporation PO Box 9954 San Antonio, TX 78204
Prueda Del Desarrollo Initial Del Lenguaje (W. Hresko, D. Reid, and D. Hammill) (Tests speakers of Spanish)	Measures spoken language, expressive and receptive syntax, and semantics in Spanish.	Pro-Ed, Inc. 8700 Shoal Creek Blvd. Austin, TX 78757-6897
Receptive One-Word Picture Vocabulary Test-Spanish-Bilingual Edition (R. Brownell, Ed.)	Offers an assessment of receptive vocabularies of individuals who are bilingual in Spanish and English. By permitting examinees to respond in both languages, this test assesses total acquired vocabulary. The test is co-normed on a national sample of Spanish-bilingual individuals ages 4-0 through 12-11. Record forms include acceptable responses and stimulus words in both languages.	Academic Therapy Publications 20 Commercial Blvd. Novato, CA 94949
Scales of Independent Behavior-Revised (SIB-R) (R. Buininks, R. Woodcock, R. Weatherman, and B. Hill) (Available in Spanish)	Assesses four adaptive behavior clusters: motor skills, social and communication skills, personal living skills, and community living skills. Ages birth to adult.	Riverside Publishing Company 425 Spring Lake Dr. Itasca, IL 60143
Screening Kit of Language Development (SKOLD) (L. Bliss and D. Allen)	Assesses preschool language development and aids in early identification of language disorders/delays in speakers of Standard English and AAVE.	Slosson Educational Publications PO Box 280 East Aurora, NY 14052
Screening Test of Spanish Grammar (A. Toronto)	Used to identify Spanish-speaking children with grammatical difficulties who need further evaluation.	Northwestern University Press 1735 Benson Ave. Evanston, IL 60201
Spanish Articulation Measures-Revised Edition (L. Mettes)	A criterion-referenced measure using spontaneous and elicited tasks to assess speech sound production and use of phonological processes. For school-age Spanish-speaking children.	Academic Communication Associates Publications Division Department 2C PO Box 6044 Oceanside, CA 92056

Name	Description	Available from
Spanish Assessment of Basic Education, Second Edition (SABE-2) (CTB Macmillan/ McGraw Hill)	Grades 1-8. Norm-referenced measure of Word Attack, Vocabulary, Reading Comprehension, Mechanics, Expression, Mathematics Computation, Mathematics Concepts and Applications, Total Reading, Total Mathematics, Total Battery, Spelling, Study Skills.	CTB Macmillan/McGraw-Hill 2500 Garden Rd. Monterey, CA 93940
Spanish Language Assessment Procedures: A Communication Skills Inventory-Third Edition (Revised) (L. Mattes)	Criterion-referenced measures for assessing vocabulary development, speech sound production, sentence structure, listening, pragmatics, and other aspects of a child's communication.	Academic Communication Associates Publications Division Department 2C PO Box 6044 Oceanside, CA 92056
Spanish Oral Language Screening Instrument	A screening instrument for examining language skills in Spanish-speaking children; grades K-6.	The National Hispanic University 255 E. 14th St. Oakland, CA 94606
Spanish Test for Assessing Morphologic Production (STAMP) (T. Nugent, K. Shipley, and D. Provencio)	Assesses production of plurals, verb endings, and other structures as children complete sentences related to the action in pictures. Ages 5-11 years.	Academic Communication Associates PO Box 566249 Oceanside, CA 92056
Spotting Language Problems: Pragmatic Criteria for Language Screening (J. Damico and J. Oller)	A language-screening instrument with a pragmatic focus; for use with English-speaking, bilingual, or LEP children. In-service training suggestions for teachers also are provided.	Los Amigos Research Associates 7035 Galewood, Suite D San Diego, CA 92120
Structured Photographic Expressive Language Test-II and P (E. Werner and J. Krescheck) (Available in Spanish)	Test of expressive language for Standard English or AAVE speakers. Available for preschoolers or elementary age children. Spanish version also available.	Janelle Publications PO Box 12 Sandwich, IL 60548
Test de Vocabulario en Imagenes Peabody (L. Dunn, D. Lugo, E. Padilla, and L. Dunn)	Contains items from PPVT-R, selected for universality and appropriateness is Spanish.	American Guidance Service 4201 Woodland Rd. Circle Pines, MN 55014
Test for Auditory Comprehension of Language: English and Spanish Forms-3 (E. Carrow-Woolfolk)	Designed for use with children 3-6 years to measure receptive language in English or Spanish.	Pro-Ed, Inc. 8700 Shoal Creek Blvd. Austin, TX 78757-6897
Test of Auditory Perceptual Skills-Revised (TAPS-R) (M. Gardner) (Available in Spanish)	Used with children who have diagnoses of auditory perceptual difficulties, imperceptions of auditory modality, language problems, and/or learning problems.	Academic Therapy Publications 20 Commercial Blvd. Novato, CA 94949
Test of Auditory Reasoning and Processing Skills (TARPS) (M. Gardner) (Available in Spanish)	Age range 5-14 years. Assesses ability to think, understand, reason, and make sense of what a child hears. Evaluates how children understand, interpret (process), draw conclusions, and make inferences from auditory information.	Slosson Educational Publications PO Box 280 East Aurora, NY 14052
Test of Phonological Awareness in Spanish (TPAS) (C.A. Riccio, B. Imhoff, J. E. Hasbrouck, and G.N. Davis)	Measures phonological awareness skills in Spanish-speaking children ages 4-10; 11 years. Normed on over 1000 Spanish-speaking children. Internal consistency reliabilities from 0.87 to 0.98, test-retest reliability for composite scores are above 0.80.	Pro-Ed, Inc. 8700 Shoal Creek Blvd. Austin, TX 78757-6897

Name	Description	Available from
Vineland Adaptive Behavior Scales-II (S. Sparrow, D. Balla, and D. Cicchetti) (Available in Spanish—interview forms and reports to parents/caregivers only)	Assesses performance of daily activities required for personal and social self-sufficiency. Ages birth-90 years.	American Guidance Service 4201 Woodland Rd. Circle Pines, MN 55014
Woodcock-Munoz Language Survey-Revised (R. Woodcock and A. Muñoz-Sandmal) (Available in Spanish)	Measures cognitive, academic, and language proficiency. Assesses picture vocabulary, verbal analogies, letter-word identification, and dictation as measures of oral language, reading, and writing domains.	Riverside Publishing Company 425 Spring Lake Dr. Itasca, IL 60143
Woodcock Language Proficiency Battery-Revised (R. Woodcock) (English and Spanish forms available)	Measure of oral and written language skills, receptive and expressive semantics.	Riverside Publishing Company 425 Spring Lake Dr. Itasca, IL 60143
Zuni Articulation Test	Alphabet book adapted for use as a stimulus for articulation testing. Picture and word stimuli for sounds in initial and medial positions are provided. Several pictures are presented for each sound. Training in test administration procedures is required.	Zuni Public School District Speech and Language Therapy Program PO Box Drawer A Zuni, NM 87327
Zuni Language Screening Instrument	Assesses language proficiency in the Zuni language for children in grades K-12. Both receptive and expressive language are measured, and a language sample can be obtained. Instructions have been taped in Zuni; age-appropriate language samples obtained from the test's picture sequence stories are provided for comparison with assessment data collected. Training is required in test administration procedures.	Zuni Public School District Speech and Language Therapy Program PO Box Drawer A Zuni, NM 87327

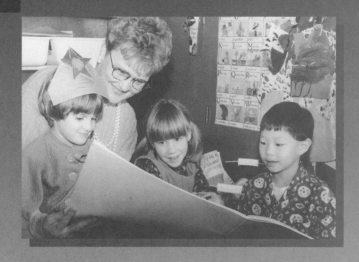

FROM BIRTH TO
BROWN'S STAGE V

ASSESSMENT AND INTERVENTION IN THE PRELINGUISTIC PERIOD

CHAPTER

6

CHAPTER OBJECTIVES

Readers of this chapter will be able to do the following:
- Discuss the principles of family-centered practice for infants and newborns.
- Describe the elements required for service plans for prelinguistic clients.
- List risk factors for communication disorders in infants.
- Discuss the principles of assessment and intervention for high-risk infants and their families in the newborn intensive care nursery.

- Describe methods for assessment and intervention for preintentional infants and their families: 1 to 8 months.
- Describe assessment and intervention for infants at prelinguistic stages of communication: 9 to 18 months.
- Discuss the issues relevant to communication programming for older prelinguistic clients.

Janice was born with Down syndrome (DS) 8 weeks before her due date. She weighed less than 4 pounds and had to spend 1 month in the hospital before she was able to go home. She developed respiratory distress syndrome and needed to be intubated and placed on a ventilator for 2 weeks. Her mother had to travel back and forth every day from her home outside the city to visit her, and she had to find someone to care for her other two preschoolers each time. She had arranged for a 6-week maternity leave at her job; as the end of the leave grew nearer, she became more and more worried that she would lose her position if she couldn't go back on time. She was able to get another 6 weeks to allow her to get the baby settled at home, but she didn't see how she could manage to go back to work even then. Janice's father worked in a glass factory and was working double shifts to keep up with the family's co-pays on the doctor bills. He hardly saw Janice when she was in the hospital.

When she came home, Janice weighed just 5 pounds. The tube had been removed and she was able to breathe without a ventilator, but she seemed so tiny and fragile and had been so sick that her mother was frightened to be away from the medical setting, even though she was glad to be able to stop running back and forth between there and home. Janice had trouble sucking; feeding her took close to 1 hour, and even so she needed a bottle every 3 hours or so. Her mother was frazzled with trying to get enough milk into Janice to keep her growing and still pay some attention to the other two children. She found she was hardly doing

anything with Janice but giving her bottles and trying desperately to get other things done in the short time she had between feedings. And always in the back of her mind was the question: Janice was going to be retarded—how could this have happened? Could she love a child who was so different? How would she and her family manage to raise a handicapped child? Would she grow like the other children and learn to walk and talk and play? Her husband was anxious about the expenses at the hospital and resentful that Janice's mother was so exhausted that she could barely talk to him the few hours a day he was home, let alone cook a meal or get the laundry done.

FAMILY-CENTERED PRACTICE

Janice is one kind of baby who is at risk for language and communication disorders. There are many kinds of risk; what they have in common is their impact, not only on the infant but also on the family. The burden of caring for and fostering the development of infants at risk for communication disorders falls on their families, who may already be experiencing a great deal of stress. Even caring for a healthy newborn is hard work. Imagine how much harder that work becomes when it is done in the context of constant anxiety about the infant's well-being and future. When we deal with infants at risk for communication disorders we are dealing with the family in which the infant finds a home. Although this is true for every client we see, it is especially true for the very youngest of our charges, who depend on the adults in their environment for every aspect of their existence. When thinking about the needs of the high-risk infant, we need to think about the needs of the family, too, to provide that infant with the best environment for growth and development. A variety of resources are available to help clinicians develop family-centered practice skills. Crais (1991) and Bruns and Steeples (2001), for example, made some suggestions for strategies to be used in family-centered practice. These strategies are summarized in Table 6-1. Additional resources include Andrews and Andrews (1990), Crais and Calculator (1998), Dinnebeil and Hale (2003), Donahue-Kilburg (1992), and McWilliams (1992).

TABLE 6-1	Developing Family-Centered Clinical Practice		
SITUATION	**GUIDELINES FOR PRACTICE**	**INTENDED OUTCOMES**	**COMMUNICATION STRATEGIES**
First encounter with family	1. Allow and encourage family members to describe interests before describing services. 2. Provide choices and allow family to make decisions. 3. Avoid being too nosy. 4. Let family know what information you have received from other professionals and ask whether they feel it is accurate and unbiased. 5. Reaffirm confidentiality. 6. Respond quickly and don't push families off until "later."	1. To convey to families that you respect them 2. To offer immediate assistance if it is wanted (information, resources, emotional support, services, skills) 3. To give family members control over entry into services (decision making, choices) 4. To let family members know who you are and what you do (e.g., philosophy, qualifications, services) 5. To understand the family's major areas of concern and priorities	1. How are things going with (client)?
Gathering client and family data	1. Requires continuous opportunities for gathering, exchanging, and interpreting information. 2. Families should have the opportunity to be present for all discussion. 3. It should be convenient for the family to participate. 4. The language used in communicating with families should be readily understood (e.g., jargon-free, using the family's own words).	1. To identify what families hope to achieve through involvement with you and your agency 2. To determine how families define the issues related to the client's handicapping condition within the context of their family values, structures, and daily routines 3. To establish yourself as a family ally	1. What have you been told about (client's name) (hearing, vision, motor skills, etc., using words of family members)? 2. How does this fit with what you know and believe about (client's name)? 3. What else do you know about (client's identified disability)? 4. In what ways has this information been helpful? Or not helpful?
Involving family in assessment process	1. Assessment should be shaped by family priorities and information needs. 2. Assessment should meet the needs of the family rather than the needs of the program or staff. 3. Preferences for family involvement should be identified and honored.	1. To request and use information provided by family members to understand the client's abilities and plan intervention 2. To promote the building of consensus about the nature of the presenting client and family needs 3. To underscore the client's and family's abilities and potential	1. For what areas do you need or want more information concerning (client's name)? 2. What kinds of information would be most useful to you regarding (client)? 3. Where and what would be the best place and time to assess (client)? 4. Are there other people who you might like to be involved in the assessment? 5. How have you been involved in assessment activities previously? 6. Was that type and level of participation satisfactory to you?

TABLE 6-1	Developing Family-Centered Clinical Practice—cont'd		
SITUATION	**GUIDELINES FOR PRACTICE**	**INTENDED OUTCOMES**	**COMMUNICATION STRATEGIES**
			7. Are there additional ways you would like to be involved?
			8. If so, which activities would you like to be a part of (e.g., stay with client, sit outside and observe, fill out checklist or survey, perform actual testing)?
Reporting assessment information to family	1. Assessment information should be shared at a time and place that are suitable for family members.	1. To promote the building of consensus on the nature of the needs of the client and family and the need for treatment	1. Where and when would you like the assessment information shared?
	2. Families should decide who will be present and how the information will be shared.	2. To provide family members with information about the client so that they may be able to make informed decisions regarding further assessment and intervention	2. Who would you like to be present when the information is shared?
	3. Families should decide what type of assessment information will be helpful to them.	3. To promote and support family decision making regarding further assessment and/or intervention	3. What part in the information sharing would you like to take?
	4. Families should determine when intervention planning will take place.	4. To promote the building of consensus on the course of action that follows	4. How would you like the information to be shared (e.g., face to face, in writing, in detail, just in an overview, citing age levels)?
			5. If face-to-face interaction, whom would you like to go first in presenting information?
			6. Are there particular topics you would like discussed first?
			7. What would you like to take place after the information sharing (e.g., talk about future plans, wait and talk later, follow-up call)?
			8. How did you feel about the assessment activities performed with (client)?
			9. Do you think that what we saw today was typical of (client)? If not, what kinds of differences did you observe and how are things typically?
			10. Were there any areas that we did not assess that you feel would be helpful to assess?
			11. What did you think overall of (client's) interactions with the assessors?
			12. Were there things that happened today that surprised you? If so, what?
			13. How do you feel about the assessment results?
			14. What would you like the next step to be?
Planning intervention program with the family	1. Parents should have the opportunity to be involved in all planning meetings related to the client and family.	1. To identify priorities and to promote solution development with families related to their priorities	1. If you were to focus your energies on one thing for (client's name), what would it be?
	2. Intervention plans should be designed to fit within the family's daily routine.	2. To support family decisions	2. If you could change one thing about (event of importance), what would that be?

TABLE 6-1	Developing Family-Centered Clinical Practice—cont'd		
SITUATION	GUIDELINES FOR PRACTICE	INTENDED OUTCOMES	COMMUNICATION STRATEGIES
	3. Families should be the ultimate decision makers regarding intervention planning; individualize practices to match parent needs and preferences. 4. The written plan should be easy for families to understand and use, and flexible enough to allow ongoing changes.		3. Imagining 6 months down the road, what would you like to be different in terms of (event or area of importance)? Are there some things that you would like to be the same? 4. What would you like to accomplish in 6 weeks? 6 months? 5. What are some ways of getting to where you want to go? Who would need to be involved in accomplishing what you want to do? 6. What would each of you need to do to accomplish what you want? 7. How will you know when you've done what you want to do? 8. How will you know when (client's name) has made progress in the ways you described? 9. How long do you think it will take to get to where you want to go?
Throughout all contacts	1. Support, trust, and respect parents. 2. Use a strengths-based approach. 3. Understand and accept parents' perceptions and experiences. 4. Coordinate professional team.	1. To maximize receptiveness and effective bonds 2. To support parents' perceptions of child 3. To overcome past negative experiences and form partnerships with professionals 4. To avoid confusing or overwhelming families	

Adapted from Crais, E. (1991). *A practical guide to embedding family-centered content into existing speech-language pathology coursework.* Chapel Hill, NC: University of North Carolina; and Bruns, D., & Steeples, T. (2001). Partners from the beginning: Guidelines for encouraging partnerships between parents and NICU and EI professionals. *Infant-Toddler Intervention, 11,* 237-247.

SERVICE PLANS FOR PRELINGUISTIC CLIENTS

Recent changes in federal policy have helped to move clinicians in the direction of family-centered practice. Public Law 99-457, part of the Education of the Handicapped Act Amendments of 1986 (Part H), was the landmark legislation that established a discretionary program to help states set up early identification and intervention services for infants, toddlers, and their families. These were incorporated into the 1997 reauthorization of the Individuals with Disabilities Education Act (IDEA; PL 105-17) and into the 2004 reauthorization. This legislation establishes the requirement for an Individual Family Service Plan (IFSP) for children in the birth-to-3 age range that must include services needed not only to maximize the development of the child but also to optimize the family's capacity to address the

child's special needs. The IFSP is similar to an Individual Education Program for a school-aged child, but instead of focusing on the child alone, the IFSP focuses on the child within the context of the family. In addition, the IFSP is a plan for comprehensive services to support the child's development in the context of the family; the IEP is focused exclusively on educational programming. The IFSP should include information about the family's resources, priorities, and concerns for the child's development. The plan, then, also may include some services for the family, such as skilled child care to provide respite for them, or other social services that the family feels are necessary to help them cope with the stress of raising a handicapped child.

The elements that are required by law to be included within an IFSP, according to the 2004 reauthorization of IDEA, include the following:

1. Information about the child's present level of physical, cognitive, social, emotional, communicative, and adaptive development, based on objective criteria.
2. A statement of the family's resources, priorities, and concerns related to enhancing the development of the child, with the concurrence of the family.
3. A statement of the major outcomes expected to be achieved for the child and family, and the criteria, procedures, and timelines used to determine progress and whether modifications or revisions of the outcomes or services are necessary.
4. A statement of the specific early intervention services necessary to meet the needs of the child and the family to achieve the specified outcomes including (1) the frequency, intensity, and method of delivering the services and (2) the environments in which early intervention services will be provided and a justification of the extent, if any, to which the services will not be provided in a natural environment, the location of the services, and the payment arrangements, if any.
5. A list of other services such as (1) medical and other services that the child needs and (2) the funding sources to be used in paying for those services or the steps that will be taken to secure those services through public or private sources.
6. Projected dates for initiation of the services as soon as possible after the IFSP meeting and anticipated duration of those services.
7. The name and discipline of the service coordinator who will be responsible for the implementation of the IFSP and coordination with other agencies and persons.
8. A plan for transition to preschool services.

Johnson, McGonigel, and Kaufmann (1989) and Nelson and Hyter (2001) provided guidelines for developing IFSPs. They reported that no official form or format has been approved for these plans in order to give teams the freedom to develop whatever works best for an individual family. Some teams use only handwritten IFSPs to allow for immediate recording and to keep them dynamic and easy to revise. Other teams create model formats that can be adapted to individual families by the team members. An example of one possible format for an IFSP appears in Appendix 6-1.

For some infants who are identified at birth as high risk, an IFSP may be implemented very soon after the baby leaves the hospital. For others, a decision may be made to wait and watch the child's development before instituting a plan. The decision to provide services also depends on the particular family and the team of professionals with whom they work. A single, teenage, drug-abusing mother living in poverty may herself feel, and be considered by the team of professionals, to be in need of supportive services for her premature infant when she leaves the hospital for the first time. On the other hand, a middle-class married woman in her 20s, with a mother living nearby who has offered to help, may be able to cope on her own for a time, as long as follow-up assessment is provided to ensure that the infant is developing.

Other children in the prelinguistic stage of development may be identified some time after birth. Some will be discovered through Child Find and other screening programs. Child Find programs are mandated by the IDEA and are targeted at early identification of children with special needs who might not otherwise come to the attention of agencies who could serve them. These children may have conditions that are not identified at birth, nonspecific forms of mental retardation that have no obvious physical signs, or autism that does not become apparent until later in infancy when communication skills emerge in normal development. As Nelson (1998) pointed out, finding these children is not as easy as it sounds; even many professionals are unaware of the need for and appropriateness of intervention in this very early part of life. Public education of both parents and professionals is an important component of Child Find efforts, to increase the likelihood that children will be referred for diagnostic services. Multiple observations are often needed to establish special needs in early development, since infant behavior changes so dramatically during the first year of life.

Other children functioning at prelinguistic levels of development are those with severe to profound handicaps, who will be considerably older than the at-risk infants whom we've been discussing. These clients may have been identified at birth or early in life and may have received intervention for some time. They will, though, continue to have needs related to the development of basic preverbal communication skills. We'll talk about services for these clients in the last section of this chapter.

Many of the instruments used for screening and diagnostic assessment in the prelinguistic period are listed in Table 6-2. Using instruments with strong psychometric properties is just as important in early assessment as it is for any client, for all the reasons we talked about in Chapter 2. Clinicians choosing assessment instruments for prelinguistic children should apply all the same psychometric standards in making this judgment that would be used in selecting tests for older children. Similarly, we will always need to supplement standardized instruments with more flexible and ecologically valid measures. Crais (1995) and American Speech-Language-Hearing Association (ASHA) (2005) discussed the importance of including caregivers as significant partners in the assessment and using culturally sensitive procedures and naturalistic observations of play and other daily routines within the assessment process. These measures, which go beyond traditional instruments, will always contribute important information to the data that we collect.

When providing services to high-risk infants and their families, the language pathologist will be an integral part of the team of professionals developing the IFSP. Language disorders are the most common developmental problem that presents in the preschool period (Rossetti, 2001), so any infant at risk for a developmental disorder in general is at risk for language deficits in particular. These babies do not have communication disorders yet; work with high-risk infants and their families is a preventive form of intervention. We've talked about primary and secondary prevention as important aspects of the role of the speech-language pathologist (SLP). When

TABLE 6-2	Tools for Assessing Infant Development

SCALE	AREAS ASSESSED	COMMENT
Ages and Stages Questionnaires (ASQ): A Parent-Completed Child-Monitoring System (ed. 2) (Bricker & Squires, 1999)	4-60 mo. Developmental questionnaires sent to parents of at-risk children. Areas screened include gross and fine motor control, communication, personal-social, and problem solving.	Involves parents in the assessment process. Questions available in Spanish, French, and Korean.
Albert Einstein Scales (Escalona & Corman, 1966)	Tactile exploration activities not readily available in other scales	Provides a qualitative assessment of behaviors.
Assessing Linguistic Behavior (ALB) (Olswang, Stoel-Gammon, Coggins, & Carpenter, 1987)	Birth to 2 yr; observational scales to assess the performance of cognitive antecedents, play, communicative intention, language production and comprehension.	Provides a developmental level comparison and detailed instructions for administering assessments.
Assessment in Infancy: Ordinal Scales of Infant Psychological Development (Uzgiris & Hunt, 1989)	Follows Piagetian sequences to measure infant development in communicative and social domains.	Used during the sensorimotor period of development; helpful in the development of functional, generative, instructional objectives; useful as a tool to explain the child's level of achievement across developmental domains to parents.
Assessment, Evaluation, and Programming System (AEPS): *For Infants and Children* (ed. 2) (Bricker, 2002)	B–6 yr. Assessment and evaluation of fine and gross motor movements and adaptive, cognitive, and social communication.	Criterion-referenced assessment and evaluation; also includes a Family Report Measure for parents to assess their child.
Battelle Developmental Inventory (ed. 2) (Newborg, Stock, Wnek, Guidubaldi, & Svinicki, 2004)	B–8 yr. Cognitive, perceptual, discrimination, memory, reasoning, academic, conceptual behaviors; personal-social, motor, communication, and adaptive.	Specific adaptations for specific handicapping conditions; very comprehensive standardization data for normally developing children; provisions for testing directly, by observation, and by interview; sparse number of items provided for each age range; a good screening tool.
Bayley Scales of Infant Development (ed. 3) (Bayley, 2005)	Sensorimotor skills; cognitive, psychomotor, social, visual, and auditory. Motor scale can be administered separately.	Used with handicapped infants and children; excellent standardization properties; measures a large number of behaviors; some items may be scored based on observations, omissions, refusals, and caregiver reports; not appropriate for children with moderate to severe sensory and motor deficits; most appropriate with children who exhibit mild cognitive delays or mild sensory communication impairments.
Birth to Three Checklist of Language and Learning Behaviors (BTC-3) (Ammer, 1999)	A criterion-referenced tool that measures five categories of early skill acquisition, including language comprehension, language expression, avenues to learning, social behaviors.	Results yield IFSP for the family and child.
The Brigance Infant and Toddler Screen (Brigance & Glascoe, 2002)	B-23 mo. Fine motor, receptive language, expressive language, gross motor, self-help, and social-emotional.	Parent report and direct elicitation versions. Spanish direction booklets available.
Carolina Curriculum for Infants and Toddlers with Special Needs (ed. 3) (Johnson-Martin, Attermeier, & Hacker, 2004)	B-24 mo. Cognition, language, self-help, fine motor, gross motor; includes daily routine integration strategies.	Criterion-referenced procedure for developing intervention targets.
Casati-Lezine Scales (Casati & Lezine, 1968)	Searching for hidden objects; use of intermediaries, exploration of objects, and the combination of objects	Offers additional Piagetian items not included on the Dunst scales.

TABLE 6-2	Tools for Assessing Infant Development—cont'd	
SCALE	**AREAS ASSESSED**	**COMMENT**
Denver Developmental Screening Test (DDST-II) (Frankenburg et al., 1990)	Assesses four developmental areas: personal-social development, fine motor–adaptive development, language development, gross motor development.	Determines whether a child, ages birth to 6 yr, performs within normal range on various tasks in the areas of personal-social, fine motor–adaptive, language, and gross motor skills; identifies whether a child is likely to have delays in any of those areas.
Developmental Assessment of Young Children (DAYC) (Voress & Maddox, 1999)	Communication, cognition, social-emotional development, physical development, adaptive behavior	Normed on 1269 children. One subtest for each of the five domains listed at left. Administration time: 10-20 min. for all 5 subtests
Developmental Assessment for Students with Severe Disabilities (DASH-2) (Dykes & Erin, 1999)	Assesses language, sensorimotor function, activities of daily living, pre-academic and social-emotional performance.	Determines developmental functioning age.
Developmental Diagnosis (Knobloch, Stevens, & Malone, 1980)	Adaptive, gross motor, fine motor, language, and personal-social behaviors	Provides examples of developmental skills.
Developmental Profile II (DP-II) (Alpern, Boll, & Shearer, 1997)	Used to evaluate a child's functioning and risk of delayed development in five key areas: physical age, self-help age, social age, academic age, and communication age.	Assesses development in the following areas respectively: muscle coordination and sequential motor skills; ability to cope independently; interpersonal abilities, emotional needs; intellectual abilities and prerequisite skills; expressive and receptive communication skills.
Developmental Programming for Infants and Young Children (Moersch & Schafer, 1981)	Assesses function and facilitates development of children in five areas: perceptual and fine motor, cognition, language, social and emotional skills, and gross motor skills.	Provides direct transition to intervention goals and programming.
Early Intervention Developmental Profile (Rogers et al., 1981)	Perceptual and fine motor, cognition, language, social-emotional, self-care, and gross motor domains	The motor scales are strengths of this scale; comprehensive developmental coverage, intended for use in a team approach; graphic profile of children's abilities; limited number of items at each age range; desirable for screening.
Early Learning Accomplishment Profile (Glover, Preminger, & Sanford, 1988)	Cognition, language, communication, adaptive behavior, social and emotional, motor skills	Criterion-referenced assessment; especially useful in educational settings.
Early Screening Profile (Harrison, Kaufman, Kaufman, Bruininks, Rynders, Ilmer, Sparrow, & Cicchetti, 1990)	Screens development in cognitive language, motor, self-help/social, articulation, health, development, and home environments.	Helps identify children at risk for learning problems.
Griffiths' Mental Developmental Scale (Griffiths, 1954)	Locomotor, personal-social, hearing and speech, eye and hand coordination and performance	Designed for use with children who have delays and deficits; contains the Abilities of Babies Subtest for assessment during the first 2 yr; includes information on performance of children with various handicaps; comparisons of client can be made to children with similar deficits; practical items relate to everyday activities; a general intelligence quotient may be derived; test administration may be limited by the many perceptual motor items that are timed; normed on a British population.

TABLE 6-2	Tools for Assessing Infant Development—cont'd	

SCALE	AREAS ASSESSED	COMMENT
Hawaii Early Learning Profile (Furuno, O'Reilly, Inatsuka, Husaka, Allmon, & Zeisloft-Falbey, 1994)	Cognitive, language, fine and gross motor, self-help, and social	Performance is rated on four levels of mastery, rather than pass-fail; provides sequential approach to a Piagetian assessment of cognition particularly during the first 2 yr; sensitive to attachment and bonding behaviors; provides a good number of behaviors to assess; readily integrates into intervention programs.
Infant Developmental Screening Scale (Proctor, 1995)	Screens for developmental delays in six domains: habituation, attention, interaction, motor, physiological movements, and reflexes.	Useful for hospital-based practice with infants.
Infant Intelligence Scale (Cattell, 1960)	Sensorimotor skills, cognitive, psychomotor, and social	Very similar to the Bayley although not as comprehensive; additional items are provided if one item is administered in error; designed to be administered by teachers and instructional personnel.
The Rossetti Infant-Toddler Language Scale (Rossetti, 1990)	Areas assessed include play, interaction, . attachment, gesture, pragmatics, language comprehension, and expression	Developed for ages birth to 3; includes parent questionnaire and test protocol to gather observed, elicited, and parent report information; also includes a vocabulary checklist for comprehension and production.
Mehrabian and Williams Scale (Mehrabian & Williams, 1971)	Denotation and representational ability, linguistic and nonverbal communication abilities, domains of denotation and representation, observing response, reciprocal assimilation, object stability, imitation, and causality	Gives level of cognitive development in months; provides assessment framework for the development of nonverbal behaviors and for the cognitive relationship between early "motor gestural" and later linguistic development.
Mullen Scales of Early Learning (Mullen, 1995)	Five brief scales that measure gross motor skills, visual-reception skills, fine motor skills, expressive and receptive language	Provides examiner with a good picture of early cognitive and motor development; for each scale there is a T-score, percentile, and an age-equivalent score.
The Portage Guide: Birth to Six (Portage Project, 2003)	General development	Set of tools for assessment and curriculum planning. One set of materials for B-3 yr. Each set of materials includes Tool for Observation and Planning (TOP) Assessment, spiral bound set of Activity and Routines Resource book corresponding to each TOP item, and User's Guide.
Schedule of Growing Skills (ed. 2) (Bellman, Lingam, & Auckett, 1996)	Assesses a range of areas for identification of normal or delayed development.	A rapid and reliable standardized assessment of child development; based on recent data from UK health surveillance.
Syracuse Dynamic Assessment for Birth to Three (SDA) (Ensher, Bobish, Gardner, Michaels, Butler, Foertsch, & Cooper, 1997)	Evaluates development of neuromotor sensation, perception, cognition, language, communication, social emotional behavior, and adaptive behavior, with priority to an integrated assessment of the whole child in the most familiar and natural contexts.	Play-based assessment of early development.
Test of Pretend Play (TOPP) (Lewis & Boucher, 1999)	Measures a child's ability to play symbolically in structured play conditions and in free play conditions.	Measures conceptual development, ability to use symbols, emotional status, and imagination and creativity.

TABLE 6-2	Tools for Assessing Infant Development—cont'd	
SCALE	**AREAS ASSESSED**	**COMMENT**
The Vulpe Assessment Battery—Revised (VAB-R) (Vulpe, 1997)	Object, body, shape, size, and space concepts; visual memory; auditory discrimination; auditory attention; comprehension; memory; cause-effect or means-ends behaviors; categorizing and combining schema	Comprehensive, process-oriented, criterion-referenced assessment that emphasizes children's functional abilities; the VAB-R provides a systematic interactive assessment/analysis of several key developmental domains to identify children who may be at risk of educational failure.
Vineland Adaptive Behavior Scales (ed. 2) (Sparrow, Balla, & Cicchetti, 2005)	Expressive and receptive communication, socialization, daily living, motor	Extremely well-standardized with norming groups containing normal and handicapped individuals. Structured interview format.

working with high-risk infants, primary and secondary prevention are the predominant goals. We hope that by working with these families to enhance the baby's communicative environment, we can ward off some of the deficits for which they may be at risk or minimize the extent of these deficits.

Many high-risk infants present with feeding problems, hearing losses, and neurological and behavioral difficulties that can influence communication development. For these reasons and to prevent later deficits, the language pathologist is very likely to be called upon to participate in the planning and delivery of services for the high-risk infant. Bear in mind that this enterprise must always be a team effort that involves professionals from a variety of disciplines and viewpoints, as well as the infant's family. The language pathologist needs to be ready to lend expertise on communication acquisition and its disorders in a collaborative spirit.

RISK FACTORS FOR COMMUNICATION DISORDERS IN INFANTS

Who are high-risk infants? Any condition that places a child's general development in jeopardy also constitutes a risk for language development. The March of Dimes (2003) estimates that 12% of newborns can be considered as high risk. In this chapter, we'll discuss some of the conditions that place an infant at risk and talk about strategies for serving at-risk infants and their families at three different developmental stages: the newborn period, the preintentional period from a developmental level of 1 to 8 months, and the period of prelinguistic communication from a developmental age of 9 to 18 months. First, let's look at some of the conditions that place an infant at risk for communication disorders.

PRENATAL FACTORS

As we've discussed, anything that could lead to a developmental disorder can constitute a risk for the development of commu-

nication in infants. Certain prenatal factors place an infant at risk. These factors include maternal consumption of excessive alcohol, which may result in fetal alcohol syndrome—a pattern of deficits including small size, developmental delay, and facial abnormalities—as well as abuse of other drugs, which often occurs in conjunction with alcohol abuse. Exposure to environmental toxins such as lead, mercury, and other heavy metals, and in utero infections such as rubella, cytomegalovirus (CMV), and toxoplasmosis also place a child at risk.

PREMATURITY

Prematurity is defined as birth prior to 37 weeks' gestation, with low birth weight. Low birth weight is defined as less than 2500 grams, or $5^1/_2$ pounds; very low birth weight (VLBW) is considered less than 1500 grams, or $3^1/_3$ pounds. Seriously premature birth and its consequent low birth weight can constitute both medical and developmental risks; low birth weights have been found to be associated with increased risk of developmental delay (Farnoff, Hack, & Walsh, 2003; Taylor, Burack, Holding, Lekine, & Hack, 2002). Premature infants are also more susceptible to a range of illnesses and conditions that produce developmental disabilities, such as respiratory distress syndrome, apnea (interrupted breathing), bradycardia (low heart rate), necrotizing enterocolitis (a serious intestinal disorder), and intracranial hemorrhage (Rais-Bahrami, Short, & Batshaw, 2002; Rossetti, 2001). Respiratory distress in premature babies can sometimes lead to the need for intubation and the use of ventilators to aid breathing, as it did in Janice's case. This can, in a minority of instances, lead to *bronchopulmonary dysplasia,* a thickening of the immature lung wall that makes oxygen exchange difficult (Rais-Bahrami, Short, & Batshaw, 2002). For children suffering from this condition, long-term tracheostomy may be necessary, which can affect both speech and language development (McGowan, Bleile, Fus, & Barnas, 1993; Woodnorth, 2004). Further, treatment of the premature child may have negative consequences, even though it is necessary to save the child's life. Newborn intensive care nurseries can be noisy and overstimulating (Aucott, Donohue, Atkins, & Allen, 2002); in the past, some infants even suffered noise-induced hearing losses (Kellman, 1982). The communicative environment also presents risks. Infants there undergo painful procedures such as suctioning and intubation, which can cause tactile defensiveness and trauma or tissue damage to the larynx (Comrie & Helm, 1997). Parents are unable to spend as much time interacting with very small newborns as do parents of larger babies, because of the infants' need for hospitalization and medical treatment. Further, the parents' perception of the baby as weak and sick may result in less willingness to hold, handle, and play with the child.

The first hurdle that the premature infant faces is to survive the premature birth. The smaller and younger the baby is at birth, the greater the chances for mortality. Survival rates for very small (1000 to 1500 grams) or very young (more than 10 weeks' preterm) babies are increasing, though, because of advances in intensive care for newborns. As recently as 1960, only about 50% of these babies survived, whereas by the mid-1990s survival rates were more than 90% (Rais-Bahrami, Short, & Batshaw, 2002). As more of these tiny babies—who would not have lived 40 years ago—mature, the rate of developmental delays seen in the population of children with a history of prematurity also may increase. Current estimates place the risk of developmental delays at 30% to 50% for all infants born prematurely (Rossetti, 2001), and, on average, full-term infants have significantly higher cognitive scores compared with children who were born preterm (Bhutta, Cleves, Casey, Cradock, & Anand, 2002). The good news is that early intervention clearly makes a difference. Bleile and Miller (1993) reported significant IQ differences between preterm infants who received intervention and those who got only routine follow-up. Rauh, Achenbach, Nurcombe, Howell, and Teti (1988) also found significant IQ differences at age 3 in low-birth-weight babies who received home visits during the first 3 months of life. Blair and Ramey (1997), in reviewing a large number of intervention studies for this population, report that low-birth-weight infants who receive intervention consistently show benefits over untreated groups in terms of IQ. Burchinal et al. (1997) validated this finding for children of low-income African-American families; Ment et al. (2003) showed that early intervention had its greatest effect on infants whose mothers had less than a high school education. These findings suggest that a relatively small investment in intervention can have important long-term effects for children who have risks associated with prematurity and low birth weight.

Genetic and Congenital Disorders

Many congenital and inherited disorders also place children at risk for developing language and cognitive deficits. Inborn errors of metabolism, such as Hurler syndrome, Hunter's syndrome, and Morquio syndrome, are one example. Craniofacial disorders, which have adverse effects on the morphology of

the auditory mechanism, as well as congenital forms of deafness, put a child at risk because information from the auditory channel is lost. A variety of chromosome abnormalities also can influence communicative development. These include DS (trisomy 21; three members of chromosome 21, instead of the normal two) and cri du chat syndrome (5p-, absence of the short arm of the fifth chromosome). Disorders of the sex (X and Y) chromosomes present with fewer physical stigmata than other genetic disorders. As a result, they are often undetected during infancy and may only be diagnosed later, when the child starts to exhibit delays. Sex chromosome disorders include Klinefelter's syndrome (usually an XXY chromosome complement in males, instead of the usual XY), Turner's syndrome (X0 in females, instead of the usual XX), and fragile X syndrome. Batshaw (2002b) provides a detailed discussion of chromosomes and hereditary disorders.

Other Risks Identified After the Newborn Period

Not all children with special needs are identified at birth. As discussed earlier, others will be identified through parent or physician referral or through Child Find efforts later in infancy. Hearing impairment is one condition that may not be identified at birth. Many, but not all, states provide newborn hearing screening. In states where screening is not available, children with hearing impairments are not identified until sometime after the newborn period. Disorders without physical stigmata, such as autism, nonspecific mental retardation, and specific language disorders, also are identified later in the prelinguistic or emerging language period. Children who experience abuse or neglect, too, are identified only after the newborn period has passed. All these children, though, have clear risks for communication development.

Any infant known or suspected to be subject to these conditions, then, would be considered at risk for communication disorders. Now that we know something about what these risk factors are, let's see what we as language pathologists can do about them.

Assessment and Intervention for High-Risk Infants and their Families in the Newborn Intensive Care Nursery

Each year approximately 250,000 infants begin life in the neonatal intensive care unit (NICU) (Bruns & Steeples, 2001). ASHA has recently outlined the roles that SLPs can play in the NICU (ASHA, 2004a). An SLP may be called in to consult on the management plan of an infant being cared for in the NICU. The language pathologist can assist in several areas in assessing and providing for the needs of these at-risk newborns. These areas include feeding and oral motor development, hearing conservation and aural habilitation, infant behavior and development, and parent-child communication.

FEEDING AND ORAL MOTOR DEVELOPMENT

Assessment

The ability to take nutrition orally is one of the criteria for discharging infants from the NICU (McGrath & Braescu, 2004). As such, promoting oral feeding is an important aspect of helping prepare the child and family for life at home. Evaluating feeding and oral motor development in the high-risk newborn involves two components: chart review and bedside feeding evaluation. Alper and Manno (1996) suggest that chart review should yield information on adjusted gestational age, excess amniotic fluid at delivery that could signal a lack of intrauterine sucking and swallowing, type and duration of intubation, respiratory disorders, and degree of family involvement.

Bedside feeding evaluation can be used to observe the infant's behavior and state during feeding, the effects of environmental stimuli on the infant's feeding behavior, vocalizations and airway noises during feeding, and reflex patterns. According to Jaffe (1989), reflexes that should be observed in the infant during feeding include the following:

1. *Suckling.* This involves a primitive form of sucking that includes extension and retraction of the tongue as well as up-and-down jaw movements and loose closure of the lips.
2. *Sucking.* This more mature pattern differs from suckling in that more intraoral negative pressure is generated, the tongue tip is elevated rather than extended and retracted, lip approximation is firmer, and jaw movement is more rhythmic.
3. *Rooting.* This reflex causes the infant to turn the head toward the source of tactile stimulation (gentle rubbing) of the lips or lower cheek.
4. *Phasic bite reflex.* When teeth or gums are stimulated, usually by placement of the bottle or nipple in the mouth, the baby exhibits a rhythmic bite-and-release pattern that can be observed as a series of small jaw openings and closings.

When looking for these reflexes in the high-risk newborn, it is important to remember that they are typically seen in full-term babies. If a seriously premature infant does not exhibit them, we should not be too surprised. The presence or absence of these reflexes, though, will both determine the need for further assessment and contribute to the development of the feeding plan for the infant.

Ziev (1999) and McGrath and Braescu (2004) provide guidelines for determining whether a baby is developmentally ready to begin nipple feeding. Using a developmental evaluation, such as Brazelton and Nugent's (1995) *Neonatal Behavioral Assessment Scale,* we can estimate developmental level and determine whether the premature infant has developed sufficiently to engage in some form of nipple feeding. Additional considerations for beginning oral feeding are presented in Box 6-1.

In addition to observational assessment, several formal procedures are available for collecting information on feeding and oral skills. These are outlined in Table 6-3; Thoyre, Shaker, and Pridham (2005) developed the *Early Feeding Skills Assessment,* a checklist for assessing infant readiness for oral feeding, which may also assist in this evaluation. Jelm (1990), Kedesdy and Budd (1998), Lowman, Murphy, and Snell (1999),

---

BOX 6-1	**Considerations for Readiness for Oral Feeding**

Gestational age: Generally at least 35-37 weeks.

Severity of medical condition: Respiratory disorders contribute to delays in readiness for oral feeding.

Respiratory/cardiovascular stability: Infants needing oxygen support, with apnea, or periodic breathing are more delayed in readiness for oral feeding.

Motoric stability: Oral tone, posture, and quality of oral movements should be evaluated.

Coordination of sucking, swallowing, and breathing: Mature suck consists of ten or more sucking bursts with breathing interspersed with suck/swallow; consider evaluating in non-nutritive sucking.

Behavioral state organization: Infant must be able to maintain an alert state long enough to complete feeding.

Demonstration of hunger: Exhibits rooting, may exhibit non-nutritive sucking, crying may be weak.

Adapted from McGrath, J., & Braescu, A. (2004). State of the science. *Journal of Perinatal and Neonatal Nursing, 18,* 353-368.

Morris and Klein (2000), and Wolf and Glass (1992a) provide additional information on childhood feeding disorders. If formal assessment procedures are unavailable, informal interviews also can be used to gather data about the infant's feeding and oral skills. Box 6-2 provides some of the questions that could be asked in an informal interview.

Children with disabilities or those with tracheostomies often experience *gastroesophageal reflux,* or the backward flow of contents of the stomach up into the esophagus. This condition can seriously interfere with nutritional intake (Eicher, 2002). Special diagnostic procedures, which will be described a bit later, are often undertaken by the physician when this condition is suspected.

Management

The results of the feeding and oral assessment provide the clinician with information necessary to make decisions about whether feeding therapy is needed and what aspects of the feeding and oral behavior ought to be addressed. Very often, though, because of the neurological immaturity of the infant in the NICU as a result of failure to thrive on oral feeding or for other medical reasons, oral feeding may not be an option. In these cases, tube feeding may be initiated. The decision to tube feed is usually made by the physician, and the SLP may not be consulted. But, as Imhoff and Wigginton (1991) pointed out, the SLP can be an important advocate for the parents in understanding the tube feeding decision and its consequences, in helping them to ask appropriate questions of the medical staff, and in making the eventual transition from

TABLE 6-3	Infant Feeding Assessment Instruments

INSTRUMENT	DESCRIPTION
Clinical Feeding Evaluation of Infants (Wolf & Glass, 1992a)	Provides a checklist for recording behaviors and a description of normal oral movement patterns.
Early Feeding Skills Assessment (Thoyre, Shaker, & Pridham, 2005)	A checklist for assessing infant readiness for oral feeding
Feeding Flow Sheet (VandenBerg, 1990)	Used to document feeding progress during NICU stay
Feeding Assessment (Morris & Klein, 2000)	Provides a questionnaire in both English and Spanish that the clinician can use with whoever is feeding the infant, whether parent or medical staff, and also provides guidance in developing a treatment plan.
LATCH (Jensen, Wallace, & Kelsay, 1994)	Consists of a scale for evaluating breastfeeding.
Neonatal Oral-Motor Assessment Scale (Palmer, Crawley, & Blanco, 1993)	Includes both oral-motor evaluation and checklist for scoring normal and disordered feeding movements.
Newborn Individualized Developmental Care and Assessment Program (NIDCAP) (Als, 1995)	Provides procedures for observing and summarizing natural infant behavior before, during, and after caregiving, and provides guidelines for developing behavioral goals on the basis of the observation.
Oral Motor Assessment (Sleight & Niman, 1984)	Developed for use with Down syndrome babies, but may be used with infants who have a variety of handicaps.
Preschool Oral Motor Examination (Sheppard, 1987)	Involves clinical direct assessment of motor and feeding behaviors.
Pre-Speech Assessment Scale (Morris, 1982)	Assesses a range of behaviors in addition to feeding, including respiration and vocalization, and provides an extensive questionnaire to be used with parents; also contains a wealth of information on normal and atypical prespeech and feeding development.
Preterm Infant Breastfeeding Behavior Scale (Nyquist, Sjoden, & Ewald, 1999)	Assesses breastfeeding behaviors in preterm infants.

BOX 6-2	Questions for Informal Assessment of Feeding and Oral Skills

Who is the baby's primary feeder?
What positions have you tried for feeding?
Does one type of nipple seem to work better than another?
Can the baby suck vigorously?
How much milk can the baby take in one feeding?
How long does the feeding take?
How long does the baby go between feedings?
How many feedings a day is the baby getting?
Does the baby seem to be alert during feedings? Does he or she look at the feeder?
How well does the baby control the jaw, head, and trunk during feeding?
Does the baby gag, choke, cough, or bite during feeding?
Does the baby have trouble or seem to delay swallowing?
Can the baby coordinate sucking, swallowing, and breathing?
Does drooling interfere with feeding?

tube to oral feeding. To serve in this advocate role, the SLP should be familiar with the various forms of tube feeding.

Three options currently are in use for nonoral feeding, and each has certain advantages and disadvantages for the baby and the family. The *nasogastric*, or *N-G*, tube is inserted through the nose and descends down the pharynx and into the stomach, whereas the *orogastric*, or *gavage*, tube is inserted through the mouth; a *nasojejunal* tube might also be used; this is inserted into the second part of the intestine. These methods preclude oral feeding while they are in place and can lead to hypersensitivity of the oral cavity. They also are visible and remind the parents every time they see the child about how sick the baby is. Physicians generally prefer these methods because they do not involve the surgical risk of the third option, the *gastronomy*, or *G-tube*. The G-tube brings food directly into the stomach and frees the oral cavity for exploration as well as for supplementary oral feeding and is typically used when nonoral feeding will be needed for an extended period of time.

Infants who need nonoral feeding for extended periods, particularly if they need endotracheal tubes to help them breathe as well, may show decreased sucking and oral motor development (Comrie & Helm, 1997). An important contribution that the SLP can make to this situation is to encourage parents and medical personnel to offer the baby a pacifier, nipple, or finger to suck on during the tube feeding. This will help strengthen the sucking reflex and also help the baby learn to associate sucking with feeling contented from feeding. Other oral stimulation, such as stroking the cheek, lips, and gums, may also help make the child ready for oral feeding (Fucile, Gisel, & Lau, 2005). The SLP also can take the time, which medical personnel will not always be able to do, to explain why the feeding tube is needed and to reassure the family that normal feeding will eventually be achieved. Further, the SLP can encourage the family to ask about supplementary oral feedings and may encourage the parents to ask the physician about using a G-tube to minimize effects on oral development if prolonged nonoral feeding (more than 1 month) is necessary.

If our assessment suggests that the baby is ready to graduate from nonoral to oral feeding, or is able to feed orally from the first, the SLP can use several techniques to help the infant succeed. Spatz (2004) discusses ways to promote breastfeeding for premature infants. These include working with nurses to help mothers maintain their milk supply by pumping and to safely store and track each mother's milk, encouraging the mother to hold the baby skin-to-skin during nonoral feeding and to provide non-nutritive sucking experiences while holding the baby at the breast. When making the transition to breastfeeding, the SLP can help with positioning the infant, using a "football" hold to support the head and neck. Although hospitals are more likely to encourage breastfeeding for premature infants than they were only a few years ago, since breast milk contains many nutrients and antibodies that are beneficial to the baby's health, some premature or high-risk infants may be unable to nurse, and their feeding times will be long and closely spaced, making nursing very difficult for the mother. Some mothers may still want to pump breast milk for the baby to drink from a bottle, and many NICUs provide breast pumps for this purpose. When the mother feels she wants to contribute to her infant's well-being in this way, she should certainly be encouraged to do so. Fletcher and Ash (2005) discuss the importance of working with other professionals to support mothers who wish to breast feed babies in the NICU. However, mothers should also be helped to understand that the infant can thrive on formula as well. Interaction is just as important, and perhaps more important to the babies' development, as the milk they drink. In counseling the mother of a baby in NICU, the SLP will want to help her to do for the baby what she can do best and to feel that she is making a contribution to the baby's overcoming of a difficult start. If the mother can nurse or express milk, fine. If a particular mother cannot or feels uncomfortable with these options, she can help her baby in many other ways. The SLP can play a crucial role in helping the mother to understand the importance of interaction and communication in the baby's development and in making her see that these are her most crucial contributions to her child's well-being. It is especially important to stress to these mothers that meals must be communicative as well as nutritional activities and to encourage mothers to develop interaction and communication early in the feeding process.

Feeding is almost as important to the mother's development as it is to the infant's. If a mother cannot feed her baby, her sense of herself as the primary source of nurture in the baby's life is seriously threatened. The SLP developing a feeding plan for a baby in the NICU can help the mother to feel her way toward this nurturing role. Specific techniques and instruction for facilitating feeding by either breast or bottle can be provided, such as the following:

1. *Positioning.* Jaffe (1989) suggested that the premature baby be placed in a flexed position, with the chin tucked into the neck and the shoulders and arms pressed forward. This is an ideal "cuddling" position and can aid in bonding as well as feeding. Ideal positioning also can be achieved by placing the baby in an inner tube, infant seat, or beanbag chair. Hall, Circello, Reed, and Hylton (1987) advocated keeping the child's face near the feeder's to encourage eye contact and social interaction. Comrie and Helm (1997) provide additional detailed positioning alternatives. The mother's comfort and the baby's success are most important in deciding on a position for feeding. Trial and error may be necessary to find the best position.

2. *Jaw stabilization.* The mother can place her thumb or finger on the baby's chin, just below the lower lip, another finger on the temporomandibular joint, and a third finger under the chin. This support allows her to stabilize the head and jaw and to provide more control as the infant sucks. This control on the mother's part should be gradually faded as the infant's feeding skills develop.

3. *Negative resistance.* Comrie and Helm (1997) suggest using negative resistance to help infants who bite rather than suck or have an inefficient sucking pattern. As the infant pulls on the nipple during sucking, the feeder tugs gently back. This often stimulates a longer and stronger suck.

4. *Using specialized feeding equipment.* Comrie and Helm also suggest that nipple characteristics can influence sucking patterns, and suggest that if breastfeeding is not possible, nipples with various characteristics of flow rate, suction, and compression should be tried, as well as angled bottles. Spatz (2004) advocates using a nipple shield for breastfeeding mothers, to increase milk intake.

5. *Modifying temperature and consistency.* Alper and Manno (1996) point out that chilling liquids has been tried to increase swallowing rate and decrease pooling of liquid in the pharynx. However, the main effect of this change may be to thicken the liquid, which may make it easier to swallow. Formulas also can be thickened by adding rice cereal.

6. *Oral stimulation in feeding.* McGowan and Kerwin (1993) suggested providing oral stimulation during feeding. They advised having parents use the following sequence to introduce bottle feeding:
   a. Stroking the nipple on the side of the baby's cheek to elicit a rooting reflex.
   b. Touching the nipple to the center of the lips and gum surface to produce mouth opening.
   c. Allowing the baby to close on the nipple and start sucking, then stroking upward on the palate in a rhythmic motion with the nipple to encourage continued sucking.

7. *Nonfeeding oral stimulation.* In addition to being encouraged to touch and stroke their babies' bodies in the NICU, mothers also should be encouraged to provide gentle stimulation to the baby's face, rubbing it gently with fingers or soft toys and providing non-nutritive sucking of a pacifier or finger whenever possible (Fucile, Gisel, & Lau, 2005). McGowan and Kerwin (1993) gave some specific suggestions for oral stimulation activities, including the following:

   a. Putting a finger (nail down) in the baby's mouth and rubbing the palate with an upward motion (midsection to front) to stimulate non-nutritive sucking.
   b. Rhythmically stroking the midsection of the tongue, front to back.
   c. Rubbing the infant's cheeks, one at a time, with a circular motion.
   d. Tapping around the baby's lips in a complete circle.
   e. Placing a finger or toothbrush in the mouth and massaging the upper and lower gums.

Additional resources for assessing and managing infant feeding problems include Alper and Manno (1996), Arvedson and Brodsky (1993), Eicher (2002), Johnson-Martin, Hacker, and Attermeier (2004), Kedesdy and Budd (1998), Lowman, Murphy, and Snell (1999), McGrath and Braescu (2004), Morris and Klein (2000), Spatz (2004), Tuchman and Walter (1993), and Wolf and Glass (1992a).

HEARING CONSERVATION AND AURAL HABILITATION

Federal law now requires hearing screening for all newborns in the NICU. But, as we discussed earlier, the NICU itself may be hazardous to the baby's health. Clark (1989) reported that the incubators, cardiorespiratory monitors, and ventilators present in the NICU can generate noise levels of more than 85 dB, which not only interferes with sleep but may result in hearing loss by means of cochlear damage. This risk to hearing is in addition to the high incidence of hearing loss associated with many of the syndromes and conditions that resulted in the child being placed in the NICU in the first place. As we saw earlier, many congenital and genetic syndromes affect the development of the auditory structures, and hearing loss is one of the most important causes of the language disorders we see in such children. The SLP can play a crucial role in conserving the hearing of the high-risk newborn. Language clinicians should be sure that aural habilitation is part of the management plan if screening indicates hearing loss. Further, the SLP should encourage the parents to have the infant's hearing tested by an audiologist periodically throughout the child's early years, even if losses are not identified during the newborn period. In this way a loss that occurs for whatever reason can be treated at the earliest possible time.

CHILD BEHAVIOR AND DEVELOPMENT

Assessment

Sparks (1989) emphasized that the purpose of assessment for infants should *not* be to predict future behavior, but to determine the infant's *current* strengths and needs. First, it is important to know as much as we can about what risks the infant faces. This knowledge can help us decide how much and what kind of intervention to propose. If the child has DS, for example, we know that the risk for future speech and language delays, as well as for middle-ear dysfunction, is high. This knowledge may lead us to argue more strongly for early communication intervention than we might in the case of a child with prematurity alone. Careful interviewing of family and medical staff, as well as medical chart review, can provide this information.

Second, we need to evaluate the infant's level of physiological organization. The premature infant's functioning is immature in every way. Even the simplest ability to maintain physiological stability is affected. Premature infants experience irregular respiration; color changes; bodily instability, including jitteriness and flaccidity; and disorganized patterns of alertness. The infant's level of behavioral organization and homeostasis will, in large measure, determine his or her ability to participate in interactions. So an important part of the assessment of the at-risk newborn involves evaluating the extent to which the baby can maintain physiological and attentional states.

The *Neonatal Behavioral Assessment Scale* (Brazelton & Nugent, 1995) and the *Assessment of Preterm Infant Behavior* (Als, Lester, Tronick, & Brazelton, 1982) grew out of the realization that earlier instruments were not sufficiently sensitive for the less-well-organized premature infant. These instruments were designed to look at a range of abilities for infants at 28 to 40 weeks gestational age. They help the clinician to identify the conditions under which the baby functions best, what places stress on the baby, how much handling and stimulation the baby can tolerate, how easily the baby's homeostasis is disrupted, what supports are useful to the baby in maintaining self-control, and how much endurance the baby has for interactive functioning. Many NICUs use these instruments routinely to evaluate patients. When this evaluation has been done by medical staff, the SLP should carefully review the results for information that will help in the planning of a communicative intervention program. If no formal instrument is routinely used, the SLP should consider administering the *APIB, NBAS* or another developmental assessment. *The Newborn Behavioral Observation* (Nugent, Keefer, O'Brien, Johnson, & Blanchard, 2005) and *the Neurological Assessment of the Preterm and Full-Term Newborn Infant* (Dubowitz, Dubowitz, & Mercuri, 1999) are additional tools that may be considered.

Management

According to Gorski (1983), the goal of intervention for the baby in the NICU is to achieve stabilization and homeostasis of physiological and behavioral states and to prevent or minimize any secondary disorders that might be associated with the child's condition, rather than to attain milestones appropriate for full-term babies. The best way for us to achieve these goals is to become a member of the NICU team and to earn the respect of the medical staff for our in-depth knowledge of early communicative and oral-motor development. When this has been achieved, the SLP can offer suggestions that will benefit communicative development. Gorski (1983), Griffer (2000), and VandenBerg (1997) advocated developmentally supportive care that uses strategies like the following:

1. Encourage careful monitoring both of noise levels and infant hearing within the NICU.
2. Develop staff awareness of the dangers of ototoxic effects of medications.
3. Foster sensitivity to laryngeal damage from endotracheal tubes (Sparks, 1984).
4. Work to alleviate sensory overstimulation because of constant bright light.
5. Suggest ways to counteract the dangers of low language and interactive stimulation that can result from infrequent handling in the NICU.
6. Encourage consideration of the oral-motor consequences of continued use of N-G and gavage tube feeding, bearing in mind the surgical risks that G-tube feeding entails. The SLP can help families and medical staff to work together to consider how these risks can be balanced.
7. Advocate for the importance of non-nutritive sucking and oral stimulation to aid in the baby's oral-motor development.
8. Educate staff about the efficacy of early intervention (Rossetti, 2001).
9. Provide information about services offered by other disciplines (e.g., SLP, occupational therapy, physical therapy, counseling) that may be of help to families of babies in the NICU.
10. Support parents in achieving their goals for the child during the NICU stay.
11. Encourage parents to talk to, touch, and hold the baby; help with positioning.
12. Help parents recognize, understand, and interpret the infants' signals; help time caregiving and interaction to promote the infants state regulation and allow for natural sleep-wake cycles.

PARENT-CHILD COMMUNICATION

As we've seen, the newborn in the NICU is at risk for an inadequate interactive experience because medical needs and the appearance of frailty make it difficult for parents to respond to the baby in the usual way. Further, the infant's neurological immaturity may render the baby less able to take advantage of the interactions that the parent offers. Let's see how the language pathologist can facilitate the parent-infant interaction in the NICU.

Assessment

Assessing Infant Readiness for Communication. Information gathered from an instrument, such as the *APIB*, will help identify the level of interactive, motor, and organizational development that the infant in the NICU is showing. This information is crucial for deciding whether the infant is ready to take advantage of communicative interaction. Gorski, Davison, and Brazelton (1979) defined three stages of behavioral organization in high-risk newborns. The child's

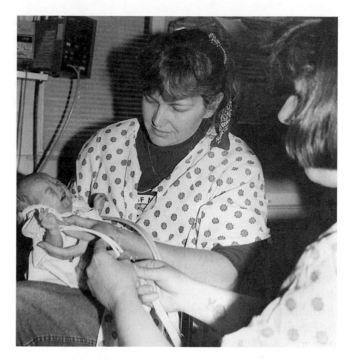

Communication intervention for at-risk infants can begin in the newborn intensive care unit.

state of organization determines when he or she is ready to participate in interactions. These states include the following:

1. *Turning In* (or physiological state). During this stage the baby is very sick and cannot really participate in reciprocal interactions. All the infant's energies are devoted to maintaining biological stability.
2. *Coming Out.* The baby first becomes responsive to the environment when he or she is no longer acutely ill, can breathe adequately, and begins to gain weight. This stage usually occurs while the baby is still in the NICU, and this is the time when he or she can begin to benefit from interactions with parents. It is essential that the SLP be aware when this stage is reached so that interactions can be encouraged.
3. *Reciprocity.* This final stage in the progression usually occurs at some point before the baby is released from the hospital. Now the infant can respond to parental interaction in predictable ways. Failure to achieve this stage, once physiological stability has been achieved, is a signal that developmental deficits may persist.

An important function that the SLP can serve in fostering communicative development in an infant in the NICU is to acquaint the parents with this progression and help them to learn from the medical staff when the child turns the corner from the first to the second stage. At this time, more active parental involvement with the infant should be encouraged by the SLP.

Assessing Parent Communication and Family Functioning. Several instruments are available to assess parent-child communication. These may be used once the baby is ready to participate in communicative interactions. The *Parent Behavior Progression* (Bromwich, Khokha, Fust, Baxter, Burge, & Kass,

1981) is an instrument that provides a clinician with guidelines for observing a parent's behavior with the infant to assess what the parent needs in order to improve or maximize the value of the interactions. This instrument rates the parent's apparent pleasure in the interaction; the sensitivity of the parent to the child's behavioral cues; the stability and mutuality of the interactions; and the developmental appropriateness of the parent's choice of actions, objects, and activities. The *Observation of Communicative Interaction* (Klein & Briggs, 1987) and *Parent-Infant Relationships Global Assessment Scale* (Aoki, Iseharashi, Heller, & Bakshi, 2002) are similar instruments.

There also are formal assessment procedures to address family strengths and needs. These assessments are often included in the development of an IFSP because of IDEA's emphasis on family-centered intervention. Formal instruments include the *Family Needs Survey* (Bailey & Simeonsson, 1988), the *Family Needs Scale* (Dunst, Cooper, Weeldreyer, Snyder, & Chase, 1988), the *Family Strengths Profile* (Trivette, Dunst, & Deal, 1988), the *Measurement of Family Functioning* (Fewell, 1986), the *Family Environment Scale* (Moos, 1974), and the *Family Resource Scale* (Leet & Dunst, 1988).

Some danger exists, though, in using formal procedures to assess parent-child communication and family functioning. Although communication is, of course, a two-way street, we do not want to convey to the family in any way that we think they are the problem. As Slentz and Bricker (1992) pointed out, when parent-child interactions or family function are assessed, the implication to family members is often that they have a problem that needs assessing or that their child has a problem because they have a problem. Slentz, Walker, and Bricker (1989) found that the most threatening aspect of early intervention for parents of handicapped children is the assessment of the family. Mahoney and Spiker (1996) discuss similar concerns. The intent of IDEA, through the IFSP, is to provide support to the family in promoting the infant's development. Although the IFSP mandates participation of the family and identification of *their* "priorities and concerns," it does not specifically mandate formal assessments.

A simple and effective way to find out about family priorities and concerns is to ask. Slentz and Bricker (1992) suggested that the time it would take to do extensive formal assessment of family functioning is better spent developing a relationship with the family and giving them the opportunity to talk at length with the clinician about the frustrations and joys of raising their baby. This formation of an alliance with the family is more likely to lead to valid insights into their strengths and needs than will misguided attempts at pseudoscientific assessment. Cripe and Bricker (1993) have developed the *Family Interest Survey,* not to evaluate the family, but to simply find out what they think about their child's needs. It is intended to be a nonjudgmental means of identifying areas of the family's interest in both intervention goals and social services and can help the SLP see the family's perspective on the child's needs and the services required to provide for them. The *How Can We Help* survey (Child Development Resources, 1989) is a similar instrument. This survey appears in Appendix 6-2.

What about the truly dysfunctional family? The one that presents a danger to the infant or appears unable to meet the baby's needs in an even minimally adequate way? Here the SLP's responsibility is referral to appropriate social services and advocacy for the services the family needs to provide for the baby. Even if formal assessment were needed to identify such a family, the SLP would not be able to provide the financial assistance, drug and alcohol counseling, and other services that would be required to set this family on the right track. A straightforward statement of the SLP's concerns about the family to the appropriate agency is enough to alert social service personnel to the family's situation. In truth, we should be aware that the family's needs will not always be adequately addressed. Since this is the case, the justification for intrusive and threatening probes into the family's psyche seems even less compelling. Again, the role of the SLP as advocate and ally is most important to preserve, to get the parents to cooperate to any extent they can in enhancing the baby's learning environment.

As we've discussed, one of the best ways to find out about family members' priorities and concerns is to talk with them. In discussing how a family can best cope with a handicapped or at-risk child, it is a good idea to remember that the family is probably experiencing a good deal of shock, grief, guilt, confusion, and a feeling of loss of the perfect baby they dreamed of having. They also may be experiencing information overload as a result of the well-meaning efforts of the hospital staff to keep them up-to-date on their baby's condition and prospects. The language pathologist is uniquely suited to give the family the opportunity to express these conflicting feelings and to be a model for the family in listening to and responding to their needs, as we hope the family will do for the infant.

The feelings the family is expressing may not be pretty. They may be angry at the medical staff or at no one in particular at the blow they have been dealt and the burden they will have to carry, perhaps for the rest of their lives. Who wouldn't be angry and frightened? The notion of family-centered intervention dictates that we acknowledge and respect both the unrelenting difficulties parents of babies in the NICU are experiencing and the ways in which they are able to cope. Our goal is to support the family, not to engineer them; to give them the information they need at the present time and to be ready to provide more information when it is wanted; and to respond to the family's needs and desires rather than to dictate what they should do. Thus a family-centered approach involves not a complicated psychology, but rather a simple, human attempt to treat others as we would wish to be treated if we were experiencing the difficult transition that the NICU infant's family must face.

Management

A recent innovation in the care of the medically stable infant in the NICU is "kangaroo care" (Rossetti, 2001; Ruiz-Palaez, Charpak, & Cuervo, 2004). This technique involves skin-to-skin contact between parent and child during the NICU stay. Parents are encouraged to swaddle the infant to their unclothed chest for about 30 minutes each day. The method has been shown to be associated with decreased length of hospital stay;

shorter periods of assisted ventilation; increased periods of alertness; and, perhaps as importantly, with an enhanced sense of nurturance of the child on the parent's part (Dodd, 2005; Ruiz-Palaez, Charpak, & Cuervo, 2004). This technique seems to have great potential for improving parent-child interactions during the infant's first days, and can be used as part of the preparation for oral feeding, as we discussed earlier.

Still, the very sick neonate may not be ready to take advantage of interactions with parents during the period of acute illness for some time after birth. When this is the case, SLPs can still encourage one important activity in parents: we can help parents to learn to observe their babies and, specifically, to identify states the baby is exhibiting. Learning to identify the

baby's state will be very useful for parents when the time arrives to begin communicative interactions with the baby. Babies are only receptive to interactions in certain states. A parent who can recognize these states and use them as interactive opportunities will have a better chance to engage the baby's attention and elicit reciprocity. Brazelton (1973) gave a description of the various states seen in the healthy newborn. Each state carries implications for the kinds of caregiving activities that can go on when the infant is in that state (Blackburn, 1978). These states and their implications are summarized in Table 6-4.

We can facilitate parents' identification of the infant's state by encouraging them to observe their babies and by talking with them about what they see. We can use the behaviors

TABLE 6-4	**Infant States***

STATE	BEHAVIORS	IMPLICATIONS FOR INTERACTION
Deep sleep	1. Body still, except for occasional twitch 2. Eyes closed 3. Still face 4. Breathing smooth 5. Threshold to stimuli high—only very intense stimuli will cause arousal	Little possible; adults will do better to wait to feed or interact until child arouses naturally.
Light sleep	1. Some body movement 2. Eyes flutter beneath closed lids 3. May smile or cry briefly 4. Breathing irregular 5. More responsive to stimuli; may arouse to drowsy state if stimulus occurs	Makes up largest part of newborn sleep pattern; brief fuss sounds may cause adults to try to feed, rouse, or interact with babies before they are ready.
Drowsy	1. Variable activity, usually smooth 2. Eyes open and close, appear dull 3. Face often appears still 4. Breathing irregular 5. React to stimuli, but reactions are delayed; this state often changes after reaction	Infants left alone in this state may return to sleep, but if parents provide something for the baby to look at, listen to, or suck on, baby may be aroused to a more responsive state.
Quiet alert	1. Little bodily movement 2. Eyes brighten and widen 3. Face appears bright 4. Breathing regular 5. Attends to environmental stimuli	Providing something for baby to look at, listen to, or suck may maintain this state, which is ideal for interaction.
Active alert	1. Much bodily movement 2. Eyes are open and bright 3. Much facial movement 4. Breathing irregular 5. Increasingly sensitive to disturbing stimuli (e.g., hunger, noise)	Parents can cuddle and console to bring baby to a less aroused state.
Crying	1. Increased motor activity, color changes 2. Eyes may be tightly closed or open 3. Facial grimaces 4. Breathing irregular 5. Highly responsive to unpleasant stimuli	Tells parents the child has reached his or her limits; needs to be fed or consoled.

*"State" is a group of behaviors that regularly occur together, including (1) bodily activity, (2) eye movement, (3) facial movement, (4) breathing pattern, and (5) responses to stimuli.

Adapted from Blackburn, S. (1978). State organizations in the newborn: Implications for caregiving. In K.E. Barend, S. Blackburn, R. Kang, & A.L. Saetz (Eds.), *Early parent-infant relationships. Series 1: The first six hours of life, module 3.* White Plains, NY: The National Foundation/March of Dimes.

listed in Table 6-4 to distinguish deep sleep from light sleep, for example, and discuss what the parent would do differently, depending on which type of sleep was observed. We also can encourage parents to learn to distinguish among the various waking states and ask similar questions about these. Although the very sick neonate may exhibit few states of alertness, the parent can be encouraged to observe alertness in other babies in the NICU and to identify the fleeting alert states that do occur in the baby who is still in the Turning In stage. When more frequent alert states do emerge, the parents will be ready to recognize and take advantage of them.

Once the infant has progressed to the Coming Out stage and can take advantage of parental communication, our most important job is to get parents to start communicating with their babies. By keeping in close touch with medical staff, we can be sure that parents are alerted to their baby's transition to this stage. Once it occurs, we will be in a position to encourage the parents to use their knowledge of the baby's states to tune in on when the baby is alert and able to interact. We can encourage the parents to look at, handle, talk to, sing, and show things to the baby during this state. A second important aspect of these interactions is to help the parent identify when the infant can no longer interact and allow the baby to recoup his or her resources so that further interaction will be possible later.

Parents can be helped to identify the infant's signs of stress, such as averting the gaze, turning the head away, spreading the fingers, arching the back, and grunting. Parents can be encouraged to see these signs of stress as a natural part of the baby's transition from one state to another, rather than as a rejection of their efforts to interact. We can teach parents to give the baby "time out" to reorganize. They can be asked not to try to re-establish mutual gaze if the baby has broken it. Instead, they should be counseled to wait for signals, such as bodily quieting and a reinitiation of mutual gaze by the baby, that he or she is ready for more interaction. These same skills can be fostered during feedings, helping the parent to become aware of the baby's readiness both to feed and to interact in this very important communicative context.

Rossetti (2001) suggests that another way to increase the parents' role with the newborn in the NICU is to encourage the parent to participate in charting the child's behavior. The SLP can discuss this option with other staff and try to make them understand the advantages of enlisting the parents' help in the big job of keeping the copious records required in the hospital. Not only will the parents feel more a part of the baby's care team, but charting can help them learn to be better observers of the child's behavior, a skill that will serve them well throughout the child's development.

ASSESSMENT AND INTERVENTION FOR PREINTENTIONAL INFANTS AND THEIR FAMILIES: 1 TO 8 MONTHS

Although life with a baby in the NICU is difficult, taking that baby home for the first time can be just as daunting. Whereas in the hospital the parents may have felt isolated and shut out

of the baby's care, at home the same parents may feel overwhelmed by the responsibility that they must now face alone. If the IFSP includes follow-up by the SLP during this difficult period, there are many ways in which we can support the family in its new capacity.

Before learning what they are, though, let's make sure we understand the terminology used to describe this period of development. Infants in this phase are referred to as *preintentional* because they have not yet developed the cognitive skills to represent ideas in their minds and to pursue goals through planned actions. Bates (1976) referred to this stage of development as "perlocutionary." This term implies two important things: first, infants do not intend any particular outcome by their behavior, and secondly, that adults act as if they do. Adults' willingness to attribute intentionality to the young infant's behavior is one way babies are "taught" how to have these intentions, which will eventually lay the basis for communication later in the first year of life. Let's examine the same four areas that we looked at for the newborn to see how the SLP can provide effective services to preintentional infants and their families.

FEEDING AND ORAL-MOTOR DEVELOPMENT

Feeding Assessment

The same instruments that we discussed using to assess feeding and oral-motor development in the newborn are relevant here. Similarly, informal interviews that include questions such as those given in Box 6-2 also can be used to gather information about the child's feeding ability. Toward the middle of the first year of life, though, the normally developing infant begins to acquire new feeding patterns that facilitate the introduction of solid foods into the diet. These patterns include integrating the front-to-back movement of the tongue used in sucking with rhythmic up-and-down jaw movements to produce the "munching pattern" that enables the child to eat solids (Eicher, 2002). During the next year or so, additional patterns develop. These are summarized in Table 6-5. Informal oral-motor assessment of the preintentional infant can include attempts to observe these patterns during feeding at the appropriate developmental level.

For infants with tracheostomies or neurological involvement, some specialized assessments may be necessary to evaluate the safety of oral feeding, particularly for solid foods. ASHA (2004a) holds that some of these studies can be carried out by SLPs, such as the following:

Cervical auscultation detects changes in upper aerodigestive tract sounds and is the most noninvasive of these measures.

Videofluoroscopic swallowing function studies, similar to those used with adults who have acquired dysphagia, also can be used to examine oral and pharyngeal movement during feeding and to assess risk for aspiration in children with neurological involvement.

Ultrasound studies allow for the visualization of relations between movement patterns and oral/pharyngeal structures.

TABLE 6-5	Development of Feeding and Oral-Motor Skills		
AGE (MO)	**FOOD TYPE**	**ORAL-MOTOR SKILL**	**DEVELOPMENTAL SKILL**
0–4	Liquid	Suckle on nipple	Head control acquired
4–6	Purees	Suckle off spoon Progress to sucking	Sitting, hands to midline
6–9	Soft chewables	Vertical munching "Sippy" cup drinking Limited lateral tongue movements	Hand-to-mouth reach, grasp Finger feeding; assist with spoon
9–12	Lumpy textures	Independent "sippy" cup drinking	Pincer grasp Grasps spoon
12–18	All textures	Lateral tongue action Straw drinking	Scoops food to mouth Increased independence in feeding
18–24	More chewable food	Rotary chewing	Independent walking Can obtain food/nonfood objects on own
24	Tougher solids	Mature chewing	Total self-feeding Use of fork, open cup

Adapted from Arvedson, J., & Lefton-Greif, M. (1996). Anatomy, physiology and development of feeding. *Seminars in Speech and Language, 17,* 261-268; and Jaffe, M. (1989). Feeding at-risk infants and toddlers. *Topics in Language Disorders, 10(1),* 13-25.

Endoscopy involves passing a fiberoptic tube through the mouth down the esophagus and into the stomach while the child is sedated.

Other procedures are completed by medical personnel. Eicher (2002) and Lefton-Grief and Loughlin (1996) described additional tests that may be used to assess danger of aspiration or gastroesophageal reflux (GER):

The *upper gastrointestinal study (upper GI)* involves the child's ingesting a liquid containing barium that is visible on x-ray. This allows a radiologist to observe structural abnormalities or reflux into the esophagus.

The *milk scan* also uses a radioactively marked fluid. Here the radiologist sees where the marker fluid settles. If it is seen in the lungs, aspiration can be inferred.

Additional assessments that might be required include the following:

Radionuclide imaging studies (scintigraphy) help to quantify esophageal and gastric emptying and aspiration and provide multiple static images of concentrated regions of tracer residue over prolonged periods.

The *pH probe* measures acidity by placing a nasogastric-like tube at the junction of the stomach and esophagus. The probe at the end of the tube can detect acid that refluxes through an incompetent valve from the stomach. Results of this assessment can help to determine positioning needs during feeding to avoid reflux. The physician can then visualize the tissues and take small biopsy specimens to examine for inflammation.

Methylene blue screening is used to determine whether a child with a tracheostomy is aspirating food into the lungs, which can lead to recurrent pneumonia. In this procedure, food is dyed and evidence of emission of dye in the tracheal stoma, which would indicate aspiration, is monitored.

The pH probe and gastroesophageal endoscopy are considered the "gold standards" in the evaluation of feeding and swallowing (Eicher, 2002).

Vocal Assessment

In addition to concern about feeding, we also have concerns at this stage of development about the infant's vocal ability. Proctor (1989) has provided a detailed instrument for assessing the baby's vocal skills from birth to 12 months. Bleile and Miller (1993) and Mitchell (1997) also provided guidelines for this assessment. Figure 6-1 presents a worksheet for assessing early vocal development adapted from these sources. Mitchell (1997) suggests that the sample consist of what she calls "comfort state" vocalizations. These include sounds the child makes when in an alert and contented state and are typically heard during familiar caretaking routines, such as changing, feeding, or playing. Her findings indicate that 20 minutes is usually adequate to collect a sample of up to 70 vocalizations and that this constitutes a reasonably representative sample. If the infant becomes fussy, however, she suggests collecting the sample over several observations, until 50 to 70 comfort state vocalizations have been produced. Vocalizations included in the sample are those that contain a vowel-like and/or consonant-like element, are produced with an egressive air stream, and sound speech-like. Mitchell advocates practicing the analysis with a colleague until 80% to 90% agreement is reached on the classification of vocalizations.

To record the child's performance, the SLP begins by observing the child and parent and listening carefully to each vocalization produced by the child. Vocalizations are divided either by intonation contours, pauses, or an inhalation by the infant. If the child is vocalizing frequently, it may be necessary to audiorecord the session for later analysis. In many cases, though, it will be possible to do the assessment in real time, especially when the clinician is familiar with the assessment recording form. The clinician then codes each vocalization heard during the observation according to the criteria on the form and notes it with a checkmark in the corresponding box in the "observed directly" column. For vocal behaviors listed at the child's developmental level (in the first column of Figure 6-1) that are not observed directly, the clinician can demonstrate the behavior for the parent and ask whether the child ever produces that behavior. If so, a checkmark can be recorded in the "parent report" column on the form. If the parent reports that the behavior does not occur at home and the clinician does not observe it, a (—) should be recorded for that vocal behavior. If most behaviors at the child's level are observed, the clinician can ask the parent about behaviors at subsequent levels. If the direct observation indicates few behaviors at the child's developmental level, the clinician can ask parents about behaviors typical of earlier levels. The clinician also can indicate on the form the vowel-like or consonant-like productions heard, using phonetic transcription, in the "phonetics/comments" column. The number of vocalizations produced in the time frame of the observation also can be recorded there.

Although this is not a norm-referenced assessment, it may be used to help determine whether vocal development appears to be progressing appropriately and whether intervention ought to include stimulation of vocalization. The number of checkmarks and (—)s on the form can be used to determine the general stage of vocal development. The stage at which at least one appropriate type of vocalization occurs can be seen as the stage of vocalization in which the child is emerging. If this stage corresponds to chronological age, then vocal development can be considered as progressing adequately.

One particularly important benchmark to be aware of is the emergence of what Oller and colleagues call *canonical babbling*. Oller, Levine, Cobo-Lewis, Eilers, and Pearson (1998) define canonical babbling as the production of well-formed syllables that consist of at least one vowel-like element and one consonant-like element that are connected in quick transition and are recognized to contain sounds similar enough to speech to be transcribable. Examples include /baba/, /dIdI/, /iba/, and /ta/. Oller et al. have shown that the failure to produce these syllables by 10 months of age predicts delays in the acquisition of words and word combinations in the second year of life. These forms are, then, an important benchmark to monitor as the child reaches the last quarter of the first year. Oller, Eilers, and Basinger (2001) report that parents can reliably report whether or not these forms are present in children's speech, so that for children over 10 months of age, parents should be asked if they hear these forms if the infant does not produce them during the assessment.

Other important features to note in the child's babbling are the rate of vocalization, proportion of consonants, and multisyllabic babbling (Mitchell, 1997). Rate of babbling is computed by counting the number of vocalizations (not syllables) and dividing by the number of minutes the sample includes. Although there are no norms for rate in infants younger than 12 months, in general the rate should increase with age. If rate fails to advance for 6 months or so, some stimulation of vocal production should be considered as part of the management program, and hearing should be assessed. Percentage of consonants to vowels also should increase during the first year. By 16 months, the sample should include more consonants than vowels. Babbling that contains more than one syllable also should increase during the first year and a half, and vocalizations that include more than one type of consonant should begin to appear by the end of the first year (Mitchell, 1997). An additional milestone is the beginning of the imitation of the intonation contour of the ambient language (Rothganger, 2003). The babble of children toward the end of the first year should begin to mimic the melody, or prosodic contour, of sentences. These milestones, too, can help determine whether vocal development is proceeding typically. This assessment can be repeated periodically to ensure that vocal development is continuing and to determine the efficacy of any intervention that is initiated.

For children with a history of prematurity, corrected gestational age (CGA) should be used as the standard for comparison during the first year of life (Rossetti, 2001). CGA is computed by subtracting the number of weeks of prematurity from the child's chronological age. If, for example, Janice were assessed at 3 months after birth, her 8 weeks of prematurity would be subtracted from her chronological age of 12 weeks. Her CGA, then, would be 4 weeks, and vocal behaviors typical of a 4-week-old would be considered appropriate for her developmental level.

Managing Feeding

For the nursing or bottle-feeding infant, the same strategies we discussed earlier can be used to improve sucking and feeding behavior. Oral stimulation in the form of gentle touching, encouragement of non-nutritive sucking, and presentation of safe items for the baby to mouth, such as soft rubber toys, a toothbrush, or teething ring, also can be encouraged. Care should be taken to help parents become aware of what items should and should not be mouthed. Balloons, coins, and toys with small parts are particularly dangerous.

As the baby approaches the second half of the first year, feeding of solid foods may be introduced, if assessment indicates that this will be safe for the infant. Babies with orofacial anomalies or conditions involving depressed muscle tone, such as DS, may have difficulty making this transition. Jaffe (1989) offered a series of suggestions for improving feeding skills, summarized in Box 6-3. In addition, many of the suggestions presented in Box 6-4 for feeding older prelinguistic clients also can be adapted for feeding at-risk preintentional infants. The resources we mentioned earlier for assessing and managing feeding in the newborn also will be helpful for addressing feeding issues at the preintentional stage of development.

Managing Vocal Development

For infants whose vocal behavior appears to be less frequent or less mature than would be expected for their age (or age corrected for gestational age in the case of premature babies),

Child's name: _____ Birthdate: _____

Address: _____ Phone: _____

_____ Parents: _____

	Observed directly	Parent report	Phonetics/comments
Stage 1 (birth to 2 months)			
Vocalization Types			
Crying with sudden pitch shifts, extremely high pitch			
Fussing or discomfort			
Vegetative sounds (burps, sounds accompanying feeding)			
Neutral sounds (grunts, sighs)			
Vowel-like sounds: (i, I, e, ∧, u, U, o, a]			
Stage 2 (2 to 4 months)			
Vocalization Types			
Vowel sounds predominate, but a few consonants emerge (primarily velars and glottals)			
Marked decrease in crying (after 12 weeks)			
Begins consonant plus vowel; mostly " coo" and "goo"			
Begins to produce pleasure sounds, such as "mmmmm"			
Stage 3 (4 to 6 months)			
Vocalization Types			
Consistent production of consonant-vowel (CV) (syllabic) combinations			
Imitation of sounds in back-and-forth babbling games with others			
More variations in vowel production			
Number of consonant segments increases to include front stops and nasals			
Laughter emerges(arounds 16 weeks)			
Front sounds begin to predominate, including blowing "raspberries," bilabial trills (lip smacks)			
Begins variation of intonational (pitch) contours, often when playing alone with toys			
Extreme pitch glides, such as yells, squeals, and low-pitched growls			
Stage 4 (6 to 10 months)			
Vocalization Types			
Canonical, repetitive, or reduplicated babbling (CV or CVCV-like structure) begins to appear (|mama|, |dada|, and |n∧n∧|)			
Consistent variation of intonational contours			
Early nonreduplicated CV sequences appear			
Parent may report hearing first word around 10 months			
Utterances produced with full-stop consonant (p, b, t, d, are most common)			
Short exclamations such as "ooh!" begin to appear			
Stage 5 (10 to 12 months)			
Vocalization Types			
Variegated babbling (successive syllables not identical) appears			
Variety of CV and CVC combinations with sentence-like intonation			
Syllables other than CVs produced			
Use of jargon, protowords, or phonetically consistent forms emerges			
Increased development of prosodic contours to match intonation patterns of ambient language			
Approximations of meaningful single words; phonological processes may operate on word approximations			

FIGURE 6-1 ✦ Developmental vocal assessment form. (Adapted from Proctor, A. (1989). States of normal noncry vocal development in infancy: A protocol for assessment. *Topics in Language Disorders, 10(1),* 26-42; used with permission of Aspen Publishers; Bleile, K., & Miller, S. (1993). Infants and toddlers. In J. Bernthal [Ed.], *Articulatory and phonological disorders in special populations.* New York: Thieme; McCune, L., & Vihman, M. (2001). Early phonetic and lexical development: A productivity approach. *Journal of Speech, Language, and Hearing Research, 44,* 670-684.)

| BOX 6-3 | Suggestions for Improving Feeding Skills |

Vary texture–Use applesauce, cereal, cracker crumbs, wheat germ, or yogurt to vary consistency until an optimal form is found.

Use single-consistency foods–Foods with more than one consistency, such as soups or packaged cereal with milk, may present problems resulting from lack of discrimination and coordination.

Identify preferred tastes–Finding foods that the baby likes may be more important than a balanced diet in the early stages.

Avoid foods that are lumpy or extreme in temperature–Infants with oral hypersensitivity may reject foods that are very hot, very cold, or lumpy. Experiment until foods that child will accept are found.

Improve chewing–Use crunchy foods, such as dry cereal, crackers, and cookies.

Control overproduction of mucus–Control intake of milk; control overproduction of saliva by controlling intake of sugar.

Sit below the baby's eye level to feed–This will help to control head flexion.

Present small amounts of food on the spoon in early spoon feeding–Present the spoon from just below mouth level and withdraw it straight out to prevent hyperextension of the neck; press on the center in the front part of the tongue to inhibit bite reflex and encourage lip closure around the spoon.

Cut food into strips–Use foods such as cooked carrots, fishsticks, and cold cuts, and place them on the biting surfaces to teach chewing.

Place food directly between gums and molars–This will help stimulate chewing.

Wrap cooked meat or fruit in gauze attached to a string–This prevents swallowing but gets the client to practice chewing.

Place finger food on the center of the tongue–Press down to encourage tongue lateralization. Finger food also may be placed on the nonpreferred side.

Place a cup on the baby's lower lip–Use downward pressure while controlling the flow of liquid to encourage cup feeding; thicken liquids with cereal at first, if necessary.

Adapted from Jaffe, M. (1989). Feeding at-risk infants and toddlers. *Topics in Language Disorders, 10,* 13-25.

| BOX 6-4 | Considerations in Feeding Older Prelinguistic Children |

Food Choice

1. Sweet, sour, salty, or citrus foods tend to increase saliva; may be avoided for children with excessive drooling.
2. Milk tends to thicken saliva; broth tends to thin it.
3. Thin liquids are hard to manage orally; thicker liquids such as shakes or "smoothies" are easier to swallow.
4. Combinations of textures, such as soup with noodles, are hard to handle; they should be blended.
5. Slightly cooked vegetables are easier to chew than raw ones.
6. Avoid foods that could block the airway, such as hot dogs, foods with skin, unmashed grapes, and food in chunks.
7. Keep cold foods cold and hot foods hot so that the child can experience temperature differences; be careful not to overstimulate child with foods that are very hot or very cold.
8. A balanced diet is a must for any child's health. Vitamin supplements may be necessary and can be added to food.

Equipment for Feeding

1. Towels and washcloths for cleaning child.
2. Teflon-coated spoon with a shallow bowl to prevent pain if child bites hard.
3. Cup with soft plastic rim; cup should be as big around as child's mouth is when open.
4. Equipment to maintain food temperature if feeding takes a long time.

Positioning

1. Hips and knees at 90-degree angles when seated.
2. Feet supported.
3. Shoulders slightly forward and arms supported.
4. Spine straight.
5. Head at midline and slightly forward.
6. Knees slightly apart.

BOX 6-4   **Considerations in Feeding Older Prelinguistic Children—cont'd**

Developing Cup-Drinking Skills

1. Introduce cup outside of mealtime in playful situations.
2. Let child play with empty cup.
3. Rub a preferred taste on rim of cup and allow child to mouth it.
4. Introduce thickened liquid in cup, resting cup on lower lip in front of teeth; do not tip at more than a 20-degree angle. Be sure lips are closed before beginning.
5. Let child use upper lip to suck liquid from cup; be careful not to dump liquid in the child's mouth.
6. To increase stability and facilitate mouth closure and upper lip movement, place middle finger under chin and gently push up while placing index finger or thumb on bottom edge of lower lip and gently pushing up.

Developing Spoon-Feeding Skills

1. Use adaptive positioning for comfort and stability.
2. Introduce spoon outside mealtime in playful situation, such as pretending to feed doll.
3. Let child play with empty spoon.
4. When child tolerates spoon, dip it in food with a preferred taste.
5. Present spoon to lips or front of mouth. Let child use upper lip movement to remove food from spoon. Do not dump food in child's mouth.
6. If tongue protrudes or child shows low facial tone, apply pressure down on middle of tongue with the spoon and withdraw it at a neutral angle, being careful not to scrape the spoon upward.
7. Use support to jaw or chin to increase stability, permit graduated jaw movement, and allow child to use upper lip movement to close on spoon.
8. When child accepts food from spoon, gradually increase textures presented.

Developing Chewing Skills

1. Stimulate a munching pattern by presenting crunchy solid foods between molar surfaces. Look for up-and-down movement of the jaw.
2. Facilitate lateral tongue and jaw movements by stroking the side of the tongue with a solid food, then place the food between the molar surfaces.
3. Stimulate chewing during eating by rubbing the child's cheeks, one at a time, in a circular motion.
4. Provide jaw and chin support (as previously described) to reduce tongue protrusion and facilitate graduated jaw movement.
5. As child develops more control, place food closer to front of mouth.

Cautions

1. The possibility of choking is always present. Practice feeding techniques, use care in choosing foods that will be easy for child to manage orally, and know first aid procedures in case choking occurs.
2. Seizures may occur during eating. If they do, stop feeding and wait until seizure is under control. Check to see whether any food is in mouth during and after seizure.
3. Look for abnormal feeding behaviors, such as those identified by Jaffe (1989) and listed in the following:
   a. **Tongue thrust:** abnormal protrusion of tongue.
   b. **Tongue retraction:** strong pulling back of tongue to pharyngeal space.
   c. **Jaw thrust:** abnormally forceful downward extension of mandible.
   d. **Lip retraction:** drawing the lips back so that they make a tight line over the mouth.
   e. **Lip pursing:** a tight protrusion of the lips.
   f. **Tonic bite reflex:** an abnormally strong closure of the teeth or gums when stimulated.
   g. **Jaw clenching:** an abnormally tight closure of the mouth.

If these occur, specialized physiological feeding assessments may be necessary.

Adapted from Hall, S., Circello, N., Reed, P., & Hylton, J. (1987). *Considerations for feeding children who have a neuromuscular disorder.* Portland, OR: CARC Publications; McGowan, J., & Kerwin, M. (1993). Oral motor and feeding problems. In K. Bleile (Ed.), *The care of children with long-term tracheostomies* (pp. 157-195). San Diego, CA: Singular Publishing Group.

hearing should always be assessed. In addition, encouraging vocalization should be part of the intervention plan. As with any intervention developed for the infant, the family must be involved and will probably be the ones to deliver the intervention. Encouraging vocalization in an infant is an activity in which all family members, even siblings, can engage. The family should be encouraged both to talk and to babble to the baby. The clinician can demonstrate the kinds of vocalizations that the infant is ready to learn to produce. These can be identified from the form in Figure 6-1 by choosing vocal behaviors that are produced rarely or not at all but are at the stage into which the child is emerging. For a child emerging into stage 2, for example, who is currently producing only /a/ and /u/ vowels, the clinician can demonstrate the other vowels that are appropriate at this level, such as /I/ and /i/, and can encourage everyone in the family to babble and sing these vowels to the baby.

If the baby is producing a very low frequency of comfort vocalization in general, the clinician can encourage everyone in the family to imitate any comfort vocalization the baby produces, anywhere, anytime. McGowan et al. (1993) also suggested encouraging parents to greet the child each time they come together and to say good-bye each time they part. Babies can be encouraged to make eye contact during these greetings. McGowan et al. also suggested using rattles, tickling games, and mirrors to elicit infant vocalization. For any baby with deficits in vocal development, all family members can be encouraged to talk "baby talk" to the baby as often as possible. If family members are uncomfortable with or not proficient in baby talk, the clinician can teach baby-talk register—including high-pitched speech; exaggerated intonation; simple words; and short, repetitive sentences—directly through modeling. Alternatively, some of the parent education sources discussed in the next section can be used.

HEARING CONSERVATION AND AURAL HABILITATION

It is important to monitor hearing closely in the high-risk infant. Hearing should be evaluated by an audiologist every 3 to 6 months during the first year. Further, parents should be counseled to be aware of signs of otitis media, such as pulling on the ear or jaw, fever, or unexplained fussiness accompanying a cold. They should be encouraged to have the baby visit the pediatrician if any of these signs occur so that otitis media can be treated early and aggressively. If the otitis becomes chronic, the SLP should encourage the parents to ask the physician about additional treatments, such as antibiotic prophylaxis or myringotomy tubes, to control the episodes. For infants with identified hearing impairments, use and maintenance of hearing aids is, of course, crucial to optimal communicative development. Some of these children will be candidates for cochlear implants. According to Chute and Nevins (2003) good candidates for cochlear implants are children who meet the following criteria:

▶ Have profound hearing loss in both ears
▶ Can receive little or no useful benefit from hearing aids

▶ Have no other medical conditions that would make the surgery risky
▶ Have families who are involved in all aspects of the informed consent process, understand their roles in successful use of cochlear implants, have realistic expectations for cochlear implant use and are willing to be involved in intensive rehabilitation services
▶ Have support from their educational program to emphasize the development of auditory skills

Research has demonstrated that for children with appropriate candidate status, cochlear implantation before 2 years of age promotes the efficient acquisition of expressive language (Ertmer et al., 2002), as well as receptive language and speech intelligibility (Peng, Spencer, & Tomblin, 2004). Some studies suggest that these children's language development approximates the normal rate (Ertmer, Strong, & Sadagopan, 2003). For these reasons, it is important that SLPs discuss implantation with families of young children with severe hearing losses. Implantations, as of this writing, are frequently done between 14 and 24 months of age. Detailed information on cochlear implants can be obtained from ASHA's (2004b) *Technical Report on Cochlear Implants.*

CHILD BEHAVIOR AND DEVELOPMENT

Assessment

For many high-risk infants, the management plan contains ongoing follow-up assessment of behavior and development. For some babies, ongoing assessment is the sole component of the intervention. When we assess infant development we need to remember, again, that the goal is not to predict future status but only to identify current strengths and needs. A variety of instruments are available for assessing early development. The *Bayley Scales of Infant Development-III* (Bayley, 2005) and the *Mullen Scales of Early Learning* (Mullen, 1995) are perhaps most widely used. These scales sample behavior in several domains: cognitive, language, motor, social-emotional, and adaptive behavior on the *Bayley*, and verbal, nonverbal, and motor on the *Mullen*. Infants can receive credit for behaviors observed directly or reported by parents. The *Vineland Adaptive Behavior Scales—II* (Sparrow, Cicchetti, & Balla, 2005), a parent-interview instrument, can be used with children from birth to assess communicative, social, self-help, and motor development areas. Areas identified in the assessment can be used to develop intervention plans that are suggested in the expanded form of the interview. The *Denver II* (Frankenburg et al., 1990) is a direct assessment often used by pediatricians in their offices to assess development. The WILSTAAR screener (Alston & James-Roberts, 2005; Ward, 1999) is another instrument with some potential for this purpose. A more comprehensive list of infant assessment instruments appears in Table 6-2. In addition to general developmental assessment instruments, several instruments are designed to look more specifically at early communicative and vocal behavior. A sampling of these is presented in Table 6-6.

TABLE 6-6	**A Sample of Language Assessment Tools for Infants in the Prelinguistic Period**

TITLE	COMMENTS
Assessing Linguistic Behavior (ALB) (Olswang, Stoel-Gammon, Coggins, & Carpenter, 1987)	Ages birth to 2 yr; observational and structured scales; includes assessment in cognitive antecedents, play, communicative intention, language production, and comprehension
Assessment, Evaluation, and Programming System for Infants and Children (ed. 2) (Bricker, 2002)	Criterion-referenced assessment, evaluation and family participation components; measures abilities in the following areas: fine and gross motor skills, adaptive, cognitive, and social communication development; also includes a Family Report Measure for parents to assess their children.
Birth to Three Assessment and Intervention System (ed. 2) (Ammer & Bangs, 2000)	Comprehensive program that allows examiners to identify, measure, and address developmental delays; includes a norm-referenced screening test and a criterion-referenced checklist; measures receptive and expressive language, avenues for learning, social-emotional development and motor ability.
*British Picture Vocabulary Scale—*2nd Edition (BPVS II) (Dunn, Dunn, Whetton, & Burley, 1997)	Quick, easy measure to assess a child's understanding of English vocabulary; individually administered picture-based test of receptive vocabulary; does not require reading, writing, or spelling.
Clinical Linguistic and Auditory Milestone Scale (Capute, Palmer, Shapiro, Wachtel, Schmidt, & Ross, 1986)	Assessment of behaviors and infant communication skills
Communication and Symbolic Behavior Scale (CSBS) (Wetherby & Prizant, 1993)	Used to provide early identification of children at risk for having or developing communication impairment; examines and measures communication, social-affective, and symbolic abilities; results are used to monitor changes in behavior and plan treatment.
Early Language Milestones Scale (ed. 2) (Coplan, 1993)	Assesses auditory, receptive language, expressive language, and visual skills and development; passing criterion for this test is noted as liberal, and failure of this test is recognized as severe impairment.
MacArthur-Bates Communicative Development Inventories (Fenson, Dale, Reznick, Thal, Bates, Hartung, Pethick, & Reilly, 1993)	Parent-report instruments used to determine child's comprehension and production vocabularies for children using words and gestures, and production vocabulary for children using word combinations; assessment of early child language from first nonverbal gestural signals through expansion of early vocabulary and the beginning of grammar.
*Pediatric Language Acquisition Screening Tool for Early Referral—*Revised (Shulman & Sherman, 1996)	Designed to identify potential communication problems in at-risk children; uses parent report.
*Receptive-Expressive Emergent Language Scale—*3rd Edition (REEL-3) (Bzoch, League, & Brown, 2003)	Designed to identify major receptive and expressive language problems in infants and toddlers.
Rossetti Infant and Toddler Language Scale (Rossetti, 1990)	Developed for birth to 3-year-olds; includes parent questionnaire and test protocol to gather observed, elicited, and parent-report information; areas assessed include play, interaction-attachment, gesture, pragmatics, language comprehension and expression; also includes questionnaire and addresses parental concerns regarding interaction and communication development.
*Sequenced Inventory of Communicative Development—*Revised (SICD-R) (Hedrick, Prather, & Tobin, 1995)	Designed to evaluate expressive and receptive communication abilities of children with and without retardation who are functioning between 4 mo and 4 yr of age; SICD-R can also be used in remedial programming for children with language disorders, mental retardation, and specific language problems.

Any of these instruments can be used to get a picture of where the child is functioning in terms of general and communicative development. For children whose general developmental level or level of communication appears to be behind what would be expected for chronological age (or for corrected gestational age in the case of premature babies), a general stimulation program to enhance motor and cognitive development may be initiated. Such a program would be implemented in collaboration with a team of professionals that might include a physical therapist, occupational therapist, special educator, and nurse.

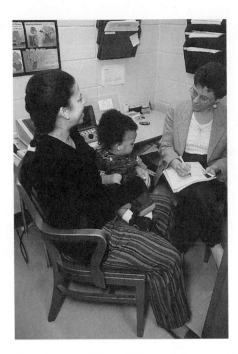

Parent interviews provide useful information about infant communication and development.

Management

The management of behavior and development is, again, a team effort focused on the family as well as the child. Some localities provide center-based infant stimulation programs that place the baby in a setting with other handicapped or at-risk infants. These programs provide general motor and cognitive stimulation as well as more specialized services designed to target gross motor, fine motor, and oral-motor behavior. When these programs are used, the SLP may be called upon to develop a plan for oral-motor development, including some of the elements already discussed, as well as to provide communicative intervention, which focuses on the interaction patterns discussed in the next section.

Most services for infants at this stage will be home-based, however. Rossetti (2001) discussed the efficacy of home-based treatment for infants and reported the Infant Health and Development Project finding that highly positive outcomes result from this model. When services are home-based the SLP will, again, be a member of a team providing counseling and advice to the parents of the at-risk infant. When the team uses an interdisciplinary or multidisciplinary approach, SLPs may visit homes themselves and provide direct consultation to families. In settings using a transdisciplinary model, the SLP may provide information to another professional who will work directly with the family to implement the SLP's plan. Either way, the SLP can play an important role in emphasizing the relatedness of motor, cognitive, and communicative development. The language pathologist can stress to the parents that all the activities the other specialists suggest should be presented in the context of back-and-forth, warm, affectionate communication. If this communicative aspect of the intervention is lost, it can become a lifeless exercise for both parents and child. The SLP can help to remind everyone on the team, parents and professionals alike, that babies develop within the context of human communication and that this communication is what makes entrance into the human community possible.

Another important function the SLP can fulfill in the home-based interdisciplinary program for the at-risk infant is to serve as coordinator and parent advocate. The team approach provides a broad range of expertise to the family. It also can mean that the family must deal with a lot of different people, each with a different personality and style and each offering different advice. Imagine how a new mother of a handicapped or at-risk baby must feel in this situation. She's just brought her sick baby home from the hospital. The physical therapist visits her and tells her to do exercises with the baby. The nurse tells her to be sure to give the baby medication on time. The occupational therapist tells her to position the baby a certain way for feeding. The physician has told her to watch for a set of danger signs. She's worried and frightened and wonders how she can follow everyone's prescriptions and still care for her other children, manage her household, and do whatever else she did before the baby came. The multitude of professionals inundating her with advice and assignments can be overwhelming, especially in a situation already fraught with worry.

SLPs can take on the role of putting this all in context. We can help the parents sort through the advice; decide on an overall schedule for delivering therapy and medication to the baby; and help the mother seek support from her network of resources, including family, neighbors, and friends, to get her through the difficult first few months. Most importantly, perhaps, the SLP can remind the mother that what the baby needs most is the same thing every other baby needs—to be loved and played with. Further, the baby needs a family that is healthy and rested. If that means skipping the baby's exercises once in a while so that the mother can take a nap, there is always tomorrow. The SLP's awareness of the importance of affective communication as the basis of the baby's development can help us to integrate the information the family receives about their at-risk baby and to put it in perspective. In a transdisciplinary team setting, the SLP can emphasize this perspective to team members and encourage the case manager to communicate it to the family.

PARENT-CHILD COMMUNICATION

Assessment

The *Parent-Infant Relationships Global Assessment Scale* (Aoki, Iseharashi, Heller, & Bakshi, 2002), the *Parent Behavior Progression* (Bromwich et al., 1981), and the *Observation of Communicative Interaction* (Klein & Briggs, 1987) were discussed earlier as means of assessing parent-child interactions. The *Parent-Child Play Scale* (Dunst, 1986a), the *Parent-Child Interaction Scale* (Farran, Kasari, & Jay, 1983), and the *Caregiver Styles of Interaction Scale* (Dunst, 1986b) are additional instruments that can be used to rate parental communication. These are somewhat formalized means of looking at how parents interact with the young baby who is not yet initiating much communication but is beginning to be able to respond consistently to the interactions of the family.

Parent-child interaction also can be assessed informally. When observing parents interacting with their at-risk babies, we can look for the following:

1. Pleasure and positive affect.
2. Responsiveness to the child's cues of readiness and unreadiness to interact.
3. Acceptance of the baby's overall style and temperament.
4. Reciprocity and mutuality—the degree to which the parent and infant seem to be in tune with each other.
5. Appropriateness of choice of objects and activities for interactions; the parent's awareness of safety issues and choice of activities and objects that interest and engage the baby.
6. Language stimulation and responsiveness; the degree to which the mother talks to the baby appropriately, engages in back-and-forth and "choral" babbling activities.
7. Encouragement of joint attention and scaffolding the baby's participation, the extent to which the mother is effective in directing the baby's attention to objects of mutual interest, and the ways she evokes progressively more elaborated responses from the baby.

Establishing which aspects of parent-child interaction can be improved can serve as the basis for the intervention program designed to facilitate parent-infant communication. It is crucial to remember, though, that when assessing parent-child interaction patterns, we must show respect and appreciation of the parent's attempts to get through to the child. If we behave as if we know better than the parents how to interact with this baby, we will be undermining rather than supporting them.

But it is important to know, as Whitehurst et al. (1988) pointed out, that even normal parent-child interactions may not be optimal. In other words, it is always possible to intensify and increase the frequency of parental input, even when the parent is doing everything right. The stance we want to project to the parents of a handicapped or at-risk infant is that of maximizing the parents' effectiveness, rather than correcting their mistakes. We want the parents to feel that they are partners in providing an enhanced communicative environment for their child and that we are simply making some suggestions for that enhancement. Using data from the assessment of parent-child interactions can help us to identify *with the parent* the aspects of the interaction that can be enhanced. This approach is greatly preferable to using the assessment to identify what the parent is doing wrong. Everything we discussed in the newborn section about the dangers of formal assessment of parent-child communication and family function applies to the older baby, too.

Management

Intervention in the area of parent-infant communication, in either a home- or center-based setting, involves three components. First, we need to make parents and other caregivers aware of the normal communicative patterns of infants and how to tune in to the baby's communicative capacities. Second, we need to provide instruction and modeling of adult-infant communi-

cation. Third, we need to help the parents develop self-monitoring skills so that they can evaluate and modify their own performance.

Awareness of Infant Communication Patterns. Communication with babies is a two-way street. Mothers tend to interact more frequently with and respond more consistently to babies who smile and vocalize at them more often (Clarke-Stewart, 1977; Rossetti, 2001). So if a parent seems unresponsive to the baby, our first task is to remind ourselves that the mother's earlier communicative attempts may have been extinguished by a lack of consistent response from the child. Communication may have to be reinvigorated, no matter whose behavior is extinguishing whose. But we should refrain from being too quick to blame the parent for the dyad's failure to achieve optimal communication. Parents are more likely to cooperate if they feel that we understand the difficulties of communicating with an at-risk baby, who may not be normally responsive and interactive. If the parents feel they are being blamed for the child's problem, collaboration is more difficult.

Remember, too, that we don't always have to say out loud that we blame the parents. Even unspoken censure can be perceived by parents. However, by reassuring the parent explicitly and repeatedly that we know that communicating with this baby can be hard, we can protect against the potential of this unspoken disapproval to interfere with our relationship with the parent. By acknowledging the difficulty of communicating with the child, we tell parents that we know they are not to blame, that the child participates in forming the quality of the interaction, that it takes two to tango. With this acknowledgment, we can get on cooperatively with the difficult job of providing a mutually positive communicative environment for the parent and child.

Helping parents become aware of basic interactive patterns of preintentional infants can be part of a general program of parent education, involving direct instruction about infant development and directed observation of videotapes or live interactions between infants and caregivers. Many parent education materials, including videotapes, are available for this purpose. Some of these are listed in Tables 6-7 and 6-8. Parent education also can be a more circumscribed exercise, in which the SLP provides information specifically about communication to the infant's family. Either way, we want parents to know several things about how babies communicate. First, we want them to know that although the infant participates in structuring the interaction, the infant—because of his or her immaturity—has very little choice about how to interact. The infant is not choosing to be difficult or consciously rejecting the parents' advances. Infants are simply expressing their inborn style, as well as their physiological and neurological immaturity in these behaviors. The preintentional infant does not "mean" to be naughty. The parent, though, as a mature adult, has choices. Parents need to know that they are the ones who need to adapt for the interaction to succeed, even when it is the infant who is causing the problem by being difficult or unresponsive.

Second, the parents need to know that the most important thing they can do for their babies is to enjoy them. Whatever they and the baby like to do together is what constitutes an

TABLE 6-7   Training Resources for Parents of Preintentional Infants

RESOURCE	SOURCE	COMMENTS
Baby Signals (book)	Lynch-Fraser, D., & Tiegerman, E. (1987). New York: Walker and Co.	Helps parents learn to identify infant states and learning styles.
The Carolina Curriculum for Infants and Toddlers with Special Needs (ed. 3) (book)	Johnson-Martin, N., Hacker, B., & Attermeier, S. (2004). Baltimore, MD: Paul H. Brookes	Provides comprehensive information on facilitating feeding and communicative development for infants and toddlers with a variety of handicapping conditions.
Curriculum Guide: Hearing-Impaired Children—Birth to Three Years—and Their Parents (book)	Northcott, W. (1977). Revised Edition. Washington, DC: Alexander Graham Bell Association for the Deaf	Comprehensive infant program focuses on home-centered, parent-guided, natural language approach to learning that is based on child's daily activities.
Developmental Communication Curriculum (book)	Hanna, R.M., Lippert, E.A., & Harris, A.B. (1982). Columbus, OH: Charles E. Merrill	Curriculum intended to help extend prelinguistic communication skills on which language is based; uses play as natural context for learning; includes parent information.
Developmental Play Group Guide	Browne, B., Jarrett, M., Hvey-Lewis, C., & Freund, M. (1997). Austin, TX: Pro-Ed	Manual contains group-lesson plans to give parents the information they need to guide the development of their birth to 12-month-old infants; lessons cover communication, cognition, and developmental play intervention.
Ecological Communication Organization (Becoming partners with children: From play to conversation) (book)	MacDonald, J. (1989). San Antonio, TX: Special Press	Helps parents establish a balanced, responsive, and matched social relationship with preverbal children.
Exceptional Children Conference Papers: Parent Participation in Early Childhood Education (collection of papers)	Council for Exceptional Children. (1969). Reston, VA: Author	One area covered is programs for training mothers to instruct their infants at home.
"Family Administered Neonatal Activities" (journal article)	Cordone, I., & Gilkerson, L. (1989). *Zero to Three, 10,* 23-28	Involves parents in observing and interpreting newborn's actions and reactions.
"Hanen Early Language Parent Program" (journal article)	Girolametto, L., Greenberg, J., & Manolson, H. (1986). *Seminars in Speech and Language, 7,* 367-382	Teaches families to develop dialogue skills by responding contingently to children and to increase opportunities for communication by planning play activities with communication goals in mind.
Illinois Early Learning Project Tip Sheets: Language Arts	Illinois Early Learning Project http://www.illinoisearlylearning.org	Easy-printing pages are available as Web pages and as PDF files. Tip sheets related to promoting pre-literacy skills and conversation.
Infant Learning: A Cognitive, Linguistic Intervention Strategy (book)	Dunst, C.J. (1981). Allen, TX: DLM/Teaching Resources	Intended for use by teachers, therapists, and child-care workers; three phases are response-contingent behaviors, sensorimotor abilities, and early cognitive-linguistic abilities.
It Takes Two To Talk: A Practical Guide for Parents of Children with Language Delays (ed. 3) (book)	Pepper, J., & Weitzman, E. (2004). Toronto, Canada: The Hanen Centre	Helps parents of children with language delays to promote their child's communication and language development in everyday conversations, daily routines, play activities, music, book reading, and art activities.
Learning Language and Loving It (ed. 2) (book)	Weitzman, E., & Greenbar, J. (2002). Toronto, Canada: The Hanen Centre	Provides guidelines for developing language in everyday activities. French and Korean version available for 1st ed.
Making the Connections that Help Children Communicate (workbook)	Hanen Centre. (2000). Toronto, Canada: Author	Summarizes the Hanen approach in a workbook format. Teaching aid to support a one-day workshop for parents awaiting speech-language pathology services.

TABLE 6-7	Training Resources for Parents of Preintentional Infants—cont'd

RESOURCE	SOURCE	COMMENTS
More Than Words: Helping Parents Promote Communication and Social Skills in Children with Autism Spectrum Disorder (book)	Sussman, F. (1999). Toronto, Canada: The Hanen Centre	Guidebook for parents of children with autistic spectrum disorder. Contains descriptions of strategies drawn from current research, which are known to help children with autism develop more advanced communication skills. See accompanying videos listed in Table 6-8.
Parent Articles for Early Intervention (book)	Dunn Klein, M., ed. (1990). Austin, TX: Pro-Ed.	102 articles that provide parents with practical information on therapeutic ways to interact with their special-needs child.
"Parenting a Hearing-Impaired Child" (journal article)	Northcott, W. (1973). *Hearing and Speech News, 41*, 10-12, 28-29	Systems approach to parental participation, aids for parents.
Parent-Infant Communication (ed. 4). (book)	Schuyler, V., & Sowers, J. (1998). Hearing and Speech Institute: Portland, OR	Curriculum for hearing-impaired with objectives in auditory development, presymbolic communication, and receptive and expressive language; helps parents become accurate reporters and coordinate services for their child.
Promoting Communication in Infants and Young Children (book)	Quick, J., & O'Neal, A. (1997). Vero Beach, FL: The Speech Bin	500 activities and suggestions for promoting communication development in infants and young children.
Reach Out and Teach (book)	Ferrell, K. (1985). New York: American Foundation for the Blind	Two volumes: *Parent Handbook* and *Reach*; contains chapter on "Daily Living and Communicating" (eating skills are a topic in this chapter).
Since Owen: Parent-to-Parent Guide for Care of the Disabled Child (book)	Callanan, C. (1990). Baltimore, MD: The Johns Hopkins University Press	Discusses raising a disabled child from before birth through life in the adult world.
Speech and Language Handouts Resource Guide (ed. 2)	Brooks, M., & Hartung, D. (2000). Austin, TX: Pro-Ed	Tear-off sheets that clinicians, physicians, speech pathologists, pediatricians, and others can give to parents who are concerned about their child's speech and language development. Spanish edition also available.
Talk to Me: A Language Guide for Parents of Blind Children *Talk to Me II: Common Concerns*	Kekelis, L., Chernus-Mansfield, N., & Hayashi, D. (1984). Los Angeles, CA: The Blind Children's' Center	Two pamphlets with some suggestions to encourage language development.
Talk! Talk! Talk! Tools to Facilitate Language	Muir, N., McCaig, S., Gerylo, K., Gompf, M., Burke, T, & Lumsden, P. (2000). Eau Claire, WI: Thinking Publications	Birth to 10 yr. Strategies for listening and talking to teach to caregivers.
Take Home: Preschool Language Development (book)	Drake, M. (1998). East Moline, IL: LinguiSystems	Designed for parents of children from 1 to 6 yr of age who have communication disorders. Includes lesson plans and activities.
Teach Your Child to Talk (revised ed.) (book)	Pushaw, D. (1976). New York: Dantree Press	Manual; slide; cassette tape; movie; parent handbook; and *Teach Me to Talk*, a booklet for parents of newborns.
The Exceptional Parent (magazine)	Johnstown, PA	Practical information for parents of handicapped children. Also see www.eparent.com.
The Portage Guide to Early Education (revised ed.) (kit)	The Portage Project (2003). Portage, WI: Cooperative Educational Services (CES)	For mental ages birth to 5 yr; two parts: checklist of behaviors and card file; five developmental areas: cognitive, self-help, motor, language, socialization. Also available in Spanish.
"Tips for Parents" (magazine column)	Lawrence, G. (1991). *Exceptional Parent, 21*, 54	Tips for feeding disabled children who have a G-tube or who are developmentally delayed.
"Training Prerequisites to Verbal Behavior" (chapter)	Bricker, D., & Dennison, L. (1978). *Systematic instruction of the moderately and severely handicapped* (pp. 155-178). Columbus, OH: Charles Merrill	Gives behaviors preliminary to formal language development; strategies included for on-task behavior, imitation, discriminate use of objects, and word recognition.

TABLE 6-7	Training Resources for Parents of Preintentional Infants—cont'd	
RESOURCE	**SOURCE**	**COMMENTS**
Transactional Intervention Program (book)	Mahoney, G., & Powell, A. (1986). Farmington, CT: Pediatric Research and Training Center, University of Connecticut Health Center	A home-based program that helps parents to develop a responsive style of interaction with children with developmental delays from birth to 3 yr.
You Make The Difference: In Helping Your Child Learn (book and video)	Manolson, A., Ward, B., & Dodington, N., (1995). Toronto, Canada: The Hanen Centre	Helps parents connect in encouraging a child's self-esteem and learning.
Your Child's Speech & Language	Brooks, M. (1978). Austin, TX: Pro-Ed	Provides information about speech and language development from infancy through 5 yr.
When Your Child Has a Disability: The Complete Sourcebook of Daily and Medical Care, revised ed. (book)	Batshaw, M. (2002). Baltimore, MD: Paul H. Brookes	Offers expert advice on a range of issues, including doctors, care techniques, and fulfilling educational requirements.

TABLE 6-8	Videos for Training Parents of Infants	
TITLE	**SOURCE**	**COMMENTS**
Baby Speech: An adult's Guide to Helping Your Little One Communicate	Chatterbox Communications Available through Speech Bin	Produced in 2001 and written by Castillo, G.R., & Ramsay, J. 40 minutes. Teaches parents simple techniques to promote speech.
Communicating Effectively with Young Children	Communication Therapy Skill Builders (A Division of the Psychological Corporation) 555 Academic Court San Antonio, TX 78204	Gives families effective communication strategies for use with children who have communicative, physical, social, or cognitive impairments. Teaches, illustrates, and models routines and communication strategies for parental interaction with the child.
Family-Guided Activity-Based Intervention for Infants and Toddlers	Brookes Publishing PO Box 10624 Baltimore, MD 21285	Will help parents with daily routines and activities to foster skill development in young children with special needs.
Feeding Skills: Your Baby's Early Years	Churchill Films 662 North Robertson Blvd. Los Angeles, CA 90069	How and why babies feed as they do; breastfeeding, transition to spoon feeding, home preparation of food, finger feeding.
Growing Together	American Guidance Service 4201 Woodland Rd. Circle Pines, MN 55014	Designed to provide teen parents with practical information on understanding and caring for infants.
Human Development: The First Two-and-One-Half Years: Program 7—Language	Concept Media PO Box 19542 Irvine, CA 92713	Stages in child language development are illustrated: cries of hunger, discomfort, fear; cooing, babbling, first words.
Human Development: A New Look at the Infant: Program 4—Infant Communication	Concept Media PO Box 19542 Irvine, CA 92713	Describes process of communication, three components that form basic structure of communication, and forerunners of full-fledged communication.
Human Development: The First Two-and-One-Half Years: Program 3—The Development of Understanding	Concept Media PO Box 19542 Irvine, CA 92713	Piaget's observations of infant development are discussed; infants actively seek information and absorb information gained.
Making the Most of Early Communication: Strategies for Supporting Communication with Infants, Toddlers, and Preschoolers Whose Multiple Disabilities Include Vision and Hearing Loss	Deborah Chen & Pamela Haag Schachter AFB Press American Foundation for the Blind PO Box 1020 Sewickey, PA	This 37-minute video demonstrates selected interventions to assist infants and toddlers with multiple disabilities, including vision and hearing loss, in developing early communication and other skills.

TABLE 6-8	**Videos for Training Parents of Infants—cont'd**	
TITLE	**SOURCE**	**COMMENTS**
More Than Words (introductory video and teaching tape)	Hanen Centre Suite 515, 1075 Bay Street Toronto, Ontario Canada M5S 2B1 www.hanen.org	Demonstrations of techniques described in the guidebook (see Table 6-7). Introductory video is 20 minutes, teaching video is 120 minutes.
Observing and Enhancing Communication Skills: For Individuals with Multisensory Impairments	Concept Media PO Box 19542 Irvine, CA 92713	Teaches parents how to observe, analyze, and enhance communication skills in children who have vision and hearing impairments or multiple disabilities.
On This Journey Together (4-video set)	Family First and Ohio Department of Mental Retardation and Developmental Disabilities	Parents speak about their experiences in raising a child with developmental disabilities.
Premie Potential: Improving the NICU Environment of the Premature Infant	Communication Skill Builders 3830 E. Bellevue PO Box 42050-P93 Tucson, AZ 85733	Gives how-to's on approaching the infant, determining levels of stimulation, teaching parents interaction skills, making the infant's world as pleasant and nurturing as possible.
Sharing Books with Babies: Promoting Early Literacy in Early Care and Education	Margot Kaplan-Sanoff Boston Medical Center One Boston Medical Center Place Maternity 5 Boston, MA 02118	The video demonstrates the following: (1) the developmental stages of early literacy growth in the first 5 yr of life, (2) examples of early literacy-promoting activities which can be used throughout the day, and (3) literacy rich home- and center-based environments for infants, toddlers, and preschoolers.
Successfully Parenting Your Baby with Special Needs: Early Intervention for Ages Birth to Three	Produced by Grace Hanlon, M.S. 1999 Brookes Publishing PO Box 10624 Baltimore, MD 21285	Gives first-time parents of infants with special needs a full introduction to the early intervention process. Covers diagnoses and referral, evaluation criteria, IFSPs, community resources, and transitions.
Your Baby and You: Understanding Your Baby's Behavior	Communication Skill Builders 3830 E. Bellevue PO Box 42050-P93 Tucson, AZ 85733	Helps parents understand and respond to their infant in the NICU; shows parents what to expect as their baby develops and how they can provide a sensitive environment; available in English and Spanish.

ideal interactive context. If they enjoy making silly faces or funny noises or swinging the baby around, these activities should be encouraged. Similarly, if the baby's siblings like jostling the baby and the baby giggles and coos, these activities, too, should be fostered, even if they make the parents a little nervous. A bit of extra watchfulness, rather than a prohibition on these sibling interactions, may be needed.

The third thing we want parents to know is that communication that enhances development has two major characteristics: it is *enriching* and *responsive* (Clarke-Stewart, 1973; Poehlmann & Fiese, 2001). This means that as they interact with their high-risk babies, parents should think about providing visual, auditory, and tactile experiences that engage the baby's attention and allow the child to explore novel stimuli that have been carefully chosen for safety and interest. They also should attempt to make their interactions responsive to and contingent on what the infant is doing. This involves needing to tune in to the baby to observe and learn to recognize the baby's signals of need for attention and readiness for interaction. Some parents may need to be educated about the

impossibility of "spoiling" the preintentional infant. Parents need to know that being consistently responsive to the infant's cries and moods at this stage can only enhance development.

Modeling Interactive Behaviors. Four types of interactive behaviors should be encouraged in parents to foster communication with their infants. These are: *turn-taking, imitation, establishing joint attention,* and *developing anticipatory sets.* Gazdag and Warren (2000) showed that adult contingent vocal imitation, particularly, increased the amount of imitation produced by babies with developmental disabilities. These behaviors can first be observed by the parents, using videotapes if they are available. If not, the clinician can provide models directly.

Effective modeling of turn-taking, imitation, and establishing joint attention and anticipatory sets involves, first, being sure that the parent is sensitive to the infant's readiness to interact. It will not be possible to set aside a particular time of day for these activities. The parent must be prepared to engage in them whenever the infant signals readiness through a state of alertness, gaze at the parent, and the expression of comfort vocalizations. When these signals are perceived, the interactions should be initiated. So it is important to be sure parents can recognize and respond to these signs when they occur. Parents should be reminded that these signals can come at any time—during meals, diapering, at bath time, or during a myriad of ordinary daily living routines. Parents can be encouraged to take advantage of the baby's alertness whenever they observe it and can be helped to learn to integrate ordinary caretaking activities with interactive stimulation.

Once parents can recognize the baby's readiness to interact, the four aspects of interaction can be modeled by the clinician. We can use the acronym TIPS to help with this modeling (Box 6-5). To model *turn-taking* and *imitation,* we can demonstrate observing the infant; using smiles and vocalization to elicit infant behavior; and waiting while the infant performs some behavior, whether it be vocalizing, moving the limbs, or making a face. Once the infant does something, the clinician can imitate it, then wait for the infant to do something else. MacDonald's ECO program (see Table 6-7) for example, encourages parents to use a "match and wait" strategy in developing turn-taking and imitation skills. Parents are advised to imitate or "match" something the child does, then wait for the child to provide a response that the parent can "match" again. The parent can be encouraged to try this turn-taking and imitation while the infant remains in an alert state. Vocalization to the infant and imitation of infant vocalization should be particularly encouraged, since these are especially helpful techniques for encouraging infant vocal development.

In addition to fostering turn-taking and imitation skills, it is important to help parents learn to develop *joint attentional routines* with their babies. Bruner (1981) emphasized the importance of establishing joint attention to help the baby learn to share focus on a topic and elaborate on it. This ability to share a topic and make additional comments upon it lays the basis for the topic-comment structure of mature conversation, in which a shared topic is established, then elaborated on by additional comments from the participants.

The establishment of joint attention can begin by modeling for the parent how to identify the infant's focus and share

attention to that. The clinician can show the parent how to follow the infant's line of regard, look at what he or she is looking at, and then make a comment about it or a gesture toward it. For example, we can demonstrate looking at the baby's hands as the baby focuses on them. We can then say, "Hands. You have such little hands!" and gently stroke them as the baby continues to regard them. If the baby's gaze then shifts to the clinician's face, we can return the gaze and remark, "I see you, too!" The clinician can then introduce an attractive toy and demonstrate showing it to the baby to engage his or her attention. When the baby looks at it or reaches for it, the clinician can demonstrate commenting on it or using it in a new way. In this way the clinician can model establishing joint attentional activities with the infant. "Choral" vocalization, saying what the infant says at the same time he or she says it, as if singing together, also can be encouraged as a joint attentional activity.

Another joint attentional activity that can be fostered is the use of baby games. These games also are useful in *establishing anticipatory sets.* Anticipatory sets are expectations that actions that have been repeated often for the baby will occur in a particular sequence, so that the infant "gets ready" to observe them when part of the sequence is enacted. These anticipatory sets provide the baby with predictable series of sound and action that lay the basis for the development of knowledge of scripts or schemata. It is thought that these scripts help organize knowledge and the acquisition of language used to encode this knowledge (see Milosky, 1990, for further discussion). "Peek-a-boo," "gonna getcha," and other games that foster predictable series of actions and words are especially useful in laying the groundwork in this process. By observing the parent repeatedly reenact the same actions using the same words, the infant learns to anticipate the climax of the routine. This pleasurable anticipation not only intensifies the baby's interest in the joint action, but also heightens awareness of the sequence, making it more salient and "learnable." Once the baby learns the routine as a script, it becomes available for the child to manipulate, as when, for example, the child spontaneously uses an action in the routine as a request for the

---

BOX 6-5 | **TIPS for Working with Parents of Preintentional Infants to Optimize Parent-Child Communication**

T: *Take turns:* Coach parents to engage in back-and-forth interactions with babies through songs, games such as peek-a-boo, and play with toys. Encourage parents to do something the baby enjoys, then wait for the child to do something (anything!) before the adult takes another turn.

I: *Imitate:* Coach families to play "monkey see, monkey do" or "copy cat" by mirroring any infant actions or sounds.

P: *Point things out:* Coach families to engage the baby in joint attention routines by bringing things the child likes within view, and monitoring that the child is looking at them before making them move, sound, or operate. Later, when the child is 6 to 10 months, use gestural pointing to establish joint attention to objects at a distance in addition to bringing objects near the child.

S: *Set the stage:* Coach parents to establish anticipatory sets by repeating simple games and songs the child likes. When the child has become very familiar with these, encourage parents to stop momentarily in the middle to allow the child to anticipate and request the next part of the action.

parent to play the game. Predictable joint action sequences also foster in the baby a sense of trust and reliability, a feeling of knowing what one can expect from people. This sense has obvious consequences for socioemotional development, but it has consequences for communication, too. A child who feels others are dependable and predictable, particularly if they are predictable in providing fun and interesting things for the baby to see and do, is more likely to think that communicating with these people is worthwhile and worth the effort to learn.

It is important for the clinician to determine which games are culturally appropriate for the family. Not all cultures play "peek-a-boo" exactly the same way, and each culture has its own set of baby games that the parents learned from their own parents. The family should be encouraged to recall and to ask older family members if they recall what baby games are traditionally used. These games will have the greatest affective value for the parent and so are likely to be more engaging for the child than games taught by the clinician. If the family is really unable to come up with games that have been used traditionally in their social group, only then should the clinician offer to introduce baby games from the mainstream culture.

Developing Self-Monitoring Skills. Once parents have learned the basics of communication development in the preintentional infant and have had the opportunity to observe the clinician demonstrate appropriate interactive techniques, they need to develop confidence in their own ability to communicate with the baby. One very effective way to achieve this result is through the use of videotaping to monitor communicative interactions and allow the parent to self-monitor. If videotaping equipment is available, parents can be encouraged to interact with their babies, and later, when the baby is no longer alert, review the tape to observe themselves with the baby.

The clinician must be very careful to do this training in a nonthreatening atmosphere. It is essential to give the parent a feeling of acceptance and safety. Doing so requires establishing an atmosphere in which both the clinician and parent are attempting to learn about what works best with this baby, rather than one in which the clinician is dictating behavior to the parent. In this accepting atmosphere, parents can learn to observe their own and the baby's behavior, determine whether they have made a good match between the two, and develop strategies for assessing the effectiveness of the interactions and modifying them when necessary. Allowing parents to view videotapes and analyze their own performance, rather than having it analyzed by the clinician, can facilitate this process. The clinician can comment on the positive aspects of the interaction. If the parent fails to note some changes that the clinician feels should be made, the SLP can ask the parent how the interaction might be conducted differently or whether there were any times when the baby seemed to be unresponsive. These episodes of unresponsiveness can be used as a springboard for discussing how the interaction might have been made more effective.

After several videotaping sessions, parents will probably benefit from watching a tape of the earliest interactions. They can observe how much the baby has grown, as well as how their own interactions have changed and become more attuned to the child. The clinician can use these occasions to praise and appreciate the efforts the parents have made. The development of confidence in their own ability to do what is best for the baby is what will encourage parents to further progress in providing an optimal environment for their child's growth. The *Hanen Early Language Parent Program* (Girolametto, Greenberg, & Manolson, 1986) is one commercially available program that incorporates many of these principles we've been discussing. Other programs include MacDonald's (1989) ECO program, Bricker's (2002) system, and the *Carolina Curriculum for Infants and Toddlers with Special Needs* (Johnson-Martin, Hacker, and Attermeier, 2004). Additional resources can be found in Table 6-7.

ASSESSMENT AND INTERVENTION FOR INFANTS AT PRELINGUISTIC STAGES OF COMMUNICATION: 9 TO 18 MONTHS

In the last quarter of the first year of life, infants undergo an important transition. They move from being participants in interactions to being intentional communicators. Children in this developmental stage, in Halliday's (1975) terms, "learn how to mean." In Bates's (1976) parlance, these children are in the *illocutionary* stage of communication, when they express intentions through signals to others but do not yet use conventional language. At this level children need interactions that both acknowledge and enhance their growing understanding of the functions and meanings of communication. The techniques used in the preintentional period to evaluate and encourage vocal and oral-motor development, as well as those for assessing and enhancing general cognitive growth and monitoring hearing, are still applicable to the prelinguistic communicator. However, the needs of the child in the 9- to 18-month developmental level will change in terms of the types of communicative interactions that will best foster development. It is important to remember that we are talking about children whose *developmental* level is 9 to 18 months. For children with a history of prematurity, CGA will still determine expectations for performance at this stage. Ten months after Janice's birth, for example, her CGA would be 8 months (40 weeks CA minus 8 weeks prematurity), and she would not be considered delayed if intentional communicative behavior had not yet emerged. Other children with disabilities who are 9 to 18 months old chronologically also may remain in the preintentional stage of development for some time. When cognitive assessment suggests that this is the case for children in the first 2 years of life, intervention should continue at the preintentional level. Only when a toddler evidences through play and other behavior that intentionality is emerging should the intervention begin to "up the ante," to require more initiation of communication and more conventional forms of communicative behavior from the child.

Assessment

How do we know that the infant has made this transition to intentionality? This question can be answered either formally or informally. The formal assessment procedures outlined in Box 6-2 can be used for the older infant. When the child achieves a developmental level of 9 to 10 months or more on one of these instruments, readiness for intentional behavior can be inferred.

Intentionality also can be assessed through observation of the child's play. This can be done using one of the formal play assessments listed in Chapter 2, such as the *Symbolic Play Test* (Lowe & Costello, 1976), Carpenter's (1987) *Play Scale*, Casby's (2003) *Developmental Assessment of Play*, or the *Communication and Symbolic Behavior Scales* (Wetherby & Prizant, 2003). It also can be done informally, by providing the child with common objects that invite conventional and pretend play, such as dolls, child-sized common utensils, and familiar household objects. The observation can be used to determine whether the child is demonstrating some recognition of common objects and their uses, such as using a comb to comb hair or putting a toy telephone to the ear, and can engage in simple pretend play schemes, such as pretending to eat from an empty spoon. More detailed information on informal play assessment is provided in Chapter 7. If these conventional uses of objects and early representational behaviors are observed during the play session, the clinician can be confident that the child is ready to engage in intentional communication.

Alternatively, we can use a parent-report instrument to elicit information about early communicative behavior. The Words and Gestures form of the *Communicative Development Inventory* (Fenson et al., 1993), for example, provides a checklist that parents can fill out to answer questions about early communicative and symbolic gestural production. The *Vineland Adaptive Behavior Scales-II* (Sparrow, Cicchetti, & Balla, 2005) also contains items on play development. This information, too, can be used to help determine whether the child is demonstrating behaviors that imply intentionality.

If intentional behaviors are neither observed nor reported, the clinician can attempt to elicit them by modeling conventional use of objects and engagement in simple pretend schemes and observing whether the infant can use the models in his or her own play. If the infant can produce these behaviors in response to a model, some intentionality is likely to be present and the infant could probably benefit from intervention focused on eliciting intentional communication. At least it can't hurt to try. If repeated attempts to elicit conventional and early pretend play do not succeed, however, the clinician may decide to postpone moving to a program for eliciting intentional communication. Instead, we can continue to encourage the parents to engage in turn-taking, imitation, building anticipatory sets and joint attentional activities in their interactions with the baby, and we can look for evidence of intentional behavior as time progresses.

Once it has been established that the infant can benefit from a program focused on intentional communication,

assessment may be useful in determining the frequency and types of communication that the baby is demonstrating. The *Communication and Symbolic Behavior Scales* (Wetherby & Prizant, 2003) is a formal instrument for assessing infant and toddler communication skills. This procedure involves videotaping the baby engaged in play interaction and using a standard format for examining the child's means of communicating, speech production capacity, receptive language, related cognitive abilities and social-affective behavior. Paul (1991*b*) provided a less formalized approach that uses direct observation rather than videotaping to examine intentional communication. We will discuss procedures for assessing early intentional communication in detail in Chapter 7.

The point of assessing communicative behavior in the child with a developmental level of 9 to 18 months is simply to determine whether any functional communication is present. When the intentional underpinnings, as evidenced by the appearance of conventional and early pretend play, are observed in children at this level, functional communication should begin to enter their behavioral repertoire. We simply want to find out whether a play interaction with a familiar adult elicits any communicative behaviors, whether they are gestural, vocal, or verbal. We also would like to know what kinds of intentions are being expressed. Typical functions expressed at this level include requesting objects or actions; attempting to get the adult's attention on what the child is interested in; and initiating social interactions through greeting, calling, or showing off. If any intentional communication on the child's part is observed, we can infer that a child in the 9- to 18-month developmental range is progressing adequately. If intentional communication does not appear to be present in a child functioning at a 9- to 18-month level and parents confirm that the child's behavior during the observation was typical, we can infer that communication development is beginning to lag.

Management

If the child's communication development does seem on target, this does *not* imply that we can stop providing advice or support to the family of an at-risk infant. On the contrary, we want to foster the communication the child is showing, and primary and secondary prevention of later language disorders is still our main concern. For the at-risk child at a 9- to 18-month developmental level who is expressing some communicative intent, we need to encourage parents to learn how to scaffold or support the child's move toward more conventional communication. Brady, Marquis, Fleming, and McLean (2004) showed that parent responsiveness is a significant predictor of language development in children with disabilities. "Upping the ante" is Bruner's (1981) term for the techniques parents normally use to elicit a higher level of response from a child, once a response of some kind has been evoked.

For example, suppose a baby at a developmental level of 9 to 18 months has been playing peek-a-boo for some time with his mother, consistently showing joint attention to her when she covers her face to start the game and demonstrating antici-

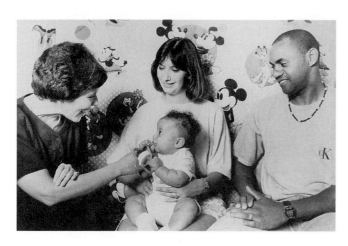

SLPs can work with parents of at-risk infants to optimize interaction for the purpose of secondary prevention.

pation of her revealing her face again. The mother can "up the ante" by keeping her face covered until the child does something. At first, she can keep her face covered until he reaches up and pulls her hands away. When the baby does this consistently, she can refuse to move her hands until he vocalizes along with his reaching toward her. By requiring increasingly more mature and sophisticated behaviors on the baby's part to complete the routine, the mother is shaping his behavioral repertoire to include more conventional ways of expressing his intents.

Rossetti (2001) suggested helping parents of infants in this stage to demonstrate contingent relations between words and actions. For example, parents can be asked to produce a verbal accompaniment to their response to a child's signal to be picked up. They can say, "Up!" when they pick up the child in response to the child's raising arms as a signal. Rossetti also encouraged teaching parents to amply reward any gesture or vocalization used as a communicative signal during this stage.

Warren and Yoder (1998) advocate the use of *prelinguistic milieu teaching (PMT)* to help in making the transition to intentional behavior. You may remember that we discussed milieu teaching as one of the hybrid forms of intervention in Chapter 3. In the prelinguistic period, it involves, first, arranging the environment by putting things the child will want in view but out of reach or by violating the order of events the child has come to expect. So we might put a new stuffed animal on a shelf where the child cannot reach it or offer the child juice before we have given a cup. The next step is to follow the child's attentional lead and focus on the child's item of focus. If the child looks at the new stuffed animal, we can look at it, too, then at the child, and wait expectantly for the child to do something (almost anything!) we can interpret as a request. Warren and Yoder stress that it is important to adapt our expectations to the child's initiation rate, which may be lower than we would like. It is more important to wait for the child to do something, then make our actions contingent on the child's, than it is to get the child to do something as a response to our own action. For children who just do not initiate, Warren and Yoder

suggest two contingent strategies. *Contingent motor imitation* is an exact, reduced, or slightly expanded imitation of a child's motor act performed by the adult immediately after the child does it. *Contingent vocal imitation* occurs when the adult follows a child's vocalization with a partial, exact, or modified vocal imitation. Both these techniques allow the child to regulate the amount of social stimulation and may encourage him or her to produce more behavior for the adult to imitate.

Once the child has established some initiation of communication, Warren and Yoder suggest using some additional techniques to increase the frequency of initiation, so long as the teaching episodes are brief, positive, and embedded in ongoing natural interactions. These techniques include using three types of prompts: *time delay, verbal,* and *gaze intersection. Time-delay* prompts involve interrupting an ongoing turn-taking activity or routine and withholding the continuation until the child initiates some form of request to resume. For example, if the adult and child are rolling a ball back and forth, the adult can hold onto the ball during one turn, look at the child, and wait expectantly until the child does something (again, almost anything) to initiate a request to continue. *Verbal* prompts can be open-ended questions ("What?") or directions ("Look at me"). *Gaze intersection* involves the adult's moving into the child's gaze when the child does not make eye contact. This prompt is gradually faded as the child begins to use eye contact more consistently for regulating interaction. Another technique is *modeling.* Models are used to increase the child's use of vocal and gestural communication. Vocal models of sounds that the adult has heard the child use are matched to communicative events to show how vocalization can express intentions. For example, if the child has been heard to produce /ba/, the adult can use this syllable when blowing bubbles, saying /ba/, /ba/ as each bubble pops. Gestural models can be used in a similar way to encourage the child to imitate communicative actions. For example, if the child has been seen to reach for an object, the adult can point to it. An additional technique that can be used to encourage communication is *natural consequences,* in which the child's communication is rewarded with its intended goal. If the child points to a cookie jar, the child is given a cookie, even if it is just before dinner. In addition to the natural consequence, though, the adult can provide a simple linguistic mapping ("You want a cookie!") as well as an acknowledgment that an appropriate form of communication was used ("I can tell because you pointed. Nice job!"). Yoder and Warren (2002) showed that PMT did accelerate growth in frequency of child-initiated comments, frequency of child-initiated requests, and lexical density in some, though not all children in an experimental study of the technique.

Book-reading situations are particularly apt settings for encouraging communication. Elliott-Templeton, Van Kleeck, Richardson, and Imholz (1992) showed that parents begin reading books to babies when the children are as young as 6 months. Snow (1983) has documented how parents of children with typical development use book-reading situations to scaffold language acquisition, and Bedrosian (1997) discussed this context for use with children with disabilities. Book-reading interactions have been shown to be effective in fostering both language and literacy development (Chomsky, 1972; Whitehurst et al., 1988). Parents of at-risk youngsters should be encouraged to begin engaging babies in looking at simple picture books as soon as the child can sit up. They can first have the babies sit with them and look at the pictures as the parent names each page with a simple label. Girolametto and Weitzman (2002) identify behaviors that can facilitate communication development in this setting, which include the following:

▶ Waiting for the child to initiate interest in something in the book by looking or pointing
▶ Being face-to-face during book sharing
▶ Asking questions
▶ Verbally inviting children to interact
▶ Labeling and talking about pictures in the book

The child's first level of response is simply to share joint attention to the pictures. Once the child has seen the book and heard it read several times, the parent can stop on one page and wait for the child to do something. If the child points to the picture, the parent can name it. Later the pointing gesture can be "upped" to a vocalization. Eventually the child will be expected to name or approximate the names of some of the pictures. Upping the ante in this way comes naturally to some parents and caregivers. They spontaneously recognize when the baby is ready to be nudged to a higher level of response or will do so readily once the clinician points out the baby's readiness to

them. Other parents may need more explicit instruction. Yoder and Warren (2002) showed that training parents to use responsive strategies in communicative interactions does result in positive changes in their ability to respond to child communication. Again, direct modeling by the clinician, showing the parents ways to up the ante in familiar day-to-day routines and activities, is helpful. Parents should then be encouraged to follow the clinician's example in the same routines. Monitoring, discussion of the effectiveness of the techniques, and self-monitoring using videotape are, again, useful adjuncts in this enterprise.

Another technique used to foster the development of communication at this level is *communication temptations*. These involve creating situations in which the child is strongly motivated to try to get a message across to the adult, who then responds swiftly and positively when the child does attempt to communicate. Wetherby and Prizant (1989) and Warren and Yoder (1998) presented some examples of communication temptations, which are listed in Box 6-6. These temptations can be used to increase the frequency of communication in at-risk children and to give them practice with using intentional behavior and seeing its positive results. In these activities, the focus is not on the form of communication. Any gesture or vocalization that is clearly intended to send a message receives the desired response. Communication temptations also can be used to elicit initial communicative behaviors from children at this level who are not yet demonstrating such behavior spontaneously.

| **BOX 6-6** | **Suggestions for Communication Temptations** |

- Eat a desirable food item in front of the child without offering any to him or her.
- Activate a wind-up toy, let it run down, then hand it to the child.
- Give the child several blocks, one a time, to drop in a can, then give the child a small toy figure to drop in.
- Initiate a familiar game, play it until the child expresses pleasure, then wait. Look expectantly at the child, and give a prompt ("What do you want?").
- Open a jar of bubbles, blow some bubbles, then close the jar tightly, and hand it to the child.
- Blow up a balloon, and let the air out. Then hand the deflated balloon to the child.
- Hold a food item the child does not like near his or her mouth.
- Place a desired toy or food item in a clear container with a tight lid that the child cannot open. Give the child the container and wait.
- Put the child's hand in a cold, wet, or sticky substance such as pudding or paste.
- Roll a ball to the child. After several rolls back and forth, substitute a car or other wheeled toy.
- Put a toy that makes noise in an opaque bag. Shake the bag and hold it up to the child.
- Bring the child a new toy, or initiate a silly or unusual event (wear a clown nose). Wait for the child to do something. When he or she does, map the child's action onto a linguistic form ("You think my nose is silly!").
- Pay less attention than usual to the child; back away or turn your back during an ongoing game. Wait for the child to try to elicit your attention.
- Give the child the run of the room for a few minutes. Wait for the child to direct your attention to an object he or she finds of interest.

Adapted from Warren, S., & Yoder, D. (1998). Facilitating the transition from preintentional to intentional communication. In A. Wetherby, S. Warren, & J. Riechle (Eds.), *Transitions in Prelinguistic Communication* (pp. 365-384). Baltimore, MD: Paul H. Brookes; and Wetherby, A., & Prizant, B. (1989). The expression of communicative intent: Assessment guidelines. *Seminars on Speech and Language, 10*, 77-91.

In addition to fostering the child's expression of communicative intents, we want to provide experiences in which the child can develop comprehension of language. Rossetti (2001) suggested using baby games to pair words with gestures and referents. Parents can start out demonstrating meaning for the infant by saying, for example, "Show me your nose" and taking the baby's hand and placing it on the nose. Later, the ante can be "upped" by having the parent say, "Show me your nose" and then waiting until the baby produces some gesture. In addition to developing communicative skills, these kinds of routines are ideal for expanding the child's comprehension repertoire, by adding new items (eye, ear, mouth) to the game. The same modeling, monitoring, and self-monitoring techniques used to work with parents of younger babies, including use of videotape to facilitate self-monitoring, can be used as part of these kinds of interactions. Some of the published programs in Tables 6-7 and 6-8 also can be useful at this stage.

These suggestions outline a prevention program for the at-risk child at a 9- to 18-month developmental level who appears to be developing adequately in terms of communication. What about the child who functions at a 9- to 18-month level but who has not yet evidenced intentional use of communication? I would suggest that for this child, intervention should focus on providing intensified input using a "motherese" speech style (Newman, 2003); focusing on developing comprehension skills; encouraging vocalization; and making the adult's communication contingent on what the child does, rather than on eliciting communication just yet. Providing a responsive atmosphere and a range of models of intentional communication is, in my view, a sufficient goal at this stage. There will be time for more intensive efforts to increase the frequency and maturity of communication when the child moves on to the next developmental stage. For now, both parent and child can benefit from what enriched, contingent input has to offer: for the parent, practice in providing responsive and contingent language stimulation, and for the child, the opportunity to experience its benefits for understanding language and providing a reliable scaffold toward linguistic production. Parents and caregivers ought to be encouraged to respond consistently to any initiation on the child's part, of course, even if it is in the form of gestures or nonconventional vocalizations. Focusing on the linguistic environment seems to me to be the most sensible approach for the infant who has not yet figured out the purpose of communication. Although there are no empirical data to support this position, I offer it to you as my best clinical hunch.

Some of the activities outlined in the preceding paragraphs for the emerging communicator can certainly be tried with the 9- to 18-month-level noncommunicator as well. Book reading is clearly an appropriate activity, as are the continuation of joint attention routines and baby games, whether or not the ante gets upped in this context. Some communication temptations can be tried to elicit intentional communication. However, if they don't elicit the desired behaviors, I advocate returning to basic joint attention activities and enriched contingent input, rather than continuing the temptations for

now. They can be tried again when the developmental level moves closer to 2 years. Activities to encourage oral and vocal imitation, including imitating the child's vocal behaviors and providing simple, conventional single words in response to the baby's vocalizations, also can be suggested to parents of these reluctant communicators.

The key, in my opinion, is to keep the focus on responding to the baby's needs and interests, making the parent's communication contingent on the infant's actions, and making sure that the parents and baby are still enjoying each other. Insisting too soon on particular behaviors from infants instead of responding contingently to all their behaviors runs the risk of teaching babies the opposite of what we want them to learn. We want to teach that communication is an effective, pleasurable way to influence those around us and to exert some control over our environment. This is the message that we need to bring home to the baby who is emerging as a communicating human being. I believe we do this best by example, by providing babies with models of communication that respond to their wants and needs.

CONSIDERATIONS FOR THE OLDER PRELINGUISTIC CLIENT

Some clients who function at prelinguistic levels of communication are older than the infants we've been discussing. Who are these clients? Some are severely or profoundly impaired with cognitive deficits that limit their ability to develop symbolic communication skills. Many of the syndromes of retardation that we discussed in Chapter 4 can present this picture. Some older children with autism may function at prelinguistic levels of communication, with very little use of words. Young hearing-impaired children who were not identified or amplified early and who did not receive early introduction to sign language can communicate at prelinguistic levels beyond the age of 18 months. Children with severe speech impairments who have not been provided with alternative forms of communication also can function at this level beyond the first 2 years of life. Finally, children who suffer severe or profound acquired brain damage through trauma or disease can lose their ability to communicate with language.

Let's clarify one important distinction, though. A child can be nonspeaking yet still be a linguistic communicator. Children with cerebral palsy, for example, may be unable to speak because of neuromotor difficulties but can communicate linguistically through spelling on a communication board with a headlight or by means of an electronic device that prints out or speaks messages the client creates on a keyboard. These children with severe speech production impairments were discussed in Chapter 4. In this section we are concerned with children who have deficits that extend beyond the neuromotor act of speaking to include limitations in the ability to understand and use words or symbols to communicate. These children, who function within the first 2 years of cognitive development, are considered *prelinguistic* communicators. Let's examine the same issues for this group of clients that we looked at for prelinguistic infants:

feeding and oral-motor development, hearing conservation and aural habilitation, behavior and development, and communication.

FEEDING AND ORAL-MOTOR DEVELOPMENT IN OLDER PRELINGUISTIC CLIENTS

Many older children with prelinguistic communication skills have difficulties feeding because of neuromotor involvement. For these children, feeding and swallowing issues clearly need to be addressed. Although an in-depth discussion of feeding and swallowing is beyond the scope of this text, many of the references cited earlier for use with infants in these areas also are useful for addressing feeding issues in older clients. Pressman and Berkowitz (2003) emphasize that before initiating a feeding program, any associated medical problems must be addressed. McGowan and Kerwin (1993) discussed these issues in detail for children with long-term tracheostomies, with suggestions that can apply to children with a variety of types of feeding disorders. Alexander (2001), Bricker (2002), Eicher (2002), and Hall et al. (1987) provided discussions of feeding issues for children with neuromuscular disorders that are helpful in working with parents on developing children's feeding skills. Box 6-4 summarized some of the suggestions of these writers. Arvedson (2000) provides comprehensive guidelines for conducting the major portions of the evaluation of children with feeding and swallowing disorders, which include the following:

▶ Review of medical, developmental, and feeding history.
▶ Physical examination, including growth and nutrition, neurodevelopmental, oral-facial, cranial nerve, respiratory, and gastrointestinal elements.
▶ Prefeeding assessments, such as posture and position, oral-motor structure and function, and social and affective aspects of feeding.
▶ Direct observations of chewing, biting, swallowing, and interactions during feeding.
▶ Assessment of food preferences.
▶ Deciding whether to employ instrumental assessments, such as the videofluoroscopic swallow study.

Pressman and Berkowitz suggest that feeding issues, like others, can often be addressed with behavioral approaches, involving new skill acquisition, generalization, and reinforcement. In addition, Jaffe (1989) and Lowman, Murphy, and Snell (1999) are careful to point out the importance of helping parents learn not only the physical skills involved in feeding a child with a disability, but also of emphasizing the communicative aspects of feeding. Eating is a social experience; a pleasant, interactive atmosphere is essential to developing a good feeling about food and eating. If the parent (or therapist) treats eating as a mechanical exercise, this crucial social component can be lost. As a result, both child and parent may come to see eating as a purely biological function, rather than an event in which people participate and interact. Hall et al. (1987) suggested that parents be encouraged to maintain a pleasant, positive facial expression and voice during feeding; that they give lots of praise and verbal encouragement; and that they speak to

children during feeding, being careful to time remarks so that they don't excite abnormal patterns of chewing or swallowing. For older children in school programs, developing social opportunities during eating times also is important. Morris (1981) suggested setting up "lunch clubs" for children with feeding problems. These would give the child with a disability the opportunity to eat with small groups of mainstream children, who are chosen as a special privilege, to eat with the client in a special place (such as a classroom or teachers' room), perhaps on a rotating basis. This approach provides social opportunities and reduces the distractions present in a large cafeteria. Lowman, Murphy, and Snell (1999) provide additional suggestions.

Hall et al. (1987) emphasized the role of developing feeding skills as a foundation for vocalization and speech. As Nelson (1998) pointed out, though, it is important to be aware that oral-motor skills such as those used in feeding are necessary, but not sufficient, for learning to talk. Morris (1981) found that many children who make gains in oral-motor skills do not necessarily translate these skills into speech production. In other words, developing oral-motor skills through feeding is important because eating is important, but it will not guarantee that these skills will generalize to speech. To develop speech skills in children at risk for speech impairment, speech must be addressed directly in an intervention program. We cannot assume that work on the vegetative function of eating will ensure the development of the voluntary function of speech.

For older prelinguistic clients, the development of vocal skills for speech must, as we've said, be addressed explicitly. Several approaches are available. Ling (1976) developed a sequenced approach to acquiring vocal skills that was designed for children with impaired hearing but can be adapted for children with other types of impairments. Windsor, Doyle, and Siegel (1994) described a program that used both auditory and written input to develop speech skills in a nonverbal client with autism. This program is of particular interest because the client was 10 years old and had been mute before the intervention, suggesting that speech is a possibility even for clients who remain mute into middle childhood. Hayden (1984) advocates the use of a program of tactile stimulation, derived from work with adults with apraxia, the PROMPT program.

Yoder and Warren (2002) found that production of canonical (CV) syllables was predictive of speech development; clinicians can encourage families to stimulate the production, through modeling and enthusiastic imitation, of these syllables as they play with prelinguistic children. Because the development of consonant production in early childhood has been shown to be a good predictor of speech outcome (Whitehurst, Fischel, Arnold, & Lonigan, 1992), working on expanding consonant repertoires in prelinguistic children is also important. Bleile and Miller (1993) presented a series of contexts that can help facilitate consonant production in children in the earliest stages of speech production. These contexts are summarized in Box 6-7. Augmentative and alternative forms of communication are also, of course, important considerations for these clients.

BOX 6-7	**Contexts for Facilitating Consonant Production in Early Speech**

1. Stressed syllables facilitate consonant production (*baby* to facilitate /b/).
2. Velar consonants are facilitated at the ends of syllables (*talk* to facilitate /k/) and when they come before a back vowel (*good* to facilitate /g/).
3. Alveolar consonants are facilitated when they precede a front vowel (*tea* to facilitate /t/).
4. To facilitate production of a consonant at a new place of articulation, use a word that contains another consonant at the same place of articulation (*toss* to facilitate /s/).
5. Position facilitates the production of voicing distinctions. Use beginning contexts to facilitate production of voiced consonants (*dough* to facilitate /d/) and ending contexts to facilitate production of voiceless consonants (*eat* to facilitate /t/).
6. Fricatives are facilitated in contexts between vowels (*taffy* to facilitate /f/).

Adapted from Bleile, K., and Miller, S. (1993). Infants and toddlers. In J. Bernthal (Ed.), *Articulatory and phonological disorders in toddlers with medical needs* (pp. 81-109). New York: Thieme.

HEARING CONSERVATION AND AURAL HABILITATION

Older children at prelinguistic levels of development can't tell their parents when they have an earache or if they aren't hearing as well as usual. For these reasons, it is especially important to assess hearing regularly in these populations and to be aggressive, as Roland and Brown (1990) suggested, in identifying and treating otitis media. For children who are found to have impaired hearing, early identification and amplification are two of the most important factors in determining good outcomes. If a hearing impairment is identified in an older prelinguistic child, amplification needs to be introduced immediately. Even a child with hearing impairment (HI) who has significant impairments in cognitive and motor areas can benefit from amplification. If amplification can boost auditory stimulation and increase prespeech vocalization in a prelinguistic client, there will be more vocalization that the clinician can work with and shape into speech-like communication. Parents and teachers also need to learn how to manage and maintain the child's aids in good working order. In addition, as with any child with HI, the older prelinguistic client may benefit from assistive listening devices, such as auditory trainers, to improve signal-to-noise ratio and maximize the benefit the child can receive from the auditory environment. For children who are good candidates, cochlear implantation can also be considered.

CHILD BEHAVIOR AND DEVELOPMENT

Older prelinguistic clients may become frustrated over the difficulty of getting their messages across to others. For this reason they sometimes display aberrant or maladaptive behaviors such as aggression or self-abuse. Donnellan, Mirenda, Mesaros, and Fassbender (1984) showed that these behaviors can be understood as a form of communication for clients who do not have more conventional, comprehensible means at their disposal. These behaviors are sometimes inadvertently reinforced

by parents and teachers, who pay a great deal of attention to a child who is engaging in them. In these cases, one goal of intervention is to provide clients with more acceptable means of expressing their intentions, as we discussed in Chapter 4. If, for example, analysis of a child's maladaptive behavior indicates that it is being used to signal frustration with an intervention activity, the child can be given a conventional means of expressing the same idea. A client might, for example, be taught to use the sign for "stop" to signal that he or she has had enough. When the client uses this signal, it must, of course, be respected to reinforce its communicative value. The teacher or clinician will have to do something else with the client once he or she has asked in this more conventional way to have the activity cease. Bopp, Brown, and Mirenda (2004) discuss the use of positive behavioral support to achieve this end; more detail on their discussion can be found in Chapter 9.

Another approach to coping with maladaptive communication in older prelinguistic clients is to use what LaVigna (1987) called *differential reinforcement of other behavior (DRO)*. If clients are using maladaptive forms of communication to secure attention from adults, these behaviors can be decreased by systematically paying attention to other behaviors deemed more acceptable. In this way the client learns that it is not necessary to be disruptive to gain adults' attention.

In addition to maladaptive forms of communication, a second area of concern for the older prelinguistic client's development has to do with the progression of cognitive and communicative skills. You'll remember that we talked earlier about perlocutionary and illocutionary stages of communication. In these stages, the child's interaction is communicative, though not mediated by language. Bates (1976) referred to a third stage of communication, the *locutionary* stage. This occurs in normal development at 12 to 18 months of age, when the child begins to use conventional forms, such as words, signs, or symbols, to communicate intentions that were encoded with idiosyncratic gestures and vocalizations during the illocutionary phase. For older prelinguistic clients, ongoing assessment is necessary to detect whether a shift from illocutionary to locutionary communication is taking place or could take place with a "push" from the environment. Evidence presented by Windsor et al. (1994) suggested that there is no absolute age limit on the ability to acquire locutionary communication. For prelinguistic clients, even when a nonsymbolic AAC system is used, continual probes should be used to investigate whether symbolic skills, including linguistic communication, can be acquired. Ongoing cognitive and play assessment using instruments such as the *Developmental Assessment for Individuals with Severe Disabilities—2nd Edition (DASH–2; Dykes & Erin, 1999)* can help to identify the point at which cognitive skills capable of supporting more symbolic communication—in forms such as speech, sign, or Blissymbols—can be added to the client's communicative repertoire. For clients with autism particularly, written language may be a useful augmentative modality for aiding in the acquisition of symbolic language.

INTENTIONALITY AND COMMUNICATION

Although clients in the prelinguistic stage may not communicate by conventional means, they do communicate, as Siegel-Causey and Guess (1989) pointed out. However, these communications may be difficult to interpret. We need to be prepared to search for and identify any such nonconventional forms, whether they appear in guise of *echolalia*, the echoing of others' speech; aggressive or self-abusive behaviors; touching or manipulating others; bodily orientation; generalized movements; or changes in muscle tone (Seigel-Causey & Guess, 1989). Johnson, Baumgart, Helmstetter, and Curry (1996) suggest looking for a behavior that tends to precede the maladaptive one and attempting to use that as a communicative gesture. For example, if the client protests by hitting, the clinician can interrupt the hitting and prompt the client to simply raise an open hand as an alternative. Some formal assessment procedures for guiding this process have been developed by Coggins, Olswang, and Guthrie (1987), Johnson et al. (1996), Linder (1993), Lund and Duchan (1993), Kleiman (2003), Norris and Hoffman (1990a), and Wetherby and Prizant (2003). Giving children acceptable, readable means to express the intentions they have, whether the form is spoken or through AAC, is a primary goal of intervention for older prelinguistic clients.

In addition to helping older prelinguistic clients map intentions onto acceptable forms of expression, we may need to expand the frequency and range of intentions they express. Wetherby, Yonclas, and Bryan (1989), for example, showed that children with various types of disorders showed different patterns of communication. Children with DS showed communicative skills that were similar to those of normal children. Children with autism showed a normal frequency of communicative acts but an abnormal preponderance of regulatory acts (e.g., requests and protests), unlike normal children, who use predominantly joint attentional acts (e.g., showing, directing attention, showing off). Paul and Shiffer (1991) found that toddlers with slow language development also showed a dearth of joint attentional conversational acts when compared with normally developing toddlers. Mirenda and Santogrossi (1985)

discussed the fact that clients with severe disorders often don't communicate much at all without prompting, even when they have communicative means available. These studies suggest that differences in the frequency and range of communicative function need to be addressed in older clients at the prelinguistic stage. Such clients may need to develop a broader base of preverbal intentions as a modality of conventional communication, speech or AAC, is being acquired. Several commercially available programs can address this issue, including the Ski-Hi curriculum developed for children with HI (Clark & Watkins, 1985), the INSITE program (Clark, Morgan, & Wilson-Vlotman, 1984), and the ECO Model (MacDonald, 1989). Romski and Sevcik's (1996) System for Augmenting Language (SAL) also is a useful model.

Mirenda and Santogrossi (1985) suggest using a "prompt-free" approach as a way to elicit beginning intentional communication. The client can be rewarded with a piece of cereal each time he or she accidentally touches a picture of the cereal box that has been set in his or her view, for example. As these touches become more frequent and intentional, the ante can be "upped" by requiring that the child not only touch the picture but look at the adult to accomplish a request. More pictures can then be added, until a communication board or a book with a variety of pictures and symbols can be used by the client to get messages across. In this way the frequency of communication can be expanded and a functional AAC system can be introduced. Communication temptation activities adapted to the client's physical abilities also can be an important part of this process.

Bondy and Frost (2002) have introduced the Picture Exchange System (PECS), based on principles from applied behavioral analysis (ABA), to teach functional communication initiations. Here, too, the goal is to avoid prompts or directives, but to get the client to communicate spontaneously. The client is presented with a desired object (e.g., a cookie) and its picture. When the client reaches for the cookie, an aide standing behind him directs his hand to the picture and guides him to give it to the clinician. When she receives the picture, she exchanges it for the cookie. This procedure is continued, through backward chaining (Sulzer-Azaroff & Mayer, 1991), until the client hands the picture to the clinician spontaneously. The program then focuses on enhancing spontaneity, discriminating among symbols, and acquiring other functions of communication beyond requesting. Bondy, Tincani, and Frost (2004) provided detailed guidance on these steps in the program. Kravits, Kamps, Kemmerer, and Potucek (2002) reported on a case study in which PECS training resulted in increases in spontaneous communication in a girl with autism. Tincani (2004) showed that both PECS and Sign were effective for increasing communication and vocalization in school-aged children with autism at the prelinguistic stage, but different children benefited more from one approach or the other.

Halle, Brady, and Drasgow (2004) and Keen (2003) discussed the fact that the prelinguistic communications of children with severe disabilities are often misunderstood, so that frequent communication break-downs occur. Halle et al. suggested guidelines for programs to help clients repair these breakdowns.

Using strategies for repairing communicative breakdowns can help to decrease frustration and provide more effective communication for these individuals. These appear in Box 6-8. Kevan (2003) reminds us also that communication difficulties may arise not only from expressive limitations, but from inability to comprehend language spoken to these clients. She emphasizes the importance of careful and thorough assessment of receptive language as part of the evaluation of these students.

A final consideration in organizing a communication system for children with severe impairments involves helping to create more supportive environments for their communicative attempts. Several methods are available for assessing the interactive environment, in order to determine how to make it more congenial for the client's communication. McCarthy et al.'s (1998) *Communication Supports Checklist* and Rowland and Schweigert's (1993) *Analyzing the Communicative Environment* and the *Functional Communication Profile—Revised* (Kleinman, 2003) are instruments to assist in doing these evaluations. Duchan (1997) presents the Situated Pragmatics approach, which is designed as a means to optimize functional communication in natural settings. Situated pragmatics takes advantage of the systems model of language disorders. As such, it focuses not only on the client but also on the interaction between the client and the environment. It uses two approaches to achieve its

goals: preparing the environment to ensure successful inclusion of the client and providing various kinds of ongoing support. Box 6-9 presents the kinds of support that can be provided to increase opportunities for a client to participate in everyday activities. Once we have described the environment, we may need to find ways to improve opportunities and rewards for communication. Falkman, Sandberg, and Hjelmquist (2002), for example, showed that nonspeaking children with cerebral palsy used fewer linguistic communications than would be expected, based on their normal cognitive levels. They concluded that environmental supports for linguistic communication via AAC were lacking. When developing AAC systems for clients, it will be important to work with parents, teachers, and other caregivers to be sure they are responsive to the use of these systems in real communicative situations.

■ CONCLUSIONS

Although infants and other children at prelinguistic levels of communication may look like two very different groups of clients, our goals for these two categories are in some ways very similar: helping caregivers learn to read and respond to the child's signals and supporting the family in providing an enhanced communicative environment for the child, improving feeding

---

| **BOX 6-8** | **Guidelines for Teaching Repair of Prelinguistic Communication Breakdowns** |

- Identify (1) situations in which communication breakdowns are occurring or are likely to occur, (2) function of the communicative behavior associated with the breakdowns, and (3) the responses of social partners in those situations.
- Select AT LEAST two new forms to teach as repairs. Focus intervention on teaching replacement forms that produce a good contextual fit with the demands of the situation.
- Select forms that have wide application and are more efficient than existing repairs. For example, if a child is at the one-word stage, a socially appropriate alternative response might be to point to the desired object. Be sure the new behavior has immediate, consistent, and positive responses from the communication partner.
- Teach the new forms by creating situations that replicate the natural situations in which break-downs are likely to occur. Have team members agree upon a prompting system, such as graduated guidance or verbal prompts that they can use to ensure that the child will use the new forms. Use a milieu teaching approach, in which adults observe the child carefully and then insert teaching trials at motivating moments. Help the child learn to use an alternate repair strategy if the first fails. This can be accomplished by responding quickly to most opportunities when the child uses a new repair form and, on some small number of occasions, waiting and prompting a second new repair form when the child has already attempted repair. Be sure social partners do not respond to any existing socially unacceptable communication. When it is not possible to ignore unacceptable communication, attempt to ensure that the consequence is less immediate, less consistent, and of lesser quality than consequences for socially appropriate communication.
- Encourage social partners to be responsive to the new forms. Select communication forms that are easily recognized and understood by a variety of social partners. Model the forms for the social partners, and alert them to the situations in which the new forms are most likely to occur. Encourage social partners to respond quicker, more often, and with greater magnitude to the new repair forms.
- Monitor use of new repair forms. Look for instances of new repairs in the child's everyday settings under communicative breakdown situations. This information can be used to guide and refine instructional strategies because it provides ongoing assessment information about the progress of the interventions.

Adapted from Halle, J., Brady, N., & Dragsow, E. (2004). Enhancing socially adaptive communicative repairs of beginning communicators with disabilities, *American Journal of Speech-Language Pathology, 13,* 43-54.

BOX 6-9	Providing Ongoing Support to Enhance Communication

Social Support: Helping others (with and without disabilities) to understand and expand on their assigned roles, to create a positive role identity, to understand their roles in relation to others, and to relate well with one another

Emotional Support: Helping partners to respond to the emotional state of one another, to develop conventional emotional responses, to feel empowered, and to help one another "save face"

Functional Support: Helping partners to achieve their communication goals and to understand and support their partner's goals

Physical Support: Providing access to communication and physical support for enhancing communication

Event Support: Scaffolding events to provide contextual support for communication, to establish participation patterns and roles, and to let participants know what to expect

Discourse Support: Providing scaffolds, discourse markers, and discourse support to expand on and encourage communication of others

Reprinted with permission from Duchan, J. (1998). A situated pragmatics approach for supporting children with severe communication disorders. *Topics in Language Disorders, 17* (2), 14.

and vocal skills, conserving and making best use of hearing, and developing functional communication that has the potential to grow into symbolic language. The language pathologist has two unique goals in working with at-risk infants and their families: primary and secondary prevention of communication disorders in the infant. The vehicle by which we accomplish these goals in the first years of life is the IFSP. Remember Janice? Box 6-10 gives an example of an IFSP that might have been developed for her and her family. An additional IFSP sample format appears in Appendix 6-1.

The IFSP in Box 6-10 exemplifies several of the critical elements discussed with regard to work with high-risk infants and their families. First, it looks at the baby in the context of the family. Notice that the intervention services outlined in the plan are exactly the ones that the family identified as their priorities and concerns in their discussion with the IFSP team. Second, the goal of the IFSP is not concerned with prediction of the baby's ultimate outcome but provision of what the baby needs now to achieve maximal potential. Goals are not chronologically age-appropriate milestones, but simply those behaviors that Janice's family feels are important for her to develop now. Finally, the IFSP integrates services from a variety of providers under the watchful eye of a case manager, who develops a real relationship with the family and advocates for them and their concerns.

The language pathologist has a unique opportunity when working with the family of an at-risk infant. Very often in our profession we are trying to fix what is already broken. With a baby who starts out with risk factors, though, we may have the chance to prevent things from getting broken in the first place. This is a rare opportunity and one that we ought, as a profession, to embrace. Despite our best efforts at primary and secondary prevention, many of the babies we work with will develop communicative problems that we will need to address with rehabilitative methods. However, for some infants, we may be able to ward off the effects of early difficulties. A detailed and comprehensive understanding of infant development and communication, as well as knowledge of the techniques to enhance that development, will ensure that we can take advantage of this invaluable opportunity.

We have some special opportunities when we work with older prelinguistic clients as well. These children may have spent a good part of their lives in enforced isolation because of their inability to find ways to express their interests and desires. Developing a conventional communication system for a child who has never had one can make a tremendous difference in the quality of that child's life. Giving the gift of communication to such a child is also an achievement in which we can take a good deal of pride.

STUDY GUIDE

I. Family-Centered Practice
   A. What is IDEA?
   B. Describe the Individual Family Service Plan. Name its required elements. How is it used to provide family-centered services to handicapped infants?
   C. Discuss the uses and dangers of family assessment.
   D. Discuss communication strategies that can be used in family-centered practice.
   E. Why is a language pathologist needed on the team that plans services for the at-risk infant?

II. Risk Factors for Communication Disorders in Infants
   A. Discuss some of the prenatal factors that can place a child at risk for developmental and communicative disorders.
   B. How does prematurity influence communicative development?
   C. Name and describe six genetic conditions that place an infant at risk for communication disorders.

III. Assessment and Intervention for High-Risk Infants and Their Families in the Newborn Intensive Care Nursery

| **BOX 6-10** | **Example of an IFSP for Janice** |

Name: Janice XXX
Date of Birth: May 22, 2005
Chronological age: 71/2 weeks, uncorrected
Sex: Female
SSN: 000-00-000
Case Manager: Kay Jones, CCC-SLP
Assessment date: July 14, 2005
Legal Guardian: Mary and Henry XXX
Siblings: Jenna, 2.6, Harry, 4.8
Address: 6500 S. 36th Ave.
Phone: (205) 555-3788
Referred by: University Hospital

History

This is the first follow-up assessment for Janice after she left the NICU. She was the product of an otherwise uneventful pregnancy and was identified as having DS at birth. She was born at 32 weeks, weighing 3 lb. 2 oz. Ventilator treatment was needed for respiratory distress syndrome. She was intubated and received gavage tube feeding for the first 2 weeks in the NICU, then graduated to bottle feeding. Initially, feeding was difficult, but her mother was very determined to make the bottle feeding succeed, which it soon did. Janice was removed from the incubator after 3 weeks and did well in the NICU until discharge, at which point she weighed 5 lb. 3 oz.

Current Status

The *Brazelton Neonatal Behavioral Assessment Scale* was administered to Janice just before discharge from the NICU. Janice's performance on three of the Brazelton scales—motor capacities, organizational capacities (state), and organizational capacities (stress)—was considered within normal limits. Her score on the interactive capacities scale, however, indicated reduced ability to attend to and process environmental events and to respond to faces and voices.

Hearing status was found to be normal on auditory brainstem-evoked response testing. Vision screening could not be accomplished and should be performed at the next assessment. Hearing status should be monitored regularly because of risks associated with DS.

Family Resources, Priorities, and Concerns

Extensive discussion with Janice's mother and some less extensive conversations with her father revealed the following:

Resources

Janice's mother says she is determined to do the best she can for this baby, even if she has to give up her job; she will stay home with Janice as long as she feels Janice needs it. The mother reports that she was frightened about Janice's retardation, but now that she's seen how far Janice has come in the last few weeks, she feels confident that she can help Janice to achieve her potential.

Priorities

Janice's mother has been expressing breast milk throughout her stay in the NICU and would like very much to breastfeed Janice now that she is home. She is willing to do so even on a supplementary basis and to continue bottle feeding to maintain weight gains. The mother also is very interested in having Janice interact with her brother and sister, so that they can "get to know the baby." Janice's father wants life at home to return to some semblance of normal and hopes now that Janice is home he will see more of his wife and have things run more smoothly. He would like to give Janice's mother some help at home but cannot afford to hire help.

Concerns

Janice's mother is worried about her job and wonders whether she will be able to keep it and still give Janice what she needs. She and her husband are both concerned about the financial repercussions of Janice's hospitalization. They are concerned about their ability to care for a child with retardation over the long term. Their main concern now is to be sure that Janice gets everything she needs to grow and develop, but they also are worried that their other children will feel slighted or abandoned because of all the flurry around Janice.

BOX 6-10 **Example of an IFSP for Janice—cont'd**

Outcomes

1. Encourage breastfeeding. SLP will work with mother on positioning to maximize baby's intake during breastfeeding. *Criteria/timeline:* Mother will report on success of breastfeeding at next IFSP meeting; weight gain will be monitored by a pediatrician.
2. Effect of vision on Janice's difficulty in attending to faces will be evaluated. *Criteria/timeline:* Vision check at next pediatrician visit.
3. Provide emotional and financial support to family. Social work service will explore supplementary insurance issues as well as visiting nurse and home health aide services for Janice. *Criteria/timeline:* Check with family at next IFSP meeting; home health aide should be provided within the next month, if at all possible.
4. Provide home visits to develop Janice's interactive skills, particularly with siblings. SLP will meet with both parents to discuss interactive activities and will focus particularly on ways that the siblings can play with the baby. *Criteria/ timeline:* SLP will meet monthly with the family to teach and monitor interactive activities. Janice's communicative development will be evaluated formally at 6 months to decide what further intervention is needed at that time.

Early Intervention Services and Dates of Initiation of Services

1. Monthly meetings with SLP to develop breastfeeding and interactive activities. Begin July 21, 2005.
2. Social work services to explore financial and other assistance. Meet with social worker before the end of July 2005.
3. Visiting nurse or home health care to provide help to the mother as soon as can be arranged by social work service.
4. Explore possibility of classroom-based program for Janice with Regional Early Intervention Collaborative when Janice reaches eligibility age for program (12 to 18 months).

   Case Manager

SLP Kay Jones will coordinate services, do monthly home visits with family, contact social work services, and arrange next IFSP meeting after Janice's 6-month developmental assessment by the pediatrician.

Transition to Preschool Services at Age 3

SLP will coordinate multidisciplinary developmental evaluation at 30 months and arrange for coordination and transfer of information to school system Child Find team and oversee their evaluation and recommendations for preschool services. Case manager will argue for need for early intervention services in light of Janice's DS diagnosis.

A. Discuss the formal and informal methods available for assessing feeding and oral-motor development in infants.

B. Discuss the pros and cons of three major types of nonoral feeding used in the NICU.

C. Describe three ways the SLP can facilitate oral feeding in at-risk newborns. What instruments can be used to assess feeding skills?

D. How and why should the SLP promote hearing conservation in the NICU?

E. What is the purpose of assessment of infant behavior and development?

F. What information can the SLP gather in the NICU to assess infant development? What are some of the ways the SLP can contribute to the infant's development in the NICU?

G. When is a newborn ready to take advantage of interaction? Discuss the signs of readiness. How can we help families recognize them?

IV. Assessment and Intervention for Preintentional Infants and Their Families: 1 to 8 Months

A. Discuss methods for improving feeding skills in a 6-month-old baby.

B. Describe how you would use the assessment of vocal behavior to evaluate an 8-month-old baby. What could be done to enhance vocal production during the first year of life for a baby showing poor vocal skills?

C. List several instruments that can be used to assess infant development. What instruments are available for assessing early communicative development?

D. How can the SLP work to coordinate services for infants and their families?

E. How can assessment of parent-child communication be made family-centered?

F. Discuss the three areas in which the SLP can work to enhance parent-infant communication.

G. Name four interactive behaviors the SLP can encourage parents to use with their babies.

H. To what cultural issues must the SLP be sensitive in teaching baby games to parents?

V. Assessment and Intervention for Infants at Prelinguistic Stages of Communication: 9 to 18 Months
  A. How do the infant's communicative needs change in the last quarter of the first year of life?
  B. How can play assessment be used to evaluate the cognitive level in the prelinguistic infant?
  C. Discuss the terms *scaffolding* and *upping the ante*. How do they apply to intervention for the prelinguistic infant?
  D. How and when should communication temptations be used?
  E. How is language comprehension fostered in the prelinguistic infant?
  F. What parent training programs are available for the SLP to use in fostering parent-infant communication?
VI. Considerations for the Older Prelinguistic Client
  A. Describe techniques that can be helpful in developing feeding skills in prelinguistic clients.
  B. How do communication issues relate to feeding? Give examples of some strategies to deal with these issues.
  C. How are the development of feeding and speech related?
  D. Describe five methods used to assess feeding skills in infants or older prelinguistic clients.
  E. How can maladaptive forms of communication be addressed?
  F. How can we find out whether a client is ready to move from illocutionary to locutionary communication?
  G. Describe the PECS and talk about clients for whom it might be appropriate.
  H. Discuss methods of helping clients with prelinguistic communication to repair communicative breakdowns.
  I. Define *situated pragmatics*, and discuss assessment and intervention procedures associated with it.

SAMPLE INDIVIDUALIZED FAMILY SERVICE PLAN

Date of Referral: _____   Sample Format
Beginning IFSP Date: _____
Review Dates: _____

Child's Name: _____
   County of Residence: _____
   Date of Birth: _____
   School District: _____
   Current Placement/Services: _____
Mother's Name: _____
   Address: _____
Father's Name: _____
   Address: _____
   Phone (home): _____
         (work): _____
Case Coordinator: _____
   Phone: _____
Diagnosis: _____

Medical Information

Vision: _____
Hearing: _____
Medication: _____
Precautions: _____

IFSP Committee Signatures   **Date** _____

Parents(s): _____
Teacher: _____
Therapist: _____
County Representative: _____
Local Educational Agency Representative: _____
Speech-Language Pathologist: _____
Nurse/Pediatrician: _____
Social Worker: _____
Case Manager: _____

Adapted from Johnson B., McGonigel, M., and Kaufmann, R. (1989). *Guidelines and recommended practices for the Individualized Family Service Plan.* Washington, DC: Association for the Care of Children's Health; Fewell, R., Snyder, P., Sexton, D., Bertrand, S., and Hockless, M. (1991). Implementing IFSPs in Louisiana: Different formats for family-centered practices under Part H. *Topics in Early Childhood Special Education, 11,* 54-65.

DEVELOPMENTAL HISTORY

Date: _____

Child's Name: _____

   DOB: _____

   Address: _____

   Phone: _____

Family Composition

Mother: _____

Father: _____

Step-Parent: _____

Foster Parent: _____

Other Children: _____

Others Living in Home: _____

Grandparents, Relatives: _____

Pregnancy

Pregnancy was _____ normal _____ problem

   If problems, what kind: (please circle)

chronic disease	viral infection	Rh incompatibility
vaginal bleeding	toxemia	hypertension
trauma	other _____	

Birth History

Child's birth weight: _____

Length of labor: _____

Special considerations: (please circle)

cesarean	cord around neck	premature (# of weeks) _____
jaundice	breech	transfused
baby rotated	Rh negative	twin (1st born, 2nd born)
other _____		

Length of child's hospital stay: _____

List any special cares that were needed (e.g., oxygen, incubator, tube feedings, surgery): _____

CHILD'S PRESENT LEVELS OF DEVELOPMENT
Physical Development

   Vision: _____

   Hearing: _____

   Health Status: _____

Area	Test/Obs. Used	Date	Chron. Age/ CGA Age at Testing	Age Equivalent Score*
Cognitive	_____	_____	_____	_____
Speech/Lang.	_____	_____	_____	_____
Motor: Gross	_____	_____	_____	_____
Psychosocial	_____	_____	_____	_____
Self-Help	_____	_____	_____	_____
Additional Information:	_____	_____	_____	_____

*Age-equivalent score is reported only if test standard score indicates performance is significantly below age level. Otherwise WNL (within normal limits) is reported.

Continued

Family Resources, Priorities and Concerns/Outcome Statements

| Child/Family Needs and/or Concerns (present status) | Outcome Statement (includes criteria timelines) | Resources/Who's Responsible |

EARLY INTERVENTION SERVICES/DATES OF INITIATION AND DURATION OF SERVICES

Suggested Early Intervention Services

_____ Family Service Coordination   _____ Speech-Language Pathology

_____ Health Services   _____ Occupational Therapy

_____ Special Instruction   _____ Physical Therapy

_____ Family Training, Counseling, and Home Visits   _____ Audiology

_____ Medical Services (for diagnostic/evaluation purposes)

Services Parent(s) Feel Are Necessary to Meet Needs

Service Provided by	Frequency	Time	Location	Method	Begin	End	Payor	Contact Person	Phone No.

Case Manager/Transition Services

Case Manager/Family Service Coordinator:

    Name: _____

    Title: _____

    Agency: _____

    Phone: _____

Transition Plan (if applicable):

Date	Plan of Operation	Who's Responsible	Time Line	Date Achieved

How Can We Help?

Family Name: _____ Date: _____

Each child and family receiving early intervention services has their own strengths and needs. Please use this form to help us know how we can be most useful to your family. We know that your needs will change from time to time and that this will be just a beginning in helping us to plan together. Answer only those questions that you think will help us to know how we can be most helpful to you and your family.

What pleases you most about your child?

What worries you most about your child?

What kind of help or information about your child do you need?

Are there things that you feel are going well for your family and child right now?

In the next several months, I would like my child to be able to . . .

Besides my family, other people I would like to include in the assessment and planning meeting for my child and family are . . .

In the next several months, I would like my family to . . .

Continued

OUR FAMILY WOULD LIKE . . .

	We Have Enough	We Would Like More	Not Sure
Information about:			
Child development	_____	_____	_____
Child behavior	_____	_____	_____
Nutrition/feeding	_____	_____	_____
Our child's health problems	_____	_____	_____
Our child's developmental problem	_____	_____	_____
Toys or books for our child and how to get them	_____	_____	_____
Other: _____			
Help with child care:			
Finding daily child care	_____	_____	_____
Finding babysitters or respite care	_____	_____	_____
Finding a preschool for my child	_____	_____	_____
Teaching the care provider how to take care of my child	_____	_____	_____
Finding ways to pay for child care	_____	_____	_____
Evaluating child care settings or determining appropriate child care settings	_____	_____	_____
Other: _____			
To know about community services for my child and family:			
GED and other adult education	_____	_____	_____
Transportation to services	_____	_____	_____
Public transportation	_____	_____	
Who can help with transportation to doctor's appointments and other special services for my child	_____	_____	_____
Food, food stamps, WIC, or other nutritional programs	_____	_____	_____
Housing	_____	_____	_____
Fuel	_____	_____	_____
Clothing	_____	_____	_____
Finding a job or job training	_____	_____	_____
Financial assistance	_____	_____	_____
Individual or family counseling	_____	_____	_____
Other: _____			
To know about getting medical and dental care for my family:			
Finding a doctor or dentist	_____	_____	_____
Getting help paying for health care	_____	_____	_____
Getting and using special equipment and supplies for my child	_____	_____	_____
Training in how to give first aid/CPR for my family and others	_____	_____	_____
Family planning/birth control	_____	_____	_____
Other: _____			
Help talking about my child:			
To nieces, nephews, and to other children	_____	_____	_____
To friends and other relatives	_____	_____	_____
To doctors and nurses to get the information and help we want	_____	_____	_____
To other professionals (social workers, teachers, others) about my baby and ourselves to get the information and help we want	_____	_____	_____
To other people I meet	_____	_____	_____
Other: _____			
Help planning for the future/transition:			
Eligibility and the public school special education process	_____	_____	_____
Eligibility, legal rights, parent's role	_____	_____	_____
Visiting other service settings	_____	_____	_____
Determining the best setting for my child	_____	_____	_____
Other: _____			

Please tell us the other ways we might be able to help:

The early intervention program can provide services to help you help your baby grow and develop.
Families often need many services we cannot provide. When that happens, your case manager will help you find out how to get other community services.

ASSESSMENT AND INTERVENTION FOR EMERGING LANGUAGE

CHAPTER OBJECTIVES

Readers of this chapter will be able to do the following:

- Discuss the principles of family-centered practice for toddlers.
- Describe the communication skills of typical toddlers.
- Discuss methods of screening, evaluation, and assessment for emerging language.
- Describe strategies for using assessment information in treatment planning at the emerging language stage.

- List appropriate goals, procedures, and contexts for treatment of children at the emerging language stage.
- Discuss the issues relevant to communication programming for older, severely impaired clients with emerging language.

Joey had been a difficult baby. He'd cry inconsolably for hours on end, and the only way his parents could calm him was to put him in his car seat and drive around. Even at 6 months, when most babies have outgrown their colicky stage, Joey continued to be extremely irritable and unable to find comfort in his parents' cuddling and attention. He sat up at only 4 months, walked at 11 months, and at that time began to take an interest in objects that bounced or sprang. He spent long periods playing with rubber bands. He was quiet, too, and didn't seem to babble as much as his parents' friends' babies. When he was 18 months old, he said a few phrases, usually echoes of what he'd heard before, such as "Go, dog, go," or "Is it in you?" He didn't seem to be learning a lot of new words, though. Still, he was very good at letting people know what he wanted. He would take adults' hands and lead them to things. It didn't seem to matter much who the adult was, though. Once he got what he wanted, he was content to play with it alone for long periods. Everyone told his parents there was nothing to worry about; Joey was just a "late bloomer." When he had his second birthday, Joey's mother took him to the pediatrician for a checkup. The doctor asked about Joey's speech, and his mother reported that he said a few things. She commented that Joey's brother Bobby had talked a blue streak when he was 2 and said she remembered taking him to an amusement park for his second birthday present. She recalled that he'd known the names of all the animals on the merry-go-round and had labeled each one as it went past. She knew that all children were different, but maybe Joey really was

slow in his speech. She expressed her concern to the doctor. Her pediatrician recommended that Joey have his hearing tested. When the test came back within normal limits, the pediatrician reassured her that Joey would probably grow out of his slow start in speech.

Joey's story probably sounds familiar. Everyone knows a toddler who was late to begin talking, and everyone knows that most of them do eventually "catch up." We've all heard stories about how Einstein didn't start talking until he was 4. Popular wisdom, common sense, and most people's experience support Joey's pediatrician's claim that Joey will grow out of his early delay. However, for some toddlers, early lags in the development of speech foretell more long-lasting problems. Some of the other behaviors Joey has displayed throughout his development, such as his early inconsolability, his inordinate interest in particular kinds of objects, his lack of social awareness, and his use of echoed phrases, may suggest greater risk for long-term disability. How can we decide which toddlers with slow language development are at risk for long-term deficits? What should we do about them? These are some of the questions this chapter addresses.

This chapter also discusses assessment and management issues for youngsters identified as at-risk for communication disorders during infancy. These children will probably begin to evidence their delays during the 18- to 36-month period that comprises the toddler age range. This is the time during which children normally begin speaking, producing single words, and soon beginning to combine words into two-word utterances and simple sentences. If a child is going to have problems developing language, those problems will probably become evident in the toddler stage.

Finally, the approaches and principles discussed in this chapter will be appropriate for assessing and treating children of any age whose language is just emerging. Preschoolers with language disorders and older children and adolescents with severe deficits in language learning also can be seen to function in this stage. In summary, then, this chapter addresses methods of assessment and intervention for any client just beginning to use symbolic forms of expression.

Remember that when we discuss children at this beginning language level we mean children whose *developmental level* is 18 to 36 months. Some toddlers who do not talk, particularly those identified as at-risk during infancy, will not yet function at this developmental level. Using the general developmental assessment tools outlined in this chapter, a toddler's developmental level can be described. When developmental assessment indicates that a child is functioning below a 12- to 18-month level, even if he or she is chronologically older, management should continue to follow the guidelines given in Chapter 6. Only when general developmental level reaches 18 months or so should the direct communication intervention that is discussed in this chapter be considered.

We'll refer to this period as the *emerging language* (EL) stage, to suggest that this is the period in which conventional words are just beginning to appear as viable forms of communication. Children may enter the emerging language stage at any age, of course, just as the child with prelinguistic communication can be of any age. For normally developing children, this stage corresponds to the "toddler" age range, or an 18- to 36-month developmental level. Let's look first at issues in assessment and intervention for children who are chronologically close to this age range. Then we'll discuss issues for older children functioning as emerging communicators.

ISSUES IN EARLY ASSESSMENT AND INTERVENTION

SCREENING AND ELIGIBILITY FOR SERVICES

IDEA 2004 provides for the development of programs for infants and toddlers with disabilities, as we saw in Chapter 6. One of the intents of this law is to affect both primary and secondary prevention by allowing children with disabilities to be identified as early as possible and to receive prompt intervention. Evaluations of early intervention efforts, such as the Guralnick (1997), McLean and Cripe (1997), the National Research Council (2001), and Reynolds, Want, and Wahlberg (2003) comprehensive reviews, have concluded that early intervention is effective, often resulting in faster gains than those seen in normal development, so the justification for intervening in these cases is quite compelling. The law's impact on clinical practice for speech-language pathologists (SLPs), then, is that

more and more children younger than 3 are being identified and referred for communication evaluation, assessment, and intervention. SLPs employed in a variety of settings—in hospitals, schools, nonprofit agencies, and private practice—will be seeing this birth-to-3 population.

Children we will serve include those born with known risk factors who were referred for speech and language services during infancy. These are children with identifiable syndromes of developmental disorder, such as Down syndrome or fetal alcohol syndrome; those with hearing impairments identified in infancy; and those with neurological involvement, such as cerebral palsy or prenatal drug exposure. For these children, no screening or evaluation for eligibility will be necessary.

Other children, though, may also present as toddlers with apparently specific language delays. These children may come to us through Child Find or other referral sources or simply because parents are concerned about their development. Some of these toddlers may turn out to have related disorders, such as hearing impairment, that were not previously detected, or less obvious forms of developmental disorder, such as fetal alcohol effects or fragile X syndrome. Some may have suffered from early acquired disorders secondary to diseases such as encephalitis or from trauma or abuse. Some, like Joey, will have disorders on the autism spectrum. Some will have no evident correlates of their slow language development, but present with circumscribed deficits in language skills that place them at risk for specific language impairment or learning disabilities at school age. For these children, screening may be the first step in the evaluation process.

In recent years, several screening instruments have been developed and refined to help clinicians make a general determination about whether further evaluation for communication is needed. Two parent report measures, which focus primarily on vocabulary size, have been prominent. The *MacArthur-Bates Communication Development Inventory* (Fenson et al., 1993) has been shown in a variety of studies (e.g., Girolametto, Wiiigs, Smyth, Weitzman, & Pearce, 2001; Heilmann, Weismer, Evans, & Hollar, 2005; Lyytinen, Eklund, & Lyytinen, 2003; Weismer & Evans, 2002) to be effective in identifying toddlers with low language skills, and to be valid for both English- and Spanish-speaking toddlers (Marchman & Martinez-Sussman, 2002). *The Language Development Survey* (LDS; Rescorla, 1989) has also been shown to be valid, reliable, sensitive, and specific for this purpose (Klee, Pearce, & Carson, 2000; Rescorla & Achenbach, 2002; Rescorla & Alley, 2001). Klee et al. (2000) also reported that the number of false positive results decreased when questions about ear infections and whether parents were concerned about the child's language development were added to the LDS criterion of less than a 50-word expressive vocabulary or no word combinations for 24-month-olds. Although there are no current mandates for universal screening for toddlers for language delay, these instruments can be given to parents who have concerns about their children's language development, as a first step toward deciding whether further evaluation is needed. Clinicians can also distribute these instruments to local pediatricians. Their patients who have some concern about a toddler's language can be encouraged to complete them. The SLP can periodically review these to decide whether any referrals to birth-to-three services should be made.

For toddlers who have delays in cognition, motor, and other areas besides language, evaluation is clearly warranted. But not all would agree that an otherwise typical child of 18 to 36 months who fails to begin talking or who talks very little is evidencing significant delay. Many professionals both in and outside the field of language pathology would hesitate to label a child with no other difficulties outside of speech development as "language disordered" before the third or even the fourth birthday (Rescorla & Lee, 2001), for just the reasons mentioned earlier—that many children who are slow to start talking eventually catch up. Providing intervention at the 18- to 36-month level for such children would not be cost-effective. Early intervention, although known to be effective when necessary, is expensive. It is wise to conserve such resources for children who really need them.

So who needs them? Both Whitehurst and Fischel (1994) and Paul (1996, 1997a) have argued that for children in the 18- to 36-month age range, the decision to intervene should be based on an accumulation of risk factors. These researchers suggested that children with cognitive deficits, hearing impairments or chronic middle ear disease, social or preverbal communicative problems, dysfunctional families, risks associated with their birth histories, or family history of language and reading problems (Bishop, Price, Dale, & Plomin, 2003; Lyytinen, Poikkeus, Laakso, Eklund, & Lyytinen, 2001) should receive highest priority for intervention. Brady, Marquis, Fleming, and McLean (2004), Campbell, Dollaghan, Rockette, Paradise, Feldman, Shriberg, Sabo, and Kurs-Lasky (2003), McCathren, Yoder, and Warren (1999), and Olswang, Rodriguez, and Timler (1998) suggested that additional factors, listed in Box 7-1, also be considered. In light of these suggestions, a detailed case history and comprehensive direct assessment of all these areas are important for any toddler referred for failure to begin talking. When a toddler with slow language

---

| **BOX 7-1** | **Predictors and Risk Factors for Language Growth in Toddlers** |

Predictors of Need for Intervention

Language

1. Language Production
   Small vocabulary for age
      Few verbs
   Preponderance of general verbs (*make, go, get, do*)
      More transitive verbs (that take a direct object: *hit ball*)
      Few intransitive verbs (without direct object: *lie down*) and bitransitive verbs (that take both direct and indirect object: *give* the *ball* to *me*)

2. Language comprehension
   Presence of 6-month comprehension delay
   Comprehension deficit with large comprehension-production gap

3. Phonology
   Few prelinguistic vocalizations
   Limited number of consonants
   Limited variety in babbling
   Reduced rate of babbling
   Fewer than 50% consonants correct (substitution of glottal consonants and back sounds for front)
   Restricted syllable structure
   Vowel errors

4. Imitation
   Few spontaneous imitations
   Reliance on direct modeling and prompting in imitation tasks

Nonlanguage

1. Play
   Primarily manipulating and grouping
   Little combinatorial or symbolic play

2. Gestures
   Few communicative gestures, symbolic gestural sequences, or supplementary gestures (gestures that add meaning to words produced)

BOX 7-1   Predictors and Risk Factors for Language Growth in Toddlers—cont'd

3. Social skills
   Reduced rate of communication
   Reduced range of expression of communication intentions
   Behavior problems
   Few conversational initiations
   Interacts with adults more than peers
   Difficulty gaining access to peer activities

Risk Factors for Language Delay

1. Males more vulnerable to delay than females
2. Otitis media
   Prolonged periods of untreated otitis media
3. Family history
   Family members with persistent language, reading, and learning problems
4. Parent characteristics:
   Low maternal education
   Low SES
   More directive than responsive interactive style
   Produces less talk contingent on child's productions
   High parental concern

Adapted from Brady, N., Marquis, J., Fleming, K., & McLean, L. (2004). Prelinguistic predictors of language growth in children with developmental disabilities. *Journal of Speech, Language, and Hearing Research, 47,* 663-677; Campbell, T., Dollaghan, C., Rockette, H., Paradise, J., Feldman, H., Shriberg, L., Sabo, D., & Kurs-Lasky, M. (2003). Risk factors for speech delay of unknown origin in 3-year-old children. *Child Development, 74,* 346-357; McCathren, R., Yoder, R., & Warren, S. (1999). The relationship between prelinguistic vocalization and later expressive vocabulary in young children with developmental delay. *Journal of Speech, Language, and Hearing Research, 42,* 915-924; and Olswang, L., Rodriguez, B., & Timler, G. (1998). Recommending intervention for toddlers with specific language learning difficulties. *American Journal of Speech-Language Pathology, 7,* 29.

development shows significant risk factors, intervention is clearly warranted. The goal of that intervention is secondary prevention—minimizing the effects of the delay on the acquisition of language.

There are a variety of standardized instruments that can be used to evaluate toddlers for eligibility for birth to three services. Generally, regulations require that children show impairments in at least two areas in order to be eligible for services; whether expressive and receptive language constitute two areas varies from state to state. Clinicians will need to be familiar with the guidelines for their particular locality. However, informed clinician opinion is always part of the evaluation process, so test scores alone will not be adequate to establish eligibility. Because more than one area of deficit is typically required for eligibility, instruments that sample several areas of development are often used for this purpose. Some procedures that can be part of this evaluation are listed in Box 7-2.

For toddlers without other known risk factors who are simply slow to start talking, deciding whether to intervene is more difficult. Intervention for this group may accomplish facilitation, hastening development that would eventually

happen on its own, rather than induction. Children who have learning disabilities are known to have histories of delayed language development (Butler & Silliman, 2002; Catts, 1997; Catts & Kamhi, 1986; Maxwell & Wallach, 1984; Steele, 2004; Tallal, 2003; Weiner, 1985). Even late talkers who perform within the normal range in language and literacy measures by age 5 or 6 (Paul & Fountain, 1999) begin to show deficits in literacy skills later in development (Rescorla, 2002), and there is a risk that these will persist into adolescence (Rescorla, 2005; Snowling, Adams, Bishop, & Stothard, 2001; Snowling & Bishop, 2000). Early language intervention may serve a secondary preventive function, then, helping to minimize later effects on learning even when the more basic oral language problems resolve. In addition, Robertson and Weismer (1999), for example, showed that intervention for late talkers not only increased their language skills but resulted in improvements in social skills and reductions in parental stress, so there may be other important secondary effects of supplying early intervention to these children. Paul (2000b) has argued that perhaps the best approach for late talkers without additional risk factors is to provide parent training in language facilitation techniques, rather than direct intervention. Girolametto, Pearce, and

---

BOX 7-2 **Instruments for Evaluating Children Under Three**

Mullen Scales of Early Learning (Mullen, 1995)
Vineland Adaptive Behavior Scales—II (Sparrow, Cicchetti, & Balla, 2005)
Assessment, Evaluation, and Programming System (AEPS): For Infants and Children (ed. 2) (Bricker, 2002)
Battelle Developmental Inventory (ed. 2) (Newborg, Stock, Wnek, Guidubaldi, & Svinicki, 2004)
Bayley Scales of Infant and Toddler Development—III (Bayley, 2005)
Birth to Three Assessment and Intervention System (Ammer & Bangs, 2000).
Cognitive, Linguistic, and Social-Communicative Scales (ed. 2) (CLASS; Tanner, Lamb, & Secord, 1995)
Developmental Assessment of Young Children (DAYC; Voress & Maddox, 1998)
Developmental Profile II (DP-II) (Alpern, Boll, & Sheare, 1997)
Hawaii Early Learning Profile: 0–3 (HELP; Furuno, O'Reilly, Inatsuka, Husaka, Allmon, & Zeisloft-Falbey, 1994)
The Vulpe Assessment Battery—Revised (VAB-R) (Vulpe, 1997)

Weitzman (1996) and Peterson, Carta, and Greenwood (2005) showed that parents of late talkers could be trained to produce positive effects on the amount of child speech, the size of child vocabulary, and the number of multi-word combinations.

TRANSITION PLANNING

Hadden and Fowler (2000) discussed the importance of developing active coordination among agencies serving young children with disabilities in order to smooth their transition from early intervention to preschool programs. SLPs can play an important role in developing these interagency relationships. Prendeville and Ross-Allen (2002) outlined a variety of ways SLPs can be effective members of transition teams. These include the following:

▶ Providing families with information and support to participate in transition planning
▶ Setting aside time to work with team members from both early intervention and preschool service providers to prepare a timely transition plan
▶ Sharing information about adaptations, accommodations, resources, and developmentally appropriate activities with preschool staff
▶ Actively helping preschool staff prepare the necessary services and supports to promote successful preschool placement

FAMILY-CENTERED PRACTICE

Like children at the prelinguistic stage of development, children with emerging language still function primarily in the context of the family. Practice for this developmental level, too, must be family-centered in order to succeed. Many of the same principles we discussed for infants apply to our work with toddlers. Dinnebeil and Hale (2003), Dunst, Boyd, Trivette, and Hamby (2002), and Polmanteer and Turbiville (2000) discuss some of the considerations that are primary in working with families in early intervention. These include the following:

▶ Spending time with the family to learn about their vision for the child and discussing what parents would like to see their child do as a result of intervention
▶ Finding out what families expect from the program at the outset and discussing expectations in order to come to a consensus about what is reasonable to expect
▶ Including the family's assessment of the child in the assessment report; writing the report in the words used by the family
▶ Including multiple ways for families to be involved in the child's program; providing choices and options
▶ Working together with families to choose natural environments as a source of learning opportunities; reviewing progress with families to make sure new skills are used consistently across natural environments; identifying important people with whom the child needs to practice communication skills
▶ Working with families to find ways to use children's interests to involve them in everyday learning opportunities
▶ Providing families with opportunities to be involved in both direct work with their child and acquiring new knowledge and skills for interacting with their child; enabling parents to decide on the correct balance for their family

COMMUNICATIVE SKILLS IN NORMALLY SPEAKING TODDLERS

What do we mean by "normal language development" in toddlers? Considerable research in recent years has allowed us to flesh out the picture of what constitutes normal language skills in very young children, so that we can determine when development is falling behind. Wetherby, Cain, Yonclas, and Walker (1988) and Paul and Shiffer (1991) reported that children at about 18 months of age produced an average of two communicative acts per minute in interactive samples. The functions of these acts are usually to request objects or actions, to establish joint attention, or to engage in social interaction (Hulit & Howard, 2002; Wetherby, Woods, Allen, Leary, Dickinson, & Lord, 2004). During the second year of life, many of these intentions are expressed not with words, but with gestures (Capone & McGregor, 2004) and vocalizations (Oller, 2000). By 24 months, children produce an average of five to seven communicative acts per minute (Chapman, 2000). The majority of these communicative acts consists of words or word combinations, although some nonverbal acts are still used. Between 18 and

24 months of age, then, children significantly increase their frequency of communication, both verbally and nonverbally, and move toward more frequent verbal expressions of intent.

Nelson (1973) showed that most middle-class toddlers were combining words into simple two-word sentences by 18 months; Roulstone, Loader, Northstone, and Beveridge (2002) reported that 78% of typically developing 25-month-olds were using multiword utterances. Grove and Dockrell (2000) reviewed literature that demonstrates that there are predictable patterns in the ways words are first combined, with stable word orders that follow patterns in the adult language, and that the meanings expressed by children in their first "telegraphic" sentences conform to a small set of semantic relations. Stoel-Gammon (1987, 2002) indicated that normally developing 24-month-olds produced at least 10 different consonants and were 70% correct in their consonant productions. Speech samples of these toddlers included a variety of syllable shapes, including CV and CVC, in virtually every child, and two-syllable words in the majority; the most frequent two-syllable form was the CVCV reduplicated syllable. McLeod, van Doorn, and Reed (2001) also showed that 2-year-olds are beginning to produce consonant clusters, although they may not always be correct relative to adult targets.

Detailing changes in expressive vocabulary size in the second and third years of life has been the focus of much recent research (e.g., Dale, 2005; Feldman et al., 2005; Rescorla & Achenbach, 2002). Fenson, Dale, Reznick, Hartung, and Burgess (1990) reported that average expressive vocabulary size at 18 months is about 110 words. Dale, Bates, Reznick, and Morisset (1989) have shown that by 20 months, average productive lexicon size reaches 168 words. By 24 months, Fenson et al. found mean vocabulary size to be 312 words, and at 30 months, 546 words. Stoel-Gammon (1991) pointed out that there is a great deal of variability in lexicon size in young children, but that this variability decreases dramatically during the third year of life. At 18 months, the variability in vocabulary size is larger than the mean, so that more than 16% of children still have very few words at this age. However, by 24 months the average variation in vocabulary size is only half as large as the mean and 84% of children at this age have vocabularies larger than 150 words. At 30 months the standard deviation in vocabulary size is only 18% of the average lexicon size. This means that 84% of children at this age have vocabularies larger than 450 words. The degree to which a small expressive vocabulary represents a significant deficit increases drastically between 18 and 30 months of age.

Traditional wisdom has been that comprehension precedes production. Receptive vocabulary size is always larger than the size of the productive lexicon; this is true even for adults. For example, if you read the sentence, "Her proclivity for using long sentences in lectures drove her students to distraction," you would no doubt comprehend the word *proclivity*. But if you were asked to come up with a synonym for *tendency* you might not be so likely to produce *proclivity*. The child's comprehension of a first word is usually about 3 months ahead of the production of a first word, and comprehension of 50 different words usually occurs about 5 months before the productive lexicon reaches this size (Benedict, 1979).

In terms of sentences, though, comprehension is probably not so far ahead of production. Chapman (1978) argued that children in the 18- to 24-month age range probably understand only two to three words out of each sentence they hear (that is, about the same number of words per sentence that they are producing in their own speech). The appearance of more sophisticated comprehension skills that they often achieve is related to their ability to use nonlinguistic information to supplement their knowledge of language. These comprehension strategies allow the child to combine cues from gestures, facial expressions, and the way they know things usually happen with their understanding of words. The result is that children can appear to comprehend a long sentence such as, "Why don't you go close that door for me?" by combining their knowledge of the meaning of *close* and *door* with their understanding that adults usually ask children to do things (Paul, 2000a; Thal & Flores, 2001).

The information presented here can help to guide us in determining whether a toddler is significantly behind in communicative skills. In some ways, the recent research may lead us to intervene more quickly than we might have earlier. The demonstration that children as young as 24 months communicate frequently, have large vocabularies, and are accurate in their phonological productions the great majority of the time may emphasize and make more obvious the deficits seen in children with slow communicative growth. In addition, Thal and Clancy (2001) show that the interaction between biological development and environmental input plays an important role in language acquisition, so that providing high-quality input can have significant effects on early development. Still, we want to use caution and remember the large variations seen in normal development. In this chapter we'll look at some procedures that can be used to assess the various areas of communicative development in children with emerging language: symbolic play and gestural behavior, intentional communication, comprehension, phonology, and expressive language. We'll then look at some guidelines for integrating these assessment data into the processes of deciding when and how to intervene with children at this developmental level.

ASSESSMENT OF COMMUNICATIVE SKILLS IN CHILDREN WITH EMERGING LANGUAGE

Multidisciplinary and Transdisciplinary Assessment

When children younger than 3 years are assessed by an evaluation team, the assessment may be multidisciplinary or transdisciplinary. In multidisciplinary assessment, each professional carries out a relatively independent assessment, exploring the issues relevant to his or her own discipline. The SLP assesses communication issues, the physical therapist assesses motor skills, and so on. The team comes together at the end of the assessment to report findings, talk with parents, and plan intervention. Many of the assessment procedures outlined in this chapter could be used in this model. They provide in-depth information that can be used not only to decide whether a client is significantly impaired but also to establish baseline function and identify intervention goals.

An alternative form of assessment being used with increasing frequency for children younger than 3 is the transdisciplinary approach (Kritzinger, Louw, & Rossetti, 2001; Linder, 1993; Rossetti, 2001), sometimes called "arena assessment." Transdisciplinary or arena assessments involve the child's interacting with just one adult, a "facilitator," who performs some formal and informal assessments. The other members of the team, including the SLP, observe the facilitator's interaction with the client. They may ask the facilitator to present certain tasks to the child, and they take notes on their observations of the child's behavior in the situation, but they do not interact directly with the client. This approach is useful for looking at very young children who may have difficulty responding to a changing parade of unfamiliar adult faces. Many of the assessment techniques we discuss in this section can be incorporated into transdisciplinary evaluation by having the SLP go over them with the facilitator before the client is seen and then by having the facilitator include them with his or her interactions with the child. For example, the SLP might ask the facilitator to do a play assessment or a communicative intention assessment (both of which are described in this chapter). The SLP could teach the procedures to the facilitator, gather the necessary materials, and explain the purpose of the assessment. During the interaction with the client, the SLP would observe and score the client's responses on a prepared worksheet and also would note any other relevant behaviors the client displays. Transdisciplinary assessment is generally used for evaluation; to decide whether a young child is eligible for early intervention services. Once eligibility for speech and language services has been established, the clinician can do more in-depth criterion-referenced assessments during the course of the intervention program, if additional information is needed to establish baseline function and choose intervention goals.

Play and Gesture Assessment

Before deciding that a toddler has a communication problem, we want to be sure that the child has achieved a general developmental level consistent with the use of symbolic communication. This is a controversial area. Traditional Piagetian thinking on the relation between language and cognitive development held that children could not be expected to use symbolic language until they had achieved certain cognitive milestones, such as the understanding of object permanence, tool use, or symbolic play. A great deal of research on the relations between cognitive and language development (Tomasello, 2002; Witt, 1998) has suggested, though, that such simple prerequisite relations are not typically found in normal development. Thal (1991) explained that most current researchers in this area do not believe that there is a general relationship between language and cognition. Instead there is what researchers call *local homologies*. Local homologies are specific relationships that

occur at certain points in development. For example, Bates, Bretherton, Snyder, Shore, and Volterra (1980) have shown that in the single-word period, there is a strong relationship between the use of words as labels and the ability to demonstrate functional play, or to use objects in play for their conventional purposes, such as putting a toy telephone up to the ear. A little later, when children begin to combine words, this relationship decreases in strength. However, a relationship emerges between the ability to combine words and the ability to produce sequences of gestures in play, such as going through the series of motions to feed and bathe a doll. Later, this relationship, too, declines.

Current thinking about these findings (e.g., Casby, 2003a) suggests that although particular cognitive skills are not necessarily prerequisites for language development in general, certain behaviors that can be observed in a child's play and gestural behavior tend to go along with particular communicative developments. Brady et al. (2004) and McCathren et al. (1999) for example, showed that prelinguistic children with developmental disabilities who used symbolic play behaviors were likelier than those who did not to increase their rate of communication in an intervention program. If early symbolic behaviors are present, this would suggest that the language skill that normally appears along with them should be within the child's zone of proximal development and that it should be teachable. If the play and gestural skills are absent, as well as the language, then we might attempt to elicit both the play and language skills in tandem, since their development seems to be parallel and they may reinforce or complement each other.

Play assessment provides a specifically nonlinguistic comparison against which to gauge a child's linguistic performance. It also gives insight into particular aspects of the child's conceptual and imaginative abilities. The point of play assessment, and more generally of cognitive assessment at the 18- to 36-month level, is not to decide whether the child has the "prerequisite" cognitive skills for learning language. Language learning is more complicated than that. The main thing we have learned about the connection between language and cognition is that we cannot specify what their relationship is, except perhaps for very small segments of time, and even then there is no clear chicken or egg. The point of these assessments is to sketch a fuller picture of the equipment the child is bringing to the task of learning to talk. Knowing what play abilities the child has helps to decide, not so much the language skills the child is ready to learn, but the activities, materials, and contexts that will be most appropriate to encourage that learning and the conceptual referents on which it might focus. Play also is the most natural context for language learning. Knowing the level of play behavior that the child is able to use can help the clinician structure play sessions that will maximize the child's participation and opportunities for learning.

A variety of methods are available for assessing level of play skills in children at the 18- to 36-month developmental level. Several of these were outlined in Chapter 2. Any of these assessments can serve to identify the child's play skills to determine how they can be put in the service of language acquisition. An additional assessment tool specifically designed for the toddler developmental level is the *Communication and Symbolic Behavior Scales-Developmental Profile* (Wetherby & Prizant, 2003). This procedure analyzes videotaped samples of interactive play behavior and allows the clinician to score both symbolic and combinatory play, in order to provide a general level of symbolic development that is relatively independent of language. It has been shown to be reliable and valid for identifying children with developmental delays in the emerging language period (Wetherby, Allen, Cleary, Kublin, & Goldstein, 2002).

Another method is Carpenter's (1987) *Play Scale*. This scale was designed to assess symbolic behavior in nonverbal children who don't "talk out" their play, so that symbolic skills must be inferred from their interactions with objects. As such, the scale is useful both for nonspeaking toddlers and for older children at the emerging-language stage. To use this scale, a parent is asked to play with the child by engaging in four play scenes with appropriate props: a tea party, a farm, and scenes involving transportation and nurturing. Parents are asked to follow the child's lead in interacting with each set of toys for just 8 minutes. Parents are advised to respond to the child in a natural way, but to let the child play without continually talking or giving directions. Parents are asked not to touch the toys unless invited to by the child and not to give suggestions for play. They are given specific prompts to provide only when the child will not touch or play spontaneously with a set of toys. A detailed description of this assessment can be found in Carpenter (1987). A sample of behaviors examined by this assessment and the ages at which they are mastered by more than 90% of children with normal development appear in Table 7-1.

McCune (1995) also provided a detailed method of analyzing play behavior. Using her system, the child is given a standard set of toys including a toy telephone, dolls, a toy bed and covers, a toy tub, a tea set, combs and brushes, a toy iron and ironing board, toy cars, toy foods, and similar items. The child is then invited to play with the objects along with a familiar adult. Criteria for analyzing the behaviors observed are ordered hierarchically; they are summarized in Table 7-2. The highest level of play the child exhibits spontaneously can be taken as the child's current level of symbolic behavior. Once this has been established, an emerging level of symbolic play also can be identified by having the clinician model the next level of symbolic play. If the child imitates this model, emergence into the next level of symbolic behavior can be inferred. The types of symbolic behavior that the child can attain in assessments such as these can be used as contexts in which language intervention takes place. In addition, higher levels of play behavior can be modeled by the clinician and parents in informal interactions with the child. These models can help the client evolve toward more advanced modes of symbolic thinking that will, in time, provide even richer contexts for language acquisition.

Casby (2003b) provides guidance for conducting these assessments. He suggests presenting the child with a set of toys

TABLE 7-1	Play Scale Items		
PLAY BEHAVIOR*	**DEFINITION**	**EXAMPLE**	**AGE**
Semiappropriate toy use	Uses object in appropriate but fleeting way; object need not be correctly oriented.	Touches comb to hair with tines facing up; puts blanket on doll in crib but only covers doll's face.	12 mo
Nesting	Object(s) placed or stuffed into a container; need not be correctly oriented or topic-related	Crams all toys into crib; tosses all cars into cowboy hat.	15 mo
Multiple play episodes with different actions	Two or more appropriate or semiappropriate toy uses that are thematically related and involve different actions; object may or may not be the same.	Pushes truck, loads blocks in truck; feeds doll with spoon, gives cup to parent to drink.	18 mo
Multiple play episode with same action	Two or more appropriate or semiappropriate toy uses that are thematically related; the actions are the same but the objects differ.	Feeds doll with spoon, feeds self with spoon; pushes truck, Jeep.	21 mo
Extended multiple play episode	Three or more appropriate or semiappropriate toy uses that are thematically related. There must be three different actions; objects may or may not be the same.	Dials telephone, puts telephone to ear and talks, hangs up; takes doll out of truck, puts truck in garage, puts doll on motorcycle and "drives" away.	24 mo

*Play behaviors for which three examples were produced by more than 90% of children at given age in a play session in which children interacted with parent during four play scenes for 8 min each. Play scenes: tea party (dolls, table, chairs, eating and cooking utensils); farm animals; nurture (dolls, crib, toy comb, brush, bottle, telephone, hat); transportation (garage, cars, trucks, boats).

Adapted from Carpenter, R. (1987). Play scale. In L. Olswang, C. Stoel-Gammon, T. Coggins, & R. Carpenter (Eds.), *Assessing prelinguistic and early linguistic behaviors in developmentally young children* (pp. 44-77). Seattle: University of Washington Press.

TABLE 7-2	Guidelines for Play Assessment		
APPROXIMATE DEVELOPMENTAL LEVEL	**SYMBOLIC PLAY LEVEL**	**McCUNE (1995) AND NICOLICH (1977) CRITERIA**	**EXAMPLES**
<18 mo	1	Presymbolic scheme: the child shows understanding of conventional object use or meaning by brief recognitory gestures. There is no pretending. Properties of present object are the stimulus. Child appears serious rather than playful.	Picks up a brush, touches it to hair, drops it. Picks up the toy telephone, puts it to ear, sets it aside. Swishes broom on floor briefly.
18–24 mo	2	Autosymbolic scheme: the child pretends at self-related activities. Pretending is present. Symbolism is directly involved with the child's body. Child appears playful, seems aware of pretending.	Pretends to drink from toy teacup. Eats from an empty spoon. Closes eyes, puts hands by cheek, pretending to sleep.
24–36 mo	3	Single-scheme symbolic games: the child extends symbolism beyond own actions by including other agents or objects of actions. Pretending at activities of other people or objects such as dogs, vehicles, etc.	Feeds doll. Brushes doll's hair. Pretends to read a book. Pretends to sweep floor. Moves a block or toy car with appropriate sounds of vehicle.
24–36 mo	4	Combinatorial symbolic games: 4a. Single-scheme combinations: one pretend scheme is related to several actors or pretend receivers of action.	Combs own, then mother's hair. Drinks from toy bottle, then feeds doll from bottle. Puts empty spoon to mother's mouth, then experimenter and self.
		4b. Multischeme combinations: several schemes are related to one another in sequence.	Holds telephone to ear, dials. Kisses doll, puts it to bed, puts blanket on. Stirs in the pot, feeds doll, washes dish.
24–36 mo	5	Hierarchical pretend: 5a. Planned single-act symbolic games: the child indicates verbally or nonverbally that pretend acts are planned before being executed. 5b. Planned multischeme symbolic acts.	Finds the iron, sets it down, searches for the cloth, tossing aside several objects. When cloth is found, irons it.

Adapted from McCune, L. (1995). A normative study of representational play at the transition to language. *Developmental Psychology, 31* (2), 206; Nicolich, L. (1977). Beyond sensorimotor intelligence: Assessment of symbolic maturity through analysis of pretend play. *Merrill-Palmer Quarterly, 23,* 89-99.

that lend themselves to pretend. These include blocks, balls, rattles, and paper and crayons, dolls or stuffed toys, feeding utensils (cup, spoon, etc.), hygiene utensils (brush, washcloth, etc.), nurturing toys (blanket, bottle), and a toy telephone. The clinician can then begin playing out a theme, such as feeding the doll, in parallel play with the child, modeling a range of play behaviors. The highest level of behavior the child demonstrates in response to these models can be scored. Casby also suggests that the child should be allowed to play alone with the materials for part of the time, in order to look for differences in play when a model is absent.

Use of gestures is an additional aspect of symbolic behavior. Several studies have shown that gestures are highly related to language in early development (Bates & Dick, 2002; Goldin-Meadow & Butcher, 2003). Goldin-Meadow and Butcher (2003) discuss the fact that young children often rely on gestures to express meanings when they are still very limited in their verbal abilities, and that word-gesture combinations often lead the way to multiword speech. Evans, Alibali, and McNeil (2001) showed that children with language disorders, too, use gestures to express meaning that is beyond their linguistic capacity. Moreover, Goodwyn, Acredolo, and Brown (2000) showed that children whose parents used word-gesture combinations in interactions when they were infants outperformed control groups on language measures when they were toddlers. Capone and McGregor (2004) also showed that for children with a variety of communication disorders, early use of gestures tends to predict language development. Gesture use, then, may be an important prognostic indicator for children with delayed language. Capone and McGregor (2004) discussed the types of gestures that can be assessed and the general sequence of gestural development. This discussion is summarized in Table 7-3. Assessment of gestural use can take place in the context of play assessment. Additional notations can be made when gestures appear, using a form like the one in Figure 7-1. Alternatively, the *Communication and Symbolic Behavior Scales-Developmental Profile* (Wetherby & Prizant, 2003) and the *McArthur-Bates Communicative Development Inventory* (Fenson et al., 1993) contain scales for assessing the use of gestures.

Communication Assessment

A variety of scales are commercially available for assessing a range of communicative skills in children younger than 3. These measures can be used to provide a broad picture of communicative functioning and to decide whether, in general, it is commensurate with the child's current functioning in other areas. Many of the general developmental assessments outlined in Box 7-2 provide a scale or subtest of language ability or contain some items that tap language skills. The *Transdisciplinary Play-Based Assessment* (Linder, 1993), for example, provides opportunities for observing social-emotional, cognitive, communicative, and sensorimotor skills. It is particularly useful for clinicians working within transdisciplinary assessment settings. However, it is often useful to look at language and communication skills more specifically in a child in the emerging language stage who is suspected of a delay in language development. In this way we can avoid confounding the child's nonverbal abilities with any deficits in communication that might exist. This is particularly useful for toddlers suspected of having specific communication deficits rather than more general developmental delays.

One strategy for assessing a child with emerging language follows. First, a general developmental level could be ascertained by a psychologist or developmentalist, using one of the general scales outlined in Box 7-2, or by a transdisciplinary team using *Transdisciplinary Play-Based Assessment (TPBA)*. If developmental level is near or greater than 18 months, the language pathologist can use the developmental level to guide a more in-depth comparison of language and nonlinguistic skills. To achieve this end, the SLP can first administer a play assessment (or use data from the TPBA to evaluate play behavior) as a nonverbal index of cognitive development. This index can be used to decide whether the child with emerging language appears to be at or near the level of symbolic development

TABLE 7-3	**Gestures and Gestural Development in the Prelinguistic and Emerging Language Stages**			
GESTURE TYPE	**10–12 MO**	**12–13 MO**	**15–16 MO**	**18–20 MO**
Deictic (showing, giving, pointing, ritualized requests such as reaching)	Deictic gestures emerge; use of pointing predicts first word use		Gestures complement spoken forms; children show preference for either gestural or vocal expression	Increased pointing in combination with spoken words
Symbolic (play schemes, including recognitory gestures: actions carried out on an object to depict the object and its function; e.g., holding a toy telephone to the ear)		Play schemes emerge, recognitory gestures first, then self-directed symbolic play; e.g., "feeding" self from empty spoon	Other-directed play schemes emerge; e.g., pretending to "feed" doll	Transition to play schemes w/out object; e.g., holding hand to ear instead of toy telephone to pretend "talking" Multischeme symbolic play emerges; e.g., "stirring" then "feeding"
Representational (do not manipulate objects; a form is used to stand for a referent; e.g., flapping arms to represent a bird)		Representational gestures emerge; e.g., puts hand to mouth to indicate wants bite of Mom's cookie.	Gestures complement spoken forms; children show preference for either gestural or vocal expression	Gesture-plus-spoken word combinations emerge; increase in word use; preference for words over gestures

Adapted from Capone, N., & McGregor, K. (2004). Gesture development: A review for clinical and research practices. *Journal of Speech, Language, and Hearing Research, 47*, 173-187.

	10-15 mo. level	15-18 mo. level	18-21 mo. level	21-24 mo. level
Deitic	Show——— Give——— Point——— Ritualized request———		Deictic gesture accompanies word———	
Symbolic	Recognitory gesture———	Self-directed play———	Other-directed play——— Play scheme w/o object——— Sequence of play schemes———	Planned multischeme play———
Representational	Representational gestures———		Representational gestures accompany speech———	Gesture-plus-word combinations used to express two-word meaning———

FIGURE 7-1 ✦ Sample form for recording play and gestural behavior.

that would ordinarily accompany symbolic communication. The clinician can then assess language and communication specifically and compare them to nonverbal abilities. If nonverbal symbolic and communicative abilities are both very low, then intervention may focus on providing play contexts that can elicit early symbolic behaviors while providing simple language input around the emerging levels of play. If, on the other hand, symbolic play is more advanced but communication and language are found to be at lower levels, more focused language elicitation techniques in appropriate play contexts may be used.

We will talk more about decision-making strategies for planning communicative intervention for this developmental level shortly. For now the important point to be made is that we want to have a relatively independent assessment of nonverbal cognitive or symbolic ability and language or communication. One effective way to meet this goal is to assess play behavior and to use some additional means of assessing communication level as well.

There are two approaches to accomplishing the communication portion of this assessment. One is to use a formal assessment instrument. Table 7-4 lists several instruments available either commercially or in the research literature. Some, such as the *Language Development Survey* (Rescorla, 1989) and the *MacArthur-Bates Communicative Development Inventories* (Fenson et al., 1993), use a parent report format. Others use direct assessment or a combination of direct observation and parent report. The *Communication and Symbolic Behavior Scales-Developmental Profile* (Wetherby & Prizant, 2003) provides an example of one form of direct assessment, and also has parent report components. Wetherby and Prizant (2003) also provided normative data at the 6- to 24-month developmental range. The instrument can be used with children who function at the emerging language stage but are as old as 6 years in chronological age. It also has been demonstrated to be valid with children from culturally different backgrounds (Roberts, Medley, Swartzfager, & Neebe, 1997). Some additional assessment procedures appropriate for this developmental level can be found in *Preschool Functional Communication Inventory* (Olswang, 1996), *Interdisciplinary Clinical Assessment of Young*

Children With Developmental Disabilities (Guralnick, 2000), *Alternative Approaches to Assessing Young Children* (Losardo & Notari-Syverson, 2002), and the *Assessment, Evaluation, and Programming System for Infants and Children* (Bricker, Capt, & Pretti-Frontczak, 2002). All these sources include dynamic, criterion-referenced procedures that use developmentally appropriate approaches for evaluating young children.

A second method of assessing communication involves using informal methods to examine communicative functioning in several domains independently. This strategy, advocated by Crais and Roberts (1991) and Paul (1991b), has the advantage of integrating assessment and intervention activities and allowing more detailed intervention planning. This is possible because, instead of a general level of communication, the procedure allows several areas of communicative behavior to be examined separately and a level of development established in each. In this way, a profile of communication and related abilities can be derived, and specific intervention targets in nonverbal communication, expressive language, receptive language, and phonology can be readily identified. In addition, informal methods allow the clinician to interact more directly with the child and to use more "child-initiated" (Norris & Hoffman, 1990a) activities for observation and evaluation.

Paul (1991b) outlined informal procedures for profiling early communicative skills. These procedures make use of real time rather than videotaped interactions, as well as analysis of audiotaped and interview data. Many areas assessed in this procedure are very similar to those examined in the *Communication and Symbolic Behavior Scales* (Wetherby & Prizant, 2003). This procedure is described in some detail here, not as an endorsement, but to give the student clinician a detailed idea of what is involved in informal assessment of the various areas of communication at this developmental level.

ASSESSING COMMUNICATIVE INTENTION

Even before they begin to talk, children with emerging language attempt to communicate with those around them. This commu-

TABLE 7-4	**General Communication Assessments for Children Younger Than 3**

INSTRUMENT	COMMENT
Assessing Prelinguistic and Early Linguistic Behaviors in Developmentally Young Children (Olswang, Stoel-Gammon, Coggins, & Carpenter, 1987)	Provides assessments of phonology, expressive language, preverbal communication, play, and cognitive antecedents to word meaning; norm-referenced data from relatively small sample.
Birth to Three Assessment and Intervention System—2nd Edition (Ammer & Bangs, 2000)	Provides examiners with an integrated, three-component system for screening, assessing, and intervening with children ages birth–3 yr; the three component parts are the *Screening Test of Developmental Abilities, Comprehensive Test of Developmental Abilities,* and the *Manual for Teaching Developmental Abilities.*
Carolina Curriculum for Infants and Toddlers—3rd Edition (Johnson-Martin, Attermeier, & Hacker, 2004)	Provides an in-depth, whole child assessment and intervention covering 26 domains of development for children ages birth–24 mo; looks at areas of cognition, communication, social skills, fine- and gross-motor skills; excellent sections on preverbal and verbal communication.
The Capute Scales: Cognitive Adaptive Test and Clinical Linguistic and Auditory Milestone Scale (CAT/CLAMS) (Capute et al., 2005)	Norm-referenced 100-item screening and assessment instrument; surveys broad range of communicative behaviors and visual-motor functioning; designed for use by pediatricians with infants 1–36 mo of age.
Communication and Symbolic Behavior Scales (CSBS) (Wetherby & Prizant, 1993)	Includes assessment of symbolic play, nonverbal communication, and expressive and receptive language; requires videotaped observation; uses communication temptations.
Communication and Symbolic Behavior Scales—Developmental Profile (CSBS DP) (Wetherby & Prizant, 1993)	Norm-referenced screening tool for identifying infants at risk for developmental delay or disability. Includes assessment of symbolic play, nonverbal communication, and expressive and receptive language. Contains a checklist, caregiver questionnaire, and behavior sample.
Early Language Milestones Scale—2nd Edition (Coplan, 1993)	Designed for pediatric screening; pass/fail criterion only; evaluates expressive, receptive, and visual skills; best for identifying severe delays.
Early Learning Accomplishment Profile (E-LAP) (Glover, Preminger, & Sanford, 1995)	Developed to assess gross- and fine-motor skills and social, cognitive, and language areas; designed to identify the developmental level of functioning.
Environmental Prelanguage Battery (MacDonald & Carroll, 1992)	Assesses early prelinguistic communication skills such as play, gestures, imitation, and following directions.
Expressive One-Word Picture Vocabulary Test—2000 Edition (Brownell, 2000)	Offers an in-depth assessment of a child's speaking vocabulary by asking the child to make word-picture associations; comprehensive manual provides standard scores, scales scores, stanines, percentiles, and age equivalents.
Interaction Checklist for Augmentative Communication—Revised (Bolton & Dashiell, 1984)	Developed for clients with physical barriers to speech, but provides assessment of interactive behaviors useful with developmentally young clients.
Language Development Survey (Rescorla, 1989)	Screening tool for evaluating expressive language; parent-report instrument; good validity for identifying language delay in toddlers.
MacArthur-Bates Communicative Development Inventories (Fenson et al., 1989)	Parent-report instrument with scales for assessing expressive and receptive vocabulary sizes and early grammatical production; reports good validity when compared with direct observation measures.
Preschool Language Scale—4th Edition (Zimmerman, Steiner, & Pond, 2002)	Measures a broad range of receptive and expressive language skills; provides standard scores and percentile ranks in addition to age equivalents for auditory comprehension, expressive communication, and total language; PLS tasks are ordered to reflect acquisition of sequential developmental milestones in language.
Receptive One Word Picture Vocabulary Test—2000 Edition (Brownell, 2000)	Provides an assessment of receptive vocabulary; child indicates (from four possible alternatives) the picture that represents a word spoken by the examiner; test is individually administered and can be administered and scored in 20 min.
Receptive-Expressive Emergent Language Scale—3rd Edition (Bzoch, League, & Brown 2003)	Parent-interview instrument; tends to overestimate comprehension level.
Reynell Developmental Language Scales-III (Edwards et. al., 1999)	Designed to measure language skills in young or developmentally delayed children; the verbal comprehension scale measures receptive language skills and the expressive language scale assesses production skills using three sets of items (structure, vocabulary, and content).

TABLE 7-4	General Communication Assessments for Children Younger Than 3—cont'd

INSTRUMENT	COMMENT
Rossetti Infant and Toddler Language Scale (Rossetti, 1990)	Used to assess preverbal and verbal communication skills and interaction in children from birth-3 yr; criterion-referenced measure looks at language comprehension, language expression, interaction, attachment, gestures, pragmatics, and play.
Sequenced Inventory of Communicative Development—Revised (Hedrick, Prather, & Tobin, 1984)	Diagnostic test that evaluates the communication abilities of children with and without retardation who are functioning between 4 mo and 4 yr of age.
Symbolic Play Test—2nd Edition (Lowe & Costello, 1988)	Assessment provides an objective indication of child's early concept formation and symbolization; includes a format for informal data collection of play features.
Test of Early Language Development—3rd Edition (Hresko, Reid, & Hammill, 1999)	Yields an overall spoken language score and includes scores for subtests of receptive and expressive language; psychometric qualities include demographics, reliability, validity, and limited bias.
Test of Pretend Play (TOPP) (Lewis & Boucher, 1999)	TOPP is designed to assess the three different types of symbolic play: substituting one object for another object or person; attributing an imagined property to an object or person; or making a reference to an absent object, person, or substance; TOPP also is designed to assess whether the child can incorporate several symbolic actions into a meaningful sequence, and a child's level of conceptual development.
The Nonspeech Test (AAC) (Huer, 1988)	Standardized on preschoolers and children with multiple disabilities in schools and institutions; this test of receptive and expressive language is popular for children who are nonspeaking; test yields an age equivalency score in monthly increments from 0 to 48 mo.
Transdisciplinary Play-Based Assessment: A Functional Approach to Working with Young Children—Revised (Linder, 1993)	A dynamic, comprehensive instrument that provides information to conduct play sessions that combine insights of parents with the expertise of a transdisciplinary team; uses specific observation guidelines to assess a child's cognitive, social, emotional, communication, and language development during play time.

nication can take several forms. It can be verbal, through the use of single words or combinations of words, or it can be nonverbal, through the use of a variety of gestures and sounds. Children can get their messages across by pointing, reaching, whining, babbling, or vocalizing a variety of protowords that don't sound like adult targets but do have speech-like components. Many of these nonverbal forms can be recognized by adults as attempts to communicate. Very often an adult familiar with the child with emerging language can discern the child's intention in these nonverbal forms.

There are several ways in which communication changes over the course of the second and third years of life. One way is that it becomes more verbal, with nonverbal means of communication gradually giving way to more conventional verbal forms. Another way is that attempts increase in frequency, with rates of communication more than doubling over the 18- to 24-month period. A third way is that the range of intentions the child is trying to express broadens. The result of all these changes is that by the third birthday, the normally developing toddler is more like an adult speaker than like his or her 1-year-old counterpart. Paul and Shiffer (1991), Pharr, Ratner, and Rescorla (2000), and Rescorla and Mirren (1998) showed that late-talking toddlers generally show lower rates of communication, vocalization, initiation, and joint attention, even nonverbally, than their typical peers.

When toddlers are referred for evaluation, it is usually because they have failed to begin talking or are talking very little. One of the things we need to learn about such toddlers, or about an older child with emerging language, is whether this failure to speak is accompanied by a more pervasive deficit in the ability to communicate generally or whether it is restricted to the oral symbolic modality of speech. That is, we need to know whether and how the child is sending messages nonverbally. Children with little speech who attempt to communicate with those around them by other means have a potentially strong foundation that can support the growth of functional language. On the other hand, children with both sparse speech and little or no nonverbal communication have less motivation to acquire symbolic forms, since they are not so actively engaged in attempting to send messages to others. These children may need to learn the purpose of communication in order to lay the communicative grounding on which language can be built.

To assess communicative function in this age range, we need to observe the child playing with some interesting toys and a familiar adult. Westby (1998b) and Casby (2003b) emphasize the importance of providing low-structure interactions in which toys are accessible and the adult follows the child's lead. This encourages the child to call the adult's attention to himself and his actions and prevents an over-representation of request acts. The same toys used in the play assessment can be used here. In fact, if the play assessment is videorecorded, as Wetherby and Prizant (2003) suggest, it can be viewed again as a sample of communicative behavior. Because the rate of communication is generally quite low at this developmental level, though, it also is possible to observe communicative behavior without recording but by simply watching a client interact with a parent. After some practice, most clinicians can learn to score communicative behavior in real time (Coggins & Carpenter, 1981), so long as this is the only behavior they are trying to observe. If play assessment also is to be done from a real-time observation, it will have to be done in a separate session, even if the same materials and participants are involved.

Three aspects of communication can be examined as part of this assessment: the range of communicative functions expressed, the frequency of communication, and the means by which the child attempts to convey his or her messages. Let's look a little more closely at each of these areas.

RANGE OF COMMUNICATIVE FUNCTIONS

There are a variety of schemes for summarizing the communicative functions typically seen in normally developing toddlers (see Chapman, 1981; Paul & Shiffer, 1991; and Wetherby et al., 1988, for review). Perhaps the most accessible system, though, is the one outlined by Bates (1976) and elaborated by Coggins and Carpenter (1981). Bates divided early communication into two basic functions: *proto-imperatives* and *proto-declaratives*. Proto-imperatives are used to get an adult to do or not do something. They include the following:

Requests for objects: Solicitation of an item, usually out of reach, in which the child persists with the request until he or she gets a satisfactory response.

Requests for action: Solicitation of the initiation of routine games or attempts to get a movable object to begin movement or reinitiate movement that has stopped.

Rejections or protests: The expression of disapproval of a speaker's utterance or action.

Proto-declaratives are preverbal attempts to get an adult to focus on an object or event by such acts as showing off or showing or pointing out objects, pictures, and so on, for the purpose of establishing social interaction or joint attention. By far the most frequent proto-declarative function seen in normally developing toddlers (Paul & Shiffer, 1991) is the *comment*, which is used to point out objects or actions for the purpose of establishing joint attention. Comments are very important in the development of mature language because they establish the framework for the topic-comment structure of adult conversation. Social-interactive intentions, such as showing off or calling attention to self, can also be included in this category. Both proto-imperative and proto-declarative intentions appear in normally developing toddlers between 8 and 18 months of age.

Beyond these earliest appearing intentions, several new communicative functions appear for the first time at about 18 to 24 months in normally developing children. These new intentions are evidence of more advanced levels of communicative behavior. They have what Chapman (1981, 2000) called *discourse functions* (that is, they refer to previous speech acts rather than objects or events in the world). They indicate that the child has now incorporated some of the basic rules of conversation into a communicative repertoire, such as the conversational obligation to respond to speech. These discourse functions include the following:

Requests for information: Using language to learn about the world. At the earliest stages, the requesting information function can take the form of requests for the names of things. Later, they may include a *wh-* word, a rising intonation contour, or both.

Acknowledgments: Providing notice that the previous utterance was received. In young children this is often accomplished verbally by imitating part of the previous utterance or nonverbally by mimicking the interlocutor's intonation pattern. Head nods also can communicate this intention.

Answers: Responding to a request for information with a semantically appropriate remark.

These more advanced intentions, then, are evidence of a higher level of communicative function than the use of the earlier set alone. All seven of the communicative functions we've discussed are listed on the Communication Intention Worksheet in Figure 7-2.

When looking at the range of intentions expressed, we try to determine, first, whether the full range of the early developing intentions is being used. This is because various kinds of disabilities show different profiles of expression of communicative intentions. Mundy and Crawson (1997) and Mundy and Burnette (2005) report, for example, that children with autism are likely to produce proto-imperative functions but less likely to produce proto-declaratives. Children with Down syndrome, on the other hand, show more proto-declarative intentions but have deficits in proto-imperatives. Similarly, Paul and Shiffer (1991) reported that toddlers with slow language development produced significantly fewer proto-declarative comments, even nonverbally, than their normally speaking peers. So failure to produce the full range of early intentions, particularly comments, may be an important indicator of diagnostic category and prognosis in children with delayed language development.

If the full range of early intentions is observed, we then want to determine whether any of the higher-level intentions are being expressed. If so, the client would clearly be ready to learn words for mapping these intentions. If not, conventional words for the early intentions expressed could be targeted. In addition, the clinician could provide simple one-word models of the more advanced intentions. The SLP might, for example, acknowledge client utterances consistently, saying "Yes!" before going on to comment on the child's remark. Clinicians also can model seeking information by stating simple questions for the client, then answering them (that is, when looking at the client's shirt, the SLP can say, "What color? Green!").

I. Early intentions

Form: →	Gesture (8-12 mo.)	Vocalization (12-18 mo.)	Word (18-24 mo.)
Function Expressed: ↓			
Request action			
Request object			
Protest			
Comment			

II. Later intentions (18-24 months)

Form: →	Gesture	Vocalization	Word
Function Expressed: ↓			
Request information			
Answer			
Acknowledge			

FIGURE 7-2 ✦ Communication intention worksheet.

FREQUENCY OF EXPRESSION OF INTENTIONS

We've talked about how the frequency of communication changes over the age range in which language normally emerges. We expect 18-month-olds to produce about two instances of intentional communication per minute, whereas we generally see more than five per minute in 24-month-olds (Chapman, 2000). If a prelinguistic client produces fewer than 10 total communicative acts within a 15-minute observation (and if the parent affirms that the behavior during the observation was more or less typical of the child), this rate would be considered significantly low. In addition, Yoder, Warren, and McCathren (1998) reported that children with mild to moderate retardation in the prelinguistic period were unlikely to develop functional speech if they produced fewer than one proto-declarative communication act every five minutes. This suggests that if a nonspeaking client produces fewer than three proto-declarative acts within a 15-minute observation period, there is a risk for development of functional speech. In both these cases, intervention would focus not only on eliciting single-word productions, but also on increasing the frequency of nonverbal communication, particularly proto-declaratives. Communication temptations, such as those outlined by Prizant and Wetherby (1989), may be useful for this purpose.

FORMS OF COMMUNICATION

As children progress through the emerging language period, they increase the sophistication of the forms of communication they use. Chapman (1981, 2000) summarized the progression this way:

1. Gestural means of communication are predominant at approximately 8 to 12 months of age.
2. Gestures are combined with word-like vocalizations containing consonants at 12 to 18 months.

3. Conventional words or word combinations are used with increasing frequency to express a range of intentions at 18 to 24 months.

So another aspect of the child's communication that we would note is the form used. Purely gestural forms would be considered less advanced than vocalizations, which are in turn less mature than conventional words. These stages of communicative form are included in Figure 7-2.

Yoder, Warren, and McCathren (1998) demonstrated that prelinguistic children who produced fewer than one vocal communication act every four minutes were significantly less likely to develop functional speech 1 year later. If fewer than four vocal communications are produced in a 15-minute communication interaction, then an attempt ought to be made to elicit vocalizations for functions the child is already expressing with gaze and gestures. We may need to help children understand that we must do something relatively specific with our mouths to communicate effectively, and this effort may need to precede elicitation of particular words. If, on the other hand, four or more functions are expressed with vocalizations in a 15-minute sample, words should be taught first in the context of those functions. Later the same words can be taught to express other functions currently expressed with gestures alone.

USING A COMMUNICATION INTENTION WORKSHEET

A worksheet such as the one in Figure 7-2 can be used to summarize the child's performance during an assessment of intentional communication. Column heads list the form of the communicative act: gesture, vocalization, or conventional word. For the earliest-appearing intentions or functions (proto-imperatives and proto-declaratives), the form of the communication determines its level. For any of these early appearing functions, a gestural form is taken as evidence of performance comparable to that of a normal 8- to 12-month-old. A gesture plus a speech-like vocalization ("dada") or nonconventional word-like vocalization alone is considered evidence of 12- to 18-month-level performance. An intelligible word or word approximation is assigned to an 18- to 24-month level. For the later-developing intentions—such as requesting information, acknowledging, and answering—the form, whether gesture, vocalization, or word, is noted in much the same way as it is for the earlier set. However, here the form does not determine communicative level. Form is merely noted for intervention planning. All the later-developing intentions are considered evidence of 18- to 24-month communication performance.

Clinicians who devote time to learning the coding system for communicative intents can score a 15-minute interaction involving a nonverbal or minimally verbal child, using Figure 7-2, during short interactions without resorting to videotaping or other recording schemes. The most common mistakes made in using this coding system involve being too generous in attributing communicative intent to the child (that is, beginning clinicians are likely to score any action of the child's as some form of communication). To qualify as communicative act, though, a child's behavior must satisfy the following criteria:

1. It must be directed, primarily by means of gaze, to the adult. The child must look at, refer to, or address the adult directly in some way as part of the act.
2. It must have the effect, or at least the obviously intended effect, of influencing the adult's behavior, focus of attention, or state of knowledge. The child must be obviously trying to get a message across to someone.
3. The child must be persistent in the attempt to convey a message if the adult fails to respond or responds in a way the child had not intended.

A clinician can become skillful in this kind of observation by coding videotaped interactions with another clinician, learning to recognize the communicative acts as a team, then coding independently until their reliability reaches a 90% level.

This form of communication assessment is not based on standardized, quantitative procedures. So it is not crucial to score every single communicative act within an observation period. Instead, a clinician should attempt to note and score the general—not the precise—frequency and function of communication by recording as many acts as can be coded with a reasonable degree of certainty. Note can be taken of the diversity both of functions expressed and of the forms used to express them. Such assessment data have the potential to yield an index of the three dimensions of communicative behavior we have been discussing: (1) *frequency of communication,* (2) *diversity of functions* expressed, and (3) *diversity of forms* used to express the functions. This index can serve as a guide to planning an intervention program that helps the child to expand the frequency and range of intentions expressed and increase the maturity of the means of expression.

In addition to assessing the child's communication, there also are instruments for assessing parent communication, which we looked at in Chapter 6. Another example is *The Infant-Toddler Family Assessment Instrument* (Apfel & Provence, 2001). As we discussed before, though, it is very important to avoid any appearance of blaming the parent for the child's communication problem. Research on language-disordered children in general (Leonard, 1989) and on toddlers with slow expressive language development in particular (Paul & Elwood, 1991) indicates that parental input is generally well-matched to the child's language level, although there are some subtle differences in the input to late-talkers (Vigil, Hodges, & Klee, 2005). This is not to say that there won't be some parents who are poor communicators. But in general, the great majority of parents are doing the best they can to get through to an often hard-to-reach child. They don't need to be made to feel that they are at fault if their child is not developing normally. They probably aren't at fault, and even if they are, feeling bad about themselves won't help. Rather than subjecting parents to an intimidating assessment of their own communication skills, we would be better off just to ask them what makes communicating with their child hard for them. We can then offer suggestions to address the concerns they raise. These suggestions will probably be the same ones we would offer in any case: following the child's lead, modeling talking about ongoing experiences with self-talk, expanding on what the child says or indicates interest in, limiting initiating new topics and giving the child time to respond, and using other indirect language stimulation techniques and communication temptations (Girolametto, Weitzman, Wiigs, & Pearce, 1999; Vigil et al., 2005). Isn't it better to offer these suggestions in a spirit of helping the parent with needs he or she identifies than as a correction of the parents' mistaken attempts?

We also need to be sensitive to cultural differences in communication styles. Parents from all cultures do not talk to toddlers the way middle-class contemporary American parents do (Garrett, 2002; Rodriques & Olswang, 2003; Westby, 1998b). We in mainstream America tend to use a very contingent form of interaction, making our remarks depend on what the child contributes. However, many other cultures use a more routine style: providing, in a variety of settings, repetitive, predictable language that is initiated by the parent rather than the child. Some cultures use child-rearing patterns that involve encouraging children to listen and observe interactions, rather than speaking themselves. And in many cultures young children spend most of their time with multiple caregivers, including older siblings, rather than with their own mothers. Toddlers in all these cultures learn to talk, at about the same rate as toddlers in our own. Our way is one way that works to teach language to children, but there are other ways. If we see parents using these more routine styles, we need to be aware that these styles are not "wrong." They may, in fact, be more "right" for a child who will eventually function within that cultural group than the styles we prefer.

There are some clues, though, that parent interactional style has an effect on how children respond to intervention. Yoder and Warren (1998) and Brady et al. (2004) showed that prelinguistic children with more responsive mothers were more likely to increase the frequency and maturity of their communication in structured intervention. Children with less responsive mothers did better with a small group intervention program that incorporated a more child-centered, facilitative play method. These data suggest that rather than judging parental style as "good" or "bad," we may want to understand it in order to help decide what intervention approach will be most effective for a particular child from a particular family.

To summarize the communicative intention assessment, then, we want to evaluate communicative behavior independent of conventional language use. Looking at the frequency of communicative behavior and the diversity of forms and functions the child has available helps us decide what the client is most ready to learn. If little communicative behavior is present, we need to get clients to see what communication is for and to find ways of getting messages across to others. We can then help them find more conventional means for expressing the intentions they are developing. Parents must see us as allies in this enterprise, since they will be doing much of the communication with the child. It is crucial that we respect their concerns and individual styles of interacting, then try to choose an intervention that complements their style.

ASSESSING COMPREHENSION

As Chapman (1978) long ago pointed out, parents often claim that children as young as 12 months "understand everything" said to them. However, researchers have found receptive language skills to be quite limited at this age. Normally developing children accomplish this "deception" by the use of a series of strategies for comprehending linguistic input. These strategies change with development to incorporate new linguistic knowledge as it is acquired and to integrate it with knowledge of the way things usually happen. The use of comprehension strategies not only enables the child to "look good" in receptive

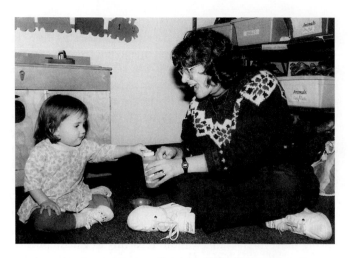

Assessing expression of communication intentions.

language activities, but also provides children with stepping-stones to the next level of development by allowing them to participate successfully in interactions and get feedback on their performance. For example, a mother playing with a 10-month-old girl might point to a ball on the floor while saying to her, "Get the ball!" The child would not have to comprehend a single word to comply with the instruction. All she would have to do is to follow the point gesture and then act in the most customary way on the object noticed. A strategy like "Look at what mother looks at; then do something about it," would allow her to appear to interact successfully without really knowing the meaning of the words. The child would at the same time be learning to make a connection between the word *ball* and the thing for which it stands. Table 7-5 summa-

	TABLE 7-5	**Summary of Comprehension Abilities in Children Up to 3 Years Old**

AGE	COMPREHENSION ABILITY	COMPREHENSION STRATEGY
8–12 mo	Understands a few single words in routine contexts	1. Look at same objects as mother 2. Act on objects noticed 3. Imitate ongoing action
12–18 mo	Understands single words outside of routine, but still requires some contextual support	1. Attend to object mentioned 2. Give evidence of notice 3. Do what you usually do
18–24 mo	Understands words for absent objects, some two-term combinations	1. Locate objects mentioned, give evidence of notice 2. Put objects in containers, on surfaces 3. Act on objects in the way mentioned (child as agent)
24–36 mo	Comprehends three-term sentences, but context or past experience determines meaning; little understanding of word order	1. Probable location, probable event 2. Supply missing information

Adapted from Chapman, R. (1978). Comprehension strategies in children. In J.F. Kavanaugh & W. Strange (Eds.), *Speech and language in the laboratory, school, and clinic* (pp. 308-327). Cambridge, MA: MIT Press; Edmonston, N., & Thane, N. (1992). Children's use of comprehension strategies in response to relational words: Implications for assessment. *American Journal of Speech-Language Pathology, 1,* 30-35.

rizes the strategies identified by Chapman (1978), Edmonston and Thane (1992), and Paul (2000a) that are used in the 1- to 3-year age range.

When evaluating very young children with delayed language, then, we need to be careful about relying totally on parental impressions of children's receptive skills. Like normally developing children, children with delayed linguistic development may use strategies that make them appear to understand language when in fact their comprehension is based on attention paid to nonlinguistic behaviors and cues, such as gaze, gestures, and situations, or event probabilities (Coggins, 1998; Miller & Paul, 1995; Paul, 2000a). It is important, then, to assess the status of receptive language skills in any child at risk for delayed language development.

Very few standardized tests of receptive language for children younger than 3 years are available. Many of those that are, such as the *Peabody Picture Vocabulary Test—Revised (PPVT-4)* (Dunn & Dunn, 2006) or *Communication and Symbolic Behavioral Scales-DP* (Wetherby & Prizant, 2003), assess only single-word vocabulary. Parent checklists designed to assess receptive vocabulary have been shown to be less reliable than those assessing expressive skills at the emerging language level (Dale, 1991; Thal, O'Hanlon, Clemmons, & Fralin, 1999). General scales, such as the *Receptive-Expressive Emergent Language Scale, 3rd Edition* (Bzoch, League, & Brown, 2003), the *Sequenced Inventory of Communicative Development* (Hedrick, Prather, & Tobin, 1995), and the others listed in Table 7-4, look at a range of responses to both verbal and nonverbal auditory stimuli. While these general measures can be quite useful for assessing listening skills, more specific information about how children process word combinations and sentences is helpful for deciding what a child is able to discern from the language in the environment. Miller and Paul (1995) provided a broad range of comprehension assessment activities for this developmental level. We'll outline a sampling of them here.

The major questions to be answered about the comprehension skills of children in the emerging language stage first involve whether words are understood at all without the support of nonlinguistic cues. If so, we will want to know whether words within a sentence can be processed and semantic relations understood. These questions can best be answered observationally, not only because there are few standardized tests for children at this level, but also because, as Coggins (1998) and Paul (2000a) pointed out, comprehension in very young children is highly context-dependent. As a result, the ability to manipulate context, disallowed in standardized tests, is an important aspect of the assessment. Also, the vocabularies of these children may be somewhat idiosyncratic. The words they understand may not be those routinely tested on standardized instruments. They may, instead, be words for the family pet, for a particular toy, for a favorite game, and so on. It is often useful, when planning an assessment session, to interview parents briefly on the telephone about their child's comprehension skills. They can then be asked to bring to the evaluation several items whose names the child might know.

In the first phase of comprehension assessment, the clinician determines whether the child understands any single words without the support of nonlinguistic cues. A collection of six to eight objects (the names of which the parents indicated the child may know) is placed before the child. Single words are then presented in a simple sentence frame ("Give me…"). The clinician must be careful not to look at the item being named, point toward it, or name an item the child already is handling or reaching toward. Since only the word for the object is being tested in this procedure, a gesture, such as holding out the hand, can be used to indicate "Give me… ." Several other words, such as person names (e.g., Mommy, child's name) and nouns for body parts and locations (e.g., table, chair, floor, door), can be tested using a "Where's (object)?" sentence frame. These instructions can be modeled by first asking the parent, "Where's the table?" and having the parent demonstrate answering the question by touching or pointing to the named object. The *Communication and Symbolic Behavioral Scales—DP* (Wetherby & Prizant, 2003) uses body part names ("Show me your nose!") to accomplish this portion of the assessment.

If the child can identify several nouns in this way, verbs can be tested next. Words for actions that the parent indicated the child is likely to know, such as *kiss, hug, bite, push, pat, throw,* and *hit,* can be tested by offering the child an object (since only the verb is being tested here) and saying "Hit it. Throw it. Pat it." and so on. It is necessary in both the noun and verb assessments to have the child demonstrate comprehension of each word two to three times at random intervals during the initial phase of the comprehension assessment. Comprehension of single words without the support of nonlinguistic cues is taken to indicate performance expected at the 12- to 18-month level in normally developing children (Chapman, 1978).

If the child fails to show reliable signs of any lexical comprehension, an attempt can be made to step back and see whether the child makes use of 8- to 12-month-level comprehension strategies outlined in Table 7-5. After the initial phase of the assessment is completed, the same words can be tested again, but this time paired with gestural cues. If performance is better with the addition of these nonverbal cues, the child can be said to be using 8- to 12-month strategies. The worksheet seen in Figure 7-3 can be used to record these data.

If the child demonstrates linguistic comprehension of three to five nouns and three to five verbs at the 12- to 18-month level, testing for 18- to 24-month-level comprehension performance can proceed, as indicated in Figure 7-3. Here the primary goal is to assess understanding of two-word instructions. One such instruction is the *action-object* semantic relation. Because children functioning at 12- to 18-month levels of comprehension use a "Do what you usually do" strategy to respond to such instructions, it is necessary to present *unusual* two-term combinations to assess whether an individual child is responding to the word combinations themselves. Combinations should be generated from the words on which the child succeeded in the first part of the assessment. Using a worksheet like Figure 7-3, we can list words comprehended during the first phase of the assessment in the 12- to 18-month

Age	Comprehension activity	Linguistic stimuli	No. of trials	Strategy observed From previous level
8-12 mos	Routine games without gestural cues	_____	_____	
12-18 mos	Single words	_____ _____ _____ _____	_____ _____ _____ _____	Look at what examiner looks at; act on objects noticed; imitate ongoing action
18-24 mos	Two-term instructions	_____ _____ _____ _____	_____ _____ _____ _____	Attend to object mentioned; give evidence of notice; do what you usually do
24-36 mos	Three-term instructions: probable	_____ _____ _____ _____	_____ _____ _____ _____	Locate objects mentioned and give evidence of notice; child-as-agent

FIGURE 7-3 ✦ Informal comprehension assessment worksheet.

section. In the 18- to 24-month section, the *action (verb)-object (noun)* combinations of these words that we use to test understanding of word combinations can be recorded. Unexpected combinations would include instructions such as "Kiss the apple," "Hug the shoe," and "Push the baby." Each action-object combination should be tested several times, as in the individual noun and verb assessments.

If a child fails to respond correctly to a majority of the two-term combinations presented, then probable combinations can be presented to assess whether the more basic 12- to 18-month level strategy "Do what you usually do" is operative. Clients can be asked to "Bite the apple" or "Push the car." If they respond correctly to these instructions but not to the unusual ones, a "Do what you usually do" strategy can account for this performance. (Some children may demonstrate a reliance on this strategy when responding to the unusual combinations in the assessment [that is, when told to "Kiss the apple," they may bite it, or when told to "Hug the car," they may push it]).

If the child succeeds on a majority of the 18- to 24-month items, demonstrating linguistically-based comprehension of two-term relations, we can move on to the next phase of the comprehension assessment, in which we try to determine the presence of appropriate behaviors at the 24- to 36-month level. Typical children at this level are able to process *agent-action-object* instructions, but they still rely on a "probable event strategy" for deciding which noun represents the agent and object of action. When presented with a sentence such as "The mommy feeds the baby," children in the 24- to 36-month period typically perform successfully on object manipulation tasks. But if asked to act out the sentence, "The baby feeds the mommy," they are likely to interpret it in the more probable direction (mommy feeds baby). To test for basic 2- to 3-year-level comprehension skills, then, a series of probable agent-action-object sentences should be presented, first using the same vocabulary items that were used in the earlier phases of

the assessment. Children who get this far in the assessment process generally have larger vocabularies. More nouns (such as *girl, boy, baby, dog*) and verbs (such as *lick, pull, chase*) can be pretested in the same manner as the earlier single words. These words can then be used in constructing probable three-term combinations to be acted out with toys. If children use a "child-as-agent" strategy by performing the requested actions on the named object themselves, we can interpret this behavior as evidence of an 18- to 24-month-level comprehension strategy.

Because these procedures are not standardized, there are no hard and fast criteria for deciding when a child "passes" or "fails" a particular level. If a child is performing correctly on a majority of items at one level, credit for that developmental level of comprehension can be given, at least provisionally, even if the child uses some lower-level strategies. If a client is getting the majority of items wrong, we must then ask whether the child is using a comprehension strategy appropriate to the previous developmental level, which is listed in the last column of the worksheet in Figure 7-3. If this is the case, then the previous level of strategy used ought to be attributed to the child. For example, a client may be able to act out unusual two-word combinations, such as "Bite the fish." When asked to act out three-term combinations such as "Make the horse bite the cow" (24- to 36-month level), though, the child may bite the cow himself or herself. If this happens, failure on the 24- to 36-month-level items is noted on the worksheet. In addition, the "child-as-agent" strategy is circled in the last column of the worksheet at the 24- to 36-month level. This indicates that, although the child is not functioning at a 24- to 36-month stage of comprehension, he or she is using appropriate strategies that would be expected to lead to this level in time. If the child fails the majority of items and does not use strategies from the previous level, comprehension is then ascribed to the highest level at which items were passed.

Children who succeed at the 24- to 36-month level of nonstandardized comprehension assessment can next be tested using formal comprehension measures such as the *PPVT-4* (Dunn & Dunn, 2006), the *Test of Auditory Comprehension of Language—3* (Carrow-Woolfolk, 1999a), the *Miller-Yoder Test of Grammatical Comprehension* (Miller & Yoder, 1983), *Receptive One-Word Picture Vocabulary Test* (Brownell, 2000), or the *Token Test for Children* (DiSimoni, 1978) to name a few.

If comprehension level is on par with communicative intention level, as assessed by the methods in the previous section, a nonspeaking child can be said to have a relatively isolated language production deficit. If, on the other hand, comprehension skills lag behind communicative intentions, a more pervasive language disorder is present. Longitudinal studies of children with language disorders (Paul, Cohen, & Caparulo, 1983) and toddlers with slow language development (Olswang, Rodriguez, & Timler, 1998; Yoder & Warren, 1998) suggest that children with poorer comprehension skills have poorer outcomes. Comprehension skills in children with little or no speech, then, may be indicators of prognosis. Analysis of these skills can contribute to the decision as to whether to initiate intervention or continue to monitor language development. Children who have poor comprehension skills but make use of developmentally appropriate strategies may have a better outlook for acquiring receptive skills than children who not only do not comprehend, but also do not make systematic attempts to respond to language. Thal and Flores (2001), for example, showed that the use of comprehension strategies in late-talkers, who generally go on to show more or less normal oral language development, was similar to that of younger typical children. Again, information about strategy use in children with receptive problems will help in planning an intervention program.

For children with little or no speech who also have receptive deficits, it is important to build a strong input component into the intervention plan. Focused language stimulation, verbal script activities, and child-centered approaches such as indirect language stimulation, are especially important adjuncts to eliciting expressive language for these clients. Those with limited use of strategies and limited comprehension need additional practice in observing how language maps onto objects and events. Facilitative play and modeling of play behaviors—using both conventional and symbolic uses of objects—along with simple descriptive language should be added to these clients' programs.

ASSESSING PRODUCTIVE LANGUAGE

ASSESSING SPEECH-MOTOR DEVELOPMENT

One piece of information we would like to have about a client who is not talking concerns speech-motor development. It would be very useful to know whether slow speech development is related to deficits or delays in motor speech abilities. This information is particularly hard to get from children at the 18- to 36-month developmental level, because so much of the speech-motor assessment requires imitation, which

children at this developmental level may be unwilling to do. We talked in Chapter 2 about some hints for doing the speech-motor assessment for very young children, such as pretending to make clown or fish faces together, letting the child examine your intraoral cavity with a flashlight first then letting you take a turn, pretending to look for strange creatures in the mouth, and so on. Even the most creative clinician may fail to get the cooperation of a 2-year-old in this phase of the assessment, though. When the child is completely unwilling to imitate oral gestures or let the clinician examine intraoral structures, all we can do is get to know the child better in the course of the intervention program and try again later.

In this case, it is especially important to refrain from jumping to conclusions about relations between speech-motor behavior and speech development. In a 2-year-old who is not talking, there is just not enough information available to determine whether or not speech-motor deficits or childhood apraxia of speech (CAS) contribute to the speech delay. Diagnostic criteria for CAS, as we saw in Chapter 4, include inconsistent speech errors, reversing sounds in words, more errors as utterances become more complex, and errors in stress production (Betz & Stoel-Gammon, 2005; Forrest, 2003; Shriberg, Campbell, Karlsson, Brown, McSweeny, & Nadler, 2003). Toddlers who do not talk simply do not produce enough speech to judge whether these symptoms are present, and their imitation skills are too immature to accurately assess oral motor imitation. The best approach to use for a child who is suspected of CAS at this level is to provide the kinds of focused, developmentally appropriate speech and language intervention that we would use for any nonspeaking toddler (Davis & Velleman, 2000), and monitor progress. Children who show substantial growth in speech production by age 3 probably did not have true CAS. If the kinds of symptoms outlined above begin to appear as the child begins to produce more speech, more focused CAS assessment and intervention methods can be considered.

One aspect of speech-motor development we can accomplish in children in this age range, though, is the feeding assessment. All the instruments and procedures suggested for feeding assessment of infants in Chapter 6 are relevant for children with emerging language, too. The feeding assessment can be used to look for muscular weakness, paralysis, or dysarthric-like conditions that might interfere with speech development. Feeding assessment, though, does not rule out other types of neuromotor disorders that affect only voluntary functions. For these, a more specific speech-motor assessment is needed. Again, we may not be able to be as thorough as we would like in accomplishing a speech-motor assessment of a child at this level. When we cannot, the best approach is to gather as much information about present and early feeding skills and early babbling behavior as we can. The vocal development assessment in Figure 6-1 can be very helpful in the assessment of babbling behavior. If feeding and babbling history appear normal, then neuromotor involvement is probably not the primary cause of the slow speech development. If feeding and babbling skills do appear to be problematic, some motor involvement may be implicated. In this case, we would want to try especially hard to do a more thorough speech-motor assessment as we get to know clients better and win their trust and cooperation. But again, we really cannot assess the degree of speech-motor involvement until the child produces enough speech to manifest the characteristic symptoms of CAS. For many late-talking children, this may not be until 3 or 4 years of age, and, in my opinion, no diagnosis of CAS should be made before this point. Nothing is lost in simply providing traditional speech and language intervention to the young child with limited speech. These techniques will help to develop the conceptual and symbolic foundation for language that will then be in place when the child is developmentally ready for more focused speech therapy to begin.

COLLECTING A SPEECH SAMPLE

Children with emerging language being assessed for communication disorder probably don't talk much, so collecting a speech sample may seem an unimportant part of the evaluation. Trying to collect a free speech sample in the clinic setting may, in fact, not be very successful. However, we would like to get some idea of what words and sounds the child is producing. There are two ways we can gather these data: from a sample audiorecorded in the home and from a parent diary.

Perhaps the simplest way to collect a vocalization sample is to send a good audio recorder home with a family and ask them to turn it on during several periods in which the child usually produces a lot of sounds. Playtime with a sibling or during dressing, feeding, or bath time (remind parents to be sure to keep the recorder away from the water!) are often such times. This method allows us to hear the child's vocalization in natural settings and will probably paint a more valid picture of productive skills than will trying to elicit words in an unfamiliar environment. Problems can arise, though, if there is too much background noise or if parents forget to make the tape or return it. Providing a self-addressed stamped mailer or, if possible, going to the home to make the recording may increase the chances of getting it back.

Another way to collect information about the child's spontaneous vocalizations is to ask parents to keep a diary of the child's productions, again during times when the child normally vocalizes. Miller (1981) provided guidelines for collecting a parent diary. He suggested asking parents to record everything their child produces during several 10- to 15-minute intervals over the course of 1 week. A form such as the one in Figure 7-4 is provided to the parent. Miller suggested that the parents keep a form and pencil with them during several activities when the child usually produces a lot of sounds. Then they simply record as much as they can of both what the child means and how it actually sounds. Miller's method asks parents to note whether the vocalization was an imitation, if it was directed to a particular person, and what was going on when the child said it. This kind of record also can be very helpful in determining the words, sounds, and communicative skills the child is showing. However, it does require a fairly dedicated parent. Clinicians will have to use judgment to decide which families can keep an accurate record. When this task seems to be too much to ask of a family, sending home an audio recorder may be a better alternative.

Once a speech or vocalization sample has been collected, we want to examine several aspects of the child's production. These include phonological skills—the sounds and syllable types the child produces—as well as the frequency and types of conventional words the child uses and how the child combines words. Let's look at each of these areas.

ASSESSING PHONOLOGICAL SKILLS

Stoel-Gammon (1998, 2002) and Williams and Elbert (2003) talked about the close relationship between the development of words and sounds in very young children. Although it is possible for a child to have a rich phonological repertoire in babbling but to fail to use that repertoire in meaningful words, this scenario is not usually what we see. Typically, children with small expressive vocabularies also show small phonetic inventories of consonants and a restricted number of syllable shapes in both meaningful speech and in nonverbal vocalizations (Mirak & Rescorla, 1998; Paul & Jennings, 1992; Rescorla & Ratner, 1996; Williams & Elbert, 2003). Children with autism spectrum disorders may be one exception to this rule

---

Child's name _____

Age _____

Date _____

Activity observed _____

Word(s) child meant	How it sounded	Imitated?	Spoken to?	What was happening?
baby	baba	no	Mom	reached for doll
blanket	baki	no	Mom	Mom took blanket from dryer
cookie	googi	no	Mom	reached for cookie jar
cookie	googi	yes	Dad	He asked if she wanted a cookie
no night-night	no ni	no	Mom	bedtime

FIGURE 7-4 ✦ Sample parent diary form.
(Adapted from Miller, J. [1981]. *Assessing language production in children: Experimental procedures*. Needham Heights, MA: Allyn and Bacon.)

(Paul et al., 2006). Generally, the development of words and sounds seems to be very closely linked in both normal and delayed language development (Fletcher et al., 2004). Further, the development of consonants specifically is closely related to the development of words. Whitehurst, Fischel, Lonigan, Valdez-Menchaca, Arnold, and Smith (1991) have shown that there is a strong correlation between the amount of vocalization containing consonants and language outcome in late talkers. What's more, the amount of vocalization that contained only vowels was negatively related to expressive language growth. Williams and Elbert (2003) presented a list of phonological behaviors that predict long-term speech delays in late-talkers. These appear in Table 7-6.

Assessing phonological production in children with emerging language is very useful, then, both as a prognostic indicator and as an aid in choosing words to be included in the child's first lexicon. As Schwartz and Leonard (1982) have shown, children are more likely to add words to their productive lexicons if the words contain consonants already in their phonetic repertoire.

Since consonant production seems to be an important aspect of phonological development at this level, one viable form of phonological assessment is the compilation of a consonant inventory (Shriberg & Kwiatkowski, 1980). This can be done by listening to a live or recorded vocalization sample and simply writing down each consonant used in the sample at least once, regardless of whether it appears in a conventional word, word approximation, or nonconventional vocalization. If a diary has been provided by the parents, a consonant inventory can be gathered from the "what it sounded like" column of the diary form. The consonant inventory can be used in two different ways:

1. Consonants already in the inventory can be used to select words to be included in the first lexicon to be taught to the child. Although there are other considerations, too—such as concepts the child has available for mapping onto words and the familiarity and communicative value of the words to be taught—choosing words that have sounds already in the child's repertoire greatly enhances the chances that the child will add the word to the productive lexicon. The

consonant inventory should be used primarily to select *words* to be taught, rather than as a way to identify *sounds* we should try to get the client to say. Children of this age have little phonological awareness, and there is not much evidence that children can learn sounds in isolation at this developmental level. Rather than trying to increase the consonant inventory at this stage, I would suggest using the consonant inventory to help choose words that will be easy for the child to learn. Later, after the child reaches a developmental level of 3 or so and has more cognitive awareness, focused work on the acquisition of additional consonant sounds can be undertaken.

2. The number of consonants present in the inventory can be used as an index of severity of phonological delay. Paul and Jennings (1992) found that normal 18- to 24-month-olds produced an average of about 14 different consonants in a 10-minute communication sample, whereas 24- to 36-month-olds produced an average of 18. Children with small expressive vocabularies, however, produced significantly fewer consonant types: an average of six at 18 to 24 months and 10 at 24 to 36 months (Williams & Elbert, 2003). Comparing a client's consonant inventory size with these data can help a clinician decide whether the child more closely resembles a normally speaking peer or a child with a significant language delay. This information can be useful in deciding whether to recommend early intervention.

One other measure that may be helpful in phonological assessment is the syllable structure level (SSL), which was developed by Paul and Jennings (1992), based on Olswang, Stoel-Gammon, Coggins, and Carpenter's (1987) Mean Babbling Level. This measure examines both intelligible words and nonconventional vocalizations. It is derived by rating 20 to 50 child vocalizations, each at one of the following three levels, in terms of canonical (syllable) structure:

Level 1: The vocalization is composed of a voiced vowel (/a/), voiced syllabic consonant (/lll/), or CV syllable in which the consonant is a glottal stop or glide (/ha/, /wi/).

Level 2: The vocalization is composed of a VC (/up/) or CVC with a single consonant type (/kek/), or a CV syllable that does not fit the criteria for level 1. Voicing

TABLE 7-6   Predictors of Long-Term Speech Delay in Late-Talkers at 30-35 Months.

PHONOLOGICAL CHARACTERISTIC	DESCRIPTION/EXAMPLES
Limited phonetic inventory	Order of acquisition of phonemes is delayed, not deviant; at 30–35 mo, late-talkers have only 6–9 different consonants
Simple syllable structures	Fewer syllables with more than one consonant or consonant clusters (Pharr et al., 2000)
More sound errors	Percent consonants correct <0.45
Greater inconsistency in substitution errors	Individual phonemes are produced in a variety of ways
Atypical errors	Unusual substitutions (/d/ / /h/); vowel errors
Slow rate of resolution	Little change over the 24- to 36-mo time period

Adapted from Williams, A., & Elbert, M. (2003). A prospective longitudinal study of phonological development in late talkers. *Language, Speech and Hearing Services in Schools, 34,* 138-154.

differences in CVCs are disregarded (*toad* would be considered a level 2 vocalization).

Level 3: The vocalization is composed of syllables with two or more different consonant types, disregarding voicing differences (/pati/ would be considered a level 3 vocalization; /dati/ would be considered level 2).

The SSL is then computed by averaging the levels assigned: adding up all the ratings given to each vocalization and dividing by the number of vocalizations rated.

Paul and Jennings (1992) found that SSLs for normally developing 24-month-olds were about 2.2, indicating that most utterances were at level 2 and some were at level 3. SSLs for toddlers with small expressive vocabularies, on the other hand, were about 1.7, showing that many of their utterances were at levels 1 and 2, but very few at level 3. Pharr et al. (2000) found that at 24 months, most syllables produced by late talkers were at level 1 and fewer syllables had a final consonant, more than one consonant, or a consonant cluster. The ability to include more than one consonant within an utterance seems to be an important phonological milestone that 2-year-olds with slow language development are missing.

Computing an SSL from a communication sample or diary may be useful for determining whether a client is seriously limited in phonological skill. This can be done by simply rating each of the client's vocalizations according to the three levels described and averaging these ratings. If the average is less than 2, we can conclude that the child with emerging language is showing limited syllable structures. Alternatively, we might simply want to inspect the communication sample or diary form for any evidence of level 3 structures, those containing more than one consonant type. If more than 25% of syllables are at level 3 structures, we would be less likely to conclude that the child has a limitation in the development of canonical form. If fewer than 25% of the syllables are at level 3, however, and if we believe the sample we are inspecting is a valid reflection of the child's phonological performance, a deficit in syllable structures might be inferred.

Whether we compute an SSL or just look for the presence of level 3 syllable structures, a deficit in syllable structure would lead us to try to elicit more advanced productions, first in imitative babbling and only later in conventional words. Data from Paul and Jennings (1992) indicated that the most common level 3 syllable types produced by normally speaking toddlers are C1VC2 (/pat/) and C1VC2V(C) (/baki/, /patIt/, or /pati/). These kinds of productions can be elicited in back-and-forth babbling games. First the clinician can simply imitate the child's vocalization. Next, the clinician can expand the child's vocalization to include one of these more advanced syllable forms. If the child says /baba/, the clinician can respond with /bata/. If the child imitates this expansion, the clinician can imitate it again, encouraging the child to repeat the more advanced syllable form. If not, the clinician can continue to produce the more advanced structure in response to the child's simpler one, giving additional opportunities for the child to take advantage of the model. It is important to remember that the goal of these activities is *not* to elicit particular sounds, but

only to get the child to try to produce two different sounds within an utterance. If the child produces *any* two different sounds, lavish praise ought to be the consequence, regardless of whether the two sounds are the ones the clinician produced.

The two methods of phonological assessment we have been discussing are both examples of what Stoel-Gammon (1991) called *independent analyses.* That is, they look only at the child's productions themselves, not in relation to adult targets. *Relational analyses,* on the other hand, compare what the child produces with an adult form and identify whether it is right or wrong. Stoel-Gammon (1987, 1998), for example, showed that normally developing 24-month-olds are close to 70% accurate in their production of consonants, relative to adult target words, whereas late talkers have been found to be less than 50% (Paul & Jennings, 1992; Williams & Elbert, 2003). Stoel-Gammon (1991) also reported limited vowel repertoires in children with language delays. Stoel-Gammon (1991) and Roberts, Rescorla, Giroux, and Stevens (1998) have shown, though, that many of these errors resolve spontaneously between 2 and 3 years of age. For this reason, Stoel-Gammon recommends using only independent analysis to evaluate phonology in children with developmental levels younger than 3 years. Relational analyses, such as examination of phonological process use (Preisser, Hodson, & Paden, 1988) or analysis of Percent Consonants Correct (Shriberg & Kwiatkowski, 1982b), are best reserved for children who function above 3 years of age. At 18- to 36-month developmental levels, clients in the emerging language phase produce few words anyway. Our goals are to increase their vocal production and to expand their vocabularies. Phonological accuracy and the relational assessments needed to attain it can wait. The two independent analyses we've talked about—collecting a consonant inventory and looking at the sophistication of syllable structures produced by the client—will be sufficient for most clients at the emerging language level. Both these measures are relatively easy to compute from live, recorded or diary samples, and each contributes information that is useful for assessing prognosis, designing a program to increase the sophistication of the child's vocalizations, and for choosing words that the child will be likely to incorporate into a first lexicon.

ASSESSING LEXICAL PRODUCTION

Children at the 18- to 36-month developmental level who are referred for communication evaluation will probably be producing few intelligible words. There are, though, several ways to get an idea of the size and range of vocabulary these clients do produce. One is through language sampling, using the methods we have already discussed, such as observation of a play session, recorded communication samples, or parent diary recordings. These methods give us some notion of the words the child produces but are unlikely, because they are samples, to show us all the words the child says. Some of the screening measures we discussed earlier, including Rescorla's (1989) *Language Development Survey* and the *MacArthur-Bates Communicative Development Inventory* (Fenson et al., 1993) are well-constructed parent-report measures that can be used for this purpose (Klee, Carson, Gavin, Hall, Kent, & Reece, 1998; Rescorla, Mirak, & Singh, 2000; Thal, O'Hanlon, Clemmons, & Fralin, 1999). Parent report of expressive vocabulary size is, then, an easy-to-collect and useful index of the number of different words that a child with emerging language can produce. Both these instruments also divide words into semantic classes. This semantic class information can be used to decide what concepts and meanings the child is currently talking about and to aid in determining the concepts and categories for words that are available to be added to the child's lexicon.

A variety of general expressive communication measures also are given in Table 7-4. Direct assessments of expressive language in this age range have, like the language sample procedures we discussed, the problem of representativeness. When a child fails to produce a form, we don't know whether that failure is a reflection of the fact that the form is really absent from the repertoire or whether the child just didn't feel like producing it. This problem is especially acute for children with emerging language for two reasons. First, their rate of communicative behavior is relatively low, so the samples we get from them are fairly sparse. Second, children in the emerging language stage often just don't comply with requests from adults, particularly with requests to talk or name things. For these reasons, parent-report instruments or those that allow parent report as one source of data are especially useful for this age group. The *Vineland Adaptive Behavior Scales II—Communication Domain* (Sparrow, Cicchetti, & Balla, 2005) is, like the vocabulary checklists we have been discussing, a parent-report instrument. It displays high correlation with direct measures of language use (Rescorla & Paul, 1990; Paul, Spangle-Looney, & Dahm, 1991) and is another measure that can be considered in examining expressive language in this age group.

ASSESSING SEMANTIC-SYNTACTIC PRODUCTION

Most clients with emerging language have little to show in the way of productive syntax. If they are verbalizing at all, it is likely to be in the form of single words. In normal development, children do not begin to combine words until vocabulary size reaches about 50 words. Therefore, if a client is producing fewer than 50 words, we would be wiser to work on increasing expressive vocabulary size before trying to get the child to produce word combinations. When the productive lexicon reaches 50 words, syntactic intervention becomes appropriate, if word combinations have not appeared spontaneously. Detailed productive syntactic assessment, then, is not likely to be an important part of our evaluation in the emerging language stage. Computing an MLU is fairly easy for this age group; it will generally be either 0 or 1. But there may be some children with emerging language who have productive lexicons larger than 50 words or who are beginning to combine words into sentences. When this is the case, we want to look at two aspects of these combinations: the relative frequency of word combinations within a communication sample and the range of meanings or semantic relations expressed. Let's see how we might examine each of these parameters.

Relative Frequency of Word Combinations

To look at the relative frequency of single-word versus two-word utterances, we need to collect a relatively large sample of verbal production from the client. This may not be so easy to do. If a communication sample is being collected to look at expression of intents, a separate portion of the session needs to be reserved for recording the interpretable one- and two-word combinations. The recording collected from a home with sample by the family or from a clinic play or communication sample also can be transcribed and inspected for two-word combinations. If we use the diary method, we can note the relative proportions of one- and two-word utterances recorded by the parents from the several sessions during which they took data. We might ask the parents to be especially careful to record word combinations.

If the rate of word combinations is too great to be recorded easily from either a sample or by parents keeping a diary, it may be that the child is moving out of the emerging language stage into the next phase of language development. If this is the case, we need to do a more detailed assessment of syntactic skills, using methods such as those we'll discuss in the next chapter for children with developing language. Lahey (1988) also provided a detailed method for assessing the semantic and syntactic skills of children at this level. Children with a history of risk factors at birth who are being followed for communication development may present this happy picture. Rescorla, Dahlsgaard and Roberts (2000) found that 30% to 40% of late talking toddlers had moved into the normal range of syntactic production by age 3. If an at-risk toddler's MLU exceeds 1.5 at about 24 months, or if half the utterances contain word combinations, we are justified in feeling that a major hurdle toward normal development has been overcome. Further monitoring may be necessary, but the client is well on the way toward normal language acquisition.

For most clients with emerging language, though, frequency of word combinations is much lower. We can compute a proportion of word combinations by simply dividing the number of utterances containing more than one word by the total number of interpretable verbal utterances in any speech sample we can collect. This proportion gives us an idea of how frequently the child combines words. If the proportion is close to or exceeds 50%, we can conclude that the client is functioning at least at a 24-month level in terms of syntactic production. If the proportion of word combinations is much less than 50%, we can conclude that the client is functioning below this level. It would be surprising if a child with a very small expressive vocabulary (fewer than 50 words) used a lot of word combinations. Like the connection between lexical and phonological acquisition, the link between the acquisition of syntax and vocabulary size is usually quite close, too. Typically, all these aspects of early language acquisition proceed in tandem. However, there may be the unusual client for whom some separation of developmental strands has taken place. For this reason, we want to look at each of the areas of language individually.

Semantic Relations Expressed

When children begin combining two words in sentences, these combinations result in new meanings that are not present in the meaning of either of the words alone. For example, there is nothing about the word *doggy* or the word *bed* that means possession. But when the two words are combined into the utterance *doggy bed,* this utterance can convey a meaning of possession (it's the doggy's bed) if spoken in the right context. Further, children do not combine their words randomly but use consistent word order to denote the relations. This ability to combine words syntactically to produce new *semantic relations* that are not part of the meaning of either of the component words in the utterance is one of the accomplishments of normally developing children in the 18- to 36-month age range.

When children are producing some word combinations, it makes sense to examine the meanings expressed in these combinations. Generally, normally developing toddlers express a relatively small range of semantic relations in their speech. Eight to 11 major ones (depending on which researcher's coding system you use) can usually account for the great majority of relations used by children in this age range. Table 7-7 gives the semantic relational categories used by Brown (1973) that are typically found in the speech of normally developing toddlers who are learning a variety of languages and dialects (Stockman & Vaughn-Cooke, 1986). Haynes and Shulman (1998b) reported that children with language disorders have been shown to produce these same relations when they begin to combine words.

One assessment method appropriate for this developmental level is Lahey's (1988) content/form assessment. This approach uses both semantic and syntactic information, gathered from the analysis of a spontaneous speech sample, to target goals in emerging content-form-use interactions. This method can provide a rich source of data for planning intervention targets and charting the progress of children in the emerging language stage. Detailed instructions for this method can be found in Lahey's (1988) text. Lee's (1974) Developmental

Sentence Types (DST) procedure is another method of speech sample analysis appropriate for this stage.

Alternatively, we can look more narrowly at the expression of semantic relations in children with emerging language. Using this approach, we would first attempt to code each multiword utterance in our language sample (derived from an observation, recording, or parent diary) into one of the categories in Table 7-7. Utterances that did not fit any of these would be placed into an "other" classification. One way to start the analysis would be to look at the proportion of utterances we had to call "other." Normative research indicates that this should be about 30%. If it is more than 50%, we would want to inspect the "other" utterances to see whether they are encoding higher-level semantic relations having to do with concepts such as time (go now), manner (go fast), sequence (eat [then] drink), or causality (cry [because] hurt). If these higher-level relations are being conveyed frequently, they would suggest to us that the child is exhibiting some advanced cognitive development in the presence of delayed expressive language. We would want to foster this advanced development with appropriate play contexts and attempt to provide the child with more conventional means for expressing these sophisticated notions.

If the proportion of "other" utterances is less than 40% or 50%, we then look at the distribution of relations expressed within the set of utterances coded according to Brown's (1973) categories. If a client is encoding a range of these relations, we conclude that the child is moving toward normal semantic and syntactic development. Intervention, if needed, would focus on increasing the vocabulary available for combining into multiword utterances. Even if the range of relations expressed is somewhat restricted, we would not necessarily conclude that the child is showing a deficit. Lahey (1988) discussed the fact that children sometimes show preferences for encoding certain semantic relations in early language development. Until developmental level exceeds 36 months, we should not try to discourage the client from these preferences. Rather, we should teach

---

TABLE 7-7 | **Semantic Relational Categories Used by Brown (1973) to Account for the Majority of Word Combinations in Toddlers' Spontaneous Speech**

SEMANTIC RELATION	EXAMPLE
Attribute-entity	Big shoe
Possessor-possession	Mommy nose
Agent-action	Daddy hit
Action-object	Hit ball
Agent-object	Daddy ball
Demonstrative-entity	This ball
Entity-locative	Daddy chair [Daddy's in the chair.]
Action-locative	Throw chair [Throw it onto the chair.]
Recurrence	More milk
Nonexistence, denial, rejection	No cookie
Disappearance	Allgone cookie

Adapted from Brown, R. (1973). *A first language, the early stages.* Cambridge, MA: Harvard University Press.

more words that the child can use to express them and provide increased opportunities in play contexts for the client to encode these relations with the new words. In addition, we can supply models in appropriate play contexts for the child to hear other relations expressed and give opportunities, through indirect language stimulation, for the child to imitate these models.

Box 7-3 provides a sample transcript from a 28-month-old child in the emerging language stage. You might like to try some of the semantic and syntactic analyses we've been discussing on this transcript. You can compute the relative frequency of word combinations. Then assign each word combination to one of the categories in Table 7-7 or to the "other" category. Compute the proportion of utterances rated "other" and examine the range of semantic relations expressed. My analysis is given in Appendix 7-1.

BOX 7-3 **Sample Transcript from a 28-Month-Old Child (C) Collected During Free Play with Parent (P) Using Dollhouse Toys**

P: Do you see the kitchen?
  C1: Yeah.
P: What's this doll's name?
  C2: Name, Mom
  C3: Name Cinderella.
P: Oh, that looks like a changing table.
  C4: Yeah.
P: For the baby.
  C5: No, Mom, no.
P: Can you find a bed for the baby?
  C6: Yeah.
  C7: No, here is.
P: Where's the living room?
  C8: What?
P: Where is it, the living room?
  C9: Here is.
P: Can I sit in the living room?
  C10: Yeah.
  C11: Here Daddy.
P: What is this?
  C12: What that?
P: I think it's a stove.
  C13: Yeah.
P: There's the kitchen.
  C14: Mommy cook.
P: Are you making spaghetti for dinner?
  C15: Yeah.
P: Maybe lasagna?
  C16: Yeah. [Holds up small, white plastic box.]
P: Is it a cake?
  C17: No, that bed.

BOX 7-3 **Sample Transcript from a 28-Month-Old Child (C) Collected During Free Play with Parent (P) Using Dollhouse Toys—cont'd**

P: Oh, should you put it in the bedroom?
  C18: Yeah.
P: Where's the bedroom?
  C19: Right here.
  C20: Oh, don't fit.
P: Too big.
  C21: Mom.
P: What is it?
  C22: Baby.
P: Oh, what's the baby's name?
  C23: Name.
P: We know some new babies, don't we?
  C24: Yeah.
P: Auntie Barbie's gonna have a baby?
  C25: Yeah.
  C26: Baby go in bed.
P: Where's Daddy's clothes?
  C27: Mine upstairs.
P: Oh, in the closet?
  C28: Yeah.
P: OK.
  C29: Daddy cowboy! [Holds up doll in cowboy suit]
P: What's this?
  C30: (um) window.
P: How many windows are in your room?
  C31: What?
P: How many windows are in your room?
  C32: No.
  C33: Hey, baby.
P: Is Baby crying?
  C34: No.
P: Is Baby hungry?
  C35: Yeah.
  C36: Baby me hold.

In summary, assessing production in a child with emerging language involves looking at phonological skills, vocabulary size and content, and semantic-syntactic combinations. Typically, all these areas are closely related. Some children may show disconnections, though. Children with hearing impairment, for example, may have semantic relations and pragmatic intents that are more advanced than their syntax and phonology. Children like Joey may show just the opposite pattern, with relatively strong skills in language form and less development of semantic and pragmatic skills. For clients like these, clearly, it is important to have a complete picture of language skills in each area. Even when clients show the normal interrelatedness of these areas, though, we need to know something about each to plan the most effective program for improving expressive skills. Because lexical development is closely tied to phonology, we need to know what sounds and syllables the child can produce so that we can choose words appropriately. Because syntax usually does not begin until vocabulary size reaches 50 words, we need to look at the productive lexicon before making decisions about teaching word combinations, and so on. Even when there is little productive language to assess, it is our responsibility to find out as much as we can about what expression there is.

DECISION MAKING BASED ON ASSESSMENT INFORMATION

The essence of the model of assessment of emerging language involves comparing a child's functioning in various areas of communicative development and using this information in developing a prognosis that will help us decide whether a child would benefit most from direct intervention or continued monitoring, as well as to help in devising a treatment plan. The model is schematized as a decision tree represented in Figure 7-5. Crais and Roberts (1991) and Whitehurst and Fischel (1994) also provided decision trees for planning intervention for children with emerging language. Olswang, Rodriquez, and Timler (1998) provided an alternative means of evaluating the need for intervention. In the model I've proposed, the decision process begins with the question of whether the child demonstrates functional or symbolic play behavior that would normally accompany the use of conventional language. If a nonspeaking client is not using these play behaviors, then intervention should focus not only on developing communication but also on modeling the use of objects for conventional and pretend play schemes. If these kinds of symbolic play are present, we then look at nonverbal communicative behavior. If the frequency

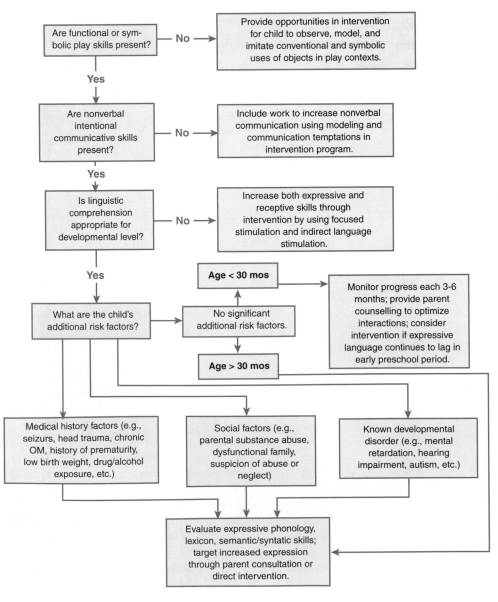

FIGURE 7-5 ✦ Decision tree for intervention planning in the emerging language stage.

and/or range of communicative behavior is found to be limited, we would use modeling and communication temptations to try to increase the frequency of intentional behavior in addition to heightening the rate of vocal production. These activities could either precede or accompany the development of early vocabulary. If the child appears to be a good nonverbal communicator but to lack the conventional verbal forms of communication, the issue of level of language comprehension is raised next. If comprehension skills are found to be below those expected for the level of communication demonstrated, then activities to foster receptive language skills, such as the focused stimulation activities and indirect language stimulation, should be an important component of the management program.

If receptive language is considered adequate for developmental level, then we need to take the child's level of accumulated risk factors into account. Children without any other risk factors who are slow to start talking have a good chance of "catching up" with their normally speaking peers by school age, if their deficits are limited to expressive language; they begin to use some speech by 30 months; and their cognitive, symbolic, receptive, and communication skills are developing normally (Capone & McGregor, 2004; Girolametto et al., 2001; Paul, 1996a; Thal, 1991; Whitehurst & Fischel, 1994). These children with circumscribed expressive language delays should be monitored closely throughout their third and fourth years of life. If expressive deficits persist through the preschool period, intervention options can be carefully discussed with parents (see Paul, 2000b; Whitehurst & Fischel, 1994, for suggestions.) For children who have known developmental disorders or other risk factors such as those listed in Figure 7-5 or Box 7-1, though, early intervention seems appropriate even if only expressive language is delayed. The consequences of language delay for a child's social and cognitive development can be pervasive and language is one of the most vulnerable functions in young children's development. Providing help to children who are slow to learn to talk serves an important secondary preventative function and ought to be considered if the child is known to be at risk. For children with severe language deficits who are older than 3 years but still in the phase of emerging language, intervention or tertiary prevention is always appropriate, of course.

▮ FROM ASSESSMENT TO INTERVENTION

The decision tree in Figure 7-5 can be used to help us decide when to recommend intervention for a child with emerging language. Once we have decided to provide intervention, of what should the intervention consist and how should it be delivered? I have already given some suggestions about what I would consider appropriate targets and methods of intervention for this developmental level, but let's address these issues more directly now.

FAMILY-CENTERED PRACTICE

Most clients in the emerging language stage will, like their prelinguistic counterparts, be served through an Individual

Family Service Plan (IFSP) designed by a team of professionals, as mandated by IDEA. Unless the SLP is designated as the case manager, we provide just one part of that plan: the data on language assessment and the family-based services in communication development. The form of the IFSP for a child with emerging language is very similar to the one designed for a prelinguistic child (see Chapter 6 for examples), except that the section on planning for transition to preschool services is more detailed. The issues discussed in developing an IFSP for a child with emerging language are very similar to those discussed in Chapter 6.

One issue we'll need to consider in the development of the intervention plan is the parent's role. When fostering communication at the prelinguistic stage for developmentally young children, we definitely want to involve the parent as the primary agent of the intervention. The communicative routines that the young prelinguistic child needs are not hard to learn; in fact, they come naturally to most parents. The management program for children at the emerging language stage is somewhat more focused and specific. Are parents still the ideal primary agents of intervention at this stage?

Many programs have been developed for addressing communication disorders in children with emerging language that use parents as the primary agents of intervention. Some of these programs involve teaching parents clinician-directed or behaviorist approaches to eliciting language (Kemper, 1980; MacDonald, Blott, Gordon, Spiegel, & Hartmann, 1974; MacDonald, 1978; Whitehurst, Fishel, Lonigan, Valdez-Menchaca, Arnold, & Smith, 1991). Others teach parents to use hybrid approaches (Cheseldine & McConkey, 1979; Clezy, 1979; Girolametto, Pearce, & Weitzman, 1996; Lederer, 2001; Peterson, Carta, & Greenwood, 2005; Wulz, Hall, & Klein; 1983; Yoder & Warren, 1998, 2002) or child-centered methods (Chandler, Christie, Newson, & Prevezer, 2002; Fey, Newhoff, & Cole, 1978; Hubbell, 1981; Kaiser & Hemmeter, 1996; MacDonald, 1989; Manolson, 1992; Norris & Hoffman, 1990b; Seitz & Marcus, 1976; Yoder & Warren, 1998). The rationale for parent involvement includes the notion that parent-implemented intervention will promote more generalization and may improve

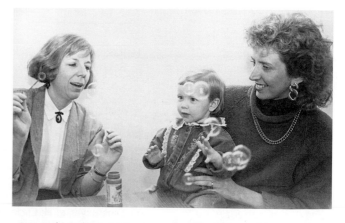

Parental involvement increases the effectiveness of intervention for children with emerging language.

other aspects of functioning, such as social skills, in addition to improving communication (Kaiser, 1993; Paul, 2000b). It also grows out of the concept of family-centered practice, which encourages family involvement in all aspects of service delivery (Crais & Calculator, 1998; Rini & Hindenlang, 2006). Unfortunately, the rationale sometimes includes the notion that part of the child's communication problem resides in the parent's communication style. Many people, even language pathologists, believe that children fail to start talking because people in their environment anticipate their needs and the child has no incentive to learn language. From this point of view, the way to improve the child's communication is to improve the parent's.

But remember: *normally* speaking children don't *need* to talk either, in the sense that their needs, too, are anticipated and their nonverbal communications are consistently responded to and rewarded. They learn to talk because it is part of their biologically programmed development (Locke, 2005; Pinker, 1994). Data on mother-child interactions (Paul & Elwood, 1991; Vigil et al., 2005) shows very few differences in linguistic input to normally speaking toddlers and their late-talking peers. Still, it is possible, as Whitehurst et al. (1991) and Girolametto et al. (1996, 1999) have shown, to maximize the quality of parental input to a child in the emerging language period. Maximizing their input does not mean that they were doing anything wrong in the first place, nor does it mean that the entire burden of intervening in their child's communication disorder should fall on the parent's shoulders. There may be times when parents should *not* be teachers but should instead make their child feel understood and accepted, even if his or her speech is not working well. However, helping parents provide the most beneficial input to their child is certainly an attainable goal. Much of the intervention we will provide to children in the emerging language period can be done successfully by parents with some training and monitoring from the SLP. Family-centered practice dictates that we encourage parents to do as much of the intervention as they feel is appropriate for them and their child. However, as Robertson and Weismer (1999) showed, clinician-delivered intervention can also have important secondary effects, such as improving overall social skills and reducing parental stress. In cases in which parents do not feel comfortable doing so, it is appropriate for the SLP or another intervention agent to be provided. We need to keep both the costs and benefits of parent-delivered intervention in mind when we plan programs for these children.

Table 7-8 lists printed materials that clinicians can use to help parents maximize the communicative and cognitive value of their interactions with their children. Table 7-9 lists videotaped presentations that have been developed to help parents understand their toddlers' development and to communicate more effectively. *Exceptional Parent* magazine also contains a

	TABLE 7-8	**Training Resources for Parents of Toddlers**

RESOURCE	**SOURCE**	**COMMENTS**
"Learning Through (and from) Mothers"	P. Levenstein; in *Childhood Education, 48* (December), 130-134, 1971	"Toy Demonstrators" use verbal interaction techniques with mothers and their 2-yr-old children.
"Pre-Computer Skills for Young Children"	L. Symington; in *Exceptional Parent, 20*, 36-38, 1990	Suggests activities to train young disabled children skills for using the computer.
"Taking Turns"	J. MacDonald & Y. Gillette; in *Exceptional Parent, 15* (September), 49-52, 1985	Focuses on turn taking as a primary approach to language learning.
Adaptive Play for Special-Needs Children: Strategies to Enhance Communication and Learning	C.R. Musselwhite; San Diego, CA: College-Hill Press, 1986	Intended for professionals, paraprofessionals, and parents; has information on early communication through speech: parent-child dialogues, puppetry; early augmentative communication; annotated bibliography on adaptive play.
Beautiful Beginnings: A Developmental Curriculum for Infants and Toddlers	H. Raikes & J. McCall Whitmer; Baltimore, MD: Brookes Publishing	Activity-based approach to enhancing infant and toddler development in communication, gross motor, fine motor, intellectual, discovery, social, self-help, and pretend.
Beyond Baby Talk	K. Apel & J. Masterson; New York: Prima Publishing, 2001	A book for parents that answers questions about their baby's speech and language development.
Developmental Therapy for Young Children with Autistic Characteristics	A.W. Bachrach, A.R. Mosley, F.L. Swindle, & M.M. Wood; Baltimore, MD: University Park Press, 1978	Samples of techniques and materials, routines and environments, activity periods, learning experiences, and home programs designed for 0–3 yr; for teachers and parents; organized from "stage one" through normal developmental sequences.
Early Childhood STEP	D. Dinkmeyer, et al; Circle Pines, MN: American Guidance Service	Kit including parent guide, videos, posters; Spanish version available.

TABLE 7-8	Training Resources for Parents of Toddlers—cont'd	
RESOURCE	**SOURCE**	**COMMENTS**
Early Communication Games: Routine Based Play for the First Two Years	A. Casey-Harvey; Austin, TX: Pro-Ed	Examines and provides examples of play for children birth–24 mo, developing initial communication skills.
Ecological Communication System	J.D. MacDonald & Y. Gillette; Columbus, OH: The Ohio State University, 1986	Two treatment modules available: (1) turn-taking with actions—functional interactive play and (2) turn-taking with communications (initial conversation).
Everybody's Different: Understanding and Changing Our Reactions to Disabilities	N. Miller & C. Sammons; Baltimore, MD: Brookes Publishing Co., 1999	Discusses ways in which personal thoughts, feelings, and questions about disabilities can obstruct effective communication between people; offers strategies, activities, and exercises that enhance development and social relationships.
Every Day Matters: Activities for You and Your Child	Washburn Child Guidance Center; Circle Pines, MN: American Guidance Service, 1997	Simple, easy-to-use suggestions for parent-child learning experiences; covers five developmental areas: discipline, self-esteem, infant care, language, and coordination.
Games to Play with Toddlers— Revised Edition	J. Silberg; Beltsville, MD: Gryphon House, 2002	Games that develop areas important for the growth of a 12- to 24-mo-old: language, creativity, coordination, confidence, problem-solving, and gross motor skills.
Games to Play With Two Year Olds—Revised Edition	J. Silberg; Beltsville, MD: Gryphon House, 2002	Games that develop areas important for the growth of a 2-yr-old: language, coordination, social interactions, and problem-solving skills.
Helping Babies Learn: Developmental Profiles and Activities for Infants and Toddlers	S. Furuno, K. O'Reilly, C. Hosaka, T. Inatsuka, & B. Falbey; San Antonio, TX: Communication Skill Builders, 1998	Shows parents how to help children ages birth–3 yr realize their fullest potential; emphasizes parent-child partnerships by focusing on developmental activities occurring in daily life; provides parents with reproducible activities to integrate all aspects of development.
It Takes Two to Talk: A Practical Guide for Parents of Children with Language Delays	J. Pepper & E. Weitzman; Toronto, Ontario, Canada: The Hanen Centre, 2004	Parent handbook focuses on the child's attempts to communicate; guides parents to respond in ways that facilitate interaction; "You Initiate Opportunities for Language Learning" (the second part of the guide) suggests ways to increase opportunities for communication.
Learning Through Play: A Resource Manual for Teachers and Parents	R. R. Fewell & P.F. Vadasy; Hingham, MA: Teaching Resources Corp., 1983	Contains activities to stimulate learning targeted at birth–3 mo, 4–6 mo, 7–9 mo, 10–12 mo, 13–18 mo, 19–24 mo, 25–30 mo, and 31–36 mo, specific sections on language.
Learning to Talk Is Child's Play	C. Ausberger, M. Martin, & J. Creighton; Tucson, AZ: Communication Skill Builders, 1982	For parents, nursery school teachers; stresses use of responsive language teaching through adult-child dialogues.
Parent Articles for Early Intervention	M. Dunn-Klein; Austin, TX: Pro-Ed, 1977	Compilation of articles for parents of children, ages birth through 3 yr, who have communication and physical disorders; articles are grouped by 12 major topics, including communication, cognitive development and play, family support, and personal care; each article answers commonly asked questions, includes detailed instructions and additional resources for further reading, and suggests related activities and materials.
Parent-Child Habilitation	Infant Hearing Resource Publications; Portland, OR: IHRP, 1987	Uses play as teaching milieu, gives techniques for teaching speech and language to hearing-impaired toddlers.

| TABLE 7-8 | Training Resources for Parents of Toddlers—cont'd |

RESOURCE	SOURCE	COMMENTS
Preparing Children to Learn: Parent Letters	V. McNay, E. Kottwitz, S. Simmons, & M. McLean; San Antonio, TX: Communication Skill Builders, 1996	Covers assessment, planning, and implementation for children ages 1 mo–5 yr, addressing the full span of developmental objectives in interpersonal interactions and communication, cognition, receptive language, expressive language, and movement.
Puppetry, Language, and the Special Child: Discovering Alternative Languages	N. Renfro; Austin, TX: Nancy Renfro Studios, 1984	Describes activities to integrate visual and verbal aspects of puppetry to enhance language and communication.
Read, Play, and Learn	T. Linder (1999)	Uses popular children's books to promote early learning.
Systematic Training for Effective Parenting (books and videos)	D. Dinkmeyer, L. McKay, & S. Dinkmeyer; Windsor, Berkshire, SL4 1DF, UK: NFER-Nelson Darville House, 1997	Available in book and video form.
Talking with Your Baby	A.S. Honig; Syracuse University Press, 1996	How to help low-literacy parents, and parents for whom English is a second language, enhance the literacy and cognitive development of their children in the home environment through daily activities.
Teach Me Language	S. Freeman & L. Dake; New York: SKF Books, Inc., 1998	Program designed for teaching parents with a step-by-step manual of instructions, explanations, examples, games, and cards to attack language weaknesses common to children with PDD and other disabilities.
The Home Stretch	D. Cansler; Winston-Salem, NC: Kaplan Early Learning Company, 1982	Encourages parents to use unit topics at home (e.g., body parts, people, family, clothing).
When Your Child Has a Disability	M. Batshaw; Baltimore, MD: Brookes Publishing Co., 2002	Comprehensive volume offers advice on a wide range of issues, such as finding the right physician, learning important care techniques, and fulfilling educational requirements. Detailed chapters explore behavior management, treatment, nutrition, therapy services, and medicines.
You and Your Small Wonder: Parent Books of Learning Activities for Infants and Toddlers	M. Karnes; Circle Pines, MN: American Guidance, 1997	Includes two books full of playlike learning activities, building skills in natural ways; clear instructions and photos for demonstration; includes mealtime, changing, bath time, and indoor/outdoor activities.

| TABLE 7-9 | Videos for Training Parents and Teachers of Toddlers |

RESOURCE	SOURCE	COMMENTS
Activity-Based Intervention (1995)	Executive Producer: D. Bricker Co-Directors: P. Veltman and A. Munkres Brookes Publishing Co. PO Box 10624 Baltimore, MD 21285	Intervention techniques provide daily routines and activities to foster skill development in children with special needs. 14 min.
Beginning Language Connections (1995)	Educational Productions 7412 SW Beaverton-Hillsdale Highway, Suite 210 Portland, OR 97225	The first in a 4-video series called *First Steps*. 30-min video, practice exercises, trainer's manual, overheads, handouts, and activities. Shows how adults' interactions with infants and toddlers are key to their language learning. Available in Spanish.

TABLE 7-9	Videos for Training Parents and Teachers of Toddlers—cont'd	

RESOURCE	SOURCE	COMMENTS
Building Conversations (1995)	Educational Productions 7412 SW Beaverton-Hillsdale Highway, Suite 210 Portland, OR 97225	The fourth in a 4-video series called *First Steps*. 30-min video, practice exercises, trainer's manual, overheads, handouts, and activities. Shows how animated exchanges with verbal and nonverbal children continually enhance their emerging communication and social skills. Available in Spanish.
Learning Language and Loving It, Teaching Tape (1993)	The Hanen Centre 1075 Bay St., Suite 515 Toronto, ON M5S 2B1	Provides an overview of typical development from birth to 3 yr; designed to accompany Hanen Early Language Parent Program.
Let's Talk (1988)	Educational Productions 7412 SW Beaverton-Hillsdale Highway, Suite 210 Portland, OR 97225	33-min video, Facilitator's Guide. Describes communication skills that invite children and encourage talking, how to avoid asking questions that stop conversations, and how to correct a child's speech/language errors in a positive way.
Now You're Talking (1988)	Educational Productions 7412 SW Beaverton-Hillsdale Highway, Suite 210 Portland, OR 97225	30-min video, Facilitator's Guide. Describes how to add to the child's topic and extend conversation, how to ask questions that stimulate thinking and problem solving, how to support all of a child's efforts to communicate.
Oh Say What They See (1985)	Educational Productions 7412 SW Beaverton-Hillsdale Highway, Suite 210 Portland, OR 97225	Methods used in indirect language stimulation: self-talk, parallel talk, reinforcement, and expansion methods.
Reading the Child's Message (1995)	Educational Productions 7412 SW Beaverton-Hillsdale Highway, Suite 210 Portland, OR 97225	The second in a 4-video series called *First Steps*. 30-min video, practice exercises, trainer's manual, overheads, handouts, and activities. Takes a close look at messages babies and toddlers are sending from birth. Available in Spanish.
Successfully Educating Preschoolers with Special Needs: Ages 2½ to 5, A Guide for Parents, A Tool for Educators (2002)	G.M. Hanlon; Baltimore, MD: Brookes Publishing	30-min video, offers practical information about preschool education and special education services for children ages 2½–5.
Successfully Educating Preschoolers with Special Needs: Early Intervention for ages Birth to Three (1999)	G.M. Hanlon; Baltimore, MD: Brookes Publishing	60-min video; gives parents an introduction to the early intervention process.
Talking with Young Children (1995)	Educational Productions 7412 SW Beaverton-Hillsdale Highway, Suite 210 Portland, OR 97225	Part of a 4-video series called *First Steps*. 30-min video, practice exercises, trainer's manual, overheads, handouts, and activities. Demonstrates how children must understand what words and concepts mean before they can begin to use words or signs to communicate. Available in Spanish.
The Handicapped Child: Infancy Through Preschool; Program 5—Cognitive/ Language Development (1978)	Concept Media PO Box 19542 Irvine, CA 92714	Elements for fostering language development are discussed; sequence of language development briefly described.

wealth of helpful information for parents of children with disabilities. These resources can be used by the clinician to involve parents in fostering their child's growth, in understanding the complexity and wonder of development, and in providing the most appropriate forms of play and interaction of which their child can take advantage.

The family can and should be actively involved in setting goals for their child's intervention program, and the clinician should consult the parents as to what they most want the child to learn and how much of the intervention they would like to deliver themselves. Parent training that incorporates materials such as those in Tables 7-8 and 7-9 can be used by the clinician in a consultative role to maximize the impact of parent-child communication on the child's development. In addition, teaching or encouraging parents to use indirect language stimulation techniques, using either video or printed materials that address this area (some can be found in Tables 7-8 and 7-9), will be particularly useful for optimizing the linguistic input the child with emerging language receives. However, I believe that there also is a role for more focused, direct intervention for a child with emerging language who meets the criteria we've discussed for entrance into early communication intervention. Let's look at some of the specific goals and methods that might be used in this intervention.

PRODUCTS, PROCEDURES, AND CONTEXTS OF INTERVENTION FOR CHILDREN WITH EMERGING LANGUAGE

INTERVENTION PRODUCTS: GOALS FOR EMERGING LANGUAGE

We want to address several areas of communicative development in children with emerging language. We select these areas based on the results of our assessment, following our decision tree structure. Depending on these results, we will decide to address one or more of the following areas in the intervention plan: the development of functional and symbolic play and gesture; the use of intentional communicative behavior; language comprehension; and production of sounds, words, and word combinations. As we discuss each of these areas, suggestions for procedures and contexts for the intervention program also will be presented.

Developing Play and Gesture

If the child is not demonstrating any appropriate or semiappropriate use of objects or symbolic play and gestures listed in Tables 7-2 and 7-3, a more basic foundation in reciprocity and anticipatory sets may need to be established. Using techniques outlined in Chapter 6 can help to establish this basis. What if observation of play and gesture indicates that the child is already showing reciprocal behavior, such as turn-taking in back-and-forth babbling games, and anticipates actions in baby games, such as peek-a-boo, but is not yet using the functional and symbolic behaviors? This child is probably ready to be encouraged to use the next levels of symbolic behavior, such as early conventional and symbolic play and deictic gestures. In this situation, the clinician can use either a direct or consultative approach. The goal is to model the early forms of conventional and symbolic play (e.g., Nicolich's levels 1 and 2 in Table 7-2) and gestures (see Table 7-3) and give the child opportunities to imitate them. Accompanying these gestures and actions with simple language also can help foster receptive language development. For example, to encourage early autosymbolic play the adult might present the child with some child-care toys (bottle, bed, spoon, cup, comb, etc.). If the child looks at or touches the cup, the adult might say, "Nice cup! Let's have a drink" and pretend to drink from the empty container. The adult would then encourage the child to imitate the autosymbolic action: "Now you try a drink. Mmm! It's good, isn't it?" More advanced play behaviors from subsequent levels also can be modeled in the context of

pretend play scripts involving routines that are familiar to the child, such as pretending to give a doll a bath, feed it a meal, take it to the store, and so on. Deictic and representational gestures can be modeled in a similar way. For example, if the child bangs a cup, the clinician can imitate the banging, then hold the cup up to the child's face to show it, saying "Cup!" If developing conventional and symbolic play and gesture is one goal of the intervention, this is an ideal context for parent involvement. Parents can easily be shown how to model these play and gesture behaviors, and engaging in them provides an ideal setting for positive, facilitative parent-child interactions.

Using Intentional Communicative Behaviors

You'll remember that we evaluated the frequency, form, and functional range of expression of communication intentions in the child with emerging language. Intervention aimed at increasing the frequency of intentional communication bumps us up against what Hubbell (1981) called the "be spontaneous paradox" (p. 250). We want children to *initiate* communication, but we have to somehow *get* them to do it. Here we can use communication temptations, such as those of Wetherby and Prizant (1989) in Box 6-6. In providing communication temptations, we are using a hybrid method of intervention. We do not require a specific response (although there is one we are hoping for), but we do structure the situation and provide multiple opportunities and models for the child. An excellent way to involve parents in this aspect of the intervention is to demonstrate the communication temptation to the parent and ask the parent to respond as we want the client to respond. If we hand the parent the clear, closed container, for example, we can let the parent know that we want her to hand it back and use a direct gaze, questioning expression, or simple single-word request ("Help"). After modeling this several times, we can hand the container to the client.

Another hybrid approach to increasing the rate of communication is to use the milieu teaching techniques discussed in Chapter 3. Warren and Yoder (1998) and Yoder and Warren (2002) trained parents to use what they called prelinguistic milieu teaching (PMT) to increase intentional communication in children with developmental delays. The method follows the basic principles of milieu teaching. It involves arranging the environment to elicit child communication, focusing on and following the child's attentional lead, embedding instruction in ongoing interaction, focusing on specific target behaviors, and using prompts and reinforcement to elicit and maintain communicative behaviors. An important component of this approach is to provide a long time for the client to provide a response (Olswang & Bain [1991] suggested 15 seconds). Warren and Yoder found the method to be highly effective, particularly for children with mothers who were already quite responsive to the children's communicative attempts. Some specific methods used in this approach appear in Box 7-4.

Routine or script therapy also can be used. Here we would establish routines in games or day-to-day activities and then playfully violate the routine in the hope of eliciting a protest or correction from the client. Social games such as "peek-a-boo" and

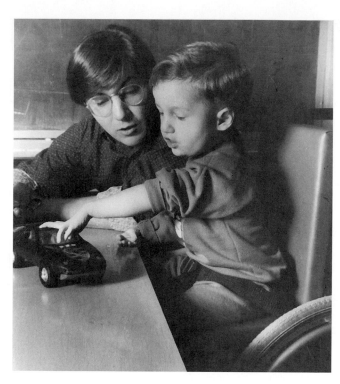

Eliciting intentional behavior is often a communication goal in the emerging language stage.

"Gonna getcha" work well. Sussman's (1999) book and accompanying video provide a variety of ideas for these activities that can easily be taught to parents. Other resources available from the Hanen center can also be useful in parent education. Parents can also observe the clinician engage in these kinds of activities and be encouraged to try them during routines in the home.

If the child is showing low rates of communication overall and our goal is simply to increase the frequency of any kind of intentionality, we must be prepared to accept any form of behavior as conveying an intention. In fact, if the child does not give us any clear sign of communication, Prizant (1991) suggested that we impute intent to some behavior we do observe, treat it as communicative, and respond accordingly. In this way we can begin to shape the child's behavior into communication.

Another aspect of expression of communicative intent that we addressed in assessment involved the range of intentions expressed. If assessment indicates that a child is expressing a restricted range of intentional functions, it is important to remember to work toward eliciting both proto-imperative and proto-declarative functions in an intervention program. Proto-imperatives are often addressed first because they are easier to elicit. We can use many of the techniques in Box 7-4 for arranging the environment to encourage their production. Warren and Yoder (1998) also suggest establishing social routines, then having the adult withhold a turn and look expectantly at the child or provide a verbal prompt, such as "What do you want?" to encourage the child's production. If this fails, the adult might use gaze intersection or a gestural model (see Box 7-4) to assist the child.

While the proto-imperatives are often targeted first, it is the proto-declaratives that more closely resemble the great majority of conversational speech acts. These acts also are less frequent in the communication of children with a variety of disabilities (Adamson & Chance, 1998; Rescorla & Mirren, 1998; Wetherby et al., 2004; Wetherby, Yonclas, & Bryan, 1989), although they are much more frequent than requests in typical children (Paul & Shiffer, 1991). For these reasons, it is especially important that we encourage the production of proto-declarative acts when attempting to broaden the range of expression of intentions. Warren and Yoder suggest that, because proto-declaratives involve sharing states of feeling and attention, it is important to develop a strong positive relationship with the child. Once this relationship is established, they advocate introducing novel events or objects to the child to encourage comments. New toys can be placed within established routines (rolling a car instead of a ball). Routines also can be sabotaged with silly or unusual events, such as pouring juice into a bowl, instead of a cup, at snack time. Adults also can pay less than the normal amount of attention to the client by backing away or facing away from the child during an interaction. This forces the child to do something to regain the adult's attention. Adults also can pretend not to notice something the child has directed our attention to or can begin to comply with a request and fail to finish. Then the child needs to get our attention back to complete the task or game. These kinds of activities can help children learn how to direct other people's attention to topics on which they are focused. Warren and Yoder suggest continuing these kinds of activities until the child produces more than one communicative act per minute. When this milestone is reached, we can begin to focus on initial symbolic communication.

For children who show relatively frequent expressions of a range of proto-imperative and proto-declarative functions but use only gestures as the form of their expression, we want to increase the maturity of the mode of communication. With children for whom speech seems a reasonable goal, we will attempt to elicit vocalizations, and eventually conventional words. Here our approach must be somewhat different than the one we used to encourage intentional communication. In this case, instead of responding to all the child's actions as if they were communicative, we want to "up the ante" and withhold responding until the child produces some vocal behavior. Capone and McGregor (2004) suggest that we first identify concepts and intentions the child is already expressing with gestures. Since these are early symbolic behaviors, they should be within the child's zone of proximal development for expression with a more mature form. They suggest we present higher level forms along with an imitation of the child's gesture, to help make the connection between the child's current symbolic representation and the new word we would like to become a symbol for the same idea. We don't want to ignore gestures, though, as they may be the only way the child has at present to express wants and needs. Rather than trying to "extinguish" gesture use, we would be wiser to help children augment their gestural communication with increasingly mature vocalization. Using manual signs may be a bridge from gestures to symbolic

BOX 7-4	**Prelinguistic Milieu Teaching Methods**

Arranging the Environment

- Place desired materials in view but out of reach.
- Place materials where adult assistance is necessary to obtain them (such as in a tightly closed, clear plastic jar).
- Violate the expected order of events (e.g., give the child a shoe to put on before giving a sock).

Following the Child's Attentional Lead

- Attend to and talk about toys selected by the child from an array.
- Reduce adult behavior to child's rate of initiation, even if this means long periods of silence.
- Use contingent motor imitation—an exact, reduced, or slightly expanded imitation of a child's motor act immediately after the child's production to establish early turn-taking.
- Use contingent vocal imitation—following a child's vocalization with a partial, exact, or modified adult vocal production (e.g., if the child says "aaah," the adult can say, "aah" or "baa").

Building Social Routines

- Engage the child in repetitive, predictable games, such as "patty-cake" or "peek-a-boo"; encourage parents to play the game at least once a day with the child.
- Vary the game slightly (e.g., if the child has learned "patty-cake," change it to "Bake me a cake as S-L-O-W as you can," with a corresponding change in the pace of the song).

Use Specific Consequences

- Provide the following specific consequences in teaching episodes that are brief, positive, and embedded within the ongoing interaction:
  Prompts
  - *Time delay prompts:* Nonverbal prompts that interrupt an ongoing turn-taking routine (e.g., if the child and adult are rolling a ball back and forth, the adult can hold onto the ball instead of returning it and wait with an expectant look for the child to initiate a request to continue).
  - *Gaze intersection:* To establish eye contact, the adult moves his or her head into the gaze of the child. This is faded out as the child begins to engage in eye contact more regularly.
  - *Verbal prompts:* Attempts to elicit communication, such as an open-ended question ("What?") or directive statement ("Look at me.").
  Models
  - *Vocal models:* Delayed imitations of sounds that the adult has heard the child use. If the child is heard saying "ba," for example, the adult can use "ba" at another time to try to elicit a vocalization from the child.
  - *Gestural models:* Encourage the child to use presymbolic gestures by modeling them at appropriate times (e.g., if a plane passes overhead, the adult can point up to it, as a model of nonverbal commenting).
  Natural Consequences
  - Be sure the child achieves any intent expressed. If the child expresses a protest, honor it by ceasing the protested action.
  - Provide any object the child requests and attend to anything on which the child is seeking joint attention.
  - Provide acknowledgment of communication. Smile, look at, or comment on any intentional behavior of the child. Make sure the child knows the message was received.
  - Provide linguistic mapping. Use simple language to "translate" a child's nonverbal intention to words. If the child holds up a cup, respond, "It's a cup! I'm glad you showed me!"

Adapted from Warren, S., & Yoder, D. (1998). Facilitating the transition from preintentional to intentional communication. In A. Wetherny, S. Warren, & J. Reichle (Eds.), *Transitions in prelinguistic communication* (pp. 365-384). Baltimore, MD: Paul H. Brookes.

communication. DiCarlo, Stricklin, Banajee, and Reid (2001) showed that teachers' use of manual signs along with speech in an inclusive preschool was accompanied by increases in communicative interactions by toddlers with and without disabilities.

Whitehurst et al. (1991) suggested, further, that vocal forms of communication containing only vowels actually compete with the development of linguistic forms of communication. In other words, one type of vocalization is not as good as another. Only those vocalizations that contain consonants help to move the child in the direction of speech. This would suggest that vowel-only forms of vocalization, such as grunts, whines, and "uh-uh"s, ought to be treated no differently from gestures. When the child produces these forms of communication, we should first acknowledge that we perceive the child's intention by saying something such as, "You want it. Tell me." As a first step, any vocal behavior will be acceptable as long as it contains a consonant. As soon as clients produce a vocalization including a consonant, we can give them what they want or engage in joint attention. If they continue only to gesture or produce a vowel-only vocalization, these attempts can be ignored and further prompts for speech-like productions can be given. Once some consonant productions have been elicited, we can "up the ante" again and require a closer approximation to a conventional word.

There is one exception to this general series of procedures. That involves clients who use maladaptive means of expressing their intentions. Some clients, for example, use self-abusive behavior to get attention or to express boredom with a task. Others may use aggressive behavior to request objects. These forms of behavior are certainly communicative and ought to be understood as such. But because of the inherent danger of such behaviors, we will not be able to simply accept or ignore the maladaptive form of expression. Again, we always want to acknowledge to the client that the message was received; however, in the case of maladaptive forms of communication, we need to provide an alternative means quickly and to make clear that the form the client used was not acceptable. If a client, for example, requests a snack by grabbing food from another client, we can say, "I see. You want it. Point to it, and I'll give you one. Like this. Now you show me." If the child uses self-injurious behavior to request the end of an intervention session, the clinician might say, "No. Don't scratch. You're tired. Show me (demonstrate a gesture, like putting face on hands as if sleepy). Then I'll know you're tired. We can stop then. You show me." It is important, of course, once these more acceptable forms of expression have been acquired, that we honor them. If the child uses the new signal we've taught to request an end to an activity, then we need to end it. Otherwise, the signal will not have been an effective means of communication and the old maladaptive means will reappear.

All the approaches we have been discussing for increasing the frequency, range, and maturity of communicative behavior involve, to some extent, a refusal on the adult's part to antici-

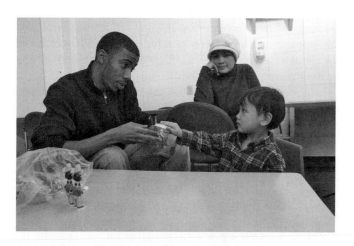

Communication temptations can increase expression of intentions in clients with emerging language.

pate the child's needs and a delaying of the adult's provision of goods and services to the child. Should parents be providing this kind of intervention? Family-centered practice dictates that parents be involved in the decision about who should deliver this and any other form of intervention. We should discuss this issue with parents and ask whether they are comfortable behaving this way with their child. These discussions also should emphasize that it was not the parents' willingness to respond to the child's immature forms of communication that caused the problem. I would suggest, too, that regardless of who provides the intervention, parents should be encouraged to continue to anticipate and respond to the child's needs, at least some of the time, and to feel that they do not have to provide this aspect of the intervention if that is their preference. Again, we want the child to feel that the parent can be relied on to understand and accept the child's attempts to get messages across. Occasional playful violations of routines and communication temptation games are appropriate activities for parents, but children also should be able to feel that their parents will respond when they communicate with them, even if the attempts are immature. This is one area in which direct service by a clinician may be appropriate, until the child establishes a repertoire of consonant-containing vocalizations that are used for communication. Once this repertoire is established, parents can take over and up the ante to requiring these more speech-like forms in their own communication with the child.

Not all practitioners accept this view. Whitehurst et al. (1991), for example, argued that parents should be taught to ignore all gestures and vowel-only communication in these children. They advocated giving parents structured activities to do with the child to elicit speech. As in many areas of language pathology, this is an issue about which experienced clinicians disagree. Whitehurst et al.'s suggestions for parent activities are detailed later, in Table 7-11.

Developing Receptive Language

In Chapter 3, we said that intervention should focus primarily on productive skills, but that an input component ought to be included in the intervention program when comprehension deficits are identified. Indirect language stimulation (ILS) is one form of this structured input. ILS is especially appropriate for clients in the 18- to 36-month developmental range and can be used to provide multiple opportunities for the child to observe how language works to map the nonlinguistic context onto words. It provides great opportunities for the client to try out comprehension strategies and to develop expectations about conversational structure. It also can be combined with efforts to develop play skills by providing ILS in the context of facilitative play interactions. This aspect of the intervention is, in my view, particularly well suited to using parents as intervention agents. ILS is an ideal vehicle for giving the child a clear set of examples for how language can be used to describe experience. It allows, but does not require, clients to try out this new understanding in their own production.

Parents can be trained to use ILS techniques by taking advantage of some of the materials in Tables 7-8 and 7-9. The

Hanen Program has been particularly successful in providing this kind of training and publishes books for parents (Manolson, 1992, 1995) in English, Spanish, and French. Prizant (1991) suggested that training for parents in ILS should focus on helping the parent learn to follow the child's lead by imitating actions, sounds, and words the child produces and providing words to match the child's actions and activities. Parents need to be made aware of the importance of letting the child choose the topic, activity, or material and of being sure to comment on something the child is already doing.

The standard ILS techniques outlined in Chapter 3—such as expansion, extension, recasts, and open-ended and verbal reflective questions—can be taught to parents through modeling. Although parents normally supply these kinds of input to their toddlers, we want to encourage parents of clients with emerging language to provide *super-normal* levels of these facilitative stimuli. Explaining to the parents that we are trying to provide very high levels of facilitative input can help to allay any lingering suspicion parents may have that we feel they have failed to provide adequate stimulation to the child. Our research on maternal linguistic input to toddlers (Paul & Elwood, 1991) suggested that one of the few ways that parents' interactions with normally developing toddlers differ from those with children who have slow language development is that the mothers of normally developing toddlers get more speech from their children. This in turn gives them more opportunities to expand and extend the child's remarks. You may remember that we said in Chapter 3 that these expansions and extensions are some of the most efficient types of input for encouraging language acquisition. So one important way we can influence the child's linguistic environment is to ask the parents to expand or extend just about anything the child says. Further, we can instruct parents to provide simple one-word labels for whatever the child is focusing on or referring to with preverbal communication. They can then expand or extend their own one-word label, modeling how simple language can be built upon and used. For example, if the child is looking at a doll, the parent can say, "Doll. Pretty doll! It's a pretty doll." Fey (1986) provided guidelines for training parents to understand the goals and methods of ILS. These are summarized in Box 7-5. The relations between receptive and expressive language also are important to emphasize to parents. Although lexical production in clients with emerging language may be quite limited, we want to provide a broad range of models in play and other facilitative contexts to build receptive vocabulary. Getting a child to say words is not the only goal of ILS.

Developing Sounds, Words, and Word Combinations

Increasing Phonological Skills. The primary goal of phonological intervention in the earliest stages of language development should be the enlargement of the consonant inventory and the range of syllable shapes the child can produce. For the child with fewer than 50 words in expressive vocabulary, this enlargement can take place in the context of back-and-forth babbling games. These games involve, first, having the clinician

---

BOX 7-5	Guidelines for Parent Training

1. Be sure parents understand specific goals before beginning training.
2. Involve as many family members and caregivers as are willing to participate in the intervention.
3. Delineate parent and clinician responsibilities clearly.
4. Explain the purpose of all procedures.
5. Collect baseline data.
6. Model procedures for the parent; observe parent using procedures.
7. Provide feedback to parent, using videotape or group-training procedures.
8. Monitor the parent's use of the procedures, using direct observation or audiotapes recorded by the parent during intervention sessions in the home.
9. Encourage parents to make incidental use of the procedures in natural day-to-day activities.
10. Maintain regular contact with families.
11. Monitor the effectiveness of the intervention.

Adapted from Fey, M. (1986). *Language intervention with young children.* San Diego, CA: College-Hill Press.

---

simply imitate the child's vocalization. Once a back-and-forth imitation pattern is established, the clinician can introduce a new consonant into the babble and produce it for the child to imitate. New consonants that are added would be selected on the basis of the order of acquisition of consonants by normally developing children. Paul and Jennings (1992) found that late-talking toddlers acquire consonants and syllable shapes in the same order as normally developing children do, but at a slower rate. By 18 to 24 months we found the late talkers to be producing most stop, nasal, and glide consonants, but few fricatives or liquids. So a clinician working to increase the phonetic inventory of a child with emerging language would first attempt to fill out the stop and nasal inventory, providing models for the child of any stops or nasals that were currently absent. If, for example, the client were producing only front stops in babble, the clinician would respond to the child's /bababa/ with /gagaga/. Once the full range of stop and nasal consonants is present in the child's babbling repertoire, the clinician can begin introducing some fricatives. I should emphasize again that even though we are modeling sounds in developmental order, the goal of these activities is *not* to get the child to produce particular sounds, but only to increase the consonant inventory. Any new consonant produced, even if it is not the one modeled by the clinician, should be rewarded. Work on expanding the range of syllable shapes would proceed in an analogous way.

When speech is a goal for children at the 18- to 36-month developmental level, phonological work should focus primarily on expanding the repertoire of sounds and syllable shapes, rather than on correcting errors relative to adult target words. Normally developing children at this developmental level still use a variety of phonological processes to simplify their speech (Bernthal & Bankson, 2004; McLeod et al., 2001; Roulstone et al., 2002). Any conventional word approximations that children with developmental delays are producing ought to be rewarded, not corrected. When expressive vocabulary and sentence length increase, there will be ample opportunity to work toward correct articulation. At the emerging language stage of development, the goal is to get the child talking and to increase the range of phonological structures available to support this talk.

Developing a First Lexicon. In Chapter 3 we discussed some of the considerations in choosing the first words to teach to children with small expressive vocabularies. These considerations include choosing words that are similar to those used first by normally developing children. Nelson (1973) found that close to one half of normally developing children's first words are nouns. These nouns include the child's own name and names of pets and family members, names for objects the child acts on directly *(shoe, spoon)*, names for body parts *(nose, belly button)* and preferred foods *(cookie, juice)*, labels for objects that move and change *(ball, light)*, and for social games and routines *(hi, bye-bye,* and *patty-cake)* (Owens, 2004).

Nelson's data, though, suggested that the other half of children's first words are *not* nouns. Lahey and Bloom (1977) also emphasized the importance of teaching first words not just as labels for objects but also for other kinds of communication. They stressed the need to teach not just substantive words, or nouns, but also words that can be used to talk about the relations among objects. In fact, Banajee, DiCarlo, and Stricklin (2003) found that none of the most commonly used words in toddlers vocabularies were nouns; instead they consisted of pronouns, (I, you), function words (that, the), verbs (help, is) and relational words (more, alldone). Teaching these kinds of words gives the child the opportunity to express more communicative functions than simply naming. It also provides a set of words that can be readily combined with others into two-word utterances when the child is ready to make that step, and a whole new set of vocabulary items would not have to be taught when the time arrives to make the transition to syntax. Table 7-10 presents the words found to be most common in children's early lexicons. These would be good words to include when teaching first words to children with emerging language.

An important consideration in choosing words for a first lexicon is that first words are functional and fulfill a broad range of communicative purposes (Owens, 2004). We want to teach children words that they can make use of often to accomplish their social goals. We don't want word training to consist of the clinician asking the child, "What is this?" since this kind of format is unlikely to teach the child how to use the word in the real communicative world.

MacDonald (1989) suggested further that words be chosen that encode ideas and interests children already have. These ideas and interests can be identified through analysis of play behavior. If, for example, a child demonstrates driving cars during the play assessment, *drive* would be an accessible word, although simplified pronunciation (/dai/) should be expected.

One further consideration in choosing a first lexicon has already been mentioned: the phonological shape and composition of the words to be taught. You'll notice that most of the words in Table 7-10 have simple, one-syllable CV or CVC shapes. These restrictions are appropriate for an early lexicon. In addition, when planning a lexicon for a particular client, it is important to match the words taught to the child's consonant

TABLE 7-10	**Words for a First Lexicon**

COMMUNICATIVE FUNCTION TO BE SERVED	RELATIONAL WORD	SUBSTANTIVE WORD
Rejection, nonexistence, or disappearance	*No, allgone, away*	
Cessation or prohibition	*No, stop, alldone*	
Recurrence	*More, again*	
Existence	*This, that, there, what*	
Action on objects	*Get, do, make, throw, eat, find, draw, fix, wash, kiss, bump, help*	
Locative action	*Put, take, up, down, out, fit, sit, fall, go, dump, turn, in, on, here, out, off*	
Attribution	*Big, hot, pretty, dirty, some*	
Naming	*I, it, you*	Objects child acts on (*shoe, cup*) Objects that move (*dog, car*) Familiar people (*mom, dad,* sibling names)
Possession, commenting	*My, mine, want*	
Social interaction		*Hi, bye-bye, night-night, yes*

Adapted from Lahey, M., & Bloom, L. (1977). Planning a first lexicon: Which words to teach first. *Journal of Speech and Hearing Disorders, 42,* 340-350; Lahey, M. (1988). *Language disorders and language development.* New York: Macmillan; Banajee, M., DiCarlo, C., & Stricklin, S. (2003). Core vocabulary determination for toddlers. *Augmentative and Alternative Communication, 19,* 67-73.

inventory. If only stops /b/, /p/, and /g/ and the glides /h/ and /w/ are present in the inventory, then first words ought to contain those sounds primarily, at least in initial position. *Hi* and *bye-bye* would be good choices. So would *go, get, put, allgone,* and *bump.* Later, as new sounds enter the inventory by means of phonological work in back-and-forth babbling activities, new words containing those sounds can be added.

What are the best procedures for increasing early vocabulary? As with any language goal, we have clinician-directed, child-centered, and hybrid methods available to us. Many clinicians (Lahey, 1988; Owens, 2004) favor a child-centered (CC) approach involving natural play contexts. This involves introducing activities and objects to which the targeted words can refer and having the clinician provide numerous models of the use of the target words to refer to these objects, activities, and their relations. Choice of target words, again, would be influenced by play assessment. Words chosen on the basis of the child's current knowledge and interests would be included. Play contexts that give opportunities for incorporating these words into the interaction would allow the client to learn words for ideas already being expressed through play. As in all our CC approaches, clients would not be required to imitate the adult's model in these activities, but would be generously praised if they do.

A hybrid approach, such as milieu teaching, using either the mand-model or incidental teaching format (see Chapter 3 for details), also can be used to elicit words from the child. Milieu teaching, you'll remember, involves organizing the environment so that desired objects and activities must be requested or commented on by clients for them to get the goods and services that they want.

Weismer (2000) advocates another hybrid approach, script therapy. In this approach the clinician and child engage in a verbal routine or a ritualized pattern of actions that involves the use of words targeted for the child's early lexicon. At first the clinician does all the talking. If a verbal routine is used, it can be accompanied by a mime or finger play that the child performs. Alternatively, action routines can be used. For example,

the clinician can go through a series of steps to place the child's nametag on a board to indicate that he or she is present each day at the intervention session. The clinician can accompany each action in the sequence with a simple utterance (for example, "You're here. Your coat. Take it off. Put the tag on. You put your tag on!"). When the routine is over-learned, the clinician can violate an aspect involving one of the target words. Or the SLP can use a cloze technique, providing the routine language but leaving a blank for the child to fill in the target word ("Your put your tag. . . ?"). Whitehurst et al. (1991) also have devised a hybrid program for stimulating the early stages of language development that was intended to be used by parents of children with specific language disorders. The methods they suggested for eliciting first words are described in Table 7-11. Lederer (2001) showed that a focused stimulation approach delivered by parents was also effective in increasing overall and target vocabulary acquisition.

It is, of course, also possible to use clinician-directed (CD) approaches, such as drill, drill-play, or CD modeling, with required imitation, to elicit early words. For some clients, this may be an appropriate tack to take. Friedman and Friedman (1980) reported that elicited imitation techniques such as these were more effective with minimally verbal children with low IQs than were more naturalistic approaches, whereas the more naturalistic approaches worked better for children with higher IQs. Connell and Stone (1992) showed that children with specific language impairment were more likely to learn to produce new grammatical morphemes if they were required to imitate during instruction than if modeling alone were used. Kouri (2005) reported that approaches using both CD elicited imitation ("Say, shoe") and hybrid focused stimulation, in which children listened to multiple models of target forms during play interactions without being required to imitate, were equally effective in producing increased use of target words in natural, home settings for toddlers with developmental delays. This suggests that, like older children, toddlers with language delays can benefit from a range of approaches, so long as focused attention to language is present in the activities; whereas CD approaches to early lexical development may be better-suited

TABLE 7-11	**Suggestions for a Parent-Administered Program of Early Language Intervention: First Words**

BIWEEKLY ASSIGNMENT	ACTIVITY
1	Forced choice: Ask the child to choose between a liked and disliked object. Give the desired object only if the child tries to label it or imitates parent labeling it.
2	Develop vocabulary: Clinician chooses 20 words to begin vocabulary; parent asks *wh-* questions when child is attending to the referent for one of these words. Parent gives item or complies with child request only if child tries to label item or imitates parent's label.
3	Incidental teaching: Parent asks child to label or imitate parent's labeling any object or activity child is attending to or requests and over which parent has control.

Adapted from Whitehurst, G., Fischel, J., Lonigan, C., Valdez-Menchaca, M., Arnold, D., & Smith, M. (1991). Treatment of early expressive language delay: If, when, and how. *Topics in Language Disorders, 11,* 55-68.

to the older, developmentally delayed child at an emerging language developmental level. Like all choices about processes of intervention, though, hard and fast rules rarely apply. We need to determine which approach, or mix of approaches, works best for the particular client. Whatever approach is used, the same considerations we have discussed for choosing lexical items should apply. Even in a CD approach, words taught ought to have potential communicative value and appropriate phonological shapes.

Issues concerning receptive language also should be kept in mind when developing a first lexicon. Receptive vocabulary is typically in advance of expression in the emerging language period (Owens, 2004). Children with language impairments in this stage should not be deprived of hearing a rich mix of words, even though we may concentrate on eliciting only a few of them in production. Beyond the specific language elicitation procedures we use with these children, we should encourage parents *not* to limit their word use to the lexical items the child can say (Hart, 2004). Instead we should urge parents to provide a range of labels for objects, events, and relations in clear, here-and-now contexts. If they see that the child is looking at a truck, for example, we should encourage them to label it for him not only as *truck,* but with more specific terms, as well, such as *flatbed, cherry-picker,* or *pick-up.* In this way, receptive vocabulary can continue to move ahead even when production is limited.

Developing Word Combinations. Children's first word combinations are used to talk about the semantic relations they already have been encoding with single words (Bloom & Lahey, 1978). As we've seen, most early two-word sentences convey a small range of semantic relations that are common across children and related to their current knowledge and interests, regardless of the language they are learning (Brown, 1973; Grove & Dockrell, 2000). When we try to elicit first two-word utterances, we want to encourage children to talk about these typical early semantic relations. The semantic relations listed in Table 7-7 can serve as a framework.

As with all our language goals, CD, hybrid, and CC approaches can be developed to elicit two-word utterances. CC approaches involve the use of indirect language stimulation. Here the adult engages the child in a play situation. Whenever the child produces a one-word utterance, the clinician expands it to encode the same relation the child intended, using a two-word phrase. For example, if the child were playing with a spoon to feed a doll and said, "Eat," the clinician might reply, "Yes, the doll eats!" If the child were playing with a car and bumped it into another one, saying, "Bump!" the clinician could remark, "Yes, the cars bump!" or "You bump the cars!" As with all types of ILS, no imitation would be required. The child would be praised for imitating a two-word combination and the clinician could imitate the child's two-word production once again. Play contexts for ILS aimed at two-word productions would, again, be chosen on the basis of play assessment for appropriate level and for content that matched the client's current knowledge and interests. Our goal would be to provide models of two-word utterances that map ideas the child is

already expressing in play. Frome-Loeb and Armstrong (2001) showed that indirect language stimulation techniques aimed at increasing word combinations were effective in eliciting longer utterances from toddlers with language delays.

Hybrid approaches also can be used at this stage. Schwartz, Chapman, Terrell, Prelock, and Rowan's (1985) vertical structuring technique is one example. Here, the clinician responds to a child's incomplete utterance ("doggy") with a contingent question ("Where is the doggy?"). If the child then responds to the question with another fragmentary remark ("bed"), the clinician takes the two pieces produced by the child and expands them into a more complete utterance ("Yes, the doggy is in the bed."). Since this is a hybrid approach, the child is *not* required by the clinician to imitate this expansion. If the client does spontaneously imitate, lavish praise is given. If not, the clinician simply goes on to elicit another set of related utterances from the child and offers the vertically structured expansion again.

Whitehurst et al. (1991) also have developed a hybrid program intended to be used by parents to elicit two-word utterances. This program is an extension of the activities described in Table 7-11 for eliciting single words. The steps in this program are outlined in Table 7-12.

Milieu teaching also can be used to elicit two-word sentences (Warren, Yoder, & Leew, 2002). If an incidental teaching context is used, for example, the clinician might place some stuffed animals on the top ledge of a chalkboard out of the child's reach or hang them above the child's reach using "window hooks" (plastic hooks attached to clear plastic suction cups designed to hang decorations in windows). If the child looks at, points to, or names one of the animals, the clinician can say, "*Get the duck?* You want me to *get the duck?* Tell me, '*Get the duck.*'" Wilcox and Shannon (1998) report that research has demonstrated that milieu teaching increases the frequency of communication, use of vocabulary, and use of language structures in clients with a variety of disabilities.

In a script therapy approach (Weismer, 2000), the clinician might teach a finger play, such as "Where is Thumbkin?" After the child has done the finger play with the clinician singing the song numerous times, the clinician might violate it by singing, "*What* is Thumbkin?" or by holding up one of the fingers ("pinky" is probably easiest to pronounce) and delaying the production of the line in the song. If the child corrects the clinician, ("No! *Where* pinky?") or produces an appropriate two-word utterance when the clinician delays ("Where pinky?"), lavish praise can be used as a reward, and additional violations or delays can be used later. If the child does not correct or fill in, the clinician can continue to provide the language routines and try again another time. Focused stimulation is another hybrid technique that has demonstrated efficacy in eliciting both early words and word combinations (Bunce, 1995; Kouri, 2005; Wilcox & Shannon, 1998).

CD approaches also have been used to elicit early two-word utterances. Leonard's (1975a) modeling procedure has been used successfully to elicit two-word utterances. As you'll recall from Chapter 3, this method involves a confederate of the clinician's, such as a parent or puppet, who is used as a model.

TABLE 7-12	Suggestions for a Parent-Administered Program of Early Language Intervention: Word Combinations

BIWEEKLY ASSIGNMENT	ACTIVITY
1	Introduce word combinations: Begin to require child to produce two-word versions of requests used in earlier activities. Reward with verbal praise ("Good talking!").
2	Shift reward from verbal to social: Have the child label objects and activities in which the reward is attention and praise, rather than receipt of the object or activity.
3	Storybook reading: Parent asks the child to label pictures during book reading. Parent responds to child's label with a *wh-* question ("What does the cow say?").
4	Open-ended questions: Parent uses open-ended prompts during storybook reading ("Tell me about this page."). Parent is taught to expand on child's remarks.

Adapted from Whitehurst, G., Fishel, J., Lonigan, C., Valdez-Menchaca, M., Arnold, D., & Smith, M. (1991). Treatment of early expressive language delay: If, when, and how. *Topics in Language Disorders, 11,* 55-68.

The clinician, after pretesting the client on the target structure, gives the model a set of pictures not used in the pretest and asks the confederate to "Tell what's happening here." The confederate provides a two-word utterance that describes each picture presented by the clinician (e.g., "boy drink," "girl eat," "cat walk"). After 10 or 20 of these descriptions, the client is asked to "talk like" the model and to describe a similar but not identical set of pictures. The model and client alternate their productions until the child produces three consecutive correct versions. Then the child is asked to continue until a criterion (say, of 10 consecutive correct responses) is reached. At this point the pretest stimuli would be post-tested without models.

MacDonald et al. (1974) developed the Environmental Language Intervention Strategy (ELI), which is summarized in Box 7-6. This is a CD approach that has some naturalistic modification in that it involves some extensions into semi-controlled versions of conversation and play. This approach has been used widely in eliciting early language. Because of its tightly controlled, well-laid out, adult-directed format, it has been especially attractive for parent training programs. Parents are taught to work on the same language goal, usually a particular semantic relation, for 15 minutes in each of the three conditions—imitation, conversation, and play. Sessions take place three times a week in the child's home. The SLP visits the family monthly in a consultant capacity to review progress and make any changes necessary in the child's program. As semantic relations are added to the child's repertoire, new ones are introduced into the intervention program.

One issue that commonly comes up when we attempt to elicit early two-word utterances is whether the linguistic input should be well-formed or contain the deletions that children are likely to make in these utterances, resulting in telegraphic productions. In other words, we need to decide whether we will say, "Pat bunny," or "Pat the bunny." We discussed this issue in Chapter 3, but let me reiterate my position here. Leonard (1995) and Fey, Long, and Finestack (2003) have argued that the sentences children hear should contain all the required

grammatical elements, even if we expect that the child will delete them in his or her own production. And Kouri (2005) showed that reduced models were not more effective than grammatical models in eliciting longer utterances from toddlers with delayed language. It may be that hearing a full sentence can help the child to build up an accurate auditory image of what well-formed sentences are supposed to sound like. Leonard (1995) suggests that it helps to focus on the weak-strong syllable pattern that is prevalent in English and appears to facilitate children's identification of important units in the speech stream. The rhythmic frame of the utterance that is created by the inclusion of grammatical morphemes may eventually help the child to fill in the slots created by the rhythm. If the child does not comprehend the morphemes and inflections, Chapman (1981) argued that they will simply be filtered out by the child's comprehension strategies and so will not get in the way of understanding the message. Well-formed, grammatical input cannot do any harm, and it may do the young child some good. It also is a more naturalistic form of input, and parents who are involved in delivering intervention will probably feel more comfortable speaking to their child "correctly." As always, the decision as to the method of intervention, whether it is CD, CC, hybrid, or some combination of the three, will be based on the needs of the individual client. But whatever approach we use, I would argue that the linguistic input ought to be complete and well-formed.

Preliteracy Development. It may seem early to be thinking about literacy, but the emerging language period is a time in which typically developing toddlers are acquiring important experiences with books and print (Dodici, Draper, & Peterson, 2003). Rosenquest (2002) and Scheffell and Ingrisano (2000) described ways to use storybooks in working with toddlers and their families in order to build early language and literacy skills. She suggests the following:

▶ Working collaboratively to select books that are developmentally appropriate and attractive to toddlers and being sure families have access to these books

| BOX 7-6 | Three Phases of the Environmental Learning Intervention Strategy |

Phase One: Imitation

A linguistic and nonlinguistic stimulus are paired. The child is told to imitate the adult; e.g., the adult pets a stuffed animal and says, "Pet the bunny. You say it: 'Pet the bunny.'"

If the child responds correctly, the adult repeats the child's utterance, gives praise and a token reinforcement (e.g., "Pet the bunny. Good talking!" and presents a plastic chip).

If the child fails to respond or responds incorrectly, the adult looks away for 3 seconds, then repeats the stimuli.

Phase Two: Conversation

The nonlinguistic stimuli are the same as in the imitation phase.

The linguistic stimulus is a question, rather than a request for imitation (e.g., "What am I doing?").

Response to correct productions is the same as in the imitation phase.

If the child fails to respond or responds incorrectly, an imitative prompt is given, followed by a repetition of the linguistic stimulus (e.g., "Say 'Pet the bunny.' What am I doing?"). This may be repeated.

Phase Three: Play

While the child is playing with the materials used as nonlinguistic stimuli in the imitation and conversation phases, the adult asks for the conversational response in an appropriate context (e.g., if the child pets the toy bunny, the adult can ask, "What are you doing?" Or the adult can pick up one of the toys and ask, "What shall I do?").

If the child gives a correct response containing a two-word expression of the target semantic relation, a confirming response is given (e.g., "Yeah, you pet the bunny!").

If the child does not respond or responds incorrectly, the adult does not confirm the response or comply with the request. Instead, a 3-second pause is followed by a request for an imitation of the target utterance.

Adapted from MacDonald, J., Blott, J., Gordon, K., Spiegel, B., & Hartmann, M. (1974). An experimental parent-assisted treatment program for preschool language-delayed children. *Journal of Speech and Hearing Disorders, 39,* 395-415.

▸ Teaching parents routine interactive reading strategies, such as pointing out connections between pictures and text, stopping to let children "fill in" elements after they have heard the story a few times, etc.

▸ Encouraging parents to use exaggerated intonation and stress during reading to highlight important elements in the text

▸ Encouraging parents to develop play activities around the themes from storybooks read; e.g., after reading *One Fish, Two Fish*, children can be encouraged to find red and blue things in their house

▸ Exposing children to decontextualized talk relating the stories they have heard to their own day-to-day activities; e.g., talking about times the child has seen fish

Zeece and Churchill (2001) discuss additional strategies for choosing and using books with toddlers. For SLPs, preliteracy development at the emerging language stage will consist primarily of encouraging families to expose their children to interactive storybook reading, and helping parents develop book sharing strategies that fit in with their parenting style and schedule. We know that children with disabilities tend to have less exposure to books during their early years than typically developing children do (Goin, Nordquist, & Twardosz, 2004), so anything we can do to enhance toddlers' opportunities to get experiences with literate language and literacy artifacts will be helpful in improving their readiness for school success.

CONSIDERATIONS FOR OLDER CLIENTS WITH EMERGING LANGUAGE

Some children with severe disabilities remain in the emerging language stage for an extended period. Children with severe mental retardation, those with autism, and children who suffer severe effects of acquired neurological damage are examples of clients who may present this picture. Many of these children have feeding and swallowing problems; these can be addressed with all the techniques and resources we discussed in Chapter 6. Older clients at this stage of development have some rudimentary form of symbolic communication but have not progressed beyond the one- or two-word (or symbol) stage in their expression of communicative intents. Our responsibilities with these clients are threefold: to maximize the effectiveness of the emerging communicative forms they express, to provide opportunities for them to expand the sophistication of their communication to as great an extent as possible, and to work on expanding the opportunities for and responsiveness to their communication by people in their environment.

MODIFYING ASSESSMENTS FOR OLDER CLIENTS WITH EMERGING LANGUAGE

When assessing communication skills in the older client with emerging language, we address the same issues we talked about for children at this stage with mild to moderate disabilities: play and symbolic skills; intentional communicative abilities; comprehension; and expressive capacities in the areas of phonology, vocabulary, and word combinations. When speech is not an option for these clients, the viability of augmentative and alternative forms of expression also need to be explored. We may have to modify some of our assessment procedures to gain the information we need, though. Let's take a look at how this might be done.

Play and Gesture

The first point to remember in developing play and symbolic assessments for children in the emerging language stage is that the purpose of these evaluations is *not* to determine whether the child has the "prerequisites" for a communication system. Instead, we use this information to help us decide how best to implement communication intervention for these clients. The other thing to remember is that when we evaluate children with motor impairments, they may have trouble demonstrating the symbolic behaviors we usually look for, such as use of objects for pretend or the use of conventional gestures. If this is the case, we may need to turn to other types of nonverbal assessment that can be demonstrated without so much motor involvement. Object permanence skills are one example of cognitive skill that can be demonstrated with eye pointing. Some assessment of object permanence ability, using methods such as those outlined in Dunst (1980), might serve as an index of cognitive skill in severely motorically involved clients. Traditional Piagetian assessments also can be modified by the clinician. For example, we can fit the child with a Velcro mitt to allow him to use a support (pillow or cloth) to obtain a toy out of reach, or attach string toys to switches to allow the child to operate the switch in order to use the string to obtain the toy. Guerette, Tefft, Furumasu, and Moy (1999) have validated a cognitive assessment battery for use with individuals with physical disabilities. Robinson, Bataillon, Fieber, Jackson, and Rasmussen (1985) have developed a parent-interview form to assess sensorimotor skills in children with physical disabilities. These procedures can be helpful in making an estimate of symbolic ability in children with severe speech-motor impairments. In addition, Byrne et al. (2001) reported on the development of new tools that measure brain activity during tasks such as looking at sets of pictures that do and do not match. These emerging protocols do not require either verbal or motor responses; they may be helpful in the future for getting a more accurate picture of the cognitive function of children with severe motor disorders.

Intentional Communication

In assessing intentional communication skills in older clients with emerging language, we want to look at *all* expressions of intent, including nonconventional and maladaptive forms. For clients without functional speech, it is especially important to assess the use of other communicative signals, such as gestures, sounds, limb actions, facial expressions, body postures, and orientation. We need to know what and how the client is attempting to communicate in order to provide more mature means for expressing these intentions that are already present. When we observe maladaptive behavior in these clients, it is especially important to attempt to identify the communicative intent of these behaviors. Rather than ignoring or extinguishing them, we may want to attempt to shape them into more conventional forms. It is important to observe the client in natural settings, such as the home or classroom, to see when these behaviors occur, what precedes them, and how adults in the environment react to them. These observations help us understand what intents the client is communicating by the behavior, what environmental events trigger the behavior, how the contingencies the client receives as a result of the behaviors tend to reinforce rather than reduce them, and the degree to which breakdowns in communication contribute to maladaptive behavior (Halle, Brady, & Drasgow, 2004). With this information we can work to give the client conventional ways to express the intents once we understand them. In addition, we can work toward modifying the environment so that acceptable behavior is reinforced while maladaptive behavior is not. Prizant and Rydell (1984), for example, discussed communicative functions that children with autism expressed by means of echolalia. A sample of these functions is listed in Table 7-13. This list would be a useful starting point for understanding and managing echoic behaviors in autistic clients with emerging language.

Halle et al. (2004) remind us that we need to use both naturalistic observations and structured probes in assessing the communication of AAC users. Naturalistic observations can show us how often communication occurs, how it is responded to, when breakdowns occur, and their relations to maladaptive behavior. This kind of functional assessment is crucial to understanding the communicative needs of clients with emerging language. But it may take a long time to gather all the information we need if we wait for it to happen naturally. That's why we can also learn a lot by using structured communication temptations to elicit particular kinds of communication. For example, if we want to know how a child will clarify a message if it is misunderstood, we can offer the child two objects, see which one s/he chooses, then pretend to misunderstand and give the wrong one. This probe elicits the child's strategies for clarifying communication without having to wait until a natural misunderstanding occurs.

Comprehension

When we assess comprehension skills in older clients with emerging language, we may again be faced with motor impairments that limit a child's ability to respond. If a child cannot point, we can have the client use eye pointing for picture or object identification. Eye-pointing behavior may need to be taught explicitly during the assessment session to maximize its use. Yes/no responses are another alternative to pointing or

TABLE 7-13	Some Communicative Functions of Echolalia

FUNCTION	DESCRIPTION AND EXAMPLE
Turn-taking	Adult: How was your weekend? Client: Weekend.
Verbal completion	*Completes a familiar routine initiated by an adult.* Adult: What do you do first? Client: Hang up coat (echoed from adult's completion of routine on previous occasions).
Declaration	*Labels using an echo.* Adult: What kind of ice cream do you have? Client: Ice cream.
"Yes" answer	Adult: Do you want a cookie? Client: Cookie.
Request	Adult: There's a car in the toy garage here. Client: Car in garage (used with gesture toward car).
Protest	*Delayed echolalic remark used to protest or prohibit others' action.* Adult: Let's do our speech work now. Client: Don't you dare! (echoing remark parent made earlier).
Directive	*Delayed echolalia used to direct others' actions.* Client: Time to clean up now (echoed from teacher's previous remark; used to tell fellow student to pick up blocks).
Calling	*Delayed echolalia used to get attention.* Client: All eyes up here (echoed from teacher's use of same phrase; used to get peer to pay attention to client during play interaction).
Provide information	*Delayed echolalia used to give new information not in the immediate environment.* Client: Dog's loose again (echoed from parents' use of same remark; used to inform teacher that something anxiety-producing has happened).

Adapted from Prizant, B., & Rydell, P. (1984). Analysis of functions of delayed echolalia in autistic children. *Journal of Speech and Hearing Research, 27,* 183-192.

object manipulation for assessing comprehension. Instead of asking a child, for example, to "Show me, 'The horse pushes the truck,'" we might demonstrate a toy truck pushing a toy horse, and ask "Is the horse pushing the truck?" Any yes or no response the child has available (head nod, sign, pointing, or eye pointing to a yes or no signal on a communication board) can be accepted. Miller and Paul (1995) provided additional suggestions for modifying informal comprehension assessments for children with a variety of disabilities.

We need to be careful in using pictures for assessing comprehension in clients at this level. As Glennen (1997) discussed, we should not assume that children understand that a picture is a representation of a concept. Before using pictures to test language comprehension, we need to pretest the child's ability to associate pictures with their referents. This can be accomplished by pretesting the child's ability to identify line drawings of common objects with which we know the child is familiar. If the child is unable to do this, Glennen suggests trying the same task with color photographs. If the child is still unable to associate common objects with their photographic representations, we may need to use objects themselves in the comprehension assessment. We also should remember that children with severe impairments might have more difficulties than younger, less impaired children in choosing from an array of several items or pictures. If a child has difficulty in selecting a named object from an array of four pictures, for example, we may try reducing the array to a choice between just two.

Phonological and Lexical Production

Looking at productive skills in older clients with emerging language should include examining both phonological and lexical skills. Reports have appeared in the literature of nonspeaking adolescents who have developed speech skills (Romski & Sevcik, 1996; Windsor, Doyle, & Siegel, 1994), so speech need not be eliminated as a goal, even if a client with emerging language currently uses some AAC system to communicate. Ongoing assessment of phonological production can help identify whether speech will become a possibility for some of these clients. Periodically assessing spontaneous vocalizations for phonetic inventory and syllable structure level can be part of the ongoing evaluation plan for older clients with emerging language. When new sounds or syllable shapes appear in the repertoire, they can be incorporated into speech targets, using facilitating contexts like those outlined in Box 6-7. If an AAC system is already in use, it need not be abandoned. Some clients may be able to produce some communication by means of speech and continue to use the AAC system for the remainder of their communication. Adding some speech to the repertoire of these clients or increasing the amount of speech they produce can expand their communicative range and make their AAC system even more efficient.

To assess lexical knowledge in these older clients with emerging language, the parent checklists we discussed earlier can be very beneficial. The *MacArthur-Bates Communicative Development Inventories* (Fenson et al., 1993) are especially helpful because they contain scales that address symbolic play, words produced, words understood, and word combinations produced. Detailed information in this broad range of areas obtained from parents with intimate knowledge of their child's abilities can provide a very useful picture of the client's skills. Spanish, French, and Italian language forms of this assessment also are available. The *Vineland Adaptive Behavior Scale—II* (Sparrow, Cichetti, & Balla, 2005) is another parent-report instrument that can be very effective for clients at this developmental level. It has excellent psychometric properties and gives an in-depth picture of adaptive uses of both receptive and expressive communication.

Motor Skills Assessment. For clients with severe speech and physical impairments, the choice of an AAC system is strongly dependent on the physical abilities of the client to manipulate the aspects of the system. Signs may be a viable system for children with relatively good motor skills, but if a child's Signs are as unintelligible as his or her speech, another form will have to be investigated. Although this complex issue cannot be explored in detail here, DeCoste (1997) outlined the basic questions that need to be asked and emphasized that the goal of this assessment is *not* to identify motor deficits but rather to discover motor capabilities that *can* be used to access a system. This assessment involves examination of the following five major components:

Movement: Here we try to find the client's best movement pattern; one that is reliable and accurate and can be performed without undue effort and minimal abnormalities of tone and overflow movement. Finger, hand, arm, and head movements are used most often. Chin, mouth, and shoulder movements are used if these others are not available. Lower extremity movements are used as a last resort. Emerging technologies also use eye blink and eye movement. This evaluation is best conducted in collaboration with other professionals, such as occupational and physical therapists, who can assist with the motoric assessment, as well as with teachers and family members who need to facilitate the client's use of the system in everyday settings.

Control site: This refers to the point of contact with the communication device. It may be a body part, such as a fingertip or hand, or an aid, such as headstick or light beam from a laser pointer.

Input method: The communication aid itself provides a method by which the client inputs intentions to communicate. It may be a computer keyboard, touch window, or cardboard with pictures or symbols on it. The device also may include some type of switch or joystick by which the client indicates a selection. Input can take place by means of *direct selection,* where the client indicates directly (by pointing, touching or using a headstick or laser beam) what he or she wants to choose. If direct selection is not possible because of movement limitations, *scanning* may be used. Here the device goes through a series of choices and when the one the client wants is indicated, he or she hits a switch to indicate a choice.

Positioning: The optimal placement of the communication device needs to be considered in light of the client's movement abilities, choice of control site, and input method. This often involves trial and error to determine the best arrangement of the device and switching equipment.

Targeting: The number, size, position, and spacing of symbols on the communication array needs to be assessed in order to maximize its accuracy and reliability for the client.

Beukelman and Mirenda (2005), Bridges et al. (1999), DeCoste (1997), and Lloyd, Fuller, and Arvidson (1997) provide detailed guidance for doing this assessment.

INTERVENTION TARGETS AND PROCEDURES FOR OLDER CLIENTS WITH EMERGING LANGUAGE

Play and Gesture

It's important to foster symbolic ability in older clients with emerging language. The nice part about this obligation is that it encourages us to engage these clients in play. Because we want to adhere to the principle of using chronologically age-appropriate activities for these older students, the kinds of play we set up will be different from the pretend situations with dolls and toys that we use for children closer to the normal chronological age range for emerging language. Nelson (1998) suggested using practical jokes as play activities with older clients with emerging language. A clinician can model placing a rubber slug on her shoulder and can collude with clients to see how it affects another teacher in the room. Students can then be allowed to communicate requests to play similar tricks on each other and other staff members. Using vocational and daily living props for unconventional, silly uses is another way to encourage play. A clinician might, for example, conclude a lesson on making pudding by putting the mixing bowl on her head (after the designated dishwasher has done his job!) and commenting, "Nice hat!" Students also can be allowed to play similar tricks with other materials they use in group activities, so long as they frame their silliness as a "joke" by producing a comment about it. Similarly, we want to encourage gestures in children who have the motor ability to produce them. Accompanying our own speech with gestures, using the hierarchy in Table 7-3, can encourage children to incorporate gestures into their communicative repertoires. Using songs and rhymes that incorporate finger plays can also serve as a basis for helping children learn to use gestures symbolically.

Intentional Communication

Regardless of the form of a client's communication, whether it be speech, Sign, or some other AAC system, most clients with emerging language need to increase the frequency of their communicative acts. Many also need to expand the range of intentions they express. When these needs are evident from the assessment, communication temptations will again be a useful technique. As with other methods for older clients, we want to adapt these temptations to make use of age-appropriate materials. Instead of a wind-up toy, for example, we might turn a radio on to a rock music station for a moment, then turn it off and wait for a request to turn it on again. Instead of blowing bubbles, then closing the jar lid tightly, we might put a favorite item in a clear glass jar, close the lid tightly, and hand the jar to the client, waiting for a request for help to open the jar. The practical jokes and tricks we talked about in our discussion of play skills also can be very useful contexts for developing joint attentional and commenting behavior.

For clients using or being introduced to AAC systems, we want to expand the frequency and range of communication expressed by means of the AAC modality. Here we may use prompt-free approaches, such as the ones discussed in Chapter 6, to shape behavior into communication and continually up the ante to require more conventional forms of expression. We can reward a random touch to a picture of a radio on a client's communication board by turning on the radio for a moment. Later we can require more purposeful pointing or eye pointing before we turn on the radio. Still later, we can up the ante to requiring a point at the picture on the communication board and a glance at the clinician.

In addition, we need to find ways to increase the effectiveness of our students' communicative acts. Halle et al. (2004) discuss the role of *Functional Communication Training* (FCT) in providing this kind of support to students with emerging language. FCT goes beyond simply teaching students to express needs; it is aimed at providing strategies for a range of situations in which communication can serve to reduce problem behavior and support integration. FCT involves identifying the purpose of maladaptive behavior, finding out what triggers it, and providing the student with new, more adaptive ways to solve the problems with which they are confronted. Sigafoos et al. (2004), for example, discuss ways of teaching students with emerging language how to reject objects and activities in a socially acceptable and effective way. These are summarized in Box 7-7. Halle et al. (2004) discuss specific techniques to teach for repairing communicative breakdowns. We discuss these aspects of FCT in more detail in Chapter 9.

Comprehension

Encouraging the development of language comprehension in older clients with emerging language involves many of the ILS techniques we discussed in Chapter 3 (expansions, extensions, buildups and breakdowns, recasts, parallel talk, and self-talk). Cross (1984) suggested further that parents of children with disabilities should be encouraged to make their remarks closely tied in meaning to those of the client, to reduce their directiveness and increase their responsiveness, to speak slowly and clearly, and to talk with their children as often as possible. These activities are helpful to any client in the emerging language stage, regardless of age. For older clients with severe impairments, though, it is especially important to remember that we also want to provide models of talk about objects and events outside the "here and now." Lucariello (1990) referred to these kinds of topics as *displaced talk*. They are crucial for showing clients how language is used to go beyond the immediate context to provide new information. First steps in this direction can include talk about familiar, highly "scripted" events that happened in the recent past (for example, talking about what a client had for breakfast when he arrives at school) or will happen in the near future (for example, talking just before a client leaves school in the afternoon about what will happen at dinner time). Parents, too, should be encouraged to engage in these kinds of simple "there-and-then" displaced talk activities around events with which the client is familiar.

Harris and Riechle (2004) showed that aided language stimulation is especially effective in increasing language comprehension and production in this population. Aided language stimulation involves the adult's using both speech and the child's

---

| **BOX 7-7** | **Steps to Teaching Communicative Rejection** |

1. Identify behaviors used to avoid or escape events.
2. If behavior is unacceptable, inefficient or hard to interpret, replace old form with newer, more efficient and acceptable form.
3. Define new replacement behavior in objective, measurable terms; e.g., "when presented with an unwanted object, student will select the 'don't want' symbol on communication board within 15 seconds."
4. Ensure new form is efficient by making sure the new form is easy to perform and leads to consistent reinforcement. Be sure everyone who interacts with the student knows this.
5. Provide instruction in new form when student is highly motivated to reject. Use incidental teaching techniques to provide extra practice.
6. Create extra opportunities for practice by offering objects or activities, and giving the nonpreferred choice, even when student requests the other.
7. At first use prompts to elicit the new behavior; provide immediate and consistent reinforcement for new behavior, no reinforcement for maladaptive behavior. Gradually fade prompts.
8. Be sure the new behavior is always rewarded with stopping the unwanted object or activity consistently by all who interact with the student.

Adapted from Sigafoos, J., Drasgow, E., Reichle, J., O'Reilly, M., Green, V., & Tait, K. (2004). Tutorial: Teaching communicative rejecting to children with severe disabilities. *American Journal of Speech-Language Pathology, 13,* 31-42.

augmentative system when directing input to the child. For example, if an adult is telling a child who uses a picture communication board to eat his cereal, the adult would not only say, "Eat your cereal," but would simultaneously point to the appropriate picture(s) in the child's communication book. Providing this enriched input appears to encourage children not only to learn the meaning of their augmentative symbols, but to use them more frequently, as well.

Production

One of the crucial decisions to be made for children with severe impairments concerns whether to focus on an AAC system for expression or to provide structured speech training. Yoder, Warren, and McCathren (1998) showed that there are three factors that most strongly affect a developmentally disabled preschooler's prognosis for speech development. Functional speech development is significantly related to the child's number of consonant-vowel (CV) vocalizations in a 15-minute communication sample (more than one CV production per 4 minutes predicted the development of functional speech 1 year after the assessment); the rate of proto-declaratives produced (more than one comment per 5 minutes predicted functional speech); and the receptive-to-expressive vocabulary ratio, as assessed by parent report on Fenson et al.'s (1993) *Communicative Development Inventory* (more than four words said for every 100 understood predicted functional speech). These findings can be helpful in differentiating which children have the highest likelihood of developing speech skills from those for whom AAC should be the main focus of intervention.

The means of deciding what AAC modality will be most effective to facilitate communication in clients at emerging language levels is, again, too complex an issue to discuss in detail here. Beukelman and Mirenda (2005), Bridges et al. (1999), Millikin (1997), and von Tetzchner and Grove (2003) provided detailed discussions of the considerations that go into making this decision. Light and Drager (2002) discuss AAC issues that pertain particularly to young children. For starters, though, there are a few rules of thumb we can use to guide us.

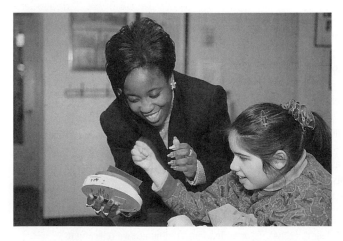

Clients in the emerging language stage can use AAC devices to produce their first expressive language forms.

For clients with severe speech and physical impairments, motor access to the system is a central issue. The choice of an AAC system is strongly dependent on the physical abilities of the client to manipulate the aspects of the system. DeCoste's (1997) assessments will provide important input into making the choice of the AAC system. This process is best conducted in collaboration with other professionals, such as occupational and physical therapists who can assist with the motoric evaluation, as well as with teachers and family members who need to facilitate the client's use of the system in everyday settings. The SLP should not try to make this decision in isolation.

The choice of a symbol system for the communication aid must be considered carefully, too. Even pictorial systems have varying degrees of transparency (how close the icon is to the thing it represents) and complexity (how many aspects of the symbol need to be processed and decoded), as we discussed in Chapter 3. Millikin (1997) and Bridges et al. (1999) discussed this issue in detail. Moreover, Preissler (2003) found that children with severe disabilities often fail to understand that pictures represent objects, and simply make associations between pictures and objects without knowledge of their referential function. This means that if we use a picture system, such as the Picture Exchange Communication System (PECS; Bondy, Tincani, & Frost, 2004), we need to make sure that children develop the understanding that a picture stands for a class of objects.

As a general guideline, we will want to provide more iconic systems (such as pictures or drawings) for children with developmental levels less than 18 months, although a small set of more symbolic items can be learned even at low developmental levels (Romski & Sevcik, 1996). More symbolic representations, such as Sign or Blissymbols, are appropriate for children with developmental levels greater than 18 months. In general, written systems are used with clients whose developmental levels are at least school age, although preliteracy experiences and instruction in alphabet letters should be provided at much earlier points in development for all clients. Children with autism often benefit from some visually cued modality, whether it be signs, pictures, or writing (Quill, 1998). It is important to know, though, that Grove and Dockrell (2000) found that children with severe disabilities who are taught signs rarely go beyond the one-word stage of language development. A picture-based system, such as PECS, may also be helpful at this developmental level. Ganz and Simpson (2004) showed that children with autism increased their use of words, utterance length, and grammatical complexity with PECS instruction. Sutton, Soto, and Blockberger (2002) discuss issues in moving children with AAC from one-word to grammatical productions.

Systems that include a voice output component have been shown to encourage not only increases in communicative expression but in vocalization as well (Mirenda, 2003; Paul, 1998; Romski & Sevcik, 1996; Sigafoos, Didden, & O'Reilly, 2003). Brady (2000) showed that using Voice-Onset Communication Aids (VOCAs) in joint attention routines also increased children's understanding of the words being introduced. Whenever possible, clients who need AAC—even those with low cognitive levels—should be provided with electronic VOCAs.

Even clients with emerging language who are provided with an AAC system should still be encouraged to vocalize. Any vocalizations that can be used communicatively will be useful, even if they are simply calls for attention. If a client can use vocalizations to get an adult to attend to the client's AAC communication, the vocalizations serve an important communicative purpose and should be fostered even if they never evolve into intelligible speech. Heim and Baker-Mills (1996) remind us that communication in AAC is always a multimodal proposition. We should encourage the client to use any means at his or her disposal to get messages across. If, at some point, vocalizations with consonants and more complex syllable shapes begin to occur, we can attempt to shape some intelligible speech from these raw materials.

In choosing symbols to include in a first lexicon for older clients, we will want to include words (or signs, Blissymbols, or other symbols) for the functions that are typically expressed in early speech, but we also want to consider words for other functions that are more appropriate for the daily living situations in which the client operates. These might include symbols for the objects the client uses in vocational activities, for chores that are part of the daily living curriculum, or for recreational activities that are part of the leisure-time program. Fried-Oken and More (1992) discussed in detail the issues surrounding selecting a first lexicon for AAC users. Beukelman and Tice (1990) developed a software program (the Vocabulary Tool Box) that allows for the development of a customized lexicon to be used in conjunction with a computer-assisted AAC system. Fallon, Light, and Paige (2001) developed a questionnaire method that enlists parents' help in selecting the most appropriate first vocabulary for children beginning an AAC system that clinicians may wish to use in this endeavor.

For children with severe hearing impairment (HI) who are at the emerging-language stage, use of a total communication (TC) system is especially appropriate. Although TC is not, as we discussed earlier, appropriate for teaching grammatical aspects of language because of the mismatch between the syntactic rules of English and American Sign Language (ASL), it is ideal for demonstrating the early symbolic aspects of language, using single words and two-word combinations. TC can be used to introduce symbolic communication to children with severe HI and to get them to express early semantic relations with single signs and two-sign combinations. When language level moves beyond the two-word stage, the clinician will be in a good position to observe the aspect of the TC signal, auditory or visual, for which the client shows a preference. This information is very helpful in deciding, in conjunction with other information about the client and family, whether to concentrate further instruction in the oral modality or whether ASL will be a more accessible system for this client.

When older clients with emerging language produce close to 50 different lexical items, using whatever communication system was developed for them, we should begin to encourage them to combine symbols to express the semantic relations typical of this period. Vertical structuring and milieu teaching, using both the mand-model and incidental teaching approaches

we discussed in Chapter 3, can be adapted to clients who use AAC systems. Many of the other programs listed in Tables 6-7 and 7-8 also can be useful for helping parents encourage clients to make the transition to multisymbol productions. Again, in working with older clients with emerging language we want to use age-appropriate materials, topics, and scripts to encourage this transition. Instead of using dolls and toys to do vertical structuring activities, for example, we can use daily living or recreational contexts. If a client is learning to shelve groceries as a vocational activity, we might do some vertical structuring of object-location relations in this context. As the client works, we might say, "You put soap there. You put the soap on the shelf. Tell me your job." If the client says "soap," we can reply, "Where are you putting it?" If the client says "shelf," we can respond, "Yes, you put the soap on the shelf." We can then wait for a response from the client. If it contains the target two-word phrase ("soap shelf"), we can praise lavishly. If not, we can model the two-word utterance again and go on to another vertically structured model. These procedures also can be adapted for clients using AAC modalities.

As we saw when talking about providing clients with AAC in Chapter 6, teaching the client to use the system is only half the battle. The other half is getting communication partners to interact with the client around the AAC. Johnston, Reichle, and Evans (2004) described the barriers communication partners face in interacting with AAC users. The important point to remember, however, is that in developing an effective AAC system, we will need to go beyond teaching it to the client; we will also need to work directly with parents, teachers, and peers to encourage and support them in making the system work for the client.

EMERGENT LITERACY

Normally developing toddlers engage in a variety of preliteracy activities around book reading and storytelling during the emerging language period (Snow, Burns, & Griffin, 1998). Children with disabilities who function in this stage need similar opportunities to develop basic preliteracy skills. If even minimal reading and writing skills can be developed, they greatly enhance a client's opportunities for communication and independent living. We talked about some techniques for doing so in Chapter 4. In working with clients who are functioning in the emerging language stage, we want to emphasize to parents the importance of book reading and storytelling and remind them that their child can benefit from such opportunities. Books chosen for these clients should contain simple pictures that can be labeled or described with a few words. Real stories with plots and multiple characters will probably be too advanced for children at this stage to comprehend. Showing children simple, attractive pictures in books and labeling them with one- and two-word descriptions will be appropriate for now. Parents can be encouraged to do this kind of simple book "reading" whenever they have time on their hands with their child, such as when they are waiting for transportation or for a professional visit. Even if only a magazine is available in the waiting room, rather than a real children's book, parents can be advised to find attractive pictures in it (such as pictures of babies or animals in ads) and to provide simple labels as they show the pictures to the child. In this way the time the parent spends with the child can be used productively, and other times during the family's busy day will not have to be set aside.

Other literacy-related activities also can be suggested for both home and school. Parents can be encouraged to talk about writing and its functions by showing the shopping list when they go to the store, leaving written messages for family members on the refrigerator, and reading aloud the signs they encounter on the street or at the doctor's office. Parents also can invite clients to "write" letters and thank-you notes to friends and family, even if they begin by only drawing or scribbling. Teachers can be urged to display print—in the form of alphabet posters, signs displaying classroom rules and routines, labels for objects, and so on—around the classroom at the client's eye level (not the teacher's!). We also can advise that teachers give clients access to "literacy artifacts," such as letters for felt boards and magnetic boards; paper stapled into books for drawing, writing, and pasting labeled pictures; and ample materials for writing and drawing that are adapted to the clients' physical limitations. These simple opportunities can provide an easily taken path toward the development of reading and writing skills. These skills, in turn, can make a great deal of difference in the communicative ability and potential for independence in clients with severe disabilities. Wood and Hood (2004), Sturm and Clendon (2004), and Pebly and Koppenhaver

(2001) discuss ways to include book sharing and literacy activities in intervention programs for children who use AAC. Some of these recommendations are outlined in Box 7-8.

For children such as these who come from culturally different backgrounds, we want to encourage the development of emergent literacy skills, but we'll need to be sensitive to the different ways in which parents from these cultures traditionally interact with their children. Many will be more comfortable telling stories orally than reading to their child from a book. When this is the case, we should encourage parents to tell their children as many stories as they can and to tell the same stories again and again. We can help parents find library books that contain pictures of culturally relevant items and events that they can label and discuss with their child. As described in Chapter 5, we'll want to encourage parents to read to their children in the language in which the parents are most comfortable, even if that is not English. If reading is not an activity in which parents want to engage, we can urge them to provide some of the other kinds of early literacy experiences we talked about instead. The point is to find the kind of activity the parent likes and feels good doing with the child, even if it is not the one we would prefer. By collaborating with the parents to develop an emergent literacy program that works for their family, rather than telling them what they "should" do to develop preliteracy skills, we have a better chance of ensuring cooperation and success. This issue actually pertains to the whole enterprise of supplying an AAC system (Parette, Huer, & Wyatt, 2002). We

---

| **BOX 7-8** | **Emergent Literacy Intervention Strategies for Children with Emerging Language who use AAC** |

Model literacy activities: encourage parents and teachers to demonstrate their use of books to get information and entertainment, writing lists, labeling objects in the environment with signs, and so on.

Make literacy artifacts attractive and accessible: print menus for school lunches and song sheets for favorite songs, label photos of favorite people and activities, make sure children have opportunities to write and draw with interesting materials, such as MagnaDoodle, EtchASketch, alphabet letters made from felt, plastic, etc.

Provide opportunities to request specific books and reading activities: include pictures of favorite books and several reading-related options ("pick a book," "read to me," "read it again," "turn the page") on communication boards.

Provide adapted writing opportunities: for example, put a marker through a hole cut in a tennis ball or a pencil on a headstick.

Use multimedia: Interactive storybooks on CD-ROM can be used to increase interactions with texts.

Increase story participation: Put a series of pictures copied from a favorite book on a communication board overlay and have the client 'retell' the story by pointing to the pictures, or program a VOCA to emit story elements so the student can 'retell' it.

Build from these routine productions to develop concepts (if an overlay for "Over the River and Through the Woods" has been made, use the "over" symbol in other contexts, such as Simon Says, in which the client instructs peers to go *over*, *under* and *through*) and multiword expressions (encourage client to pair "over" symbol with another to describe events, such as *over the river, over the bridge, over the barn*).

Encourage the development of phonological awareness: pair known pictures on the communication board with their written form in which first or last letters are underlined. Make a page of all /b/ words and talk with child about how all the words on the page start with the same sound; encourage the child to point to other objects in the environment that begin with the same sound; provide a "sounds like" symbol on the communication board, and help children identify words that "sound like" boat (e.g., coat, float, goat) using pictures or yes/no responses.

Adapted from Pebly, M., & Koppenhaver, D. A. (2001). Emergent and early literacy interventions for students with severe communication impairments. *Seminars in Speech and Language, 22,* 221-232.

need to work with families to find a way to make the AAC system a viable means of communication for the client within the context of their values and preferences.

■ CONCLUSIONS

Assessment and intervention for the child functioning at the 18- to 36-month level will always be family-centered, since the family is the social system that has the greatest impact on the life of a developmentally young child. Being family-centered, as we have seen, means being responsive to the interests and concerns of the family; being sure that they are involved in all the decisions made about assessment and intervention for the child; and respecting their culture, traditions, and personal style. When assessing communication in a child at the level of emerging language, we need to make use of a variety of informal procedures that allow us to look at how the child uses and understands communication in natural settings. The goal of the assessment of communication is to learn not only what clients can say in terms of sounds, words, and sentences, but also what they understand, what nonverbal means of communication are available to them, and what play and gestural abilities are present. Integrating information from the assessment of all these areas allows us to develop an intervention program that makes the best use of the skills the child has to build more mature communication. Parents may participate as agents of this intervention but do not have to be the only agents. As always, we want to provide an appropriate mix of services that best meets the needs of the particular child and family.

Let's see how this approach might work for the little boy we met at the beginning of the chapter, Joey.

When Joey went to the doctor for his next checkup and was still talking very little, the pediatrician recommended a speech and language evaluation. Ms. Bauer, after reviewing his medical records and audiological report, interviewed the parents about Joey's feeding, babbling, and social skills. Joey's parents told Ms. Bauer that Joey did not have any trouble with feeding, but he had been a somewhat "unhappy" baby, crying more and babbling less than they remember his brother doing. They reported that he made some sounds now, but most sounded like "aa-aa" instead of like the /bababa/ they heard from most babies. He seemed so uninterested in people and didn't babble back and forth the way his brother had.

Ms. Bauer talked with them about what they thought Joey understood, asked the parents to describe how Joey did get his messages across, and how the parents felt about his communication. She then explained that she wanted to observe how Joey played and how he communicated with familiar people and that she also would like them to make a tape-recording at home so she could hear the kinds of sounds Joey made. She suggested that a comprehensive developmental assessment might be helpful and that they consider starting this process by taking Joey to a psychologist who could do a cognitive evaluation before she did the communication evaluation.

Ms. Bauer also talked with the parents about their concerns for Joey's ability to take part in a preschool program and about their

worries for his success in school when the time came. Joey's parents told her that they had a lot of concerns about his ability to get along in preschool, especially since his mother was planning on going back to college in the fall and needed to have him in day care several days a week. His father especially worried that Joey would not be able to make it in school and might be put in a special class. They were very eager for Ms. Bauer to assess speech and language, but they did not want Joey to have an IQ test. They thought he was too young and didn't want him labeled "retarded." They would be happy to make a tape at home, though.

Ms. Bauer told them that she appreciated their willingness to make an audiotape and respected their desire not to have him labeled too early. She talked with them about what they wanted most for him to get out of any intervention program she developed. She explained that many children with slow speech development do "grow out of" their slow start, but she agreed with the parents that it was wise not to take chances with such an important part of development. She stated again her concern that Joey might need a more comprehensive assessment, but agreed to do a preliminary evaluation. She said she would also like to do an informal assessment of cognitive skills that was not an IQ test. Joey's parents agreed to this approach. Ms. Bauer devised an assessment plan for Joey (Table 7-14).

After gathering the assessment data, Ms. Bauer concluded that Joey's play skills were restricted to nonappropriate uses of objects with little evidence of symbolic play, even in response to a model. He showed a restricted range and limited frequency of communicative intents and showed poor comprehension and a lack of comprehension strategy use. He had a phonetic inventory of only six consonants. He rarely put more than one consonant in an utterance, had an expressive vocabulary of 16 words, and almost never combined words spontaneously into sentences, although he did produce some longer utterances that appeared to be frozen chunks he'd heard, usually from TV commercials. The communicative intent of these utterances was often difficult to interpret. Ms. Bauer explained these results to the parents. She let them know that she thought Joey's problems might extend beyond language to a more pervasive disorder. She reiterated her preference for a multidisciplinary evaluation to explore his problems more fully.

Joey's parents were not ready for this step. They wanted Ms. Bauer to "teach him to talk." They felt if he would just begin talking normally, his other problems would go away. They begged Ms. Bauer to work with him. Ms. Bauer explained that she didn't believe she could teach Joey to talk normally, at least not in a short period of time, and she felt strongly that he had other needs. She offered a compromise. She would agree to see Joey for 3 months and would attempt to teach him, not to talk per se, but to increase his communication. At the end of the 3 months, if she still felt his needs were more pervasive, the parents would be asked to have a full evaluation done. If the full evaluation indicated the need, continued intervention would use a more integrated approach, incorporating findings from the entire team.

Ms. Bauer's interim intervention plan focused on using communication temptations to increase the range of communication. She planned to use a milieu teaching approach to increase use of consonants in communication and eventually to add expressive

TABLE 7-14	Assessment Plan for Joey

AREA TO BE ASSESSED	ASSESSMENT TOOL
Nonverbal cognitive skill	Dunst procedures for assessing sensorimotor development
Symbolic play activity	Nicolich play assessment from observation of a structured parent-child play session
Vocal skills	Vocal assessment from audiotape made during home play session
Nonverbal communication	Communication Intention Worksheet assessment from observation of an unstructured parent-child play session
Receptive language	Informal comprehension procedures
Phonological skills	Phonetic inventory and SSL derived from audiotape made during home play session
Productive lexicon	*Language Development Survey* filled out by parents
Productive semantics and syntax	Speech-sample analysis of audiotape made during home play session if LDS vocabulary is larger than 50 words

vocabulary items to his repertoire. Ms. Bauer also wanted to work on developing conventional and symbolic play skills. She used part of each session to model this behavior with toys Joey was most interested in and asked the parents to carry over these modeling activities at home. She encouraged the parents to continue to model a wide range of words to Joey as he played. The parents and Ms. Bauer worked together to figure out what intents Joey was conveying by his use of frozen phrases from TV. When they discovered his intentions, they provided a simple one- or two-word conventional utterance to use to express the same idea.

Joey continued to use some of his inappropriate language and still was content to play alone with his rubber bands a lot of the time. He still showed limited pretend play, although he could imitate more appropriate use of toys in structured play sessions. At the end of the 3-month trial period, Ms. Bauer discussed progress with Joey's parents, and they agreed to the multidisciplinary assessment they had discussed earlier. They were glad to see the growth Joey had shown. They saw more clearly now, from the observations Ms. Bauer discussed with them and from their understanding of Ms. Bauer's work with Joey, what he could do, as well as the areas in which he remained different from other children.

STUDY GUIDE

I. Early Assessment and Intervention
   A. Discuss the pros and cons of early intervention for slow language development in toddlers.
   B. What is meant by "children with emerging language" in this chapter?
   C. What is involved in "family-centered" intervention for toddlers? Why is it important?
   D. Describe the communication skills seen in normally developing 18-month-olds in terms of comprehension, vocabulary size, sentence structure, and phonology. Do the same with 24-month-olds and 30-month-olds. How does this information affect practice in early assessment and intervention?
   E. What is the purpose of a symbolic play assessment? Describe Nicolich's levels of play and how they can be used to conduct a play assessment.
   F. What are the components of a communication assessment for children with emerging language?
   G. What formal tools are available for assessing the 18- to 36-month age range?
   H. What is the rationale for using informal assessment procedures for children with emerging language?
   I. How can nonverbal communication be assessed? What are the three dimensions of the assessment?
   J. Discuss the role of cultural differences in assessing parent-child communication.
   K. Describe formal and informal methods available for assessing comprehension in children with emerging language. Why is it important to look not only at what the child understands but at what comprehension strategies he or she uses?
   L. How can speech-motor development be assessed in children with emerging language?
   M. Give three methods of collecting a speech sample from children with emerging language. What are the pros and cons of using speech samples to assess vocabulary size in children with emerging language? Of using parent report?
   N. Describe two methods of assessing phonological skill in children with emerging language. Why are independent phonological assessments more appropriate than relational methods for children with emerging language?
   O. Describe the methods you would use to assess semantic-syntactic development in children with emerging language.
   P. Describe the decision process for determining whether and in what areas children with emerging language can benefit from communication intervention.
   Q. How does family-centered practice affect decisions about intervention for toddlers? What are its implications for who will deliver the intervention?

R. Under what circumstances would you attempt to develop symbolic play skills in a child with emerging language? How would you do it?

S. What methods would you use to increase nonverbal communication skills in a child with emerging language?

T. How can maladaptive forms of communication be handled?

U. Under what conditions would you include work on receptive language in the communication program for a child with emerging language? What methods would you use?

V. Would you work on diminishing phonological process use by a child with emerging language? Why or why not? If not, what phonological skills would you target?

W. What considerations go into choosing a first lexicon?

X. What methods would you use to increase the vocabulary size of a child with emerging language?

Y. Describe one CD, one hybrid, and one CC approach to developing two-word combinations in the speech of a child with emerging language.

Z. Do you think adult speech to children with emerging language should be telegraphic? Why or why not?

II. Considerations for Older Clients with Emerging Language

A. Discuss adaptation of assessment methods that can be used to evaluate communication skills in older clients at the emerging language stage.

B. What aspects of intervention are unique to older, severely impaired clients with emerging language?

C. Describe the role of emerging literacy skills in older clients with emerging language. What functions can emergent literacy serve for these clients?

D. Define Functional Communication Training and its role in AAC provision for children with severe disorders.

E. Talk about considerations in developing emergent literacy for children from culturally different backgrounds.

ANALYSES OF TRANSCRIPT IN BOX 7-3

Proportion of Multiword Utterances
Number of single-word utterances: 20
Number of multiword utterances: 16
Proportion: 44%
Semantic Relations Expressed in Multiword Utterances
Attribute-entity: #29
Possessor-possession: —
Agent-action: #14, #26, #36
Agent-object: #36
Action-object: #36

Demonstrative-entity: #17
Entity-locative: #7, #9, #11, #26, #27
Action-locative: #26
Recurrence: —
Nonexistence, denial, rejection: #5, #7, #17, #20
Disappearance: —
Other: #2, #3, #12, #19, #33
Proportion of Multiword Utterances in "Other" Category
5/16 = 31%

ASSESSMENT OF DEVELOPING LANGUAGE

CHAPTER OBJECTIVES

Readers of this chapter will be able to do the following:
- Describe family-centered assessment procedures appropriate for preschool clients.
- List areas outside of communication abilities that are necessary to assess in young children.
- Discuss issues and methods for screening for communication disorders in preschool children.
- Discuss the uses and abuses of standardized tests for communication

assessment during the preschool period.
- Describe a range of criterion-referenced and observational methods for assessing speech and language development.
- Analyze samples of communication including conversation and narration.
- Discuss the application of assessment methods for children at early stages of language development to older students with severe communication disorders.

Jerry was the third child in the family, so when he was a little slower than his sisters to get started talking, no one thought much about it. But when he entered preschool at age 4, his teacher, Mrs. Hamilton, noticed that his speech seemed immature. He made mistakes that other 4-year-olds in the class didn't make, such as leaving out the little words and endings in sentences. He'd say, "Me a big boy," and "I want two cracker." He seemed not to know the words for many things other children could name, and he often used vague or idiosyncratic labels to refer to common objects. He called a pineapple a "spiky," for example. Some of his words were hard to understand, too. He made some errors, such as saying /fʌm/ for thumb, that were like those made by lots of 4-year-olds, but he also left out sounds and parts of words in ways that weren't typical of children his age. He said 'mato' for tomato and /bʌ/ for bug. All these errors combined made his speech difficult to understand at times. Mrs. Hamilton noticed that when Jerry had trouble making himself understood, he often became angry, sometimes hitting or pushing the child who did not get his message.

At the parent conference that fall, Mrs. Hamilton told Jerry's parents that she felt Jerry was a bright child but that he was having some trouble with his communication skills. She explained that these problems might go away by themselves in time, but at present they were causing Jerry some frustration and interfering with his ability to get along with other children and succeed in the

classroom. She recommended that Jerry's parents consider having a speech-language pathologist (SLP) evaluate Jerry's language skills and determine whether some intervention would help him navigate this period of his development.

Jerry is a preschool child with a specific disorder of language learning. Like many such children, his problem includes several aspects of language development; these problems often affect his ability to get along in the social situations he encounters when he ventures outside the family circle. Jerry exemplifies just one of the many kinds of pre-school children a practicing SPL encounters. Other such children have hearing losses. Some may be developmentally delayed or have autistic behaviors. Others have accompanying emotional disturbances or a history of experiential problems, such as parental substance abuse. Still others may have suffered acquired neurological damage. Some, of course, are older than the typical preschool-age range. Whatever other conditions surround the language disorder, though, the children we will consider in this and the next chapter share certain language characteristics:
1. They have expressive vocabularies larger than 50 words.
2. They have begun combining words into sentences.
3. They have not yet acquired all the basic sentence structures of the language.

For children who are of preschool age but have expressive vocabularies smaller than 50 words or are not yet combining words, more appropriate assessment and remedial strategies can be found in Chapter 7, which deals with the emerging language period when first words are beginning to appear and a few two-word combinations may be used. Children who are functioning at the emerging-language level, even if they are of preschool age or older, benefit most from procedures aimed at this early phase of language development.

The period we'll call the "developing language" stage is the one that occurs when normally speaking children are between 2 or 3 and 5 years of age. Another way to describe this period is to say that it refers to language levels in Brown's stages II through V. That is, children with developing language have mean lengths of utterance (MLU) of more than two but less than five morphemes. These children are in the most explosive stage of language development, the period in which they move from telegraphic utterances to the mastery of basic sentence structures. For children with typical development, this process begins a bit after 2 years of age and proceeds rapidly during the preschool period. For children with disorders of language learning, though, the process is more protracted. They may be a good deal older than 2 when they start it, and they may be well into school age before they complete it. When we discuss language assessment and intervention at the developing language level here and in Chapter 9, we are referring to those children whose *language* functions in the period between Brown's stages II and V. The children themselves, though, may be chronologically older than preschool age. The principles of this and the following chapter can be applied to children of any age who have started combining words but have yet to develop the full set of forms for expressing their intentions.

■ Family-Centered Assessment

The first thing we need to know when we begin an assessment is that the Individuals with Disabilities Education Act (IDEA) makes specific requirements for the inclusion of the family in the evaluation and intervention processes. IDEA reminds us that we need to enlist parents as partners in the assessment process from the very beginning for any child with a disability. Recent IDEA regulations stipulate that parents must be specifically included as members of the Individualized Educational Planning (IEP) team. They require that parents' concerns be considered during the evaluation process and that all evaluations be disclosed to families at least 5 school days before any hearing process takes place. The regulations state further that the parents must be notified about any services delivered to the child and given progress reports at least as often as parents of typical children are. They must be told of their right to see any records or reports about their child and of their right to seek an evaluation outside the local educational agency, if they choose. A preassessment conference is often very useful to allow parents to meet members of the assessment team, to explain families' legal rights to them, and to give parents enough information and answer their questions so that they can give informed consent to the assessment procedures.

Family-centered practice means more than complying with these legal requirements, though. In addition, it means that we rely on parents as an important source of information about the child. We discussed interviewing parents on developmental and history information in Chapter 2. Standardized interview formats, such as the *Vineland Adaptive Behavior Scales—II* (Sparrow, Cicchetti, & Balla, 2005), can be used to help establish general developmental level. Questionnaires about general and medical history, like the one in Appendix 2-1, can be used to gather information from parents as well. But family-centered practice also means that from the first encounter with the family, we convey to them a sense of "being in this together," a desire and intention to address the family's concerns about the child and to respect the family's point of view.

As discussed in Chapters 6 and 7, family involvement does not necessarily mean that the family must be evaluated along with the child. This is often both off-putting and threatening to families. It does mean that we need to seek the family's perspective on the child's strengths and weaknesses, identify the family's concerns for the child, and find out what priorities the family has for the skills the child needs to learn to function most effectively. Let's take Jerry as an example. Suppose the family takes Jerry to the preschool assessment center of the local educational agency. The parents talk with the assessment team leader and the SLP there about Mrs. Hamilton's recommendation. They express some dismay that Jerry seems to be having so much trouble, since they haven't experienced difficulties with him at home. They say Mrs. Hamilton thinks he is bright, but now they wonder whether he might be retarded. Their main concern is helping Jerry get along better in school and avoid any problems when he reaches kindergarten. They don't want him labeled a "troublemaker."

How would we use a family-centered approach to assessment to deal with these concerns and use them to structure the assessment plan? First, we should try to assure parents that our evaluation reflects the "real" child. Assessment should be completed over a period of time in a variety of contexts, using naturalistic activities (Rini & Hindenlang, 2007). We want to ensure that the family is confident the team truly has a sense of who their child is. Second, we want to gather extensive information about the child from family members, so that they are assured that their perspective on the child is being included in the appraisal. Whether we used structured measures, like the *Vineland* or more informal interviews, we want to acknowledge that parents have the broadest and deepest knowledge about their child, and that we hope to draw on that knowledge as we conduct the evaluation. Third, all of the parents' anxieties should be addressed. If the parents are worried that Jerry might be retarded, even if the assessment team does not believe this is very likely, his cognitive and adaptive skills ought to be assessed. Referral can be made for a psychological evaluation to assess cognitive level. Alternatively, the SLP might ask the family whether they would be comfortable with her doing an informal cognitive assessment based on play behavior. She might assure the parents that if the child performs within the normal range on this measure, further assessment might not be necessary, but if she has any concerns at all about cognitive functioning, a referral for testing in greater depth can be made. The SLP also can offer to use the *Vineland Adaptive Behavior Scale—II* (Sparrow, Cicchetti, & Balla, 2005) to assess adaptive behavior, since a child must function below the normal range in *both* cognitive and adaptive areas to qualify for a diagnosis of mental retardation. In any case, a family-centered approach requires that we take the parents' concerns seriously and incorporate them into the assessment plan.

Next, the clinician would need to address the discrepancy between the parents' perceptions and those of Mrs. Hamilton. The assessment team might ask the parents to talk about how they see Jerry in relation to the family, how he gets along with his sisters, and whether and how he plays with children in the neighborhood. They might then ask the parents to review some of Mrs. Hamilton's concerns, to have them check their thoughts about Jerry's social skills with what the teacher told them to see whether the two seem to be in line in any areas. We want to give the parents the impression that we trust their viewpoint and at the same time help them to see that everyone—including children—acts differently in different situations. A clinician might explain that seeing Jerry interact with several different people through the course of the evaluation helps both the parents and the assessment team to get a fuller picture of Jerry's language and social skills. The team might request permission to observe Jerry playing with his mother or sister, either in their home or at the center, and also to go to Jerry's preschool and do an observation there.

The team also would want to work with the parents to plan the evaluation to include not only areas in which problems are currently obvious, such as his immature speech and language skills, but also areas about which parents have other concerns. Jerry's parents expressed doubts about his ability to succeed in kindergarten. In this case, the team might suggest including a special education evaluation in the assessment. This would give the team a chance to look at his readiness skills and give the parents more information about the skills Jerry has that will equip him for kindergarten, what skills he is lacking, and what skills they might be able to help him acquire. The team also can assure the parents that the recommendations that come out of the assessment will not only address basic oral language but also will provide information about ways the parents can help get Jerry ready for school. The team could then check with the parents to be sure (1) that what they have heard makes sense to them, (2) that it addresses the concerns they have about Jerry, and (3) that any other questions they forgot to ask or that came to mind during the discussion are addressed and considered in the evaluation plan.

What if, after the assessment takes place, conflicts arise between the family and the clinician or team about the recommendations based on the assessment? Suppose, for example, that the team evaluating Jerry believes that he needs a special preschool program that would overlap with the hours of his neighborhood preschool program, so that he was unable to attend both. Suppose further that the parents feel very strongly that they want him in the neighborhood program. How would a family-centered approach address such a problem? Again, the key is an attitude of respect and accommodation for the family on the part of the assessment team. Can a compromise solution be reached that would meet both the team's need to feel Jerry was receiving adequate services and his parents' need to see him in a "normal" preschool setting? Can a discussion with the parents allow both parties to express their concerns in a context of mutual respect so that either the parents or the assessment team might modify their views about what is best for Jerry? If no mutually acceptable solution can be reached, can the team defer to the parents' decision and cordially invite them to bring Jerry back at a later time so that everyone can reconsider his situation? These tactics would convey to the family that the team understands that the parents have Jerry's best interests at heart and that they are doing the best they can to provide for his needs as they perceive them. Such an attitude allows disagreements to take place without alienating the families of the children we hope to be able to serve. There may be rare cases in which we suspect serious abuse or neglect, which might make us less comfortable with deferring to parental decisions. Even in these situations, though, we want to be able to maintain a relationship with the family. This is the only way we will be able to serve the child. In such cases, it is incumbent upon us to make referrals to the appropriate social service agencies that can address the caretaking problem. However, we would still want to take a family-centered stance in trying to set up services to meet the needs of the child.

Family-centered assessment, then, does not mean assessing families, trying to identify their weaknesses. Instead it means including families in the process of deciding why, what, and how to assess each child. Moreover, it means taking the family's concerns seriously and treating parents as a valid and reliable source of information about the child. It also means respecting the parents' decisions about their child, even when we disagree with them. While it is always appropriate to try to resolve disagreements through compromise and courteous persuasion, we will not always succeed. When we do not, family-centered clinicians defer to the family's judgment and try to maintain a relationship with the family that will make them feel welcome to come back another time, when the child's problems, or their feelings about them, change. Bruce, DiVenere, and Bergeron (1998), Dunst, Trivette, and Deal (1988), and Rini and Hindenlang (2007) provided additional discussion on family-centered practice.

ASSESSING COLLATERAL AREAS

When we talked about assessment in Chapter 2, we discussed the importance of assessing every client referred for a speech or language disorder in the areas of hearing and speech-motor ability. This principle, of course, holds true for the child with developing language. Audiometric screening and, if necessary, full evaluation should be conducted, even if hearing problems have never been mentioned in the child's medical history.

Similarly, any child in the developing language phase who has difficulty talking should receive a thorough speech-motor assessment, following the guidelines given in Chapter 2.

Some language clinicians, particularly those in private practice settings, function independently in their assessment activities, making referrals to other professionals for information on collateral areas outside their own field of expertise. The majority of clinicians who do assessment in school, hospital, or nonprofit agency settings, though, usually conduct their assessments as part of a multidisciplinary or transdisciplinary team, as we discussed in Chapter 2. It could be, though, that information on collateral areas of particular interest will not be within the expertise of anyone else on the team. When this is the case, a referral to an outside agency may be necessary. Alternatively, the clinician might decide to do some informal evaluation in these areas to get a sense of how they relate to the child's language functioning.

We've talked before about the dangers of requiring that certain cognitive skills be present before language skills are taught. If we see a child of preschool age who is unable to accomplish any object permanence tasks, for example, we do not want to conclude that the child cannot learn language. We know such simple prerequisite relationships do not capture the complexity of the interactions of cognitive and linguistic development (Johnston, 1994; Nelson, 2000; Whitmire, 2000b). Still, we do need to know something about the child's general level of development, to help both in planning appropriate contexts and materials for intervention and in deciding on appropriate language goals. If, for example, a 7-year-old with a developmental delay is found to have a general developmental level of 15 to 18 months, we would want to focus on acquisition of single symbols, and stimulating language growth, using the goals and approaches advocated for children with emerging language (see Chapter 7) for some time. If, on the other hand, another developmentally delayed 7-year-old had a general developmental level of 30 to 36 months, we would focus more on approaches appropriate for children with developing language (that is, we would move more quickly from single words to two-word combinations and on to three- and four-word sentences and might consider more focused, clinician-delivered intervention). The point is that knowing something about general developmental level does not necessarily dictate what language skills are targeted, but it may influence the context, pace, and intensity of the intervention.

If general developmental level has not been assessed formally by a psychologist or special educator on the team, the speech-language clinician can use several informal approaches to get a picture of overall developmental status. Play assessment is one. In Chapter 7, we gave examples of procedures for assessing play skills as an index of general cognitive level. This type of assessment also is appropriate for children at the developing language stage. Table 2-2 provided some additional measures that can be used to assess nonverbal cognitive skills.

Table 2-3 also provided some more formal measures of nonverbal intelligence assessment. Some of these require administration by a licensed psychometrist. The revised *Leiter International Performance Scale* (Royd & Miller, 1997) is used on occasion by SLPs to get a picture of nonverbal cognitive functioning in children with language disorders. The *Columbia Mental Maturity Scale—Third Edition* (Burgemeister, Blum, & Lorge, 1972) and the *Draw-a-Person Intellectual Ability Test for Children, Adolescents, and Adults* (Reynolds & Hickman, 2004) are additional measures that can be considered.

If the *Leiter, Columbia,* or other cognitive assessment is used by a speech-language clinician to evaluate nonverbal cognition, it is important not to interpret the scores as IQs, but rather as indices of nonverbal developmental level. Knowing a child's nonverbal developmental level can be useful for language programming, as we have seen. As speech-language pathologists (SLPs), we are not qualified to assign an IQ, which is often perceived as a fixed, immutable trait. Findings from nonverbal cognitive assessments, if they are not administered by a psychologist, should be used solely to approximate a general level of nonverbal cognitive function for comparison with language skills. Reports of these procedures by the SLP should be given only in terms of nonverbal developmental level, not as IQ scores.

SCREENING FOR LANGUAGE DISORDERS IN THE PERIOD OF DEVELOPING LANGUAGE

Remember that *screening* is deciding whether a child is significantly different from other children in terms of language skills. To make this decision, we want a procedure that is relatively quick yet psychometrically sound, so that it is a fair measure of whether the child performs within the normal range. The point of screening is not to assess all areas of language but to get an idea about the child's general level of functioning in both of the major modalities: comprehension and production. Screening measures should always be standardized instruments; deciding whether a child is significantly different from other children is just what standardized tests do best.

Many standardized instruments are commercially available for screening purposes with preschool populations. A sampling of these is presented in Tables 8-1 and 8-2. One example is the *General Language Screen* (Stott, Merricks, Bolton, & Goodyer, 2002), a parent report screening measure for 3-year-olds. This instrument, which has demonstrated high reliability, validity, and reasonable accuracy, appears in Figure 8-1. Choosing which instrument to use should not be based on random factors, such as what happens to be on the shelf or what was advertised in a recent catalog. As clinicians, we have a responsibility to review all testing instruments and to choose those that are the most efficient and fair. For screening, that means that we want a test that is short and psychometrically sound. Reasonable levels of sensitivity and specificity have been reported for some preschool language screeners, including the *Early Language Milestone Scale—2* (Coplan, 1993), the *Language Development Survey* (Klee, Pearce, & Carson, 2000; Rescorla, 1989), the *Clinical Linguistic and Auditory Milestone Scale* (Clark, Jorgensen, & Blondeau, 1995), the *Levett-Muir Language Screening Test* (Levett & Muir, 1983), the *Screening Kit of Language Development* (Bliss & Allen, 1984), the *Fluharty Preschool Speech and Language*

TABLE 8-1	A Sample of Articulation Screening Tools for the Developing Language Level

TEST (NAME, AUTHOR[S], DATE, PUBLISHER)	DEVELOPMENTAL RANGE	COMMENTS
Arizona Articulation Proficiency Scale—Third Edition Fudalla, J. (2001). Western Psychological Services	1:6–18 yr	Identifies misarticulations and total articulatory proficiency Provides intelligibility descriptions Administration time: 10 min
Hodson Assessment of Phonological Patterns–Preschool Phonological Screening Hodson, B.W. (2004). Austin, TX: Pro-Ed	Preschool	See HAPP-3 in Table 8-3 Yields pass/fail score Uses objects rather than pictures Administration time: 2–5 min
Denver Articulation Screening Exam Drumwright, A.F. (1973). Denver, CO: Denver Developmental Materials	2:6–7 yr	Administration time: 5 min
Fluharty Preschool Speech and Language Screening Test, 2nd Ed. Fluharty, N.B. (2000). Austin, TX: Pro-Ed	3–6:11 yr	Standardized on multiracial, multiethnic group of 705 standard English-speaking children Uses common objects for naming Administration time: 10 min
Kaufman Speech Praxis Test for Children Kaufman, N. (1995). Detroit, MI: Wayne State University Press	2–5:11 yr	Identifies the level of breakdown in a child's ability to speak Assists in assessment of dyspraxia of speech in preschool children
Photo Articulation Test, 3rd Ed. (1997)		Can be adapted for screening See Table 8-3
Preschool Language Scale—4 Screening Test Kit Zimmerman, I.L., Steiner, V., & Pond, R. (2005). San Antonio, TX: Harcourt Assessment	3–6:11 yr	Screens a variety of skills including articulation and language Administration time: 5–10 min
Screening Test for Developmental Apraxia of Speech, 2nd Ed. Blakely, R. (2000). Austin, TX: Pro-Ed	4–12 yr	A screening instrument to assist in the differential diagnosis of developmental apraxia of speech Areas assessed include expressive language discrepancy, vowels and diphthongs, oral-motor skills, verbal sequencing, and articulation
Slosson Articulation, Language Test with Phonology (SALT-P) (1994) Slosson Education Publications	3–5:11 yr	Incorporates screening of articulation, phonology, and language into a single score that shows a child's communicative competence
Templin-Darley Tests of Articulation Templin, M.C., & Darley, F.L. (1969). Iowa City: Bureau of Education Research and Service, University of Iowa		Has a 50-item screening test See Table 8-3

Screening Test (Allen & Bliss, 1987) and the *Sentence Repetition Screening Test* (Sturner, Funk, & Green, 1996). When we look for a screening measure, we should examine test manuals for information on sensitivity and specificity, as well as other psychometric properties (see Chapter 2). It is important to know the properties of the tests we use and to choose tests with properties that are the best match for the assessment question that we are trying to answer. In practice, this means we have an obligation to read the statistical sections of the manuals of all the tests we use and to base decisions about their use not only on their efficiency and attractiveness, but also on how well their measurement properties stack up. There ARE such

things as bad tests: tests that are poorly constructed and do not give enough psychometric information for us to decide whether they test fairly and accurately. But there are very few tests that are so good that they are right for every situation. Clinicians need to match tests to their needs on the basis, at least to some extent, of the tests' statistical properties.

USING STANDARDIZED TESTS IN ASSESSING DEVELOPING LANGUAGE

Everything we just discussed about choosing screening instruments for children with developing language applies to

TABLE 8-2	A Sample of Language Screening Tools at the Developing Language Level

TEST (NAME, AUTHOR[S], DATE, PUBLISHER)	DEVELOPMENTAL RANGE	AREAS ASSESSED	COMMENTS
Bankson Language Screening Test—2nd Ed. Bankson, N.W. (1977). Baltimore, MD: University Park Press	4–7 yr	Receptive and expressive: semantics, morphology, syntax; auditory and visual perception	Lists 38 of the most discriminating items as appropriate for quick screen, but gives no norms for this screen Standardized on 637 children, all socioeconomic levels Test-retest reliability = 0.94 Concurrent validity: with PPVT = 0.54 with Boehm = 0.62 with TACL = 0.64
Battelle Developmental Inventory Screening Test Newborg, J., Stock, J., Wnek, L., Guidubaldi, J., & Svinicki, J. (2004). Itasca, IL: Riverside Publishing	Birth–8 yr	Communication, cognitive, personal-social, adaptive-motor	See Table 8-4 Standardized on 800 children nationwide Administration time: 10–30 min
Denver II Frankenburg, W.K., et al. (1990). Denver, CO: Denver Developmental Materials	2 wk–6 yr	Language, expressive-receptive vocabulary, concepts, personal-social, fine and gross motor	Gives age range for percentage of children who pass each item Standardized on 1032 children in Denver who varied socioeconomically and racially Interrater reliability = 0.62–0.79 Administration time: 15–20 min
Early Screening Profiles (ESP) Harrison, P., Kaufman, A., Kaufman, N., Bruininks, R., Rynders, J., Ilmers, S., Sparrow, S., & Cicchetti D. (1990). Circle Pines, MN: American Guidance Service	2–6:11 yr	Profiles cognitive, language, self-help and social, motor; surveys articulation, home health behavior	ESP claims link with K-ABC, Vineland, and Bruininks-Osteretsky Test of Motor Proficiency Nationally standardized on more than 1100 children Yields standard, age-equivalent, and percentile scores Administration time: 15–30 min
Fluharty Preschool Speech and Language Screening Test—2nd Ed. Fluharty, N.B. (2000). Circle Pines, MN: AGS Publishing	3–6:11 yr	Articulation, receptive and expressive language, composite language	Allows assessment of Black English Dialect. Provides standard scores and age equivalents. Standardized on 705 children from varied racial, ethnic, and socioeconomic status (SES) and from 21 states. Administration time: 5–10 min
Joliet 3-Minute Speech and Language Screen (Revised) Kinzler, M.C., & Johnson, C.C. (1993). San Antonio, TX: Harcourt Assessment	K, 2nd, and 5th grades	Expressive syntax, receptive vocabulary, articulation, voice and fluency	Has computer program for record-keeping. Provides pass/fail, cutoff score for each grade. Standardized on 2587 children from three different SES and ethnic backgrounds. Administration time: 3 min
Kindergarten Language Screening Test—Second Edition (KLST–2) Gauthier, S., & Madison, C. (1998). Austin, TX: Pro-Ed	3:6–6:11 yr	School readiness	Identifies children who need further diagnostic testing to determine whether they have deficits that will impede academic achievement Administration time: 5 min

Child's Name _____ Parents' Name _____

DOB _____ Age _____ Phone# _____

Please circle the answer below that best describes your child's use and understanding of language at the present time.

1. When your child speaks can he or she be understood by you?   YES   NO

2. When your child speaks can he or she be understood by other members of your family?   YES   NO

3. When your child speaks can he or she be understood by other strangers?   YES   NO

4. Can your child string three or more words together in a meaningful way?   YES   NO

5. Can your child follow two-step instructions; e.g., "Pick up the block and put it on the table?"   YES   NO

6. Can your child answer "where" questions; e.g., "Where is your teddy?"   YES   NO

7. Can your child make a choice when asked; e.g., "Would you like milk or orange juice to drink?"   YES   NO

8. Can your child place objects in, under or on when asked; e.g.,   YES   NO

     "Put the toys in the box."

     "Put the cup on the table."

     "Put the shoes under the chair."

9. Does your child enjoy listening to simple stories?   YES   NO

10. Is what your child says usually meaningful and relevant to the ongoing conversation or situation?   YES   NO

11. Can your child say more than fifty words?   YES   NO

12. Are you confident that your child has never had a hearing loss, including one that came and went over a period of weeks or months?   YES   NO

If the answer to one or more of the above questions is NO, in your view is there any obvious, known reason why this should be so?

_____

_____

FIGURE 8-1 ✦ *General Language Screen* for 3-year-olds. A *NO* response on any item is a trigger for further evaluation. (Reprinted with permission from Stott, D., Merricks, M., Bolton, P., & Goodyer, I. (2002). Screening for speech and language disorders: The reliability, validity and accuracy of the General Language Screen. *International Journal of Language and Communication Disorders, 37,* 133-150.)

choosing more in-depth standardized tests as well. Remember that the thing standardized tests do best is to show whether a child is significantly different from children in their norming samples, so every standardized test we use has a screening component. That means that when we choose a standardized instrument, we need to be sure that it provides us with some more information than we got from the initial screening test. If the standardized test only tells us again that the child is different from other children in general language skills, we have wasted our time and the child's in giving it. Let's look at what information is provided by standardized tests available for assessment of this stage of language development and see how they might enhance our evaluation of the client with

developing language. A sample of standardized tests designed for use with children in the developing language phase is given in Tables 8-3 and 8-4.

If you recall the four "whys" of assessment that we listed in Chapter 2, you may remember that one of our goals is to identify targets for intervention. Here is the place that standardized tests can be very useful. Once we have established that clients are generally less skilled in language than others at their developmental level, we can look more closely at specific classes of language behaviors and construct a profile, such as the one in Figure 2-2, which portrays language skills across a range of components of the linguistic system. We can use standardized tests to establish whether a child who failed a

Text continued on p. 330.

| TABLE 8-3 | A Sample of Articulation Assessment Tools at the Developing Language Level | |

TEST (NAME/AUTHOR(S)/DATE/ PUBLISHER)	DEVELOPMENTAL RANGE	COMMENTS
Arizona Articulation Proficiency Scale—Third Edition Fudala, J.B. (2001). Los Angeles: Western Psychological Services	1:6–18 yr	Standardized on 5500 children from nationwide sample Reliability (interrater) = 0.68–0.99 (test-retest) = 0.96 Internal consistency = 0.77–0.94 Concurrent validity = 0.82–0.89 (with Photo Articulation Test, Goldman-Fristoe Test of Articulation, Templin-Darley Tests of Articulation) Administration time: 2–10 min
Articulation Testing for Use with Children with Cerebral Palsy Irwin, O.C. (1961). A manual of articulation testing for children with cerebral palsy. *Cerebral Palsy Review*, 22, 1–24	3–16 yr	Scores: percentile, T-score, standard score Administration time: 5–10 min
Assessment Link Between Phonology and Articulation—Revised (ALPHA) Lowe, R.J. (1995). East Moline, IL: LinguiSystems	3–8:11 yr	Assesses phonetic repertoire through sound-in-position analysis, and assesses deviant use of phonological processes Assessment time: 15 min Scores: standard, percentile
Hodson Assessment of Phonological Patterns—3rd Ed. (HAPP-3) Hodson, B.W. (2004). Austin, TX: Pro-Ed	Preschool	Normative data for 3–8 yr Uses objects and some pictures Administration time: 15–20 min
Bankson-Bernthal Test of Phonology Bankson, N.W., & Bernthal, J.E. (1990). Austin, TX: Pro-Ed	3–9 yr	Tests 23 consonants, clusters Scores by phonological process or phoneme Provides consonant inventory, phonological process inventory Yields percentile ranks and standard scores Normed on a sample of 1000 children similar to national average in ethnic composition High reliability (0.95 internal consistency, 0.89 test-retest) Administration time: 15 min.
Bzoch Error Pattern Diagnostic Articulation Test Bzoch, K.R. (1971). Introduction to Section C: Measurement of parameters of cleft palate speech. In W.C. Grabb, S.W. Rosenstein, & K.R. Bzoch, (Eds.). Cleft lip and palate: *Surgical, dental, and speech aspects*. Boston: Little, Brown.	3–6 yr	Useful for clients with structural abnormalities of the oral mechanism
CID Phonetic Inventory Moog, J. (1988). St. Louis, MO: Central Institute for the Deaf	3–15 yr	Evaluates phonetic aspects of speech, primarily in the context of syllables, typically elicited through imitation of spoken model Phonetic Skills Profile summarizes scores Useful for establishing objectives and documenting progress Administration time: 30 min
Compton Phonological Assessment Compton, A.J., & Hutton, J.S. (1978). San Francisco, CA: Carousel House	3 yr–adult	Uses sentence completion
Deep Test of Articulation McDonald, E. (1968). Pittsburgh, PA: Stanwix House	3–12 yr	Tests articulation of sounds in various phonetic contexts to determine contexts that will facilitate correct production
Fisher-Logemann Test of Articulation Competence Fisher, H.B., & Logemann, J.A. (1971). Austin, TX: Pro-Ed	3 yr–adult	Has screening form available Sentence portion for 3rd grade and above Provides distinctive feature analysis

TABLE 8-3	A Sample of Articulation Assessment Tools at the Developing Language Level—cont'd

TEST (NAME/AUTHOR(S)/DATE/ PUBLISHER)	DEVELOPMENTAL RANGE	COMMENTS
Goldman-Fristoe Test of Articulation— Revised Goldman, R., & Fristoe, M. (1999). Circle Pines, MN: American Guidance Service	2–21 yr	Can be used with Khan-Lewis Phonological Analysis Yields percentile rank by age Administration time: 10–15 min for single-word portion
Iowa Pressure Articulation Test (IPAT) Morris, H.L., Spriestersbach, D.C., & Darley, F.L. (1961). An articulation test for assessing competency of velopharyngeal closure. *Journal of Speech and Hearing Research, 4,* 48-55.	3–8 yr	Consists of 43 items from Templin-Darley Tests of Articulation; assesses velopharyngeal closure
Kaufman Speech Praxis Test for Children (KSPT) Kaufman, N. (1995). Vero Beach, FL: The Speech Bin	2–5:11 yr	Assists in the developmental diagnosis and treatment of apraxia of speech in preschool children Identifies the level of breakdown in a child's speech
Khan-Lewis Phonological Analysis, 2nd Ed. Khan, L., & Lewis, N. (2002). Circle Pines, MN: American Guidance Service	2–21 yr	Use with Goldman-Fristoe Test of Articulation Yields percentile ranks, age equivalent; percentage occurrence of processes Standardized on 1175 males + 1175 females at 11 age groups; groups contain mix of genders, races, ethnic and geographical distributions Test-retest reliability = .94 across all phonological processes Administration time: 10–30 min
Natural Process Analysis (NPA) Shriberg, L.D., & Kwiatkowski, J. (1980). Natural process analysis: A procedure for phonological analysis of continuous speech samples. NY: John Wiley & Sons	All ages	Requires 90 words from spontaneous speech sample Yields phonetic inventory; data on use of eight phonological processes
Phonological Process Analysis (PPA) Weiner, F.F. (1979). Baltimore, MD: University Park Press	2–5 yr	Uses spontaneous and elicited production Looks at words in sentence context
Photo Articulation Test—Third Edition (PAT-3) Lippke, S., Dickey, S.E., Selmar, J.W., & Soder, A. (1997). Austin, TX: Pro-Ed	3–12 yr	Can be adapted for screening Provides means and standard deviations for age Normed on 684 children 3–12 yr Concurrent validity = 0.82 with Templin Darley Tests of Articulation Administration time: 25–30 min
Structured Photographic Articulation Test II Featuring Dudsberry: Articulation and Phonological Assessment (SPAT-DII) Dawson, J., & Tattersall, P. (2001).	3–9 yr	Uses 48 photographs to assess 59 consonant singletons and 21 consonant blends Identifies phonological processes used by preschool and school-age children Administration time: 10–15 min
Templin Darley Tests of Articulation Templin, M.C., & Darley, F.L. (1969). Iowa City: Bureau of Educational Research and Service, University of Iowa	3–8 yr	Has 50-item screening test plus Iowa Pressure Articulation Test for assessment of velopharyngeal closure Uses words, sentences, and sentence completion Provides means and standard deviations for age Test-retest reliability = 0.93–0.99
Test of Articulation in Context (TAC) Lamphere, T., & Menard, R. (1998). Austin, TX: Pro-Ed	Preschool– elementary	Based on the premise that articulation skills are most accurately represented in spontaneous speech; uses pictures to elicit all common consonants, consonant clusters, and vowels Administration time: 20–30 min

TABLE 8-3	A Sample of Articulation Assessment Tools at the Developing Language Level—cont'd

TEST (NAME/AUTHOR(S)/DATE/PUBLISHER)	DEVELOPMENTAL RANGE	COMMENTS
Test of Minimal Articulation Competence (TMAC) Secord, W. (1981). San Antonio, TX: Harcourt Assessment	3 yr–adult	Has 24-item quick screen Yields developmental articulation index Test-retest reliability = 0.94
The Apraxia Profile Hickman, L. (1997). San Antonio, TX: Harcourt Assessment	2–12 yr	Helps identify the presence of oral apraxia, diagnose developmental verbal apraxia, and determine oral motor movement and sequence disorders
Weiss Comprehensive Articulation Test Weiss, C.E. (1980). Austin, TX: Pro-Ed	Preschool–adult	Based on studies by Prather, Hendrick, and Kera (1975), Pendergast et al. (1966), and Templin (1957) Yields age-equivalent, intelligibility, stimulability score Standardized on 4000 children (ages 3–8) Test-retest reliability = 0.96 Administration time: 20 min

TABLE 8-4	A Sample of Language Assessment Tools at the Developing Language Level

TEST (NAME/AUTHOR(S)/DATE/PUBLISHER)	DEVELOPMENTAL RANGE	AREAS ASSESSED	COMMENTS
Assessment, Evaluation, and Programming System for Infants and Children (AEPS), 2nd Ed. Bricker, D., Ed. (2002). Baltimore, MD: Paul H. Brookes Publishing Company	Birth–6 yr	Assesses the skills and abilities of children who are at risk or who are functioning at a developmental age of birth-6 yr	Curriculum-based assessment/evaluation system that provides a framework for developing goals and objectives in intervention Measures functional skills and abilities, gathers data by observing in familiar environments, refers to IFSP/IEP goals
Batelle Developmental Inventory—Second Edition Newborg, J., Stock, J.R., & Wnek, L. (2004). Chicago, IL: Riverside Publishing	Birth–8 yr	Speech and language, social/emotional, cognitive, motoric skills, learning, and hearing	Normative data gathered from over 2500 children Includes optional scoring software so data can be input to a Web-based program or on a Palm Pilot Scoring includes standard scores, age equivalents, and cut-off scores Administration time: 1–2 hr
Boehm 3—Preschool Boehm, A.E. (2001). San Antonio, TX: Harcourt Assessment	3–5:11 yr	Receptive concepts: space, time, quantity	Yields age equivalent, percentile, T-scores Standardized on 433 children in 17 states; stratified by sex, race, region, SES Test-retest reliability = 0.87–0.94 Internal consistency = 0.88 Administration time: 20–30 min
Clinical Evaluation of Language Fundamentals—Preschool, 2nd Ed. (CELF-Preschool) Wiig, E.H., Secord, W., & Semel, E. (2004). San Antonio, TX: Harcourt Assessment	3–6 yr	Concepts, syntax, semantics, morphology	Downward extension of Clinical Evaluation of Language Fundamentals—Revised Yields standard, percentile scores, receptive and expressive composites Standardized on 1500 children Administration time: less than 1 hr

TABLE 8-4	A Sample of Language Assessment Tools at the Developing Language Level—cont'd

TEST (NAME/AUTHOR(S)/ DATE/PUBLISHER)	DEVELOPMENTAL RANGE	AREAS ASSESSED	COMMENTS
Communication Abilities Diagnostic Test (CADeT) Johnston, E.B., & Johnston, A.V. (1990). Austin, TX: Pro-Ed	3–9 yr	Syntax, semantics, pragmatics	Normed on 1000 nationwide
Coordinating Assessment and Programming for Preschoolers (CAPP) Karnes, M.B., & Johnson, L.J. (1991). Tucson, AZ: Communication Skill Builders	3–5 yr	6 domains: language, social, general knowledge, school readiness, fine and gross motor	Includes classroom and home activities program
Detroit Test of Learning Aptitude-Primary—3 Hammill, D.D., & Bryant, B.R. (2005). Austin, TX: Pro-Ed	3–9:11 yr	Domains: linguistic, cognitive, attentional, motoric	Has software available for scoring Has articulation measure Includes items measuring conceptual matching, design reproduction, digit sequences, following directions, word opposites, motor directions, visual discrimination, and other skills Yields standard score, percentile, developmental quotient (DQ), age equivalent Normed on 1976 children Construct validity and reliability date available Administration time: 15–45 min
Developmental Sentence Score (DSS) Lee, L.L. (1974). Evanston, IL: Northwestern University Press	2–7 yr	Expressive language: indefinite pronouns, personal pronouns, main verbs, secondary verbs, negatives, conjunctions, interrogative reversals, wh- questions	Speech-sample analysis Use for Standard American dialect only Yields developmental sentence score and scores for 10th, 25th, 75th, 90th percentiles for each age Standardized on 200 children in Illinois; mostly middle-class; 10 each at 3-mo intervals, ages 2 yr-6:11 yr
Evaluating Acquired Skills in Communication—Revised (EASIC-R) Riley, A.M. (1991). Austin, TX: Pro-Ed	3 mo–8 yr	Semantics, syntax, morphology, pragmatics	For evaluation of severely language impaired
Expressive One-Word Picture Vocabulary Test—2000 Edition Brownell, R., Ed. (2000). Novato, CA: Academic Therapy	2–18 yr	Expressive vocabulary	Spanish version available Norming sample related to ROWPVT Yields standard, percentile, age-equivalent scores Administration time: 20 min
Expressive Vocabulary Test–2 Williams, K.T. (2006). Circle Pines, MN: AGS	2:6–adult	Naming, synonyms	Normed on same children as PPVT Designed as a companion expressive assessment to PPVT
Grammatical Analysis of Elicited Language Moog, J.S., & Geers, A.E. (1985). St. Louis, MO: Central Institute for the Deaf	2:6–5 yr	Syntax: articles, adjectives, possessives, demonstratives, conjunctions, *wh-* questions, copula, prepositions, negatives	Video available for training administrator Yields profile, not standard scores Standardized on 200 hearing-impaired and 200 normal-hearing children

| TABLE 8-4 | A Sample of Language Assessment Tools at the Developing Language Level—cont'd | | |

TEST (NAME/AUTHOR(S)/ DATE/PUBLISHER)	DEVELOPMENTAL RANGE	AREAS ASSESSED	COMMENTS
Illinois Test of Psycholinguistic Abilities (ITPA)—Third Edition Hammill, D., Mather, N., & Roberts, R. (2001). Austin, TX: Pro-Ed	5–13 yr	The Global Composites scores are: General Language, Spoken Language and Written Language Specific Composites scores include: Semantics, Grammar, Phonology, Comprehension, Spelling, Sight-Symbol Processing, and Sound-Symbol Processing	Standard scores, percentiles, age and grade equivalents The ITPA-3 Scoring Software and Report System, sold separately, automatically converts raw scores into standard scores, percentile ranks, and age equivalents. Administration time: 45–60 min
Miller-Yoder Language Comprehension Test (MY) Miller, J.F., & Yoder, D.E. (1984). Baltimore, MD: University Park Press	4–8 yr	Receptive grammar and morphology	Normed on 120 preschool and kindergarten children Scores yield developmental profile Yields percentage correct with pass/fail criteria Administration time: 15–30 min
Peabody Picture Vocabulary Test—4th Ed. (PPVT-4) Dunn, L., & Dunn, L. (2006). Circle Pines, MN: American Guidance Service	2:6 yr–adult	Receptive vocabulary	Spanish version available Yields standard score, percentile, age equivalent, stanine, standard error of measurement Standardized on 4012 children ages 2-18 years Administration time: 10–20 min
Porch Index of Communicative Ability in Children (PICA) Porch, B.E. (1981—revised edition in preparation). Albuquerque, NM: PICA Programs	3–12 yr	Verbal, gestural, graphic abilities	Scores responses qualitatively Yields percentile rank, gives means for age Standardized on several hundred children representative of U.S. population Administration time: 30–60 min
Preschool Language Assessment Instrument— Second Edition (PLAI-2) Blank, M., Rose, S., & Berlin, L. (2003). Austin, TX: Pro-Ed	3–6 yr	Matching perception, analysis of perception, reasoning about perception	Assesses ability to use and understand the "language of learning" at varying levels of abstraction Available in Spanish Provides numerical and qualitative scores Gives reliability and validity data Includes family information form
Preschool Language Scale—4 (PLS-4) Zimmerman, I.L., Steiner, V., & Pond, R. (2002). San Antonio, TX: Harcourt Assessment	Birth–6:11 yr	Language precursors; expressive and receptive semantics, syntax, morphology; integrative thinking; auditory comprehension	Spanish version available Articulation screening included (see Table 8-1) Can be used as criterion-referenced test for older child Yields standard scores, percentile, age equivalent Standardized on 1500 children nationwide
Receptive One-Word Picture Vocabulary Test—2000 Edition Brownell, R., Ed. (2000). Novato, CA: Academic Therapy Publications	2:11–12 yr	Receptive vocabulary	Spanish version available Yields standard, percentile, age-equivalent score Similar to norming population for Expressive One-Word Picture Vocabulary Test Administration time: 20 min

TABLE 8-4	A Sample of Language Assessment Tools at the Developing Language Level—cont'd		
TEST (NAME/AUTHOR(S)/ DATE/PUBLISHER)	**DEVELOPMENTAL RANGE**	**AREAS ASSESSED**	**COMMENTS**
Sequenced Inventory of Communication Development—Revised (SICD-R) Hedrick, D.L., Prather, E.M., & Tobin, A.R. (1984). Seattle, WA: University of Washington Press	4 mo–4 yr	Receptive language (speech sound awareness and understanding); expressive language (imitating, initiating, responding)	Incorporates speech sample Age norms for receptive and expressive scales Has adapted version for older clients with physical disabilities Standardized on 252 white children from varied socioeconomic backgrounds Administration time: 30–45 min, longer to score
Structured Photographic Expressive Language Test 3 (SPELT-3) Dawson, J., Eyer, J., & Stout, C. (2003). DeKalb, IL: Janelle Publications	4–9:11 yr	Syntax and morphology	Has guidelines for scoring Black English dialect Spanish version available (second edition) Yields standard, percentile, age-equivalent scores Standardized on more than 1800 children nationwide Administration time: 15–20 min
Test for Auditory Comprehension of Language (TACL–3) Carrow-Woolfolk, E. (1999). Austin, TX: Pro-Ed	3–9:11 yr	Receptive language: word classes and relations, grammatical morphemes, elaborated sentence constructions	Spanish version available Yields percentile standard score, age equivalent Normed on 1003 children Administration time: 15–25 min
Test of Early Language Development—Third Edition (TELD-3) Hresko, W.P., Redi, K., & Hammill, D.D. (1999). Austin, TX: Pro-Ed	2:7–11 yr	Receptive and expressive syntax, semantics	Yields standard scores, percentile, age equivalent Normed on 1184 children in 30 states Administration time: 15–20 min
Test for Examining Expressive Morphology (TEEM) Shipley, K.G., Stone, T.A., & Sue, M.B. (1983). Austin, TX: Pro-Ed	3–7:11 yr	Present progressive, plurals, possessives, past tenses, third-person singular, derived adjectives	Uses sentence completion Has companion program—Teaching Expressive English Morphology Yields age equivalent, means, and standard deviation for 6-month intervals Normed on 540 children Construct validity = 0.87 Intrarater and interrater reliability = 0.94 Administration time: 7 min
Test of Language Development—3: Primary (TOLD-3:P) Newcomer, P.L., & Hammill, D.D. (1997). Austin, TX: Pro-Ed	4–8:11 yr	Receptive and expressive semantics and syntax	Has graph for visual representation of scores Uses imitation, sentence completion, picture pointing Yields standard scores, percentile, and equivalent quotients Nationally standardized on more than 2000 children in 28 states and Canada Administration time: 40 min
Test of Relational Concepts Edmonston, N., & Thane, N.L. (1993). Tucson, AZ: Communication Skill Builders	3–8 yr	Receptive semantics	Normed on 1000 children

TABLE 8-4	A Sample of Language Assessment Tools at the Developing Language Level—cont'd		
TEST (NAME/AUTHOR(S)/ DATE/PUBLISHER)	**DEVELOPMENTAL RANGE**	**AREAS ASSESSED**	**COMMENTS**
Test of Pragmatic Skills (Revised) Shulman, B.B. (1986). Tucson, AZ: Communication Skill Builders	3–8 yr	Pragmatics: verbal, and nonverbal, naming and labeling, reasoning, denying	Uses structured elicitation format
Test of Pragmatic Language (TOPL) Phelps-Terasaki, D., & Phelps-Gunn, T. (1992). Austin, TX: Pro-Ed	5–13:11 yr	Comprehensive assessment of student's abilities to use pragmatic language effectively	TOPL test items provide information within six core subcomponents of pragmatic language: physical setting, audience, topic, purpose (speech acts), visual-gestural cues, and abstraction
Test of Semantic Skills— Primary (TOSS-P) Bowers, L., Huisingh, R., LoGiudice, C., & Orman, J. (2002). East Moline, IL: LinguiSystems	4–8 yr	Receptive and expressive semantics: labels, categories, attributes, functions, definitions; has 6 themes: learning and playing, shopping, household, working, meals and health, and fitness	Yields standard, percentile, age-equivalent scores Standardized on 1500 students nationwide Administration time: 25–30 min Previously called *Assessing Semantic Skills Through Everyday Themes* (ASSET)
Token Test for Children DiSimoni, F. (1978). Austin, TX: Pro-Ed	3–12 yr	Auditory comprehension, temporal and spatial concepts	Yields age- and grade-equivalent score Standardized on 1300 children (urban and rural) Administration time: 10–15 min
Utah Test of Language Development—4 Mecham, M.J. (2003). Austin, TX: Pro-Ed	3–9:11 yr	Receptive and expressive language, auditory comprehension	Yields standard scores and language quotient Administration time: 30–45 min
Wiig Criterion-Referenced Inventory of Language Wiig, E.H. (1990). San Antonio, TX: Harcourt Assessment	4–13 yr	Semantics, pragmatics, syntax, morphology	No norm-referenced scores; use as criterion-referenced procedure
Woodcock Language Proficiency Battery— Revised Woodcock, R.W. (1991). Chicago, IL: Riverside Publishing	2–95 yr	Oral language, vocabulary, antonyms and synonyms, reading and writing	Compuscore software for scoring Spanish form available Yields standard, age- and grade-equivalent scores Nationally standardized on 6300 students Reliability coefficients = 0.95 Administration time: 20–60 min

general language screening scores significantly lower than peers in the areas of articulation, semantic comprehension, syntactic comprehension, semantic production, and syntactic production. By identifying the specific areas in which the language-impaired child is different from peers, we can begin working toward targeting our intervention goals.

Let's take Jerry as our example again. Suppose Jerry, after failing a screening measure given by the SLP, is given the *Test of Language Development—3: Primary* (TOLD-P:3) (Newcomer & Hammill, 1997) to explore his profile of language skills across a range of components of language. This test provides

a standardized measure of several areas of expressive and receptive language and allows us to construct a profile such as the one in Figure 8-2, which displays Jerry's scores on the TOLD-P:3. The profile tells us that Jerry is performing adequately in several areas of receptive language, but that his expressive skills, and particularly his articulation, are low for his age. This profile suggests that we need to focus on expressive areas of language development, including the area of phonology.

Another strategy for obtaining similar information would be to choose several tests, each of which focuses on one area. For example, we might select the *Test of Auditory Comprehension*

TOLD-P:3

Profile/Examiner Record Booklet

Test of Language Development–Primary
Third Edition

Section I. Identifying Information

Name _Jerry G._   Female ☐   Male ☑   School _Day Bright_   Grade _Pre-K_

	Year	Month		
Date tested	06	10	Examiner's name	_N. Dieterle_
Date of birth	02	6		
Age	4	4	Examiner's title	_SLP_

Section II. Record of Scores

Subtests

Core

	Raw Score	Age Equiv.	%ile	Std. Score
I. Picture vocabulary (PV)	9		50	10
II. Relational vocabulary (RV)	5		37	9
III. Oral vocabulary (OV)	0		16	7
IV. Grammatic understanding (GU)	13		63	11
V. Sentence imitation (SI)	1		9	6
VI. Grammatic completion (GC)	1		16	7

Supplemental

	Raw Score	Age Equiv.	%ile	Std. Score
VII. Word discrimination (WD)	12		63	11
VIII. Phonemic analysis (PA)	25		1	8
IX. Word articulation (WA)	8		9	6

Composites

	PV	RV	OV	GU	SI	GC	Sums of SS	Quotients
Spoken language (SLQ)	10	9	7	11	6	7	50	89
Listening (LiQ)	10			11			21	104
Organizing (OrQ)			9			7	16	88
Speaking (SpQ)					7	7	14	82
Semantics (SeQ)	10	9	7				26	91
Syntax (SyQ)				11	6	7	25	87

Other test data

Name	Date	Std. Score	TOLD-P;3 Equiv.
1.			
2.			

Section III. Profile of Scores

FIGURE 8-2 ✦ *Test of Language Development—3: Primary* record form. (Reprinted with permission from Newcomer, P., & Hammill, D. [1997]. Austin, TX: Pro-Ed.)

of Language—3 (Carrow-Woolfolk, 1999a) to look at receptive vocabulary and syntax, the *Goldman-Fristoe Test of Articulation—Second Edition* (GFTA-2) (Goldman & Fristoe, 2000) to examine single-word pronunciation, the *Expressive Vocabulary Test* (Williams, 1997) to investigate productive semantics, and the *Structured Photographic Expressive Language Test—Third Edition* (Dawson, Stout, & Eyer, 2003; Perona, Plant, & Vance, 2005) to explore expressive sentence structures. We could use the results from this test battery, too, to construct a profile that outlines strengths and weaknesses in language skills.

Now let's be clear about what tests such as these would tell us. Like the screening measures, standardized tests tell us whether a child is different from other children. A battery similar to the ones we've outlined here would tell us in what aspects of language a child performs significantly below his or her peers. This information, in turn, would alert us to the areas we would need to address in a remedial program. However, the results of the standardized tests would *not* necessarily tell us what specific forms, functions, and structures to target. They identify areas in which the child is deficient, but they don't pinpoint the specific deficiencies. Why not?

Well, for one thing, they are designed to sample a variety of behaviors within a domain so that they can get a valid comparison across children. That means there won't be many examples of any particular structure. *The Test of Auditory Comprehension of Language—3* (Carrow-Woolfolk, 1999a), for example, has only one item that tests comprehension of plural forms. If Jerry fails that item, would you target plural forms as part of your remedial program? It's hard to say. It's possible that he really doesn't understand the meaning of the plural marker, but there might be other reasons why a child might fail that item. Maybe he wasn't paying very close attention at that moment. Maybe he didn't know the words in the sentence. Before deciding to target plurals, we would want to see more of a *pattern* of performance. A standardized test is not designed to provide that kind of information.

Here's another reason that standardized tests don't give us all the information we need for remedial planning. Take the *Goldman-Fristoe Test of Articulation—Second Edition* (2000) or the *Patterned Elicitation of Syntax Test* (Young & Perachio, 1993). These measures will be very effective for showing us whether Jerry is different from other children in articulating single words and imitating grammatical sentences, respectively. However, research shows that although children's scores on standardized and naturalistic language procedures are related, children do not make the same errors on both types of assessment, so we cannot identify forms for remediation from the standard test items (Morrison & Shriberg, 1992; Shriberg & Kwiatkowski, 1980; Prutting, Gallagher, & Mulac, 1975). Moreover, some children do better on tests than on naturalistic measures (Condouris, Mayer, & Tager-Flusberg, 2003), suggesting that the tests may not be fully tapping their difficulties in real life communication. Standardized tests, particularly those designed to measure expressive skills, tend to use elicited production formats. Standardized tests of expressive syntax usually require children to imitate sentences spoken by the examiner. Standardized tests of articulation require children to produce single words in response to pictures. Both these formats tend to elicit performance from the child that is substantially different from the performance of the same children in spontaneous speech. Not only do children produce different frequencies of errors in these imitation and citation formats, they make different kinds of errors, too. So knowing the errors Jerry makes on one of these measures doesn't tell us what errors he will make when he actually tries to talk to someone. It's the errors that children make when they actually try to talk that we need to address in intervention, so we need to know what those are. Standardized tests do not necessarily give us this information. Criterion-referenced measures, such as language sampling, are much more valid and effective for gathering information on the errors children make in real communicative situations.

Does this mean that we should not use standardized tests in assessment? Should we go directly from screening to criterion-referenced measures and language sampling? My opinion is that we should not. Standardized testing is valuable for doing exactly what it was designed to do, pointing out the areas in which the child is performing significantly more poorly than peers. Using standardized tests to identify general areas of deficit is more efficient than doing in-depth criterion-referenced probing in every area. Standardized tests can narrow down the range of areas we need to evaluate with criterion-referenced procedures.

Let's take Jerry as our example again. Standardized testing told us that Jerry's receptive skills, as well as his word discrimination skills, are within normal limits. This suggests that we do not need to do any further assessment in these areas. His expressive syntax and phonology do exhibit mild deficits, though. Now we need to know specifically and in detail what his expressive syntactic and phonological errors are like when he tries to communicate in real interactions. That's where criterion-referenced procedures and language sampling come in. But remember: standardized testing was very efficient both in documenting broad areas of deficit and in narrowing the focus of our criterion-referenced evaluation. Using standardized testing in this way to sharpen the focus of the criterion-referenced assessment saves a good deal of time. It also provides the norm-referenced documentation required by many educational and service agencies to qualify the client for intervention. Standardized testing, then, is one aspect of an assessment plan. Used wisely and appropriately, with an understanding of its functions and limitations, it makes the assessment process efficient and economical.

CRITERION-REFERENCED ASSESSMENT AND BEHAVIORAL OBSERVATION FOR CHILDREN WITH DEVELOPING LANGUAGE

Standardized testing is not enough, though. As we have seen, standardized tests don't tell us what mistakes the client makes in real conversation, and these are the mistakes we need to address in intervention. Nonstandardized assessments are needed to complete the picture. Nonstandardized or informal evaluation does not mean the assessment is spontaneous or unplanned, though. On the contrary, nonstandardized assessment requires *more* planning than use of standardized tests, since the clinician must decide on the linguistic stimuli, specify a developmentally appropriate response, and choose materials and context for gathering the data, all without instruction from a standardized procedure. An effective approach to nonstandardized assessment is to compile all the information from the standardized portion, evaluate it, decide what informal assessments are needed, plan them, and collect the data in a subsequent session with the client. This suggests that nonstandardized assessment may not always take place during the formal "evaluation" session with the client, but may happen in the early part of the intervention phase. In other words, assessment may not be complete when the one or two sessions we label as "assessment" are completed.

For clinicians working in diagnostic settings, where assessment and making recommendations for intervention are their only tasks, this means that one assessment session is not usually enough. We should plan to see each client at least twice, once for formal assessment and once to do some nonstandardized evaluations that are indicated by the results of the formal procedures. For clinicians who do both assessment and intervention as part of their jobs, this means we should not feel constrained to get all the assessment data during the first evaluation session. Assessment can continue into the early part of the intervention period, as it is an ongoing part of the intervention that we use to decide when targets have been met.

PHONOLOGY

A clinically useful approach to analysis of a child's speech production is to start out just talking with the child for 5 to 10 minutes to get a sense of general intelligibility. Gordon-Brannan (1994) and Morris, Wilcox, and Schooling (1995) discussed issues in assessing intelligibility. Morris et al. advocate using the *Preschool Speech Intelligibility Measure* (PSIM), which consists of having children repeat a list of words. The child's productions are recorded and listeners are asked to judge which word a child says on each trial from a group of similar sounding words (e.g., *warm, store, swarm, for, horn, corn, door, torn, born, floor, storm,* and *form*). This measure can be very useful for documenting changes in intelligibility over the course of an intervention program. As a more informal measure, it is useful for making an initial determination about whether intelligibility is impaired. The clinician can also rate intelligibility in a short conversation by estimating the proportion of intelligible words. Gordon-Brannan and Weiss (2006) advocate collecting a conversational sample and counting 200 consecutive words within the sample. The clinician then listens to this portion of the sample again, counts the number of unintelligible words, and divides by the number of words in the sample. This figure is then subtracted from 100 to get a percentage of unintelligible words. Weiss et al. and Coplan and Gleason (1988) provide

guidelines for judging when children in the developing language period show a lower level of intelligibility than would be expected for their age. These are summarized in Table 8-5. *The Children's Speech Intelligibility Measure* (Wilcox & Morris, 1990) is another method available. Coplan and Gleason have shown that children whose intelligibility is below age expectations are at increased risk for the presence of a range of developmental disorders, not just speech delay. In fact, 46% of the children in their study who were identified on the basis of failing an intelligibility screen turned out to have developmental difficulties beyond speech and language, so identifying poor intelligibility in a preschooler should lead to a more intensive assessment of the child's abilities in a range of areas of development.

If the short speech sample indicates that a client is hard to understand, the next step in our clinical procedure would be to do an articulation test. We also might do an articulation test if the child is intelligible but makes more articulation errors than we would expect on the basis of developmental level. Although, as Morrison and Shriberg (1992) showed, articulation tests do not always identify the pronunciation errors children will make in spontaneous conversation, they do reliably show whether a child is significantly different from other children. Articulation tests are relatively quick and easy to administer and score. As such, they are sensible approaches to the problem of deciding whether phonology is an area that needs to be addressed in an intervention program. An articulation test can be given to decide whether more information is needed about the child's phonology. If the child scores within the normal range on the articulation test *and* intelligibility in conversation appears adequate, further assessment of phonological skill is probably not necessary.

If a child scores below the normal range on an articulation test or conversational speech is judged hard to understand, we want to decide whether the child is showing a primarily *articulatory* deficit or has a more *phonologically* based disorder. To make this determination, we can analyze the errors made on the articulation test. Shriberg (1994) has suggested identifying a speech problem as articulatory if it involves errors that are primarily *distortions*. When deletion and substitution errors are present, the disorder is considered primarily *phonological*.

TABLE 8-5	Expected Relations between Age and Intelligibility in Typically Speaking Children

AGE (MO)	PERCENT INTELLIGIBLE WORDS
24	50
36	80
48	100

Adapted from Coplan, J., & Gleason, J. (1988). Unclear speech: Recognition and significance of unintelligible speech in preschool children. *Pediatrics, 82,* 447-452.

Bauman-Waengler (2004) advocates using a traditional articulatory approach to intervention, such as that described by Bernthal and Bankson (2004), Creaghead, Newman, and Secord (1989) and Van Riper and Emerick (1987), when errors are primarily phonetic distortions or when a speech sound is completely absent from the phonetic inventory. Traditional approaches focus on individual sounds, include activities directed at discriminating and identifying target sounds, and begin by having children produce the target sound in isolation making use of visual, motor, and acoustic cues. However, if a client shows errors such as inconsistent substitutions and deletions that suggest a phonological disorder, or if the client is significantly unintelligible in conversational speech, we may need to know more about the patterns of errors before initiating an intervention program. The best way to look for these patterns is to collect a sample of the child's spontaneous speech and analyze it for its sound change properties by means of phonological analysis. Figure 8-3 schematizes these guidelines for deciding whether phonological analysis is a recommended part of the speech assessment.

When the phonological analysis indicates phonological errors, or a combination of phonetic and phonological issues, a phonological, or language-based approach is recommended (Bernthal & Bankson, 2004). This type of intervention will typically target production of sounds in words using contrastive word pairs to highlight the meaningful content of the speech change targeted. For example, if children are having trouble with dropping final consonants, they will be asked to practice saying names of pictures such as *toe* and *toad*. These approaches also target groups of sounds that experience the same simplification pattern, rather than individual sounds; so children who drop final consonants will work on word pairs with a variety of final sounds, rather than focusing on just one (e.g., *toe/toad; sew/soap; me/mean*).

Suppose we decide that a phonological analysis of a continuous speech sample is needed to get a true picture of the

child's phonology and to select intervention targets. What do we look for? Williams (2001) suggested that there are two ways to analyze children's speech: *independent analyses,* which attempt to describe what the child produces, regardless of whether it is correct by adult standards, and *relational analyses,* which compare the child's production to adult targets and look for error patterns. When we assessed phonological production in the emerging language stage, we used primarily independent analyses. Let's look at examples of the most common approaches to each of these types of analysis for children in the developing language period.

Independent Analysis: Phonetic Inventory

A phonetic inventory tells us what sounds a child says without comparing the child's production with an adult target. To collect a phonetic inventory we simply write down, or check off on a checklist, each consonant a child produces, regardless of whether it is the correct one for that context by adult standards. The articulation test results can be used to collect phonetic inventory information. Each consonant that the client produces in response to the articulation test stimuli, whether correctly or incorrectly used, can be listed. Alternatively, the phonetic inventory can be derived from a sample of conversational speech. All the consonants the client produces can be taken to comprise the phonetic inventory. Each consonant needs to be recorded only once, regardless of how many times it appears. The result is a list of the set of consonants the child produces. This tells us that these are the consonants the child knows "how" to say and suggests that these consonants will not need to be taught by means of a traditional articulatory approach.

Suppose, for example, that Jerry never produces a /z/ in the appropriate context. We might be tempted to try to teach him "how" to say /z/, with an articulatory approach, perhaps using isolated sound drills and nonsense words. But suppose further that we find /z/ does appear in his phonetic inventory. Perhaps he uses it in one or two words where /d/ is required. Clearly, then, he knows "how" to say /z/. What we need to teach him is not *how* to say it but, as Shriberg (1987) has argued, *when* to say it. In this case, a more phonological approach to intervention, focusing on whole words and meaningful contrasts, is appropriate. If /z/ never appeared at all in the phonetic inventory, then Jerry really does need to learn "how" to say the /z/ sound and a more articulatory approach would be appropriate.

Shriberg (1993) has grouped consonants by their normal order of acquisition. He divided the 24 consonant phonemes of English into three groups: the early eight (those that are used first in development), the middle eight (the group that appears next), and the late eight (the group that appears latest in normal acquisition). Shriberg's assignment of consonants to these groups is given in Box 8-1. This scheme can be useful in deciding where in the process of acquiring sounds a client is, based on the phonetic inventory. If the inventory contains only sounds from the earliest group, some articulatory and motor training work may be necessary to elicit later-developing sounds. If the inventory contains sounds from both the early and middle groups, more emphasis might be placed on getting

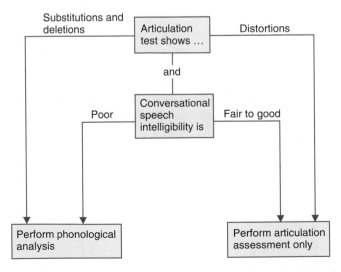

FIGURE 8-3 ✦ Guidelines for deciding to do phonological analysis of continuous speech.

BOX 8-1	**Groups of Sounds Ordered Developmentally**

Early 8: /m/ /b/ /j/ /n/ /w/ /d/ /p/ /h/
Middle 8: /t/ /ŋ/ /k/ /g/ /f/ /v/ /tʃ/ /dʒ/
Late 8: /ʃ/ /θ/ /s/ /z/ /ð/ /l/ /ʒ/

Adapted from Shriberg, L. (1993). Four new speech and prosody-voice measures for genetics research and other studies in developmental phonological disorders. *Journal of Speech and Hearing Research, 36,* 105-140.

the client to produce these sounds in their correct contexts. If sounds from all three groups are present but speech still contains many errors, then, we would want to concentrate on getting the child to use the sounds he or she already has in appropriate contexts. If middle and later sounds are present, but many early sounds are missing, we might conclude that this child is showing atypical phonological development and might look for speech-motor or other organic bases of the disorder.

Phonetic inventories are easy to collect from continuous speech samples, by simply listening to a recording of the sample and writing down or checking off the first appearance of each consonant the client uses. They can be very helpful in deciding which sounds are in the inventory and need not be approached with motor training or articulatory procedures. They also can help identify sounds that are truly absent, suggesting that the child needs to learn "how" to say them. Looking at the distribution of sounds and comparing them with Shriberg's (1993) scheme also can be helpful in deciding whether phonological acquisition is delayed or proceeding along a deviant course. Williams (2001) also suggested conducting a distributional analysis of the phonetic inventory to determine in what word positions (initial, medial, final) the child's sounds appear.

Relational Analysis: Simplification Process Assessment

Since the 1970s, speech researchers and clinicians have been interested in describing not just individual errors in child speech, but also the patterns or rules that govern these errors. One particular approach to analysis of error patterns has been productive in this research: the use of simplification processes to describe sound changes. Simplification processes have been described in detail by many authors, including Ball and Kent (1999), Bauman-Waengler (2004), Bernthal and Bankson (2004), Creaghead, Newman, and Secord (1989), Gordon-Brannan and Weiss (2006), Grunwell (1987), Hodson and Paden (1991), Ingram (1976), and Shriberg and Kwiatkowski (1980). Detailed definitions and discussion can be found in these writings. For our purposes, let's just say that simplification processes are a way of describing sound changes that appear to be rule-governed attempts, which apply across a class of sounds or syllable

structures, to make pronunciation easier. One example of a phonological simplification process is *unstressed syllable deletion*. It applies across the class of words containing more than two syllables and results in productions in which the least stressed syllable is dropped (*mato* for *tomato*). *Velar fronting* is another example. It applies across all sounds produced in the velar position (in English /g/, /k/, and /ŋ /) and results in the production of each one as the corresponding sound produced with the same manner, nasality, and voicing in the alveolar position (/d/, /t/, and /n/, respectively).

There are many ways to conduct process analysis. Some methods resemble articulation testing. These elicit single words or single sentences from children and apply phonological analysis procedures, analyzing errors according to the type of simplification process used. The *Clinical Assessment of Articulation and Phonology* (Secord & Donohue, 2000), the *Bankson-Bernthal Test of Phonology* (Bankson & Bernthal, 1990), and the *Hodson Assessment of Phonological Patterns—Third Edition* (Hodson, 2004) are some examples. Other approaches provide guidelines for reanalyzing data gathered from an articulation test by means of phonological analysis procedures. Khan and Lewis (2002) have developed one such procedure. All these instruments, though, suffer from the same limitations as traditional articulation testing. They use elicited production, usually in citation format, and do not give a valid picture of what pronunciation is like in spontaneous speech. Morrison and Shriberg (1992) have argued that the only valid way to examine phonological production in general, and simplification process use in particular, is to look at them in conversational speech.

Several procedures are available in the literature for organizing this analysis. Bauman-Waengler (2004), Grunwell (1987), Ingram (1981), Lund and Duchan (1993), Owens (2004), Shipley and McAfee (2004), and Williams (2001) provided guidelines for approaches to phonological analysis of continuous speech. Andrews and Fey (1986) suggested procedures for applying Hodson's analysis scheme for single words to spontaneous speech. The most extensive, well-documented, and clearly set-out method, though, is Shriberg and Kwiatkowski's Natural Process Analysis (NPA) (1980). I'll give you a brief overview of the NPA procedure simply as an example of one approach to phonological analysis. I don't mean to imply that this is the only analysis procedure that can be used effectively. I want only to give you a flavor of what phonological analysis of continuous speech can be like, using one of several possible analysis approaches. Remember that clinical use of any procedure requires that a clinician study the guidelines provided by the authors in much greater detail than can be given here.

The *NPA* encourages the clinician to obtain a sample of 100 different words produced in spontaneous speech and to analyze those words for their phonetic inventory and for the appearance of eight of the most common simplification processes in children's speech. Shriberg and Kwiatkowski suggested that the sample may come from either an audio-recorded segment of the child's conversational speech or from a transcription of the first 100 different words the child produces in a continuous speech sample. This would generally involve about 15 minutes of continuous speech on the part of the child. Since many children with phonological disorders are difficult to understand, Shriberg and Kwiatkowski suggested that instead of using an open-ended conversational format for eliciting the speech sample, as we did when we got our initial general measure of intelligibility, we use a more structured task. We can give the child a complex picture with lots of different items in it to describe, such as the pages found in a "big" Richard Scary book. These kinds of stimuli elicit a sample in which the referents are known and the gloss of the child's speech is much easier to determine. Whether you use a conversational or picture description format to elicit your sample, you can reanalyze the same sample later for syntactic, semantic, pragmatic, and phonological information. So here's how a clinician might proceed:

1. Give the child a complex picture book, and ask him or her to tell about some of the things in the picture. Or ask the child to engage in conversation around common play materials with the parent.
2. Audio record the sample.
3. While the child is talking, quickly get down the gloss and phonemic transcription of the first 100 different words. (Have a piece of paper already labeled with two columns [gloss, phonemic transcription] and 100 numbered rows, or use the forms provided by Shriberg and Kwiatkowski [1986].)

4. Later, check the recording for any glosses or transcriptions you aren't sure about. You also can collect your phonetic inventory during the same pass through the recording. Save the recording for later analyses of other language areas.
5. Do the phonological process analysis on the 100 transcribed words.

Shriberg and Kwiatkowski's procedure yields data on both independent and relational analyses. It contains both a phonetic inventory and a summary of the use of the eight simplification processes most common in children's speech. To obtain the phonetic inventory, we can use the form provided by Shriberg and Kwiatkowski, which is displayed in Figure 8-4, or we can simply inspect our 100 words and make a list of each consonant that appears at least once in the phonemic transcription.

Next we do the relational analysis, analyzing the child's 100 words for error patterns. Shriberg and Kwiatkowski provided detailed guidelines and abundant worksheets for performing this analysis. Basically, they are looking for the appearance of the eight most common simplification processes seen in development. They identify these as the following:

1. Final consonant deletion (leaving off the last sound in a CVC word, such as saying /da/ for *dog*).
2. Velar fronting (pronouncing /k/, /g/, and /ŋ/ as /t/, /d/, and /n/, respectively, such as saying /tʌb/ for *cub*).

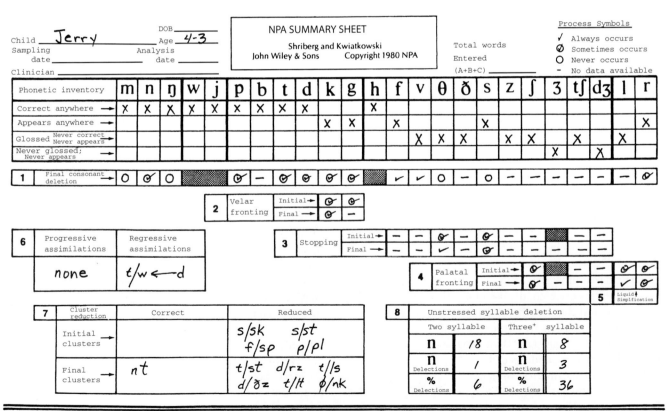

FIGURE 8-4 ✦ NPA summary sheet. (Reprinted with permission from Shriberg, L., & Kwiatkowski, J. [1980]. *Natural process analysis: A procedure for phonological analysis of continuous speech samples* {p. 110}. NY: Macmillan.)

3. Stopping (pronouncing fricatives as the corresponding stops, such as saying /to/ for *sew*).
4. Palatal fronting (producing palatal sounds in the alveolar position, such as saying /su/ for *shoe*).
5. Liquid simplification (substituting another sound for one of the liquids [/l/ and /r/], such as saying /wawi pap/ for *lollipop*).
6. Assimilation (making two sounds in a word more alike, such as saying /dadi/ for *doggy*).
7. Cluster reduction (dropping one or more sounds from a cluster or making substitutions within the cluster, such as saying /pe/ for *play*).
8. Unstressed syllable deletion (leaving off the least stressed syllable in a multisyllablic word, such as saying /næ næ / for *banana*).

Using the information provided in the NPA manual, the clinician assigns each error in the 100 transcribed words to one of these processes, or to a miscellaneous "other" category, using a summary worksheet such as that in Figure 8-4. This information tells us several things, including (1) which sounds are subject to simplification; (2) what typical simplification strategies apply to these sounds; (3) whether atypical processes appear (as indexed by a large number of errors that need to be assigned to the "other" category); and (4) how consistent the use of each process is for each sound, as noted by the "always," "sometimes," "never," and "no data" codes on the summary worksheet.

The NPA also has a computer-assisted format, called the *Programs to Examine Phonetic and Phonological Evaluation Records* (PEPPER) (Shriberg, 1986). This procedure requires the clinician to key in, in phonetic transcription and gloss form, the information on the 100 words to be used in the analysis. The program then automatically computes percentage of consonants correct and gives the percentage of occurrence of each of the eight processes.

Let's see what a phonological process analysis tells us about a child like Jerry. Suppose the data presented in Figure 8-4 were derived from a sample of Jerry's spontaneous speech. How would we use it to understand his phonological disorder and select intervention targets? First, Figure 8-4 tells us that the sounds that are absent from the inventory are all in the middle or late groups, according to Shriberg's scheme. This suggests that Jerry's phonological development is delayed rather than deviant. Second, the phonetic inventory tells us that some of the sounds on which Jerry makes errors, such as /k/, /g/, /s/, /f/, and /r/, do appear in the inventory, suggesting that he knows "how" to say these sounds. These findings tell us that a process approach to intervention is appropriate for Jerry, since what he needs to learn is "when" to say some of these sounds.

The process analysis shows us that most of Jerry's processes are used inconsistently. This suggests that he can sometimes "tune up" his pronunciation to make it more accurate. Only /f/ and /v/ are dropped consistently at the ends of words, and only /θ/ is consistently stopped. Only initial clusters are consistently simplified; at least one final cluster appears in correct form. Jerry does produce some multisyllabic words, with better accuracy in two syllables than in three. The processes he uses are all typical in development; no "other" processes are listed in the Notes section. This again suggests delayed phonological development.

Jerry uses all the processes that the NPA measures. Combined, they can have a devastating effect on intelligibility, as his teacher noted. How would we decide where to start in trying to change that picture? Another way to ask this question is to inquire how we can set priorities among possible intervention targets, since we probably do not want to target all eight processes at once. One approach would be to target the processes that disappear first in normal development. Grunwell (1987) provided information on the ages at which these processes are used by normally developing children. Information based on her findings is presented in Figure 8-5.

FIGURE 8-5 ✦ Developmental sequence of phonological processes. (Adapted from Grunwell, P. [1987]. *Clinical Phonology* [ed. 2], p. 229. Baltimore, MD: Williams & Wilkins.)

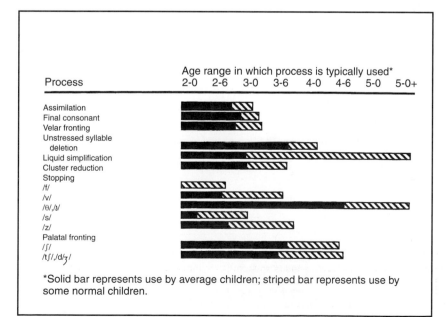

*Solid bar represents use by average children; striped bar represents use by some normal children.

If we were using a developmental criterion to target processes, we might decide to try to get Jerry to stop using final consonant deletion, assimilation, unstressed syllable deletion, cluster reduction, velar fronting, and stopping on /s/ and /f/. These processes are not typically used by 4-year-olds, according to Grunwell's data. We might decide that at his age, palatal fronting, liquid simplification, and stopping of interdentals would not be appropriate targets since some normal 4-year-olds still use them. Even eliminating these latter three processes, we're still left with quite a few to address. If we wanted to reduce the list somewhat more, we might try to target first those processes that have the most detrimental effect on intelligibility. Deletions reduce intelligibility more than substitutions, so final-consonant deletion might top this list. One of the most frequently appearing phonemes in English is /s/, so getting Jerry to pronounce it correctly more often also could increase his ability to be understood. Targeting final consonant deletion and stopping, particularly on the /s/ phoneme, then, might be our highest-priority goals for Jerry, with other processes targeted as the first set of targets resolves.

Jerry's example points out the general principles involved in assessing speech and determining intervention targets for clients with phonological problems. Figure 8-6 summarizes these principles in a decision-tree form.

Shriberg and Austin (1998) reported that 30% to 40% of children with language disorders also have speech problems. Further, 15% to 20% of children with speech delays also have problems in vocabulary, grammar, or both. This suggests that we must be careful not to let the child's unintelligibility blind us to possible language components of the disorder. Every child who presents with unintelligible speech should receive a thorough language assessment, to identify any areas of linguistic disorder that might not be obvious because the child's speech is so hard to understand. Let's talk now about how to do this assessment for a child in the developing language phase.

CRITERION-REFERENCED LANGUAGE ASSESSMENT

Just as the standardized assessments of phonology do not always answer all our questions about a child's speech, standardized assessments of language skill, although able to point out general areas of deficit, do not tell us everything we need to know about a client's linguistic functioning. To get a fuller picture, we need to use some nonstandardized measures to tell us what kinds of errors the child makes in more naturalistic contexts. In general, standardized assessments for children with developing language can detect deficits in several broad areas. Depending on the tests used, the following areas can usually be examined:

▶ Receptive vocabulary (by responding to names by picture pointing)
▶ Expressive vocabulary (by naming pictures or defining words)
▶ Receptive syntax and morphology (by pointing to one of several pictures, including contrasting foils, that depicts a sentence spoken by the examiner [Point to: "The *boys* are here."]).
▶ Expressive syntax and morphology (by imitating sentences or filling in blanks with words containing grammatical morphemes ["I have a dress; you have two . . . ."])

Several areas of language function are usually *not* covered by standardized tests. These include pragmatics and semantic areas other than associating words with pictures. A standardized test battery, then, can usually point out whether a child has deficits in each of the broad areas outlined in the preceding list. Once the areas of deficit have been identified, though, we want to look at each one more closely, using informal assessment proce-

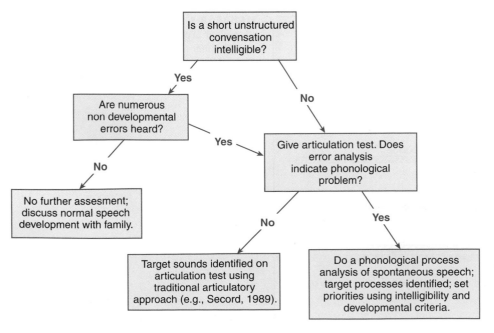

FIGURE 8-6 ✦ Decision tree for child speech assessment.

dures to examine specific error types and pinpoint targets for intervention. We also want to look at pragmatic and semantic areas not covered by standardized tests, if history and discussions with the family indicate that the child might be having any trouble in these areas. That's where nonstandardized, criterion-referenced procedures come in.

Vocabulary

Guidelines for Vocabulary Assessment and Intervention. Generally speaking, the size of receptive vocabulary is larger than that of expressive vocabulary in children, and children can commonly recognize a pictured item by name, even though they may not be able to come up with the label for the same item in a confrontation naming task. The conventional wisdom is that if a child can produce a word, he or she must understand what it means. This is not entirely true, though. Research on children's word-learning strategies (Bloom, 2001; Dollaghan, 1985; Rice, Buhr, & Nemeth, 1990) suggests that preschoolers can pick up some notion of a word's meaning from very brief exposure, but that the meaning will be quite limited until the child acquires additional experience with the word. Researchers call this strategy "fast mapping" (Carey, 1978). What it implies for us as clinicians is that children's understanding of word meaning, even when they produce the word themselves, may be more limited than the adult's understanding of the meaning of the same word. The result is that it is difficult, with children in the developing language phase, to make a clear differentiation between the knowledge required to understand a word and the knowledge required to use it. It is not entirely true to say that "comprehension precedes production," because a word may very well be produced even when comprehension of the word is very limited, by adult standards. This implies, to my mind, that clinicians should handle receptive and expressive vocabulary knowledge in an integrated way.

What does this mean in practice? It implies that we should not worry too much about assessing vocabulary separately in each modality and then treating each modality separately. If a child does poorly on a receptive vocabulary test, such as the *Peabody Picture Vocabulary Test—4* (Dunn & Dunn, 2006), the logical next step in assessment is to use criterion-referenced methods to look at what words the child has difficulty understanding. But there would not seem to be a need to teach these words receptively first, before trying to get a child to say them. Since children normally say words with only limited knowledge of their meaning, production can be targeted from the beginning of the intervention program. In short, I would recommend a strategy, following Lahey (1988), of focusing on comprehension during assessment but on production during intervention.

There are two exceptions. First, for children with very limited phonological skills, words should be selected for production that the child can pronounce or at least approximate. Schwartz and Leonard (1982) showed that children in the early stages of phonological acquisition are selective about words that they try to produce, attempting only those that have at least a beginning sound that is already in their repertoire. For clients who are still in this very early stage of phonological development,

then, pronounceability should be a consideration in choosing words that we are trying to get the child to say. Intervention for vocabulary might focus on receptive skills while work is going on to increase the child's phonological repertoire.

The second exception has to do with word retrieval. It may be that a child has a normal receptive vocabulary size on a standardized test but uses very few words in spontaneous speech or does very poorly on a naming test such as the *Expressive One-Word Picture Vocabulary Test—Revised* (Brownell, 2000). We may suspect that the problem is the inability to recall words when needed for production rather than lack of knowledge of the words. Word-retrieval skills are often assessed in test batteries for learning-disabled children of school age, since word retrieval problems commonly coexist with reading deficits (Brackenbury & Pye, 2005; Wolf, Bally, & Morris, 1986). Retrieval is not typically included in the assessment of the child with developing language. However, if word retrieval appears to be a problem—because of a large decrement on an expressive vocabulary test when compared with the score on a receptive measure or because the child seems to have trouble recalling words in spontaneous conversation—intervention should focus more sharply on helping the child to recall and produce the words he or she already knows, in addition to increasing vocabulary size.

Let me summarize my suggestions for working with vocabulary at the developing language level. Because of the issue of fast mapping and the complicated relationship between comprehension and production of word meaning in the developing language period, I would advocate the following strategy for handling vocabulary issues:

Assess receptive vocabulary skills with a standardized instrument.

▶ If the child scores below the normal range, do criterion-referenced assessment of word classes that are important in the child's communicative environment. Target words identified in this assessment, using both receptive and expressive intervention activities, with the emphasis on production. Control for pronounceability with children in the early stages of phonological acquisition.

▶ If the child scores within the normal range on the receptive vocabulary test, but history or parent or teacher report indicates concern about word use, assess expressive vocabulary with a standardized naming test. Watch for signs of word-finding problems, such as circumlocutions, overly general labels *(thingy),* or inability to name items responded to correctly on the receptive test. If there is evidence of a retrieval problem, focus intervention on practicing the recall and production of already known words, providing strategies such as using phonetic and semantic cues for retrieval (see details in Chapter 11).

Methods of Criterion-Referenced Vocabulary Assessment. Standardized measures of vocabulary typically tell us whether a child's ability to recognize and produce the names of items pictured in the test is similar to that of other children. Sometimes we want to know what a child knows about a particular category of words. We may need this information because this set of words is important for the child's success in preschool.

Colors or spatial terms (*in, on, under, beside, in front, behind, next to,* and so on) needed for following directions might be examples. Perhaps the child needs a set of word meanings for getting along better in social situations. One example of the latter might be the child with autism who uses a lot of echolalia when answering questions. We might want to know whether this child comprehends the meaning of the question words, since research on echolalia (Prizant & Duchan, 1981) suggests that children with autism often use echoing as a response when they don't know a more appropriate way to answer a question. Another example is verbs, which are known to be especially difficult for children with language disorders (Windfuhr, Faragher, & Conti-Ramsden, 2002), and are not frequently assessed on standardized tests. These kinds of word classes are reasonable targets for criterion-referenced assessment.

Suppose we (or the client's parents or teachers) identify a set of words that are important for a child who scored low on a vocabulary test to know. We can look at knowledge of these words by using a nonstandardized assessment protocol. A variety of games and informal procedures can be used to probe children's knowledge of word meanings. For example, the understanding of question words can be assessed. James (1990) provided an order of acquisition of the understanding of question words. This order is given in Figure 8-7. One means of assessing the comprehension of these question words is to read the child a short, simple story and ask questions about it during the reading (for example, if reading *Chicken Little*, the clinician might read the first page, where Chicken Little tries to tell her friends the sky was falling, then ask, "What was falling?"). We would use this procedure to avoid testing memory rather than the question words of interest. The clinician can choose questions so that each question word is used at least three times. Using a checklist such as the one in Figure 8-7, the clinician

Spatial preposition	Age that normally-developing children comprehend (years-months)	Number of trials	Number of correct placements
Beside	3-0	_____	_____
In	3-0	_____	_____
In front of	3-0	_____	_____
Next to	3-0	_____	_____
On	3-0	_____	_____
Over	3-0	_____	_____
Out	3-0	_____	_____
Under	3-0	_____	_____
On top	4-0	_____	_____
Between	4-0	_____	_____
Behind	5-0	_____	_____
Below	5-0	_____	_____
Above	6-6	_____	_____

FIGURE 8-8 ✦ A checklist for evaluating understanding of spatial terms. (Adapted from Boehm, A. [1989]. *Boehm resource guide for basic concept teaching.* San Antonio, TX: Psychological Corp.)

can record the child's responses to each trial of each of the question words used in the procedure. This alerts the clinician to the question words the child can answer appropriately and identifies the question words the child has trouble answering accurately. These may be targeted for the intervention program.

Here's another example: the "hiding game." This procedure can be used to assess understanding of spatial prepositions. Normative data come from Boehm (1989). In the hiding game the clinician arranges two identical cups on the floor or table so that one is inverted and one is right side up. The clinician gives the client a raisin to hide from a somewhat backward puppet. The catch is that the child must hide the raisin in the place the clinician indicates. The clinician then tells the child to hide the raisin in locations such as *in, on, under, beside,* or *next to* a cup or *between* the cups. The child hides the raisin and the puppet then "looks" for it in the place the clinician said to put it. If the puppet finds the raisin where the clinician said it should go, the puppet wins the raisin. However, this puppet is a picky eater and does not like raisins, so he always offers the treat to the client. The game continues until each spatial preposition has been tested three times. Using a checklist such as the one in Figure 8-8, the clinician can assess the level of the child's understanding of spatial terms and identify those that the child has trouble comprehending. These might be included as intervention targets.

These are just two ideas. Clinicians can come up with a variety of "games" and activities such as these to get more information about a child's comprehension of certain classes of words. Miller and Paul (1995) provided additional ideas. The point is this: when a child scores poorly on a standardized measure of receptive vocabulary, specific content categories can be probed with informal techniques when necessary. This kind of assessment allows us to evaluate a client's understanding of meanings that are important in his or her communicative

Question word	Age that normally-developing children response appropriately (years-months)	Number of trials	Number of correct responses
What . . . ?	2-0	_____	_____
Where . . . ?	2-6	_____	_____
Who . . . ?	3-0	_____	_____
Whose . . . ?	3-0	_____	_____
Why . . . ?	3-0	_____	_____
How many?	3-0 (response with a number, though not necessarily the right one, is acceptable)	_____	
How . . . ?	3-6	_____	_____
When . . . ?	4-6 or older	_____	_____

FIGURE 8-7 ✦ A checklist for evaluating comprehension of question words. (Adapted from James, S. [1990]. *Normal language acquisition.* Boston, MA: College-Hill Press.)

interactions. These meanings can, if found to be problematic, be included as targets of intervention.

Syntax and Morphology

Receptive Syntax and Morphology. Unlike vocabulary, syntax and morphology need to be carefully assessed in each of the receptive and expressive modalities. The reason is this: children commonly produce sentence forms, such as agent-action-object constructions, even when they fail to perform correctly on comprehension tests of these same forms in settings where nonlinguistic cues have been removed (Chapman, 1978; Paul, 2000c). Knowing that a child produces a sentence type does not necessarily mean that the child fully comprehends the same sentence if it is spoken to him in a decontextualized format. We do need, then, to be careful about assessing comprehension and production of syntactic forms separately.

Some writers (Lund & Duchan, 1993; Rees & Shulman, 1978) have raised the question of whether the difference between *contextualized* and *decontextualized* comprehension invalidates the use of standardized tests in this area. In real communicative situations, they argue, it is rarely necessary to get all the information needed for a response from the words and sentences. Many other cues are available, including knowledge of what usually happens in situations (often called "scripts" or "event knowledge"); facial, intonational, and gestural cues; and objects and events in the immediate environment that provide nonlinguistic support, to name a few. Most children can take advantage of all these additional cues to assist their understanding of the words and sentences they hear. But if these cues are removed, a child is likely to do more poorly. This is as true for normally developing preschoolers as it is for children with language problems (Naito & Kikuo, 2004; Paul, Fisher, & Cohen, 1988). Of course, most of our standardized and many of our nonstandardized methods of assessing receptive syntax and morphology use decontextualized settings. Children typically perform more poorly on these than they would if the same

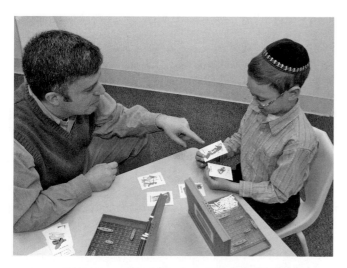

Games can be incorporated into informal criterion-referenced assessments.

forms were used in a more normal communicative context. Is this a bad thing?

As you might guess, my answer would be, "It depends." It depends on how we interpret the results of the decontextualized assessments and whether we include some contextualized assessments for contrasting information. We can look at the decontextualized results as a window onto how much *linguistic* comprehension a child displays and as a way to identify linguistic forms than can cause problems when few other cues are available. This information is very useful for contrasting with performance on production tasks. It can help us determine whether the child can demonstrate linguistic comprehension for forms he or she is not using at all in speech; whether linguistic comprehension and production are about on par; or whether, as normally developing children do in some stages of development (Chapman & Miller, 1975), the child is producing some forms that he or she does not comprehend in decontextualized formats. Knowing how comprehension contrasts with production can help us to decide whether to focus strictly on production skills in the intervention program or whether activities that foster both comprehension and production—such as focused stimulation and verbal script approaches (see Chapters 3 and 9 for details)—might be more appropriate. In this way, looking at comprehension skills in decontextualized formats can be useful.

Contrasting this performance not only with production but also with performance in more contextualized activities also can be very useful. Lord (1985) advocated this approach for looking at comprehension skills in children with autism. I believe it can be helpful for evaluating comprehension skills in any child at a developing language level who has trouble with decontextualized comprehension. Here's why: if a child can take advantage of the nonlinguistic cues in the environment, he or she is in a good position to benefit from intervention activities such as child-centered approaches that provide enriched language carefully matched to the nonlinguistic context. Child-centered activities would be an important component of intervention for such a child. But suppose a client does no better on a contextualized assessment than on a standardized test. Some research (Paul, 1990; Paul, Fisher, & Cohen, 1988) on children with autism and specific language disorders suggests that these children are not as efficient as normally developing preschoolers at integrating information from linguistic and nonlinguistic sources. For clients such as these, approaches that make use of naturalistic nonlinguistic context may provide too complex a mix of cues. These clients may need to have the input scaled down, with very clear, simple connections made between the forms being taught and their meanings. For these clients a less naturalistic, more structured form of input may be needed to increase receptive skills.

The following is a general strategy for assessing syntactic and morphological comprehension at the developing language level:

1. Use a standardized test of receptive syntax and morphology to determine whether deficits exist in this area.
2. If the client performs below the normal range, use criterion-referenced decontextualized procedures to probe forms that appear to be causing trouble.

3. If the client performs poorly on the criterion-referenced assessments, test the same forms in a contextualized format, providing familiar scripts and nonlinguistic contexts; facial, gestural, and intonational cues; language closely tied to objects in the immediate environment; and expected instructions.

   a. If the child does better in the contextualized format, compare performance on comprehension to production. Target forms and structures that the child comprehends well but does not produce as initial targets for a production approach. Target structures that the child does not comprehend well for child-centered, focused stimulation, or verbal script approaches to work on comprehension and production simultaneously.

   b. If the child does not do better in the contextualized format, provide more-structured, less-complex input using more hybrid and clinician-directed activities for both comprehension and production.

Criterion-Referenced Methods for Assessing Receptive Syntax and Morphology. Remember that one reason we may need to do criterion-referenced assessment of receptive syntax and morphology is that standardized tests generally provide very few items per structure. This means that, when a child fails, it is hard to know how significant that failure is. Criterion-referenced assessment can help us to decide, for example, whether a child really doesn't know what a structure means or whether he or she just wasn't paying much attention to that particular item on the test. What we want to do on criterion-referenced assessment, then, is to use the standardized test data to point out structures the child may be having trouble

understanding. We can then probe these areas in more depth with criterion-referenced procedures. Let's look at some examples of criterion-referenced methods for assessing understanding of language structure in both contextualized and decontextualized formats.

Decontextualized Formats. Recall from the discussion of comprehension assessment in Chapter 2 that we have several means available to evaluate comprehension, including picture pointing, behavioral compliance, object manipulation, and judgment. We would choose one of these methods based on the child's developmental level and on how well each matches to structures we want to test. It would be fairly easy to use pictures or object manipulation to test understanding of plurals, for example ("Show me the apple/apples."). Behavioral compliance might be a better procedure for testing understanding of *is (verb)ing* constructions ("Show me: the girl is jumping."). Judgment tasks are usually not appropriate for preschoolers.

Just as we could construct games and activities to test receptive vocabulary, we can follow a similar procedure for probing the comprehension of those structures that were identified as possible sources of errors on a standardized test. Sentences containing past and future tense might be one example. Suppose a client missed the past- and future-tense items on a standardized test. We would want to find out whether comprehension of these items is really impaired. We might construct an activity such as the one in Box 8-2.

This is just one example of a method for probing a client's understanding of specific syntactic and morphological forms. Clinicians can devise simple activities such as these for any form on which additional information is needed. Miller and

---

BOX 8-2	**Decontextualized Criterion-Referenced Activity for Probing Understanding of Past and Future Tense**

Clinician: This is my friend Sammy (display a puppet). Sammy likes to help people, but he doesn't always do it right away. I'll ask Sammy to help me. Sammy, please set the table. In puppet voice: I will set the table. In normal voice: He said he will, but he's not going to do it right now. It's not done yet. I'll try something else. Sammy, please clean your room. Puppet voice: I cleaned my room. Normal voice: Good! I didn't have to wait for that one. Sammy cleaned his room! It's done! Give several additional examples. Then say: You listen now. Listen to Sammy. Then tell me if the job is done.

Clinician	"Sammy"	Correct Client Response	+/_
Please make the bed.	I will make it.	not done	_____
Please tie your shoe.	I tied it.	done	_____
Please eat your soup.	I will eat it.	not done	_____
Please help me.	I helped you.	done	_____
Please hop to it!	I hopped to it!	done	_____
Please stand still.	I will stand still.	not done	_____
Please stop jumping.	I stopped jumping.	done	_____
Wash your face.	I washed . . .	done	_____
Dry your hands.	I will dry . . .	not done	_____
Please get my hat.	I will get . . .	not done	_____
Please call Dad.	I called Dad.	done	_____
Please go away.	I will go . . .	not done	_____

Paul (1995) provided additional activities. Notice that activities such as these, although not standardized, still remove most of the nonlinguistic context and require the child to understand the message from just the words and sentences. We can, as we've seen, contrast performance on decontextualized assessments such as these to performance in more naturalistic comprehension situations. Let's see how.

Assessing Comprehension Strategies. In Chapter 7 we talked about some methods of assessing comprehension and comprehension strategies in children with emerging language. We said it was important to look at what children do when they *don't* understand all the words and sentences in decontextualized activities. If they use strategies such as those used by normally developing children, we can feel more confident that comprehension skills are proceeding along a normal course. Naturalistic approaches such as indirect language stimulation and verbal script therapy will be useful for increasing receptive skills. If, on the other hand, clients are not using typical strategies, we might conclude that they are not able to take advantage of naturalistic communicative cues for comprehending and may need more structured input. The techniques outlined for assessing comprehension strategies at the emerging language stage in Chapter 7 also can be used with children at a developing language level. Here we would be looking for use of strategies such as "child as agent" and "probable events."

Remember that normally developing children at the 2- to 3-year level of comprehension are able to process *agent-action-object* instructions, but also they still rely on a "probable event strategy" for deciding which noun represents the agent and object of action. That is, when presented with a sentence, such as "The mommy feeds the baby," children in the 24- to 36-month period typically perform successfully on an object-manipulation task. But if asked to act out the sentence, "The baby feeds the mommy," they are likely to interpret it in the more probable direction (the mommy feeds baby). To test for basic 2- to 3-year-level comprehension skills, then, a series of probable agent-action-object sentences could be presented for a child to act out with some toys. If the child uses a "child-as-agent" strategy by performing designated actions on the named object himself or herself, he or she is demonstrating an 18- to 24-month-level comprehension strategy.

If the child performs correctly on the probable sentences, we can move to the next level of receptive language development. Correct comprehension of both probable and improbable simple sentences is typical of normally developing children at the 3- to 4-year level of comprehension (Chapman, 1978). We can present more agent-action-object sentences for the child to act out, interspersing probable ("The boy pushes the wagon.") and improbable sentences ("The wagon pushes the boy."). If the child performs correctly on both types, we can conclude that linguistic comprehension of agent-action-object sentences is present. If the child gets the probable sentences correct but the improbable ones wrong, we can suspect the use of a probable-event strategy. This client is showing comprehension that is following the normal path. However, if the client does not do any better on the probable than improbable types, we

might conclude that the client was not taking advantage of nonlinguistic background information to help in processing sentences. A client like this, who has comprehension deficits, might benefit from more structured input that matches language very clearly and simply to ongoing events. Such a child also might need to develop a fuller set of "scripts" or event expectations to aid in comprehension. Work on play scripts around familiar events, in which the clinician and child re-enact a set of recurring actions over and over, also might be useful. The clinician could include such scripted play as part of every session, carefully choosing simple language forms to match each action in the script and being careful to repeat each action and its accompanying language exactly during each re-enactment.

Comprehension strategies also can be examined by looking at the errors in the other nonstandardized assessments conducted. For example, if spatial prepositions are assessed, the clinician can look at the child's errors to see whether the child tended to place objects "in" containers when told to put them "on," or "on" surfaces when told to put them "under." These types of errors would be representative of a "probable location strategy" (Chapman, 1978), which is typical of 2- to 3-year-old children. If a child at a 4-year developmental level uses them, they would be evidence of comprehension that is delayed but is nonetheless developing along a normal course.

Information from nonstandardized assessments, then, can be useful not only for probing specific forms and structures, but also for looking at children's strategies for comprehending difficult language. These strategies can give a clinician additional information about how a child deals with language input. Such information can be useful, as we've seen, in developing an intervention program.

Assessing Comprehension in Contextualized Settings. We've talked about using nonstandardized assessment both to probe comprehension of specific forms and to look at strategies for comprehending difficult input. For both these purposes we are looking at comprehension in somewhat contrived situations. If we want to know more about how a child responds to language in a more naturalistic setting, we can set up some communicative situations and observe the child's responses. The reason for doing so, again, is as a contrast to the performance on the decontextualized situations. If a child does just fine on a standardized comprehension test, there is no need to assess comprehension further in a naturalistic setting. However, if the child is not so good at responding to language in formal contexts, it would be nice to know whether he or she does better in more natural ones.

One way to do this is to look at clients' responses to speech addressed to them in ordinary conversation. We can use the sample of speech collected for phonological or expressive syntactic analysis. Besides looking at what the child said, we can look at how it related to what was said to the child. We can, for example, compute a percentage of *contingent responses* on the child's part. Contingent responses are those that relate semantically to the previous speaker's utterance. If you say, "Would you like an ice cream?" and I say, "Yeah, I'm in the mood for chocolate," my utterance is clearly related to and contingent upon yours. But if you said, "Would you like an ice cream?" and I answered, "The Kentucky Derby is run in May," the relation between your utterance and mine would not be very clear. According to Bloom, Rocissano, and Hood (1976), children's proportion of contingent utterances rises from less than half at 24 months to more than 75% at 42 months. Looking at contingent responses in spontaneous speech can give us some notion of whether the child is processing the linguistic input well enough to respond contingently.

Lund and Duchan (1993) suggested examining children's language samples to look for a variety of comprehension errors. They suggested, for example, examining responses to questions in the speech sample for understanding of the question words. They suggested further looking at responses to adult requests to determine whether the request was understood. Analyzing spontaneous speech samples for information about comprehension is another way to make use of the conversational samples we collect during the nonstandardized phase of assessment.

Criterion-Referenced Methods for Assessing Productive Syntax and Morphology

Speech-Sample Analysis. We've talked about a variety of ways to use samples of conversational speech to fill out our picture of a client's language skills. Perhaps the most prevalent use of speech-sample analysis is for the purpose of assessing productive syntax and morphology. Spontaneous speech provides the most valid look at how a client uses words and sentences in natural situations. So if we really want to know how a client produces language forms, the best way to find out is to take a sample of the use of these forms in real communication.

The first decision we need to make when we do speech-sample analysis concerns how we *collect the sample.* Quite a bit of research has focused on how the sampling context affects the quality of language samples. Schmidt and Windsor (1993), for example, showed that there was little difference in MLUs of both normally developing children and those with Down syndrome (DS) when samples were gathered from conversations during structured or unstructured activities. Sedey, Miolo, and Miller (1993) demonstrated that the degree of linguistic complexity produced by both normally developing children and those with DS did not differ in conversations with a parent as opposed to a clinician, although more speech overall and more lexical diversity were found in the parent-child samples. Wagner, Nettelbladt, Shalen, and Nilholm (2000) found that intelligibility and fluency were higher in conversational samples than in narration among preschoolers with language impairments. In addition, children used more complex verb forms in conversation than narration at this age. This research suggests that when using a language sample to evaluate expressive syntactic and morphological skills, a conversational sample based either on a relatively unstructured free-play situation or on a more structured activity with either parent or clinician is an appropriate method at the preschool level, although we will need to consider other contexts for children at higher language levels.

Table 2-5 gave some suggestions from Miller (1981) for eliciting a representative speech sample from children of various ages. Duchan (1991) pointed out that, for children at developing language levels, event descriptions of what is going on in the here and now are better sampling contexts than narratives or reports of past events. Event descriptions can include back-and-forth conversation about ongoing play or descriptions of pictures, as were suggested in the section on phonological assessment. However, Longhurst and File (1977) showed that more complex language is elicited in conversation, as opposed to picture description. Perhaps picture description should be reserved for samples collected from unintelligible children and conversational samples should be preferred from children who are easier to understand. In any case, children at the level of developing language need some contextual support to give their best performance in speaking situations. The materials used also can make a difference. O'Brien and Nagle (1987) reported that play with dolls produced more complex language than play with vehicles, for example, for both boys and girls. For preschoolers, generally situations, people, activities, materials, and topics that are familiar will elicit the most representative sample (Owens, 2004).

Both Hubbell (1988) and Owens (2004) emphasized the importance of the adult's interactive style in collecting these samples. They suggested placing few limits on the child's behavior within the interaction, choosing topics of interest and familiar to the child, and attempting to give the child some measure of control over the conversation. These kinds of interactions are most likely to elicit optimal communication from a client with developing language.

How long a sample do we need? Most writers (e.g., Lahey, 1988; Miller, 1981; Nelson, 1998) suggest 50 to 100 utterances. Cole, Mills, and Dale (1989) showed that a 50-utterance sample yields about 80% of the information available in a sample twice as long. For efficient-yet-valid clinical data gathering, then, a 50-utterance sample is usually adequate. For children in the developing language stage, a sample of this length can generally be obtained from 15 to 30 minutes of conversation (James, 1990).

Many researchers (e.g., Cole, Mills, & Dale, 1989; Nelson, 1998) have advocated collecting several samples for analysis of productive language, arguing that multiple samples yield more representative information. Cole, Mills, and Dale suggested that two short samples (say 10 minutes each) taken on two different days would provide a more valid picture of productive language than a single longer sample. Here's my opinion on this issue: language sampling is one of the best methods we have available for establishing productive language baseline function, targeting intervention goals, and evaluating progress in the intervention program. The most important thing about language sampling is to *do it.* If it is possible to collect two or more short samples for analysis, great! The danger arises when we feel we have to collect and analyze more than one sample and therefore decide not to do language sampling at all. If the alternative to collecting multiple samples is not do any analysis of spontaneous speech, then it is better to take just one sample that is as representative as we can make it. Doing an imperfect language sample analysis is better for clinical purposes than not doing any at all.

When we collect a speech sample, we usually want to *record the sample* in some way. This allows us to examine it in more detail than we could if we had to get all the information from it in real time. It lets us go back later and pick up information we may have missed the first time around and also allows us to analyze the same sample for several different purposes on several different passes through it. As discussed in Chapter 2, audio recordings are usually used when speech itself is the focus of the assessment and when there is enough intelligible speech present that other information is not needed to figure out what the client is talking about. Video recording can be used when nonverbal context is necessary to decipher the child's meanings or when nonverbal aspects of communication are of interest. The recorded sample is then transcribed at whatever level is appropriate for the analysis being done. Syntactic analyses require only word-by-word transcriptions of the client's speech, probably with the linguistic context of the other speaker's remarks included. If we plan to do phonological analysis on the same transcript, this requires phonemic transcriptions and, in some cases, phonetic level information as well. Pragmatic analysis necessitates some information about the nonlinguistic context and perhaps about paralinguistic cues that accompany the speech.

Several formats are available for transcription. Miller (1981) provided one example, which involves writing each child and adult utterance on a separate line, with one speaker's utterances indented so it is easy to identify visually who is talking. The child and adult utterances are each numbered consecutively; the child's are numbered C1, C2, and so on, the adult's A1, A2, and so on. Using this method, we also provide columns for morpheme counts, nonlinguistic context, and any comments the transcriber wishes to make. Several symbols are used to indicate questionable transcription, unintelligible utterances, pauses within the utterance, and phonetic transcription. These conventions, along with Miller's transcription format, are shown in Figure 8-9.

One of the most important decisions we make when transcribing is how to separate speech into utterances. Since we transcribe the sample with one utterance per line and often compute morpheme length and do syntactic analysis utterance by utterance, making reliable judgments about when an utterance ends is important. Owens (2004) presented a set of rules that can be used for segmenting utterances in transcripts at the developing language phase. These are summarized in Box 8-3.

One way language level is often assessed in a sample of spontaneous speech is by computing MLU in morphemes. Instructions for computing MLU can be found in Box 8-4. Brown (1973) inaugurated this measure as a means of indexing syntactic development and demonstrated that MLU was a much better yardstick of syntactic development than was age. Brown showed that there was lots of variation in the age at which preschoolers achieved certain syntactic skills, but much less variation in the MLU they displayed when each milestone was reached. For example, some children produced adult question forms at age 2, whereas others did not produce them until close to age 4. But no matter how old the children were when they produced adult question forms, their MLU was always around 3 to 3.5. There has been a good deal of research on the validity of MLU as an index of language development over the years (Klee, 1992; Lahey, Liebergott, Chesnick, Menyuk, & Adams, 1992; Miller, Freiberg, Rolland, & Reeves, 1992). The current consensus would appear to be that MLU alone should never be used to determine whether a child has a delay in

Name of child: _____

Clinic number: _____

Chronogical age: _____

Date of evaluation: _____

Examiners: _____

Child MLU: _____

   Numbers of utterances: _____

   Number of intelligible utterances: _____

   Sources of transcription: _____ Audiotape _____

Adult MLU:
   1.
   2.
   3.

Key:

C = Child   [   ]   Gloss or contextual notes

E = Examiner   (   )   Questionable transcription

XXX = Unintelligible   /   /   Phonetic transcription

... = Pause

Situation variables:

Time of day:

Setting:

Materials used:

Length of interaction:

Participants/Type of interactions:
   1.
   2.
   3.
   4.

Pragmatics		Speaker	Utterance number	Dialogue	Morpheme count		Syntax	Semantics
Child	Adult				Child	Adult		

FIGURE 8-9 ✦ Transcription format. (Adapted from Miller, J. [1981]. *Assessing language production in children.* Needham Heights, MA: Allyn and Bacon.)

BOX 8-3 **Rules for Segmenting Utterances in Preschool Speech Samples**

1. A sentence is an utterance:
   Mommy will go to the store yester… tomorrow = 1 utterance.
2. A command is an utterance:
   Go home! = 1 utterance.
3. Run-on sentence with *and* should contain no more than one *and* joining clauses. Sentences with more than one *and* should be separated into additional utterances:
   We went on the bus and we got to the zoo and we saw lots of animals and we had ice cream =
   We went on the bus and we got to the zoo
   (and) we saw lots of animals
   (and) we had ice cream
4. Other complex and compound sentences are treated as one utterance:
   He was sad because his daddy yelled at him because he broke the cup and spilled the baby's food.
5. Pauses, inhalations, and falling intonation mark the ends of utterances:
   Eat (drop in intonation; pause)…oatmeal cookie = 2 utterances: Eat. Oatmeal cookie.
   Eat (momentary delay, no fall in intonation)…oatmeal cookie = 1 utterance: Eat oatmeal cookie.

Adapted from Owens, R. (2004). *Language disorders: A functional approach to assessment and intervention* (4th ed.). Boston, MA: Allyn & Bacon.

---

language development (Eisenberg, Fersko, & Lundgren, 2001), but it does have some value as one aspect of the description of a child's language level, especially when combined with other information about language production, such as the number of different words (NDW) in a speech sample (Klee et al., 2004; Leonard & Finneran, 2003). Table 8-6 gives the normal range for MLU for children in the developing language period, based on data from Brown (1973), Miller (1981), Miller, Freiberg, Rolland, and Reeves, (1992) and Owens (2004).

MLU can be computed from a free-speech sample to compare other areas of language development to it. This comparison can be used to determine whether some areas of language

---

BOX 8-4 **Rules for Computing MLU from a Sample of Spontaneous Speech**

1. Segment the child's speech sample into utterances.
2. Transcribe the sample, putting each utterance on a new line.
3. Identify the first 50 consecutive fully intelligible utterances in the transcript. (Eliminate any utterances that are unintelligible or partially unintelligible from the count.)
4. Count the number of morphemes in each utterance, using the following counting rules:
   a. Count each free morpheme (word) and each bound morpheme or inflection (such as plural *-s*, possessive *-'s*, third-person singular *-s*, past-tense *-ed*, present progressive *-ing*, and so on) as one.
   b. In stuttering or false starts, count each word only once. If a word is repeated for emphasis ("No, no, no!"), count each occurrence of the word.
   c. Count compound words *(birthday)*, proper names *(Mickey Mouse)*, and reduplications *(night-night)* as only one morpheme.
   d. Count irregular past-tense forms *(went, saw, came)* as one morpheme. If a child overgeneralizes a past-tense form, such as *goed* or *comed*, count this as two.
   e. Count words with diminutive endings *(doggie, toesie)* as one morpheme.
   f. Count auxiliary verbs *(is, are, was, were, have, had, has, will, could, can, would, must, might, shall, should,* and others) as one, even if they are contracted (*He/'s* is two morphemes; *are/n't* is two morphemes), except for *can't* and *don't,* which count as one.
5. Add up the total number of morphemes in the sample. Then divide by the total number of utterances (usually 50). The result is the MLU.

Adapted from Brown, R. (1973). *A first language: The early stages.* Cambridge, MA: Harvard University Press; Chapman, R. (1981). Exploring children's communicative intents. In J. Miller (Ed.), *Assessing language production in children.* Needham Heights, MA: Allyn and Bacon.

TABLE 8-6	Typical Values for MLU (Morphemes) and NDW in Preschool Children	
AGE (MO)	NORMAL RANGE OF MLU	AVERAGE NUMBER OF DIFFERENT WORDS/50 UTTERANCES
18	1.0–1.6	36
21	1.1–2.1	41
24	1.5–2.2	46
27	1.9–2.4	51
30	2.0–3.1	56
33	2.2–3.5	61
36	2.5–3.9	66
39	2.7–4.2	71
42	3.0–4.6	76
45	3.2–5.0	81
48	3.5–5.3	86
51	3.7–5.7	
54	3.8–6.1	
57	3.9–6.5	
60	4.0–6.8	117

Adapted from Brown, R. (1973). *A first language: The early stages.* Cambridge, MA: Harvard University Press; Miller, J. (1981). *Assessing language production in children.* Boston, MA: Allyn & Bacon; Miller, J., Freiberg, C., Rolland, M., & Reeves, M. (1992). Implementing computerized language sample analysis in the public school. *Topics in Language Disorders, 12(2),* 69-82; Owens, R. (2004). *Language disorders: A functional approach to assesment and intervention* (4th ed.). Boston, MA: Allyn & Bacon.

development are further behind than MLU would suggest, even when the MLU itself is less than would be expected for developmental level. Although we know that the relationship between MLU and grammatical development is not a simple one (Leonard & Finneran, 2003), knowing a child's MLU can help guide the remaining portions of the analysis. For example, if the MLU is less than 3, we may wish to concentrate on semantic analyses, such as the analysis of semantic relations discussed in Chapter 7 or Lahey's (1988) semantic-syntactic analysis procedure. These methods would identify meanings expressed and the basic forms used to express them. The clinician could use this information to target additional meanings for expression or to encourage the child to express all meanings with the most advanced forms currently in the repertoire before attempting to expand syntactic complexity. If the MLU is between 3 and 4.5, further analysis might focus on basic morphological and syntactic markers in simple sentences, since such forms typically develop during these MLU stages. If MLU is greater than 4.5, complex sentence development might be the primary area of assessment, since basic morphological and syntactic structures are usually mastered at this MLU level and more advanced structures are beginning to emerge.

MLU also is a useful way to chart change in productive language. If we track MLU taken from a free-speech sample each semester in an intervention program, we have a valid means of showing change in spontaneous speech in response to our intervention. You might like to try computing an MLU on the short transcript in Box 8-5. (Remember that we ordinarily want to use at least 50 utterances to compute an MLU.) Cover the answers in the morpheme column and try your hand. Then check against the morpheme counts given in Box

8-5. Use the data in Table 8-6 to decide whether the MLU you found is appropriate for a child of this age.

There are some disadvantages to using MLU as a speech-sample-analysis procedure, though. First, it is too global, in itself, to highlight areas of syntactic deficit. If only one syntactic analysis can be done on a sample, MLU is probably not the best choice, since it gives too general a picture and does not pinpoint specific targets for intervention. Second, as we've discussed, MLU may not be our most trusted guide to grammatical level (Eisenberg et al., 2001). Finally, MLU computation requires full transcription of a speech sample—a time-consuming process.

One issue in using speech sample analysis concerns *increasing the efficiency of the sampling and analysis* procedures. Should we compute MLU for every speech sample collected for the purpose of syntactic and morphological analysis? I would say probably not. Other analysis techniques, given limited clinical time and resources, yield more information relevant to intervention planning. We might do these more detailed analyses for initial assessment purposes. Then we might use MLU to track progress in intervention without doing more detailed analyses, but rather probing for specific forms using elicited production contexts and using MLU changes to show that these forms are generalizing to spontaneous speech. This would be a more economical allocation of clinician effort than doing an MLU for every speech sample we analyze.

Many practicing SLPs say that speech-sample analysis is impractical for real clinical situations because of the time it takes to transcribe and analyze the sample. Let me give you my view on this issue. Speech-sample analysis *is* more time-consuming than scoring a standardized test, but it also provides much richer and more valid information. How can we recon-

BOX 8-5	Sample Transcript from a Child Aged 4 Years, 2 Months for Morpheme and Sentence-Structure Analysis

Key

( ) = questionable transcription
[ ] = gloss or contextual notes
/ / = phonetic transcription
XXX = unintelligible
. . . = pause
C = Child
A = Adult

Utterance	Nonlinguistic Context	Morpheme Count
C1: What this thing?	[point to tape recorder]	3
A: I think it's a tape recorder.		
C2: I can (touch) it?		4
A: I don't think you'd better, honey.		
C3: I talking on it?		5
A: I think so!		
C4: It hearing me?		4
A: Yup.		
C5: It the lady's tape?		5
A: Yes, it is.		
C6: It not like /gæ miz/ [Grammy's].		5
A: No, Grammy has a bigger one, doesn't she?		
C7: Grammy's don't have buttons on.	[touching buttons]	7
A: No, that's right, hers has dials.		
C8: They got toys in here?		6
A: Sure. Here are some. . . . Let's look at these.		
C9: Yeah, cars in blue box.		6
A: Um-hm, there are some cars in the blue box here.		
C10: I want XXX green car.		4
A: OK, here's the green one.		
C11: Hey, it went under there!		5
A: Well, go get it.		
C12: Got it!		2
A: Good. Is it running OK?		
C13: Yeah, it run good.		4
A: Good. Let's see what else is in here.		
C14: Look, red car.		3
C15: Donny have red car.		4
A: Yes, Donny's car is red, but it's a lot bigger than this one, isn't it?		
C16: Yeah, Donny always drive his car too fast.		8
A: He does! How do you know?		
C17: Daddy say so last time.		5
A: Oh-oh. I better not let you ride in his car again.		
C18: No, I'll tell him go slow.		7
C19: You seed him last time?		6
C20: He hitted a wall!	[jumps up and down]	5
C21: The cop yelled at him!		6
A: Oh, no!		

cile this conflict? My opinion is that we need (1) to be very judicious about choosing when to do a speech sample and what analyses to perform and (2) to learn to do speech-sample analyses more quickly and efficiently.

In deciding when to use a speech sample, we should remember that standardized tests are designed to tell whether a child is different from other children. Dawson et al. (2003), for example, showed that the SPELT-3 is very sensitive and specific in identifying children with language disorders. For the purposes of initial identification of expressive language deficit, using a valid tool like the SPELT-3 is certainly recommended. Speech-sample analysis, on the other hand, is not constructed psychometrically for this purpose. Speech-sample analysis should only be done when it has already been established, by means of standardized testing of expressive language, that the child has a productive language deficit.

The efficiency of speech-sample analysis can be increased in two ways. The first is to shortcut some of the steps involved in traditional analysis methods. I talked about doing some of the phonological process assessment of connected speech in real time, rather than transcribing the whole sample phonemically. We can take a similar approach to analyzing syntactic and morphological production from a speech sample. The second way is to make use of computer-assisted procedures.

Let's look at the second alternative first. Several computer programs for language sample analysis are available. Some examples are listed in Table 8-7.

Long (1999) and Long and Channell (2001) provided detailed descriptions of several of these programs. What all these programs have in common is that they require transcription of a speech sample into a computerized data file. The software

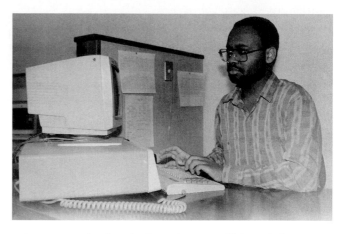

Computer-assisted methods can increase efficiency in language sample analysis.

for each program then identifies and counts features from a list of available options that the clinician chooses. The clinician also can insert special codes into the transcription that allow for the identification and counting of items not on the program's existing menu, or that allow the program to perform various pre-programmed analyses on the coded transcripts. Long (2001) showed that computerized analyses were completed faster and with equal accuracy when compared with manual analysis, when coded transcripts were used. Still, the data entry time required to type in transcripts and insert all appropriate codes can be considerable, especially for those just learning the systems. However, as Long points out, new "intelligent" software is rapidly being combined with these basic counting programs to enable clinicians to have the software perform predetermined analysis

TABLE 8-7	**Examples of Computer-Assisted Language Sampling Analysis Software**
PROCEDURE	**DESCRIPTION**
Automated LARSP (Bishop, 1985)	Based on *Language Assessment, Remediation, and Sampling Procedure* (LARSP; Crystal, Fletcher, & Garman, 1976).
Computerized Profiling (Long & Fey, 2004)	Includes routines for calculating MLU, Conversational Act Profile (Fey, 1986), Developmental Sentence Score (DSS; Lee, 1974), Profile of Semantics-Lexical Forms (Crystal, 1982), Profile of Phonology (Crystal, 1982), narrative analysis, and Type-Token Ratio (TTR) on coded transcripts.
DSS Computer Program (Hixson, 1985)	Computes DSS on coded transcripts.
Lingquest (Mordecai, Palin, & Palmer, 1985)	Computes MLU, TTR on coded transcripts.
Parrot Easy Language Sample Analysis (Weiner, 1988)	Calculates MLU on coded transcripts.
Pye Analysis of Language (PAL; Pye, 1987)	Provides options for analysis categories on coded transcripts.
Systematic Analysis of Language Transcripts (SALT; Miller & Chapman, 2003)	Calculates MLU, NDW, Total Number of Words (TNW), allows user to count words/forms in specific categories and create categories and codes. Includes routines for comparing multiple transcripts.
CHILDES, CHAT and CLAN (MacWhinney, 2000)	Includes a database of transcripts, tutorials on data entry, programs for computer analysis of transcripts, methods for linguistic coding, and systems for linking transcripts to digitized audio and video.

routines on uncoded transcripts, thus reducing the need for the insertion of special codes as the sample is entered. Figure 8-10 provides an example of a transcript of Jerry's speech as it would be coded in SALT (Miller & Chapman, 2003) and analyzed with the standard SALT profile analysis, comparing Jerry's data to that of children of his age in the SALT database.

In addition, newer methodologies are beginning to take advantage of more powerful software solutions to simplify the clinician's job in performing language sample analysis. Channell and Johnson (1999) reported on a program that uses probability algorithms to automatically tag words within a speech sample as examples of particular parts of speech, such

A

```
$ CHILD, EXAMI                          : :02                                  : :03
+C: Jerry                               C COKE UP.                             C WHAT DO YOU X.
+GENDER: M                                E HEY LOOK WHO I HAVE.                 : :11
+CA: 4;3                                 C YEP.                                 - 3:00
+CONTEXT: CON+                           C TWO OF THEM?                           E OK.
[EW] ERROR AT THE WORD LEVEL+             E TWO OF THEM.                        C WHAT?
[EU] ERROR AT THE UTTERANCE LEVEL       C OH.                                    E WHOA THAT GUY/'S GONNA FALL!
- 0:00                                    E TWO MONKEY/S.                       C GET THIS.
                                        C OH.                                  C ME GET IT [EU].
  E <OK>.                                : :03                                   E IS HE OK?
C <WHAT IS> THIS RIGHT HERE?            C THIS GO[EW:GOES] RIGHT <THERE> RIGHT? C YEAH.
  E IT LOOK/3S LIKE A LITTLE TABLE WITH AN UMBRELLA.  E <OH>.                    : :16
C HERE.                                   E YEAH THAT GO/3S RIGHT THERE.        = C PLAYING WITH SOMETHING, MAKING NOISE.
C RAIN/3S.                                E LOOKIT.                             C WHAT *IS THIS?
  E FOR WHEN IT RAIN/3S.                  E THE GORILLA.                        C GO.
  E THAT/'S <RIGHT>.                     C YEP.                                 C THEM.
C <YEP>.                                  = E "ROARS", LAUGHS.                   : :05
C MORE PEOPLE                            : :03                                    E OH THE MONKEY HANG/3S BY HIS TAIL.
  .E <MORE PEOPLE>.                      C THIS GO?                              : :04
C <ELEPHANT GO>?                           E WHERE SHOULD WE PUT THAT SEAL?     C TAIL.
  E ELEPHANT GO/3S WHERE?                C <YEAH>.                              C OH.
C RIGHT HERE.                             E <I BET HE> WANT/3S TO BE BY WATER.  C WHERE *DO THESE G0 THEN?
  E OH.                                   E IS THERE ANY WATER TO PUT HIM BY?   C MONKEY/S.
C XX FIT HERE.                           C YEAH.                                C MONKEY/S.
  E HE DOES/N'T FIT THERE DOES HE?        E WHERE?                                E WHERE DO THOSE MONKEY/S GO?
C RIGHT HERE.                            C <WATER>.                             - 4:00
  E OH OK.                                 E <OH> MAYBE THIS IS WATER UP HERE HUH? C YEAH.
  E THAT LOOK/S LIKE A GOOD IDEA.        - 2:00                                  : :04
  E <OH>.                                 : :03                                 C THERE?
C <HERE>.                                C GO UP.                                 E THERE!
C WHAT <IS> THAT?                         : :06                                  : :10
  E <LOOK>.                                E UP!                                   E THERE WE GO.
  E IT/'S A HIPPOPOTAMUS.                 : :03                                 C MORE?
C OH.                                      E OK WHAT ELSE?                       C IN HERE?
C X HERE TOO.                             E HERE/'S A BIRD.                       E IS THERE MORE IN THERE?
  E PUT HIM RIGHT THERE TOO?             C <YEAH>.                              C MHM.
C YEAH.                                    E <IT/'S> A PARROT.                  C BEER.
  E OK.                                  C MORE?                                  E BEER?
  E WHAT ELSE DO WE HAVE IN HERE?          E HERE/'S ANOTHER PARROT.             E ANIMAL/S DON'T DRINK BEER.
C (THIS) THIS GUY.                       C (THIS GUY) <THIS>^                    : :02
C *AND THIS GUY.                           E <HERE/'S A> VULTURE.              C YEAH.
  E THAT GUY AND THAT GUY.                 E HE LOOKS^                            E DO THEY?
C MORE?                                  C THIS *IS YOUR/Z.                     C YEP.
C WHAT (IS TH*) IS THAT?                   E THAT/'S MINE?                       : :06
- 1:00                                   C YEP.                                 C XX THIS.
  E THIS IS A OH :03 <I/'M> NOT QUITE SURE.  E THANKS.                          : :05
C <CAR>.                                   E WE/'LL EACH HAVE A BIRD HUH?       C WHAT *ARE THESE?
 : :02                                   C RIGHT HERE.                            E THAT/'S COCACOLA.
  E <IT ALMOST LOOK/3S> LIKE A BUFFALO OR  E OH YOU/'RE GONNA PUT YOUR/Z RIGHT UP THERE?  E POP BOTTLE/S.
SOMETHING.                               C THERE/'S TWO RIGHT?                  C OH.
C <XXX>.                                   E THERE/'S TWO.                       : :02
C POP.                                     E YOU/'RE RIGHT.                       E <X>.
  E HERE/'S THE SEAL.                     : :02                                 C <PEAR/S> GO <HERE>.
C YEP.                                   C THIS.                                  E <HERE/'S>>
  E YOU SAW POP BOTTLE/S HUH?             : :02                                   E WHAT?
C YEP.                                     E OK THAT/'S A GOOD IDEA.            C PEAR/S GO *HERE.
  E THOSE ARE PRETTY CUTE.                 E TAKE THAT OFF.                     - 5:00
```

FIGURE 8-10 ✦ A, SALT coded transcript of Jerry's speech sample.

B

DATABASE PROFILE COMPARISON:STANDARD MEASURES TRANSCRIPT INFORMATION

Speaker: JEREMY (CHILD)   Database: WisconsinCon.sdb
Sample date: 2/2/07   Subjects: 18 females, 17 males
Current Age: 3;3   Age range: 2;9 - 3;9
Context: Conversation   Context: Conversation
63 C&I Verbal Utts   63 C&I Verbal Utts

STANDARD MEASURES

Language measure	Child		Database				
	Score	+/-SD	Mean	Min	Max	SD	%SD
Current Age	3.25	0.26	3.19	2.75	3.75	0.23	7%
Transcript length							
Total Utterances	69	-0.31	70.17	64	78	3.78	5%
# C&I Verbal Utts	63	0.00	63.00	63	63	0.00	0%
No. Complete Words	120**	-2.73	243.11	179	348	45.05	19%
Elapsed Time (5:00)	5.00	-0.83	6.81	4.18	15.05	2.18	32%
Syntax/morphology							
# MLU in Words	1.62**	-2.72	3.23	2.16	4.46	0.59	18%
# MLU in Morphemes	1.73**	-2.74	3.52	2.37	4.97	0.65	19%
Semantics							
# TTR	0.37*	-1.60	0.44	0.33	0.54	0.04	10%
# No. Diff. Word Roots	38**	-3.16	89.37	66	136	16.25	18%
# Total Main Body Words	102**	-2.72	203.51	136	281	37.34	18%
Discourse							
% Responses to Ques	89%*	1.04	74.90	38	94	14.02	19%
Mean Turn Length (wds)	2.27**	-2.09	4.09	2.63	6.06	0.87	21%
Utts. with Overlaps	13**	2.45	6.54	1	12	2.64	40%
Intelligibility							
% Intelligible Utts.	93%	-0.55	94.94	86	100	4.16	4%
Mazes and abandoned utts							
# Utterances with Mazes	2*	-1.71	10.77	3	22	5.13	48%
# No. of Mazes	2*	-1.64	12.20	3	27	6.21	51%
# No. Maze Words	3*	-1.35	22.97	3	70	14.76	64%
# % Maze Wds/Total Wds	3%*	-1.39	9.73	2	24	4.94	51%
Abandoned Utterances	0*	-1.25	2.40	0	7	1.91	80%
Verbal facility and rate							
Words/Minute	24.00*	-1.29	38.28	12.82	62.33	11.05	29%
Between Utt Pauses	20	-0.14	22.60	0	101	19.09	84%
Between Utt Pause Time	1.57	0.10	1.43	0.00	6.35	1.32	92%
Within Utt Pauses	0	-0.61	0.71	0	5	1.18	165%
Within Utt Pause Time	0.00	-0.57	0.03	0.00	0.28	0.06	176%
Omissions and error codes							
# Omitted Words	6*	1.61	2.31	0	7	2.29	99%
# Omitted Bound Morphemes	0	-0.71	1.17	0	7	1.65	141%
Word-level Error Codes	1	-0.85	3.54	0	14	3.00	85%
Utt-level Error Codes	1	-0.54	1.86	0	7	1.59	86%

\# Calculations based on C&I Verbal Utts; * at least 1 SD (** for 2 SD) from the database mean.

Database selection criteria: age +/- 6 months

FIGURE 8-10 ✦—**cont'd B,** SALT Analysis of Jerry's transcript; compared with age-matched database sample.

as nouns, verbs, and pronouns. They found accuracy to range from 60% to 95% and suggested further improvements were needed before the system is appropriate for clinical use. More recently, Channell (2003) reported on a fully automated *Developmental Sentence Score* (DSS; Lee, 1974) program in the Computerized Profiling system, which requires only transcript entry without coding. Channell found that the automated DSS produced overall scores that were highly correlated with manually scored samples, although agreement on particular categories between the automatic and manual analyses was still only 78%. Long and Channell (2001) had reported good agreement between automatic or manual coding for global (normal/not normal) clinical decisions, although Channell's (2003) results suggest that we still have a way to go before obtaining highly accurate descriptions of performance in individual semantic and syntactic categories from uncoded transcript entry, which is necessary in using automated language sample analysis for intervention planning. Still, with the speed at which technology changes, it probably will not be long before clinicians can rely on "intelligent" software to do a substantial amount of the work involved in clinical language sampling. In addition, advances in automated speech recognition may, before too long, allow us to play an audiosample directly into a computer program that would automatically transcribe it orthographically, so that the clinician would only have to either enter semantic, syntactic, and discourse codes or input the basic transcript into another program that provided them automatically and did a prescribed analysis (Paul, 2003b).

In the meantime, let's not forget our other option. To analyze morphological and syntactic production, we also can listen to an audiorecorded speech sample, perhaps the same one we collected for phonological analysis, and analyze it without transcription. Instead, we could record data gathered from listening onto a worksheet developed from one of the speech-sample analysis procedures we will discuss. We could stop the recording periodically to process the data and listen again to segments about which we were unsure. However, we would not need to transcribe the entire sample to record the morphemes and syntactic patterns that we heard. These could simply be recorded on the score sheet as we listened to the recording.

This approach has some disadvantages, of course. We would not have a written transcription to put into a client's file. We might miss some morphemes while we were listening for sentence structures or vice versa. It would not be easy to compute an MLU using such an approach. However, this method would make speech sampling for morphological and syntactic production more practical in a clinical setting, and this, to me, seems a sufficient justification. The recording could always be transcribed later, if a written record is needed or an MLU calculation becomes necessary. It can be listened to again by another clinician if reliability information is wanted. Furthermore, Furey and Watkins (2002) showed strong positive correlations between online recordings and those obtained from transcription when analyzing verb productions. This analysis suggests that online analysis can be a viable alternative to transcription procedures and can reduce the time required for language analysis.

However, we should note that this study supported accuracy in online recording for one relatively focused aspect of language production. This should emphasize to us that when analyzing language data from a recording rather than a transcript we need to focus on just one aspect of the analysis at a time.

Three key elements are involved in being able to do speech-sample analysis without transcription: practice, practice, and practice! The only way to achieve competence and make speech sampling valid and efficient is to be completely familiar with the procedure you are using, to the point of having it memorized. This way, your brain becomes the computer that does the analysis. What you need to make this method work are a firm and detailed knowledge of the normal stages of syntactic acquisition, complete familiarity with the structures assessed in the procedure that you are using, and an organization of the analysis firmly in mind before you start. There is no way to achieve this level of knowledge and familiarity except by doing a lot of practice analyses.

These two approaches to speech-sample analysis—nontranscribed and computerized—save time on the opposite ends of the process. The former allows the clinician to listen for features in the sample without writing down every word the child says. The computerized methods require us to transcribe the sample, but the computer does the searching and counting automatically. Both methods are faster than transcribing and analyzing by hand, but both require the clinician to—again—practice, practice, practice to make the process efficient. Clinicians committed to doing speech-sample analysis can choose their weapon. If you like working with computers, by all means get one of the speech-sample analysis packages and learn to use it. The investment of time will pay off in a greatly enhanced ability to sample and analyze your clients' speech. Miller et al. (1992) suggested using laptop computers that can be carried into clinical situations to allow not only language sample analysis but also ongoing monitoring of progress in intervention.

Perhaps, though, you are not a "technophile." If you prefer to work with a pencil, devote some time to studying one of the speech-sample analysis methods we'll discuss next. If you choose one procedure and—you guessed it—practice, practice, practice, you can greatly reduce the time it takes to perform the analysis by hand. When you know one procedure well enough, you'll find you don't need to transcribe every sample but will be able to score it directly from your recording. Either way, you will have performed a great service to your clients. You will have learned to make efficient use of the most valid means of assessing a child's productive language.

One more thing: any speech-sample analysis procedure requires a fairly elaborated knowledge of English grammar and of normal language development. Hubbell (1988), Justice and Ezell (2002), Quirk, Greenbaum, Leech, and Svartick (1990), and Parker (1986) all supply helpful background information on the basics of English linguistics. Gleason (2001), Haynes and Shulman (1998b), Hoff (2001), Hulit and Howard (2002), Miller (1981), and Owens (2001, 2004) provided detailed accounts of the acquisition of English syntax and morphology. Retherford (2000) and Owens (2004) provide step-by-step guides to analyzing language transcripts and provide information on semantic and pragmatic as well as syntactic and morphological procedures. Extensive information on collecting and transcribing samples also is included in Retherford (2000) and Owens (2004). Retherford provided sample transcripts and audiotapes for guided practice and feedback that are very useful in developing the expertise necessary to accomplish language sampling efficiently. These sources are useful references for any clinician beginning the process of speech-sample analysis.

Let's look at some of the *speech sample analysis procedures* available for examining spontaneous speech. Hubbell (1988), Lahey (1988), Lund and Duchan (1993), Owens (2004), and Retherford (2000) provided guidelines for analyzing spontaneous speech using informal, descriptive approaches. Crystal, Fletcher, and Garman (1976) and Tyack and Gottsleben (1977) provided somewhat more formalized approaches that allow the clinician to use the analysis to determine presence of disorder and intervention targets. I will give you some more detailed information on the procedures devised by Miller (1981), Scarborough (1990), and Lee (1974). This is not intended as an endorsement of these procedures over the others. They are simply chosen as a sample of some of the more commonly used procedures. Use of *any* speech-sampling analysis goes a long way toward making our assessments of children with developing language more valid measures of real communicative skill.

Miller's (1981) Assigning Structural Stage Procedure is a two-step process. The first involves the analysis of Brown's (1973) grammatical morphemes. The second looks at sentence types and structures. Much of the analysis is available in a computer-assisted form, the SALT program. If you do the analysis by hand, you may transcribe the sample and compute MLU from the transcription, then use the transcription for further analyses. As I suggested earlier, for MLUs less than 3, semantic relational analysis or Lahey's (1988) content-form analysis may be most

informative. For samples with MLUs between 3 and 4.5, analysis might focus on basic morphological and syntactic markers in simple sentences. For MLUs greater than 4.5, complex-sentence development might be the primary area of assessment. Alternatively, you can do each step of the two-step analysis on a separate pass by listening to the recorded sample without transcribing or computing MLU. Figures 8-11 and 8-12 provide sample worksheets to use for each step in the analysis.

Miller has assigned each of Brown's (1973) grammatical morphemes to the stage of syntactic development in which it is acquired (contractible and uncontractible forms of the copula and of the auxiliary *be* have been collapsed in Figure 8-11, so the total number of morphemes examined is 12, not the traditional 14). According to Brown, a morpheme is *acquired* when it is used correctly in 90% of its obligatory contexts. An *obligatory context* (OC) is a place in the sentence that requires the morpheme to make the sentence grammatically correct. "I have two new shoe_," for example, is an obligatory context for the plural morpheme. These stage assignments are based on Brown's stages indexed by MLU, although you do not need to compute MLU to do the analysis. You'll notice that some morphemes are acquired in Stages II, III, V, and V+, but none in Stage IV. That's because many forms emerge in IV but are not acquired until later (that is, they are not used correctly 90% of the time in Stage IV). We'll see these emerging forms when we do the second step of the Assigning Structural Stage Procedure.

To do the morpheme analysis, note when each morpheme is used and also when it is required. This allows us to look at correct usage in obligatory context. That's why there is a column for "obligatory context" and one for "morpheme appears" on the form in Figure 8-11. As we listen to the sample, we note when a particular morpheme is required in context (with a "" in the "obligatory context" column, for example). Then in the "morpheme appears" column, we put a "+" if a morpheme is

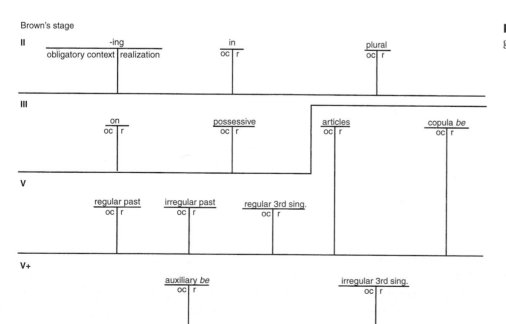

FIGURE 8-11 ✦ Worksheet for analyzing grammatical morpheme use.

Name _____ Developmental level _____ Age _____ Date _____

Stage	NP	S*	A†	VP	S*	A†	Negative	S*	A†	Question	S*	A†	Complex	S*	A†
I	NP alone (not in sentence context) with modifier Pronouns: *I, me*			Unmarked V Absent copula Absent auxiliary			*No* or *not* + *NP* or *VP*			Routines: *What . . .? What . . . doing? Where . . . going?*					
II	Noun modified in object position Pronouns: *my, it*			Main V marked occasionally *-ing* w/o *be* Catenative alone w/o NP Copula appears occasionally			*NP* + {*No, not, can't,* or *don't*} + *VP*			*What* or *Where* + (N) + V					
III	Modified NP may appear in subject position Demonstratives *(this, that, these, those)* and articles *(a, an, the)* appear Pronouns: *you, your, she, them, he, we, her*			Auxiliaries: *can, will* Overgeneralized past tense			*Won't*			Aux. Vs appear in Wh-Qs, W/o inversion Yes-no Qs produced w/ rising intonation only Q words: *why, who, how, whose*					
EIV	Subject NP is obligatory; appears in all sentences			Past modals: *could, should, would, must, might* Catenative + NP			*Isn't, aren't, didn't, doesn't*			Auxiliary Vs and "dummy do" forms appear in wh- and yes/no Qs and are inverted Q words: *when*			*Let's, Let me* Simple infinitive Full proposition Simple wh- Conjoining Conj.: *and*		
LIV-EV	NP can contain three elements Pronouns: *his, him, us, they, our, its*						*Wasn't weren't, couldn't wouldn't, shouldn't*						Double embedding Conjoining and embedding w/in one S		
LV	Pronouns: *myself, yourself, their*												Infin. w/ diff. subj. Relative clause Conj.: *if*		
V+	Pronouns: *herself, himself, themselves, ourselves*			have + *en*									Gerund Wh- infinitive *Help, make, watch, let* Conj.: *because*		
V++													Conj.: *when, so*		

*Successful use.
†Attempt; incorrect use.

FIGURE 8-12 ✦ Form for scoring Miller's (1981) *Assigning structural stage procedure.* (Based on Miller, J. [1981]. *Assessing language production in children.* Needham Heights, MA: Allyn and Bacon.)

used and a "–" if it is not. When we have listened to the whole sample, we count the number of checks in the "obligatory context" column for each morpheme and divide that number into the number of "+"s that appeared in the "morpheme appears" column. This would give us the percentage of appearance of each morpheme in obligatory context. We could then use this information to help decide which morphemes should be targeted in the intervention program. Balason and

Dollaghan (2002) warn us, however, that even typical preschoolers do not routinely produce multiple examples of OCs for all of these morphemes in short speech samples. When interpreting data on grammatical morpheme production, we may need to supplement information from free speech samples with data from probes that attempt to elicit the production of morphemes for which OCs did not appear in a spontaneous sample.

Let's practice what I've been preaching. Take the short transcript in Box 8-5. (Remember, we ordinarily want to use at least 50 utterances to do a grammatical morpheme analysis.) Try doing a grammatical morpheme analysis on it, using a worksheet such as the one in Figure 8-11. You'll find my analysis in Appendix 8-1.

The second step in Miller's procedure involves analysis of sentence structures. Miller's procedure for this part of the analysis draws on research from normal language acquisition. His manual (Miller, 1981) provided normative data in a set of charts. The child's performance is compared with the data in these charts and assigned to the Brown's stage at which normally speaking children typically first use each form. Again, the stages are indexed by MLU, although it is not absolutely necessary to compute MLU to do the analysis. Rather than using an acquisition (or mastery) criterion, as the grammatical morpheme analysis does, the sentence-structure procedure uses an emergence criterion (that is, stage assignment is based on the appearance of just one instance of a structure). The assumption made is that one or two instances in a relatively brief speech sample indicate that a form is emerging into the repertoire.

Miller's procedure looks at the following five aspects of sentence structure development:

NP: The elaboration of noun phrases (with articles, demonstratives, pronouns, and quantifiers)

VP: The elaboration of verb phrases (with auxiliary verbs, catenatives, copulas, past-tense marking, and subject-verb agreement marking)

NEG: The production of negative sentences

Q: The production of questions (both yes/no and *wh-*)

COMPLEX: The use of complex sentences

Miller (1981) provided explicit instructions for scoring each form examined in the analysis, with definitions and examples of each of the forms included. Figure 8-12 provides a form that can be used in the Assigning Structural Stage Procedure, showing how forms can be assigned to the stage of development at which each typically appears.

To use Figure 8-12 to accomplish Miller's (1981) Assigning Structural Stage Procedure, we would listen again to our recorded speech sample, utterance by utterance, stopping the tape at the end of each utterance to score it in all appropriate categories. Alternatively, we could score each utterance in a transcription, if we did one. Each utterance would be given the highest score possible in each of the areas (columns in Figure 8-12) for which a score could be given.

To score for NP, each utterance is given the highest score possible for each noun phrase (subject, object of the verb, or predicate nominative) it contained. For example, if a client's utterance 1 is "See big girl," this would receive an NP score of Stage II, because a modified noun occurred in object position in the sentence. The number "1" would be written in the NP/Stage II "S" section of the worksheet. If utterance 2 is "That girl," this utterance would be placed at Stage I of NP elaboration, since the modified noun occurs alone, not in a sentence context. A "2" would be written in the "S" column of that section of the form. Noun phrases in subject position are

obligatory at Brown's Stage IV. Since this is the case, any sentence that contained a *two-word* noun phrase *as subject* would be scored as Stage IV, regardless of the type of modification, because Stage IV would be the highest stage assignment that could be given to such a sentence. If the client's third utterance were "That girl run," this utterance would be scored at Stage IV of NP elaboration, and a "3" written in the "S" column of that section of Figure 8-12. Any sentence containing a noun phrase of three or more words (*great big dog, a nice girl*) would be scored at Stage late IV to early V.

Similarly, the verb phrase in each sentence would be given the highest score possible. Utterance 3, "That girl run," which was scored as Stage IV of NP elaboration, would be scored in the VP elaboration column at Stage I, since the verb is unmarked. A "3" would be written in the "S" column of "unmarked V" on Figure 8-12. If the client's fourth utterance were "I wanna go," a VP score of Stage II would be given because the catenative *gonna* was used without a noun phrase complement. A "4" would be recorded in the "S" column of "catenative alone w/o NP."

Any sentence containing a negative form would be given the highest "neg" score possible, in addition to whatever scores were appropriate for NP and VP elaboration. If the client's fifth utterance were, "I won't stay," the score would be Stage III, since *won't* appears at Stage III on the chart. A "5" would be written in the "S" column of that section of Figure 8-12. Each yes/no question would be scored according to whether it was produced with rising intonation only ("You wanna go?"—Stage III) or with an inverted auxiliary verb or *do* ("Do you wanna go?"—Stage IV). *Wh-* questions would be scored according to both the form of the question and the question word used. For example, if the client said, "When you are going?", he would receive a score of Stage III for the uninverted auxiliary (are going) and Stage IV for the question word *when*.

If any complex sentences, either embedded or conjoined, occur in the transcript, these would be scored in the complex sentence column. Miller (1981) provided detailed descriptions of the types of complex sentences typically seen in the speech of normal preschoolers. The types of embedding the child uses are scored in the complex sentence column. If, for example, the client said, "He's the one that I played with," a score of Stage late V would be given for the relative clause ("that I played with").

Certain conjunctions appear on the worksheet because they are used frequently by normal preschoolers. If these appear in a client's sample, they can be scored appropriately. If a client says, "I like it because it's chocolate," a score of early Stage IV can be given in the complex sentence column for a conjoined sentence, and a score of V can be given for the conjunction *because.* You also can note in the Attempt (A) column when forms are unsuccessfully attempted. By this we mean when a context for a form occurs but the correct one does not appear. For example, for utterance No. 3 (*That girl run*), you *also* could put "3" in the "A" column for the VP Stage II (main V marked occurs occasionally), since a marker (third person singular) should have been there. At this point you might like to try doing a sentence-structure analysis on the sample in Box 8-5.

(Remember that we ordinarily want to use at least 50 utterances to perform sentence-structure analysis.) Refer to Miller (1981) as you go, if you have the book available. Try using a worksheet such as the one in Figure 8-12 to practice analyzing the sample for sentence structures. My analysis appears in Appendix 8-2.

Miller's procedure is descriptive in nature and does not yield a quantitative score. When we have completed both steps in the analysis, we can look across all the categories we have analyzed and identify the stage at which most of the child's scores are falling. This would be considered the child's stage of *mastery*. Any forms missing or in error (attempts) below this stage would be high-priority candidates for intervention, taking into account, of course, other considerations that we discussed in Chapter 3. We would then look for forms missing or attempted at the mastery level. These forms, too, would be candidates for consideration as intervention goals.

It's important to remember, when looking at the results of this and other syntactic analyses, that children with both normal and disordered language usually don't use structures that all score consistently at one level. Some scatter is expected. When looking for targets of intervention, though, we would want first to address forms that are missing or in error below the current baseline, or mastery level. These make appropriate short-term goals. Forms above the current mastery level would be good guides for choosing structures that could improve the child's overall level of functioning and move it closer to an age-appropriate level. This strategy would help to achieve the long-term goal of bringing the client's communicative skills more in line with developmental level.

Scarborough (1990) presented a norm-referenced extension of Miller's (1981) procedure called the *Index of Productive Syntax* (IPSyn). The IPSyn uses a "productivity criterion" of two appearances of each structure of interest within a 50- to 100-utterance speech sample. Any structure that appears twice in the sample is considered "productive," or within the child's current repertoire. The procedure is efficient in terms of time because only the first two appearances of any structure need to be counted, not the total frequency. The IPSyn orders a broad range of structures in each of Miller's five categories developmentally, so it is easy to identify emerging language levels. It includes many of the structures examined by Miller, and it adds several that Scarborough's research has shown to be diagnostic in children's speech. A sample IPSyn score sheet appears in Figure 8-13.

Although not technically standardized, the IPSyn does provide norm-referenced information from a small sample of preschool children with typical language acquisition. Of course, in general we have already decided that a child has a language disorder before analyzing a speech sample. The IPSyn's norm-referenced information can be used to track progress in an ongoing intervention program, though, as MLU can. But unlike MLU, an IPSyn score used for tracking also gives detailed information on syntactic structures used. If we can show with an IPSyn score that the child is moving closer or into the normal range on structures that we have targeted in the program, we are in a stronger position to argue for our program's efficacy. Moreover, the structural information from the procedure can help decide which syntactic goals have been met and which need additional intervention. Long and Fey's (2004) *Computerized Profiling* contains a software program to accomplish this analysis on entered transcripts.

The IPSyn also can be adapted as a criterion-referenced procedure to look at structures that are productive in a child's repertoire, to identify levels of emerging language, and to find structures currently missing from the repertoire that can be targeted for intervention. Although the procedures and scoring criteria for accomplishing an IPSyn are too extensive to be given here, clinicians who want to combine norm- and criterion-referenced assessment in speech sampling may want to locate Scarborough's (1990) paper in *Applied Psycholinguistics* and try the procedure. This method is worth investigating before you decide which speech-sample procedure you choose to study in-depth and use in clinical practice.

A third method of speech-sample analysis commonly used by clinicians is Lee's (1974) Developmental Sentence Score (DSS) procedure. Like the IPSyn, the DSS provides both norm- and criterion-referenced information. Hughes, Fey, and Long (1992) argued that despite the fact that this procedure is more than 30 years old, it is, in their words, "still useful after all these years." The reasons for its longevity include its relatively large norm-referenced data base (more than 200 children), its well-organized format that enables easy visual inspection of a variety of forms at different developmental levels, and its broad range of structures scored in a way that makes diagnostic interpretation possible. Moreover, recent work has moved toward making automated DSS analysis workable (Channell, 2003).

The DSS procedure looks at eight syntactic categories: indefinite pronouns, personal pronouns, main verbs, secondary (embedded) verbs, negative markers, conjunctions, interrogative reversals, and *wh-* question forms. In each category are eight developmentally ordered levels of complexity, which are awarded scores from one point for the simplest level to eight points for the most complex. Lee's summary of these levels, categories, and scores appears in Table 8-8. Structures in each of the eight categories are scored by assigning the appropriate number of points to each scorable structure that is present in a complete noun-verb (subject-predicate) utterance in the speech sample. In addition, a "sentence point" is added to the score of each sentence that is completely correct by adult standards. Since the DSS does require 50 complete noun-verb utterances for scoring, it is only appropriate for children whose speech contains primarily full sentences, rather than telegraphic utterances. In general, this would translate to a rule of thumb that the DSS would only be used for children whose MLUs are greater than 3.

Complete scoring instructions for the DSS can be found in Lee (1974). To do this analysis we inspect the speech sample, utterance by utterance, for structures in each of the eight categories and award points for each structure identified, according to the criteria in Box 8-6. For example, if the client said, "Don't you like ice cream?", we would inspect this sentence for

INDEX OF PRODUCTIVE SYNTAX

IPSyn Scoresheet

TOTAL IPSyn SCORE [ ]

Noun Phrases Subscale

item	cr	exemplar 1	exemplar 2	pts*
N1 noun				
N2 pronoun				
N3 modifier				
N4 2wd NP				
N5 article	N4			
N6 V+2wd NP	N4			
N7 plural				
N8 preV NP	N4			
N9 3wd NP	N4			
N10 NP adv.	V8			
N11 bound				
N12 other NP				

NOUN PHRASES TOTAL [ ]

Verb Phrases SubScale

item	cr	exemplar 1	exemplar 2	pts*
V1 verb				
V2 part/prep				
V3 prep. phr.	V2			
V4 copula	V1			
V5 caten.				
V6 pres.aux	V5			
V7 -ing				
V8 adverb				
V9 pres.mod	V5			
V10 pres.-s				
V11 past mod	V9			
V12 past -ed				
V13 past aux	V6			
V14 med. adv	V8			
V15 ellip/em	*			
V16 past cop	V4			
V17 other VP				

VERB PHRASE TOTAL [ ]

Questions/Negations Subscale

item	cr	exemplar 1	exemplar 2	pts*
Q1 inton. Q				
Q2 rout. Q				
Q3 no(t) X				
Q4 Wh-(N) V				
Q5 N not V	Q3			
Q6 Wh- aux.	Q4*			
Q7 neg aux.	Q5			
Q8 y/n aux.	*			
Q9 Why, etc.				
Q10 tag Q				
Q11 other Q/N				

*V4, V6, V11, V13 or V16

QUESTION/NEGATIVE TOTAL [ ]

Sentence Structures Subscale

item	cr	exemplar 1	exemplar 2	pts*
S1 2 words				
S2 S-V	S1			
S3 V-D.O.	S1			
S4 S-V-O	S2,S3			
S5 any conj.				
S6 any 2-VP				
S7 conj.phr.	S5			
S8 infin	V5,S6			
S9 Let's, etc.				
S10 adv.conj.	S5			
S11 pr. compl.	S6			
S12 s-conj-s	S6			
S13 Wh- cl.	S6			
S14 bitrans.	S3			
S15 3-VP sent	S6			
S16 rel. cl.	S6			
S17 infin-2	S8			
S18 gerund	V7,S6			
S19 move sub	S6			
S20 other SS				

SENTENCE STRUCTURE TOTAL [ ]

* Score 1 point for each of first two exemplars in transcript. Record 0, 1 or 2 in pts. column, depending on number of exemplars found.

FIGURE 8-13 ✦ *Index of Productive Syntax (IPSyn)* scoresheet. (From Scarborough, H. [1990]. *Applied Psycholinguistics, 11*, 6-7. Reprinted with permission from Cambridge University Press.)

structures in each of the eight categories. The *don't* would be scored in the Negative column with 4 points. It also would receive 4 points in the Main Verb column (for *don't like*), as "obligatory do + verb." (It is a peculiarity of the DSS that verbs can receive scores in several of the eight columns.) *You* would receive one point in the Personal Pronoun column. The sentence also would receive six points in the Interrogative Reversals column for the obligatory reversal of *don't* ("You don't like ice cream."/"Don't you like ice cream?"). It also would earn a sentence point for overall correctness. No points could be scored in the Indefinite Pronoun, Secondary Verb, or *wh-* Question columns for this sentence. Attempt marks (–) are used to indicate that a structure was tried but produced in error. For example, the sentence "I running" would receive an attempt mark (–) in the Main Verb column. Attempt marks receive no numerical score, but they can be inspected at the end of the analysis for error patterns.

Lively (1984) provided useful tips to improve accuracy and efficiency of DSS scoring. Hughes, Fey, and Long (1992) also provided suggestions for clarifying some ambiguous criteria

in Lee's manual and for modifying a few rules to make the procedure more clinically useful. These papers are valuable resources for clinicians who decide to make the DSS the language-analysis procedure they implement in clinical practice. Hixson (1985), Channell and Johnson (1999), Channell (2003), and Long and Channell (2001) discuss computerized scoring programs for the DSS.

Normative data on DSS scores in relation to age in typically developing children, as presented by Lee, appear in Figure 8-14. To use this graph, we identify the child's age (or developmental level) and read up to the DSS score computed for that child's transcript. If the score falls below the 10th percentile line for that age (or developmental level), we would conclude that the child had a language deficit. We also would be justified in reporting an age-equivalent score, based on the same graph. To find the age equivalent, we would simply read across from the child's DSS score to the 50th percentile line, then read down to determine the age for which that score fell on the 50th percentile. If our client is 5 years, 6 months and earned a DSS score of 5, for example, we would see that a DSS of 5 falls

| TABLE 8-8 | The Developmental Sentence Scoring Reweighted Scores | | |

SCORE	INDEFINITE PRONOUNS OR NOUN MODIFIERS	PERSONAL PRONOUNS	MAIN VERBS	SECONDARY VERBS
1	*It, this, that*	1st and 2nd person: *I, me, my, mine, you, your(s)*	A. Uninflected verb: "I *see* you." B. Copula, *is,* or *'s:* "It's *red.*" C. Is + verb + *ing:* "He *is running.*"	
2		3rd person: *he, him, his, she, her, hers*	A. −s and ed: *plays, played* B. Irregular past: *ate, saw* C. Copula: *am, are, was, were* D. Auxiliary: *am, are, was, were*	Five early-developing infinitives: "wanna *see*" ("want to *see*") "I'm gonna *see.*" (going to *see*") "I gotta *see.*" ("got to *see*") "Lemme [to] *see.*" ("let me [to] *see*") "Let's [to] *play.*" ("let [us to] *play*")
3	A. *No, some, more, all, lot(s), one(s), two (etc.), other(s), another* B. *Something, somebody, someone*	A. Plurals: *we, us, our(s), they, them, their* B. *These, those*		Noncomplementing infinitives: "I stopped *to play.*" "I'm afraid *to look.*" "It's hard *to do* that."
4	*Nothing, nobody, none, no one*		A. *Can, will, may* + verb: may go B. Obligatory *do* + verb: *don't go* C. Emphatic *do* + verb: "I *do see.*"	Participle, present or past: "I see a boy *running.*" "I found the toy *broken.*"
5		Reflexives: *myself, yourself, himself, herself, itself, themselves*		A. Early infinitival complements with differing subjects in kernels: "I want you *to come.*" "Let him [to] *see.*" B. Later infinitival complements: "I had *to go.*" "I told him *to go.*" "I tried *to go.*" "He ought *to go.*" C. Obligatory deletions: "Make it [*to*] go." "I'd better [*to*] go." D. Infinitive with *wh*-word: "I know what *to get.*" "I know how *to do* it."
6		A. *Wh*-pronouns: *who, which, whose, whom, what, that, how many, how much:* "I know *who* came." "That's *what* I said." B. *Wh-* word + infinitive: "I know *what* to do." "I know *who(m)* to take."	A. *Could, would, should, might* + verb: *might come, could be* B. Obligatory *does, did* + verb C. Emphatic *does, did* + verb	
7	A. *Any, anything, anybody, anyone* B. *Every, everything, everybody, everyone* C. *Both, few, many, each, several, most, least, much, next, first, last, second* (etc.)	*(His)* own, one, oneself, whichever, whoever, whatever: "Take *whatever* you like."	A. Passive with *get,* any tense Passive with *be,* any tense B. *Must, shall* + verb: *must come* C. *Have* + verb + *en:* "I've *eaten.*" D. *Have got:* "I've *got* it."	Passive infinitival complement with *get:* "I have *to get dressed.*" "I don't want *to get hurt.*" With *be:* "I want *to be pulled.*" "It's going to *be locked.*"
8			A. *Have been* + verb + *ing, had been* + verb + *ing* B. Modal + *have* + verb + *en: may have eaten* C. Modal + *be* + verb + *ing: could be playing* D. Other auxiliary combinations: *should have been sleeping*	Gerund: "*Swinging* is fun." "I like *fishing.*" "He started *laughing.*"

Reprinted with permission from Lee, L. (1974). Developmental sentence analysis. (Chart 8 on pages 134-135) Evanston, IL: Northwestern University Press.

NEGATIVES	CONJUNCTIONS	INTERROGATIVE REVERSALS	WH-QUESTIONS
It, this, that + copula or auxiliary *Is, 's* + *not*: "It's *not* mine." "This is *not* a dog." "That is *not* moving."		Reversal of copula: "*Isn't* it red?" "*Were* they here?"	
			A. *Who, what, what* + noun: "*Who* am I?" "*What* is he eating?" "*What book* are you reading?" B. *Where, how many, how much, what...do what...for*: "*Where* did it go?" "*How much* do you want?" "*What* is he *doing*?" "*What* is a hammer *for*?"
	And		
Can't, don't		Reversal of auxiliary *be*: "*Is he* coming?" "*Isn't he* coming?" "*Was he* going?" "*Wasn't he* going?"	
Isn't, won't	A. *But* B. *So, and so, so that* C. *Or, if*		*When, how, how* + adjective: "*When* shall I come?" "*How* do you do it?" "*How big* is it?"
	Because	A. Obligatory *do, does, did*: "*Do* they run?" "*Does* it bite?" "*Didn't* it hurt?" B. Reversal of modal: "*Can* you play?" "*Won't* it hurt?" "*Shall* I sit down?" C. Tag question: "It's fun, *isn't it*?" "It isn't fun, *is it*?"	
All other negatives: A. Uncontracted negatives: "I *cannot* go." "He has *not* gone." B. Pronoun-auxiliary or pronoun-copula contraction: "I'm *not* coming." "He's *not* here." C. Auxiliary-negative or copula-negative contraction: "He was*n't* going." "He has*n't been* seen." "It could*n't* be mine." "They are*n't* big."			*Why, what if, how come, how about* + gerund: "*Why* are you crying?" "*What if* I won't do it?" "*How come* he is crying?" "*How about* coming with me?"
	A. *Where, when, how, while, whether (or not), till, until, unless, since, before, after, for, as, as* + adjective + *as, as if, like, that, than*: "I know *where* you are." "Don't come *till* I call." B. Obligatory deletions: "I run faster *than* you [run]." "I'm *as big as* a man is [big]." "It looks *like a* dog [looks]." C. Elliptical deletions (score 0): "That's *why* [I took it]." "I know *how* [I can do it]." D. *Wh-* words + infinitive: "I know *how* to do it." "I know *where* to go."	A. Reversal of auxiliary have: "*Has he* seen you?" B. Reversal with two or three auxiliaries: "*Has he been* eating?" "*Couldn't he have been* crying?" "*Wouldn't he have been* going?"	*Whose, which, which* + noun: "*Whose* cat is that? "*Which* book do you want?"

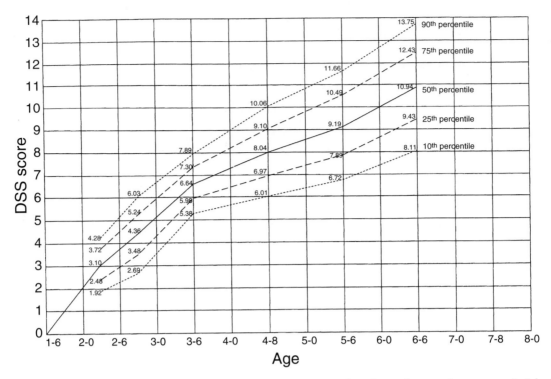

FIGURE 8-14 ✦ Age-DSS score relationships. (Reprinted with permission from Lee, L. [1974]. *Developmental sentence analysis* [p. 16]. Evanston, IL: Northwestern University Press.)

at the 50th percentile for 3-year-olds. So this client's DSS age equivalent would be 3-0. *Remember,* though, that it is only appropriate to report an age-equivalent score if the score falls below the 10th percentile for the child's age. If our 5-year, 6-month old client got a DSS of 8, we would simply report that this score fell at the 25th percentile for age and was within the normal range.

Like the IPSyn, the DSS can be used as a criterion- referenced procedure, too. Hughes, Fey, and Long (1992) suggested four ways to examine the DSS for goal selection and intervention planning. These are summarized in Box 8-6.

Figure 8-15 provides a worksheet that could be used in scoring a DSS analysis. Why not try using these criteria, along with information from Lee (1974), Hughes, Fey, and Long (1992), and Lively (1984), to score the sample in Box 8-7? Remember that you need noun-verb utterances to score in the DSS, and in a real clinical sample you would need 50 of them. If you don't find 50 noun-verb utterances in Box 8-7, do the analysis on the ones you find, remembering that you will need 50 to get a valid score from a client. My analysis appears in Appendix 8-3.

Elicited Procedures. One drawback in using speech sampling to assess productive syntax and morphology is that the child

---

BOX 8-6	**Suggestions for Using DSS Information for Goal Selection and Intervention Planning**

1. Note the frequency of attempt marks for each category. Select a grammatical target that the client is attempting to produce but producing incorrectly.
2. If many low-scoring forms are produced correctly but high-scoring forms are scarce, select forms that are at the level just above those the child is currently producing correctly.
3. Analyze sentences that did not receive a sentence point for patterns of error. If a pattern, such as leaving out articles, is found, target this grammatical class.
4. Examine the frequency of occurrence of forms for each category. Identify infrequent forms at the same level as other forms the child produces consistently and try to increase the frequency of use of the infrequent forms.

Adapted from Hughes, D., Fey, M., & Long, S. (1992). Developmental sentence scoring: Still useful after all these years. *Topics in Language Disorders, 12,* 1-12.

Name _____

Birth date _____

Recording date _____

CA:

DSS = Total score ÷
Numbers of utterances (50)

Sentence #	Indef. pro.	Pers. pro.	Main verb	Sec. verb	Neg.	Conj.	Inter. rev.	Wh- Q	Sent. pt.	Total

FIGURE 8-15 ✦ Sample DSS scoring worksheet.

BOX 8-7 **Sample Transcript from a Child Aged 4 Years, 8 Months for DSS Practice**

Child (C) 1: I got one for you.
Parent (P) : Oh, you got one, OK.
P: What else do I get?
C2: Got there.
P: What's that?
C3: I can't remember.
P: Well, what are we going to play?
C4: These cups.
P: What is this?
C5: A box to put something in.
C6: Oh two, up.
C7: Cup two fill up.
P: What did you bake, anything?
C8: It is.
P: What is it?
P: What happened?
C9: I don't spill nothing.
P: You didn't spill anything, OK.
P: What's on the plate?
C10: These.
P: Didn't you bake anything for me?
C11: I did.
P: Want to play something else?
C12: I wanna play house.
P: You want to play house?
C13: Yeah, I'm gonna do this.
C14: Play with this too.
C15: The door.
P: What's in there?
C16: Toys.
P: Do they have a bed like yours?
C17: Them don't fit in my bed.
C18: Too big for my bed.
P: Too much stuff on your bed.
P: Did you bring your dolls down?
C19: Brought my doggie.
C20: See.
C21: No play.
P: You don't want to play?
C22: No I does.

BOX 8-7 **Sample Transcript from a Child Aged 4 Years, 8 Months for DSS Practice—cont'd**

C23: I make something.
P: What are you going to make, though?
C24: Potatoes.
P: Oh I was thinking more of cookies, but that's OK.
C25: And cookies, cookie.
C26: That's the bed.
P: Oh, guess what today is?
C27: What?
P: Today's hockey.
C28: Today's hockey?
C29: I wanna put that.
P: X fix me something to eat.
P: What are we going to have?
C30: I'm thinking.
C31: Dingdong, that's the door.
C32: Now open it.
C33: Now shut it.
C34: Oh, do it.
C35: You know what this is?
P: No, what?
C36: A table.
C37: This is our lunch.
C38: A car in the garage.
C39: I opened it.
C40: This door opens.
C41: Who did that?
P: Are you making a mess?
C42: I gotta fix some.
C43: Who's that?
P: You drink coffee?
C44: In this.
C45: I'm making this.
P: How many kids have you got at your house?
C46: Only a baby.
P: What's our baby's name?
C47: You tell them.
P: OK, it's Missy.
C48: Yeah, Missy's her name.
C49: She's a big girl.
C50: She's big and she likes cookies.

may not spontaneously produce all the aspects of language in which we are interested. When talking to an unfamiliar adult, for example, a child may be unlikely to produce questions and negative forms, for pragmatic reasons. If these forms simply do not appear in spontaneous speech, how can we know what the child's skills in these areas are? The advantage of criterion-referenced assessment is that we can combine approaches as

needed to give us access to additional information. One strategy for doing a criterion-referenced production assessment would be to collect a sample of spontaneous communication, record and analyze it, and identify any structures or functions of interest that did not appear in the sample, in addition to those that appear to be in error. We could then use the strategy we discussed in Chapter 2. An elicited production procedure could be devised to try to get some evidence about these forms. If the child still failed to "take the bait" in the elicited production activity, direct elicited imitation ("Say, 'He is going.'") might be tried as a last resort.

For example, Loeb, Pye, Redmond, and Richardson (1996) provided a procedure for eliciting verb forms. They argue that verbs are an especially important part of the child's lexicon to evaluate because it is known that children with language disorders have particular troubles in acquiring verbs and in using verbs that are precise and varied (Rice & Bode, 1993). Language samples may fail to show whether the child is able to produce some of these more precise and differentiated verbs, so an elicited probe makes sense as a follow-up to speech sample analysis. Loeb et al. identified a set of verbs of various syntactic types and semantic categories and developed a task in which to elicit them. Their research showed significant differences between typical 4-year-olds and those with disordered language in the ability to produce specific verbs in the elicitation task. These differences were particularly strong for verbs that were lower in their frequency of use (70% of the low

frequency verbs were produced correctly by children with typical development, whereas only 55% were produced by children with language disorders). Table 8-9 presents the contexts used to elicit the low frequency verbs.

Questions are another good example to consider. Suppose a client did not produce any questions in a spontaneous speech sample, but use of negatives and auxiliaries suggested that questions might be a problem. A clinician might want to try a quick question elicitation, just to see what questions looked like. Here, a procedure such as the "shy puppet" activity could be used. The "shy puppet" activity is outlined in Table 8-10. Similar activities could be devised to elicit any form of interest that failed to show up in a sample of spontaneous speech. Lund and Duchan (1993), Miller (1981), and Redmond (2003) provided additional examples of procedures for eliciting particular language forms. If the child could not produce the form of interest in the elicited format, the clinician could ask the child to imitate the form directly.

Complex sentences are another important area of development during this phase. Eisenberg (2005) suggested an elicita-

TABLE 8-9	**The Verb Elicitation Probe**

TARGET VERB*	OBJECTS	DIALOGUE
Boil	Pot with water on stove	Prompt: This pan has water in it. We turn on the stove, and now the water's getting really hot. What's the water doing?
Bounce	Rubber ball	(Clinician bounces ball on table) Prompt: What's happening?
Close	Stove/oven door	(Clinician closes oven door) Prompt: What did I do?
Enter	Doll house; toy	(Clinician moves toy toward door of house) Prompt: What is he going to do?
Float	Small boat; pan of water	(Clinician places boat in water) Prompt: What is the boat doing?
Fold	Paper	(Clinician folds paper) Prompt: What am I doing?
Follow	A large and a small toy pig	(Clinician has the small pig follow the large one in a curved path) Prompt: See the pigs? What is this (small one) doing?
Leave	Doll house; toy	(Clinician puts toy in house, and begins moving it toward the outside) Prompt: He's done in his house. What is he doing?
Loosen	String around toy dog; fence	(Clinician ties dog to the fence and says, "This is too tight." Loosens.) Prompt: What did I do to the rope?
Return	Two toy animals	(Clinician has one animal wave goodbye to the other, then begin to move away. The second animal then calls the first back. The first begins to move back toward the first) Prompt: What is this one (first animal) doing?
Roar	Tiger	(Clinician has tiger stand on hind legs and says "Rahr!") Prompt: What did the tiger do?
Smash	Play-Doh	(Clinician smashes a small ball of Play-Doh with a slow motion) Prompt: What did I do?
Sweep	Doll; toy broom	(Clinician puts broom on in doll's hand and has her sweep) Prompt: What is she doing?
Swim	Pan with water; plastic toy	(Clinician puts toy in water and makes swimming motions with it) Prompt: What is he or she doing?
Tear	"Sticky" note sheet	(Clinician slowly tears sheet in half) Prompt: What am I doing?
Wind	Yoyo	(Clinician winds string around yoyo) Prompt: What am I doing?

*Verbs are alphabetized here but should be presented in random order.

Adapted from Loeb, D., Pye, C., Redmond, S., & Richardson, L. (1996). Eliciting verbs from children with specific language impairment. *American Journal of Speech-Language Pathology, 5*, 17-30.

| TABLE 8-10 | The "Shy Puppet" Activity for Eliciting Questions |

Materials: Two puppets.
Procedure: Give the client one puppet and keep the other. Tell the client, "Your puppet Shyster is shy. He wants to ask my puppet Sally some questions, but he's so shy he can't think of what to say. I'll help him. I'll tell you what he would like to ask, and you make him ask Sally the question. Try this one. Shyster, ask Sally what she likes to eat." After the client asks the question, provide an answer from Sally.
Scoring: Use the worksheet below to score the client's question productions. A sample question for each question type is provided. Give at least three opportunities for the client to produce each question type, but randomize the order in which the question types are elicited.

| | | CLIENT PRODUCTION | | |
QUESTION TYPE	EXAMPLE	NO RESPONSE	CORRECT QUESTION FORM	OTHER (TRANSCRIBE)
Yes/no	Ask whether she likes ice cream.	_____	_____	_____
What...?	Ask what she's doing.	_____	_____	_____
Where...?	Ask where she lives.	_____	_____	_____
Who...?	Ask who she plays with.	_____	_____	_____
Whose...?	Ask whose toys she wants.	_____	_____	_____
Why...?	Ask why she's sad.	_____	_____	_____
How many...?	Ask how many sisters she has.	_____	_____	_____
How...?	Ask how she play checkers.	_____	_____	_____
When...?	Ask when she is going home.	_____	_____	_____

tion technique that allows us to assess both the production and understanding of sentences with infinitive clauses, one of the first complex types to emerge. Examples are shown in Table 8-11, and the complete protocol, along with a discussion of the levels of difficulty for the tasks, can be found in Eisenberg's paper.

PRAGMATIC ASSESSMENT

Although there are tests designed to assess pragmatic skills in children, a "test" of pragmatics is almost a contradiction in terms. Since pragmatics involves the use of language for real communication, we really need to assess it in a more naturalistic context, and this implies using criterion-referenced or informal procedures.

Why do we need to assess pragmatics? In my view, the pragmatic assessment supplies two important pieces of information about our clients. First, it can tell us whether clients are stronger or weaker in pragmatic communication relative to their skills in semantics, syntax, and phonology. Bishop, Chan, Adams, Hartley, and Weir (2000), for example, showed that there is a subset of children with specific language impairments who have pragmatic difficulties over and above their problems with language form and content. Children with autism spectrum disorders (Tager-Flusberg, Paul, & Lord, 2005) and those with nonverbal learning disabilities (Volden, 2004) are additional groups for whom pragmatic skills may be a special difficulty. For children with strong pragmatic skills, the

| TABLE 8-11 | Examples of Elicitation Activities for Infinitive Verb Clause Production and Comprehension |

LEVEL/SAMPLE VERB	MATERIALS	SET-UP	ACTION/DIALOGUE	PRODUCTION TARGET	ACTING OUT TARGET
1: want (same subject)	Materials: "Barney" "Baby Bop" dolls w/ moveable arms	Barney sitting; Baby Bop standing, facing him	"Barney and Baby Bop are playing school; Barney is the teacher. Baby Bop says to Barney, 'Can I lie down?' Baby Bop wants...? You finish the story. Baby Bop...? Now show me."	Baby Bop wants to lie down.	Makes Baby Bop lie down.
2a: ask	Materials: "Barney" "Baby Bop" dolls w/ moveable arms; toy chair	Barney standing next to chair; Baby Bop, facing him	"This is Barney's chair. Baby Bop says to Barney, 'Can you sit in the chair?' Baby Bop asks...? You finish the story. Baby Bop...? Now show me."	Baby Bop asks Barney to sit in the chair.	Sits Baby Bop in chair.
2b: want (different subject)	Materials: "Barney" "Baby Bop" dolls w/ moveable arms; toy pool	Barney standing next to pool; Baby Bop in pool.	"Baby Bop is swimming in the pool. She says to Barney, 'C'mon, Barney. You swim, too!' Baby Bop wants...? You finish the story. Baby Bop...? Now show me."	Baby Bop wants Barney to swim.	Puts Barney in pool.

Adapted from Eisenberg, S. (2005). When conversation is not enough: Assessing infinitival complements through elicitation. *American Journal of Speech-Language Pathology, 14(2)*, 92-106.

clinician can target language forms in both structured and naturalistic contexts with confidence that, once learned, new skills will be incorporated into the clients' communicative repertoire. For clients who do not effectively use the language they have for communication, clinicians will be less willing to make this assumption. Language goals would be taught first in structured activities. Later, carefully scaffolded activities would work toward getting the child to use new language forms in more varied communicative contexts. The clinician would set up naturalistic situations in which the use of the new forms could be modeled for the child. Then the clinician would provide opportunities for the child to use the new form in situations similar to the model. Generalization of new forms to conversation cannot be assumed for the poor communicator, and structured generalization activities, such as those discussed in Chapter 3, are especially important.

The second purpose of assessing pragmatic skills is to identify the pragmatic contexts in which new forms should be practiced. If a child has problems with pragmatic functions, we need to teach the language necessary to achieve those functions. Then we need to provide guided practice, through hybrid and child-centered approaches, in using the newly learned forms to accomplish the pragmatic functions with which the child has trouble. A list of the kinds of pragmatic problems often reported in children with language impairments appears in Table 8-12.

There is one more purpose for pragmatic assessment: to identify the particular problems in conversation and interaction faced by the small group of children for whom pragmatic skills

are the only or primary area of deficit. At the preschool level, these children are rare, but a few with diagnoses such as Asperger syndrome, nonverbal learning disabilities or pragmatic language impairment (PLI) may be part of your caseload. For this small group of preschoolers, pragmatic assessment may constitute the main portion of the evaluation.

A variety of procedures have been proposed for looking at pragmatic skills in communicative interactions. Girolametto (1997) developed a parent-report measure for profiling pragmatic skills in preschoolers. This measure has demonstrated good internal consistency and test-retest reliability. As part of a family-centered assessment, this measure provides an opportunity to include parental perceptions in the evaluation of young children's conversational ability. The measure appears in Figure 8-16. Girolametto reports that average scores on each of the two scales (responsiveness and assertiveness) of 4.5 or greater should be considered evidence of well-developed pragmatics. Average scores between 3 and 4.4 should be considered as emerging pragmatic competence, whereas those less than 3 should be considered indicative of pragmatic weaknesses.

Many pragmatic assessments involve observation of natural communication. Rice, Sell, and Hadley (1990) developed a method that can be used to assess conversational interactions in a play setting. Prutting and Kirchner's (1983) Pragmatic Protocol is commonly used to assess general pragmatic skills in a global way on the basis of an observation of interaction. The Pragmatic Protocol appears in Figure 8-17. To use it, the clinician observes a child interacting with an adult or peer. The clinician subjectively rates each type of communicative

| TABLE 8-12 | A Profile of Pragmatic Skills of Children with Language Disorders |

COMMUNICATIVE FUNCTION	LINGUISTIC FORMS USED
Request	Less likely to be grammatically complete. Fewer indirect forms used. Less flexibility in choice of form.
Comment	Less frequent than in typical populations. May be stereotypic in form.
Presupposition	May have difficulty judging what listeners want/need to know. Marking depends more on pronouns than does that of normal speakers.
Turn-taking	More inadequate forms used in relating to preceding discourse. Turns are shorter in length and involve less speech directed to others. Utterances are less adjacent than those of same-age mates (i.e., children with language disorders take longer to follow up the previous speaker's remark with a turn of their own). Children with language disorders are less assertive about gaining turns.
Respond	Responses are variable; children with language disorders do not always provide a conversationally obligated response; do not consistently compensate for verbal limitations by using nonverbal responses. Responses to requests for clarification are less focused on the informational needs of the requester. Responses to other types of speech acts are more likely to be unrelated or inappropriate. Responses are frequently incomplete, incorrect, unresponsive to interlocutor's intent, or pragmatically inappropriate.
Speech style adjustments and register variation	Speech style adjustments are made (e.g., for younger speakers). Modifications reflect fewer questions about listeners' internal states. Adjustments of utterance length and complexity are less finely "tuned" to the needs of the listener.

Adapted from Bishop, D.V.M., Chan, J., Adams, C., Hartley, J., & Weir, F. (2000). Evidence of disproportionate pragmatic difficulties in a subset of children with specific language impairment. *Development and Psychopathology, 12,* 177-199; Craig, H. (1991). Pragmatic characteristics of the child with specific language impairment: An interactionist perspective. In T. Gallagher (Ed.), *Pragmatics of language: Clinical practice issues* (pp. 163-198). San Diego, CA: Singular.

act on the worksheet as either "appropriate" or "inappropriate" on a global basis, taking the entire interaction into account. The resulting data can give a clinician a general idea of whether the majority of the child's communicative behaviors are adequate. Such an assessment allows us to look specifically at pragmatic behaviors that are inappropriate. These behaviors can be modeled for the client in the course of using real communicative situations as contexts for intervention activities.

Roth and Spekman (1984a,b) also presented a framework for assessing pragmatic skills. They divided pragmatics into three areas: communicative intentions, presupposition, and organization of discourse. They advocated using a conversational interaction between child and adult as a basis for observing the pragmatic skills they identified. Table 8-13 gives an outline of guidelines based on Roth and Spekman (1984a, b) for analyzing a communicative interaction. Again, the results of these observations can be used to identify pragmatic behaviors that can be modeled by the clinician in the communicative interactions used to provide contexts for language intervention.

Creaghead (1984) also suggested a protocol for assessing pragmatic skills in children with developing language, which

has come to be known as the "Peanut Butter Protocol." This is a structured interaction in which the clinician attempts to elicit communication from the child, then notes whether the child rises to the communicative "bait." In addition, it looks at the form of the child's communication. The results of the "Peanut Butter Protocol," like those of the other two examples, can be used to identify communicative acts that the clinician can model for the client in the course of interactions throughout the intervention program. A worksheet based on Creaghead's "Peanut Butter Protocol" appears in Table 8-14.

Numerous other suggestions for assessing pragmatic skills in the developing language phase are available in the literature. Some useful sources are Brinton and Fujiki (1989), Chapman (1981), Lund and Duchan (1993), MacDonald and Carroll (1992), and Shipley and MacAfee (2004). Owens (2004) and Paul (2005), for example, suggested the following categories of analysis to be considered when examining conversational skills in preschoolers:

▶ *Social vs. nonsocial:* the proportion of utterances directed to the listener, rather than self-directed.
▶ *Topic initiation:* the proportion of new topics introduced by the child rather than the adults.

Instructions

The purpose of this questionnaire is to find out how your child participates in conversations, and what problems, if any, he/she has. By conversation, we mean how your child is able to start conversations, take turns, give information that is on topic, ask questions, and answer questions.

Please use the following scale to rate each statement.

1	2	3	4	5
Never	Almost never	Sometimes	Often	Always

Throughout this questionnaire, we use the words "ask" or "tell" to describe what your child does in conversation. Since children do communicate nonverbally, please interpret "ask" and "tell" to include gestures, as well as words, phrases, or sentences.

Responsiveness items

1 2 3 4 5   1. If I offer my child a choice of two things that he/she likes, my child tells me which one he/she wants.
1 2 3 4 5   2. If my child knows the name of something he/she tells me the name when I ask.
1 2 3 4 5   3. When I ask a question, my child answers.
1 2 3 4 5   4. If I ask my child to repeat something I haven't understood, he/she does.
1 2 3 4 5   5. In a conversation, my child stays on topic for two or more turns.
1 2 3 4 5   6. My child's responses follow what I am talking about.
1 2 3 4 5   7. My child's answers are connected to what I asked.
1 2 3 4 5   8. My child's sounds/gestures/words match my topic of conversation with him/her.
1 2 3 4 5   9. When I don't understand, my child keeps on trying to get his/her message across.
1 2 3 4 5   10. When I ask my child a question to check what he/she means, he/she answers me.

Assertiveness items

1 2 3 4 5   1. When something new or unusual happens, my child asks about it.
1 2 3 4 5   2. My child asks questions (using sounds/gestures/words).
1 2 3 4 5   3. When my child doesn't know the name of something we are both looking at, he/she asks me what it is.
1 2 3 4 5   4. If I am holding something my child wants, he/she asks for it.
1 2 3 4 5   5. When we are playing a fun game (e.g., tickling) and I suddenly stop, my child asks me for more.
1 2 3 4 5   6. My child asks for help when he/she can't do something and I am nearby.
1 2 3 4 5   7. My child asks me for help when he/she wants something that is out of reach.
1 2 3 4 5   8. When I say something to my child that is not a question, he/she responds.
1 2 3 4 5   9. My child comes to me to start a game or activity that we have done before.
1 2 3 4 5   10. My child starts a conversation with me during familiar routines.
1 2 3 4 5   11. My child tells me when he/she wants to change an activity.
1 2 3 4 5   12. My child asks me to join in his/her play or game.
1 2 3 4 5   13. My child comes to me to tell me about things that interest him/her.
1 2 3 4 5   14. When we are together, my child gets a game going that we have done before.
1 2 3 4 5   15. When we're playing together, my child suggests different play ideas.

Mean score for responsive items (total points/10) _____
Mean score for assertiveness items (total points/15) _____
NOTE: For a copy of the scale for parental use, please contact the author.

FIGURE 8-16 ✦ Responsiveness and assertiveness in conversational skills rating scale. (Reprinted with permission from Girolametto, L. [1997]. Development of a parent report measure for profiling the conversational skills of preschool children. *American Journal of Speech-Language Pathology, 6*[4], 33.)

▶ *Topic appropriateness*: the proportion of topics that are appropriate to the interpersonal context.
▶ *Turns/topic*: the number of turns in which the child can maintain a topic.
▶ *Discourse management*: the number of times the child interrupts another speaker or fails to take a turn appropriately.
▶ *Contingency*: the proportion of the child's utterances that relate to or are contingent on the previous speaker's remark.

The most important thing to remember about assessing pragmatics in the developing language phase is that we want to get a picture of whether clients' pragmatic communication skills are better, worse, or equal to their semantic and syntactic abilities. This information helps us choose methods of intervention. In addition, we want to know which specific communicative functions need the kind of guided practice we can provide in a carefully thought-out interention program.

		Date: _____
Name: _____		
Communicative		Communicative
setting observed: _____		partner's relationship: _____

Communicative act	Appropriate	Inappropriate	No opportunity to observe
Utterance act			
A. Verbal or paralinguistic			
1. Intelligibility			
2. Vocal intensity			
3. Voice quality			
4. Prosody			
5. Fluency			
B. Nonverbal			
1. Physical proximity			
2. Physical contacts			
3. Body posture			
4. Foot or leg movements			
5. Hand or arm movements			
6. Gestures			
7. Facial expression			
8. Eye gaze			
Propositional act			
A. Lexical selection and use			
1. Specificity and accuracy			
B. Specifying relationships between words			
1. Word order			
2. Given and new information			
C. Stylistic variations			
1. Varying of communicative style			
Illocutionary and perlocutionary acts			
A. Speech acts			
1. Speech act pair analysis			
2. Variety of speech acts			
B. Topic			
1. Selection			
2. Introduction			
3. Maintenance			
4. Change			

FIGURE 8-17 ✦ Prutting and Kirchner's Pragmatic Protocol. (Reprinted with permission from Prutting, C., & Kirchner, D. [1983]. Applied pragmatics. In T.M. Gallagher and C.A. Prutting [Eds.], *Pragmatic assessment and intervention issues in language* [pp. 29-64]. San Diego, CA: College-Hill Press.)

Communicative act	Appropriate	Inappropriate	No opportunity to observe
Illocutionary and perlocutionary acts—cont'd C. Turn-taking			
1. Initiation			
2. Response			
3. Repair and revision			
4. Pause time			
5. Interruption and overlap			
6. Feedback to speakers			
7. Adjacency			
8. Contingency			
9. Quantity and conciseness			

FIGURE 8-17 ✦—cont'd

TABLE 8-13   Suggestions for Assessing Pragmatics

AREA ASSESSED	SUGGESTED ACTIVITY
Communicative Intentions	
Expression	Communicative temptations (see Chapters 6 and 7).
Comprehension	Have client "bathe" and "dress" doll; give indirect request forms of instructions ("Why don't you wash her face?" "Could you put on her hat?"). Record client responses as compliant or noncompliant.
Presupposition	Barrier games (referential communication) in which partners cannot see each others' referents: client must encode adequate information for partner to identify referents.
	Extended discourse: Look at use of pronouns, articles, ellipsis, and conjunctions in tasks such as describing how to play a game.
	Picture description: Show client a picture and ask for description. Then show a picture that is just the same except for one obvious detail. Client's description of second picture should take into account information presupposed in first; e.g., [picture 1] "The dog is running," [picture 2] "He's eating."
Social organization of discourse	Analyze turn-taking; topic maintenance; and conversational initiation, termination, and repair in the referential communication task used to assess presupposition.
	Role-play situations in which client needs to initiate conversation (e.g., asking for directions, asking for help in a store).
	Feign misunderstanding in conversation to assess client's ability to make repairs.
	Use unclear clinician messages to assess client's ability to request clarification.

Adapted from Roth, F., & Speckman, N. (1984a). Assessing the pragmatic abilities of children: Part 1. Organizational framework and assessment parameters. (1984b); Part 2. Guidelines, considerations, and specific evaluation procedures. *Journal of Speech and Hearing Disorders, 49,* 2-11 (Part 1); 12-17 (Part 2).

CONSIDERATIONS FOR ASSESSING OLDER CLIENTS WITH SEVERE IMPAIRMENT AT THE DEVELOPING LANGUAGE LEVEL

Some children at developing language levels may be older than preschool age. These older, more severely impaired clients, who may have multiple handicaps, have probably been involved in intervention for some time. Extensive assessment data may be on file, so assessment need not start from scratch. These clients will probably already be identified as eligible for services. There may be a question, though, about their eligibility specifically for language services, particularly if nonverbal and verbal skills are more or less on par. Here the clinician may want to advocate, not necessarily for direct clinical service to the client, but for consultative or collaborative services to increase the client's

TABLE 8-14 **Worksheet for Pragmatic Assessment Based on Creaghead's "Peanut Butter Protocol"**

CONTEXT	EXPECTED PRAGMATIC ACT	CHILD BEHAVIOR		
		NO RESPONSE	RESPONSE APPROPRIATE	OTHER (TRANSCRIBE OR DESCRIBE)
Child enters room.	Greeting	_____	_____	_____
Have cookies and crackers in view, but out of reach.	Requests object	_____	_____	_____
Give child tightly closed jar with cookies in it.	Requests action	_____	_____	_____
Ask, "How do you think we can get the jar open?"	Hypothesizing	_____	_____	_____
Say, "Do you want (mumble)?"	Request clarification	_____	_____	_____
Ask whether child wants peanut butter or jelly on the cracker.	Makes choice	_____	_____	_____
Hand child the opposite of what he or she chose.	Denial	_____	_____	_____
Put the peanut butter and jelly on the table. Ask, "What are we going to do now?	Predicts	_____	_____	_____
Tell the child to put peanut butter or jelly on the cracker	Request object (knife)	_____	_____	_____
Tell child to get knife, which is out of sight.	Requests information	_____	_____	_____
Put peanut butter or jelly on cracker. Eat it. Get out an extra large toothbrush and brush teeth.	Comments on object	_____	_____	_____
Converse with child. During this, pull a hidden string so that a doll falls off the table.	Comments on action	_____	_____	_____
Ask, "What happened?"	Describes event	_____	_____	_____
Ask, "Why did it fall?"	Gives reason	_____	_____	_____
During conversation, look for:	Answering	_____	_____	_____
	Expanded answer	_____	_____	_____
	Taking turns	_____	_____	_____
	Attending to speaker	_____	_____	_____
	Acknowledging	_____	_____	_____
	Initiating a topic	_____	_____	_____
	Changing a topic	_____	_____	_____
	Maintaining a topic	_____	_____	_____
Stop leading conversation and be silent.				
Look for:	Initiating conversation	_____	_____	_____
	Asking conversational questions	_____	_____	_____
Request clarification	Clarifying	_____	_____	_____
As child leaves room	Closing	_____	_____	_____

Adapted from Creaghead, N. (1984). Strategies for evaluating and targeting pragmatic behaviors in young children. *Seminars in Speech and Language, 5,* 241-252.

access and *opportunity* (Beukelman & Mirenda, 1998) for participating to as great a degree as possible in mainstream activities with chronological-age mates. Increasing opportunities may involve changing policies that provide for separate settings for individuals with disabilities or educating the professionals in new knowledge and skills to enable the inclusion of these students in integrated settings. Increasing access consists of both providing students with compensatory skills, including assistive technology, and adapting the environment to remove barriers to their participation.

Many advocates for the disabled (e.g., Calculator, 1994a,b; Lipsky & Gartner, 1997) see full inclusion in regular education as the goal for all students with disabilities. Using a systems model, this approach would suggest assessing the mainstream environment in which the student is to be placed and identifying the demands it will make on the student. The clinician might, for example, observe a second-grade classroom language arts activity to determine what the activity requires of a multiply handicapped 7-year-old functioning at a developing language level. The clinician's role would then be to prepare the student to participate in the activity with whatever resources she or he has available (from producing three-word sentences to using an AAC device). Our role also would include work with the classroom teacher to develop strategies that allow the child's contribution to be invited and rewarded. In this type of enterprise, very little, if any, standardized testing will be needed. Criterion-referenced assessment and behavioral observation, including observation in the classroom and ecological assessment, will probably be our primary assessment tools. One tool that may be helpful in this enterprise is the *Functional Communication Profile—Revised* (Kleiman, 2003). This tool provides checklists for evaluation of communication skills in the following areas:

▶ Sensory
▶ Motor
▶ Behavior
▶ Attentiveness
▶ Receptive language
▶ Expressive language
▶ Pragmatic/social skills
▶ Speech
▶ Voice
▶ Oral structure
▶ Fluency

Clinicians can rate students' current level of functional communication in each of these areas, then use these measures as baselines for tracking changes in communicative function as a result of the intervention provided. Figure 8-18 provides a checklist for expressive language adapted from Kleiman (2003), as an example of this type of measure.

Older, severely impaired clients may never complete the developmental sequence of language acquisition, even if speech is their primary mode of communication. This fact also argues for the provision of consultative or collaborative services, with the goal of meeting the communicative needs of the important environments in which these students function.

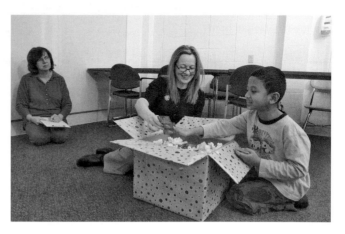

School-aged children with severe disorders may continue to function at developing language levels.

Three considerations are especially important in designing assessments that work toward this goal: assessing need for augmentative and alternative communication, using chronologically age-appropriate materials, and evaluating functional communicative needs.

Our first consideration for a child with limited language should address augmentative and alternative modalities. We've talked already about the importance of considering AAC systems for children with severe communication disorders. For some older children still functioning at emerging language levels, AAC may not yet have been tried. If it has not, we may want to consider using some of the assessment techniques we talked about in Chapters 6 and 7 to evaluate the child's need for an AAC system. If the child is obviously frustrated with his or her current level of communicative ability, produces speech that is severely unintelligible, or spontaneously uses gestures or other means to augment speech, a trial of AAC, with assessment to identify the most appropriate system, is certainly warranted.

Second, when we do criterion-referenced or observational assessments for the older, severely impaired client, we want to use situations and props that are fitting for a person of this age. We would not use dolls and toys to evaluate adolescents, even if they appear to function at the preschool level of language and cognition. We would want to use materials from the clients' occupational training program or objects from self-care and daily-living activities that they are learning to use or from leisure activities in which they like to engage. We might, for example, assess use of basic subject-verb-object sentences or use of verb + particle by asking a client to tell what is done in each step as he or she makes the bed ("I pull up the sheet. I pull up the blanket. I pull up the spread. I put on the pillow. I tuck in the spread.").

Our third consideration is the functional efficacy of communication. What do our older, severely impaired clients need to get done, and how well do current communication skills enable them to do it? One way to address this problem is to develop an *ecological inventory*. An ecological inventory allows

Language used in home_____

Verbal status: ☐ Nonverbal ☐ Verbal

Highest expressive language level:

☐ Vocalizations ☐ Single words ☐ Phrases ☐ Sentences

☐ Conversation ☐ N/a

Methods of communication (Check all that apply):

☐ Sounds ☐ Speech ☐ Signing ☐ Drawing

☐ Spelling ☐ Facial expression ☐ Gaze ☐ Nods

☐ Gestures ☐ Actions ☐ Pointing ☐ Object manipulation

☐ Manipulates others ☐ Photo book ☐ Picture book/board

☐ Word book/board ☐ Computer with pictures ☐ Computer with word prediction

Functions of communication:

☐ Basic needs ☐ Routines ☐ Preferences ☐ Interests

☐ Emotions ☐ Experiences ☐ Concerns ☐ Opinions

☐ Aspirations ☐ Humor ☐ Ideas ☐ Current events

☐ None ☐ Physical feelings ☐ Social exchanges

FIGURE 8-18 ✦ Expressive language scale of *Functional Communication Profile—Revised* (Adapted from Kleiman, L. [2003]. *Functional Communication Profile—Revised*. East Moline, IL: Linguisystems.)

us to assess the needs of particular *environments* in which the person must function, rather than the client's communication skills. The ecological inventory lets us ask the question, "What does this client need to be able to communicate successfully in this environment?" The assessment then identifies those needs, and the necessary communicative behaviors become the targets of our intervention. These behaviors may not be the next ones in the developmental sequence for this client. However, when clients are severely impaired and we know that they will probably never complete that sequence, the primary goal of intervention is to allow them to function as independently as possible within the world in which they live. For example, our developmental model tells us to follow the normal sequence of language acquisition as a curriculum guide for targeting goals. We know that the normal sequence suggests that we

would not teach reading to a child with a mental age less than 5 years or to one who had not mastered Brown's stage V of language development. But suppose an adolescent client with linguistic skills in the developing language phase had an opportunity for a paying job unloading boxes from trucks at a warehouse that required him to read some words on the warehouse shelves that indicated where certain boxes were to be placed. Should we deny the client this job because he is not developmentally ready to read? Most of us would like to help the client take advantage of this opportunity. To remove barriers to our client's ability to take advantage of this opportunity, we can use focused behavioral interventions to teach the limited amount of reading the client needs, even if he or she may not appear "ready" to read with regard to developmental level.

To compile an ecological inventory, McCormick and Goldman (1984) suggested looking at the major domains in which clients function—for example, domestic, occupational, recreational, and general community—and assessing the communicative needs of each of these settings. Do clients need to ask for help in turning on the TV in the group home? Do they have to tell their supervisor they need to use the restroom at work? Do they need to ask for a locker key at the pool at the YMCA? These needs can be identified by the ecological inventory and targeted in the intervention program.

The ecological inventory can be assembled in two ways. We can "shadow" clients for a typical day, going through each of their activities with them and noting the communicative demands of the situation. Alternatively, we can interview adults familiar with each of the major domains of the client's functioning and compile a list of the communicative needs these adults identify. Parents, of course, are important sources of information in putting this inventory together.

A more structured approach to developing ecological inventories was presented by Rowland and Schweigert (1993). They devised the *Analyzing the Communication Environment (ACE)* as a tool to guide clinicians in establishing these inventories. To use the ACE, a clinician observes one activity on at least two occasions, starting when the student makes a transition from a previous activity and ending when the activity is completed. The instrument examines six aspects of communication: the activity itself, the communication system the student uses in the activity, the way adults interact with the student in the activity, group dynamics (in group activities), the materials available in the activity, and the specific opportunities for communication that the activity affords. Under each of these aspects, the clinician considers a list of behavior statements given in the ACE and decides whether the behavior is present and whether a change in the behavior is needed. A few examples of the behaviors examined in the ACE are given in Table 8-15, just to give a flavor for the instrument. The ACE also provides

---

TABLE 8-15 **Example Items from Rowland and Schwiegert's ACE**

	CHECK IF OBSERVED	TARGET FOR CHANGE
A. ACTIVITY		
The instructional demands of the activity do not frustrate the student.	_____	_____
The student is receptive to engaging in some level of interaction at this time.	_____	_____
B. STUDENT COMMUNICATION		
The student has an effective and appropriate means of gaining attention in this activity.	_____	_____
The student is positioned so that he or she is aware that the teacher is present.	_____	_____
C. ADULT INTERACTION		
The teacher appears to enjoy the activity.	_____	_____
The teacher communicates to the student in a mode the student can understand.	_____	_____
D. GROUP DYNAMICS		
The group includes at least one peer who is a more competent communicator than the student.	_____	_____
The teacher switches easily from one communication system to another, if needed.	_____	_____
E. MATERIALS		
The materials are used for turn-taking. That is, the student and teacher take turns back and forth using the materials.	_____	_____
The student seems to enjoy this material.	_____	_____
F. OPPORTUNITIES FOR COMMUNICATION		
Teacher or peers offer choices of materials, tasks, or partners.	_____	_____
Teachers or peers ask yes/no questions for the student to confirm or negate.	_____	_____

Adapted from Rowland, C., & Schweigert, P. (1993). *Analyzing the communication environment (ACE): An inventory of ways to encourage communication in functional activities.* Tucson, AZ: Communication Skill Builders.

a videotape with example interactions and accompanying text discussing these examples and showing how each would be scored. Once needed changes are identified, the ACE also provides helpful suggestions for making the changes. These suggestions include both targeting the client's behavior and modifying the interactive environment to facilitate functional communicative success for the client. Other structured instruments for compiling ecological inventories also are available, such as McCarthy et al.'s (1998) *Communication Supports Checklist*.

Cascella and McNamara (2004) present an additional approach. They advocate that the clinician develop an individualized "communication profile" for each student, based on in-depth observation and interviews with caregivers and teachers, which lists the forms and functions the student currently uses for communication. These can include conventional forms, such as vocalizations and gestures, as well as idiosyncratic forms, such as body postures. An ecological inventory is then completed that assesses the environments in which the student must function and outlines typical discourse structures, communication expectations, and opportunities. Finally, the educational team meets to develop a support plan focused on enabling the child to use the communication strategies he or she has to meet the expectations of the classroom and other daily routines. The team's job is then to create additional communication opportunities to allow the student to use, expand, and diversify communicative acts. For example, if the team knows that a student's current communication profile includes tilting her head to the left when she needs to take a break from working, her job coach can acknowledge this communication ("I see you're tired") and encourage the student to express her need in a more conventional way that meets the expectations of the setting ("At work we need to let people know when we are stopping. Let's go to your supervisor and use our sign for 'stop.'")

The main point to remember about assessment of functional communication for students with severe-to-profound disorders is that we need not only to assess our clients' ability to communicate, but also the demands of the environment in which they function. An important part of our role for these clients is to help achieve a better match between the student's communicative ability and the expectations of their environments in order to create more opportunities for their communication to succeed in accomplishing their interpersonal goals.

■ CONCLUSIONS

Assessing the child with a language disorder at the developing language stage sounds like a big job. It is! Of course, not every single aspect of the assessment process is necessary for every child. Every assessment will, though, always be family-centered. That means, remember, being responsive to the interests and concerns of the family; being sure that they are involved in all the decisions made about assessment and

intervention for the child; and respecting their culture, traditions, and personal style. Let's go back to Jerry. Taking him as an example, we can see how to use history and referral information to develop an assessment plan. As in any plan, we will be choosing tests and procedures to use in the evaluation process based on the areas we suspect may be problematic for the client and on the need to identify specific goals for the intervention program.

Jerry's family brought him to the preschool assessment center of their local school district for an evaluation, as Mrs. Hamilton suggested. They met with the assessment team leader and the speech-language pathologist, Ms. Warren. Ms. Warren asked the parents about Jerry's medical and feeding history; asked about how Jerry had vocalized as a baby; and wanted to know more about how, from the parents' point of view, he was communicating now. She asked them what their major concerns for Jerry were and how the assessment could help them understand his needs. The parents expressed some dismay with some of the things that Mrs. Hamilton had told them. They said they did not see Jerry's problems as serious. They were clear in their desire to have Jerry take an IQ test to "prove" to Mrs. Hamilton that he was not retarded. They weren't sure what they would do if the assessment identified a language disorder in Jerry. They felt confused and somewhat overwhelmed. They said they had never had a child with a problem before. They wanted to know what Ms. Warren thought. Was Jerry behind? Would he catch up? Did he need special help?

After this discussion, Ms. Warren explained that she would like to have Jerry's hearing tested before proceeding any further. She also said she would like to have a look at how Jerry was able to use his oral structures for speech and nonspeech functions. She explained that she doubted that Jerry was retarded and asked whether the parents would feel comfortable if she did an informal assessment of cognitive skills through drawing. She explained that if there were any question of retardation she would talk with them further before taking any action. The parents agreed to this plan. When Jerry passed a hearing screening and did not appear to have any serious oral-motor problems, Ms. Warren asked whether the parents would be willing to bring Jerry back again for a more in-depth evaluation in a week or two. She explained that language learning is an extremely complex process and that many children run into obstacles along the way. She told them that even without intervention most children like Jerry eventually outgrew many of their difficulties. But she explained that, in her experience, many preschoolers were helped by the extra boost that focused intervention during the preschool period provided. She asked them not to make up their minds yet, but to consider the possibility of some short-term intervention to jump-start Jerry's language development, if the assessment indicated that it might be helpful. Jerry's parents agreed to reserve judgment until the assessment was completed.

After reviewing the referral information from Mrs. Hamilton and her notes from the pre-assessment interview, Ms. Warren devised the assessment plan.

AREA TO BE ASSESSED	ASSESSMENT TOOL
Nonverbal cognitive skill	*Draw-a-Person Intellectual Ability test for Children, Adolescents, and Adults* (Reynolds & Hickman, 2004)
Expressive vocabulary	*Expressive One-Word Picture Vocabulary Test—Revised* (Brownell, 2000)
Receptive vocabulary and syntax, expressive syntax, phonological skills	*Test of Language Development*—Primary (Newcomer & Hammill, 1997)

FOLLOW-UP CRITERION-REFERENCE PROCEDURES TO BE USED, IF JERRY SCORES BELOW THE NORMAL RANGE IN RECEPTION, EXPRESSION, OR PHONOLOGY:

Expressive language	Language sample analysis, using IPSyn procedure. If needed, use elicited production tasks to look at structures that did not appear in spontaneous speech.
Phonology	Intelligibility in short conversational sample; phonetic inventory and phonological process analysis; if needed, using NPA procedure on same sample used for IPSyn.
Pragmatics	"Peanut Butter Protocol"

Ms. Warren conducted the formal portion of the assessment and shared the results with the parents. She explained that Jerry's nonverbal cognitive skills and his receptive vocabulary and sentence structures were age-appropriate, so further testing in these areas was not needed. However, the tests suggested that his expressive vocabulary and syntax and his phonological skills were below age level. She asked the parents whether they would be willing to return and allow her to audiotape one of them playing with Jerry so she could collect a sample of his speech and to allow her to play with him for a while to get a picture of the way he participated in communicative situations. She explained that the information she got from these assessments would be helpful in determining the specific targets of an intervention program, if the parents decided Jerry could benefit from one.

The results of the criterion-referenced assessment revealed the following:

1. Jerry's speech-sample analysis, according to the IPSyn, showed that his score was significantly depressed. His noun phrase performance was adequate, but his use of verb phrases showed no structures above the level of simple copulas (V5). Questions and negatives also were limited in complexity. He produced no questions or negatives with auxiliaries (scored "0" on Q6, Q7, and Q8); no "why" questions; and no tag questions. On the sentence structure scale, he produced forms up to the conjoined phrase and simple infinitive level (S5 and S6), but none higher. Jerry's use of syntax showed deficits in the areas of verb phrase elaboration, use of negative and question forms, and use of advanced sentence structures.

2. As seen in Figure 8-4, the sounds that are absent from Jerry's inventory are all in the middle or late groups, according to Shriberg's (1993) scheme. This suggests that Jerry's phonological development is delayed rather than deviant. Some of the sounds on which Jerry makes errors, such as /k/, /g/, /s/, /f/, and /r/, do appear in the inventory, suggesting that he knows "how" to say these sounds. The process analysis shows that most of Jerry's processes are used inconsistently. This suggests that he can sometimes "tune up" his pronunciation to make it more accurate. Only /f/ and /v/ are dropped consistently at the ends of words, and only /θ/ is consistently stopped. Only initial clusters are consistently simplified; at least one final cluster appears in correct form. Jerry does produce some multisyllabic words, with better accuracy in two syllables than in three. The processes he uses are all typical in development; no "other" processes are listed in the Notes section. This again suggests delayed phonological development.

3. Analysis of Jerry's errors on the *Expressive One-Word Picture Vocabulary Test* showed that he had difficulty producing category labels, such as vegetables and furniture, even though he could produce words for individual items such as *potato* and *chair*.

4. Jerry's performance on the "Peanut Butter Protocol" showed that he performed adequately in terms of expressing communicative intentions and using conversational devices to engage in social interaction.

Ms. Warren suggested to the parents that Jerry could benefit from some intervention to improve his expressive language and articulation. She suggested that he be enrolled in the district's preschool language classroom, a language-focused preschool group taught by an SLP. However, the language classroom met at the same time as Jerry's mainstream preschool program, and the parents were reluctant to withdraw Jerry from that. Ms. Warren suggested that perhaps the parents would be willing to work with her on a consultative basis. She would talk to Mrs. Hamilton about some special activities to be done with Jerry within the mainstream preschool program and would give the parents activities to do with Jerry at home. She would make a home visit once a month to see how things were going, assess Jerry's progress, and suggest additional activities. She proposed that they try this plan for 6 months and see how things went. At that point everyone could re-evaluate the situation. The parents agreed to this plan and were very eager to do what they could to help Jerry at home. They agreed to meet again with Ms. Warren and Mrs. Hamilton to set up the ongoing consultative program.

STUDY GUIDE

I. The Developing Language Stage
   A. What is meant by "developing language" in terms of identification and assessment of language disorders?
   B. What language characteristics are seen in children at this level of language development?
II. Family-Centered Assessment
   A. What does IDEA legislation require in terms of family participation?

B. How can parents be involved in the assessment of their child with developing language?

C. What are the family's rights if conflicts arise between them and the assessment team about recommendations for services for their child?

III. Assessing Collateral Areas

A. How would a language pathologist working in a transdisciplinary team assess areas collateral to language development? How would a clinician in private practice do so?

B. Discuss three ways to assess nonverbal cognitive skills in children with developing language.

IV. Screening for Language Disorders in the Period of Developing Language

A. Discuss the important properties to look for when choosing a screening instrument for children with developing language.

B. Why is it important to read the statistical information provided when choosing a screening instrument?

V. Using Standardized Tests in Assessing Developing Language

A. What is the purpose of using standardized tests in assessment of developing language?

B. Why do standardized tests often not provide enough information for intervention planning?

VI. Criterion-Referenced Assessment and Behavioral Observation for Children with Developing Language

A. How is criterion-referenced assessment used to supplement standardized testing?

B. What is the role of intelligibility assessment in phonological evaluation?

C. Discuss methods of criterion-referenced phonological assessment.

D. What are some of the difficulties and dangers of assessing the unintelligible child?

E. How does the concept of "fast mapping" affect the assessment of vocabulary skills?

F. How can word retrieval skills be assessed in a child with developing language?

G. Describe a general strategy for assessing vocabulary skills in children with developing language.

H. Why must receptive and expressive syntax be assessed separately?

I. Discuss the assessment of contextualized and decontextualized comprehension skills.

J. Describe two methods for nonstandardized assessment of decontextualized comprehension; of contextualized comprehension.

K. Why and how do we assess comprehension strategies?

L. What is the role of speech-sample analysis in assessing productive syntax and morphology?

M. What situations, partners, and materials are best for collecting a speech sample from a child with developing language?

N. How is MLU computed, and for what purposes is it used? What are its advantages and disadvantages?

O. Discuss how the efficiency of speech sampling can be increased.

P. Compare and contrast the Assigning Structural Stage Procedure, IPSyn, and DSS procedures.

Q. What is the purpose of using elicited production procedures in criterion-referenced assessment? Give two examples of elicited production activities.

R. What is the goal of pragmatic assessment for a child with developing language? Discuss four methods of pragmatic assessment.

S. How can the results of a pragmatic assessment be used in intervention planning?

VII. Considerations for Assessing Older Clients with Severe Impairment at the Developing Language Level

A. What is meant by providing *access* and *opportunity* for older students with severe language disorders?

B. Discuss the use of an ecological inventory to assess the communicative needs of an older, severely impaired client.

C. What areas of interaction can be examined in an ecological inventory?

D. Describe the way in which an SLP develops a communication profile for a severely affected client, and how the profile can be used in supporting the student's communication in everyday settings.

Brown's stage

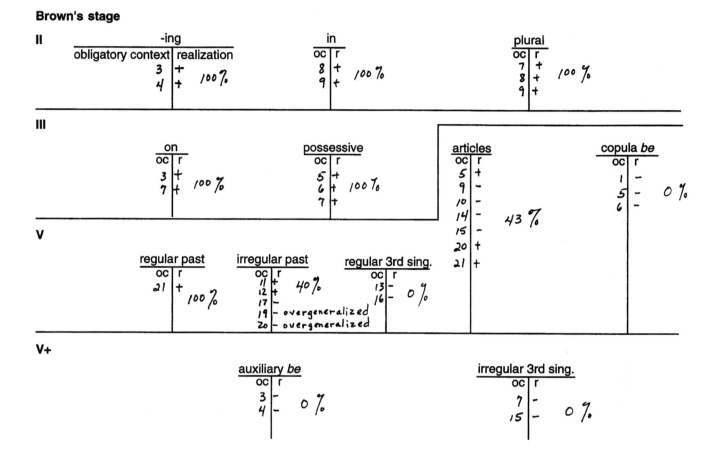

II

-ing		
obligatory context	realization	
3	+	
4	+	*100%*

in		
oc	r	
8	+	
9	+	*100%*

plural		
oc	r	
7	+	
8	+	*100%*
9	+	

III

on		
oc	r	
3	+	
7	+	*100%*

possessive		
oc	r	
5	+	
6	+	*100%*
7	+	

articles		
oc	r	
5	+	
9	–	
10	–	
14	–	*43%*
15	–	
20	+	
21	+	

copula *be*		
oc	r	
1	–	
5	–	*0%*
6	–	

V

regular past		
oc	r	
21	+	*100%*

irregular past		
oc	r	
11	+	*40%*
12	+	
17	–	
19	– *overgeneralized*	
20	– *overgeneralized*	

regular 3rd sing.		
oc	r	
13	–	*0%*
16	–	

V+

auxiliary *be*		
oc	r	
3	–	*0%*
4	–	

irregular 3rd sing.		
oc	r	
7	–	*0%*
15	–	

Sentence Structure Analysis of Transcript in Box 8-5

Name_____ Developmental Level_____ Age _____ Date_____

Stage	NP	S*	A+	VP	S*	A+	Negative	S*	A+	Question	S	A	Complex	S*	A+
I	NP alone (not in sentence context) with modifier Pronouns: *I, me*	C2 C3 C4 C10 C18		Unmarked V Absent copula Absent auxiliary	C3, C4 C9 C13 C15 C16 C17		*No* or *not* + *NP* or *VP*			Routines: *What . . .? What ... doing? What ... going?*	C1				
II	Noun modified in object position Pronouns: *my, it*	C5		Main V marked occasionally *-ing* w/o *be* Catenative alone w/o NP Copula appears occasionally	C11 C12 C21	C13 C15 C16 C17 C9	*NP* + {*No, not, can't,* or *don't*} + *VP*	C6 C7		*What* or *Where* + (N) + V					
III	Modified NP may appear in subject position Demonstratives *(this, that, these, those)* and articles *(a, an, the)* appear Pronouns: *you, your, she, them, he, we, her*	C20 C21	C9 C10 C14	Auxiliaries: *can, will* Overgeneralized past tense	C2 C18 C19 C20		*Won't*			Aux. Vs appear in Wh-Qs, W/o inversion Yes-no Qs produced w/ rising intonation only Q words: *why, who, how, whose*	C2 C3 C4 C5 C8				

Stage	NP	S*	A+	VP	S*	A+	Negative	S*	A+	Question	S	A	Complex	S*	A+
EIV	Subject NP is obligatory; appears in all sentences	C6 C8 C9 C10 C11 C13 C15 C16 C17 C18 C19 C20 C21		Past modals: *could, should, would, must, might* Catenative + NP			*Isn't, aren't, didn't, doesn't*		C6	Auxiliary Vs and "dummy do" forms appear in wh- and yes/no Qs and are inverted Q words: *when*		C2 C3 C4 C5 C8	*Let's, Let me* Simple infinitive Full proposition Simple wh- Conjoining Conj.:*and*		
LIV-EV	NP can contain three elements Pronouns: *his, him, us, they, our, its*	C16 C8 C19					*Wasn't weren't, couldn't wouldn't, shouldn't*						Double embedding Conjoining and embedding w/in one S		
LV	Pronouns: *myself, yourself, their*			have + *en*									Infin. w / diff.subj. Relative clause Conj.: *if*		
V+	Pronouns: *herself, himself, themselves, ourselves*												Gerund Wh- infinitive *Help, make, watch, let* Conj.:*because*		
V++													Conj.: *when, so*		

*Successful use.
†Attempt; incorrect use.

Name: _____

Birth Date: _____

Recording Date: _____

CA: _____

DSS = Total score ÷ Number of Utterances (50)

Sen-Tence #	Indef. Pro.	Pers. Pro.	Main Verb	Sec. Verb	Neg.	Conj.	Inter. Rev.	Wh- Q	Sent. Pt.	Total
C1	3	1,1	—						0	5
C3		1	4		4				1	10
C8	1		1						1	3
C9	—	1	—		—				0	9
C11		1	2						1	4
C12		1	1	2					1	5
C13	1	1	2	2					1	7
C17		—,1	1		4				0	9
C22		1	—						0	1
C23	3	1	1						0	5
C26	1		1						1	3
C28			1				—		0	1
C29	1	1	1	2					1	6

Sen-Tence #	Indef. Pro.	Pers. Pro.	Main Verb	Sec. Verb	Neg.	Conj.	Inter. Rev.	Wh- Q	Sent. Pt.	Total
C30		1	2						1	4
C31	1		1						1	3
C32	1		1						1	3
C33	1		1						1	3
C34	1		1						1	3
C35	1	1,6	—,1				—		0	9
C37	1	3	1						1	6
C39	1	1	2						1	5
C40	1		2						1	4
C41	1		2					2	1	6
C42	3	1	—	2					0	6
C43	1		1				1	2	1	6
C45	1	1	2						1	5
C47		1,3	1						1	6
C48		2	1						1	4
C49		2	1						1	4
C50		2,2	1,2			3			1	11

INTERVENTION FOR DEVELOPING LANGUAGE

CHAPTER OBJECTIVES

Readers of this chapter will be able to do the following:

- Discuss intervention policy issues at the developing language level.
- Describe intervention goals appropriate for developing language.
- List a range of intervention procedures with an evidence base in the developing language period.

- Describe various contexts for intervention at the developing language level.
- Discuss intervention issues and strategies for older clients with severe impairment who function at the developing language level.

Rachel was a friendly, likable little girl who loved to talk even though people sometimes had trouble understanding what she said. She was born with Down syndrome and had been enrolled in early intervention since she was an infant, first in a home program and later in a mainstream preschool, with special services in speech-language and special education provided by the local school district. Now she was close to 7 years old. Her parents were very committed to continuing mainstream education for Rachel, and her preschool teacher, special educator, and speech-language pathologist (SLP) thought Rachel could function in a mainstream kindergarten class, with some support services. Her school district and the kindergarten teacher were somewhat hesitant to go along with this plan. The kindergarten teacher was afraid Rachel would "hold her class back." The school district felt it would be more manageable logistically to provide services in a self-contained program for children with mental retardation, which was housed on the other side of town from Rachel's home. The school district developed an Individualized Educational Plan (IEP) for Rachel that included the self-contained class placement. At the IEP meeting, the parents rejected that plan, insisting that Rachel be allowed to try the kindergarten class in the neighborhood school. Reluctantly, the school-district team agreed to the plan and devised a range of special services that Rachel would receive within the classroom setting, including special education, speech-language pathology, and occupational therapy.

Ms. Snyder was to deliver the SLP services for Rachel. The IEP team had done a thorough assessment in several areas, including speech and language. The assessment report stated that Rachel's cognitive skills were close to a 5-year level, and her receptive language scores were between 42 and 54 months in most areas assessed. Her expressive skills, including vocabulary, phonology, expressive syntax, and morphology, were uniformly lower, though. She used a variety of phonological processes and was moderately unintelligible. Her sentences were primarily two or three words long with absent verb marking and grammatical morphemes and frequent errors in pronoun use. She was a good communicator, though, eager to initiate conversation, responsive to others' speech, and able to express a variety of communicative functions with the language she had at her disposal. Ms. Snyder met with the kindergarten teacher to begin to develop a program that would address Rachel's needs for language intervention and help her to succeed in the classroom.

Rachel is a child who, although older than preschool age, functions in the developing language (DL) period, the time at which words are combined in sentences but fully grammatical forms and a full range of meaning have not yet been acquired. Like children who are chronologically of preschool age, children Rachel's age or even older who have not yet mastered all the basic structures and functions of language typically acquired during the preschool years can be candidates for interventions that follow some of the principles and methods discussed in this chapter. Before looking in detail at the goals, procedures, and contexts of intervention for children with DL, though, let's look at some of the legislation and social policy issues we need to be aware of when designing intervention programs for children at this level.

INTERVENTION POLICY ISSUES AT THE DEVELOPING LANGUAGE LEVEL

INDIVIDUALIZED EDUCATIONAL PLANS

We talked in Chapters 6 and 7 about the reauthorized Individuals with Disabilities Education Act (IDEA) of 2004, the federal law that mandates free, appropriate public education (FAPE) for all children with handicaps. Part B of IDEA is concerned with school-age children, but its mandate extends to 3- to 5-year-olds as well. We talked about using the Individualized Family Service Plan (IFSP) mandated under IDEA to plan intervention services for infants, toddlers, and their families. Educational plans for preschoolers and for older children with disabilities who function at DL levels, however, may be written in a somewhat different format. This format is the Individualized Educational Program (IEP). IEPs differ from IFSPs in several ways. The content and format are somewhat dissimilar. The biggest difference is that the focus of the IEP is on the child, rather than on the family. IEPs do not by any means leave the family out of the picture, though. IDEA has some very specific requirements about how families participate in the process of developing an IEP. Family members are considered part of the IEP team. They must be notified of an IEP meeting with sufficient time for them to arrange to attend. The meeting must be at a time that is convenient for both educational staff and parents. The parents have the right to accept or reject the IEP and to request that modifications be made to it. They also must approve the plan being proposed for the child before any program is initiated. A sample IEP format is provided in Appendix 12-1.

FAMILY-CENTERED PRACTICE

The best practice for all our clients is family-centered; this is especially true for young children. Does this mean that family members must deliver the intervention? Not necessarily. As we discussed in Chapter 7 when we talked about intervention for emerging language, we need to remember that every family is different. For some families, having parents be primary agents of intervention makes sense. In these families, parents may feel they want to be centrally involved in their child's program, that they have the time and energy to devote to delivering the intervention, and that they are comfortable with the shift in role from parent to teacher.

Other families may not feel able or eager to take on that role but will want to have some supplementary part to play. They may want to do small amounts of "homework" to follow up on what is being done in the intervention setting. They may want to observe the intervention without participating directly. Other families may feel more comfortable having the large majority of the intervention done by "the pros." They may just want periodic updates on the child's progress. Family-centered intervention means respecting the family's wishes on the extent to which they want to be involved. Although we always want to encourage families to be as involved as possible and set up the intervention situation so that they can achieve this level of involvement, we never want to make families feel inadequate about the level of contribution they can make.

A second issue in family-centered intervention involves the extent to which families are involved in the choice of intervention goals and methods. As we discussed in Chapter 3, for most clients there are more potential goals than there is intervention time to achieve them. This means we must pick and choose among the potential targets. In Chapter 3, we talked about some criteria to use in making this selection, such as teachability, functionality, and so on. Another factor to be considered, though, is family preference. Families are very likely to have feelings and opinions about areas in which they would like their child to show improvement. This information is an important part of the intervention planning process. We have an obligation, in family-centered practice, both to elicit this information from parents and to take it seriously in devising the intervention program.

Take Rachel as our example again. Suppose her parents felt that an important communicative goal was to get her to use "good sentences" such as "I'm hungry" and "He's a friend" instead of "Me hungry" and "Him friend," as she currently does. They feel these kinds of usages make Rachel sound babyish and will cause her problems among her peers in the kindergarten class. Perhaps the language clinician feels that such sentences containing copula verbs that agree in person and number with nominative pronouns are not the most appropriate goal, since Rachel is still lacking developmentally earlier forms. Who's right? In family-centered intervention, being right is not necessarily the issue. Perhaps the more important question is, How can this disagreement be resolved so that Rachel's development is the foremost consideration? The clinician can communicate, in a clear, respectful, and nonthreatening way, her opinion that Rachel is not yet ready to meet the standard of these "good sentences" and needs to learn other areas of language to serve as a basis for these later acquisitions. But suppose Rachel's family continues to assert a strong desire to have Rachel work toward this goal. Family-centered practice dictates that we concede the parents' right to determine what is important for their child to learn. Even if we do not entirely agree with the family's choice of communicative goals for their child, we have an obligation to honor the family's wishes if at all possible and to use family priorities in selecting and sequencing intervention goals.

Family-centered practice for the child with DL, just as for the child at other stages of language acquisition, means actively involving the family in all levels of decision-making about the child's program. It means having meaningful and serious discussions about the assessment findings and sincerely soliciting the parents' input as we design the intervention program. It means deciding with the family how much direct involvement with the intervention program they feel able to manage and how much professional input they want. Finally, it means remembering that even our best clinical judgment must occasionally take a back seat to the parents' desires for their children.

INTERVENTION FOR DEVELOPING LANGUAGE: PRODUCTS, PROCESSES, AND CONTEXTS

In Chapter 3, we talked about three aspects of intervention that McLean (1989) suggested we consider when designing a management plan for a child with a language disorder: the *products* or intended goals of the intervention, the *processes* or methods used to achieve these goals, and the *context* or physical and social milieu in which the intervention takes place. Let's look at each of these aspects of the intervention program and see how they apply to children in the DL phase.

INTERVENTION PRODUCTS: GOALS FOR CHILDREN WITH DEVELOPING LANGUAGE

For many children who, like Rachel, are within or only a few years beyond the preschool period chronologically, goals of intervention include some of the forms and functions acquired by typical children between 3 and 5 years of age. Some special considerations are involved in planning intervention programs for older, severely impaired clients still in the DL phase, which we will discuss later. In general, though, the goals for language intervention in this phase are to help the child acquire intelligible, grammatical, flexible forms of expression for the ideas and concepts the child has in mind, to give the child the tools to make communication effective, efficient, and rewarding so that social interaction proceeds as normally as possible, and to provide the oral language basis for success in literacy. As discussed in the previous chapter, the preschool years are normally a period of exponential language growth, when children with typical development move from mean lengths of utterance of less than two words to more than five. Another way to describe this period is to say it is the interval between Brown's (1973) stages II and V+, the period of the acquisition of basic structures, functions, and meanings of the language. Table 9-1 reviews some of the major changes that take place in the language of normally developing children during the preschool years. These milestones provide a basis for establishing the goals of intervention at the DL level.

One thing you will probably notice right away about the list in Table 9-1. It's long. Not every child with DL will achieve everything on this list during the intervention period. As always, we will have to choose intervention goals judiciously. Knowing the normal sequence of acquisition is necessary to make these decisions. But it is not enough. Other considerations, such as those discussed in Chapter 3 and those we just talked about in terms of family involvement, must come into play. Later we'll talk more about the issue of choosing intervention goals for the older, severely impaired client. Let's look now at each of the major areas of intervention goals for children with DL and discuss some of the considerations necessary to establish individual targets in each one.

Phonology

We talked in the previous chapter about how to decide when and how to assess phonological production and how to distinguish between articulatory and phonological types of speech disorders. In general, children at developing levels of language are not candidates for phonological intervention unless their intelligibility is significantly impaired. Because so much phonological growth is going on in the DL period, intervention for particular sounds can usually be deferred until school age, since many speech sound problems resolve on their own by then (Shriberg & Kwiatkowski, 1994). However, if a child is seriously unintelligible, intervention is warranted. Social disvalue and even social isolation, as well as frustration and behavioral and emotional reactions, can occur in children who have difficulty in getting messages across, even if they would eventually outgrow the unintelligibility. Although the specific targets of the intervention in this area will be the acquisition of particular sounds or the suppression of particular simplification processes, we need to remember that the important long-term goal is to increase the client's overall intelligibility. All the issues we discussed in Chapter 3 about being careful to ensure that behaviors learned in intervention generalize to real conversation must be addressed to ensure that phonological production improvement leads to real gains in intelligibility. Gordon-Brannan and Hodson (2000), Kent, Miolo, and Bloedel (1994), and Morris, Wilcox, and Schooling (1995) discussed a variety of instruments that can be used to evaluate changes in intelligibility in the course of an intervention program.

We need to remember, too, that assessing syntactic and semantic skills in unintelligible children is always important; in order to avoid missing deficits in these areas that are masked by the difficulty in understanding what the client says. When assessment of an unintelligible child indicates that syntactic and semantic deficits are present, it makes sense to address those targets early in the intervention program, rather than waiting until the child is fully intelligible. One way to address them is through input, providing indirect language stimulation, focused stimulation, or auditory bombardment (see Comprehension versus Production Targets, later in the chapter) of the forms we want the child to begin learning. These activities can be supplemented with more direct production activities that control for pronounceability of target words. In general, in accordance with our principle of requiring the client to do only one new thing at a time, we will want to address phonological and semantic/syntactic targets *separately*, not within the same activity. However, Tyler, Lewis, Haskill, and Tolbert (2002, 2003) showed that when children have both phonological and morphosyntactic deficits, working on morphosyntax leads to changes in both areas. This research suggests that for children with both speech and language problems, morphosyntactic deficits should be addressed first, followed by work on whatever phonological targets have not resolved in the course of the first segment of intervention.

One further consideration in planning phonological intervention at the preschool level concerns the connection between phonology and metaphonology. *Metaphonology,* or phonological awareness (PA), is the ability to detect rhyme and

TABLE 9-1	Milestones of Normal Communicative Development: Preschool Years

AREA	GOALS
Phonology	Increase consonant repertoire.
	Increase production of closed syllables.
	Decrease use of phonological processes.
	Increase production of multisyllabic words.
	Increase accuracy of sound production.
	Increase intelligibility.
Semantics	Increase vocabulary size.
	Increase use of verbs for specific actions (sweep, slide, bend, fold, etc.).
	Increase appropriate pronoun use.
	Increase understanding and use of basic concept vocabulary (spatial terms, temporal terms, diectic terms, kinship terms, color terms, etc.).
	Increase range of semantic relations expressed within sentences (possession, recurrence, location, etc.).
	Increase range of semantic relations expressed between clauses (sequential, causal, conditional, etc.).
	Increase use of appropriate conjunctions (*but, so,* etc.).
Syntax	Increase sentence length.
	Increase sentence complexity (use of prepositional phrases, noun modifiers, verb marking, etc.).
	Increase use of a variety of sentence types (questions, negatives, conjoined and embedded, passives, etc.).
	Increase use of appropriate auxiliary verbs (*can, will, must, have, is, are,* etc.).
	Increase use of copula verbs (*is, am, was, were,* etc.).
	Increase understanding of word order in sentences.
Morphology	Increase use of simple morphemes on nouns (plural, possessives, etc.).
	Increase use of verb markers (tense, number, aspect, etc.).
	Increase use of higher-level morphemes (*-er, -est,* etc.).
	Increase appropriate use of articles (*a, an, the*).
Pragmatics	Increase use of verbal forms of communication.
	Increase use of language to achieve communicative goals.
	Increase flexibility of language forms for various contexts.
	Increase ability to initiate communication with appropriate forms.
	Expand range of communicative intentions expressed with a variety of language forms.
	Increase ability to maintain conversational topics.
	Increase ability to manage conversational turn-taking, topic-shifting.
	Begin to use various genres of language (e.g., narration).
	Increase ability to make and request conversational repair.
Play and thinking	Increase ability to use objects to represent others.
	Increase use of pretend and imaginative play.
	Increase play that involves social role-playing.
	Increase ability to use language to foster abstract thought.
	Increase ability to use language to negotiate peer interactions.
	Increase ability to use language to self-monitor and inhibit aggressive behavior.
Preliteracy	Listen to stories; talk about pictures and events in books.
	Look at books independently; orient book properly, turn pages.
	Recognize parts of books: pages, title, orientation of print.
	Recognize words in print (e.g., find first word on a page, count words on a page).
	Begin to develop metalinguistic and phonological awareness:
	Develop awareness of rhyme.
	Count syllables in words.
	Sing alphabet song; identify letters.
	Begin to be able to segment words into syllable and sound units.
	Know what a *word* is.
	Identify words that start/end with the same sound.
	Count sounds in words.
	Match sounds and letters.

alliteration; to segment words into smaller units, such as syllables and phonemes; to synthesize separated phonemes into words; and to understand that words are made up of sounds that can be represented by written symbols or letters. These PA skills develop sequentially through the late preschool period (Hodson, 1994; Swank, 1999). Several of these abilities have been shown to be closely related to success in learning to read (Scarborough, 2003; Swank, 1994, 1999) and spell (Bourassa & Treiman, 2001; Clarke-Klein & Hodson, 1995; Gillon, 2002). Bird et al. (1995), Larrivee and Catts (1999), and Rvachew et al. (2003) have shown that children with productive phonological problems during the DL period sometimes have trouble acquiring PA and are at risk for developing reading problems. This suggests that when working with preschoolers who have phonological production problems, incorporating PA activities within the speech therapy may be helpful in preventing literacy difficulties. A few studies have shown that doing so does improve both speech and PA in children with speech delays (Hesketh, Adams, Nightingale, & Hall, 2000; Van Kleeck, Gillam, & McFadden, 1998), although the interpretation of these results is still somewhat controversial (Dodd & Gillon, 2001). Since incorporating PA activities in speech therapy may help shore up preliteracy weakness in these children, clinicians can consider including PA activities in speech training for preschool children. Jenkins and Bowen (1994) provide some suggestions for doing this. They appear in Box 9-1. Noble-Sanderson (1993) and Kiewel and Claeys (1999) also provided phonology programs built around storybook activities that integrate speech-sound remediation with the development of PA for children at the DL level.

| **BOX 9-1** | **Phonological Awareness Activities for Use in a Phonological Production Program at the Developing Language Level** |

Developing Rhyming Skills

1. Using a "pocket chart," present a card with a picture of a word containing one of the client's target sounds in one pocket in each row. Have the client find a picture, from a set the clinician provides, for a word that rhymes with each, and place it in the pocket next to its "rhyming buddy."
2. Prepare a set of cards with pictures whose names contain the client's target sounds. Have some rhyming and some non-rhyming pairs in the set. Present a pair of pictures. Name each picture, and then ask the client whether the two rhyme.
3. Make up rhymes for words targeted in the speech-sound program.
4. Use rhyming words to work on sounds in final position. Point out the rhymes to clients. Encourage clients to make up new words with the same ending. Accept nonsense words.
5. Use written forms of target rhyming words as cues, along with pictures. Point out that the rhyming words have the same letters at the end in the written form.
6. Write "word family" stories with clients. Choose a rhyming-word family containing a target sound in final position (such as the -us family for work on final /s/). Have clients make a list of words in that family, and write the list on the board (e.g., us, bus, Gus, fuss). Encourage clients to make up a silly story with these words (e.g., "Gus got on the bus with us. He made a big fuss. The bus driver put us off the bus.")
7. Write down the story, and have clients illustrate it. Point out the letter for the target sound at the end of the word. Have the clients "read" the story to each other, to the clinician, and to parents.

Develop Awareness of Syllables

1. Have students tap or clap out the number of syllables contained in words targeted in the speech-remediation program.
2. Play "how many parts" with target words. Include both one- and two-syllable words with target sounds. Have cards containing pictures or cues for each target word. Have clients pick out all the cards for words with only one "part" and pronounce those. Then have clients pick all the cards for words with two "parts."

Develop Phonological Segmentation Skills

1. Use the target sound in initial position. Play an "I spy" game in which clinician and client must "spy" words that begin with the target sound (some may be "planted" around the room) and say them.
2. Display a large card with the alphabet letter or letters representing the target sound (e.g., S or SH). Have the client look through old magazines for pictures of words that begin with the target sound. Give them a bright marker to use to write the letters that represent the target sound on a magazine picture, as they say the word for the picture.
3. Prepare a set of cards with pictures whose names contain the client's target sounds. Have some pairs that begin with the same sound and some that do not in the set. Present a pair of pictures. Name each picture, and then ask the client whether the two begin with the same sound.

BOX 9-1	**Phonological Awareness Activities for Use in a Phonological Production Program at the Developing Language Level—cont'd**

Develop Phonological Segmentation Skills—cont'd

4. A puppet is introduced and named (for example his name could be Sam, if /s/ is one of the client's target sounds). The client is told the puppet likes words that begin with the same sound as his name. The client is asked to say as many words as he or she can that begin with this sound.

5. Use storybooks that include multiple examples of the client's target sound (e.g., *Hop on Pop* [Geisel & Geisel, 1963] for final /p/, or *The Very Busy Spider* [Carle, 1984] for initial /sp/, which appears on every page in the word *spin*). Read the book to the clients. Then read it again, stopping when a word with a target sound appears, allowing the client to say the target word. Point to the printed word as the client "reads" it. Later, have clients search for these "magic" words with their target sounds themselves, and have them point to the words in the book as they say them.

6. Have clients make up silly words that begin or end with target sounds. Let them use invented spelling to write the words, or the clinician can write the target sound for them and let them "guess and go" to spell the rest. Clients can draw pictures of their silly words and put the pictures together in a book that they can "read" to their family to practice their target sounds.

7. Show the client five pictures of words that begin with a target sound. Ask the client to say the first sound in each word. Do the same with five pictures that end with a target sound, and ask the client to say the last sound in each of these words.

Develop Phonological Synthesis Skills

1. Use continuent consonants (/m,n,s,r,f,h,l,v,w,z/) first for synthesis work, since they can be prolonged more naturally. Choose a word family (e.g., *am*). Write the family on a card. Then write several continuent consonants on separate cards, including ones the client is targeting in the intervention program. Place a consonant card by the word family and illustrate blending the consonant with the family to form a word or nonsense word (e.g., s-*am*). Help the client to form various words and nonsense words by combining the consonants with the word family. Let the client write the words formed, and draw pictures to illustrate them. Silly creatures can be used to illustrate the nonsense words.

2. Using several word families worked on in this way, the clinician can say a word and ask the client to find the two cards (consonant and word family) that spell the word being said. Clients can take turns saying words and having the clinician or other client spell out the word with the cards.

Adapted from Jenkins, R., & Bowen, L. (1994). Facilitating development of preliterate children's phonological abilities. *Topics in Language Disorders, 14,* 26-39; and van Kleeck, A., Gillam, R., & McFadden, T. (1998). A study of classroom-based phonological awareness training for preschoolers with speech and/or language disorders. *American Journal of Speech-Language Pathology, 7,* (3), 65-76.

Semantics

Children with language disorders appear to acquire words in comprehension much the way typically developing children do, but may need to hear a new word twice as many times as other children before comprehending and independently using the new word (Gray, 2003; Rice, Buhr, & Oetting, 1992). Children with language impairments also have particular difficulty in the acquisition of verb vocabulary (Loeb, Pye, Redmond, & Richardson, 1996) as well as the use of verb particles (pick *up*, put *down*, etc.) (Watkins, 1994). In addition, children with SLI are less able to identify semantic features than their peers with normal language. These findings suggest that children with SLI have broader difficulties with receptive vocabulary than simply a reduced ability to acquire labels. Providing enriched, repetitive input with special focus on these problem word classes will be an important part of the semantic intervention program.

Owens (2004) provided a list of likely vocabulary targets for the DL period. These appear in Box 9-2.

You'll notice from the list in Table 9-1 that this area contains targets not only in vocabulary, which is of course important, but also in the kinds of semantic relations conveyed within and between clauses of sentences. In the early DL phase, an important goal of intervention is helping children broaden the range of ideas they can talk about. Toward the end of this phase, we want to help clients make their sentences more efficient by combining ideas, or *propositions*, within a sentence to convey specific semantic relations between clauses. Assessment information collected during the standardized and informal portions of the evaluation should guide us toward the level of semantic complexity to target within the client's language.

Remember that when we're planning targets and methods of intervention for language, we artificially segment language into components such as semantics and syntax. But really, when we target a particular sentence type, that sentence is, of course, conveying a meaning. Similarly, when we target a particular

BOX 9-2	**Vocabulary Training Targets during the DL period**

Commonly Used Verbs

Ask
Begin
Break
Build
Buy
Call
Carry
Catch
Clean
Climb
Close
Cook
Copy
Count
Cry
Cut
Do
Dress
Eat
Fall
Feed
Feel
Fight
Find
Finish
Fly
Get
Give
Go
Have
Hear
Hide
Hit
Jump
Keep
Kick
Laugh
Leave
Let
Like
Listen
Look
Lose
Make
Meet
Need
Open
Pick
Play

BOX 9-2	**Vocabulary Training Targets during the DL period—cont'd**

Pull
Push
Put
Read
Roll
Run
Say
See
Shake
Shout
Sing
Sit
Sleep
Stand
Start
Stop
Take care
Talk
Throw
Touch
Wait
Walk
Want
Wash
Write

Descriptive Terms

Big, little
Long, short
Large, small, fat, thin
Soft, hard
Heavy, light
Same/alike, different
Old, young
Pretty, ugly
Blue, red, yellow…
Hot, cold, warm, chilly
Wide, narrow
Thick, thin
Sweet, sour
Nice, mean
Funny, silly, sad
Fast, slow
Rough, smooth
Angry, afraid, happy….
Clean, dirty
Empty, full
Old, new
Loud, quiet
High, low
Dark, light

BOX 9-2 **Vocabulary Training Targets during the DL period—cont'd**

Quantity Terms

One, two, three…
Many, much, lots of
Some few, couple
More, another
Nearly, almost
Less
As much/little as
Plenty
Always, never

Noun Classes

Body parts
Clothing
Foods
Animals
Tools, utensils
Furniture
Kinship terms
Colors
Shapes
Numbers
Letters
Academic items (pencil, blackboard…)

Spatial Terms

In
On
Under
Into
Over
Upside down
(in) Between
Right-side up
Inside, outside
Beside
Behind
Next to
First, last, middle
Above, below
Top, bottom
In front of
In back of
Through
Toward

Temporal Terms

Next
Soon
Later

BOX 9-2 **Vocabulary Training Targets during the DL period—cont'd**

Now
Before
After
Yesterday
Today
Tomorrow
Sometimes
Early, late
Morning, afternoon, evening
Days of week
Months of year
Seasons
Day
Week
Hour
Minute

Conjunctions

And
And then
But
Or
Because
So
If
When
Until
Before/after

Adapted from Owens, 2004.

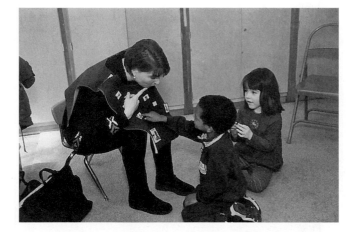

Both speech and language skills are often targeted at the developing language level.

meaning for expression, that expression takes a syntactic form. So in practice it is hard to separate the semantic and syntactic components of sentences. When we plan intervention targets and activities involving semantic and syntactic expression in sentences, the main thing to remember is the principle we talked about in Chapter 3: only one new thing at a time. When asking a child to produce a more complex sentence form, we want to be sure it encodes meanings that the child has already expressed in a simpler way. When asking the child to talk about a new meaning or combine new meanings in sentences, we need to control for syntactic complexity, making sure that the form with which the client is to produce this new meaning is already within the production repertoire.

Syntax and Morphology

Syntactic and morphological targets of intervention are perhaps the most obvious goals of the DL period. Working on production of grammatical forms is among the most traditional aims of language intervention and one most language pathologists feel comfortable targeting. We ought to be aware of two points in selecting our grammatical intervention goals for children in the DL period, though. First, although grammatical goals are virtually always appropriate for children in this period, the need to improve syntax should not lead us to ignore the other areas of intervention that also are important. Many children with grammatical deficits also have unintelligible speech, small vocabularies, word-finding problems, limited preliteracy skills, or difficulties in using language in the service of play, thinking, and conceptual development. These needs ought to be addressed, too.

A second thing we need to bear in mind is that there are some typical patterns of grammatical deficits in children with language impairments (that is, some aspects of syntax and morphology are more likely to show deficits than others). Knowing what these are can help us to zero in on these areas in the assessment process. Let's look at what these typical grammatical problems are for children in the DL period. Bound morphemes are particularly difficult for children with language problems of a variety of etiologies (Goffman & Leonard, 2000; Leonard, 1997; Rice, Warren, & Betz, 2005; Rice & Wexler, 1996). Irregular past morphemes and use of *-ing* endings seem to be a relative strength (Redmond & Rice, 2001; Rice, Warren, & Betz, 2005). Auxiliary verbs and small, closed-class morphemes, such as articles and pronouns, also seem to cause particular difficulties for children with language impairments (Bates, 2003; Beverly & Williams, 2004; Eisenberg, 2005; Rice, Warren, & Betz, 2005). Studies of children with slow expressive-language development as toddlers who show chronic delays through the preschool years (Paul & Riback, 1993; Rescorla & Roberts, 2002) substantiate this pattern. Difficulties with the elaboration of sentences through complex sentence production have also been reported (Eisenberg, 2005; Thordardottir & Weismer, 2001). It would appear, then, that verb marking with auxiliaries and inflections, closed-class morphemes, pronoun use, and the acquisition of complex sentences are areas in which children with language disorders can be expected to show particular difficulties during the DL period. These areas would be espe-

cially appropriate targets for intervention, when, of course, these deficits are documented by the assessment process. Fey, Long, and Finestack (2003) discuss some guiding principles for selecting goals for syntax and morphology during the DL phase. These are summarized in Table 9-2.

Comprehension versus Production Targets

We talked in Chapter 3 about the issue of targeting comprehension as opposed to production in the intervention program. There we said that when assessment indicates a form or meaning is comprehended but not produced, production training is indicated. Lahey (1988) emphasized the fact that equivalent comprehension and production responses are often not present in normal language learners. She argued that a child should be exposed, through multiple meaningful exemplars in the input language, to forms and meanings that are not in the comprehension repertoire. But she concluded that comprehension responses, such as pointing to contrastive stimuli, do *not* need to be trained before production of the forms is targeted. Guided production activities appear to facilitate both comprehension and production of new meanings and forms in children.

Recall, too, that Chapter 3 included some suggestions about targeting comprehension versus production performance in the intervention program. Production training should be a high priority for forms and meanings for which the child demonstrates comprehension. For forms and meanings that the child does not yet appear to comprehend but that are chosen as intervention targets on the basis of other considerations we've discussed, an input component should be part of the intervention plan. This might include focused stimulation or indirect language stimulation activities that provide multiple opportunities for the clinician to demonstrate use of the structure in context.

Auditory bombardment is another viable input option. Hodson and Paden (1991) advocated using this approach to facilitate phonological development. They argued that phonological skills are acquired, at least in part, by listening. This implies that children need to listen carefully and often to the sounds they are being asked to produce. Kouri (2005) showed that, in a vocabulary training program, auditory bombardment had effects comparable to an elicited imitation program on the use of target words in real communication. Hodson and Paden suggested having children listen to a list of target words. It is worth noting that Flexer and Savage (1993) showed that both children with language impairments and those with normal hearing showed improved attention when assistive listening devices were used to improve signal-to-noise ratios during a testing situation. There is, then, some evidence that these devices might be useful in auditory bombardment activities for children with language needs. In auditory bombardment activities, the child simply sits and plays quietly with nondistracting material such as Play-Doh as the clinician reads the list of words. Although traditional auditory bombardment uses simply a list, it might, alternatively, consist of listening to a story that contains numerous examples of target forms. Hoffman, Schuckers, and Daniloff (1989) provided poems and stories that are weighted with examples of phonological targets. Cleave and Fey

TABLE 9-2	Principles of Goal Selection for Grammatical Targets in the Developing Language Period

PRINCIPLE	EXAMPLE

1. Main goal of grammatical intervention: help the child understand and use syntax in the service of communication.
2. Goal attainment must be measured in real communication contexts (conversation or narration).
3. Producing a target at 90% correct in a clinician directed activity is not enough; form must be used in real communication.
4. Grammar is rarely the only aspect of language that needs to be targeted in an intervention program for DL children, who often have small vocabularies, social problems, and often grow to be children with reading disorders.
5. Children with most obvious errors in sentence structure are likely to need support in other areas of communication:
  • Preliteracy
  • Pragmatic skills
  • Vocabulary
6. Contexts such as guided play, mediated conversation, and storybook sharing should be considered.
7. Select goals that trigger changes both within and outside the therapy context:
  • Look for, not just single goals, but ways to change patterns of language.
8. Base goals on "functional readiness" and the communicative need for targeted forms. Target grammatical forms:
  • That the child uses correctly on occasion
  • For which obligatory contexts appear in the child's language.
  • These are more likely to show change than are forms the child does not have any experience with.
9. Children with language disorders need more experience than others to master grammatical forms:
  • Focus on emerging forms to help move them toward mastery more efficiently.
  • Provide frequent and intensive exposure and practice of these forms.
	When *is (verb)-ing* is used 80% correctly in clinician-directed formats, begin using focused stimulation or indirect language stimulation to generalize the form to more natural contexts; evaluate production in these contexts before considering goal met.
	
	For work on auxiliary verbs, use *Green Eggs and Ham* (Seuss, 1956) as one practice context. After multiple readings, allow the child to fill in verb phrases. Point to the words as the child says them. Ask him/her to identify words that rhyme.
	
	If a child says me/I, rather than working on just "I," target the distinction between subjective and objective pronouns more generally. This way, the child can learn about a broad range of forms rather than just one.
	If a language sample shows several obligatory contexts but no correct question reversals, production of occasional *be* verbs, and no contexts for *can* or *will*, target *be* and question reversals first.

Adapted from Fey, M., Long, S., & Finestack, L. (2003). Ten principles of grammar facilitation for children with specific language impairments. *American Journal of Speech-Language Pathology, 12*, 3-15.

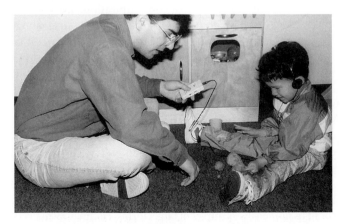

Assistive listening devices can improve signal-to-noise ratios in speech-language intervention.

(1997) discussed the development of "syntax stories" created to provide auditory bombardment of particular target forms within a story context. Box 9-3 gives an example of an excerpt from one of their "syntax stories." Regardless of whether a list or a story is read, the auditory bombardment segment generally makes up about 5 minutes of the intervention session. The child is not required to perform any discrimination activities, only to listen. Such activities also make excellent "homework" assignments for families interested in working on targets at home. They can easily be substituted for the child's usual bedtime story and don't require the parents to judge or correct the child's communication. If follow-up activities, such as illustrating the clinician's "syntax story" and rereading it with cloze procedures, are added, as Cleave and Fey suggest, even more benefit can be derived from the auditory bombardment.

| BOX 9-3 | **An Excerpt from "Dad's Bad Joke"** |

Target: ARE

Neil and Warren liked to play in the attic. It was fun up there, but it was a little scary, too. They always turned on the light so they could see. One day Neil and Warren started to go upstairs.

"Where *are* you going?" asked Dad.

"*Are* you going to the attic?"

"Yes, we *are!*" shouted Warren.

"Neil and I *are* going up now. We *are* going to play up there."

Oh you *are, are* you, thought Dad.

Reprinted with permission from Cleave, P., & Fey, M. (1997). Two approaches to the facilitation of grammar in children with language impairments: Rationale and description. *American Journal of Speech-Language Pathology, 6*, 31.

Approaches that facilitate comprehension, such as focused stimulation, indirect language stimulation, and auditory bombardment, should be presented along with activities that elicit production of target forms and meanings. Such a combination of approaches can help to ensure that clients can both understand and use the forms and meanings being taught. It is not necessary, though, to wait until the child demonstrates comprehension in pointing or discrimination activities before trying to solicit the use of target forms and meanings in production.

Pragmatics

Before we discuss intervention approaches for pragmatics, I want to clarify my view of the role of pragmatics in the intervention program for children with DL. Contemporary thought about language acquisition emphasizes the central place of pragmatic functions. That's because current thinking about language sees it not as a set of rules to be learned but as a tool for communication. Learning language, we now believe, is not just learning sounds, words, and sentence structures; it's also learning how to get things done in the real world with those sounds, words, and sentences. The study of how language is used in the context of communication is what is meant by *pragmatics*.

Pragmatics is just as important for thinking about language intervention as it is for acquisition. There are two ways to add pragmatics to our practice. The first is to generate a set of pragmatic targets or objectives for intervention. We could categorize children according to their pragmatic skills, identify their pragmatic deficits, and teach them to use whatever pragmatic behaviors they are lacking. Targets might include skills such as turn-taking, topic maintenance, and register variation. The problem with this approach is that we can't really isolate these

pragmatic skills from the syntax and semantics on which they rely. Unless we are teaching the earliest preverbal communication skills to a nonspeaking child, a client must use sounds, words, and sentences to achieve pragmatic targets.

A better way to incorporate pragmatics in the intervention program, in my view, is the method advocated by Craig (1983) and Marton (2005). They argued that rather than defining pragmatics as an additional set of rules that the child needs to learn, we are wiser to see pragmatics as the context in which intervention takes place, and to make sure that each new form learned is practiced in a variety of pragmatic contexts. That is, rather than teaching turn-taking as a separate skill, we would develop activities in which the client could take turns with the clinician using a linguistic form that was a target of intervention. Or, instead of teaching topic maintenance as a separate skill, we would give the client an opportunity to talk about a topic of interest for an extended number of turns, using newly acquired forms. We could, for example, ask a client who is working on past-tense forms to describe each step used to, for example, make the pudding now being shared with a parent who was not present during its preparation. If the child strays from the topic, the clinician could provide a prompt to return to describing the sequence, such as, "Wait a minute, weren't you saying how we made the pudding? 'We stirred the milk,' you said. Then what happened?"

Must these pragmatic contexts be present in every intervention activity? I don't think so. In fact, in my view they should not be, because that would lead us to violate Slobin's (1973) principle of one new thing at a time. If past-tense forms are just being elicited, we won't want to ask the child to use these new forms to fulfill a new function such as maintaining a topic—not until the new form has been somewhat stabilized. A more reasonable approach, to my way of thinking, is to incorporate pragmatic contexts into the intervention plan for every objective, but not for every activity. Some activities should be devoid of pragmatic context, to allow the child to focus attention on the linguistic objectives. Other activities can be designed to help clients use the new structures in real pragmatic contexts.

The real communicative contexts chosen should be based on the pragmatic assessment data. Suppose Rachel, for example, had been evaluated with Prutting and Kirchner's (1983) Pragmatic Protocol and had been found to have deficits in conversational repair. Once appropriate question forms had been added to her repertoire by means of semantic and syntactic intervention, these forms might be put to use in the context of conversational repair. The clinician might feign misunderstanding of something Rachel said, model asking a clarification question, and encourage Rachel to answer it to repair the breakdown. The clinician might then give a mumbled or otherwise unclear message and encourage Rachel to ask a question to get clarification. In this way the client can be helped to use new semantic and syntactic forms in pragmatic contexts identified as problem areas as a result of the pragmatic assessment. Brinton and Fujiki (1989, 1995) provided detailed procedures for this aspect of intervention.

Play and Thinking

A variety of studies (summarized by DeKroon, Kyte, & Johnson, 2002; Johnston, 1994; Leonard, 1997; Rescorla & Goossens, 1992) have shown that children with language problems perform less well than normally speaking peers on a broad range of cognitive tasks, including symbolic play, even when they score within the normal range on nonverbal intelligence tests. During the preschool period in normal development, as Vygotsky (1962) pointed out, language begins to help to structure thought, and thought is carried out primarily in the modality of language. One of the major accomplishments of normally developing children in the preschool period is the beginning of the integration of language and cognitive processes, each feeding off and growing out of the accomplishments of the other. Much learning about concepts, categories, and the physical world during the preschool years goes on through the medium of language, instead of through direct perception and experience, as it did in the sensorimotor period. Children structure symbolic play through language both when they play alone (often talking out loud to pretend playthings) and when they play with peers (often negotiating the roles and rules of the play by talking about them: "I'll be the baby, and you be the mommy, but be a nice mommy and don't scold me when I spill my bottle."). It should not be surprising, then, that children with language problems would begin to lag behind in some of these skills that are so intertwined with language.

When working with children at DL levels, we want to incorporate activities that encourage the child to use the language being learned to structure pretend play, solve problems, and explore new ideas. Moreover, play is an important context in which such problem solving and exploration can take place. As children develop more elaborated and flexible forms of language, these can be used for more mature and imaginative play. Again, play and thinking may not be direct targets of the intervention. Like the social skills in the pragmatics area, we can use play and problem solving as contexts in which the child can practice using new forms and meanings. By providing contexts in which the child can use recently acquired forms for new purposes, we accomplish two things. First, we help the child to generalize the intervention targets to meaningful situations. Second, we move the child into the zone of proximal development, providing a scaffold that helps the child to use language to achieve new levels of symbolic and conceptual development with our models and support. Play and problem-solving contexts are another important milieu for extending the child's use of newly emerging forms and meanings. As we proceed through the intervention program, we will want to build in some of these rich contexts, in addition to the more constrained contexts in which forms and meanings may be elicited initially.

Preliteracy

Many preschoolers with language delays or disorders later develop problems in learning to read and write, even when their oral language problems appear to resolve (Stothard, Snowling, Bishop, Chipchase, & Kaplan, 1998). And, increasingly, speech-language pathologists are being expected to promote preliteracy development in these children at risk (American Speech-Language-Hearing Association [ASHA], 2000; Justice & Ezell, 2004). When working with children in the DL phase, incorporating preliteracy goals and contexts is an important part of our direct work with clients, and can also serve as a fruitful basis for collaboration with classroom teachers and careproviders. As specialists in language development, SLPs are often the professionals with the broadest knowledge about the connections between reading and oral language and have much to offer others who work with young children when designing preliteracy programs not only for those at risk, but for all children in the preschool classroom.

Kaderavek and Justice (2004) outlined the major goals of preliteracy development during the DL period. These appear in Table 9-3. The goals can be divided into three major categories: *phonological awareness*, *print and alphabet knowledge*, and *literate language*. Phonological awareness goals should be familiar by now: they include the ability to count syllables and sounds, to identify rhymes and words that start/end with the same sounds, and to manipulate sounds in words ("What's *fun* without the /f/?"). We talked already about ways to build emerging literacy skills by incorporating PA activities within the phonological production program for children at the DL level. But PA is important for children with other language delays, as well as for children at risk for reading failure due to vulnerabilities such as limited English proficiency, cultural differences, or poverty. SLPs have important roles to play both as clinicians for children with documented language disorders, and as consultants for improving preliteracy instruction for all children in the preschool classroom.

In addition to PA, however, Kaderavek and Justice (2004) argue that skills related to print and alphabet knowledge are also crucial to emergent literacy development. These skills are sometimes called *literacy socialization* (Serpell, Sonnenschein, Baker, & Ganapathy, 2002; Snow, 1999), and involve understanding how books work and how print represents speech through written language units like letters, words, and punctuation. Activities that provide instruction and practice in literacy socialization are also important aspects of a preliteracy program.

Finally, the third aspect of preliteracy instruction has to do with the development of literate language. Literate language is the style used in written communication and is typically more complex and less related to the physical context than the language of ordinary conversation. We'll say a lot more about literate language in Chapter 10. But for now, we need to be aware that the ability to understand literate language is the "third leg" of a comprehensive preliteracy program. As we work with children in clinical sessions, with teachers as consultants, or in classrooms as collaborative interventionists, we can introduce literate language forms to preschool children by exposing them to stories, poems, plays, and other texts that exemplify this more elaborate language style, and giving them the opportunity to interact with these texts by acting them out, retelling them, and relating them to personal experiences.

TABLE 9-3	**Domains for Preliteracy Intervention**	
DOMAIN	**INSTRUCTIONAL GOALS**	**EXAMPLE ACTIVITIES**
Phonological awareness	Segment words from sentence.	Teacher has children in group clap for each word in a poem.
	Segment syllables in words.	Teacher has children stamp once for each syllable in words.
	Produce rhymes.	Teacher rereads familiar rhyming book, and has children fill in blanks ("Stop, you must not hop on ____!").
	Synthesize words from syllables.	Teacher introduces "robot" puppet who only speaks syllable by syllable ("mo tor cy cle"). Children must guess word he means.
	Synthesize words from sounds.	Teacher introduces "alien" puppet who only speaks sound by sound ("/d/ /a/ /g/"). Children must guess word he means.
	Identify words with same beginning/end sound.	Teacher has children stand up, clap, or wave each time they hear a word with a target beginning/ending sound in a story or poem being read.
Print concepts	Book reading conventions.	Teacher occasionally holds book upside down or backwards; children demonstrate correct orientation.
	Understand metalinguistic terms (word, letter sound).	Adult demonstrates elements from storybooks ("Here's a long word; Do you see this letter?")
	Link text to experience.	Teacher encourages children to make personal connections to storybook themes ("Sam-I-Am doesn't like Green Eggs and Ham. How many of you like eggs? Ham? How many don't?")
	Recognize environmental print.	Teacher shows photographs of print in the environment or from field trips; asks children to find the word that says "Stop," etc.
Alphabet knowledge	Alphabet song.	Teacher begins each day w/ choral singing of alphabet song, pointing out each letter on a chart as children sing. Eventually, children are given turns to do the pointing.
	Recognize own name in print, and the letters in it.	Children's names are used as labels throughout the classroom; they are encouraged to identify their name on their cup, coat hook, etc., and point out the letters of their name.
	Recognize letters in environmental print.	Children are given a card with a letter and encouraged to find words on a field trip or in photos of street scenes that start with their letter.
	Sort upper and lower case letters.	Toys are labeled with letters; children are encouraged to place toys in boxes with matching letters.
	Write own name.	Children are given multiple opportunities to form their names with plastic letters, tiles, letter cards, as well as to trace and write their names.
Narrative and literate language	Retell stories heard.	Children reenact stories heard, with simple costumes and props.
	Use causal conjunctions in story retells.	Children are asked to respond to questions about why events in the story took place and are prompted to use causal language, such as "because."
	Use mental and linguistic verbs in story retells.	Teacher encourages students to talk about what characters are saying and thinking in stories they have heard.

Adapted from Kaderavek, J., & Justice, L. (2004). Embedded-explicit emergent literacy intervention II: Goal selection and implementation in the early childhood classroom. *Language, Speech, and Hearing Services in Schools, 35,* 212-228.

Kaderavek and Justice (2004) review research that demonstrates that both for children with language impairments, and for those at risk for reading problems due to poverty or language differences, explicit preliteracy instruction in these areas, which is embedded in preschool classroom routines and activities, has positive effects on children's readiness for learning to read. Preschool programs that provide direct instruction and practice in name recognition and writing, alphabet recitation and recognition, awareness of book and print conventions, and PA games have been shown to lead to significantly greater growth in emergent literacy skills than programs that merely expose children to books and print (Justice, Chow, Capellini, Flanigan, & Colton, 2003; Justice & Ezell, 2004). In addition to incorporating PA within speech intervention for children with speech delays, SLPs can also consult with teachers on how to address emergent literacy for all children in the preschool classroom. SLPs can identify the relevant areas of preliteracy to address, using guidelines like those in Table 9-3; assist in designing lessons to provide instruction and practice of these skills in high interest activities tied to classroom themes; work alongside

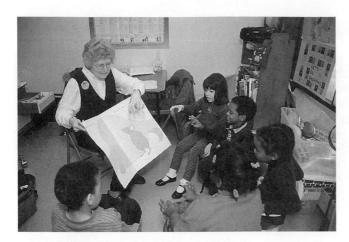

SLPs often work on preliteracy instruction in preschool and kindergarten classrooms.

the classroom teacher to present the instruction and provide extra support to children who are having difficulty; and carefully monitor children's participation in the classroom activities to identify those who might need more intensive intervention in these areas (Kaderavek & Justice, 2004).

INTERVENTION PROCEDURES FOR CHILDREN WITH DEVELOPING LANGUAGE

In Chapter 3, we discussed three major methods of intervention identified by Fey (1986): clinician-directed (CD), child-centered (CC), and hybrid. As we discussed in Chapter 3, the goal for us as clinicians is not to choose one method and use it consistently, but to have a repertoire of methods available that we can match to the needs of individual clients and the particular goals being addressed. In this way we can maximize the efficiency of our intervention and have the greatest chance that it will generalize to the client's everyday communication. Let's look at each of these methods to see how they might be applied to the child with DL.

Clinician-Directed Methods

In Chapter 3, we looked at a variety of clinician-directed approaches geared for the DL period. These included drill; drill play; Leonard's (1975a) CD modeling; and Lee, Koenigsknecht, and Mulhern's (1975) *Interactive Language Development Teaching*. There also are a variety of commercially available intervention packages, including some computer software, that use a CD approach to intervention for targets within the DL phase. Remember that CD approaches are highly effective in eliciting forms in production that the child has not used before or has used very infrequently. When initial elicitation of new forms is the goal, CD approaches make good sense for clients who can tolerate them. The weakness of CD approaches is their failure to generalize to real communication and their tendency to place the child in a respondent role. There are two ways to address these problems. One is to follow Fey's (1986) advice and use the techniques outlined in Chapter 3 to increase the

naturalness of CD activities. The second is to supplement CD approaches with other methods that give the client an opportunity to practice newly acquired forms in assertive roles and in the service of genuine communication. Let's look at some examples of CD approaches that might be used for several of the typical goals of intervention at the level of DL.

Phonology. One issue that often arises in phonological training is the question of whether to provide discrimination drills in which the child must identify pictures of words containing contrasting sounds (toe/sew) before production practice begins. This practice has been controversial, but recent research (Wolfe et al., 2003) suggests that discrimination training is helpful if the child fails to discriminate sounds on which production errors appear, prior to therapy. For these sounds, active discrimination drills worked better than auditory bombardment in increasing discrimination ability. But for sounds the child could discriminate at the beginning of training, additional discrimination training showed no positive effects. These findings suggest that assessing discrimination of sounds in error should be part of the assessment for speech delays and the use of discrimination drills should be reserved for only those sounds the child has been shown to have difficulty differentiating.

Articulation drills are a standard part of traditional intervention for speech disorders. Shriberg and Kwiatkowski (1982a) showed that drill was effective for improving phonological behavior in children in the DL period (even though neither clinicians nor preschool children liked it very much). *Contrastive drills* are one particular kind of drill often used in phonological intervention for children with DL. Contrastive drills involve developing lists of pairs of words in which the two words in each pair differ in specific ways. In a *minimal pairs* approach, two words that differ by only one feature of the target phoneme are presented for contrast (Weiner, 1981; Saben & Ingham, 1991). For example, if stopping of fricatives is a process being targeted, a list of pairs of words would be developed in which one word contained a fricative and a contrasting word contained the corresponding stop. Examples would be *sew/toe, zoo/do, fat/pat,* and *nice/night.* The client is asked to say each pair of words. The hope is that having the contrasting words in the same context will encourage the client to differentiate between them, preferably by suppressing the phonological process that would make them homonymous. The *maximal opposition* approach (Gierut, 1990) also opposes pairs of words, but this approach contrasts words that differ maximally on the target phoneme, so that the contrasting words differ not just on one feature of the target phoneme but on several. Using stopping of fricatives as our example target process again, a maximal opposition approach would contrast pairs such as *sew/no, zoo/moo, fat/cat,* and *nice/nine.* Lists of words for use in contrastive drills for various phonological process targets have been published by Elbert, Rockman, and Saltzman (1980) and Godar, Fields, and Schreiber (2004).

Drill play is often a preferred form of CD intervention at this level. The production practice segment of the approach advocated by Hodson and Paden (1991) uses a drill play format. These authors offered several possible drill play activities that can be incorporated into the production practice phase of phonological intervention. All the activities involve the use of small cards, each with a picture drawn by the client that represents one of the words containing the target phoneme or sequence that is used in the practice session. Some example activities include the following:

1. *Hide and seek.* The clinician hides the cards in obvious places around the room; the client says each word as he or she finds the card.
2. *Safari.* Each card is clipped to a picture of an animal. The client uses binoculars (which may be made from two toilet-paper tubes taped together) to find each animal and says each word on the card attached to it.
3. *Sack ball.* Large, open shopping bags, each with one of the client's cards taped to it, are placed around the room. The client throws a soft ball into a bag and then names the card on that bag. The game is continued until the client has thrown at least once into each bag.
4. *Buried.* The client's cards are buried in sand or foam peanuts. The client names each card as it is unearthed.

Drill play activities like these can, of course, be used for intervention on targets in other areas as well. "Safari" might be used to work on color words, for example. The client could be required to name the color of each animal or of a piece of construction paper it holds in its mouth as the animal is sighted through the binoculars. "Sack ball" could be used to drill the client on *is (verb)-ing* or copula sentences by attaching a picture to each sack that depicts an *is (verb)-ing* ("A boy is jumping") or copula ("It is a dog") sentence. The client would be required to say the target sentence as the ball is thrown into each sack.

One important point to consider in developing articulation drills for children in the DL was raised by Storkel and Morrisett (2002). They summarize research showing that, like younger children, children of preschool age and older show strong relationships between lexical and phonological development. This means that when working on phonological targets, the words in which those targets appear are important to consider. Storkel and Morrisett's review suggests that words used frequently in the language facilitate phonological acquisition. Clinicians can use sources like Kucera and Francis (1967) to find words with target sounds that are used frequently in everyday speech.

Shriberg, Kwiatkowski, and Snyder (1990) have presented a computer-assisted format for drilling articulation performance. They showed that although computer-assisted modes of intervention were engaging to most children, they were neither more effective nor more efficient than traditional forms of CD intervention. They suggested that computer-assisted methods are probably most useful in keeping children engaged in later phases of the intervention process when newly acquired forms are being practiced and stabilized, but that they are less effective at initial stages when new forms are first elicited. Other examples of computerized articulation programs include *The Articulation I, II, III* (San Luis Obispo, CA: LocuTour Multimedia), *Artic Games & More* (San Luis Obispo, CA: LocuTour Multimedia), *Speech Sounds on Cue* (Blacksburg, VA: Bungalow

Software); *Acorn's Gold Mine: An Interactive CD-ROM Game for Articulation and Phonological Skills* (DeKalb, IL: Janelle Publications), and *SATPAC* (Systematic Articulation Training Program Accessing Computers) (Fresno, CA: SATPAC Speech, LLC). Even at the late phases, though, the computer-assisted modes were only as good as the traditional ones, not any better. Schery and O'Connor (1995) discussed similar findings in the areas of semantics and syntax. If children like computer-assisted drill, we should by all means use it if it is available. But if intervention software is not available or if financial considerations force us to make a choice between a software package and some other useful intervention material, we should not despair. Many equally effective and engaging methods of intervention are available to us.

Semantics. Many CD programs for working on vocabulary and concepts are commercially available, such as the *Bracken Concept Development Program* (Bracken, 1986), the *Boehm Resource Guide for Basic Concept Teaching* (Boehm, 1989), Levine's (1988) *Great Beginnings for Early Language Learning: Nouns 1, Nouns 2, Concepts, Associations, Prepositions* (Pro-Ed, Inc.), and *Vocabulary with EASE* (AGS Publishing). Most computer software designed for developing vocabulary, such as the *First Words I and II* and *First Verbs, Sterling Edition* programs (Wilson & Fox, 1982-2005), *The Deciders Take On Concepts* (Interactive software. Eau Claire, WI: Thinking Publications), *Exploring Early Vocabulary Series* (Burlington, VT: Laureate Learning Systems, Wilson, M., & Fox, B.), *Words and Concepts Series* (Burlington, VT: Laureate Learning Systems), and *Basic Words for Children* CD-ROM: Version 2 (San Luis Obispo, CA: LocuTour Multimedia), use a drill or drill play format. As we've said before, many children enjoy pushing the buttons and seeing the pictures on the computer screen, and so computer-assisted intervention is often successful in motivating clients to persist with the drills the software programs contain. Schery and O'Connor (1995) discussed the *Programs for Early Acquisition of Language* (PEAL; Meyers, 1985) and the *ALPHA* programs, both designed to teach basic vocabulary to children with a variety of disabilities at early stages of language development. These programs both were found to have positive effects on word learning but did not show dramatically different results from those seen in more traditional intervention. Computers may be particularly good contexts for teaching action verbs, however. Since we know these forms are difficult for children with language disorders (Loeb, Pye, Redmond, & Richardson, 1996), finding effective intervention formats is especially important. Because computers can display action more compellingly than a static picture, they may be particularly facilitative for these forms. Schery and O'Connor emphasize that, while computer-based language programs can offer an additional tool and provide motivating contexts for language activities, they do not appear to be a replacement for an interactive environment with a responsive adult.

Syntax and Morphology. Many CD approaches to teaching syntax and morphology were developed during the 1970s, in the heyday of enthusiasm for operant approaches in our field. Fey (1986) discussed several available in the research literature. Some CD approaches to syntactic and morphological development also have been made available as commercial packages, such as the *Fokes Sentence Builder* (Fokes, 1976), the *Communication Training Program* (Waryas & Stremel-Campbell, 1983), the *Monterey Language Program* (Gray & Ryan, 1971), *Teach Me Language* (Freeman & Dakes, 1996), and *Verbal Behavior* (Carbone, 2003). An alternative to employing these operant grammar training programs is to follow the suggestions of Fey, Long, and Finestack (2003). They argue that supplementing other, more naturalistic methods with drill and drill-play activities that elicit imitation of target forms makes sense, especially when the elicited imitation activities *contrast* related forms. One such approach from the literature is presented here, both to exemplify what these kinds of programs look like and also because this particular approach has been found to be highly successful in improving grammatical production (Cleave & Fey, 1997). Connell's (1982) CD procedure for training syntactic rules with the help of contrasts, using the form, "NP is (verb)-ing," appear in Table 9-4.

Again, any CD approach, whether commercially packaged, derived from the literature, or designed by the clinician, can be modified according to Fey's (1986) guidelines to increase its naturalness. Let's look at some of the ways in which we could modify Connell's (1982) approach as an example of how this might be done. Remember that in Chapter 3 we talked about several ways to increase the naturalness of CD activities. These include making the client's contribution informative, creating intervention contexts where there is a real motivation to communicate, providing distractor items, and presenting stimuli within cohesive texts. Try to think of several ways that Connell's approach could be modified to achieve these ends.

My suggestions, which are only a sample of the many possible ways this could be done, are listed in Box 9-4.

A variety of computer software also is available for training syntactic and morphological goals using drill and drill play. The vast majority of this software targets receptive performance, however. As we've seen, receptive training is probably not necessary for most clients and does not necessarily generalize to use of the same forms in production. Production skills, on the other hand, do tend to generalize more readily to comprehension. For these reasons I would not put a great deal of time or money into the use of syntactic intervention programs that focus exclusively on receptive language. If such programs are available and clients like to use the computer, they might be used as follow-up to production training, as extra practice, and to ensure that production targets have generalized to reception. Schery and O'Connor (1997), for example, showed that special needs preschoolers who received an additional hour per week of computer training for ten weeks, over and above what they received during normal classroom instruction, showed greater gains than peers who did not receive the extra training. Computerized language instruction, then, can be a helpful adjunct to more traditional intervention. And Owens (2004) suggests that computer-assisted training works best when the child and the clinician participate together in the program. Especially at the DL level, sitting children alone in front of a computer screen may not be the best practice.

Child-Centered Approaches to Intervention for the Child with Developing Language

We talked earlier about CC intervention methods and discussed their use with children in the emerging language phase, when no specific targets of intervention are identified and the goal

---

TABLE 9-4	**Training Procedures for Teaching the Syntactic Rule "NP is (verb)-ing" through Contrasts**

Target behavior: Spontaneous production of "NP is (verb)-ing" in response to questions.
Materials: 20 pictures of assorted agents doing various actions.

STEP	CLINICIAN STIMULUS	CLIENT RESPONSE	CRITERION FOR MOVING TO NEXT STEP IN PROGRAM
1	What is the NP doing? Say, "NP is (verb)-ing."	NP is (verb)-ing.	90% correct
2	NP is (verb)-ing. Now the NP is done. What did the NP do? (Show picture, then take it away.) Say, "NP (verb)-ed."	NP (verb)-ed.	90% correct
3	What is the NP doing? (Show picture.)	NP is (verb)-ing.	90% correct
4	NP is (verb)-ing. Now the NP is done. What did the NP do? (Show picture, then take it away.)	NP (verb)-ed.	90% correct
5	What is the NP doing? (Show picture) What did the NP do? (Take it away.)	NP is (verb)-ing and NP (verb)-ed.	90% correct

Generalization training: Repeat Step 5 with different pictures, clinicians, and environments.

Adapted from Connell, P. (1982). On training language rules. *Language, Speech, and Hearing Services in Schools, 13,* 231-248.

| **BOX 9-4** | **Naturalistic Modifications of Connell's (1982) CD Procedure** |

1. Use a cohesive text. Instead of a series of unrelated pictures, use a picture book or set of sequence pictures that depicts a series of related actions, such as those involved in dressing or in preparing food. Go through all the steps in Connell's procedure in exactly the same way, using these pictures that form a cohesive unit as the stimuli.
2. Make the contribution informative. Using either unrelated picture cards or pictures that form a cohesive unit as suggested in 1, sit with the client and the pictures at a table. Place a favorite doll, action figure, or photo of someone the client knows across the table from the two of you, with its back toward you so it cannot "see" the pictures. Tell the client the doll wants to know what's going on in the pictures, so the client must "tell" the doll what's going on by answering your questions. Both to increase the communicative aspect of the activity and to provide distractor items, occasionally have the doll respond to the client's utterance by talking for it in a funny voice. Express surprise or interest in what the client is saying, and make a comment not directly related to the picture descriptions. Then tell the client the doll is so interested it wants to know more, and resume the activity.
3. Increase motivation to communicate. Use a cohesive set of pictures, and tape record each of the client's responses to the imitative set of items in Step 1 of Connell's procedure (see Table 9-4). Tell the client he or she can take the tape home and play the "story" for his or her parents, so the parents can hear how well the child tells the story. Do the same for Step 3 of Connell's procedure (see Table 9-4).

is simply improved communication. Let's look at how some of these methods can be used for children in the DL phase.

Indirect Language Stimulation. The major characteristics of indirect language stimulation (ILS), as defined by Stockman (2002), include the following:

- Contingent feedback (saying something that relates to what the child said/did; e.g., child picks up toy car; Clinician remarks, "Oh, the car! You have the car!").
- Balanced turn-taking (letting the child lead and then responding, rather than using extensive questions and initiations to get the child to talk; e.g., child is playing silently, clinician plays silently alongside, when child turns toward clinician, she remarks: "Oh, I see what you have! You have the blue car; I have the red one!").
- Extension of their child's topic (saying something that gives more information about what the child just said/did; e.g., child holds up car for clinician to see, clinician remarks, "You have the blue car! That's neat! Your blue car has big, black wheels!").

ILS can take place in a variety of contexts, including play with toys or role plays, during outdoor play, shared book reading, cooking, crafts, or other common preschool activities. In Chapter 3, we suggested that ILS in its pure form, when no specific goals are identified, is most appropriate for children with MLUs less than 3.0, when first sentences are emerging. A modified form of ILS might be used at later stages, if we incorporate some specific goals and use it as a way to provide multiple meaningful models of target forms. Instead of using primarily self-talk and parallel talk in an unstructured play setting, we can provide a more contrived play setting, one in which materials have been selected for the child, activities are suggested by the clinician, and play behaviors are modeled to make it highly probable that the need for target forms and meanings will arise. For example, suppose we are working on the use of irregular past-tense verb forms and want to provide some ILS

as an introduction to these forms, to allow the client to see how they are used. We might give the child a set of toys such as a dollhouse, garage, or play house with matching people and accoutrements. As the child manipulates the toys, we might narrate, "Oh, he *went* in the house. Uh-huh. Then he *found* a little dog. How nice. Then he *said* 'hi' to it. The dog *came* closer to him, didn't he? Then he *saw* a doghouse." We also might model talking for one of the toys—the dog, for example: "Arf, arf, I *found* a bone. I *saw* it in the yard." Although an opportunity to model irregular past-tense forms might not arise in every remark the clinician makes, each opportunity for providing these models could be capitalized on. If the child began to model the clinician's narration and role-taking, using some irregular past forms correctly or incorrectly, the expansion, extension, recast, and buildup and breakdown forms of ILS feedback could be provided. Leonard and Fey (1991) provided additional detailed examples of using modified ILS techniques to elicit grammatical forms in the DL phase. Shriberg and Kwiatkowski (1982a) also discussed this approach as a means of facilitating phonological development.

Fey (2000) advocated using recast sentences as a particularly effective form of ILS for children in the DL period. Taking a client's utterance and immediately recasting it in a different syntactic form that retains the child's meaning is thought to provide a particularly useful kind of feedback. Recasting is thought to help children see how language rules work to provide several different ways of expressing similar semantic relations. For example, if a child remarks, "Big doggy mad," the clinician might recast, "He is? Is the big doggy mad?" Research on children with a variety of disabilities has demonstrated positive effects of this kind of recasting on language growth (Nelson, Camarata, Welsh, Butkovsky, & Camarata, 1996; Yoder, Davies, Bishop, & Munson, 1994). Nelson et al. found that recast treatment was superior to a clinician-directed imitative approach. Fey and Loeb (2002), however, suggest that these techniques work best when children are producing a few of the target forms in their own speech, so careful analysis of the child's current productions is important when choosing targets for recasts.

Some additional techniques for eliciting a variety of language forms within the modified ILS approach are given by Fey et al. (2003) and Owens (2004). Examples are given in Table 9-5.

ILS can also be taught to parents, daycare providers, and other caregivers, as a way to expand the child's opportunities for language stimulation. Law, Garrett, and Nye (2004) concluded in their literature review of intervention programs for preschoolers that intervention that was administered by trained parents was, in general, as effective as intervention that was administered by SLPs. Kohnert et al. (2005) identified several components shared by successful parent training programs:

▶ Focus on specific language facilitation strategies (e.g., modeling, expansion, recasts, imitation, responsive feedback).
▶ Using multiple instructional methods (e.g., demonstration, coaching, role plays, mediated parent-child interactions, videotaped examples, written materials, and specific instructive feedback).
▶ Teaching a progression of skills and strategies embedded in specific activities.

Girolametto, Weitzman, and Greenberg (2003) also showed that day care providers could be trained to provide ILS to children in small groups. The training was aimed at helping the workers be more responsive to children's initiations, engage children in interactions, model simplified language, and encourage peer interactions. Their study showed that trained caregivers were superior to untrained staff in waiting for children to initiate, engaging them in turn-taking, using face to face interaction, and including uninvolved children. The children assigned to trained caregivers talked more, produced more word combinations, and talked to peers more often than the children in control groups. Further research by this group (DeRivera, Girolametto, Greenberg, & Weitzman, 2005) suggests that the use of questions in interactions is another important target of in-service training. Open-ended questions, those that continue the child's topic, and questions followed by a pause to allow the child's response were found to result in increases in the complexity of preschool children's responses. These strategies, too, would be helpful skills for training parents and caregivers in ILS.

Facilitated Play. An added advantage in using modified ILS in this way with children in the DL period is that, in addition to providing language models, we can provide models

TABLE 9-5   Language Elicitation Techniques

TECHNIQUE	TARGET	EXAMPLE
Violate routines	Protest, request, negative sentence	During snack, neglect to give client a cup and begin to pour juice
Violate expectations	Comment, protest, negative sentence	Clinician: "Here's your sandwich." Child: "Nothing in it." Clinician; "Oh? What should I do?"
Withhold objects or turns	Protest, request, negative sentence	Give each other child a turn to operate a toy and skip client when moving to next child
Misuse objects	Comment, verbs	Use a hairbrush to "brush teeth"
Misname objects	Comment, negative sentence, labels	Clinician: "How do you like my new hat?" (while pointing to shoes)
Misplace objects	Comment, negative sentence, spatial terms	Put paper plate on head
Provide inappropriate objects for activity	Comment, labels, negatives, word combinations	Provide noodles and cheese when activity is making a sandwich
"Pass it on"	Request for information	Clinician: "Do you know where the juice is?" Child: "No." Clinician: "Go see if Jamie does." Child: "Do you know where the juice is?"
"Strong, silent type"	Request for information	Clinician (placing interesting object before client): "This is neat." Child: "What is it?" Clinician: "A barometer" (Say nothing else until child asks for me information).
"Guess what"	Request for information, past tense	Clinician: "Guess what I did yesterday?"
Expansion invitation	Infinitive	Child: "I want crayon." Clinician: "You want a crayon to eat?" Client: "No, to color with." Clinician: "What?" Client: "I want a crayon to color with."

Adapted from Fey, M., Long, S., & Finestack, L. (2003). Ten principles of grammar facilitation for children with specific language impairments. *American Journal of Speech-Language Pathology, 12,* 3-15; Owens, R. (2004). *Language disorders: A functional approach to assessment and intervention* (4th ed.). Boston, MA: Allyn & Bacon.

of more elaborated forms of play. As we discussed earlier, play skills often lag behind in children with language disorders, and a modified ILS approach gives us the opportunity to model forms of play appropriate for this developmental period, such as role-playing and using objects symbolically. Culatta (1994) discussed the advantages of play as a format for language intervention. She argued that play is an especially appropriate context for language learning because it is highly motivating; it permits the integration of content, form, and function; and it encourages the child to bring knowledge of "scripts" for everyday events to the foreground where this knowledge can support language use. In turn, play provides opportunities for elaborating existing scripts through enacting a wider set of roles and possibilities than are present in "reality." In a doctor play scene, for example, the child can be the patient but also can play the doctor, getting a chance to use language appropriate to that role. Culatta suggested using child-centered play contexts, not only for indirect language stimulation, but also to develop a variety of language skills, such as the following:

▶ *Enhancing narrative ability* by engaging the child in direct metalinguistic planning of the roles, plans, attempts, and outcomes to be acted out in the play.

▶ *Facilitating turn-taking* by contriving reasons to communicate within the play. The clinician can require the child to communicate to multiple characters. If birthday party play is going on, the clinician can have the client tell each stuffed animal "guest" what to bring to the party.

▶ *Increasing opportunities for decontextualized language.* The clinician can use increasingly abstract props in the play, starting with real objects and moving to replicas, constructions, toys, and finally to having no props at all. The clinician also can include some discussion of events remote in space and time within the context of the play.

▶ *Enhancing the expression of communicative intentions.* The clinician can structure opportunities within the play for the child to negotiate roles and plans; project events; state rules and goals; and express the feelings, intentions, and desires of characters. The clinician can begin by modeling these functions and move to asking the child to express the functions following the model.

▶ *Increasing vocabulary.* Words specific to particular scripts can be used by the clinician multiple times within a play episode. If a shopping script is being used, the words *cashier, customer, groceries,* and *cart* might be used. Generic words important for play negotiation and enactment also can be modeled, such as *cooperate, prepare,* and *character.*

▶ *Developing emergent literacy.* Play provides many opportunities for children to pretend to write and read and to see why written forms are used. The clinician can encourage clients to make real or pretend lists, signs, and labels and to write or pretend to write notes and instructions to other characters within the play.

Patterson and Westby (1998) provided some guidelines for the kinds of play to model for children in the DL phase. These are summarized in Table 9-6. Culatta (1994) gave an extensive list of themes and events that can be used as a basis for play scenes for children with DL. Examples are given in Table 9-7.

TABLE 9-6	**Guidelines for Modeling Pretend Play**		
DEVELOPMENTAL LEVEL	**PROPS TO USE IN PLAY**	**EVENT DESCRIPTION TYPES TO USE IN PLAY**	**ROLES TO TAKE AND GIVE TO TOYS AND OTHERS**
3–3½ yr	Replica toys (dollhouse, barn, etc.); use objects to represent others (block for phone); use blocks as enclosures; use sandbox, water table for imaginative play.	Salient, memorable events in which the child has taken part (e.g., visit to doctor, losing a favorite toy).	Use doll as participant in play; talk for doll; play parent to doll.
3½–4 yr	Use language to set scene and invent some props; build city with blocks.	Familiar, observed events in which the child has not taken part (e.g., firehouse, police car, superhero from TV show).	Use dolls to act out scenes; take multiple roles in play.
4–5 yr	Use language exclusively to set action and roles.	Novel events and imaginative activities that child has not participated in or observed (e.g., pretend to be cowpunchers on the range; ride horses, set up camp, cook meal, sing around the campfire).	Use language to take roles, using different voices, etc.

Adapted from Patterson, J., & Westby, C. (1998). The development of play. In W. Haynes & B. Shulman (Eds.), *Communication development: Foundations, processes, and clinical applications* (pp. 135-164). Englewood Cliffs, NJ: Prentice-Hall.

TABLE 9-7	Themes and Events to Use as Play Contexts in Language Intervention

SCRIPT	EVENTS	POTENTIAL PROBLEMS
Getting ready for school	Get dressed, brush teeth, pack lunch, do chores, eat breakfast, get on bus.	Can't wake children, burn toast, can't find lunch box, child is sick, out of milk, miss bus.
Going on a trip	Plan and pack, load car, leave, drive to destination, arrive at hotel, go to pool.	Child doesn't want to go, no room for favorite blanket, car out of gas, child is carsick, no rooms, forgot swimsuit.
Taking care of sick baby	Take temperature, rock baby, call doctor, take in car to doctor, doctor gives baby medicine, take baby home, give juice, put to bed.	Baby still cries, line is busy, car won't start, baby throws up medicine, baby spills juice.

Adapted from Culatta, B. (1994). Representational play and story enactments: Formats for language intervention. In J. Duchan, L. Hewitt, & R. Sonnenmeier (Eds.), *Pragmatics: From theory to practice* (pp. 105-119). Englewood Cliffs, NJ: Prentice-Hall.

Hybrid Approaches to Intervention for the Child with Developing Language

Hybrid methods of intervention supply a valuable middle ground for planning language programs. More naturalistic and child-centered than CD approaches, but more structured, sequenced, and clinician-controlled than ILS or facilitated play, these techniques provide a range of alternatives for clinicians to use in improving communicative function. We talked in Chapter 3 about several hybrid techniques. Some that were discussed in detail, including *incidental* and *milieu* teaching, are extremely well suited to addressing semantic and syntactic goals of the DL period. Focused stimulation and script therapy, also outlined in Chapter 3, are likewise very useful during this phase. Let's look at some forms of focused stimulation and some extensions of the script therapy approach, as well as a few other hybrid methods that can be added to the ones we've already discussed.

Hybrid Approaches in Phonology. Hodson and Paden (1991) provided the most detailed method available for using a hybrid approach to intervention with unintelligible children. Their approach uses detailed assessment of phonological production to target sounds and processes. It is based on the principles of (1) the need to develop strong auditory models for target sounds, (2) developing kinesthetic patterns to match these auditory images, (3) the use of a phonetic environment to facilitate correct sound production, and (4) the child's active involvement in phonological acquisition. A cycling method of goal attack is used. Each intervention session has several components, including the following:

▶ Reviewing the targets from the previous session.
▶ Providing auditory bombardment for target sounds using amplification, such as an auditory training unit.
▶ Practicing production of a small number of words containing target sounds or syllable shapes in activities such as the ones described earlier under drill play.
▶ Identifying new words for the next session's or cycle's production practice by identifying two to five target words

in which the child can pronounce the target sound or syllable shape correctly.
▶ Repeating the auditory bombardment segment.
▶ Giving parents the list of words for auditory bombardment to read to the child at home between sessions.

Notice that this approach is considered hybrid even though it contains a drill play phase during the production practice segment. Hybrid programs such as this one can take advantage of several approaches and even include some CD activities within their overall plan.

Focused Stimulation. Cleave and Fey (1997) presented a detailed description of a program designed to facilitate grammar acquisition in language-impaired preschoolers. They refer to this program as a "focused stimulation" approach, because it focuses on specific forms and uses multiple models with a variety of forms of clinician feedback to stimulate language goals. As such, it combines several techniques with those we identified as pure "focused stimulation" in Chapter 3. The overall program maintains a hybrid orientation, though, with the context of natural conversation between a client and an adult. Targets for the intervention are selected from language sample data. Forms that the client used less than half the time correctly in obligatory contexts are high-priority target forms. Table 9-8 summarizes the techniques used in this approach. Lederer (2001) showed that focused stimulation was effective for increasing vocabulary in preschool children.

Script Therapy. Remember that Olswang and Bain (1991) described script therapy as a way to reduce the cognitive load of language training by embedding it in the context of a familiar routine. One way to use scripts is to develop some verbal routines with the child in the intervention context. We might, for example, have some stock phrases related to the client's targets that we say at the beginning of each session. To a client working on use of *I* and copula verbs, we could say, "I *am* glad to see you. I *am* happy you came today. I *am* ready for you. How about you?" We also talked in Chapter 3 about establishing the script and then violating it, encouraging the client to comment on or

TABLE 9-8	**Focused Stimulation Procedures**

TARGETS	EXPLANATION	EXAMPLE
Demonstrating use of targets	Targets are moved to sentence initial or final position, where they are most salient.	Child: I need a red block. Adult: *Will* you get it? Child: OK Adult: You *will*? Good, then I *will* get a blue one.
Expansion	Errors in the child's utterance are corrected.	Child: Her my dolly. Adult: Yes, *she* is yours.
Recast	Keeps child's meaning but changes the form of the sentence.	Child: This easy! Adult: *Is* it? *Is* it easy for you? It *isn't* easy for me!
Buildups and breakdowns	Demonstrate how to manipulate the elements in a sentence.	Child: I make a mess! Adult: You did! You made a big mess! A big mess! You certainly did make a mess. You made a mess, all right. Didn't you?
False assertions	Clinician makes a false remark as a prompt for the client to deny it.	Adult: This piece fits here. Child: No it not. Adult: Yes it *does*. Child: No! Adult: I guess you're right. It *doesn't* fit here.
Feigned misunderstandings	Clinician pretends not to get the message sent by client.	Child: Me need that. Adult: *He* needs it? Child: No, me need it. Adult: No, *I* do (pointing to self).
Forced choices	Provide a model of correct use of the target.	Adult: Do you want some snack? You can say "yes, please," or "no, thank you."
Other contingent queries	Used to encourage client to provide missing information.	Child: I want that one. Adult: What will you do with it? Child: Color. Adult: Oh, you want the red crayon so you can color with it.
Violating routines	Omitting or incorrectly performing a step in an established routine to encourage the child to comment.	When offering cookies, forget to provide a napkin. Child: Us need napkin. Adult: *We* do! You're right! *We* do need napkins.
Withholding objects and turns	Used to encourage requests.	Clinician skips a client's turn in a board game. Child: My turn! Adult: It *is*! Is it your turn? I guess it *is*!
Violating object function	Used to encourage use of negative forms.	Adult uses demitasse spoon to stir large bowl of pudding mix. Child: No that one! Adult: No? You *don't* want me to use this spoon? You *don't*? We *don't* use this spoon to stir?
"Syntax stories"	Clinicians and parents create stories, similar to "Dad's Bad Joke," (see Box 9-3) that give multiple exemplars of target forms.	Excerpt from "Dad's Bad Joke": Dad had a big grin on his face. Warren and Neil started to play. They were having lots of fun. Then something happened. The light went out. *We're* in the dark! said Neil. We sure *are*, said Warren. *Are* you afraid? *Are* you afraid of the dark? No, *I'm* not, said Neil. I *am* not afraid. *Are* you?

Adapted from Cleave, P., & Fey, M. (1997). Two approaches to the facilitation of grammar in children with language impairments: Rationale and description. *American Journal of Speech-Language Pathology, 6,* 23-32.

correct the violation. In addition, we discussed "playing" with the script, getting clients to ring changes on it as a way to broaden their use of the forms in the routine.

Event Structures. Script therapy also can be used in conjunction with event structures that are familiar to the client. Carrow-Woolfolk (1988) described event structures as holistic, goal-directed, sequentially organized sets of activities that have prototypic features but some internal variation. Ordering food in a restaurant would be one example; going grocery shopping is another. We can choose event structures from the "real world" that are well-known to our clients and use these as contexts for developing verbal routines. The clients and clinician can then use props to act out the event structure, with the clinician first modeling the entire verbal script. Later, cloze procedures can be used to elicit increasingly large parts of the verbal script from the clients. Eventually the clients can act out and recite the entire event structure. The clients can repeat the enactment of the event structure numerous times, trading roles so that each gets a chance to produce all the parts of the verbal script. A client who is the shopper one day may be the clerk the next. After a while, variations on the event structure and its verbal script can be imposed. Children who used a script for going grocery shopping might be asked to pretend they are shopping for pet food in a pet store. Finally, the clinician can play a role in the event structure and violate the expected events or verbal formulae that are familiar to the clients.

These scripts can serve as frames for developing both vocabulary and morphosyntax. An event script for vocabulary development might involve shopping in a clothing store. The clinician can model using a sentence frame to request items whose names the child needs to learn ("I need socks, I need a *blouse*, I need a *vest*."). Morphosyntactic targets can also be addressed (I need socks, my baby needs socks").

Using event structures in a script-based intervention program differs somewhat from using event scripts in more child-centered play. Child-centered play, as we discussed earlier, is more open-ended. The clinician can provide guidance and scaffolding but generally follows the child's lead; the focus of the activity is the play. In script therapy using event structures, the play provides a background, but the focus is using the target language. The clinician takes a stronger leadership role in the activity, modeling what the child is to say and requesting that the child say the target forms. We might use the same play scripts for each of these two types of approaches. We might, for example, use a scripted, hybrid version of "shopping" to work on specific linguistic goals, such as food vocabulary and sentences of the form, "I need X." We might use the same shopping context another time for more child-centered play, focusing on developing turn-taking skills and increasing the range of communicative intentions expressed. This time, instead of letting the child simply ask for a series of products ("I need apples, I need grapes"), as we did in the hybrid form of the activity, we could introduce some problems ("We're out of grapes") and provide opportunities and scaffolding for the child to use language to overcome these obstacles in the play.

Hybrid event structure activities using scripts can be used to target new vocabulary (for example, food words in the grocery example). They also can be used for working on syntactic forms (for instance, question production to request foods at the store: "Do you have coffee? Do you have tea?" or subject-verb-object sentences, such as "I need coffee. I need tea."). We would want to select event structures that are familiar to our clients but that also lend themselves to the goals being targeted. If spatial prepositions are intervention goals, for example, the restaurant might not be the best structure to choose. Going to a birthday party could be better (for example, "Put your gift *beside* the table; pin the tail *on* the donkey; put the candle *in* the cake; your treat bag is *under* your hat."). Script-based activities have been shown to be effective in teaching semantic relations (Kim, Yang, & Hwang, 2001) and improving social uses of language (Neeley, Neeley, Justen, & Tipton-Sumner, 2001) in preschoolers with disabilities.

Literature-Based Scripts. Snow and Goldfield (1983), Bedrosian (1997), and Wasik and Bond (2001) have discussed the advantages of joint book reading as an ideal context for language learning. Picture books are of interest to children and are a natural, familiar format for adult-child interaction. They use repetitive language closely tied to the nonlinguistic, pictured context. In addition, Kirchner (1991) pointed out that joint book reading provides an excellent opportunity for adults to scaffold the child's contribution to the interaction. With the stable, repetitive form of the text of the book, adults can encourage the child to operate in the zone of proximal development, asking the child to make a contribution to the reading that is slightly above what he or she is able to do in spontaneous speech. As the child acquires the script, the adult can "up the ante," requiring a higher level of contribution later. Ratner, Parker, and Gardner (1993) suggested further that joint book reading is an ideal context for establishing the joint attention so necessary for effective discourse and for providing a framework for semantic contingency, as the book anchors the child's and adult's remarks to a reliable, meaningful, and engaging base. Carrow-Woolfolk (1988) pointed out that both book reading and recitation of story passages provide ideal opportunities for practicing and stabilizing specific language skills. In short, much language learning normally goes on in the context of the pleasant and familiar activity of joint book reading. Research has demonstrated that shared book reading can promote vocabulary acquisition (e.g., Arnold, Lonigan, Whitehurst, & Epstein, 1994; Wasik & Bond, 2001), grammatical development (Bradshaw et al., 1998; Whitehurst et al., 1988; Yoder et al., 1995), and conversational participation (Crain-Thoreson & Dale, 1999). We can make use of this ideal context in language intervention as well.

Of course, just reading books to children with language impairments does not constitute intervention. If all they needed were to be read to, most would have learned language by now and would not be in an intervention program. We need to structure the joint book reading experience in the following three important ways:

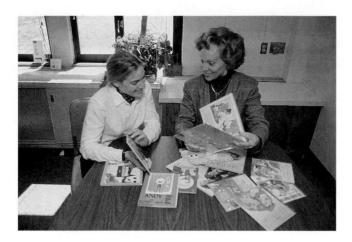

Clinicians can choose books for literature-based intervention that provide frequent examples of intervention targets.

▶ By the use of carefully planned, scaffolded language input. For example, if spatial terms are a vocabulary category to be targeted, we would choose books that provide many examples of these terms, such as *Inside, Outside, Upside Down* (Berenstain & Berenstain, 1968), reading the book repeatedly, using emphatic stress on the spatial terms, and asking the child to comment or answer questions after hearing each page ("Where is the bear now? He's..."). Eventually, cloze techniques can be used to "up the ante" on the child's contribution.

▶ By the selection of books that provide opportunities for the client to practice forms and meanings being targeted in the intervention. For example, if we are working on auxiliary verbs, we can select a book such as *Green Eggs and Ham* (Suess, 1956) and after several rereadings, ask the child to play the role of Sam-I-Am.

▶ By using these carefully selected books as an opportunity for language production practice. Using spatial vocabulary as our example again, we can, after several readings using questions and cloze techniques, ask the child to "read" *Inside, Outside, Upside Down* to the clinician and to several puppets, so the child must show each page to each "listener" and read the page over again to each.

In addition to carefully structuring these activities, though, we need to be aware, as Kaderavek and Justice (2002) caution us, that some children just don't like listening to books; in fact, unwillingness to listen to books is associated with language disorder. To use book reading as an intervention context, it is crucial that we make sure children are engaged and interested in the activity and that targets addressed in book reading are also practiced and generalized in other contexts. Kaderavek and Justice advocate using strategies like allowing children to choose a book from several that contain target forms, asking children to describe their feelings about the book being used, allowing the child to hold and control the book (by turning pages, etc.), incorporating activity and movement (such as acting out characters' antics) in the book reading, and responding to the child's interests and attentional shifts during reading. When encouraging parents and teachers to use book reading

for language enrichment and literacy development, it is equally important to alert them to these issues.

We looked at one approach to scaffolding language input in joint book reading in Chapter 7: that of Whitehurst et al. (1991). Kirchner (1991) provided another approach that is more naturalistic in its discourse structure and is suited to children in both the emerging language and DL stages. She advocated using children's books as the routine, predictable language base from which the child can learn to segment longer and more complex utterances into their constituent parts. Because children with language impairments appear to rely on using unanalyzed language forms learned through imitation, rather than generating novel utterances, more than normally developing children do (Wetherby, Schuler, & Prizant, 1997), the joint book reading situation provides an opportunity to exploit this tendency and use it to scaffold the child to higher levels of production. The fixed text of the storybook provides an ideal substrate for the child's emerging linguistic analysis. Kirchner (1991) provided a sequence of activities to be used with individuals or groups in conjunction with joint book reading. These are summarized in Box 9-5.

Books for language intervention are chosen on the basis of the forms used within their text. Not just any good children's book will do, but you may be surprised at how many classics of children's literature use repetitive semantic and syntactic forms that are commonly the targets of intervention in the DL period. Ratner, Parker, and Gardner (1993) and Owens (2004) assembled a list of classic children's books that contain repetitive use of grammatical patterns commonly targeted in language intervention. Their list forms the basis for the suggestions for books to use in literature-based script therapy that can be found in Appendix 9-1. Additional resources for using children's literature in language intervention include Gebers (1990), Kaderavek and Justice (2002), Lockhart (1992), and Owens and Robinson (1997).

In addition to classic children's books, other forms of children's literature also are very useful adjuncts to script therapy. Songs and nursery rhymes can be used in exactly the same way as books to highlight semantic and syntactic forms in reliable, repetitive formats, following Kirchner's (1991) procedures. Zoller (1991) presented some suggestions along these lines. Finger plays or songs and rhymes that lend themselves to acting out are especially helpful, as they engage clients in multimodal experience with the text. What's more, they give clients a way to participate in the activity as the clinician sings or recites, until the text has been internalized enough for them to participate through the verbal medium. Box 9-6 provides some well-known songs and nursery rhymes that contain repetitive use of forms often targeted in intervention at the DL phase. Once we have script therapy applications for children's literature in mind, it will be easy to add to these lists by visiting a children's library or bookstore to examine additional children's books and compilations of songs, rhymes, and finger plays. A clinician interested in script therapy can soon assemble an impressive array of texts to be used for any language form that a client might need to improve. A few such lists are already commercially available. Gebers (2003), Prelutshy (1986), and Sterling-Orth (2005) provide some examples.

BOX 9-5	Suggestions for Using Joint Book Reading in Language Intervention

Step 1: Read the book to the client several times over the course of a few sessions. Use prosodic cues to segment and highlight target semantic and syntactic patterns.

Step 2: After adequate exposure to the text, pause at points containing the target forms, creating a cloze condition. Let the client produce the next word, phrase, or line (in choral fashion for groups of clients). Insert pauses in linguistically specific ways to mark and select the portion of the text the client will produce. This facilitates the client's segmentation of the linguistic material for analysis.

Step 3: Read the book often enough that the client memorizes it. At each reading, segment the text in variable but explicit ways to facilitate linguistic analysis.

Step 4: Segment the text so that the client must produce increasingly long portions, until eventually the client can recite the whole book.

Step 5: Once clients have memorized the text, have them take turns "reading" it and having the clinician or other clients fill in parts left out by the "reader."

Step 6: Make up a new book using a similar linguistic pattern to encourage the child to use the learned forms in new ways. Write down each client's version, and let the clients illustrate their "books" to take home to read to family members.

Adapted from Kirchner, D. (1991). Reciprocal book reading: A discourse-based intervention strategy for the child with atypical language development. In T. Gallagher (Ed.), *Pragmatics of language: Clinical practice issues* (pp. 307-332). San Diego, CA: Singular Publishing Group.

BOX 9-6	Examples of Songs, Rhymes, and Finger Play Routines for Targeting Language Forms

Subject-Verb-Object Sentences
One, Two, Buckle My Shoe
All Around the Mulberry Bush
Old McDonald
Prepositions
In and Out the Window
Hickory, Dickory, Dock
Skidamarink-a-Dink-a-Dink
Over the River and Through the Woods
Copula
Where is Thumbkin?
Little Boy Blue
(Be)(Verb)ing
She'll Be Coming Round the Mountain
Modal Auxiliary
Mother, May I?
Jack Sprat
Third-Person Singular
The Farmer in the Dell
One He Loves, Two He Loves, Three He Loves, They Say
Past Tense
Jack and Jill
There Was an Old Woman Who Lived in a Shoe
Eensy Weensy Spider
This Little Piggy

BOX 9-6	Examples of Songs, Rhymes, and Finger Play Routines for Targeting Language Forms—cont'd

Questions
Where is Thumbkin?
Way Down Yonder in the Pawpaw Patch
***Have* Auxiliary**
Little Bo Peep
I've Been Working on the Railroad
He's Got the Whole World in His Hands
Relative Clauses
The House that Jack Built
There Was an Old Lady Who Swallowed a Fly
Conjunctions
Old Mother Hubbard
If You're Happy and You Know It

An additional plus for literature-based script therapy is that it provides an ideal "homework" activity for families interested in following up on intervention activities. Having parents read children books used in intervention is a simple and accessible activity that most parents will find enjoyable rather than taxing. Parents can be encouraged to ask the children to fill in words or phrases they leave out as they read. If songs and nursery rhymes are used, parents can ask the child to "teach" them the actions that go along with the rhymes and sing or recite them together as the parent "learns" the routine. In this way children can be made to feel that they are making an important contribution to the interaction. When encouraging parents to use literature-based scripts, whether from books or other oral texts, it will be important to be sensitive to the cultural aspects of these kinds of interactions and help parents find ways to engage their children actively and playfully around these scripts. Parents from low income or non-European backgrounds may not use the kinds of interactive strategies that clinicians expect. Family and cultural practices that are appropriate for script-based language activities should be explored with these families.

Like auditory bombardment, literature-based script therapy will probably make up a relatively small portion of the intervention session, perhaps 5 to 10 minutes. Other activities will, no doubt, use the bulk of the intervention time, but the benefits of those few minutes can be disproportionate. Not only will they contribute to the children's ability to use sophisticated language forms, they also will add to the clients' "cultural literacy," or familiarity with the classic texts of mainstream Western children's literature. Many children with language impairments have a weaker base of general information and cultural reference than normally developing children because they have limited access as a result of their language deficits. Literature-based script therapy can help fill this gap. In addition, literature-based script therapy provides excellent focused opportunities for "literacy socialization," the development of a familiarity with books and literary language style that will give the client a solid foundation for learning to read. As we use these approaches, though, we need to recall the cautions raised by Kaderavek and Justice (2002) to ensure we are maximizing children's attention and engagement with books and other literature scripts. And we must remember to provide opportunities for children to practice the forms learned within the script in a wider variety of linguistic contexts. For example, if children have learned several spatial terms from *Inside, Outside, Upside Down*, these terms should be used in other activities. The child and clinician might, for example, take turns "hiding" a raisin and giving clues that contain spatial terms so the other can "find" it (it's *inside* the drawer; it's *outside* the doll house").

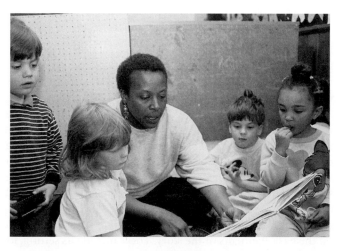

Literature-based script intervention develops cultural literacy in children with language disorders.

Structured Play. Shriberg and Kwiatkowski (1982a) also discussed using play organized by the clinician as a hybrid approach to phonological intervention. They suggested, for example, having cards with pictures representing the client's target words to be sent as letters. Each picture is named by the client as it is placed in an envelope, "stamped," and "addressed" to someone the client thinks would like to get that picture. The "letters" are then mailed in a toy mailbox. The clinician does not correct the child's pronunciation but can offer production cues if the child is receptive to them. The focus of the activity is on the fun of sending the letters, rather than on responding to the clinician's prompts to say the words. Still, the naming of the words on the cards provides opportunities for client practice and clinician feedback.

Using Conversation and Narrative in Hybrid Intervention. We

talked before about the fact that we do not generally want to add pragmatic targets to our list of intervention goals. Instead, we try to set up pragmatic contexts in which clients can use the semantic, syntactic, and phonological skills being developed. As we saw in Table 9-1, the pragmatic skills that we expect to show the greatest degree of growth during the DL stage are conversational skills and the emergence of the ability to tell and understand stories, or use narrative discourse. Let's look briefly at how we might incorporate conversational and narrative contexts into hybrid intervention activities.

Conversation. Brinton and Fujiki (1994, 1995) have presented example programs for using conversation as a context for intervention. The clinician ensures that guided conversation supports the skills being targeted. Brinton and Fujiki (1994) focused on two types of conversational behaviors identified by Fey (1986)—*assertive* and *responsive* skills—and suggested techniques for developing each set of skills in clients with language impairment.

Children with poor *assertive* skills are quiet in conversation. They take their conversational turns reluctantly or not at all and rarely initiate topics. For clients with this difficulty, Brinton and Fujiki suggested first engaging the children in entertaining interactive activities in which they must do something to sustain the interaction, although at first a child's contribution can be minimal. For example, a simple game such as "Go Fish" can be used. Here a client working on question forms might use the form "Do you have (X)?" in the game format. The game requires the client to initiate the question. If the client does not ask spontaneously, the clinician can simply wait, providing a cue only after a relatively long (10- to 15-second) pause in which the client does not initiate. As the game progresses, the clinician can use more and more truncated cues, going from "Say, 'Do you have (X)?'" to "Ask me," to simply an expectant look. Later the demands of the game can be "upped" so that more is expected of the client. For example, the rules of the game can be changed so that the client must ask a more elaborate question ("Do you have a green fish with white fins?") or a more polite form of the question ("May I please have an (X)?").

Brinton and Fujiki emphasized that the format should soon become less structured. They advocated manipulating the context so that clients are highly motivated to initiate. If questions were the structural target, again, a clinician might set up a situation in which a puppet told the clinician a "secret." Clients who wanted to hear the secret would have to ask to be told. When initiations such as these, using forms targeted in the intervention program, become frequent in conversations guided by the clinician, Brinton and Fujiki suggested having the client participate in peer conversations. Here the clinician would be present as a conversational "coach," offering advice, cues, and prompts as the client engages in conversation with first one peer, then with several. The clinician can encourage the client to be persistent about getting a turn, give hints about appropriate topic-maintaining comments the client can make, supply cues as to when it is appropriate for the client to take a turn, and help the client handle interruptions. In the context of these peer conversations, the clinician also can remind the client to use the forms learned in the intervention program to accomplish the conversational goals. Using questions as the example target again, the clinician can, for instance, remind the client to use a target form to initiate role negotiation in pretend play with peers. The clinician can coach the client to use question forms to ask who wants to play the mommy in a game of "house," who wants to be the baby, and so on.

Fujiki and Brinton (1991) showed that children who have trouble with *responsiveness* in conversation are less likely to find conversational partners responsive to them. Both peers and adults find conversations with such children difficult and unrewarding. In using conversational contexts for language intervention with unresponsive children, Brinton and Fujiki (1994) suggested some interactive games that help the child become sensitive to signals in conversation that a turn is available. They advocated setting up turn exchanges in fairly structured situations so that turn exchange points are, at first, explicitly marked. Using walkie-talkies or pretend radios, for example, the client and clinician can talk to each other and signal that their turn has ended by saying "over." The turns themselves can consist of structured talk in which forms targeted in the interaction program are used. If, for example, *[be]-[verb]-ing* sentences are intervention targets, the client and clinician can talk over their radios about what they are doing as they roam the hallway (Clinician: "I am going around the corner. Over." Client: "I am walking past our room. Over.").

Brinton and Fujiki advocated moving from these activities to more collaborative games in which the client needs to obtain and attend to information provided by the partner. They suggested that children (or puppets, if additional children are not involved in the session) can each be given different pieces of a puzzle or toy that needs to be assembled and told to hide their piece. The client can then approach each one and ask what each had and where to find it. The client would need to listen to each response before assembling the whole. The client also might "take orders" from a catalogue or fast-food menu and be required to "check back" with the customer to be sure the order was taken correctly before filling it. These games can go on at first between the client and clinician. Later, additional peers can be added, with the clinician serving again as coach,

reminding clients to signal that others can take a turn and to pay attention and respond to the talk of other participants. Brinton and Fujiki (1995) also advocate training parents, teachers, and peers to use conversational contexts to address semantic and syntactic targets, such as referring to events outside the immediate context and increasing the production of complex sentence forms.

Research is emerging that suggests that peers are especially effective agents of intervention for social and conversational skills (Paul, 2003a). We'll talk later about how to involve preschool peers in mediating social interactions for children with disabilities, in order to take advantage of the special salience that conversations with peers have for young children. DeKroon, Kyte, and Johnson (2002) showed that social pretend play, in which children played with peers using toys or objects around pretend or fantasy themes, elicited the highest levels of conversational behavior in dyads containing a child with language impairment and a typical peer. These play settings, then, would be ideal ones for the clinician to orchestrate when coaching clients in conversational contexts. Beilinson and Olswang (2003) showed that coaching preschoolers to use interesting props in order to gain entry into peer group play activities was especially helpful in increasing the opportunities for social interactions for young children with communication difficulties. Part of our conversational coaching agenda, then, could be to arm children with interesting objects in order to smooth their way into peer interactions.

Narrative. When we talk about language in the school-age period, we'll see in more detail that narrative skills—which begin to emerge during the DL period and reach their full flower during the school years—are closely related to academic success. Fey, Catts, Proctor-Williams, Tomblin, and Zhang (2004) and Paul and Smith (1993) showed that children with language disorders in the DL period were less skilled than typical peers at producing narratives. We talked just a while ago about how work on metaphonology develops emerging literacy skills and provides preventive intervention for averting later problems in learning to read. Targeting narrative skills during the DL phase can also build toward emerging literacy and effect preventive intervention. That's because narrative, too, is highly correlated with success in literacy (Bishop & Edmundson, 1987; Gillam, McFadden, & van Kleeck, 1995). Narrative contexts provide fertile ground for addressing a variety of aspects of communication, including vocabulary, syntax, morphology, verbal memory, as well as narrative structure (Swanson, Fey, Mills, & Hood, 2005).

Culatta (1994) presented some suggestions for integrating narrative contexts into language intervention at this level. She suggested using story re-enactments. These involve, first, having clients listen to simple stories. The stories can be read from classic children's books, such as those used in literature-based script activities. Familiar folktales or fairy tales also can be told orally. Before the clients listen to the story for the first time, the clinician can provide a preparatory set to focus their attention on the basic elements of the story. These include its setting, its central character, its basic problem, the characters' plans and goals, and the consequences of the characters' actions. If the story chosen is a familiar tale, clients can be asked to recall the setting, characters, and so on before it is told. If it is a new story, they can be told to listen for these elements so they can answer questions about them later. After hearing the story the first time, clients can be asked to focus on these elements by answering questions about where the story happens, who is in the story, what the character's problem is in the story, how the character tries to solve it, and what happens when the character acts on the plan. If clients hear and enact several different stories over the course of an intervention period, we can ask the same questions about each one. In this way clients can begin to internalize the story grammar structure (see Box 10-4) that these questions imply.

Clients can then assume roles to act out the story, using simple props and costumes. The language of the story can be chosen specifically to emphasize forms being targeted in the intervention. If clients are working on auxiliary *will,* for example, the "Three Little Pigs" story might be used. The client can play the wolf, who says, "I *will* huff, and I *will* puff, and I *will* blow your house in." The clinician can act as "narrator," again pointing out the critical elements in the story. The next time, the client can act as both narrator and actor, using the target language and embedding it in the narrative frame. The clinician can "coach" the client in the retelling, encouraging both the use of correct forms and attention to critical story grammar elements in the narration. Later reenactments can use paper cutouts instead of live actors, which the client can manipulate as the story is narrated. The story also can be retold with slightly different characters or by changing the language slightly to broaden the target language forms used (after using the uncontracted, "I *will* huff . . .," for example, the dialogue can be changed to the contracted, "I'*ll* huff . . ."). Swanson, Fey, Mills, and Hood (2005) provide additional suggestions for using narratives in language intervention at the DL stage.

INTERVENTION CONTEXTS FOR CHILDREN WITH DEVELOPING LANGUAGE

When deciding about the contexts for intervention for children in the DL phase, we need to answer two primary questions:
1. Who should deliver the intervention?
2. What service delivery model will be used?

Let's look at some of the options available for answering these questions in the DL period.

Agents of Intervention for Children with Developing Language

Three types of intervention agents, apart from trained clinicians, are typically considered for children in the DL period: paraprofessionals, parents, and peers.

Paraprofessionals. Paraprofessionals are individuals who deliver services to children and their families but serve under the supervision of a professional who is ultimately responsible for the intervention program. Generally, paraprofessionals provide one-to-one instruction, using methods and procedures developed by the supervising clinician. Coufal, Steckelberg,

and Vasa (1991) reported that paraprofessionals are effective in modifying both articulatory and language behavior in children. The ASHA (2000) has provided guidelines for the training and supervision of paraprofessionals in speech-language pathology; an explication of these guidelines is provided by Paul-Brown and Goldberg (2001). These documents tell us that there are several roles for paraprofessionals to assume with children in the DL period. They can be trained to use the same kind of indirect language stimulation we might teach parents to provide, for the purpose of practice and generalization, following procedures outlined in research such as Girolametto, Weitzman, and Greenberg (2003). For children in classroom-based intervention settings, the paraprofessional can supply intensive one-to-one language stimulation. This can include modeling appropriate uses of communication that the client can use to interact with peers and engage in developmentally appropriate play, and "coaching" the client within these interactions.

They can also provide structured CD or hybrid intervention to individuals or small groups, as directed by the clinician. Here the clinician designs a lesson plan in detail, including the linguistic stimuli, materials, and activities to be used; the responses to be targeted; and the reinforcement or corrective feedback to be given. Alternatively, the clinician might provide a commercially available lesson plan to address a goal that is part of the child's program. Paul (1992b) provided just one example of a commercial program that can be used in this way. In either case, the paraprofessional follows the clinician's instructions, records the client's responses, and presents the data to the clinician for evaluation and subsequent treatment planning. Use of paraprofessionals can provide helpful expansion of the amount of intervention time available to clients with language disorders. We need to remember, though, that in working with these assistants, the design and evaluation of the program remains our job, not theirs. We can make best use of paraprofessionals by training them in a small set of tasks and providing clear and explicit instruction as to what they are to do with the client, while maintaining responsibility ourselves for the bulk of the decision making and accountability in the intervention program.

There's one more issue in working with paraprofessionals. In the case of children with severe disabilities, a paraprofessional is sometimes assigned full-time to one child in order to allow him/her to function within the classroom. But, training is especially important for paraprofessionals in this role, since without it they may serve to isolate rather than integrate the child (Causton-Theoharis & Malmgren, 2005; Ghere, York-Barr, & Sommerness, 2002). SLPs should work closely with these paraprofessionals to help them develop strategies for mediating social interactions and communication between the child and peers. Methods such as those used by Causton-Theoharis and Malmgren (2005), Ghere et al. (2002), Girolametto, Weitzman, and Greenberg (2003), and Odom et al. (1999) can be used to develop this kind of training.

Parents. We've talked before about the considerations that ought to go into a decision to use parents as agents of intervention. We've heard the argument that parents make better intervention agents because they are with the child all the time and can, theoretically, do nonstop intervention. We know, too, that it may not be to the child's advantage to be in intervention all the time and that children may need the acceptance and uncritical approval that parents can offer. In the DL period, the goal of intervention moves from simply eliciting language to eliciting and elaborating specific forms. This kind of elaboration can include corrective forms of feedback that, at times, may conflict with the normal communicative patterns between parents and children, in which errors of form are accepted and only errors of meaning corrected (Brown & Hanlon, 1970).

Tannock and Girolametto (1992) and Fey, Cleave, Long, and Hughes (1993) presented evidence questioning the efficacy of intervention approaches that rely solely on parents as agents of intervention. Fey et al. showed that the effects of clinician-delivered intervention were larger, more consistent, and more likely to continue over time than were the effects of intervention delivered by parents. Tannock and Girolametto argued that parent-delivered intervention, using techniques such as ILS, is good for giving children opportunities to practice or to generalize recently learned skills but is less effective in imparting the new skills themselves. Still Law, Garret, and Nye (2004) found in a meta-analysis that parent-delivered intervention was equal in efficacy to clinician-delivered programs for preschoolers. Although parents may be effective agents of intervention, many will prefer to have a professional involved, whenever cost does not prohibit it. And concerns about the effects of too much parental responsibility for intervention on the sensitive parent-child relationship, also suggest the use of parent-delivered intervention as just one aspect of the service delivery program for language-impaired children in the DL phase, again, when other considerations permit. Tannock and Girolametto's (1992) research suggests that an ideal role for parents is to encourage generalization and provide opportunities to use newly learned forms in a facilitative context.

Peers. A third alternative for intervention agent recently has been proposed for children in the DL period: a normally speaking peer. For example, Weiss and Nakamura (1992) reported on the use of typical peers as communication models for children with language impairments in a preschool classroom setting. The idea behind this approach is that normally speaking peers provide models that are slightly above the language of the impaired child but not too far above, because of the typical peer's own still developing stage. Presumably, conversation with a peer will be more natural and engaging to a developmentally young child than will interaction with an adult, since topics of conversation and activities of interest are more likely to be shared between two speakers of similar developmental level. Moreover, the nonhandicapped peer is likely to provide models of appropriate behavior and speech that can be imitated by the child with language impairment.

Weiss and Nakamura emphasized that, if normally speaking peers are introduced into an intervention setting such as a special educational or reverse mainstream classroom or small group therapy setting, children who act as models need to be carefully selected. Not all preschoolers are equally willing or able to interact with handicapped peers. Weiss and Nakamura

suggested selecting peers as models who not only demonstrate normal language competence but also show interest in handicapped peers, willingness to engage in play with them for extended periods, and responsiveness to the conversational bids of their language-impaired peers. This selection could be accomplished by inviting several normally speaking peers to visit the language classroom or group and providing some especially engaging activities, such as water or sand play, to serve as an incentive for their participation. The visitors can be observed and models chosen from those who appear most responsive to the children with language disorders. These special visitors can be invited to return on a regular basis.

Still, simply putting a child with a disorder in a playroom with a typical peer does not constitute intervention. Peers must be supported and encouraged to provide appropriate models and opportunities for the client. Hadley and Schuele (1998) showed that adults play a critical role in supporting the development of talk between children with language impairments and their typically speaking peers (that is, the clinician may need to work with the model to demonstrate how to prolong interactions, respond to unclear messages, give time for the client to produce a conversational turn, and so on). Venn, Wolery, Fleming, DeCesare, Morris, and Cuffs (1993) showed that normally speaking preschoolers could be trained to provide very specific linguistic stimuli, using the mand-model procedure discussed in Chapter 3. Their study showed that typical preschoolers could, with some practice as well as on-line modeling by the teacher, use scripted language models to elicit appropriate requests from peers with language disorders. This study suggested that even very structured forms of peer modeling can be achieved and can help increase the use of communication by children with language disorders. Peers who model appropriate language usage can, like parents, be useful adjuncts to the intervention program. Like parents, though, peer language models will probably be most useful for providing opportunities for practice and generalization, rather than for eliciting new communicative behaviors.

One additional role for peer-mediated intervention is in the area of play and social skills. For preschoolers with communication deficits that include pragmatic and social disabilities, peers are an especially effective source of intervention (Paul, 2003a). Research has shown that training peers to engage with children with disabilities has positive effects on their social skills that generalize beyond the training period. One approach (Odom et al., 1999) uses "play organizers" in which typical peers are taught to cue the target child during play sessions to share, help, give affection, and praise others. Results of programs like this indicate positive changes in social behavior, but they do require that adults spend some time in training, modeling, and role-playing for the peer partners. English, Goldstein, Shafer, and Kaczmarek (1997) developed a peer-mediated social skills program for preschool classrooms that involves less prior training for peers and has been shown to lead to improvements in the frequency of social communication between target children and typical peers. Each child in the class is assigned a "buddy" for a specified period of time, and each day includes a "buddy time" session of 20 minutes in length, often during the "free play" period of the preschool day. All children in the class participate, so some pairs include two typical children; others have a typical child and one with a disability. The rules for buddy time are taught to the group:

▶ Week 1: STAY with your buddy: maintain physical proximity to assigned partner.

▶ Week 2: PLAY with your buddy: maintain proximity while continuing to play with your partner (partners are offered a choice of one activity each from a visual "choice board" then instructed to play with each partner's choice for half the buddy period session, usually 10-20 min.).

▶ Week 3: TALK with your buddy: say your partner's name to establish joint attention, make suggestions for playing together, talk about the play, respond to what your partner says by repeating, saying more about it, or asking a question.

Pairs who comply with the rules for a buddy session each receive a prize. This reward gives the typical child an incentive to help the child with a disability maintain contact. These kinds of peer-mediated interventions can help to integrate students with disabilities more effectively in mainstream settings. They also increase their opportunities for exposure to relevant peer models, and for using their communication skills in an authentic context.

Service Delivery Models for Children with Developing Language

Our discussion of agents of intervention answers the "Who?" aspect of intervention contexts. The following discussion of service delivery models will answer the questions "Where?" and "When?" We talked in Chapter 3 about the range of service-delivery models available to us. These include the pull-out or clinical model, the language-based classroom, the collaborative model, and the consultant model. We've seen that a variety of agents of intervention can be involved in any of these service delivery models. Paraprofessionals as well as SLPs can deliver services using a clinical model. Special education teachers in addition to SLPs can deliver services in a language-based classroom. Parents can be the agents of intervention, using a consultant model, with the clinician providing occasional input to the parent who does the actual intervention with the child. Let's look at how each service delivery model might function for a child in the DL period.

Clinical Model. Many children in the DL phase are seen for one-to-one or small-group intervention in schools, clinics, and private-practice settings using this model. If you did your training in a program that had a campus clinic affiliated with it, you probably earned some of your clinical practicum hours seeing preschool children there, using this service delivery option. Despite the many onslaughts on its primacy, it is still a common service delivery model used with children in the DL period. And there's nothing wrong with it. Roberts, Prizant, and McWilliam (1995) showed that few differences existed in interactive styles of either clients or clinicians when in-class and pull-out methods of intervention were compared. They suggested that it is premature to associate one particular service delivery model with a higher degree of treatment efficacy. Just

as we want to have a repertoire of clinical procedures available to us to match to the needs of the client, it is helpful to have a range of service delivery models we can use. The clinical model is very useful for children with attentional problems, for whom a classroom or other rich environment might be too distracting. It provides a helpfully quiet environment for children with hearing impairments or others who have difficulty screening out background noise. It can provide a safe and comforting place for children with behavioral or emotional problems who need the nurturing qualities of a one-to-one attachment to an adult.

The major shortcoming of the clinical model, aside from its high cost and labor-intensity, is that it may be less effective at achieving generalization to the natural communicative environment. For this reason, it is wise to be especially careful to build in some of the generalization activities discussed in Chapter 3 when this model is used. Similarly, we need to be sure to build in some social interactive opportunities that will facilitate peer interactions for our clients, as Hadley and Schuele (1998) have suggested. To achieve this end, the clinician must be sure to incorporate a mix of activities across the continuum of naturalness from structured CD to more naturalistic CC approaches, using multiple exemplars, involving multiple communication partners, carrying on the intervention in different places, using naturalistic reinforcers, using distractor items and intermittent reinforcement, providing coaching in peer interactions, and encouraging self-monitoring.

Language-Based Classroom. A classroom specially designed to provide intensive language stimulation and training in the context of a mainstream, reverse mainstream (typical peers invited to join a special education preschool), or special education program is a model that is used with increasing frequency to address the needs of children in the DL phase. For SLPs with little background in early education, following such a service delivery model can seem daunting. The need to address the individual needs of all the students within a common set of activities may seem difficult at first. But the advantages of the model are many. Language-based classrooms usually provide extended periods of intervention time, more than the usual 45 minutes two or three times a week. These settings also provide opportunities to work as a team to improve language and preliteracy skills for children with disabilities and those at risk (Hadley, Simmerman, Long, & Luna, 2000).

Bricker and Pretti-Frontczak's (2004) activity-based intervention program and Bunce's (1995) language-focused curriculum are two examples of language-based classroom models. These classrooms typically involve theme-based units that incorporate traditional preschool activities such as crafts, story reading, pretend play, and small-group interactions. Some may include pull-out or clinical service to some or all of the students for a portion of the day, but the bulk of the intervention is done in the context of the classroom activities, which are chosen not only for their theme and content, but for the specific purpose of fostering communicative development. SLPs often serve as lead teachers in these classrooms, or function collaboratively on a team with a special educator, and have

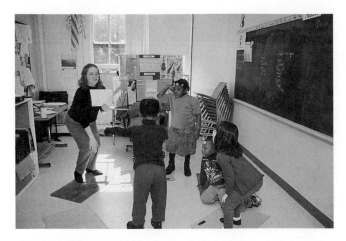

Classroom-based intervention is often used at the preschool level.

responsibility for planning the overall classroom program so that it addresses the communicative needs of all the students. Table 9-9 presents some of the strategies suggested by Bricker and Pretti-Frontczak (2004) for enhancing communicative development in these settings. The procedures can, of course, be used in a variety of other intervention settings as well. You'll probably notice that many are similar to Wetherby and Prizant's (1989) communication temptations and are not all that different from Cleave and Fey's focused stimulation. Classroom-based preschool language intervention combines a variety of approaches we've been discussing, such as milieu teaching, indirect language stimulation, script therapy, and theme-related structure. As such, it exemplifies what we mean by hybrid intervention.

Routine activities are one context for language modeling and practice in these settings. Each client's language goals can be integrated in the language used in the routines. If Rachel, for

example, were involved in this type of intervention program, a goal such as producing subjective pronouns might be addressed during snack each day. She might be asked by the teacher, "Who wants a cracker? If you want a cracker, raise your hand and say, 'I do!' Who wants a cracker?" Children with different goals would be provided with models of their own target forms during the same activity.

Theme-based units are another feature of language-based classrooms. If the theme for the week were "planting and growing," then stories, songs, and rhymes around the unit might be presented during group time. The group might play "Ring Around the Rosie" and read *The Carrot Seed* (Kraus & Johnson, 1945). Activities the children could choose from during Free Choice time might include making a plant collage with pre-cut paper shapes in the Art Center; listening to a prerecorded story with a planting theme in the Listening Center; pretending to plant a garden with appropriate props in the Dramatic Play area; and building walls, flower boxes, and a plant sale stand in the Block Center.

Again, individual goals would be addressed in theme-based activities. Using Rachel as our example, again, she might be asked to sing the line "We all fall down" when it comes up in the song. During story reading she might be asked to repeat certain parts of the story that include the pronoun *he* in response to the teacher's question. For outdoor time, the group might take a nature walk to look for things that grow. Rachel might be asked to name some of the growing things she sees as she walks along, beginning each sentence with, "I see . . ." At snack time, sunflower and pumpkin seeds might be served. Rachel could be asked to select which she wants by saying, "I want . . ." At the Art Center, Rachel could be asked to answer questions such as, "Who put a leaf on the collage?" with "I did!" A concept lesson might include planting seeds to grow in the classroom. The teacher might describe each step in the planting, then ask

TABLE 9-9	**Strategies for Activity-Based Language Intervention**

STRATEGY	EXAMPLE
Forgetfulness	Forget to give out brushes during painting; children must do something to request needed supplies.
Novelty	Introduce slightly new elements into known routine (e.g., play "Farmer in the Dell" wearing a big straw hat. Let children who comment on the hat have a turn to wear it).
In sight but out of reach	Put attractive or necessary objects where children can see them, but cannot get them without help. Encourage them to communicate a request.
Violate expectations	Omit or change a step in a routine (e.g., give a child a dish of ice cream but no spoon).
Piece by piece	Give items needed for an activity one at a time, so the clients need to communicate something to get each one. At snack time, give out one raisin at a time, or color by giving out one crayon at a time.
Assistance	Put the child's snack in a clear glass jar that he or she cannot open without help, so the child needs to communicate a request to obtain an object or activity.
Sabotage	Unplug the tape recorder, then ask child to turn it on; hide children's coats when it is time to go outside. This forces the client to do something communicative to try to correct the situation.
Delay	Pause in the midst of an activity to get the child to communicate the need to continue (e.g., pause while zipping a coat before going outdoors).

Adapted from Bricker, D., & Pretti-Frontczak, K. (2004). *An activity-based approach to early intervention.* 3rd ed. Baltimore, MD: Paul H. Brookes Publishing.

students to reiterate the sequence of actions after they were finished. Rachel, for her turn, could be asked to answer questions such as, "Who put a seed in the dirt?" with "I did! Again, children with other goals would also be presented with opportunities for modeling or practice of these forms within the same activities.

Child-initiated contexts also are used for intervention purposes in these programs, as they are in the incidental teaching approach. Any initiation by the child would receive a response that highlighted or capitalized on the child's identified intervention goals. If Rachel, for example, said, "Me cold!" to the teacher on the playground, the teacher could respond, "Are you? *I'm* cold, too. *I* am. *I* am very, very cold today. And you are too! *I* need a warmer coat. *I* need a hat. *I* need mittens. How about you?"

Another advantage is that classroom-based intervention provides ample opportunity for development not only of communicative skill but of emergent literacy. Prelock, Cataland, Honchell, and Cordonnier (1993) suggested the importance of including "literacy centers" within the preschool environment for children with language disorders. These centers would include theme-based opportunities for seeing print in labels and captions for pictures; playing with literacy artifacts such as menus, newspapers, grocery lists, and product labels drawn from classroom themes; using invented spelling to write stories and label drawings to follow up storybook experiences; and dictating class "experience stories" to record events of importance to the group. Kaderavek and Justice (2004) provide sample activities, and Watson, Layton, Pierce, and Abraham (1994) outlined additional ways to incorporate literacy events in the preschool classroom. Table 9-10 gives some examples of their suggestions.

Collaborative Model. Much of what we discussed in terms of the language-based classroom applies to the collaborative model as well. In collaborative intervention, the SLP acts as a "guest teacher," providing targeted intervention activities for clients placed in a mainstream classroom setting. This model requires the clinician to master the skills necessary to manage a classroom and to be able to work closely with a regular education teacher to plan and implement the client's program. Moreover, it requires us to come up with activities that are useful and engaging to the entire class while giving the client communicative experiences that will address the individual's targets. We discussed one example activity that might be used in this type of model in Chapter 3. Box 9-7 provides an example geared to the DL period.

Like the language-based classroom, collaborative intervention provides a great opportunity to serve our clients in a meaningful, functional setting that maximizes the potential for generalization. Further, it gives the client the chance to function in the least restrictive setting, as IDEA legislation intends. Working in the context of a mainstream or reverse mainstream classroom to address a client's needs, while at the same time supplying valuable experiences to the regular education students, goes a long way toward actualizing the spirit of the law. And it allows us to reach beyond our identified clients

to other children at risk. Hadley et al. (2000) showed when SLPs collaborate with regular teachers to "guest teach" vocabulary and PA in inner-city preschool classrooms, gains in these areas were superior to those in classrooms without SLP input. And Throneburg, Calvert, Sturm, Paramboukas, and Paul (2000) demonstrated that a collaborative model was more effective than regular instruction in teaching vocabulary both to students with identified disabilities and to other children in the classroom. Collaborative models, then, are powerful ways of improving oral language for a wide range of children.

But successful collaboration requires intensive planning, coordination, and cooperation among team members. Giangreco (2000) identified five themes that reflect successful collaborative efforts involving SLPs:

▶ *Be ready to learn from others.* It is not necessary for the SLP to present herself as the "expert." Instead, listen to the contributions of others and consider them from the perspective of the language specialist.

▶ *Take responsibility for the student as a team.* Each member of the team should feel ownership in the student's program. Rather than saying the student "belongs" to the special education or classroom teacher, the team should share their individual viewpoints on the student's needs, find points of agreement, and cooperatively assume responsibility for his/her progress.

▶ *Have a system in place for making decisions.* Build time for discussion and comparing points of view into the team process. Have established means of resolving conflicts and dealing with conflicting views.

▶ *Clarify the roles of team members.* Decide who will do what when. Not all members need to be involved in all aspects of a student's program. Make explicit joint decisions.

▶ *Support families and regular education teachers.* Include family and teachers in meetings; include family and teacher perceptions in planning. Be aware that the child will spend more time in the home and classroom than in the therapy setting; so these are the contexts in which it is most important for the child's progress to be seen.

Consultant Model. It's very likely that some part of the service delivery for children in the DL period will involve the SLP in a consulting role. If the child is in a preschool classroom, we may be called on to help the teacher individualize the client's program. If parents are agents of any portion of the intervention, we will be responsible for consulting with them on techniques to be used. The most helpful thing a clinician can do in a consulting role is to supply specific suggestions for activities that parents and teachers can use to engage the client. Many commercially available programs are useful. The clinician can select lessons, based on the client's assessment data and IEP goals, from these commercial packages and give copies to teachers and parents to use. Alternatively, the clinician can provide training in specific techniques, such as ILS or joint book reading. The point is to be as specific as possible. Teachers and parents both have enough to do without having to think up language intervention and stimulation ideas. Our backgrounds and training give us the experience and knowledge to do this, and the more

| | TABLE 9-10 | Facilitating Emergent Literacy in Preschool Classroom Activities | | | | |

	PRINT AWARENESS	BOOK AWARENESS	STORY SENSE	PHONOLOGICAL AWARENESS	MATCHING SPEECH AND PRINT	PRACTICING PREREADING AND PREWRITING
Circle time	Look for name tag	Make "book" with words of daily song; children follow along as they sing, teacher points out words in book			Match printed words in song "book" to the words they sing	"Read" job list with students' names and pictures of each classroom job
Story time	Show book during reading	Point out when pages are turned	Use well-structured stories; ask questions about story after reading	Point out rhymes, alliteration in reading; ask students to remember words that rhymed or started with the same sound from the story	Have children "read" parts of the book chorally	Have children "read" parts of the book chorally
Center time	Provide magnetic, felt, tactile letters at play centers	Provide blank paper "books" for children to write and draw in	Relate art activities to stories read; carry over story theme	Encourage invented spelling in art and play activities	Label favorite play equipment; post classroom rules for children to "read"	Label drawings, encourage children to invent spellings to label their own drawings
Snack time	Label snack supplies; have snack helpers "read" labels		Follow recipes from stories, such as "Stone Soup"	Talk about sounds in words for snacks eaten; make up rhymes for daily snack item	Encourage children to "read" labels on foods used at snack	Encourage children to "read" labels on foods used at snack
Outdoor time	Use signs, such as a "STOP" sign, in games such as "red light, green light"		Act out favorite stories in outside play		Use cards with pictures and words in addition to verbal instructions in games such as "Simon Says"	Use cards with pictures and words in addition to verbal instructions in games such as "Simon Says"

Adapted from Watson, L., Layton, T., Pierce, P., & Abraham, L. (1994). Enhancing emerging literacy in a language preschool. *Language, Speech, and Hearing Services in Schools, 25,* 136-145.

detailed and specific the information we provide to those with whom we consult, the more appreciated we will be. No one wants to devote hard-pressed time to consulting with someone purporting to be an expert who doesn't offer anything concrete in terms of what to do with the child. Box 9-8 gives an example of the kind of specific consultation suggestions that might be given to a classroom teacher to help include a client's phonological targets within the classroom setting.

The second important role we have as consultants is to do ongoing assessment and evaluation of the client's program.

BOX 9-7   **An Example of a Collaborative Intervention Activity for the Developing Language Period**

Target: Use of present-tense auxiliary verbs (*can, will*).
Theme: Neighborhood helpers.
Materials: Props for various familiar occupations (mail carrier's bag, nurse's stethoscope, teacher's chalk, dentist's floss, garbage collector's gloves, etc.).
Procedure: Assign each student to be one of the helpers the group has been discussing. Give each the appropriate prop. Ask, "Who can help us if our teeth hurt? Who will help us learn to read?" Have the student playing that role answer "I can!" or "I will." Have the student demonstrate or mime what that helper does. Then give each student a turn to ask, "Who can/will X?" After each question, the appropriate helper should answer, "I can/will!" and act out another aspect of the job (or the same one, it they can't think of another one). Give the client a turn after several other students have demonstrated the script. Then play a guessing game: "I'm thinking of someone who can/will X." Give a clue as to the job of each helper and have the students raise their hands to answer the question (e.g., "I'm thinking of someone who can bring us our mail"). Encourage them to reply, "The X (e.g., mail carrier) can/will." Again, give the client a turn after several students have demonstrated the response. After each response, have the child playing that role stand up and demonstrate. Finally, give each student a turn to say, "I'm thinking of someone who can/will X." Give the client a turn after several others have taken one.

BOX 9-8   **Consultation Suggestions for Including Phonological Targets within a Classroom Setting**

Classroom Theme: Winter.
Center: Water play.
Phonological Targets: /s/, /z/, and /s/ blends.
Activity: Cookie sheets filled with ice are placed floating in the water at the water table. Small toy people figures are placed there, too. A sign is placed over the water table that reads, "Skate, slip, and slide," which is read to the class when the activity is introduced.
Suggestions for Teacher: As you circulate among students at the table, model talking about the figures as they skate, slip, and slide. Talk with the children about safety on ice, the process of freezing and melting, how the ice feels and looks, and their own experiences with ice and skating. Introduce target vocabulary in this talk. As the ice begins to melt, give the children toothpicks and small pieces of paper to make signs that say, "Keep off ice" or "Stay off." Use target vocabulary to ask open-ended questions and comment on the changes in feel, look, and safety of the ice as it melts.
Target Vocabulary: Ice, icy, frozen, freeze, freezing, slide, slip, slippery, skate, across, start, sign, safe, safety, smooth, slick, soft, melts, cracks, slush, sink, sinking.
Evaluation: Allow the student to play at the water area for several days, providing models of target vocabulary, and encouraging peers to provide additional models. After 3 days, track the client's productions at the center for 7 minutes, using the data sheet below. Put a hash mark under "Attempts" each time the client attempts a word with a target sound and a check under "Correct Productions" each time the target sound is produced correctly. Discuss with the team at weekly meetings to decide if new target sounds and words should be added.

Data Sheet

Target Sound	#Attempts	#Correct Productions
/s/		
/z/		
/sl/		
/sk/		
/st/		
/sm/		
/ts/		
/ks/		

Adapted from Prelock, P., Cataland, J., Honchell, C., & Cordonnier, M. (1993). *Effective collaborative intervention models for the preschool and home setting*. Poster session presented at National Convention of the American Speech-Language-Hearing Association, Anaheim, CA.

We need to decide when to move on to a new goal, modify the program, or terminate intervention. This monitoring function can be fulfilled by giving the parent or teacher evaluation procedures (that is, data sheets such as the one in Box 9-8) to be filled out at specified time intervals. Alternatively, we can collect the data ourselves by spending some time directly assessing the client periodically. This approach has the advantage of keeping us in touch with the client in a more immediate way than simply reviewing written records. We can get a better "feel" not only for what but also for *how* the client is learning. It also increases our credibility with our consultees. If we are known to be willing to get down on the floor and "get our hands dirty" with the client in the DL period, we are less likely to engender resentment on the part of the people who see themselves as "really doing all the work" of delivering intervention. Such resentments are lethal to the success of a consultative form of intervention. A little direct involvement with the client can go a long way toward avoiding this dangerous pitfall.

A third role for SLPs in preschool concerns helping teachers understand and manage challenging behaviors. We talked earlier about the fact that children with disabilities sometimes turn to maladaptive behaviors, such as aggression, because they do not have more conventional means available for expressing themselves. Nungesser and Watkins (2005) report that the presence of challenging behaviors can limit a child's opportunities to participate in mainstream settings, because teachers are unwilling or feel unable to manage these difficult episodes, and that teachers are often unaware of the communicative function of these behaviors. As consultants, SLPs can help teachers to understand how communication disorders can lead to the behaviors, how language training can impact them, and how to select appropriate language-based prevention and intervention approaches. This process is often called Functional Communication Training (FCT; Bopp, Brown, & Mirenda, 2004). In working with teachers as consultants on replacing challenging behaviors with more effective forms of communication, Nungesser and Watkins (2005) and Bopp, Brown, and Mirenda (2004) made the following suggestions for SLP consultations:

▶ Help the teacher to understand that these behaviors may be used to serve a communicative function.
▶ Establish the function of the maladaptive behavior through functional behavior analysis.
▶ Use visual schedules to aid comprehension and predict events.
▶ Model dealing with the behavior within the classroom. Work with the child in a situation likely to trigger the behavior, and model how to prevent it, by providing an appropriate communication strategy to the child when aggressive behavior seems imminent.
▶ Suggest that the teacher model using language for emotions within classroom activities; show students how to talk (or communicate) about how they feel; and encourage peers to do the same.
▶ Help teachers involve families in carrying over strategies to the home setting.

INTERVENTION WITH OLDER CLIENTS WITH SEVERE IMPAIRMENT AT THE DEVELOPING LANGUAGE LEVEL

Some clients whose language is in the DL phase may be quite a bit older than preschool age. Clients with severe disabilities and developmental delays who have been in language intervention programs for a number of years may be operating within Brown's stages II to V in terms of their use of language forms and meanings. Is the goal for these clients to achieve fully adult grammar and semantics? Should we attempt to teach them all the rules and vocabulary we would choose as targets for a younger, less severely involved child? Part of this decision, of course, involves the family. Their desires and perceptions of the client's needs will play an important role in determining intervention targets. Nelson (1998) articulated several principles that we should keep in mind when designing intervention programs for older students at the DL level. These are summarized in Box 9-9.

FCT can be used with students who use some speech, or those whose primary mode of communication is augmentative or alternative communication (AAC). Task analysis, breaking the client's communicative needs down into very small "slices," also can help in planning the intervention. For example, suppose the ecological inventory identified the need to take the city bus to school each day as an important context in which communication is needed. The clinician might ride the bus with the client one day and note the communication that is required. It might be noticed that the client needs to find the correct place to wait for the bus by "reading" the sign or at least identifying the sign that says "Bus Stop" and finding the stop with the correct bus number. Then the client might need to check the number on the bus that stops; get on the right one; show the driver a bus pass; and say, "Please tell me when we get to Washington School." The client might need to sit near the front of the bus to hear the driver announce the stop. The client would need to listen for the announcement, get up when it is heard, and say, "Thank you" to the driver before getting off the bus. The clinician could record each of these steps and, using behavioral techniques, modeling, and role-playing in script therapy, teach each piece of the process, one at a time. As each is acquired, it can be "chained" (McCormick & Goldman, 1984) onto the sequence being learned, so that the sequence gets longer as each new piece is added, until the client can perform the entire sequence independently in the educational setting. Then the clinician may want to accompany the client again in the real situation to provide monitoring and feedback as the new chain of skills is used in the functional setting.

Note that, in using script therapy or behavioral techniques, a long, complex sentence such as, "Please tell me when we get to Washington School," could be taught, even though such structures might be developmentally more advanced than the client's spontaneous speech would suggest is possible. Functional intervention means teaching a few powerful scripts or

BOX 9-9	**Principles of Intervention for Older, Severely Impaired Clients at Developing Language Levels**

1. Focus intervention on helping students develop functional abilities for participating with as much independence as possible in mainstream settings.
2. Goals for older individuals in this phase of language development should be functional, rather than based on the normal developmental sequence. Instead of attempting to teach all the grammatical morphemes, choose specific language forms that are useful for particular situations selected by means of an ecological inventory.
3. Provide specific communication services for clients who:
   • Have trouble understanding instructions in their daily living activities
   • Cannot produce enough communication to function independently in a variety of mainstream settings (such as travel, school, work, shopping, leisure)
   • Violate rules of politeness and appropriateness in social interactions
   • Lack functional abilities to read important environmental signs and use functional written communication
   • Have difficulty making their speech understood, speaking fluently, or using audible voice
4. Use activities and materials in intervention that are appropriate and functional.
5. Develop early literacy skills, using specific behavioral techniques, even if cognitive levels usually associated with reading have not been achieved.
6. Develop opportunities for students to participate as independently as possible in important social contexts (athletics, church, clubs, leisure activities, etc.).

Adapted from Nelson, N. (1998). *Childhood language disorders in context: Infancy through adolescence* (ed. 2). Columbus, OH: Merrill.

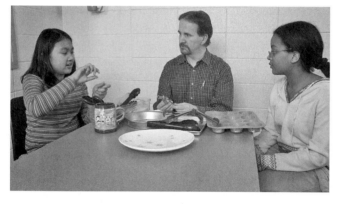

Intervention for older clients with developing language uses functional materials.

behaviors that might not be acquired as generalizable rules. Similarly, "reading" might be considered developmentally too advanced a skill for certain clients. But careful training could enable such clients to "read" several important signs and symbols that have functional significance. These might include the "Bus Stop" sign and the ability to match the numbers on the sign, the bus, and the bus pass. When working with severely impaired older clients, we don't want to impede their progress toward autonomy by requiring them to go through all the stages of normal development before attempting to teach skills that can foster independence.

Another focus for students at this level will be FCT (Bopp, Brown, & Mirenda, 2004). As we discussed when talking about our consultative role, this training is used to replace troublesome behaviors that serve a communicative function with more adaptive responses. FCT can take place either in speech or using AAC systems. Bopp, Brown, and Mirenda (2004) argue that SLPs are equipped to provide FCT, in either direct or consultative roles, because of our familiarity with AAC strategies and our depth of knowledge about communication. They provide detailed instructions for implementing an FCT program. These are summarized briefly in Table 9-11. In addition, Halle, Brady, and Drasgow (2004) emphasize the importance of helping children with severe disabilities repair communication break-downs. These, too, are a source of frustration for low-functioning students, as they may be attempting to communicate in a way that is not easily understood by their audience, and these break-downs can lead to maladaptive behaviors. They emphasize the importance of developing a larger repertoire of socially acceptable signals, so if one fails they have alternatives, and of making sure communication partners (parents, teachers, and peers) are cued in to the child's new signals and encouraged to respond to them. Research summarized by Bopp et al. also supports the use of FCT to prevent and replace maladaptive behaviors for clients with severe disabilities. Parents need to be involved in replacing maladaptive behavior with more functional communication strategies at this level, using strategies similar to the ones we discussed earlier. Tait, Sigafoos, Woodyatt, O'Reilly, and Lancioni (2004) showed that parents could be successful in helping their children replace challenging behaviors with communication and that these gains were maintained over time.

TABLE 9-11	Elements of Functional Communication Training

ELEMENT	EXAMPLE
Functional Behavior Analysis: Identify functions of maladaptive behavior	Child bites peers; observe when child bites and identify antecedent, such as inability to gain access to toy peer has
Match an adaptive response to the communicative function of the maladaptive behavior	Teach child to use sign for "want" when he wishes to gain access to a peer's toy
Establish response mastery: make sure new communication achieves desired outcome	Teach "want" sign to peers and encourage them to respond when child requests in this way, or to call a teacher if they cannot respond
Establish appropriate schedule of reinforcement	Ensure that at first desired response is achieved quickly (less than 20 sec) gradually time delay can increase; teach child to use "want" sign with clinician and adults first to guarantee quick response; later bring in peers
Provide an alternative form if first is unsuccessful	Teach child if "want" sign does not achieve goal to use "please" sign
Use mild punishment when problem behaviors occur; quickly redirect to new communication behavior	If child bites or begins to bite, use brief facial screening (hands over eyes), then hand-over-hand guidance to produce "want" sign

Adapted from Bopp, K., Brown, K., & Mirenda, P. (2004). Speech-language pathologists' roles in the delivery of positive behavior support for individuals with developmental disabilities. *American Journal of Speech-Language Pathology, 13*, 5-19; Halle, J., Brady, N., & Drasgow, E. (2004). Enhancing socially adaptive communicative repairs of beginning communicators with disabilities. *American Journal of Speech-Language Pathology, 13*, 43-54.

One additional strategy is relevant here. Visual schedules have also been shown to be helpful as a part of FCT (Bopp et al., 2004). These help students predict what will come next and can avoid maladaptive behaviors due to frustration of not understanding the rapid flow of events in a classroom. Visual schedules can be made from a variety of materials, using a variety of levels of symbols. Hodgdon (1995) provides additional examples of visual schedules.

■ CONCLUSIONS

Intervention for clients with DL requires a great deal of thought and planning, as we've clearly seen. Like intervention for any level of language development, intervention at this stage can make use of a broad range of techniques, agents, and settings. Our job as clinicians is to match this repertoire to the needs of our clients. The goals of intervention for clients in the DL period are to increase the elaboration, maturity, and efficiency of communication and to help the clients use that communication in life's important contexts, including play, problem solving, and real social interaction.

Let's go back to Rachel and see how we might address some of her needs in an intervention program. Remember that this is just one possible solution. You might like to try to devise a different program just to explore some of the many ways of attaining the same goals.

Student: *Rachel R..*   DOB: *June 5, 2001*   PPT Date. *Sept. 15, 2006*

PRESENT LEVELS OF DEVELOPMENT

Physical Development

Vision: *Within normal limits*

Hearing: *Within normal limits*

Health Status: *Within normal limits*

Communication: *Rachel's parents understand her speech for the most part, but it is difficult for those outside the family. Articulation testing on 9/10/06 with the GFTA-2 revealed performance at the 7th percentile. Errors included frequent deletions of sounds in final position, and substitution errors on /s/, /z/, /ʃ/, /g/, /k/, /ʧ/, /r/, /l/, /tʃ/, and /e/ in all positions. Phonological process analysis from a spontaneous speech sample showed frequent final consonant deletion, stopping of fricatives, fronting of palatals and velars, and gliding of liquids. Both standardized testing and speech-sample analysis revealed that Rachel is functioning significantly below age level in terms of productive syntax, with most forms at or below a 3-year level of development. Receptive skills appear about one year below general developmental level. These developmental delays often make it difficult for her to communicate her intentions in school and social settings, resulting in frustration and isolation for her.*

INDIVIDUALIZED EDUCATION PROGRAM MEASURABLE ANNUAL GOAL AND SHORT TERM OBJECTIVES

☐ Academic/Cognitive ☐ Social/Behavioral **X** Communication ☐ Gross/Fine Motor ☐ Health ☐ Self Help ☐ Other: (specify) _____

Measurable Annual Goal #1	Method of Evaluation	Performance Criteria	Report of Progress*			
			Nov.	Jan.	April	June
Rachel will improve her phonological production so that she can participate fully in the academic and social curriculum of the kindergarten class by contributing to group discussions during story time and interacting successfully with peers during dramatic play time: Use Hodson & Paden (1991) approach in individual pull-out sessions to address phonological errors identified in assessment.	1: Monthly artic. probes; 6: classroom observation	C: 80% correct in probes; J: no more than 1 misunderstanding/ observation				

Short Term Objectives/Benchmarks						
Obj# 1: By Feb. break, Rachel will produce words containing final /s/ sounds, given a list of 10 familiar CV/s/ words with 80% accuracy.						
2. By spring break, Rachel will produce CV/s/ words in spontaneous conversation with teachers and peers with 75% accuracy.						
3. By Feb. break, Rachel will produce velar sounds, given a list of 10 familiar CVC words containing /k/ and /g/ sounds, with 80% accuracy.						
4. By spring break Rachel will produce CVC words containing velars in spontaneous speech with 75% accuracy.						
5. By May 1, Rachel will produce /z/, /ʃ/, and /tʃ/ sounds, given a list of 10 familiar CVC words containing these sounds, with 80% accuracy.						
6. By the end of the school year, Rachel will demonstrate spontaneous speech that is 75% intelligible by peers and teachers in a small group activity, as indicated by three consecutive observations in which there is no more than one request for repetition or similar signs of misunderstanding.						
Alternative Bench Marks # 1. Rachel will produce CVC words accurately enough to be adequately understood by peers and the classroom teacher during group discussions around stories read at group time.						
2. Rachel will demonstrate adequate intelligibility in spontaneous speech with peers so that teacher observations reveal no more than occasional requests for repetition or clarification in dramatic play interactions.						

Measurable Annual Goal #2	Method of Evaluation	Performance Criteria	Report of Progress*			
			Nov.	Jan.	April	June
Rachel will use new vocabulary words drawn from classroom literature in mediated retelling activities and in spontaneous speech: Use collaborative lessons to focus on vocabulary items taken from classroom themes. Have the group produce vocabulary items targeted, draw pictures of scenes containing the item, do sorting activities in teams around groups of words being targeted, and similar tasks.						

Short Term Objectives/Benchmarks						
Obj#1: Rachel will retell a story heard during story time to her aide, using 6 vocabulary words pretaught from the story during language therapy session, with moderate prompting from the aide.	7: Data taken by aide	B: 90%				
Obj#2: Rachel will retell a story heard during story time to her aide, using 6 vocabulary words pretaught from the story during language therapy session, with minimal prompting from the aide.						
Obj#3: Rachel will dictate an original story to her aide that contains the the words learned in Obj. #2 in with minimal prompting.						
Obj#:						
Obj#:						

Measurable Annual Goal #3	Method of Evaluation	Performance Criteria	Report of Progress*			
			Nov.	Jan.	April	June
Increase syntactic skills in conversational contexts: ILS techniques will be taught to classroom teacher and aide; each will spend several minutes during Free Choice activity each day with Rachel, providing expansion, extension, recasts, build-ups/break-downs, focusing especially on forms of be verbs.						

Short Term Objectives/Benchmarks						
	6: SLP will take monthly speech samples to monitor responses, MLU, and syntactic errors					
Obj#1: By the end of the marking period, Rachel will imitate adult's expansions of her utterances, in Free Choice ILS activities, 70% of the time.						
Obj#2: By the end of the second marking period, Rachel will increase her MLU by 1-2 morphemes.						

Evaluation Procedures							
1=Criterion-Referenced/Curriculum Based Assessment 2=Pre & Post Standardized Assessment 3=Pre & Post Base Line Data 4=Quizzes/Tests 5=Student Self-Assessment/Rubic 6=Observation 7=Work samples/Project/Experiment/Portfolio 8=Job Performance or Products 9=Behavior/Performance Rating Scale 10=CMT/CAPT 11=Achievement of Objectives **(Note: Use with goal Only)** 12=Other: (specify) _____	**Performance Criteria**		**Report of Progress Key***				
	A=100% **B**=90% **C**=80% **D**=70% **E**=Standard Score Increase: _____ **F**=Months Growth Increase: _____ **G**=Passing Grades/Score: _____ **H**=Frequency/Trials: (e.g., 9/10) _____ **I**=Duration: (e.g., 15 min, 1 per) _____ **J**=Successful Completion of Task/Activity ____ **K**=Other: (specify) _____		**M**=Mastered **S**=Satisfactory Progress (likely to achieve) **U**=Unsatisfactory Progress (unlikely to achieve) **NP 1**=No Progress (will **Not** achieve) lack of prerequisite skills **NP 2**=No Progress (will **Not** achieve) need more time **NP 3**=No Progress (will **Not** achieve) inadequate assessment **NP 4**=No Progress (will **Not** achieve) excessive absences/tardiness **NI**=Not Introduced **O**=Other: (specify) **Indicating extent to which progress is sufficient to achieve goal by the end of the year.*				

Special Education and Related Services:
1. Rachel will have an adult educational aide present for 25% of her time in the regular classroom. The aide will be available to work with Rachel to help her accomplish fine-motor tasks that she has difficulty doing on her own (e.g., cutting, writing). In addition, the aide will monitor Rachel's interactions with peers and will prompt her to use strategies for intelligibility provided by the SLP.
2. Rachel will receive 20 minutes of direct speech-language intervention three times/week in a quiet area of the classroom. In addition, the SLP will provide consultation on Rachel's program to the classroom teacher. This consultation will consist of 30 min. per week in which the SLP updates the Teacher and Aide on Rachel's progress, makes suggestions for language activities the teacher can do in the classroom to foster Rachel's linguistic development, and shares strategies for improving her intelligibility.

Classroom Modifications:
Rachel will be given a visual schedule to assist her in making transitions throughout the school day.

Periodic Review:
As of the end Spring break, Rachel has achieved all goals listed in Annual Goal #1: "Rachel will improve her phonological production so that she can participate fully in the academic and social curriculum of the kindergarten class by contributing to group discussions during story time and interacting successfully with peers during dramatic play time." Although Rachel still makes articulation errors, her intelligibility has improved so that 80% of her speech is understandable by teachers and peers in the classroom. SLP services will now focus on language goals within the classroom setting, rather than continuing to work on pronunciation in individual therapy.

STUDY GUIDE

I. Intervention Policy Issues at the Developing Language Level
   A. What is IDEA? What kinds of service planning does it mandate for children at the preschool level?
   B. What does family-centered intervention mean for a child at the developing language level?
   C. How is the family to be involved in the development of the IEP?
II. Intervention for Developing Language: Products, Procedures, and Context
   A. Discuss some of the considerations that go into choosing intervention goals at the developing language level.
   B. Under what conditions should a child receive phonological intervention during the developing language phase?
   C. How does the principle of "one new thing at a time" apply to semantic and syntactic intervention in the developing language period?
   D. What are some of the typical patterns of grammatical difficulty seen in children in the developing language phase?
   E. Discuss the use of comprehension versus production goals in intervention at the developing language phase.
   F. Discuss the role of pragmatics, play, and problem solving in intervention at the developing language period.
   G. Discuss several clinician-directed methods of phonological intervention for children with developing language. For what kinds of clients or goals would these be appropriate?
   H. How can CD intervention methods be modified to increase naturalness?
   I. Discuss the two child-centered approaches to intervention in the developing language period.
   J. How can ILS be modified for children in the developing language phase?
   K. How can modeling of higher levels of play be integrated into ILS?
   L. Outline several extensions of script therapy for children in the developing language period.
   M. Describe an activity-based intervention program for children with developing language. What three types of activities can provide opportunities for teaching in this approach?
   N. Describe three ways to integrate emerging literacy into preschool classroom activities.
   O. Describe a hybrid approach to phonological intervention.
   P. Discuss the role of paraprofessionals in intervention for children with developing language.
   Q. What considerations go into using parents as agents of intervention? What activities are most appropriate for parents?
   R. How can peers be used in language intervention for children with developing language?
   S. What kinds of children and targets are best served with clinical models of intervention?
   T. What skills are needed by the SLP for a language-based classroom in the developing language period?
   U. What are the advantages of classroom-based and collaborative models of service delivery?
   V. Discuss ways of improving the effectiveness of a consultative model of intervention in the developing language period.
III. Intervention with Older Clients with Severe Impairment at the Developing Language Level
   A. How can an ecological inventory be used to set goals for the older, severely impaired client at the developing language stage?
   B. Describe six principles that can be used to guide intervention for older, severely impaired clients with developing language. Provide an example of applying each of these principles.
   C. Describe task analysis as it applies to the older, severely impaired client at the developing language stage.
   D. Discuss the issue of using the developmental sequence to guide intervention planning for the older, severely impaired client at the developing language stage.

TARGET	BOOKS CONTAINING TARGET PATTERN	EXAMPLE OF LANGUAGE PATTERN
-ing ending	Audrey Wood, *The Napping House*, Singapore: Harcourt Children's Books, 1984	. . . where everyone is **sleeping**.
	Bill Martin and John Auchambault, *Here Are My Hands*, New York: Henry Holt, 1995	Here are my (body parts) for *(verb)ing* and *(verb)ing*
	Marie Hall Ets, *In the Forest*, New York: Puffin Books, 1976	. . . **blowing** his horn.
	Maurice Sendak, *Alligators All Around*, New York: Scholastic, 1991	bursting balloons, **catching** colds . . .
	Maurice Sendak, *Chicken Soup with Rice*, New York: Scholastic, 1992	*(x)-ing* once, *(x)-ing* twice, *(x)-ing* chicken soup with rice
	Ruth Young, *Golden Bear*, New York: Viking, 1992	Making snowmen Watching tulips
	Steven Kellogg, *A-Hunting We Will Go*, Minneapolis, MN: Sagebrush, 2001	A-*(x)-ing* we will go.
Pronouns		
Subjective	Eric Carle, *The Very Busy Spider*, New York: Philomel Books, 1999	**She** was very busy.
	Eric Carle, *The Very Hungry Caterpillar*, New York: Philomel Books, 1994	But **he** was still hungry.
	Janet and Allan Ahlberg, *Peek-a-Boo*, New York: Penguin Books, 1984	**He** sees his (x).
	Marc Brown, *Arthur's Nose*, Minneapolis, MN: Sagebrush, 2001	**He** didn't like his nose.
	Masayuki Yabuuchi, *Whose Are They?* New York: Philomel Books, 1985	**They** belong to (animal).
	Masayuki Yabuuchi, *Whose Baby?* New York: Philomel Books, 1985	**It** belongs to (animal).
	Maureen Roffey, *Look, There's My Hat*, New York: Putnam Publishing Group, 1985	There's **my** (x).
	Nicki Weiss, *Where Does the Brown Bear Go?* New York: Greenwillow Books, 1998	**They** are on their way home.
	Robert Kraus, *Herman the Helper*, New York: Prentice-Hall Books, 1987	**He** helped (family member).
	Rod Campbell, *Oh, Dear!* New York: Philomel Books, 1994	**He** helped the (person). So **he** went to the (animal home) and asked the (animal).
Objective	Bill Martin Jr., *Brown Bear, Brown Bear, What Do You See?* New York: Henry Holt and Company, Inc., 1995	I see (x) looking at **me**.
	Steven Kellogg, *Can I Keep Him?* New York: Dial Books for Young Readers, 1976	I found an (x). Can I keep **him**?
	Craig Strete, *They Thought They Saw Him*, New York: Greenwillow Books, 1996	They thought they saw **him**.
	Mercer Mayer, *Just My Friend and Me*, New York: Golden Books, 2001	Just my friend and **me**.
	Mercer Mayer, *Just Me and My Little Sister*, New York: Golden Books, 1986	. . . **me** and my little sister.

TARGET	BOOKS CONTAINING TARGET PATTERN	EXAMPLE OF LANGUAGE PATTERN
Possessive	Bill Martin and John Auchambault, *Here Are My Hands*, New York: Henry Holt, 1995	Here are **my** (body parts) for (verb)ing and (verb)ing
	Janett and Allan Ahlberg, *Peek-a-Boo*, New York: Penguin Books, 1984	He sees **his** (x).
	Judith Viorst, *My Mamma Says*, Old Tappin, NY: Simon and Schuster, 1987	Eat **your** soup!
	Judith Viorst, *Alexander and the Terrible, Horrible, No Good, Very Bad Day*, New York: Aladdin Paperbacks, 1972	. . . **my** picture of the invisible castle.
	Marc Brown, *Arthur's Nose*, Minneapolis, MN: Sagebrush, 2001	He didn't like **his** nose.
	Merle Peek, *Mary Wore Her Red Dress and Henry Wore His Green Sneakers*, New York: Clarion Books, 1993	Mary wore **her** red dress. Henry wore **his** green sneakers.
	Nicki Weiss, *Where Does the Brown Bear Go?* New York: Greenwillow Books, 1998	They are on **their** way home.
	Noelle Carter, *My House*, New Jersey: Viking Children's Books, 1991	**My** house is a (x).
	P.D. Eastman, *Are You My Mother?* New York: Random House, 1999	Are you **my** mother?
	Robert Kraus, *Whose Mouse Are You?* New York: Simon and Schuster, 1986	What is **your** (x)?
Reflexive	Margot Zemach, *The Little Red Hen*, New York: Farrar, Straus, and Giroux, 1983	Then I'll do it **myself**, said the little red hen.
	Idries Shah, *The Lion Who Saw Himself in the Water*, Cambridge, MA: Hoopoe Books, 2001	. . . saw **himself** . . .
	Claude Lebrun, *Little Brown Bear Dresses Himself*, New York: Children's Press, 1996	I can dress **myself**.
	Mercer Mayer, *All by Myself*, New York: Golden Books, 2001	All by **myself**.
Prepositions		
	Allan and Janet Ahlberg, *Each Peach Pear Plum*, New York: Penguin USA, 1999	**In** the ditch, **over** the wood.
	Atusko Morozumi, *One Gorilla*, New York: Doubleday, 1990	Each page has a different group of animals in a new location that is preceded by a different preposition.
	Bill Martin Jr., *Brown Bear, Brown Bear, What Do You See?* New York: Henry Holt, 1995	I see (x) looking **at** me.
	Bill Martin Jr., *Polar Bear, Polar Bear, What Do You Hear?* New York: Henry Holt, 1995	I hear (animal) (sound)ing **in** my ear.
	Burton Albert, *Where Does the Trail Lead?* New York: Simon and Schuster, 1991	. . . **to** a crest of dunes **at** the edge of the sea . . .
	Ed Emberley, *Klippity Klop*, New York: Little Brown, 1974	**Across** the field. **Through** the field. **Over** the bridge.
	Eric Carle, *The Secret Birthday Message*, New York: Harper Trophy, 1986	Locative prepositions
	Gail Gibbons, *Sun Up, Sun Down*, New York: Harcourt, 1983	It rises **in** the east and shines **through** my window.
	Jonathan London, *Let's Go Froggy*, New York: Puffin Books, 1996	He looked under/in/on . . .
	Kathi Appelt, *Elephants Aloft*, San Diego, CA: Voyager Books, 1997	Locative prepositions
	Linda Banchek, *Snake In, Snake Out*, New York: Bantam Doubleday Books, 1992	Snake **in**, snake **out**.
	Mercer Mayer, *There's an Alligator Under My Bed*, Hong Kong: Dial Books, 1987	**Under, in**

TARGET	BOOKS CONTAINING TARGET PATTERN	EXAMPLE OF LANGUAGE PATTERN
	Nadine Bernard Westcott, *The Lady with the Alligator Purse*, New York: Little, Brown 1998	... *with* the alligator purse ...
	Pat Hutchins, *Rosie's Walk*, New York: MacMillan, 1997	*around* the lake, *through* the fence
	Patrician Lillie, *Everything Has a Place*, New York: Grenwillow, 1993	*In* it, *on* it.
	Robert Kalan, *Jump, Frog, Jump*, New York: Greenwillow Books, 1996	*under* the fly, *after* the frog, *into* the pond.
	Ruth Brown, *A Dark, Dark Tale*, New York: Dial Books, 1984	*In* the woods there was a house. *On* the house there was a door. *Behind* the house there was ...
	Stan and Jan Berenstain, *Bears in the Night*, New York: Random House, 1971	*Under* the bridge. *Around* the lake. *Between* the rocks.
	Stan and Jan Berenstain, *Inside, Outside, Upside Down*, New York: Random House, 1997	*in* a box, *on* a truck.
	Stan and Jan Berenstain, *The Berenstain Bears and the Spooky Old Tree*, New York: Random House, 1978	One *with* a light. One *with* a rope. One *with* a stick.
Verbs		
Present tense	Noelle Carter, *My House*, New York: Viking Children's Books, 1991	I *am* a (x).
	P.D. Eastman, *Are You My Mother?* New York: Random House, 1997	*Are* you my mother?
Past tense	Edward Lear, *The Owl and the Pussycat*, New York: Putnam Publishing Group, 1997	... *went* to sea.
	Eric Carle, *The Very Hungry Caterpillar*, New York: Putman Publishing Group, 1994	But he *was* still hungry.
	Jez Alborough, *It's the Bear*, Cambridge, MA: Candlewick Press, 1994	The bear munched. He *crunched*. He *chomped* ...
	Lois Ehlert, *Read Leaf, Yellow Leaf*, San Diego: Harcourt Brace & Company, 1991	The wind *blew*. They *twirled* and *whirled*.
	Maurice Sendak, *One Was Johnny*, New York: Harper Collins Children's Books, 1991	One *was* Johnny ... Two *was* ...
	Remy Charlip, *Fortunately*, New York: Aladdin, 1993	Fortunately/unfortunately, (x) *was* ...
	Rose Greydanus, *Double Trouble*, New York: Troll Communications, 1994	*Was* it Tim? *Was* it Jim?
	Ezra J. Keats, *Over in the Meadow*, New York: Scholastic, Inc., 1999	(Verb) *said* the Mother. We (verb) *said* the X, and they *(verb)-ed*.
	Ezra J. Keats, *Peter's Chair*, New York: Puffin Books, 1998	Peter *stretched* .... *was* finished.
	Nancy Tafuri, *The Ball Bounced*, New York: Greenwillow Books, 1989	The ball *bounced*. The (x) *(verb-ed)*.
	Ruth Krauss, *The Carrot Seed*, Mexico: HarperFestival, 1993	The dog *barked*. A little boy *planted* a seed.
	Ted Arnold, *Green Wilma*, New York: Puffin Books, 1998	She *sat* up ...; *croaked* and *started* ...
	Tommy dePaola, *Charlie Needs a Cloak*, New York: Aladdin, 1982	He really *needed* a cloak.
	Tommy dePaola, *The Knight and the Dragon*, New York: Putnam Juvenile, 1998	... had never *fought* a dragon.
(be) (verb)ing	Lydia Dabkovich, *Sleepy Bear*, New York: Puffin Books, 1985	The birds *are leaving*.
	Margaret Wise Brown, *The Runaway Bunny*, New York: HarperCollins, 2005	I *am running* away.
	Mirra Ginsburg, *The Chick and the Duckling*, New York: Simon and Schuster, 1988	I *am (x)-ing*.
	Paul Galdone, *Henny Penny* (folktale), New York: Houghton Mifflin, 1979	Where *are you going?*

TARGET	BOOKS CONTAINING TARGET PATTERN	EXAMPLE OF LANGUAGE PATTERN
	Rita Gelman, *I Went to the Zoo*, New York: Scholastic Inc., 1995	Present progressive tense
Verb Vocabulary		
	Allison Lester, *Clive Eats Alligators*, New York: Houghton Mifflin Co., 1991	Clive **eats** . . .
	Laurie Lazzaro Knowlton, *Why Cowboys Sleep with Their Boots On*, Gretna, LA: Pelican Publishing Company, 1995	Lassoed, branded, stripped, crawled
	John Burningham, *Skip Trip*, New York: Viking Children's Books, 1984	Illustrated action words
	John Burningham, *Sniff, Shout*, New York: Viking Children's Books, 1984	Illustrated action words
Modal auxiliaries	Ann Jonas, *Where Can It Be?* New York: Greenwillow Books, 1986	I'**ll look** in my (location).
	Charlotte Zolotow, *Do You Know What I'll Do?* New York: HarperCollins Publishers, 2000	I'**ll** pick you a bunch . . .
	Dr. Seuss, *Mr. Brown Can Moo, Can You?* New York: Random House, 1996	Mr. Brown **can (verb)**, can you?
	Dr. Seuss, *Green Eggs and Ham*, New York: Random House, 1999	**Would you, could you** . . .?
	Jake Wolf, *And then What?* New York: Greenwillow Books, 1993	**You'll** sail around the city . . .
	Jean Marzollo and Jerry Pinkney, *Pretend You're a Cat*, New York: Dial Books for Young Readers, 1997	**Can you** (action verb)?
	Margaret Wise Brown, *The Runaway Bunny*, New York: Harper Collins, 2005	I **will run** after you.
	Margot Zemach, *The Little Red Hen*, New York: Farrar, Straus, & Giroux, 1993	Who **will help** me (x)? "Then I'**ll do** it myself," said the Little Red Hen.
	Masayuki Yabuuchi, *Whose Footprints?* New York: Putnam Publishing Group, 1985	**Can you** guess?
	Nancy Hellen, *The Bus Stop*, New York: Orchard Books, 1988	**Can you see** the bus yet?
	Robert Lopshire, *Put Me in the Zoo*, New York: Beginner Books, 1966	I **can put** them (x).
Negatives		
	Charles G. Shaw, *It Looked Like Spilt Milk*, New York: HarperCollins Children's Books, 1993	It **wasn't** (x).
	Dr. Seuss, *Green Eggs and Ham*, New York: Random House, 1999	I **do not** like them.
	Eric Carle, *The Very Busy Spider*, New York: Putnam Publishing Group, 1999	The spider **didn't** answer.
	Ernst Ekker, *What Is Beyond the Hill?* New York, Lippincott, 1985	The world does **not** stop there . . .
	Laura Numeroff, *Dogs Don't Wear Sneakers*, Old Tappan: Simon and Schuster, 1996	X **don't** (verb)
	Marilyn Sadler, *It's Not Easy Being a Bunny*, New York: Beginner Books, 1983	I **don't** want to be a (x).
	Maurice Sendak, *Pierre*, New York: Harper Collins Children's Books, 1962	I **don't** care.
	Mirra Ginsburg, *Four Brave Sailors*, New York: Greenwillow Books, 1987	They **do not** fear.
	Nancy Carlstrom, *I'm Not Moving, Mama*, New York: Simon and Schuster, 1990	I'm **not** moving.
	Paul Galdone, *The Gingerbread Boy* (folktale), New York: Houghton Mifflin Company, 1983	They **couldn't** (x). You **can't** (x).
	Uri Shulvitz, *One Monday Morning*, New York: Simon and Schuster, 1986	But I **wasn't** home.

TARGET	**BOOKS CONTAINING TARGET PATTERN**	**EXAMPLE OF LANGUAGE PATTERN**
Questions *Wh-*	Ann Rockwell, *In Our House*, New York: HarperCollins, 1991	*What* do we do? *When … and*
	Ben Shecter, *When Will the Snow Trees Grow?* New York: HarperCollins Children's Books, 1993	
	Bill Martin Jr., *Brown Bear, Brown Bear What Do You See?* New York: Henry Holt and Company, 1995	**What** do you see?
	Bill Martin Jr., *Polar Bear, Polar Bear What Do You Hear?* New York: Henry Holt and Company, 1991	**What** do you hear?
	Diane Goode, *Where's Our Mama?* New York: Puffin Books, 1995	***Where's*** our mama?
	Janet and Allan Ahlberg, *Peek-a-Boo*, New York: Viking Children's Books, 1997	***What*** does he see?
	Jean Marzollo and Jerry Pinkney, *Pretend You're a Cat*, New York: Dial Books for Young Readers, 1997	***What*** else can you do like a *(x)*?
	John Burningham, *Would You Rather*, New York: SeaStar, 1978	***Would*** you rather (x) or (y)?
	Margaret Wise Brown, *Where Have You Been?* New York: Scholastic TAB Publishing Inc., 1990	***Where*** have you been?
	Margot Zemach, *The Little Red Hen* (folktale), New York: Farrar, Straus, & Giroux, 1993	***Who*** will (action) this (object)? ***Who*** will harvest this wheat? ***Who*** will plant this wheat?
	Margret Miller, *Who Uses This?* New York: Greenwillow Books, 1990	***Who*** uses this?
	Masayuki Yabuuchi, *Whose Baby?* New York: Philomel Books, 1985	***Whose*** baby is it?
	Masayuki Yabuuchi, *Whose Footprints?* New York: Putnam Books, 1985	***Whose*** are they?
	Mercer Mayer, *What Do You Do?* New York: Scholastic Inc., 1987	***What*** do you do with a kangaroo?
	Nicki Weiss, *Where Does the Brown Bear Go?* New York: Greenwillow Books, 1998	***Where*** does the (x) go?
	N.N. Charles, *What Am I?* New York: Scholastic, 1994	***What*** am I?
	Pamella Allen, *Who Sank the Boat?* New York: Putnam Publishing Group, 1996	***Who*** sank the boat?
	Paul Galdone, *Henny Penny* (folktale), New York: Houghton Mifflin Company, 1984	***Where*** are you going?
	Robert Kalan, *Jump, Frog, Jump*, New York: Greenwillow Books, 1996	***How*** did the frog get away?
	Robert Lopshire, *ABC Games*, New York: Harper Collins Children's Books, 1986	***Which*** one will (x)? ***Where*** is the (x)?
	Robert Lopshire, *Put Me in the Zoo*, New York: Beginner Books, 1996	***What*** can you do?
	Sue Williams, *I Went Walking*, San Diego: Harcourt Brace and Company, 1996	***What*** did you see?
	Thomas and Wanda Zacharias, *But Where Is the Green Parrot?* New York: Delacorte Press/Seymour Lawrence, 1978	But ***where*** is the green parrot?
Do insertion	Dr. Seuss, *Green Eggs and Ham*, New York: Random House, 1999	***Do*** you like them?
	Mary Serfozo, *Who Said Red?* New York: Simon and Schuster, 1992	***Did*** you say (x)?
	Shigeo Watanabe, *How Do I Put It On?* New York: Putnam Publishing Group, 1991	***Do*** I put them on like this?
	Stan and Jan Berenstain, *The Berenstain Bears and the Spooky Old Tree*, New York: Random House, 1997	***Do*** they dare (x)?

TARGET	BOOKS CONTAINING TARGET PATTERN	EXAMPLE OF LANGUAGE PATTERN
Yes/no	Eric Hill, *Where's Spot?* New York: Interlink Publishing Group, 1994	*Is* he in the (x)?
	Jean Marzollo and Jerry Pinkney, *Pretend You're a Cat,* New York: Dial Books for Young Readers, 1997	*Can you* (action verb)?
	Masayuki Yabuuchi, *Whose Footprints?* New York: Putnam Publishing Group, 1985	*Can* you guess?
	Nancy Hellen, *The Bus Stop,* New York: Orchard Books, 1988	*Can* you see the bus yet?
	P.D. Eastman, *Are You My Mother?* New York, Beginner Books, 1999	*Are* you my mother?
	Rose Greydanus, *Double Trouble,* New York: Troll Communications, 1994	*Was* it Tim? *Was* it Jim?
Have auxiliary	Shigeo Watanabe, *Where's My Daddy?* New York: Putnam Publishing Group, 1996	*Have* you seen my daddy?
	Paul Galdone, *The Gingerbread Boy* (folktale), New York: Houghton Mifflin Company, 1983	I*'ve run* from the (x).

Complex Sentences

TARGET	BOOKS CONTAINING TARGET PATTERN	EXAMPLE OF LANGUAGE PATTERN
Relative clauses	Maurice Sendak, *One Was Johnny,* New York: HarperCollins Children's Books, 1991	. . . *who lived* by himself . . .
	Nancy Tafuri, *This Is the Farmer,* New York: Greenwillow Books, 1994	This is the farmer *who kisses* his wife, *who* . . .
	P. Adams, *There Was an Old Lady Who Swallowed a Fly,* New York: Child's Play, 1989	. . . *who swallowed a fly* . . . *who swallowed spider* . . .
Wh complement	Margaret Wise Brown, *Where Have You Been?* New York: Scholastic Inc., 1989	That's *where* I've been.
If clause	Chris Riddell, *The Trouble with Elephants,* New York: HarperCollins, 1991	*If, then*
	Judi Barrett, *Cloudy with a Chance of Meatballs,* New York: Aladdin, 1982	*If* food dropped like rain . . .
	Laura Numeroff, *If You Give a Mouse a Cookie,* New York, HarperCollins Childrens Books, 1997	. . . *then* he'll want a glass of milk.
	Laura Numeroff, *If You Give a Mouse a Muffin,* New York, HarperCollins Childrens Books, 1994	. . . *then* he'll want some jam. . .
	Margaret Wise Brown, *The Runaway Bunny,* HarperCollins Children's Books, 1977	*If* you . . . *then* I'll . . .
	Tommy dePaola, *I Love You, Mouse,* New York: Harcourt, 1976	*If* I were a mouse, I'd build you a furry nest
But clause	Ann Herbert Scott, *Hi,* New York: Putnam Publishing Group, 1997	. . . *but* sentences
	Mercer Mayer, *Just For You,* New York: Golden Books Family Entertainment, 1982	I wanted to X, *but* . . .
Because clause	Laurel Portet-Gaylord, *I Love Daddy Because,* New York: Dutton Childrens Books, 1991	I love (x) *because* . . .
	Steve Zuckman & Stephen Edelman, *It's a Good Thing,* New York: HarperCollins, 1987	It's a good thing *because* . . .

Adapted from Kirchner, D. (1991). Reciprocal book reading: A discourse-based intervention strategy for the child with atypical language development. In T. Gallagher (Ed.), *Pragmatics of language: Clinical practice issues* (pp. 307-332). San Diego, CA: Singular Publishing Group; Owens, R. (2004). *Language disorders: A functional approach to assessment and intervention* (ed. 4). Boston, MA: Allyn & Bacon; Ratner, N., Parker, B., & Gardner, P. (1993). Joint book reading as a language scaffolding activity for communicatively impaired children. *Seminars in Speech and Language, 14,* 296-313.

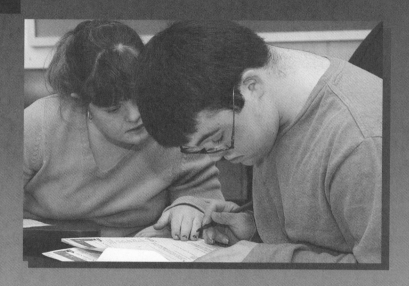

WORKING WITH LANGUAGE LEARNING DISABILITIES

LANGUAGE, READING, AND LEARNING IN SCHOOL: WHAT THE SPEECH-LANGUAGE PATHOLOGIST NEEDS TO KNOW

CHAPTER OBJECTIVES

Readers of this chapter will be able to do the following:
- Name roles and responsibilities of school-based speech-language pathology practice.
- Describe the ways in which legislation regulates this practice.
- Recognize documents critical to the school-based speech-language pathologist.

- List the characteristics of school-aged children with language and learning deficits.
- Describe connections among oral language, learning, and literacy.
- List similarities and differences in oral and written language.

Nick's mother reported she'd had a drug problem before he was born. She'd used a variety of street drugs, and Nick had been born small and showed signs of drug effects at birth. His mother enrolled in a rehabilitation program while he was an infant, overcame her addiction, and worked hard to make a good home for Nick. Nick received a variety of services during his preschool years, when he'd been somewhat overly active and slow in learning to talk. By the time he entered kindergarten, he had improved greatly and passed a kindergarten screening. He was placed in a mainstream class, and direct services were discontinued. But his third-grade teacher, Mrs. Johnson, noticed early in the year that Nick was having difficulty keeping up with the class. He seemed to be progressing adequately in first and second grade and seemed to enjoy reading the patterned picture books his teachers used for reading materials. His primary-grade teachers did note, though, that his speech was somewhat simpler than that of his classmates and he seemed to have trouble paying attention and following directions in class. Mrs. Johnson was concerned, now that more reading was required from classroom textbooks and more independent work in subject areas became part of the curriculum. Nick seemed to be falling behind. He didn't seem able to read the class texts on his own. He couldn't remember the directions she gave for completing assignments. He seemed unable to "get with" the classroom routines she'd established, such as filling out a card each day to indicate whether he was having a school hot lunch or box lunch from home. He wasn't able to learn the spelling list she assigned each week or write the simple book reports she required. He also was beginning to become disruptive, interrupting other students when they were doing their work, fidgeting and annoying others when she read to the class from the children's novels that were part of her program, and making "wisecracks" instead of contributing productively to class discussions. Mrs. Johnson felt she wanted a specialist to assess Nick's difficulties and make some recommendations for how she might help him succeed in the classroom.

Nick is a child whose oral language sounds normal to the "naked ear." He does not make many obvious errors in phonology or syntax, although he did when he was younger. Now his problems with communication are subtler and harder to define, but they seem to have a significant impact on his ability to acquire the skills needed for success in school. There are many children like Nick in our school classrooms, and they often find their way onto the caseload of the speech-language pathologist (SLP). Some, like Nick, have histories that suggest a possible root of their problem. Others have no such history, but simply have difficulty meeting the demands of the school curriculum for no apparent reason. Some have started speaking late and have shown delays in acquiring words, in combining words into sentences, and in pronouncing the sounds of speech. Others have had unremarkable preschool language histories but seem to "hit a wall" when it comes to making the transition from oral to written language. Regardless of their language history, these children are beyond Brown's stage V in terms of their vocabulary and sentence structures.

They may be classified as learning disabled, reading disabled, or dyslexic.

Here in Section III, we focus primarily on these children, referring to them under the broad rubric of *language-learning disability* (LLD). This term implies that students have difficulty with various aspects of communication that interfere with their ability to succeed in school. In this section we look primarily at children who have mastered the basic vocabulary, sentence structures, and functions of their language but have trouble progressing beyond these basic skills to higher levels of language performance in both oral and written modalities. In Chapters 11 and 12, we talk about the communicative skills needed for the elementary school years, from kindergarten through fifth or sixth grade, when normally developing children are between 5 and 12 years of age. In Chapters 13 and 14, we look at adolescents with LLD in secondary school settings.

There are, of course, children in schools whose communicative skills are still in the developing, emerging, or prelinguistic phases. Some of these students will be placed in resource rooms or special education classes, and others in inclusive settings. SLPs who work in school settings will find these children, too, included in their caseload. In fact, one of the exciting things about working in schools is the wide variety of issues and levels of functioning the SLP encounters. Thanks to legislation that mandates free, appropriate public education (FAPE) to all children, those with every type and severity of communication disorder will go to public schools along with their peers. Although specific methods for use with the broad range of disabilities seen in school settings are not addressed in this chapter, principles for addressing the needs of school children at earlier stages of communication can be found in Chapters 6 through 9. However, because SLP practice in school involves work with individuals at all points on the spectrum of communicative function, as well as knowledge of the legal and professional issues specific to school-based practice, we will preface our more focused discussion of LLD by examining some of the issues that affect practice with all our students in school settings.

SCHOOL-BASED PRACTICE IN SPEECH-LANGUAGE PATHOLOGY

SLPs, as part of the educational team that provides comprehensive services to students with disabilities, provide a wide array of services to their clients in schools. The American Speech-Language-Hearing Association (ASHA) (2001a) has defined a set of roles and responsibilities that provide the job description for SLPs whose practice includes this broad range of students in school settings. These appear in Box 10-1.

BOX 10-1	**Roles and Responsibilities of School-Based SLPs**

Required Roles

Prevention: primary and secondary prevention activities

Identification: prereferral, screening, and referral for assessments to establish eligibility

Assessment: collect data on communication functioning

Evaluation: interpret assessment data, using clinical judgment to determine nature and severity of communication disorder

Determination of Eligibility: determine, with team, whether student meets criteria for special educational services

Development of IEPs: participate with team in developing service plans

Management of Caseload: work with team to select, plan, and coordinate service delivery for students

Intervention for Communication Disorders and Differences: provide appropriate, effective services for students with disabilities; distinguish disorders from differences, collaborate to improve language proficiency in second-language learners

Counseling: provide information on prognosis and adjustment to communication disorders

Reevaluation: conduct reassessments when dismissal is considered or IEP revision is necessary

Transition Planning: collaborate with team to assist students when making a transition from one service setting to another

Dismissal Determination: weigh factors such as academic performance, state, local, or national criteria, and functional outcomes when considering dismissal

Documentation and Accountability: keep accurate, comprehensive confidential records to justify need and effectiveness of service; prepare other documents in accord with federal, state, and local requirements

Optional Roles

Collaborative Partnerships: participate in research, parent training, and other community activities

Leadership: provide mentoring, CFY and student supervision; achieve specialty certification

Advocacy: for students, programs, and legislation

Adapted from American Speech-Language-Hearing Association. (2001b). Roles and responsibilities of speech-language pathologists with respect to reading and writing in children and adolescents (Position Statement; Executive Summary of Guidelines, Technical Report). *ASHA Supplement, 21,* 17-27.

Whitmire (2002) summarizes recent trends in SLP practice in schools and finds three major changes in the way school-based clinicians function. These include an increased focus on naturalistic and context-dependent assessment procedures and less on standardized testing, the development of more educationally relevant intervention plans, and a greater emphasis on indirect service provision, including collaboration and consultation, in addition to direct service roles. A good deal of the impetus for these changes arises from the fact that SLPs who work in schools are guided by federal laws that regulate special education. The Individuals with Disabilities Education Act (IDEA) of 1997 (reauthorized in 2004) is the major piece of legislation that applies to this work. Where earlier special education laws had been concerned with insuring access to FAPE and providing Individualized Educational Plans (IEPs) for all children, the 1997 and 2004 reauthorizations shifted to emphasis on accountability for meaningful educational results by the following methods:

▶ Increasing parental participation
▶ Raising expectations for children with disabilities by relating student progress to the general education curriculum
▶ Including regular education teachers in the special educational team
▶ Including children with disabilities in district-wide assessments and public reports
▶ Supporting high standards for professionals involved in service provision

These changes have meant that SLPs are increasingly involved in classroom activities and collaborative approaches to helping children with special needs succeed in the school curriculum. Although as recently as 10 years ago, SLPs often worked on goal sequences and themes they developed themselves to address IEP objectives, current practice in schools requires us to support clients to succeed in the general curriculum, deriving communication goals and embedding activities within its scope. We have talked in earlier chapters about some of the ways in which this can be done for students with moderate to severe disorders, and this approach is especially important for the less severely impaired students who have LLDs.

Ninety percent of children in schools with disabilities are diagnosed with the following four categories (U.S. Department of Education, 1999): learning disabilities (LDs) (51%), speech/language impairments (20%), mental retardation (12%), and emotional disturbance (9%). These make up the bulk of children who receive services under IDEA; the remainder will include children with disorders such as autism, cerebral palsy, traumatic brain injury, and so on. These figures suggest that over 70% of the children on the caseloads of school SLPs will have language and/or LDs; the remainder may have more severe communication problems associated with a range of disorders. Let's talk about some of the issues and practices in which school SLPs are frequently engaged for serving this diverse population.

PREASSESSMENT AND REFERRAL

This phase of practice is not always required, but many school systems make use of this option to attempt to resolve learning problems within the regular education setting, by providing classroom modifications and accommodations that can prevent the need for special education, or for labeling a student as having a special educational need. Schools typically establish teams whose primary purpose is to assess a target student's needs, review records, engage in classroom-based assessments, design and demonstrate intervention strategies, and determine whether these strategies are successful. If the strategies are adequate, students will be monitored by the team, which will provide ongoing follow-up consultation to the classroom teacher. If however, the accommodations fail to address the student's needs, a formal referral for assessment is made. SLPs will often be a part of these "Student Success Teams" as one aspect of their duties.

DETERMINING ELIGIBILITY

School SLPs have the responsibility for deciding whether a student referred for speech-language services meets district eligibility criteria. Eligibility criteria, however, vary not only from state to state but in some cases from school district to school district. Just as we learned in Chapter 1 that there is no universally accepted definition of language disorder, there is no universally accepted criterion of eligibility for communication services in schools. Some states require a test score two or more standard deviations below the mean; others require two test scores 1.5 standard deviations below the mean, some a combination of test performance and severity rating, and so on (Moore-Brown & Montgomery, 2001). Moreover, IDEA requires that whatever impairment the child has must adversely affect academic performance if services are to be provided. This requirement is interpreted rather broadly, though. Whitmire and Dublinske (2003) show that because many state standards for academic proficiency include speaking and listening skills, children who have language problems may qualify for special educational services, even if their academic achievement is not significantly depressed by their communicative disorder. SLPs need to become familiar with the eligibility requirements and local proficiency standards of the school districts in which they are employed and learn to use these standards to find ways to provide services for all children with communicative needs.

DOCUMENTING PRESENT LEVEL OF EDUCATIONAL PERFORMANCE

The IEP includes a summary of the assessment information gathered on the child. A variety of areas are assessed by the educational team; these include intellectual functioning; readiness or academic skills; communicative status; motor ability; sensory status; health and physical status; emotional, social, and behavioral development; and self-help skills. Not every area needs to be assessed for every child, however. If deficits are restricted to speech and language, for example, present level of performance may be given in communicative areas alone. The law requires that multiple instruments be used, so that children are not identified as having a disability on the basis of only one test. Informal as well as standardized instruments can be part of this assessment, and information from previous assessment also can be used. The assessment of performance must also include information on how the child's disability affects participation and progress in academic and social environments.

WRITING INDIVIDUALIZED EDUCATIONAL PLANS

Once a child has been identified as having a special need in the area of communication, the next step is to establish goals and objectives to meet these needs, as identified in the assessment. These are incorporated into the IEP, which contains the components listed in Table 10-1.

| **TABLE 10-1** | **Required Components of the Individualized Educational Plans** |

COMPONENT	DESCRIPTION
Strengths & concerns	Parent concerns and priorities, as well as child's areas of relative strength are listed.
Evaluation results	Assessment results are reported and interpreted.
Present level of educational performance	The effect of the student's disability on participation and progress in the curriculum is reported.
Annual goals	Long-term goals related to meeting general educational curriculum or other educational needs that result from the disability are listed in each area of disability.
Short-term objective and benchmarks	Measurable, sequenced steps toward annual goals are detailed.
Amount of special education or related services	Projected beginning date, frequency and types of service, and an estimate of duration are given.
Supplementary aids and services	Describes how the regular educational program will be modified so that the child can participate, how services will contribute toward this participation in the general education curriculum, as well as in extracurricular activities. Also contains information about the types of related services needed (SLP, occupational therapy, etc.). These services may be direct, as in one-to-one therapy, or indirect, as in consultation to the classroom teacher by the SLP. Any assistive equipment the student might need to participate in the curriculum (such as a hearing aid or an AAC device) is also listed.
Participation in regular education environments (least restrictive setting; LRE)	The extent of the student's participation with students without disabilities in both educational and extracurricular settings is given. Accommodations might be included, such as support staff to help the child succeed in the setting, modifications in transportation and equipment, and behavioral interventions to manage problem behaviors in the classroom.
Test modifications	Modifications needed to participate in district-wide assessments of student achievement are given.
Transition services	Interagency responsibilities and community links to help student move toward adult placement are listed.
Notification of transfer rights	Documentation that student has been informed of his/her rights when maturity is reached.
Evaluation procedures and measurement methods	How and when student progress will be measured (progress must be reported as often as it is for general education students). Progress must be evaluated at least once every 3 years, although it can be done more often. Assessment may be relatively short and may use existing data or observational records. Parents also must be informed of how the child's progress toward goals will be measured, and they must receive progress reports as least as often as children in regular education receive report cards. The reevaluation can have three possible outcomes: (1) continuation—if the student is moving toward goals as expected, the plan can be continued without changes; (2) modification—if small changes in the IEP are needed to maximize student progress but the changes are not significant enough to warrant another IEP meeting; or (3) revision—if the IEP must be rewritten with significant changes because of lack of or greater-than-expected progress that warrants the targeting of new goals or a reduction in services needed. Parents' consent must be obtained for the program to be changed.
IEP team members	Signatures of all IEP members, including parents, general education teachers, special educators, and administrators are needed.

Adapted from Moore-Brown, B., Montgomery, J., Bielinski, H., & Shubin, J. (2005). Responsiveness to intervention: Teaching before testing helps avoid labeling. *Topics in Language Disorders, 25(2),* 148-167.

ANNUAL GOALS

IDEA requires that annual goals be designed to help the child participate and make progress in the general curriculum. The annual goals are directly related to assessment data in the Present Level of Performance section. IDEA 2004 requires that present levels of performance and annual goals be linked to the general curriculum. The goals must be measurable and be achievable within 1 calendar year. Each goal is required to have two components: the behavior being addressed and the desired end-level of achievement, or what the child will have learned. Goals are targeted for each of the areas assessed in which the child has a special educational need. Each area targeted is usually given a separate page on the IEP, and each annual goal in that area is given a section on the page. Beneath each annual goal, the short-term instructional objectives required to reach that goal may be listed. These form the basis for monitoring the student's progress.

SHORT-TERM OBJECTIVES AND BENCHMARKS

Short-term objectives (STOs) are the discrete steps toward the annual goal. They comprise the task analysis for each annual goal, and are listed sequentially in the IEP. Objectives should conform to the "SMART" acronym (PACER Center, 1990): *S*pecific, *M*easurable, *A*ttainable, *R*elevant, and *T*eachable. Each short-term objective has three components: (1) the description of a specific behavior ("Nick will complete a book report on a book chosen in collaboration between the teacher and the SLP"); (2) the circumstances under which the behavior will be performed ("after identifying its story elements with the SLP"); and (3) the criterion for measuring success or attainment of the goal ("that includes at least four of the five elements required for the class's assignment").

Benchmarks describe the amount of progress a student is expected to make during each segment of the school year. They translate grade level standards into concrete things the student should be able to do and understand and mark progress toward the achievement of curricular standards. Each benchmark may contain several indicators, which describe what students will be able to do without teacher assistance on the way toward accomplishing the goal. Both STOs and benchmarks are used to specify the sequence of specific measurable behaviors that will be observed as a student makes progress from the current level of performance to the annual goal (O'Donnell, 1999).

DELIVERING SERVICES WITHIN THE CURRICULUM

Under IDEA regulations, SLPs no longer work separately on a set of language goals and activities they develop on their own. Whether they work in individual "therapy" sessions, with a small group of students within a classroom activity, or alongside the classroom teacher in a collaborative model, language activities are drawn from the general education curriculum, and goals address helping the student progress through it, to whatever extent possible.

INCLUSION

The 1997 and 2004 regulations place a greater burden on local education agencies (LEAs) to justify any placement that is not full-time in a mainstream classroom. However, this does not mean that every child must be placed in the general classroom all the time. The law requires that there be a continuum of services to meet the needs of children who are not placed in the mainstream full time. The only alternative to full inclusion need *not* be a completely segregated program. Instead, there should be levels of involvement between these two extremes. SLPs will be involved in determining the nature and extent of inclusion for their students, and in finding ways to provide appropriate services within the mainstream setting.

These issues will be addressed again at each of the developmental levels we will discuss for the school-aged student. But for now, let's get back to Nick. How can we define and characterize the language needs of children like him? What is the SLP's role in ameliorating their problems? We'll take these questions one at a time.

STUDENTS WITH LANGUAGE LEARNING DISABILITIES

DEFINITIONS AND CHARACTERISTICS

Before we start talking about what children with LLD are like, let's make sure we understand the terms often used to discuss them. *LD* is perhaps the most general. The U.S. Interagency Committee on Learning Disabilities (Kavanagh & Truss, 1988) adopted the following definition:

> *Learning disabilities* is a generic term that refers to a heterogeneous group of disorders manifested by significant difficulties in the acquisition and use of listening, speaking, reading, writing, reasoning, or mathematical abilities, or of social skills. These disorders are intrinsic to the individual and presumed to be due to central nervous system dysfunction. Even though learning disability may occur concomitantly with other handicapping conditions (e.g., sensory impairment, mental retardation, social and emotional disturbance), with socio-environmental influences (e.g., cultural difference, insufficient or inappropriate instruction, psychogenic factors), and especially with attention deficit disorder, all of which may cause learning problems, a learning disability is not the direct result of those conditions or influences (pp. 550-551).

More recently, the U.S. Department of Health and Human Services glossary (2000) gave the following definition:

> A disorder in basic psychological processes involved in understanding or using language, spoken or written, that may manifest itself in an imperfect ability to listen, think, speak, read, write, spell or use mathematical calculations.

The term includes conditions such as perceptual disability, brain injury, minimal brain dysfunction, dyslexia, and developmental aphasia.

A more colloquial definition would be that LDs involve an unexpected difficulty, relative to age and other abilities, in learning in school. Unexpected is usually taken to mean that there is no obvious explanation for the child's difficulty. So, as the Interagency Committee states, the child may or may not have a hearing impairment, mental retardation, emotional disturbance, autistic disorder, motor deficit, or lack of opportunity or experience, but these would not be sufficient to explain the problem. Many definitions of LD have traditionally included a discrepancy criterion. That means that eligibility for the label involves a significant discrepancy (and we know how hard that is to agree upon!) between potential (usually meaning IQ) and achievement (usually measured by a standardized test of school performance) or between areas of development, such as between verbal and nonverbal IQ. The discrepancy criterion is to some degree under attack these days, for many of the reasons we talked about in Chapter 2. You'll remember that Francis et al. (1996) discussed literature indicating major conceptual and psychometric difficulties in using discrepancies between test scores to identify children with language and learning problems. That's the main reason why most current definitions use wordings such as "unexpected difficulty in relation to age and other abilities" rather than "significant difference between age and achievement," as the older definitions did. In fact, in the 2004 reauthorization of IDEA, the law specifically states that a discrepancy between test scores does not have to be the criterion for eligibility for LD. Local educational agencies (LEAs) may, under the new law, choose a different criterion, such as lack of response to scientifically-based instruction.

Not all LDs are language-based. A child could have a specific learning problem in, say, mathematics or graphomotor skills that might not be based on a language weakness. But most LDs involve deficits in the ability to learn to read, write, and spell; it is through these deficits that other academic areas, including mathematics, science, and others, are often affected. LDs that affect primarily reading, writing, and spelling are the ones we will call *language-learning disorders*. We use this term to emphasize the fact that reading, writing, and spelling are language-based skills that draw on a foundation of oral language abilities. Students with LLD have underlying weaknesses in their oral language base, even when the child's speech might sound OK to the naked ear, and often have histories of delayed language development. These children have problems beyond written word identification that affect their comprehension of both written and oral material. We can think of LLD, then, as one type—probably the most common type—of LD. That's why the LLD circle is placed within the larger LD circle in Figure 10-1.

As Figure 10-1 suggests, most children with language learning disorders (LLD) (although not all) have reading problems, as a result of the weak foundation for the development of

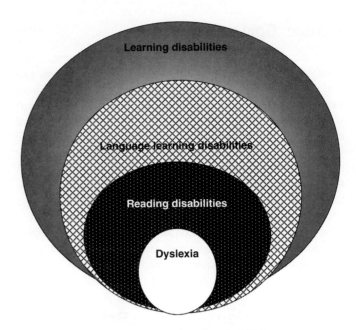

FIGURE 10-1 ✦ Relations among learning disabilities.

literacy that their shaky oral language skills provide; and many children with reading problems (though not all) will have had LLD at some point in their development. These children, who show difficulties of a variety of kinds in learning to read, are represented by the dotted circle in Figure 10-1, and are considered to have reading disabilities (RDs). Catts and Kamhi (2005b) use this term to refer to a heterogeneous group of poor readers whose weak language skills play a causal role in their reading difficulty. There is a smaller group within this category, however, represented by the white circle. This group is referred to as having dyslexia. The International Dyslexia Association adopted this definition of *dyslexia* (Lyon, Shaywitz, & Shaywitz, 2003):

> Dyslexia is a specific LD that is neurobiological in origin. It is characterized by difficulties with accurate and/or fluent word recognition and by poor spelling and decoding abilities. These difficulties typically result from a deficit in the phonological component of language that is often unexpected in relation to other cognitive abilities and the provision of effective classroom instruction. Secondary consequences may include problems in reading comprehension and reduced reading experience that can impede growth of vocabulary and background knowledge.

Dyslexia, or a specific reading disorder, is a more circumscribed instance of LLD. Vellutino, Fletcher, Snowling, and Scanlon (2004), in summarizing the current state of research on dyslexia, show that the root of this specific reading disorder has been quite firmly established as an inadequate ability in word identification due primarily to deficiencies in phonological skills. Evidence for visual processing disorders as a cause of dyslexia is very weak; children with dyslexia don't reverse words and letters visually, as has been thought in the past. Instead, their primary difficulty is in the phonological awareness, memory, and coding skills that allow children to do phonemic segmentation and synthesis tasks, and learn to use the alphabetic principle to decode print. Other deficiencies in vocabulary, knowledge, and reading comprehension stem from this basic difficulty in cracking the alphabetic code.

So what's the difference between RD and dyslexia? That's a question about which you will find some disagreement in the field. Most current thinking, represented by Vellutino et al. (2004), Snowling (1996), and Catts and Kamhi (2005a), holds that dyslexia is part of a continuum of language disorders (that's why it's placed inside the larger circles in Figure 10-1). What differentiates dyslexia from a more general LLD or RD is that dyslexia involves a specific deficit in single-word decoding that is based in a weakness in the phonological domain of the oral language base and has only a secondary impact on reading comprehension. It is a disorder affecting just one aspect of the learning process: decoding. Children with LLD, on the other hand, can have problems with both single-word reading as well as comprehension, and not only of written language, but of oral language, as well. These comprehension problems are thought to stem from difficulties the child has not only in phonological processing but in other language domains, such as syntax and semantics. Children with more general LLD often have a history of delayed speech and language development as preschoolers, whereas those with dyslexia often do not (Snowling, 1996). We can think of dyslexia as a particular subtype of RD, which is a common subtype of LLD.

For our purposes, we will be concerned with the broad category of LLD. While we understand that some of the children seen by the SLP in schools may have dyslexia, these students will often work primarily with reading specialists. It will be more common for speech-language professionals to work with students who have more broadly based LLD. What are the communicative characteristics that we'll see in these children with LLD? A great deal of research has been done in recent years to describe these characteristics. Let's look at some of the typical problems seen in students with LLD and talk about what they might mean for academic achievement.

Phonological Characteristics

Many researchers (e.g., Pennington & Lefly, 2001; for reviews, see Catts & Kamhi, 2005b; Snowling, 1996; Vellutino et al., 2004) believe that subtle phonological deficits underlie many of the problems seen in children with LLD and that dyslexia may be a very specific disorder of phonological processing. Three areas of phonological processing have proved particularly relevant: complex phonological production, phonological awareness, and phonological memory and retrieval (Snowling, 1996). In terms of phonological production, children with LLD are generally intelligible. There is, though, a higher prevalence of speech disorders in children with LLD than in the general population, with about 25% of children with LLD showing delayed speech development at school age, whereas only 4% to 6% of the general population does (Kuder, 1997). Leitao and Fletcher (2004) showed that children who entered school with significant speech impairments had substantial problems in literacy development 5 years later. Even when children with LLD

do not show obvious phonological disorders, though, they often have difficulty with complex phonological production in difficult words (such as *statistics*) or phrases ("Fly free in the Air Force") (Catts, 1986) or in repeating phonologically complex nonwords (such as /tribabli/). Larrivee and Catts (1999) found that severity of phonological disorders in kindergartners is a significant predictor of later reading skill, but that standard articulation tests were not adequate to index severity in children of this age. Instead, tests involving phonologically complex, multisyllabic words (such as *aluminum*) and unfamiliar nonsense words were needed. Snowling, Bishop, and Stothard (2000) reported that reading outcomes are poorest for children with the most severe phonological disorders. Hesketh (2004) reported that although most children with speech delays during the preschool period make adequate progress in reading once they get to school, a small number of them develop phonological awareness and literacy delays. As in other areas, phonological awareness appears to be the best predictor of literacy achievement in these children. Stackhouse (1996) reports that these speech difficulties primarily affect the acquisition of spelling.

Phonological awareness, the ability to segment words into sounds and manipulate sounds in words, is essential to learning to read in an alphabetic language such as English, in which letters are used to represent sounds (Catts & Kamhi, 2005a; Ehri, Nunes, Stahl, & Willows 2001; Snow, Burns, & Griffin, 1998). A wide range of studies (e.g., Bradley & Bryant, 1985; Liberman & Liberman, 1990; Mann & Liberman, 1984; Scarborough, 2003; Snowling & Nation, 1997; Stackhouse & Wells, 1997) have shown that phonological awareness is highly correlated with reading ability. Many investigators believe that deficits in phonological awareness are central to a majority of problems seen in poor readers (Scarborough, 2002; Snowling & Stackhouse, 1996; Snow, Burns, & Griffin, 1998; Vellutino et al., 2004). Webster and Plante (1992) and Stackhouse and Wells (1997) suggested that phonological awareness depends, at least in part, on primary linguistic ability. Children who are slow to develop primary linguistic abilities during the preschool years may have some trouble with higher-level skills, such as phonological awareness, even when the primary linguistic problems are no longer evident. For this reason, children with slow language development through the preschool period could be considered at risk for LLD, even before they actually begin to fail in school. Such children might be good candidates for preventive intervention, which we'll talk about in Chapter 12. Kamhi (2003), Schuele and Larrivee (2004), and Roth and Baden (2001) suggest that SLPs have an important role to play in helping to identify children at risk for future reading problems. Complex phonological production and phonological awareness are important areas for assessment, to identify those at risk in kindergarten and preschool.

The third area of phonology in which children with LLD have difficulty is phonological memory and retrieval. Children with LLD have consistently shown problems with short-term memory tasks (Catts, 1989; Snowling, 1996). Liberman and Liberman (1990) and Bishop (1997) reported, though, that these deficits are restricted to memory for verbal material. Students with LLD generally have no difficulty with memory tasks involving nonverbal stimuli or environmental sounds. Moreover, children with LLD have consistently been found weak in the ability to do rapid naming and nonword repetition tasks. When asked, for example, to say all the days of the week or to repeat nonsense words, such as *FLIPE* or *WID*, children with LLD perform more poorly than those with normal school achievement (Larrivee & Catts, 1999; Snowling, 1996; Wesseling & Reitsma, 2001). These problems may not sound phonological at first, but researchers believe that the source of this difficulty is in establishing and retrieving accurate phonological representations (or segmenting the words into sounds, then storing sound-by-sound auditory images and retrieving these images as a template for production) of verbal material. These same problems also are thought to be related to the word retrieval difficulties so commonly seen in children with LLD.

As we discussed earlier, some researchers, such as Tallal, Miller, and Fitch (1993), see the root of these phonological difficulties in a more basic deficit in the discrimination of the brief, rapidly changing auditory signals that need to be processed in order to perceive, categorize, and recognize speech sounds. For this reason, Tallal and colleagues have proposed their *FastForWord* (FFW) program—which uses intensive practice with computer-generated speech to teach children to gradually discriminate among increasingly brief acoustic signals—as a remedy not only for LLD but for RDs as well (Tallal, 1999b, 2003, 2004; Temple at al., 2003). The evidence on either this theory or on its application in FFW treatment of RD is not definitive. A large body of research, for instance, disputes the position of Tallal and her colleagues on the source of the deficit in speech perception that underlies the RD (e.g., Bishop, 1997; Bretherton & Holmes, 2003; Mody, Studdert-Kennedy, & Brady, 1997). Some research supports this position but suggests that the intervention will only work for children with documented deficits in temporal processing, who constitute a minority of the children with language and learning disorders (Habib et al., 2002). Troia and Whitney (2003) reported some impact on oral language skills, phonological awareness, and a reduction in problem behavior for some children with LLD who were treated with FFW, when compared to a no-treatment control group, but improvements were limited to the children with the lowest scores to begin with, and there was no comparison to intervention with something other than FFW. Hook, Macaruso, & Jones (2001) compared FFW to multisensory, structured direct instruction and found that both groups made progress in phonological awareness, but the group with standard instruction made more gains in decoding and that, after two years the two groups were similar in both spoken and written language performance. Loeb, Stoke, and Fey (2001) found that FFW delivered at home by parents led to improvements in children's performance on some structured language tasks, but broad changes in functional language use were not seen. Research has also compared changes in both auditory temporal processing and language performance in children who received FFW training when

compared to children who received comparable amounts of training with other computer-assisted language intervention programs that were not designed to improve auditory perceptual skills. Results in this study did not generally support the presence of a program-specific improvement in temporal processing, and there did not appear to be a close relationship between performance on FFW and language gains (Gillam, Loeb, & Friel-Patti, 2001). At this point, we need more objective research on these issues to be able to establish the uses of FFW and programs like it.

We can point to two important factors to remember about phonological skills in youngsters with LLD. First, phonological production may sound adequate; problems with phonological processing that appear to be related to literacy can only be tapped by specially designed tasks. Imitation of complex sound sequences is one such task. Activities that tap phonological awareness include segmenting words into constituent phonemes, counting sounds in words, producing words with one sound left out (such as *fun* without the /f/ sound), sound manipulation (such as reversing sounds in words), and sound categorization (such as identifying words that have the same last sound, like *men* and *dawn*). Several measures have been devised to tap these abilities. They include *The Test of Phonological Awareness* (Torgensen & Bryant, 2004), *Test of Phonological Skills* (Newcomer & Barenbaum, 2004), *The Phonological Awareness Profile* (Robertson & Salter, 2004), *The Comprehensive Test of Phonological Processing* (Wagner, Torgensen, & Rashotte, 1999) and *The Lindamood Auditory Conceptualization Test* (Lindamood & Lindamood, 2004), to name a few. Tasks that ask children to produce rapid sequences of names, such as naming the months of the year, or to imitate nonsense words also are useful in this regard. *The Rapid Automatized Naming and Rapid Alternating Stimulus Tests* (Wolf & Denckla, 2004), as well as subtests from language measures such as the *Clinical Evaluation of Language Fundamentals* (Wiig et al., 2003) can be helpful here. Second, the research on phonological skills in children with LLD suggests that some of the deficits that appear to be related to memory or semantic ability may actually stem from these "underground" phonological skills, particularly the ability to segment, store, and retrieve words from memory on the basis of their phonological properties. This tells us that as we think about remediating skills, such as word retrieval, we need to add phonological components to the intervention program.

Syntactic Characteristics

Deficits in comprehension of complex syntax also are widely reported in children with LLD (Catts, Fey, Zhang, & Tomblin, 1999; Gerber, 1993; Roth & Spekman, 1989; Scott, 2004; Tomblin, Zhang, Buckwalter, & O'Brien, 2003). They have particular trouble understanding sentences with relative clauses, passive voice, or negation (Kuder, 1997). Paul (1990) suggested that school-aged children with LDs tended to rely for a longer-than-normal time on comprehension strategies for processing passive sentences and those containing relative and adverbial clauses. For example, students with LLD persist in misinterpreting sentences such as "Before you brush your teeth, put away your towel," in which the order of clauses ("brush teeth," "put away towel") is the opposite of the intended order of events (first put away towel, then brush teeth). Typical children go beyond these strategies to full comprehension by 7 or 8 years. Students with LLD, though, continue to use strategies based on expectations of the way things usually happen or on word order throughout the elementary years and beyond.

Students with LLD do not make a large number of syntactic errors in spontaneous speech; error rates in children between 8 and 11 years of age decline from 11% to 3% in speech, although these rates are still significantly higher than the rates of peers (Scott, 2004). Error rates in writing are much higher, however. Moreover, their language output is often perceived as "simple" or "immature" by adults around them. They may use fewer complex sentences, less elaboration of noun phrases with multiple modifiers ("that big, red barn"), prepositional phrases ("the house in the country"), and relative clauses ("the house that's in the country") (McCormick & Loeb, 2003). Verb phrases may be less complex, containing few adverbs (such as *slowly, resentfully*) or combinations of auxiliary verbs ("could have been running"). Their sentences may actually be longer than those of peers, because they use fewer complex forms to condense their expression (Kuder, 1997). They show lower rates of subordination and embedding in speech, and fail to increase these rates in writing as typical peers do (Scott, 2004). Gerber (1993) reported that children with LLD have basic, functional syntactic skills but that their sentences are less elaborated than those of age-mates, and they may not encode all the relevant information within their utterances.

Morphological problems also are common, accounting for two-thirds of the syntactic errors in the speech of students with LLD (Scott, 2004), particularly in morphemes that are hard to hear (McCormick & Loeb, 2003; Wiig, 1990) or typically acquired late (Kuder, 1997). These errors are especially prevalent in writing (Scott, 2004). Examples of these morphemes include those with *s*, such as plurals, possessives and third-person singular; comparatives and superlatives; irregular forms; and advanced prefixes and suffixes (*-ly, un-, re-, dis-, -ment, -able, -ness*). Difficulties such as these should not be surprising in light of the morphological deficits typically seen in preschoolers with language disorders. Other error types are also seen in speakers with LLD. These include difficulty with pronoun reference and subject-verb agreement, as well as problems with coordination and subordination (Scott, 2004).

Still, many children with LLD do not exhibit any discernible problems with syntax. Doehring, Trites, Patel, and Fiedorowicz (1981) reported that only 50% of students with LLD demonstrated syntactic deficits.

Semantic Characteristics

Children with LLD have small vocabularies that are restricted to high-frequency, short words (Catts et al., 1999; Kuder, 1997). However, Snider (1989) pointed out that school-age children with normal development acquire many new vocabulary items through reading rather than through conversation. So vocabulary deficits in students with LLD are likely to be, at least in

part, the result rather than the cause of reading problems. In addition to small vocabularies, other semantic problems are commonly reported in students with LLD. Knowledge of word meanings is often restricted, with poor development of associations among words and of categorization of words into semantic classes. Difficulties with multiple-meaning words also are typical of students with LLD. Excessive reliance on nonspecific terms (*thing, stuff*) and special difficulty with relational and abstract words have been reported as well (Wiig & Semel, 1984). Word-retrieval difficulties also are widely noted (see Catts & Kamhi, 2005b; Gerber, 1993; Kuder, 1997, for review). These difficulties include decreased speed and accuracy in confrontation naming and word-finding problems, characterized by substitution and circumlocution in spontaneous speech. Again, not all children with LLD display these problems. Further, the problems may be related not only to lexical problems, but also to the difficulties with retrieval of phonological codes from memory, as discussed earlier (German & Newman, 2004).

Beyond the word level, other semantic problems are often seen in children with LLD. These include difficulties in understanding complex oral directions (Murray, Feinstein, & Blouin, 1985) and difficulties producing and understanding figurative language, such as metaphors, similes, and slang (Nippold, 1998; Roth & Spekman, 1989), and in producing narratives (Catts et al., 1999). Trouble integrating meaning across sentences (Klein-Konigsberg, 1984) also is seen. That is, some children with LLD seem to be limited in their capacity to process semantic information. They can understand information from one or two sentences as well as age-mates but have difficulty integrating information from a larger discourse unit that contains three or four sentences.

Pragmatic Characteristics

Conversation. Many children with LLD have limited verbal fluency. They don't talk much, and what they say is brief and unelaborated. Damico (1991) suggested that the speech of students with LLD is particularly prone to disruptions, such as false starts, mazes, and other forms of dysfluency. Several researchers (Brinton, Fujiki, & Sonnenberg, 1988; Donahue & Bryan, 1983; Meline & Brackin, 1987) have reported that the language used by students with LLD is often more hostile, less assertive, less persuasive, less polite and tactful, and less clear and complete than that of peers. Students with LLD are less sensitive to the needs of their listeners, often giving incomplete or inaccurate descriptions or having trouble adjusting their speech to the age or social status of their audience (Kuder, 1997). Further, these studies suggest that many children with LLD have trouble clarifying miscommunication and requesting clarification of inadequate messages (Kuder, 1997). They also are more likely to ignore the communicative bids of others and to show poor topic maintenance. Such pragmatic difficulties are seen even in students who do not have documented impairments in semantics and syntax (McCord & Haynes, 1988). In fact, conversational pragmatics may be the area of the most significant deficits in the oral language of students with LLD (Hart, Fujiki, Brinton, & Hart, 2004). These findings stress the importance of evaluating pragmatic skills when assessing communication in students with LLD.

Other Discourse Genres. Students with LLD also often demonstrate difficulties with processing and producing other types of discourse besides conversation. Westby (2005) discussed the notion that discourse genres can be thought of as falling along a continuum of formality. This continuum extends from the least formal oral, conversational style on one end to the highly formal, literate style on the other. Literate discourse styles are those found in written and other formal modes of communication, such as those used in scientific papers, essays, sermons, and lectures. Literary language differs from basic oral conversation in several ways. One is its degree of contextualization. Oral language is generally highly contextualized. Much information that supports the exchange, such as objects being discussed, facial expressions, gestures, and intonational cues, are present in the immediate environment. Literate language, on the other hand, is highly decontextualized. Virtually all the information needed for comprehension is present within the linguistic signal itself, and little support is available outside it. These two extremes also differ in function, topics, and forms. Table 10-2 describes some of these additional differences.

Westby (1991) suggested that narrative discourse falls midway between these two extremes. It does this because it relies on a very familiar structure, a "story grammar" (Box 10-2) that provides support for comprehension. Narratives differ from conversation in that they are essentially monologues rather than dyadic, but they can contain dialogue that is similar in informality to conversation. Because it covers this "middle ground" between familiar oral language styles and more difficult literate forms, Westby has argued that narrative skills can form

a bridge from oral to literate language. Research on narrative (Bishop & Edmundson, 1987; Boudreau, 2006; Feagans & Applebaum, 1986; Tabors, Snow, & Dickinson, 2001) has demonstrated that narrative skills are very important in predicting success in school. The development of narrative skills, then, would seem to be quite important in maximizing the chances for academic accomplishment in students with LLD.

Narrative discourse skills have been studied extensively in typical students and in those with LLD. These studies start from the premise that stories told by members of mainstream North American society have a more or less typical structure, which has been labeled a "story grammar." A variety of ways of schematizing this grammar have been presented in the literature. Stein and Glenn's (1979) scheme is presented in Box 10-2.

It is important to remember, though, that different cultures have different ways of telling stories (Fiestas & Pena, 2004). Chapter 5 outlined some non-Western storytelling styles. Although it is important for students in our schools to learn to use the mainstream story form, we should not assume that children from culturally different backgrounds are deficient if they tell a different style of story (O'Connell, 1997). Assessment of narrative skills in these children can follow some of the guidelines we discussed in Chapter 5. Using a Parent-Child Comparative Analysis (Terrell, Arensberg, & Rosa, 1992), for example, we can compare the story of a child from a culturally different home with a story sample from an adult in that culture to determine whether narrative deficits are present. Alternatively, we can ask an adult from the home culture to evaluate a story told by a child of the same culture. Still, even when cultural differences account for differences in narrative style, competence with mainstream story structures is nonetheless important for success in school. If a child with LLD from a culturally different background is having trouble producing

---

TABLE 10-2 **Differences between Oral and Literate Language**

	ORAL STYLE	LITERATE STYLE
Function	To regulate social interactions. To request objects and actions. To communicate face-to-face with a few people. To share information about concrete objects and events.	To regulate thinking. To reflect and request information. To communicate over time and distance. To transmit information to large numbers of people. To build abstract theories and discuss abstract ideas.
Topic	Everyday objects and events. Here and now. Topics flow according to associations of participants. Meaning is contextually based.	Abstract or unfamiliar objects and events. There and then. Discourse is centered around preselected topic. Meaning comes from inferences and conclusions drawn from text.
Structure	High-frequency words. Repetitive, predictable, redundant syntax and content. Pronouns, slang, jargon. Cohesion based on intonation.	Low-frequency words. Concise syntax and content. Specific, abstract vocabulary. Cohesion based on vocabulary and linguistic markers.

Adapted from Westby, C. (1991). Learning to talk—talking to learn: Oral-literate language differences. In C.S. Simon (Ed.), *Communication skills and classroom success: Assessment and therapy methodologies for language- and learning-disabled students* (Table 13-1, p. 337). Eau Claire, WI: Thinking Publications.

Story = Setting + episode structure.

Episode = Initiating event + internal response + plan + attempt + consequence + reaction.

Setting—introduces the main characters, the protagonist, and the context of time and place.

Initiating event—the occurrence that influences the main character to action. It may be a natural event, an action, or an internal event, such as a thought, perception, or wish.

Internal response—indicates the thoughts and feelings of the main character in response to the initiating event. It may include an interpretation of the event, formulation of a goal, or some other response.

Plan—indicates the intended action of the main character.

Attempt—indicates the actions of the main character in pursuit of the goal.

Consequence—indicates the achievement or nonachievement of the main character's goal, as well as any other events or states that might result from the attempt.

Reaction—includes any emotional or evaluative responses of the main character to the preceding chain of events.

Adapted from Johnston, J. (1982). Narratives: A new look at communication problems in older language-disordered children. *Language, Speech, and Hearing Services in Schools, 13,* 144-155; Stein, N., & Glenn, C. (1979). An analysis of story comprehension in elementary school children. In R. Freedle (Ed.), *New directions in discourse processing,* vol. 2 (pp. 53-120). Norwood, NJ: Ablex.

and understanding stories in school, attention to the standard story grammar in the intervention program can be helpful, as long as we remember to present this form as another way of telling stories, not a "better" way. If a child from a culturally different background without other language or learning problems is having the same difficulty, the clinician might work with the classroom teacher to expose the student to a series of storybooks containing increasingly mature mainstream narrative forms.

Understanding stories requires more than just repeating information heard or read. While literal comprehension involves recalling information explicitly stated, much of what it takes to make sense of a story has to be read "between the lines." For example, what if a story starts out, "She was outside riding her bike when she heard the flapping of wings under the bushes. Tears came to her eyes. She ran inside to get a shoe box"? Literal comprehension would involve remembering that the sound came from under the bushes, and the girl was riding a bike when she heard it. But most of us would also be able to infer that the story is about a girl who finds and rescues an injured bird. The comprehension skills involved in drawing this conclusion are called *inferential comprehension*, because they require us to put together information given to infer something that is not directly stated. Bishop (1997) reports that children with LLD have difficulty with both literal and inferential comprehension in narratives. Difficulties in comprehension of inferential meaning are also seen by Letts and Leinonen (2001). Westby (2005) suggests that drawing inferences is particularly difficult for these children. Roth (1986) reported that difficulty in recall of stories by children with LLD also is characterized by (1) poor understanding of temporal and causal relations, (2) dearth of detail, (3) errors in information, and (4) decreased length of retelling.

In terms of the ability to generate stories, a variety of deficits have been found in students with LLD. Ripich and

Griffith (1988) and Liles (1987) reported difficulty with cohesive devices, such as pronouns and conjunctions, although not all students with LLD had these problems. Even though students with LLD seem to have a grasp of the basic story grammar structure, such as that summarized in Box 10-2, Westby (1989b) and Gerber (1993) reported that these children tell shorter stories with fewer complete episodes, fewer complex sentences, more limited vocabulary, and less overall organization. Difficulty in the use of linguistic structures in productive narrative tasks—including utterance length and cohesive adequacy, (Bishop & Edmunson, 1987; Liles, 1985; Liles & Purcell, 1987; Paul & Smith, 1993; Pearce, McCormack, & James, 2003)—is also reported. Montague, Maddux, and Dereshiwsky (1990) also found that students with LLD used fewer internal responses and showed less attention to characters' feelings and motivations than did normally achieving students in storytelling tasks. Difficulties in the linguistic structure of narratives, including deficits in lexical diversity, correct use of morphological structures, proportion of complex syntax, and fluency have been noted (Boudreau, 2006; Reilly, Losh, Bellugi, & Wulfeck, 2004). Additionally, children with LLD also experience difficulty in constructing or retelling narratives, including recall of fewer information units, propositions, utterances, and story grammar components; as well as difficulty with text cohesion (Boudreau & Hedberg, 1999).

Applebee (1978) characterized the development of narrative skills in children as progressing through a series of stages. A modification of Applebee's system that has been used in research on children with language and learning disorders (Klecan-Aker & Kelty, 1990; Paul, Laszlo, & McFarland, 1992; Paul, Hernandez, Taylor, & Johnson, 1996) is presented in Box 10-3. Paul, Hernandez, Taylor, and Johnson (1996) found that by first grade, children with normal language development were producing stories at stage four or five in this sequence, whereas

BOX 10-3	An Adaptation of Applebee's System for Scoring Narrative Stages

Stage 1 (Heap Stories)

Heaps consist primarily of labels and descriptions of events or actions. There is no central theme or organization among the propositions. Sentences are usually simple declaratives. Stories at this level are used by normally developing children at 2 or 3 years of age.

Example: "Mercer went out his home. He got to the playground. Then he found a frog. Then he fell off the cliff. Frog is in the water. Doggy pulls on a stick. A boy is mad. Then he called the police. Then he rested. And then he goed in jail."

Stage 2 (Sequence Stories)

Sequences consist of labeling events around a central theme, character, or setting. There is nothing that could be considered a plot; rather, there is a description of what a character has done. One event does not necessarily follow temporally or causally from another. Stories at this level are used by normally developing children at 3 years of age.

Example: "Little boy. Tree, frog. Tree, person, dog, bucket, and tree that he climbing on, bucket and dog. They fell off. Then they ran down the hill and trip down. And then the frog was happy. And then the dog was swimming. Then there was a dog happy. Then there's a frog sitting on the tree. So they went to the tree that fall into the water where the frog is. And then the boy caught the dog. Lookit, the dog's in the net! And then the dog go."

Stage 3 (Primitive Narratives)

Stories have a core or central person, object, or event. They contain three of the story grammar elements: an initiating event, an attempt or action, and some consequence around the central theme. But there is no real resolution or ending and little evidence of motivation of characters. Stories at this level are used by normally developing children at 4 to 4½ years of age.

Example: "Find a frog. He sees a frog. He fell. And the frog hopped. And he catched the dog. Frog hopped again. Then he went away. The boy was angry. And the frog was pretty nervous. Then he followed the foot track."

Stage 4 (Chain Narrative)

Stories show some evidence of cause-effect and temporal relationships, but the plot is not strong and does not build on the attributes and motivations of characters. The ending does not necessarily follow logically from the events and may be very abrupt. Four story grammar elements are present. They usually include those found at the primitive narrative level: initiating event, attempt or action, and some consequence around the central theme. Some notion of plan or character motivation may be present. Stories at this level are used by normally developing children at 4½ to 5 years of age.

Example: "A boy went for a walk with his dog to fetch water and catch fish. There was a frog. He caught the frog. The boy fell in because he tripped on the dog. The dog fell in too. The frog hopped onto a lily pad. The frog fell off. And the boy tried to catch the frog. And the boy actually caught the dog. The frog climbed onto a rock. The boy called him. They went away. The frog was sad. The frog followed him. He followed him into his house. And the frog was on the dog's head."

Stage 5 (True Narrative)

Stories have a central theme, character, and plot. They include motivations behind the characters' actions, as well as logical and temporally ordered sequences of events. The stories include at least five story grammar elements, including an initiating event, an attempt or action, and a consequence. The ending indicates a resolution to the problem. Stories at this level are used by normally developing children at 5 to 7 years of age.

Example: "There was a little boy. And he wanted to get a frog. And he brought his dog. He saw a frog in the pond. He ran to catch it. But he tripped over a log. And he fell in the water. But the frog jumped over to a log. He told his dog to go try to get the frog. He almost caught the frog. But instead, he caught his dog. When he saw what he caught, he was mad. The little boy, he yelled to the frog. Then the boy went home and left the frog. The frog was sad alone. Then he followed the boy's footprints until he got into the house. Then he kept following them into the bathroom where the little boy took a bath with his dog. 'Hi,' said the frog. Then the frog jumped in the tub. And they were all happy together."

Adapted from Applebee, A. (1978). *The child's concept of a story: Ages 2 to 17.* Chicago, IL: University of Chicago Press. Modified from Klecan-Aker, J., & Kelty, K. (1990). An investigation of the oral narratives of normal and language-learning-disabled children. *Journal of Childhood Communication Disorders, 13,* 207-216; Paul, R., Lazlo, C., & McFarland, L. (Nov., 1992). *Emergent literacy skills in late talkers.* Mini seminar presented at the annual convention of the American Speech-Language-Hearing Association, San Antonio, TX; Wallach, G., & Miller, L. (1988). *Language intervention and academic success.* Boston, MA: College-Hill Publications; and Westby, C. (1984). *Development of narrative language abilities.* In G. Wallach & K. Butler (Eds.), *Language-learning disabilities in school-aged children* (pp. 103-127). Baltimore, MD: Williams & Wilkins. Examples of children's narrations from Mayer, M. (1967). *A boy, a dog, and a frog.* New York: Dial Books for Young Readers.

children with a history of language delays during the preschool period produced stories at significantly lower levels of maturity, generally around stage three. Because narrative skills are known to be related to success in school, findings such as these suggest that children with low levels of narrative development may be at risk for academic problems. This, in turn, suggests that narrative skill is one area that is important to assess in children with LLD. Although many older students with LLD produce true narratives, their progress toward this level may be slower than normal. If deficits in narrative maturity are found through narrative assessment, narrative skills could be a useful part of the intervention program. The aim would be to use narrative skills to build the bridge from oral to literate language.

Another type of discourse that can cause problems for students with LLD is the *expository* text (Scott & Windsor, 2000; Westby, 2005). Expository texts fall at the most literate end of the continuum of language styles. This genre provides the least contextual support and relies most heavily on purely linguistic processing. Expository texts don't tell a story. They are explanations and descriptions that usually contain information new to the receiver. This means that strategies of applying prior knowledge to comprehend the text ("top-down" or concept-driven strategies) are not effective. Instead, the listener or reader must attend to the individual facts and details to get the meaning ("bottom-up" or data-driven processing). This puts an extra load on memory and other information-integrating processes, since there isn't a readily available structure or framework, like a story grammar, to which to attach the information. Instead, the listener or reader has to remember all the pieces of information, organize them into some kind of schema relating to their content, then search for some kind of structure in the text to facilitate integrating the new information with what he or she already knows (Westby & Clauser, 2005).

In primary grades, most information is conveyed through narrative formats, even in content areas such as science and social studies. By the time children reach intermediate grades, however, many textbooks are written in expository rather than narrative form, and the further students progress in school, the more expository text they encounter (Otto & White, 1982). Saenz and Fuchs (2002) reported that expository texts are more difficult to comprehend than narrative for students with LLD. We will discuss the assessment and remediation of expository text deficits in the chapters on advanced language.

There is one additional text structure that students must eventually master. Scott and Erwin (1992) refer to this as the *persuasive* or *argumentative* genre. It involves the attempt to convince a listener of something and is one of the last discourse forms to be acquired. This alone suggests that it is one with which students with LLD will have considerable difficulty.

Social/Emotional Characteristics

It follows logically that children with pragmatic deficits could be expected to have difficulty with the social interactions that pragmatic skills support. In general, children with LLD have been shown to be less accepted by peers, have poorer social skills and higher levels of problem behaviors than children with typical school achievement (Weiner, 2002). These students experience rejection by peers, have difficulties in developing reciprocal friendships and gaining admittance to social groups; when they do join a group, the groups tend to be disproportionately those of companions who show high levels of problem behavior (Pearl, 2002). Fujiki, Brinton, Isaacson, and Summers (2001) showed that children with LLD were more withdrawn than peers with typical development (TD). Moreover, these children show increased levels of loneliness and depression relative to typical peers (Margalit & Al-Yagon, 2002). Clearly, work on pragmatic skills for these students will need to focus on improving their social interactive abilities.

In addition to these social difficulties, students with LLD, particularly boys, have been shown to have greater difficulties in regulating their emotions than typically achieving children (Fujiki, Brinton, & Clark, 2002).

GENERAL KNOWLEDGE

Just as much vocabulary is learned through reading during the school years, a lot of what we know about the world comes from books, too. Many areas of knowledge gained during the school years are not acquired through direct experience. Instead, students gather new knowledge from reading (Catts & Kamhi, 2005b). If students are not reading or are having trouble understanding complex verbal material so that reading comprehension is limited, how are they going to gain this new knowledge? They're not. As time goes on, students with LLD fall further and further behind peers in terms of knowledge about the world. This deficit in world knowledge in itself limits learning. Since we learn essentially by adding information to our existing background store, the smaller that background knowledge store is, the less new information can be added. It's a spiral that leads to increasing gaps in the knowledge base that students can apply to new information. Stanovich (1986) called this the "Matthew" effect, because as the gospel according to Matthew tells us, the rich get richer and the poor get poorer. This suggests that as we work with students with LLD, we want to find ways to augment their general knowledge store as we work on specific language goals. An enlarged knowledge base provides a foundation for more rapid acquisition of new information.

ATTENTION AND ACTIVITY

Unfortunately, many students who have learning problems also have behavioral and emotional difficulties that make it harder for them to take advantage of the instruction, both regular and special, that they receive (Ratner, 2004). We usually do not know whether the learning disorder is caused by these behavior problems, or vice versa, or whether something else entirely is causing both. For whatever reason, though, many students with LLD also qualify for diagnoses of behavior disorders or emotional disturbances such as those discussed in Chapter 4. The most common disorder associated with LLD is what mental health specialists call *attention deficit/hyperactivity disorder,* or ADHD (Tetnowski, 2004).

ADHD consists of a difficulty in marshaling attention, in knowing what to direct attention to and what to ignore, and in focusing on foreground information and filtering out background distractions. Children with attention disorders are easily distracted and have short attention spans, low frustration tolerance, inability to recognize the consequences of their actions or learn from mistakes, and difficulty organizing and completing tasks (Blum & Mercugliano, 1997; Damico, Tetnowski, & Nettleton, 2004). They appear forgetful, lose things, and behave impulsively. Some of these students also exhibit hyperactivity. These children are fidgety, squirm constantly, can't sit still, seem to have "ants in their pants." They are restless and run or climb excessively in inappropriate situations.

Not all students with LLD are emotionally disturbed, hyperactive, or inattentive, but a good number are. Although Tetnowski (2004) suggests it is difficult to determine the overlap of communication disorders and ADHD with any certainty, the overlap certainly exists. Forness, Youpa, Hanna, Cantwell, and Swanson (1992) estimated that 25% of students with LLD have associated behavioral or socioemotional disorders. What this means for the SLP is that working with students with LLD may not always be easy (just in case you thought it would be!). They may not always be the docile, attentive students who can pick up what we are trying to teach them the first time around. It will be important to recognize the students who have these kinds of attentional difficulties so that their special needs can be addressed in an educational program. We talked in Chapter 4 about strategies for addressing problems in attention and activity within the communication management plan. These strategies often include a combination of medication and behavioral interventions. A substantial minority of students with LLD need these special program considerations.

SUMMARY

We've seen that students with LLD commonly have problems in a variety of language areas. Many students with LLD continue to have "underground" deficits in phonological processing, even when phonological production sounds OK. These phonological processing deficits are thought by many researchers to have an important impact on learning to read. Some of the semantic deficits commonly observed in students with LLD also may be related to these higher-level phonological-processing problems. Some students with LLD have difficulties with advanced syntax and morphology, but many do not have obvious or measurable errors in this area. Rather, their language production may simply be less fluent and complex than that of their peers. For students with LLD, pragmatics may be the area in which the majority of obvious deficits reside. They may be less adept than peers at ordinary conversation and probably have difficulty comprehending and producing the discourse structures nearer the literate end of the oral-literate continuum of discourse styles. These genres, such as narratives and expository texts, are necessary for success in the classroom. The general knowledge base of students with LLD also may be limited. Some have attention deficits, are restless and overly active, or have emotional problems that affect their ability to

perform in school. These problems suggest areas of assessment and intervention beyond the traditional vocabulary, morphology, and sentence structures. To address the needs of students with LLD, then, we need to know where to look for their oral language problems to identify and remediate their difficulties. The characteristics of the LLD population that we've discussed here should help guide this process.

LANGUAGE, LEARNING, AND READING: WHAT'S THE CONNECTION?

We've seen that students such as Nick, who have difficulty succeeding in school even though they seem to have acquired basic oral language skills, commonly come to the attention of the SLP. We've talked about some of the oral language deficits typical of students like Nick as a way to answer the first question we posed: how can we characterize the language of children with LLD? Let's look now at the kinds of oral language skills that are needed for success in the classroom and how oral language skills relate specifically to the development of literacy. Then we will be in a better position to answer the second question raised in this chapter: what is the SLP's role in ameliorating the deficits of children with LLD?

THE ROLE OF ORAL LANGUAGE IN CLASSROOM DISCOURSE

Teacher Talk and the Hidden Curriculum

School talk is different from the kinds of conversations we have with friends and family (Christie, 2003). Wallach (2004) recently discussed the special requirements of classroom discourse. In school, the teacher chooses the topic and students must comment on that topic, not one of their choosing. Students who do attempt to shift the topic to their own interests often find their remarks rejected or disvalued. Turn-taking rules in the classroom are quite different from those in other settings, too. The teacher decides who gets to talk, when, and for how long. Students, to be considered successful participants in classroom discourse, must learn to read subtle verbal and nonverbal cues about when they should volunteer to speak, what they should say, and when they should relinquish

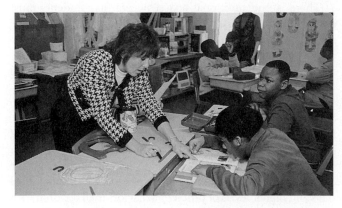

Language forms the basis for success in the classroom.

the floor. Westby (1998a) stressed that in order to succeed in school, students have to be able to draw on two sets of knowledge at the same time: their knowledge of academic content (the right answers to teacher questions) and their knowledge of the social communication rules of the classroom.

Hoover and Patton (1997) pointed out that only a small part of the structure of the classroom discourse is ever verbalized by the teacher. The rest is part of the "hidden curriculum," the unspoken set of rules and expectations about how to behave and communicate in the classroom setting. For example, Cazden (1988) reported that the typical structure of classroom discourse follows the *Initiation-Response-Evaluation* (*IRE*) format: *i*nitiation of a topic by the teacher, followed by a *r*esponse by the student, which then undergoes *e*valuation by the teacher (*I*: "What is the capital of California . . . Jose?" *R*: "Sacramento." *E*: "That's right, good job."). Students who fail to realize that adhering to this structure is part of the expectation of the classroom are often perceived by teachers as rude, difficult, or unable to learn. Yet their real problem may be an inability to grasp that this context has a different set of discourse structure rules than other contexts with which they are familiar. Donahue (1994) reported that for many students with LLD, difficulties with classroom discourse are more likely to be the trigger for referral for special education than is academic failure. This finding emphasizes the crucial role of mastering classroom discourse rules for success in school. As Donahue pointed out, inability to adapt to classroom discourse rules not only reflects but also contributes to failure in the classroom. That's because students who are not good at the "hidden curriculum" have restricted access to the kinds of learning experiences available in peer and teacher dialogues that lead to success in the academic curriculum.

Decontextualized Language

Another difficulty with classroom language is that a great deal of it is decontextualized. In ordinary conversation, we often talk about things in the immediate environment, such the ingredients we need to cook dinner, or about topics on which all the participants have a great deal of shared knowledge, such as the members of our extended families and their doings. In school, though, much of what is discussed is quite outside the direct experience of the students, not to mention its being literally outside the immediate context of the physical environment. At home, families talk about where the lunchbox is. In school, teachers talk about where Australia is. A child who comes to school without much experience of such kinds of decontextualized language will find the discourse of the classroom especially difficult.

Dickinson, Wolf, and Stotsky (1993) reported that, although children from a variety of social and economic backgrounds have ample opportunities to develop adequate semantic and syntactic skills through ordinary parent-child interactions, the same is not true of opportunities to develop the discourse skills that are helpful in school. Children from middle-class families (regardless of their racial or ethnic background) are more likely than peers from low-income groups to have participated in oral language interactions at home that contribute to the development of decontextualized language skill. These interactions include narrations about personal experiences that middle-class parents both tell to and elicit from their children, as well as extended explanations of objects, events, and word meanings.

Although middle-class families in general engage in more such interactions than low-income families, it is important to remember that there is great individual variation within each group. The important thing for us as clinicians to know is this: if children are having trouble participating in classroom discourse, in spite of marginally adequate semantic and syntactic abilities, they may need additional experience and practice with decontextualized language. If, for whatever reason, a child has not gotten such experience at home during the preschool years or was unable to take advantage of it because of slowly developing basic language skills, part of our role can be to provide such experience and practice.

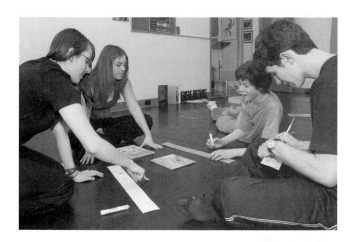

Classroom discourse patterns must be inferred for each instructional situation.

Classrooms and Culture Clash

Remember, too, that classroom discourse is a structure peculiar to our mainstream Western culture. For students entering school from culturally different backgrounds, the structure of classroom discourse is likely to be especially unfamiliar (Hammer, 2004). Differing expectations about a child's conversational role in the home do not necessarily represent a deprived environment. As shown in Chapter 5, different cultures use language for different purposes, and each culture has its own rules about how children, specifically, are to participate in linguistic interactions. A classic example comes from Phillips (1972), who described mismatches between the rules for language use in school and those of the home language of minority students. Native American children, in her example, refused to respond when a teacher asked them to correct the answer of another ("No, the capitol of California isn't San Francisco. Can you help her, Jim?"), because a display of knowledge and correction of a peer would be considered rude in their language community. Similarly, Schultz, Florio, and Erickson (1982) explained that the school requirement that only one speaker talk at a time may be very different from the norm in some children's homes, where overlapping talk by multiple speakers is the rule. The knowledge of the way to talk in school, as we've said, is often assumed by teachers and never taught explicitly. Yet this "hidden curriculum" may be vastly different from the experience of language use with which a student comes to school.

Metalinguistic Skills

In addition to the ability to understand decontextualized language and to discern and adhere to the "hidden curriculum," other special language abilities are needed for success in school. Metalinguistic skills are one example. Much of what goes on in the curriculum involves the ability to focus on and talk about language (Westby, 2005). Defining words; recognizing synonyms, antonyms, and homonyms; diagramming sentences and identifying parts of speech; recognizing grammatical and morphological errors in the process of editing writing assignments; recognizing ambiguity in words and structures with multiple meanings; and the metalinguistic skills needed to acquire reading and spelling competency all require an awareness of language beyond the ability to use words and sentences to communicate. As Webster and Plante (1992) suggested, such heightened levels of awareness may not have developed in school-age children who have just barely mastered the basics of oral language. The metalinguistic demands of the curriculum may cause problems for such children. Again, preschool experiences with talking about words and sounds at home make a big difference in the degree of metalinguistic awareness with which a child enters school (Bowey & Francis, 1991; Vellutino et al., 2004; Watson, 2003).

Metacognitive Skills

One last area of special language skill that is necessary in the classroom is the ability to reflect on and manage one's thinking processes. Succeeding in academic settings requires the student to figure out what needs to be done to accomplish a task, create a plan, carry it out, and evaluate whether the task has been completed successfully. All these actions require metacognitive ability.

Moreover, to follow the multistep, complex directions of the classroom setting, it is often necessary for students to assess their understanding of what they have heard. Comprehension monitoring is one aspect of metacognition, and it is much more central to success in the classroom than to success in ordinary dyadic conversation, which provides so many more contextual cues for the person who is doing the comprehending. Elementary school students spend more than 50% of their time in school listening to the teacher, and high school students spend more than 90% of their time doing the same thing (Griffith & Hannah, 1960). You can see, then, that listening skills and the ability to monitor their effectiveness are very necessary for school success. Teachers, particularly those who teach grades beyond the primary level, use long, complex sentences for giving instruction and directions. They might, for example, give a direction, such as "Before you start your math paper, be sure to finish your spelling work." Such a sentence in which the clause that appears first (start your math) is supposed to be done second can cause errors in interpretation for a child with language-learning problems. Children with LLD, who are unable to monitor or evaluate their ability to understand what is said to them, have difficulty in overcoming these errors. Similarly, many teachers' directions have several parts ("Put your name in the upper right-hand corner of the paper, then number from 1 to 20 down the left-hand margin, and be sure to skip a line between each number."). To ask for clarification or repetition if they need it, children must be able to evaluate whether they have comprehended and remembered the entire sequence. Comprehension monitoring in expository discourse, such as class lectures, is especially important for students to figure out whether they are getting the point of the information being presented.

The vocabulary of the teacher's talk also may include words with which a student is unfamiliar. Although many new vocabulary items can be deciphered from the context, the student needs to know when to apply these contextual strategies. Again, comprehension monitoring is essential for bringing such contextual support to bear. Moreover, some words cannot be figured out even when context is present. For these, the student must recognize the gap and ask someone, either the teacher or a peer, for a definition. Again, evaluating comprehension is a necessary part of this process. Dollaghan (1987) and Westby (2005) suggested that comprehension monitoring is likely to be less developed in students with LLD than in their normally developing peers.

THE ROLE OF ORAL LANGUAGE IN THE ACQUISITION OF LITERACY

Aside from the oral language demands of classroom discourse, oral language plays a second crucial role in school success: it lays the foundation for acquiring literacy. For many years, reading was thought of as primarily a visual-perceptual skill. But since the 1970s, when Kavanaugh and Mattingly published their seminal work, *Language by Ear and Eye* (1972), researchers in reading have become convinced of the crucial psycholinguistic aspects of the reading process. Since then, most investigators studying the reading process consider reading and writing to be language-based skills that simply use visual input as a portal into the language-processing system (Catts & Kamhi, 2005a; Snowling & Stackhouse, 1996; Vellutino, 1979; Wallach, 2004; Watson, 2003). The implication of this shift in focus is that experts in language development (like SLPs) are seen as having a great deal to contribute to the understanding of literacy development and to the promotion of its growth. Because SLPs have such a strong background in oral language development, we are in an excellent position both to influence how reading is taught, particularly to students with LLD, and to provide useful information to other educators about how oral language skills foster literacy. Let's examine the oral language skills on which literacy builds and look at some of the ways oral and written language differ. Then we can see how oral language deficits in these areas might affect literacy acquisition. This information helps us identify areas for assessment and intervention in the child with LLD, as well as providing us with ways to educate teachers about the relations of language and literacy.

Emergent Literacy

One foundation for literacy development has been termed "emergent literacy" (Justice & Kaderavek, 2004a; Sulzby & Teale, 1991; Van Kleeck, 1990; Whitehurst & Lonigan, 2003). Emergent literacy experiences are those in which children begin to develop ideas about how written language works and what it is used for before they actually begin decoding print. Emergent literacy skills develop primarily out of "literacy socialization" (Snow & Dickinson, 1991) experiences, in which the child listens to books read by adults. In these interactions, children learn a lot about books and their special language style. Children learn that if they cover up the little black squiggles on the page with their hands, the reader complains about being unable to see the words and therefore unable to tell the story, giving children the idea that the squiggles contain some meaning. Children learn which way the book opens, which page to look at first, and that the page must be turned to get to the next part. They learn that the print is consistent in telling the reader to say the same thing for each page each time that page is read, regardless of who's reading. Most importantly, perhaps, these early book-reading interactions give the child experience with the genre of literary language, which is quite different from the language used for dyadic conversation (see Box 10-3). As Westby (2005) pointed out, literary language uses more precise and abstract vocabulary and has more complex syntax and different communicative functions than language used in oral conversation. A variety of studies (reviewed by Bus, van Ijzendoorn, & Pelligrini, 1995; Goldfield & Snow, 1984) have shown that children who are read to as preschoolers have an easier time learning to read than those who weren't. These literacy socialization experiences are especially helpful if they involve an opportunity for the child to engage in extended discussion about the books (Heath, 1982). Justice and Kaderavek (2004a)

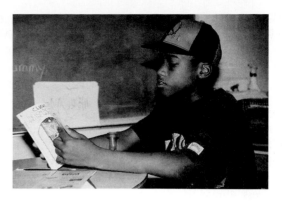

Reading is an important language skill for school-age children.

outlined four aspects of emergent literacy that research suggests are crucial to the development of reading and writing. These are summarized in Table 10-3.

In addition to parent-child book reading, other experiences also can foster literacy socialization. Watching TV shows such as *Between the Lions, Sesame Street, Blue's Clues, Wishbone,* etc., provides literacy socialization in the form of information about letter sounds, the structure of books, the communicative purposes of writing, and literary language exposure. Watching these shows, like having parent-child book reading experiences, also provides a good feeling about books and reading and a pleasant association with literary activities. This ability to feel good about books is perhaps as important as any other literacy socialization the child receives.

Oral Language Foundations for Reading Comprehension

If reading is a language-based skill, this implies that understanding meaning through reading makes use of all the same

TABLE 10-3	Aspects of Emergent Literacy that Support the Acquisition of Reading and Writing
ASPECT OF EMERGENT LITERACY	**DEFINITION**
Phonological awareness	Awareness of the fact that words can be broken down into smaller units, such as syllables (kit + ty = kitty), onset-rime units (d [onset] + og [rime] = dog), and phonemes (/d/ + /a/ + /g/ = dog); ability to blend, segment, and manipulate sounds within words.
Print concepts	Understanding that letters and print make up words and represent ideas; ability to talk about units of language, such as words and letters; understanding the structure of books such as left-to-right progression, orientation of pages, etc., understanding that print is read the same way on each repetition.
Alphabet knowledge	Knowing names and sounds of letters in upper and lower case; understanding that letters stand for sounds and can be grouped to represent words; understanding that words can be read by decoding the sounds of the individual letters within them.
Literate language	Ability to understand decontextualized language; familiarity with conventional language used in narrative genres ("once upon a time"); access to the more formal register of language typically used in print.

Adapted from Justice, L., & Kaderavek, J. (2004) Embedded-explicit emergent literacy intervention I: Background and description of approach. *Language, Speech, and Hearing Services in schools, 35,* 201-211.

processes used to extract meaning from oral language. In other words, a second foundation for understanding a written text is the linguistic knowledge about the content, form, and use of language that is required to understand speech. Both Kamhi and Catts (2005) and Scarborough (2003) pointed out that understanding the comprehension process in reading is essentially no different from understanding it in spoken discourse. Once a text has been decoded, its message is treated cognitively in just the same way as oral language input would be treated. Although the cognitive processes involved in comprehension are varied and complex (Figure 10-2), they are nonetheless similar whether the information to be comprehended came in through the eyes (read) or the ears (heard).

This means that a child with limited skills in comprehending oral discourse is going to have the same problem comprehending a written text. If basic oral vocabulary is so impoverished that students cannot recognize and associate a meaning with a large proportion of the words in a text, even if they can be decoded, the student's understanding of that text will be limited. If a student still relies on nonlinguistic comprehension strategies to understand complex sentences, that student will misunderstand such sentences in either oral or written formats. If a child has poor understanding of story grammar structure, comprehending narratives will be difficult, whether the narratives are oral or written. Nation, Clarke, Marshall, and Durand (2004) reported that children with low language abilities, even when they had not been identified as having SLI, showed poor reading comprehension, even when their phonological awareness skills were adequate. This suggests two things. First, intact, well-developed oral language skills in syntax, semantics, and pragmatics are necessary to comprehend written texts, just as they are to comprehend classroom discourse. Second, assessing a student's compre-

hension skills in oral formats and providing intervention for deficits in comprehension of oral semantic, syntactic, and pragmatic structures will build toward comprehension of both oral and written language.

Metalinguistic Awareness

A third linguistic foundation for literacy acquisition involves metalinguistic awareness. Just as metalinguistic skills are important for participating in classroom discourse, they are essential for learning to read. Learning to read requires focusing on the language itself, at least in the early stages. A beginning reader needs to notice word boundaries; to develop letter-sound correspondences; and to talk about which printed form represents what word, words, or meanings. None of these activities is necessary for oral language development, but all are necessary as the child breaks into the code of written language. Tumner and Cole (1991) reported that metalinguistic skills also are crucial for allowing students to comprehend written texts. Instruction in metalinguistic awareness was highly effective in improving reading comprehension for these students.

One additional area of metalinguistic awareness is especially important for learning to read, even though it is not necessary for other language activities; that is, phonological awareness, the realization that words are made up of sounds and that sound segments can be manipulated in words and represented by symbols (letters). We've discussed already the fact that phonological awareness, according to current thinking about the reading process, is central to learning to read in an alphabetic language like English (Brady & Shankweiler, 1991; Catts & Kamhi, 2005a; Gillon, 2000; Larrivee & Catts, 1999; Lyon, 1999; Liberman & Liberman, 1990; Snowling & Stackhouse, 1996; Torgensen, Otaiba, & Grek, 2005). To see why, let's talk about some of the differences between oral language and reading.

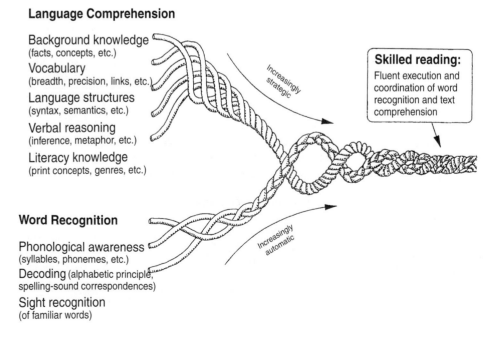

Language Comprehension

Background knowledge (facts, concepts, etc.)
Vocabulary (breadth, precision, links, etc.)
Language structures (syntax, semantics, etc.)
Verbal reasoning (inference, metaphor, etc.)
Literacy knowledge (print concepts, genres, etc.)

Increasingly strategic

Skilled reading:
Fluent execution and coordination of word recognition and text comprehension

Word Recognition

Phonological awareness (syllables, phonemes, etc.)
Decoding (alphabetic principle, spelling-sound correspondences)
Sight recognition (of familiar words)

Increasingly automatic

FIGURE 10-2 ✦ "The Reading Rope": Illustration of the many strands that are woven together in skilled reading. (Reprinted with permission from Scarborough, H. (2003). Connecting early language and literacy to later reading (dis)abilities: Evidence, theory, and practice. In S. Newman & D. Dickenson (Eds.). *Handbook of Early Literacy Research* (pp. 97-110). New York: Guilford Press.)

DISCONTINUITIES BETWEEN ORAL AND WRITTEN LANGUAGE

As we've seen, most researchers today believe that reading and writing are language-based skills. That means that reading and writing rely on a foundation of oral language ability, but they require something in addition. At first glance, it might seem that the extra piece is a visual one—the ability to process print through the visual channel. For many years, LD specialists believed that reading deficits were caused by problems in visual perception. As early as 1937, Orton noticed that children with reading problems sometimes read the word *was* as *saw*, or the letter *b* as *d*, for example, and attributed such problems to visual-perceptual deficits.

But current thinking on the question of the role of visual-perceptual deficits in reading disorders, dating back to Vellutino's (1977) review of research in this area, is that visual-perceptual problems play a relatively minor role in reading disorders. Most investigators in this area today believe that the primary deficits involved in reading disability are linguistic, not visual (Brady & Shankweiler, 1991; Catts & Kamhi, 2005a; Goldsworthy, 1996; Scarborough, 2003).

You can understand how reversals such as *was-saw* could be seen as linguistic rather than visual problems by considering the following example. Like most programs in speech and hearing sciences, the program in which I teach is predominantly female. But one year I had two men in my language disorders class, a somewhat unusual occurrence. They were both quite tall, over 6 feet in height, although the resemblance stopped there. One was dark-haired, the other was fair. One was somewhat husky, the other very slim. They always sat on opposite sides of the classroom, the dark-haired one on my left, the other on my right. Yet throughout the entire year, I consistently mixed up their names! It wasn't that I couldn't perceive the visual differences between them—I just couldn't keep straight which name went with which person. This problem in association of names and referents may be similar to the difficulties children with reading disorders have in making distinctions like the one between *was* and *saw*, or between *b* and *d*. It's possible to explain this difficulty without positing a visual-perceptual deficit. If visual-perceptual problems are not the primary impediment to reading, what skills, in addition to basic oral language competency, are needed for success in literacy?

Biological Bases for Oral Language

To answer this question, one thing we need to remember is that oral language is a primary, biologically based system with a developmental progression that is similar across cultures, specialized neural structures adapted specifically for its functioning, and universal appearance in individuals with normal development (see Kamhi & Catts, 2005; Gleason, 1993; Olson & Gayan, 2003; Snow, Burns, & Griffin, 1998, for review). Speech perception, for example, is biologically programmed. We know this because infants as young as 4 weeks can distinguish between phonemes, even when they have no comprehension of language (Eimas, Miller, & Jusczyk, 1987) and infants as young as 7 months have been shown to perceive boundaries between words and syntactic units in connected speech (Jusczyk, 1999). The ability to process and use written language does not arise from biologically based neurological systems, though (Kamhi & Catts, 2005; Liberman & Liberman, 1990). There is great variability in the age and degree of proficiency of literacy acquisition in individuals within literate societies. Some typical individuals learn to read before kindergarten, some don't learn to read until adulthood, some never learn at all. Moreover, many cultures have never developed any form of written language.

Oral language is as old as the human race. Literacy, on the other hand, is a relatively recent invention (Sulzby & Zecker, 1991; Wilford, 1999). The requirement that everyone in a society be able to read is more recent still. Until well into the 20th century, only a minority of people were literate, and there was no particular stigma or handicap attached to illiteracy. Learning to read does not come naturally to everyone, as its late development and limited penetration in human cultures suggests. For most children, learning to read does not happen as naturally and effortlessly as learning to talk does. Some direct instruction is usually needed. Why is this so? To understand fully why everyone does not learn to read naturally, we need to consider not only the lack of a biological basis for literacy but also the demands that the writing system imposes.

Writing Systems

Three kinds of writing systems have been developed in human societies. The earliest is like that used in contemporary Chinese, sometimes called *pictographic*, *logographic*, or *ideographic*. In this type of writing system, each symbol stands for a whole word. Learning to read in this writing system requires no ability to break words down into smaller units such as sounds, but does require a great deal of memory since a separate symbol has to be associated with each word in the language. It's also hard to develop a typewriter for an ideographic system! A second writing system is the *syllabary*, such as that used in the kana form of Japanese writing. In this system, each symbol represents a syllable, and syllables are combined to form words. This requires some awareness of the sound structure of words and places somewhat less load on the memory than an ideographic system. But a relatively large number of symbols must be learned, and it's still pretty hard to design a typewriter keyboard for a syllabary writing system. English uses the third type of writing system, an *alphabetic cipher*. In this system, each symbol represents a phoneme (more or less). An alphabetic writing system is extremely economical in terms of the load it exerts on the memory, since there are a relatively small number of symbols to learn. But it requires a great deal of phonological awareness, the ability to break words down into component sounds. The efficiency of an alphabetic system is obvious if you're trying to design a typewriter. But the concept of an alphabetic cipher is relatively unnatural. It developed later than either of the other writing systems and was invented essentially only once in history, by the Phoenicians about 4000 years ago. All the alphabetic systems in use today derive from that initial Phoenician alphabet.

What's the point of this digression on the history of writing? Again, it is that an alphabetic writing system is in some sense unnatural. It developed late, even within the history of writing. It was not an idea that was come upon by a lot of people in a lot different places. It was invented only once. The fact that alphabetic writing spread to many cultures is attributable to its efficiency, not to its naturalness. These facts strengthen the prediction that reading in an alphabetic writing system is not going to come naturally to every individual. There are lots of reasons to expect that it will be somewhat hard to learn, at least for some people, and that most people will need a little help, in the form of direct instruction, in breaking into the alphabetic code.

The Key to Reading in an Alphabetic Cipher

Let's get back to the question we asked at the beginning of this section. What is needed to learn to read English, over and above basic oral language skills? The answer most researchers in reading today would give is *phonological awareness*. Phonological awareness is comprised of the ability to break words down into component sounds, to realize that these units of sound can be represented by letters, to learn letter-sound correspondence rules, to analyze words into component sounds (for spelling), and to synthesize sounds represented by letters into words (for reading). Many reading researchers call this awareness of the *alphabetic principle.*

Phonological awareness is not necessarily part of normal language development. Studies of nonliterate adults show that they have limited levels of phonological awareness (Goswami & Bryant, 1990) and their phonemic awareness is clearly and strongly related to their letter knowledge (De Santos Loureiro et al., 2004). However, the following clear conclusions about the relationship between phonological awareness and reading in school children can be drawn from the research literature (Blachman, 1994; Swank, 1999; Vellutino et al., 2004):

▶ There is a significant relationship between phonological awareness and reading. Children who exhibit phonological awareness skills have been shown to learn to read more easily than children who don't (Adams, 1990; Ball & Blachman, 1988; Kamhi & Catts, 2005a; Swank & Larrivee, 1999; Snow, Burns, & Griffin, 1998).

▶ Performance on phonological awareness tasks in kindergarten and first grade is a strong predictor of later reading achievement (Scarborough, 2003; Snow, Burns, & Giffin, 1998).

▶ Direct teaching of phonological awareness and letter-sound correspondences to children who are not yet reading improves their reading and spelling development more than other forms of reading readiness instruction (Adams, 1997; Ball and Blachman, 1991; Blachman, 1989; Gillon, 2000; Snow, Burns, & Griffin, 1998). Moreover, the effects of this training persist in giving children an advantage in reading even 4 years later (Bradley, 1988), and these benefits are strongest for children whose phonological awareness skills start out lowest (Chall, 1997; Lundberg, 1994).

Phonological awareness teaching works best when combined with explicit instruction in letter-sound correspondences, especially when the two are taught in separate activities (Chall, 1997; van Kleeck, 1995).

What Does It Take to Learn to Read?

Scarborough (2003) has argued that there are two main components, or strands that need to be integrated in order for children to learn to read and write. These are represented in Figure 10-2. One strand includes various aspects of language knowledge that will support reading comprehension; such as basic vocabulary and syntax, the world knowledge children acquire through experience and instruction, higher level language skills such as verbal reasoning and metalinguistics, along with basic literary knowledge of print concepts and conventions, as well as story schemas. The second strand includes those skills that will support word recognition. These include the skills we have just been discussing, such as phonological awareness, letter-sound knowledge and, eventually, fluent and automatic recognition of an increasingly large vocabulary of sight words.

Because all these abilities need not only to be present, but to be integrated in order for fluent reading to develop, it is easy to see why disruption in any one strand can lead to difficulty in the acquisition of the entire process of learning to read. We can also see that some of these strands will be present in most children when they come to school, such as basic vocabulary and syntax; some will be present only in children who have had literacy socialization experience, such as print concepts and conventions. And we've learned that some of these skills, such as phonological awareness and letter-sound correspondence, will have to be taught directly, even to children with typical development and strong literacy socialization. Of course these things don't happen all at once. There are a series of phases through which children pass in the process of learning to read. Chall (1983) has presented a particularly useful summary of this sequence. Although some writers (e.g., Kamhi & Catts, 2005) have pointed out problems with stage theories like this one, Chall's overview does give us a sense of the kinds of reading skills generally expected at various points in the curriculum. Her sequence is outlined in Table 10-4.

In Chall's "prereading" stage, from 2 to 6 years of age, the child acquires what we've been calling literacy socialization through the natural, scaffolded kinds of interactions with adults that whole language advocates. In the first reading stage, from about the beginning of the first to the middle of second grade, decoding the print, or the processes involved in word recognition, is the focus. Most of the child's attentional resources are devoted to using letter-sound correspondence rules and phonological synthesis abilities to decipher single words. Comprehension, or attention to meaning, can be limited during this period because so much attention is going into decoding. More advanced comprehension skills emerge toward the end of this period, as the child begins to automatize some of the decoding processes. Of course, the child does not lose any of the language comprehension skills he has acquired in oral

TABLE 10-4	Chall's (1983) Stages of Reading Development

STAGE	GRADE LEVEL	ACHIEVEMENTS
Stage 0: Prereading	Pre-K	Literacy socialization
Stage 1: Decoding	1–2	Phonological analysis and segmentation/synthesis in single words
Stage 2: Automaticity	2–4	Fluent reading; greater resources for comprehension available
Stage 3: Reading to Learn	4–8	More complex comprehension, increased rate
Stage 4: Reading for Ideas	8–12	Recognition of differing points of view, use of inferencing
Stage 5: Critical Reading	College	Synthesis of new knowledge, critical thinking

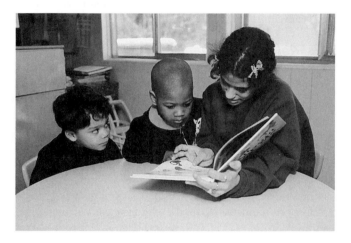

Reading acquisition proceeds through a series of stages.

activities. But decoding requires a lot of attention at first, and children in this phase will not have as many resources available to understand what they read as they have for understanding what they hear.

By stage 2, from late second to fourth grades, reading becomes more fluent, decoding is more automatic, and more attention is available for comprehension. Children's ability to take in what they read becomes more similar to their receptive ability for spoken language. Stage 3, from fourth to eighth grades, marks a major change in the child's reading ability. Now instead of learning to read, the child is reading to learn, able to get new information and derive fuller meaning from print because the decoding process has become well-learned and goes on automatically, below the level of consciousness. This frees a majority of the child's attentional resources to comprehend the text, make inferences, and so on. In Chall's later stages, more sophisticated comprehension skills evolve, in concert with the child's developing intellectual capacity and metacognitive skill. But at all the stages, lower-level decoding skills can be brought to bear when an unfamiliar word is encountered.

This sequence emphasizes the fact that children need different kinds of instruction at different points in development. In the prereading period, they need literacy socialization opportunities and lots of experience talking about words and sounds. In the decoding phase, phonological awareness activities—

breaking words into smaller parts, identifying sounds in words, finding words with the same first and last sound, associating sounds with letters, inventing spelling—and letter-sound correspondence instruction and practice are crucial. But children will continue to need to hear stories and be exposed to literate language, as well as to build a strong oral language base in terms of vocabulary, morphology, sentence, and discourse forms. In later phases, once basic decoding has been mastered, phonological awareness activities can be de-emphasized and focus shifted to explicit instruction in comprehension strategies in both oral and written texts. Catts (1999) argued against using more complex phonological awareness activities (such as sound deletion and manipulation) once basic decoding has been mastered. Instead, he suggests that most reading disabilities "occur in the context of more widespread language deficits" (p. 19). We need to continue to shore up the oral language base for these students, as well as provide them with explicit instruction in strategies for improving their comprehension of both oral and written texts they encounter in school (Mastropieri & Scruggs, 1997; Westby, 2005).

But what about our children with LLD? Don't their weaknesses in language and metalinguistic awareness dictate a different kind of instructional program? Traditional approaches to LDs, as we saw in Chapter 1, often used a specific disabilities approach to categorize children with reading problems. In this approach, areas of strength and weakness were identified, and teaching strategies attempted to build on the strengths and get around the weaknesses. The great majority of children with reading difficulties will, if assessed in this way, be found to have deficits in a variety of the language areas depicted in Figure 10-2, as we've seen (Catts, 1999; Kamhi & Catts, 2005). And, as we now know, many will be found to have deficits in phonological processing (Hesketh, 2004; Larrivee & Catts, 1999). A specific disabilities approach to this problem would avoid methods of teaching reading that rely on phonological processing, such as a decoding approach. Instead, methods would be selected that build on the child's strengths in other areas. Traditionally, whole-word ("look-say") approaches that emphasized memorizing each word as a unit (similar to the logographic system) were used with such children. In the early 1990s, whole language approaches that emphasized meaning rather than phonological analysis were advocated (Norris & Hoffman, 1993).

However, according to the National Research Council report, "Children who are having difficulty learning to read do not, as a rule, require qualitatively different instruction from children who are 'getting it.' Instead, they more often need application of the same principles . . ." in individualized, more intensive settings. This conclusion applies to children with specific reading disorders as well as to those from culturally and linguistically different backgrounds. These children are likely not to have the elaborated base in oral language, experience with decontextualized language use, exposure to literate language genres, metalinguistic skills, or knowledge of letter-sound correspondences. In fact, Warren-Leubecker and Carter (1988) showed that the area of language in which poor children differed most from those from middle-class homes was in phonological awareness, which in turn was the best predictor of reading achievement. Current research advocates tackling these problems head-on with explicit instruction and focused practice in both the basic language skills needed for strong reading comprehension and the kinds of phonological awareness and letter-sound abilities known to support word recognition in children with and without language learning problems (Adams, 1997; Chall, 1997; Gillon, 2000; Lyon, 1999; Snow, Burns, & Griffin, 1998). Gillon (2002) showed that phonological awareness training led to "sustained growth in phoneme awareness and word recognition" (p. 381) as well as in spelling in children with language impairments.

The consensus among researchers today is that teaching metalinguistic, phonological awareness, and letter-sound correspondence skills explicitly and providing practice so these skills can become automatized in word recognition activities make better readers (Ehri et al., 2001). This basic truth has been reaffirmed by Snow's committee's exhaustive review. The "Great Debate" (Chall, 1996) that resurfaced during the 1990s on the most effective way to teach beginning reading has been resolved: in the early stages, direct instruction in basic decoding skills is crucial to successful reading development for all children. Reading experts today argue for a "balanced" approach to reading instruction; one that provides lots of practice in phonological awareness and letter-sound correspondence in primary grades, but also continues to present meaningful, engaging literature and multiple opportunities for children to continue their oral language growth and their appreciation of the functions of print. Explicit teaching in comprehension and spelling strategies also is important at later stages.

THE ROLE OF THE SCHOOL SLP IN LITERACY DEVELOPMENT

Let's return to the second question we posed earlier in the chapter: What is the role of the school-based SLP in addressing written language issues? SLPs have a very important role to play in fostering balanced literacy instruction, both in our consultative role with classroom teachers and in our direct work with students who have LLD. This fact is often recognized in schools through the creation of "literacy teams;" groups of educators who support the classroom teacher in her primary

role as the individual responsible for basic literacy instruction by addressing the needs of children who are struggling to acquire literacy, and using their knowledge to create the most facilitative environments for making sure all students learn to read and write. Pressures from legislation, such as the No Child Left Behind Act of 2001 (http://www.ed.gov) have contributed to the effort to provide more resources to teachers to make sure all children acquire proficiency in literacy skills. Because of our knowledge of the oral language bases for literacy, and of the sound structure of English, SLPs are considered important members of school literacy teams. Let's discuss how we can fulfill our roles in the area of literacy, by talking first about the beginning stages of reading, and then about our roles at higher developmental levels.

SLPs' Role in Emergent Literacy and Decoding

Vellutino et al. (1996) report that with well-designed early instruction in phonological awareness and spelling-sound correspondence, all but 3% of children can become successful readers in the primary grades. Yet we know that anywhere from 10% to 40% of children are now failing to meet grade-level expectations in reading, with even higher proportions of failure in poor urban areas. Catts, Fey, Tomblin, and Zhang (2002) found the children with oral language impairments are six times more likely to have trouble learning to read than are typical peers, and that half the children who struggle with reading in primary grades have language impairments. SLPs can have a positive effect on these dismal statistics by helping both the teachers and the students we work with to participate in reading instruction that follows principles established by extensive research.

ASHA (2001) advocates two basic roles for the SLP in literacy instruction in schools. The first is in the provision of indirect services through consultation and collaboration with teachers. In these activities, the SLP works with these teachers to organize and implement activities that support literacy for all students throughout the school day (Justice & Kaderavek, 2004a). At the preschool and primary level, it is important that we help teachers get away from the idea that "phonics" instruction means worksheets and seat work. Code-emphasis reading programs do not have to be boring lectures. Children love playing with language, as their spontaneous sound and word play attests. There are lots of enjoyable approaches to developing metalinguistic and phonological awareness skills. Examples can be found in Adams, Foorman, Lundberg and Beeler (1998), Blachman (1987), Chaney and Estrin (1987, 1989), Elkonin (1973), Estrin and Chaney (1988), Gillon (2000), Justice and Kaderavek (2004b), Lewkowicz (1980), Sulzby (1980), and Yopp and Yopp (2000). Some of these methods are discussed in Chapter 12. However, because so many current teachers went through training programs that de-emphasized phonics and decoding instruction, they may have had very little training on the sound structure of our language (Fillmore & Snow, 2000). Yet, Chall (1997) cites research showing that teachers who do not themselves have adequate knowledge of phonological and phonics rules have students who do less well in reading. One way SLPs can support literacy development is to help these classroom teachers, in in-service and consultative settings, acquire a deeper knowledge of the structure of our language.

But researchers (Catts, 1999; Kamhi, 1999; Snow, Burns, & Griffith, 1998; Scarborough, 2003; Swank, 1999; van Kleeck, 1995) have reminded us that, although phonological awareness is necessary to beginning reading instruction, it is not sufficient in itself to make students fluent readers. We cannot ignore the importance of helping children learn not only to decode but to understand and appreciate what they read; to apprehend the many functions of print, and to develop their own abilities as writers. As experts in language development, SLPs have an important part to play here, too, in advocating for an inclusive and balanced approach to literacy instruction.

Justice and Kaderavek (2004a) suggest a three-tiered approach to addressing literacy for the school SLP during the preschool and primary years. First, in her indirect role, the SLP collaborates with the classroom teacher in creating a print-rich environment in which signs, lists, and labels are placed prominently throughout the classroom and referred to frequently during the day's activities. The SLP also encourages and participates in storybook reading and sharing activities that include talk about the content and structure of books and stories. SLPs can also help embed a rotating set of literacy activities within daily routines, such as having a "post office" play corner in which children are encouraged to "read" and "write," at whatever level they can, and talk about these processes is modeled and encouraged during play. The second tier involves collaborative direct instruction in activities for the entire class that focus on phonological awareness, letter-sound correspondence, and phonological analysis and synthesis. While engaging collaboratively in these lessons, the SLP can be alert to those students who seem to be having difficulty, attending less, or making less progress than others. For these students the SLP can present a third tier of instruction by supplementing classroom literacy activities with individual or small group follow-up lessons to preteach and review the literacy concepts addressed in the classroom instruction. Since at least some of the students already on the SLP's caseload will require this tier of instruction, the SLP can simply add other children who are not on IEPs, but are clearly struggling with literacy to these small group sessions. This approach makes use of dynamic assessment for identifying children at risk for literacy failure, so that the SLP does not have to screen or

assess children separately for phonological awareness or other preliteracy deficits. Instead, she does this as an ongoing part of her participation in the classroom's daily literacy instruction. As such, this method provides an efficient way for the SLP to fulfill her role on the literacy team at this level.

SLPs' Role in Later Literacy Development

Beyond the primary grades, SLPs continue to have important contributions to make to children's literacy acquisition. Four major areas of literacy beyond decoding are identified and defined in Table 10-5. In each of these areas, as in the others we've discussed, SLPs address students' literacy needs through both direct and indirect services. Schuele and Larrivee (2004) discussed the ways in which SLPs can contribute to literacy at these levels. The most familiar, of course is through individual assessments and therapeutic interventions. SLPs can identify children at risk for literacy deficits as a result of ongoing oral language problems, or through dynamic assessment during classroom collaborations, as we talked about before. We can also provide individual or small group instruction to children struggling with literacy by reinforcing reading comprehension through teaching skills and strategies for oral language comprehension, and practicing these in both oral and written contexts (see Chapters 12 and 14). In these sessions we can, as Kamhi (2003) suggested, make use of activities that involve multiple rereadings of texts the students are using in the classroom, in order to work toward fluent reading, as well as comprehension. Rereadings can take place in the context of drama activities, such as having 2-3 children at a time act out the text while the SLP and the others in the group read it aloud, having a "readers' theater" presentation in which the students take turns reading the same text aloud, as if in different moods ("Keisha can read it as if she is happy, then Hector can read it as if he is mad…") or as choral readings for recording on tape and listening to with parents as the child reads the text along with the recording at home. Combining these kinds of fluency-enhancing activities with comprehension practice can assist struggling readers in two aspects of literacy development simultaneously.

Spelling is also an area of literacy where SLPs can have an impact through direct instruction. We'll talk more in Chapter 12 about the SLP's role in spelling development, but in general we can address the spelling needs of children with LLD, as Apel (2004) suggests, using a *word study* orientation. This relies

TABLE 10-5	Aspects of Literacy beyond Decoding

LITERACY AREA	DESCRIPTION
Fluency	The ability to read smoothly with speed, accuracy, and appropriate expression (Kamhi, 2003)
Reading comprehension	The ability to understand, make inferences, draw conclusions, recall, summarize, and acquire new information from written texts
Spelling	The phonological and orthographic skills that enable conventional representations of words
Written composition	The planning, execution, and editing of written products

on our expertise in understanding the phonological and morphological structure of words, and providing metalinguistic discussion and strategies to help students move beyond basic phonological awareness to understanding the patterns in the English spelling system. SLPs can also help students at higher grade levels improve written composition skills, as we will discuss in more detail in Chapter 14, by focusing on the prewriting, or planning aspects of written communication and using oral language strategies to help students plan and organize their writing.

In our indirect service roles on literacy teams, Schuele and Larrivee (2004) advocate for helping teachers understand the connection between spoken and written language; that print is, in some sense, speech written down. As such, we can help teachers plan lessons that provide oral language activities as a bridge toward literate ones, collaborate in these lessons, and use them as opportunities for dynamic assessment to identify children who struggle with them. Again, these students can be engaged in more intensive, small group instruction in oral language activities with the SLP that will support their literacy development. SLPs can also help teachers understand that, even in intermediate and secondary grades, students continue to need direct skill instruction in areas such as learning spelling patterns, drawing inferences from texts, and planning for written composition. Lessons in skills like these are ideal opportunities for collaborative teaching and dynamic assessment. The team planning that goes into the collaborative lessons also provides opportunities for the SLP to guide the teacher in integrating oral and written language activities. It also allows an SLP to become thoroughly familiar with the instruction planned, so she can preteach and review this information in therapeutic small-group sessions. As Boudreau and Larsen (2004) have suggested, the unique role played by the SLP on a literacy team showcases our ability to provide the scaffolding, individualization, and explicit metalinguistic instruction that will help children struggling with literacy to achieve their highest potential.

■ CONCLUSIONS

We've seen that success in school, regardless of grade level, requires a vast amount of experience and proficiency with oral language. Some of these oral language skills are part of most children's natural development, but some are higher-level skills that require specialized contexts and experiences for their acquisition. As SLPs, our job is to ensure that our clients with LLD have a solid oral language basis and have moved past the developing language phase in their content, form, and use of language. Beyond this, though, we need to be aware of the special discourse requirements of the classroom and of the higher-level linguistic requirements of the curriculum. This knowledge leads us to appropriate assessment strategies; we'll know what to look for in terms of problems that can impede the child with LLD. Moreover, understanding the various ways in which oral language supports and interacts with success in school can help us develop interventions that contribute to success for our clients. SLPs are central players in school literacy teams and in providing help for students who struggle with the oral and written language demands of the school setting.

STUDY GUIDE

I. Definitions and Characteristics
   A. What is a reading disorder? Dyslexia? How do researchers today see the difference between these two disorders?
   B. What kinds of phonological deficits are seen in students with LLD?
   C. How do these relate to learning to read?
   D. How does the syntax of children with LLD differ from that of children in the developing language phase?
   E. What kinds of syntactic and morphological errors are typical of students with LLD? How prevalent are such errors?
   F. What are the vocabulary problems of students with LLD, and why do they have them?
   G. What is the role of word retrieval in LLD, and what are two alternative explanations of the problem?
   H. Describe the social interaction problems in students with LLD.
   I. Discuss narrative and expository discourse types. How do these cause problems for students with LLD?
   J. Why do students with LLD often have deficits in general knowledge?
   K. What is ADHD? What role do these disorders play in language-learning disabilities?

II. Language, Learning, and Reading: What's the Connection?
   A. Discuss some of the special properties of classroom discourse and why they may cause problems for some students.
   B. What is the "hidden curriculum?"
   C. Discuss decontextualized language. How is it acquired? Why is it important?
   D. How can classroom discourse create a mismatch for students from different cultural backgrounds?
   E. Why are metalinguistic skills needed for school success?
   F. What is metacognition? Why is it important in school?
   G. Describe the continuum of formality of language from oral to literate. Describe how the form, function, and topics of language differ along this continuum.
   H. Discuss the current conception of reading as a language-based skill.
   I. What are the implications of this conception for understanding deficits in reading?
   J. What oral language skills are needed to learn to read? Why can we not expect all children to come to school with these skills?
   K. What is the relationship between reading and language comprehension?
   L. What is phonological awareness, and how do children attain it?

M. What is literacy socialization?

N. What is the role of metalinguistic awareness in learning to read?

O. Why is learning to read an "unnatural act"?

P. Name and describe four aspects of emergent literacy.

Q. Discuss the three writing systems used throughout the world. What are the advantages and disadvantages of each?

R. Why does the SLP need to understand the reading process?

S. What oral language skills can the SLP work on to build a firm base for literacy in students?

T. What is a literacy team and who are its members?

U. Name and describe four aspects of literacy development that emerge after the primary school years.

V. Discuss Chall's stages of reading development.

W. What are the current recommendations for practices in teaching early reading, according to the report of the National Research Council?

X. What can the SLP contribute to reading instruction for clients? For all students?

ASSESSING STUDENTS' LANGUAGE FOR LEARNING

CHAPTER OBJECTIVES

Readers of this chapter will be able to do the following:

- Describe how families participate in educational planning for school-aged children.
- Define and describe methods for screening at the elementary school level.
- Discuss methods of referral and case-finding.

- Discuss the uses of standardized tests at the elementary school level.
- Describe non-standardized assessment methods for students in elementary grades.
- Carry out language analysis procedures for conversation and narratives.
- Use dynamic and curriculum-based assessment methods.
- Apply concepts discussed to assessment of students with severe disabilities.

Maria had been doing well in second grade until her bike accident. While riding without a helmet one day, she was struck by a car. She spent 3 days in a coma, and when she first emerged from it, she didn't speak at all. After several weeks in the hospital, where she received physical, occupational, and speech therapy, she was able to go home. She spent several months out of school, receiving home tutoring and more therapy. She returned to school the next year, by which time she had recovered her speech but still had some problems with her gait and small-motor skills. She continued to see the occupational and physical therapists but was thought to be doing all right with her language. She seemed quiet and never caused any trouble. On the playground, she kept to herself and didn't get involved in what the other children were doing. She was meek and somewhat shy, but always eager to please the teacher. She seemed to have regressed somewhat in her reading, which was above grade level before the accident, but she managed to follow the simple, repetitive material used in the reading program in her second-grade class, which she was repeating because she'd missed so much time the previous year. She did very well at the craft projects that went along with social studies and science units. When she spoke, her sentences were short, but that seemed to be more because of her shyness than anything else. When she got to third grade, though, she suddenly ran into trouble. She couldn't follow directions. She couldn't seem to answer the questions the teacher posed for class discussion. She was unable to read the books used for social studies and science. She began to withdraw, sometimes going for days without saying a word. She complained of stomach aches and asked to spend numerous periods of time in the nurse's office. The nurse called her family to discuss the problem. They said that Maria had started saying she was "dumb" and didn't want to go to school because she was too "stupid." They reported being very upset to find her crying in bed on school nights. The school nurse suggested to Maria's teacher that Maria be referred for an evaluation of special educational needs.

Maria is another child who seems to have difficulties making the transition from primary to intermediate grades and keeping up with the changes in the curriculum that this transition entails. Although the basic oral language she recovered after her traumatic injury seems to be good enough to get by, Maria has trouble with the more complex language of the intermediate classroom and can't manage the reading requirements of her grade level. Maria's response to these problems is different from Nick's. She retreats rather than becoming aggressive. But the reason for both responses is similar. The demands of the classroom are taxing these students' abilities and making them feel like failures.

When we, as speech-language pathologists (SLPs), assess students like Nick and Maria, we want to bear in mind the issues we discussed in Chapter 10 about the need to look not only at basic oral language skills but also at the specialized abilities that contribute to success in the classroom in general and in reading in particular. In this chapter, we'll talk about assessment issues for students who are beyond the developing language phase, with skills above Brown's stage V. We will focus on children who have mastered the basic vocabulary, sentence structures, and functions of their language but have trouble progressing beyond these basic skills to higher levels of language performance. This chapter and the next one focus specifically on clients whose developmental levels are commensurate with those of students in the elementary grades. We will be talking about the communicative skills needed for the elementary school years, from kindergarten through fifth or sixth grade when typical children are between 5 and 12 years of age or so.

Of course, some children at these chronological age levels who are served in schools or other educational settings function at lower levels. Particularly with the push toward inclusion of students with disabilities embodied by the Individuals with Disabilities Education Act (IDEA), clinicians find students in elementary schools who function at the developing, emerging, or even prelinguistic stages of communication. When these students are included in the caseload of a school SLP, assessment and intervention strategies appropriate for their level of functioning are needed. Information on assessment and intervention strategies for students at these levels of development can be found in Section II.

Although the stage of development we're considering in these chapters usually takes place when children are between 5 and 12 years of age, we may encounter some clients with language learning disabilities in middle school or even high school who function at this elementary grade level. For these students and for their younger counterparts, the assessment and intervention information presented in this chapter and Chapter 12 is germane. Let's call this phase of language development the "language for learning" period (L4L for short). The L4L stage is when many of the oral language bases for school success, including the knowledge of special classroom-discourse rules, decontextualized language, metalinguistic and phonological awareness, and literacy skills that we talked about in Chapter 10 must be acquired in order for the student to meet the demands of the curriculum.

CHILD AND FAMILY IN THE ASSESSMENT PROCESS

Although IDEA legislation mandates that families be involved in the assessment and intervention process for students with special educational needs, this ideal is not always fully met in practice. Parents may not know that their child has been having difficulty until they are told a referral has been made. Because the assessment often takes place at school, the parent may not have an opportunity to observe it and contribute a family perspective. Clinicians particularly committed to curriculum-based assessment (e.g., Nelson & Van Meter, 2002) may feel that the teacher has more relevant information to contribute about the student's needs than the family does. However, the principles of family-centered practice are just as relevant for children in the L4L stage as they are for younger clients.

These principles remind us that families need to be involved in each stage of the assessment process, from referral to remedial planning. This means contacting parents as soon as a referral is made, discussing the referral, and learning whether the family shares the referring person's perceptions about the student. A telephone conference can often be beneficial at this stage, using the same communication strategies as those outlined in Chapter 6 for parent contacts. Parental permission for the assessment must be obtained, and parents should be invited to attend any assessment sessions they wish. Parents should be kept informed periodically of the progress of the assessment, if it stretches over a period of time, and should be invited to attend a meeting when the assessment is complete to discuss the evaluation with the team and to provide input in the development of an Individual Educational Plan (IEP).

It is very helpful to families for one member of the assessment team to take on the role of case manager or parent advocate. SLPs are often excellent candidates to play this role, particularly if communication is a major area of deficit for a student. The case manager or parent advocate can ensure that the family stays informed and engaged, gets a chance to ask questions, and contributes to the planning process. The case manager also can check with the parents to make sure that they understand all the jargon being used by the professionals. It is easy for us to forget that not everyone knows all the acronyms (IEP, FAPE, LRE) and jargon that we use in our profession. A simple check with the family every now and then can give them an opportunity to say whatever they need to say. Having one person, with whom an ongoing relationship has been established, to turn to with concerns and questions is also very useful for families. Despite their best intentions, the assessment team may seem intimidating, overwhelming, cold, or uncaring to a family that is struggling to find the best way to meet their child's educational needs. If a case manager is not formally assigned to a family as part of the assessment process, the SLP can assume this role on an informal basis. Having someone that makes a special effort to express concern for the family as well as the child can make all the difference.

One other person deserves to have some input in the assessment process at the L4L stage. That's the student. By the time they are 7 or so, children have a strong need to make some of their own decisions and to function somewhat independently. Students to whom an assessment "just happens" are less likely to give their best performance than are those who feel they have some control in the situation. An SLP can talk with students before assessment begins about why it is taking place, the questions the assessment will attempt to answer, and what to expect. This can give the impression that you see students as people whose opinions and feelings matter. Asking students to talk a little about how they see the situation is another good tactic. You can ask whether they have trouble in school, what they are good at, what they find hard, and in what areas they would like some help. This conversation can serve several purposes. It gives students the feeling that you think they are mature enough to have some say about what goes on, and it provides an initial conversational sample that can help guide you to areas of communicative function that will need to be assessed.

IDENTIFYING STUDENTS FOR COMMUNICATION ASSESSMENT

SCREENING

One way children make their way to the school SLP is through screenings. These are often conducted upon entrance into the school system for the first time, or at particular grade levels. This screening sometimes includes screening for hearing, as well. Some school systems use mass screenings in which all children beginning kindergarten are screened during a few designated periods by professionals or paraprofessionals using short standardized instruments, such as the *Preschool Speech and Language Screening Test—2nd Edition* (Fluharty, 2000), the *Joliet 3-Minute Speech and Language Screen—Revised* (Kinzler & Johnson, 1993), or *Developmental Indicators for the Assessment of Learning—3rd Edition* (Mardell-Czudnowski & Goldenberg, 1998). Some districts use locally developed, informal methods. Other local educational agencies (LEAs) set aside the first week or two of kindergarten for individual screenings. Each new student meets with a teacher or team for a somewhat more intensive screening. These screenings have several possible outcomes. A recommendation to wait a year before entering kindergarten may be given, to let the child mature. Alternatively, students may be placed in a developmental kindergarten program for some preschool-level instruction with the expectation that they will enter regular kindergarten the next year. Screening also can lead to a referral for an assessment in greater depth in one area, such as communication, or by a multidisciplinary team. SLPs often participate in these screenings and may identify children who will join their caseload as a result. Whether the SLP participates directly in screenings or not, it is our responsibility to interpret screening information and make decisions about which children need further assessment.

Many school districts use informal, locally developed methods for screening, particularly for mass kindergarten screenings. Although this practice is widespread, it is not, I would argue, advisable. A screening instrument should have well-documented psychometric properties, because that is the best way to ensure its fairness. Some critics of kindergarten screening have argued that early identification through screening is unfair to minorities, culturally and linguistically different (CLD) children, and those from low-income families (Braddock & McPartland, 1990; Pavri & Fowler, 2001). Although many of these arguments may apply to standardized as well as informal procedures, the issue of unfairness is much more pronounced when screening is done using intuitive or subjective criteria. Using nationally standardized norms, or norms developed and tested locally with a relatively large normative sample, that include children from a range of ethnic and economic backgrounds helps us to guarantee that screening procedures are as fair as we can make them.

In addition to a large and representative norming sample, a screening test should have some additional properties. It should have adequate reliability and validity, cover a relatively wide range of language behaviors, provide clear scoring with pass/fail criteria, have adequate sensitivity to identify a large majority of children who have language difficulties, and take a small amount of time (Justice, Invernizzi, & Meier, 2002; Sturner, Layton, Evans, Heller, Funk, & Machon, 1994). The only way to find out whether a test meets these standards is to read the manual carefully. We need to look at the norming sample to see whether it contains children such as those on whom we will be using the test. We need to review the items to evaluate their comprehensiveness. We need to look at the scores and statistics provided to determine whether the test is valid and reliable, provides adequate sensitivity, and gives a usable pass/fail standard. We need to try it a few times to see whether it is efficient to use. When we find a test that meets these standards, we can feel confident that our screening will be fair, efficient, and accurate. Some instruments that have been developed for screening communicative skills in school-age children are listed in Table 11-1.

Still, the availability of psychometrically sound instruments is a problem. Sturner et al. (1994) found in their review of 51 standardized screening instruments that only six provided adequate validity data. Only nine were found to be adequately brief and comprehensive. Justice et al. (2002) report that none of the six early literacy screening instruments they examined contained all essential features. These findings underline the importance of being critical consumers in selecting commercial tests and screening instruments. Just because a test is published does not mean it has adequate psychometric properties. We need to review the tests we use carefully to ensure they are fair, efficient, and effective. Moreover, we should argue for careful consideration of psychometric properties in the selection of any screening instruments our schools use. This can help to ensure that we provide assessment services in a fair and appropriate way.

REFERRAL AND CASE FINDING

A second way in which school children get to the SLP for assessment is through teacher referral, because of a perception on the teacher's part that something is not quite right about the child's language. Maria and Nick are examples of these kinds of students. Some schools don't even do screening; they rely on teachers to identify children in need of assessment on the basis of their classroom performance. Teacher referral is not as simple as it sounds, though. In Maria's case, for example, the classroom teacher did not, on her own, make a referral but did so only after encouragement from the school nurse. There are lots of reasons why teachers do not refer every child about whom they have concerns. One is that they may feel these referrals are not heeded. Many teachers have the experience of waiting months before hearing from an assessment team about a child who was referred. Sometimes the whole school year goes by before the team gets to the student. Teachers who have this experience are less likely to feel the referral process benefits them or their students. Other reasons why teachers may not make speech-language referrals for students in elementary grades include the fact that the student's language sounds acceptable to "the naked ear," as we've discussed; that language deficits seem

TABLE 11-1	**A Sample of Language Screening Instruments for Grades K-5**

TEST NAME (AUTHOR[S]/DATE/PUBLISHER)	AGE RANGE	AREAS ASSESSED	COMMENTS
Bankson Language Screening Test Bankson, N.W. (1977). Baltimore, MD: University Park Press	4–7 yr	Receptive plus expressive: semantics, morphology, syntax, auditory and visual perception	Lists 38 of the most discriminating items as appropriate for quick screen, but no norms for this screen. Yields standard and percentile scores. Standardized on 637 children in rural and Washington, D.C., areas, all socioeconomic (SES) levels. Administration time: 25 min.
Battelle Development Inventory (BDI) Screening Test Newborg, J., Stock, J., Wnek, L., Guidubaldi, J., & Svinicki, J. (2004). Itasca, IL: Riverside Publishing	Birth–8 yr	Communication, cognitive, personal and social, adaptive, and motor	See BDI in Table 11-2. Administration time: 10–30 min.
Clinical Evaluation of Language Fundamentals–4 Screening Test Semel, E., Wiig, E.H., & Secord, W. (2004). San Antonio, TX: Harcourt Assessment	5–21 yr	Expressive morphology, syntax, receptive concepts and semantics, auditory comprehension, pragmatics	Yields criterion pass/fail score. Administration time: 15 min.
Compton Speech and Language Screening Evaluation–Revised Edition Compton, A. (1999). San Francisco, CA: Carousel House	3–6 yr	Expressive language, receptive language, articulation, auditory memory, oral mechanism, motor coordination	Little statistical data available. Administration time: 10 min.
Denver II Frankenburg, W.K., Archer, P., Bresnick, B., Maschka, P., Edelman, N., & Shapiro, H. (1990). Denver, CO: Denver Developmental Materials	2 wk–6:4 yr	Expressive and receptive, vocabulary, concepts, personal/social, fine and gross motor	Yields pass/fail criterion. Good concurrent validity. Interrater reliability = 0.62–0.79. Standardized on more than 2000 children in Denver (mixed SES, race). Administration time: 15–20 min.
Developmental Indicators for the Assessment of Learning–Third Edition Mardell-Czudnowski, C., & Goldenberg, D. S. (1998). Circle Pines, MN: American Guidance Service	3–6:11 yr	Motor, concepts, language, self-help, and social	Provides standard deviation and percentile cutoff points by chronological age at 2-mo intervals. Normed on 1,560 English-speaking and 605 Spanish-speaking children throughout the United States. Percentile ranks and standard scores also are provided. Administration time: 20-30 min.
Developmental Indicators for the Assessment of Learning–Speed DIAL Mardell-Czudnowski, C., & Goldenberg, D.S. (1998). Circle Pines, MN: American Guidance Service	3–6:11 yr	Motor, concepts, language	Shortened version of DIAL-3. Normed on same population as DIAL-3. Administration time: 15–20 min.
Diagnostic Evaluation of Language Variation–Screening Test (DELV–Screening Test) Seymour, H.N., Roeper, T.W., & de Villiers, J. (2003). San Antonio, TX: Harcourt Assessment	Language variation status: 4–12 yr Diagnostic risk status: 4–9 yr	Expressive language	Helps distinguish language differences from language disorders. Criterion referenced scoring that scores degree of variation and degree of risk for language disorder. Administration time: 15–20 min.

| TABLE 11-1 | A Sample of Language Screening Instruments for Grades K-5—cont'd |

TEST NAME (AUTHOR[S]/DATE/PUBLISHER)	AGE RANGE	AREAS ASSESSED	COMMENTS
Joliet 3-Minute Speech and Language Screen (Revised) Kinzler, M.C., & Johnson, C.C. (1993). San Antonio, TX: Harcourt Assessment	K, 2nd and 5th grades	Expressive syntax, receptive vocabulary, articulation, voice, and fluency	Has computer program for record-keeping. Provides pass/fail, cutoff score for each grade. Standardized on 2,587 children from three different SES and ethnic backgrounds. Administration time: 3 min.
Kindergarten Language Screening Test—2 Gauthier, S.V., & Madison, C.L. (1998). Austin, TX: Pro-Ed	4–6:11 yr	Receptive and expressive concepts, commands	Yields percentile score. Normed on 154 kindergartners. Test-retest reliability = 0.87. Construct validity given. Little information on norming sample in terms of SES and ethnic background; claims mixed cultural backgrounds. Administration time: 5–10 min.
Screening Kit of Language Development Bliss, L.S., & Allen, D.V. (1983). East Aurora, NY: Slosson Educational Publications	2–5 yr	Vocabulary, comprehension, story completion, sentence repetition, auditory comprehension (commands)	Normed for Standard and Black English. Administration time: 15 min.
Speech-Ease Screening Inventory (K-I) Speech-Ease (1985). Austin, TX: Pro-Ed	K–Ist grade	Articulation, language association, auditory recall, expressive vocabulary, concept development	Has optional section with similarities and differences and language sample. Administration time: 7–10 min.
The Wilson Syntax Screening Test Wilson, M.S. (2000). San Antonio, TX: Harcourt Assessment	Pre-K–K	Screening for children with specific language impairments	20-Item screener that uses 20 grammatical markers. Administration time: 2–4 min.

minor in comparison to behavioral, attentional, academic, or social problems the student is experiencing; or that the child's problem is considered to be primarily in the area of reading, rather than oral language.

Taylor (1992) suggested that to make best use of the teacher referral process, some in-service education of teachers is needed. Damico (1985) described his dismay at the success of this sort of effort. After giving an in-service presentation to teachers in his elementary school about the connections between language and learning disorders and the value of an SLP's contribution to the assessment and treatment of academic problems in these students, he was quickly inundated with potential clients! Although such a deluge may not be our goal, we do want to make teachers aware of the role of language skills in academic success and let them know that we are interested in working with students who are having academic problems. In-service presentations that "update" faculty on recent findings about language-literacy connections can get this message across.

Another way to optimize the efficacy of teacher referrals is to provide teachers with specific criteria or checklists to use. We can distribute these checklists to classroom teachers and ask them to fill out one for each student in the class who seems to be having difficulty or about whom they have some concern.

Damico and Oller (1980) found that encouraging teachers to use pragmatic criteria for referral, rather than criteria based on syntactic and morphological errors, resulted in more accurate referrals. Damico (1985) developed a Clinical Discourse Analysis Worksheet to analyze a speech sample of students with language-learning disorders (LLDs). This worksheet can be modified and used as a pragmatically oriented checklist to be given to teachers as a basis for referring students. One such modification appears in Figure 11-1.

Using a checklist such as this one, the SLP can evaluate whether a student having academic problems also is showing some language difficulties. Any student for whom a teacher answers "yes" to several (more than four, say) of these questions could be a candidate for assessment in greater depth. Remember that students with LLD are more likely to show deficits in pragmatic areas than in syntax and morphology, so that a pragmatic screening tool such as this one is likely to pick up students who are having difficulty with the language demands of the curriculum. Once we identify these students, of course, we can assess them in a variety of areas, including but not limited to pragmatics. Pragmatic criteria for referral, though, seem to be a valid way to identify which students are having problems with the linguistic demands of the classroom.

Student name _____ Grade _____

Teacher _____ Date _____

To the teacher: Please circle the answer to each question that best describes your student's performance in class.

Does the student:

Give insufficient information when giving instructions or directions?	Yes	No
Use nonspecific vocabulary (*thing, stuff, whatchamacallit*)?	Yes	No
Perseverate or provide too much redundancy when talking?	Yes	No
Need a lot of repetition before even simple instructions are understood?	Yes	No
Give inaccurate messages; seem to talk when he or she "doesn't know what he or she is talking about"?	Yes	No
Make rapid and inappropriate changes in conversational topic without cues to the listener?	Yes	No
Seem to have an independent conversational agenda or give inappropriate and unpredictable responses?	Yes	No
Fail to ask relevant questions to clarify unclear messages so that communication frequently breaks down?	Yes	No
Use language that is inappropriate for the social situation?	Yes	No
Produce speech that is frequently disrupted by repetitions, unusual pauses, and hesitations?	Yes	No
Use many false starts, self-repetitions, and revisions in talking?	Yes	No
Produce long pauses or delays before responding?	Yes	No
Lack forethought and planning in telling stories and giving instructions?	Yes	No
Fail to attend to cues for conversational turns, interrupting frequently or failing to hold up his or her end of the conversation?	Yes	No
Use inconsistent or inappropriate eye contact in conversation?	Yes	No
Use inappropriate intonation?	Yes	No

Please use the space below to describe any other concerns you have about this student's communication:

FIGURE 11-1 ✦ Pragmatically oriented discourse analysis to be used as a teacher referral form. (Adapted from Damico, J. [1985]. *Clinical discourse analysis: A functional language assessment technique.* In C.S. Simon [Ed.], *Communication skills and classroom success: Assessment of language-learning-disabled students* [pp. 165-206]. San Diego, CA: College-Hill Press.)

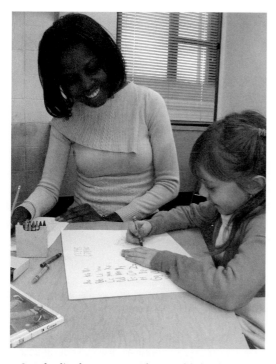

Standardized tests are used to establish eligibility for school-based services.

Ripich and Spinelli (1985) also developed a Classroom Communication Checklist (CCC) to be used by teachers in making referrals to the SLP. This appears in Figure 11-2. It can be used in a way similar to that suggested for the form in Figure 11-1. Either form can help encourage teachers to refer students with academic problems to the SLP for language assessment and intervention and help the SLP to make a relatively quick and accurate judgment about which students might benefit from these services. Bishop and Baird (2001) developed the CCC, in order to identify students with specific disorders in the area of pragmatics. Botting (2004) showed that it is sensitive to children with a variety of communication impairments. The CCC is available commercially (Table 11-2) and can also serve as a tool to help teachers make referrals for students with communication difficulties.

Additional suggestions for using checklists to identify children in primary grades who may be at risk for literacy problems come from Catts (1997) and Justice et al. (2002). A checklist based on their suggestions is shown in Figure 11-3. This can be used to help first-grade teachers identify students who may have LLD before they actually begin to fail in reading. The SLP can provide preventive intervention in early literacy skills to children identified through this assessment. We'll talk more in Chapter 12 about how this intervention can be provided on a

Child _____	SLP _____
Grade _____	
Teacher _____	Date _____

Communication Area	Effectiveness Rating* 1 2 3 4 5	Comments
Participation		
Amount		
Interruptions		
Soliciting attention		
Manner		
Frequency		
Paying attention		
Maintaining attention		
Following directions		
Questioning		
Amount		
Content appropriate		
Appropriateness		
With teacher		
With peers		
Descriptive ability		
Amount		
Organization		
Speech-language abilities		

*1 = Excellent, 2 = Good, 3 = Adequate, 4 = Fair, 5 = Poor.

FIGURE 11-2 ✦ Classroom communication checklist. (From Ripich, D., & Spinelli, F. [1985]. *School discourse problems* [p. 209]. San Diego, CA: College-Hill Press.)

TABLE 11-2	A Sample of Language Assessment Tools for Grades K-5

TEST NAME (AUTHOR[S]/DATE/PUBLISHER)	AGE RANGE	AREAS ASSESSED	COMMENTS
Assessment and Treatment of Narrative Skills: What's the Story? Apel, K., & Masterson, J. (1998). Rockville, MD: American Speech-Language-Hearing Association	School-age	Narrative	4-hr videotape and manual. This CE course examines procedures, strategies, and ideas for evaluating and treating narrative deficiencies in school-age children with language-learning impairments.
Bankson Language Test—Second Edition Bankson, N. (1990). Austin, TX: Pro-Ed	3–7 yr	Receptive and expressive language, auditory memory and discrimination	Standardized on 1,108 children. Administration time: 10–15 min.
Batelle Developmental Inventory, Second Edition Newborg, J., Stock, J.R., & Wnek, L. (2004). Chicago: Riverside Publishing	Birth–8 yr	Speech and language, social/emotional, cognitive, motoric skills, learning, and hearing	Normative data gathered from over 2,500 children. Includes optional scoring software so data can be input to a Web-based program or on a Palm Pilot. Scoring includes standard scores, age equivalents, and cut-off scores. Administration time: 1–2 hr.

TABLE 11-2	A Sample of Language Assessment Tools for Grades K-5—cont'd		

TEST NAME (AUTHOR[S]/DATE/PUBLISHER)	AGE RANGE	AREAS ASSESSED	COMMENTS
Boehm Test of Basic Concepts—3rd Edition Boehm, A.E. (2000). San Antonio, TX: Harcourt Assessment	K–2nd grade	Receptive language concepts	Spanish edition available. Group administration. Yields percentile, equivalent for grade. Normed on two samples with two different forms (E and F) in Fall of 1999 (Form E n = 2,866; Form F n = 3,189) and the Spring of 2000 (Form E n = 2,348; Form F n = 2,196). Reliability studies yielded coefficients α between .80 and .91. An alternate-forms reliability study showed that nearly 94% of students had a difference of 4 or fewer raw score points from one form to the other. Administration time: 30–45 min.
Carolina Picture Vocabulary Layton, T.L., & Holmes, D.W. (1985). Austin, TX: Pro-Ed	4–11:6 yr	Receptive sign vocabulary	Designed for deaf and hearing impaired. Yields scale scores, percentile ranks, age equivalents. Standardized on 767 children who use manual sign. Administration time: 10–15 min.
Children's Communication Checklist, Second Edition Bishop, C. (2003). London: Harcourt Assessment	4–16 yr	10 areas: speech, syntax, semantics, coherence, inappropriate initiation, stereotyped language, use of context, nonverbal communication, social relations, interests	Standard scores and percentiles for each of the 10 areas. 70-item checklist used to distinguish between children who have a specific language impairment from those who have more of a pragmatic deficit, such as autism. Administration time: 5–15 min.
Clinical Evaluation of Language Fundamentals—4 Semel, E., Wiig, E.H., & Secord, W. (2003). San Antonio, TX: Harcourt Assessment	5–21 yr	Semantics, syntax, memory, receptive and expressive, composite, pragmatics checklist	Software scoring package available (CELF-4 Clinical Assistant). Screening also available for ages 5–21. 11 subtests. Yields standard, percentile, age-equivalent scores. Normed on 2,400 students. Administration time: 30–60 min.
Communication Abilities Diagnostic Test Johnston, E.B., & Johnston, A.V. (1990). Austin, TX: Pro-Ed	3–9 yr	Syntax, semantics, pragmatics (for example, predicting outcomes)	Yields standard scores, percentile ranks. Normed on over 1000 nationwide. Administration time: 30–45 min.
Detroit Tests of Learning Aptitude—Primary 2 Hammill, D.D., & Bryant, B.R. (1991). Austin, TX: Pro-Ed	3–9:11 yr	Domains: linguistic, cognitive, attentional, motoric	Software available for scoring. Articulation measure included. Yields standard, percentile scores, and age equivalents. Normed on 2217 children. Presents construct validity and reliability. Administration time: 15–45 min.
Diagnostic Evaluation of Language Variation (DELV—Criterion Referenced)	4–9 yr	Comprehensive speech and language, including pragmatics, syntax,	Helps distinguish language differences from language disorders. Criterion referenced scoring.

| TABLE 11-2 | A Sample of Language Assessment Tools for Grades K-5—cont'd | | |

TEST NAME (AUTHOR[S]/DATE/PUBLISHER)	AGE RANGE	AREAS ASSESSED	COMMENTS
Seymour, H.N., Roeper, T.W., & de Villiers, J. (2003). San Antonio, TX: Harcourt Assessment		semantics, and phonology	Administration time: 45-50 min.
Dynamic Assessment and Intervention: Improving Children's Narrative Abilities Miller, L., Gillam, R., & Peña, E. (2001). Austin, TX: Pro-Ed	School-age	Narrative	Uses wordless picture books. Allows determination of students' responses to different types of supports.
Evaluating Acquired Skills in Communication—Revised Riley, A.M. (1991). San Antonio, TX: Harcourt Assessment	3 mo–8 yr	Semantics, syntax, morphology, pragmatics	For evaluation of severely language-impaired.
Evaluating Communicative Competence Simon, C.S. (1994). Eau Claire, WI: Thinking Publications	9–17 yr	Language processing, metalinguistic skills, functional uses of language	An informal evaluation.
The Expressive Language Test Huisingh, R., Bowers, L., LoGiudice, C., & Orman, J. (1998). East Moline, IL: LinguiSystems	5–11:11 yr	Expressive language, including sequencing, metalinguistics, grammar and syntax, concepts, categorizing, and describing	Normed on 2,666 children. Age equivalencies, percentile ranks, and standard scores. Manual includes an extensive section of remediation suggestions specific to each subtest. Administration time: 40–45 min.
Expressive One-Word Picture Vocabulary Test—2000 Edition Brownell, R. (Ed.) (2000). Novato, CA: Academic Therapy	2–18 yr	Expressive vocabulary	Spanish version available. Norming sample related to ROWPVT. Yields standard, percentile, age-equivalent scores. Administration time: 20 min.
Expressive Vocabulary Test Williams, K.T. (1997). Circle Pines, MN: AGS Publishing	2:6–90+ yr	Expressive vocabulary and word retrieval	Normed on 2725 people. Age-based standard scores, percentiles, NCEs, stanines, and test-age equivalents. Norming sample related to PPVT-III. Split-half reliabilities from .83 to .97 with a median of .91. Alphas from .90 to .98 with a median of .95. Test-retest studies with four separate age samples resulted in reliability coefficients ranging from .77 to .90. Administration time: 15 min.
The HELP Test—Elementary Lazzari, A.M. (1996). East Moline, IL: LinguiSystems	6–11 yr	Expressive language, including semantics, general and specific vocabulary, word order, question grammar, defining	Normed on 2,131 students. Correlates to the HELP series therapy materials for oral or written practice. Administration time: 25–30 min.
Illinois Test of Psycholinguistic Abilities—Third Edition Hammill, D.D., Mather, N., & Roberts, R. (2001). Austin, TX: Pro-Ed	5–12:11 yr	Spoken and written vocabulary, spelling, rhyming, sentence sequencing, grammar, phonology	Includes software scoring and report system. Provides general language, spoken language, and written language composite scores.

TABLE 11-2   A Sample of Language Assessment Tools for Grades K-5—cont'd

TEST NAME (AUTHOR[S]/DATE/PUBLISHER)	AGE RANGE	AREAS ASSESSED	COMMENTS
Language Processing Test–Revised Richard, G.J., & Hanner, M.A. (1995). East Moline, IL: LinguiSystems	5–11 yr	Associations, categorization, multiple meanings, attributes	Yields standard scores, percentile ranks, age equivalents. Standardized on more than 1500 children. Administration time: 35 min.
Lindamood Auditory Conceptualization Test–3rd Edition Lindamood, C.H., & Lindamood, P.C. (2004). Austin, TX: Pro-Ed	5–18:11 yr	Phonological analysis	Provides standard scores, percentile ranks, age and grade equivalents. Has English and Spanish versions. Administration time: 20–30 min.
Oral Communication Battery (OCB) Peins, M., & Knolmayer Glazewski, B. (1997). Oceanside, CA: Academic Communication Associates	3–8 yr	Phonology, syntax, semantics, morphology, pragmatics, following directions, storytelling, word and sentence comprehension, voice, fluency, articulation/ phonology, phonological awareness	Informal assessment tool. Vocabulary measures are included in English and Spanish.
OWLS Listening Comprehension and Oral Expresson Scales Carrow-Woolfolk, E. (1996). Circle Pines, MN: American Guidance Service	3–21 yr	Receptive and expressive language	Age-based raw scores can be converted to standard scores, percentile ranks, normal curve equivalents, stanines, and age equivalents. Administration time: LCS, 5–15 min; OES: 10–25 min.
Patterned Elicitation of Syntax Test (Revised) with Morphophonemic Analysis Young, E.C., & Perachio, J.J. (1993). San Antonio, TX: Harcourt Assessment	3–7:6 yr	Expressive syntax and morphology	Uses delayed imitation. Includes morphophonemic analysis. Provides means and standard deviation for age, percentile rank. Normed on 651 children in four states. Administration time: 20 min.
Peabody Picture Vocabulary Test–4 Dunn, L.M., & Dunn, L.M. (2006). Circle Pines, MN: AGS Publishing	2:6 yr–adult	Receptive vocabulary	Provides standard error of measurement and confidence intervals for score. Norming sample related to EVT. Yields standard scores, percentile ranks, age equivalent, stanine. Spanish version available. Standardized on 4012 children, ages 2–18 yr. Administration time: 10–20 min.
Porch Index of Communicative Ability in Children Porch, B.E. (1981). Albuquerque, NM: PICA Programs	3–12 yr	Verbal, gestural, graphic abilities	Scores responses qualitatively. 2 batteries: ages 3–5, 6–12. Provides means and percentiles. Standardized on several hundred children representative of U.S. census. Administration time: 30–60 min.
Receptive One-Word Picture Vocabulary Test–2000 Edition Brownell, R. (Ed.) (2000). Novato, CA: Academic Therapy Publications	2:11–12 yr	Receptive vocabulary	Spanish version available. Yields standard, percentile, age-equivalent score. Similar to norming population for Expressive One-Word Picture Vocabulary Test. Administration time: 20 min.

| TABLE 11-2 | A Sample of Language Assessment Tools for Grades K–5—cont'd |

TEST NAME (AUTHOR[S]/DATE/PUBLISHER)	AGE RANGE	AREAS ASSESSED	COMMENTS
Rhode Island Test of Language Structure Engen, E., & Engen, T. (1983). Austin, TX: Pro-Ed	3–20 yr	Receptive syntax	Designed for hearing impaired, but can be used for learning-disabled or English-as-a-second-language populations. Standardized on 513 children with hearing impairment and 283 hearing children. Administration time: 30 min.
Rice/Wexler Test of Early Grammatical Impairment Rice, M.L., & Wexler, K. (2001). San Antonio, TX: Harcourt Assessment	3–8 yr	Morphemes and syntactic structures that children with language disorders characteristically lack	Helps identify children with specific language impairments who might be missed by other tests. Administration time: 45–60 min.
S-MAPS, Rubrics for Curriculum-Based Assessment and Intervention Wiig, E.H., Lord Larson, V., & Olson, J.A. (2004). Eau Claire, WI: Thinking Publications	K–12th grade	Basic and advanced language and communication skills, literacy and discourse development, thinking and creativity	27 rubrics in the three categories. Student performance can be evaluated on continuum from beginner to expert. Rubrics available on CD. Helps adapt skills to curriculum.
Structured Photographic Expressive Language Test 3 (SPELT-3) Dawson, J., Eyer, J., & Stout, C. (2003). DeKalb, IL: Janelle Publications	4–9:11 yr	Syntax and morphology	Has guidelines for scoring Black English dialect. Spanish version available (2nd edition). Yields standard, percentile, age-equivalent scores. Standardized on more than 1800 children nationwide. Administration time: 15–20 min.
Test for Auditory Comprehension of Language—3rd Edition (TACL-3) Carrow-Woolfolk, E. (1999). Austin, TX: Pro-Ed	3–9:11 yr	Auditory comprehension, word classes and relations, grammatical morphemes, elaborated sentence constructions	Computer scoring available. Yields standardized scores, percentile, age-equivalent scores. Standardized on 1003 children. Internal consistency = 0.96. Test-retest reliability = 0.89–0.95. Administration time: 15–25 min.
Test of Auditory-Perceptual Skills—Revised (TAPS-R) Gardner, M.F. (1997). Novato, CA: Academic Therapy	4–13 yr	Auditory perception, including auditory word discrimination, auditory number memory, auditory word memory, auditory sentence memory, auditory interpretation of directions, auditory processing (thinking and reasoning)	Helps diagnose auditory perception deficits that could be the basis for learning problems. Spanish version available. Administration time: 15–25 min.
Test of Early Language Development—3rd Edition Hresko, W.P., Reid, K., & Hammill, D.D. (1999). Austin, TX: Pro-Ed	2–7:11 yr	Receptive and expressive syntax, semantics	Yields standard, percentile, normal curve equivalent, age-equivalent scores. Normed on 1184 children in 30 states. Reliability = 0.90. Content validity = 0.40–0.52. Administration time: 15–20 min.
Test of Early Written Language—2 Herron, S., Hresko, W., & Peak, P. (1996). Austin, TX: Pro-Ed	3–11 yr	Emerging writing skills	Helpful for identifying students with mild handicaps. Yields means, standard deviations, percentiles.

TABLE 11-2	A Sample of Language Assessment Tools for Grades K-5—cont'd		
TEST NAME (AUTHOR[S]/DATE/PUBLISHER)	**AGE RANGE**	**AREAS ASSESSED**	**COMMENTS**
Test for Examining Expressive Morphology Shipley, K., Stone, T., & Sue, M. (1983). Austin, TX: Pro-Ed	3–7:11 yr	Morphemes in sentence completion tasks	Has companion intervention program—Teaching Expressive English Morphology. Provides means and standard deviation for age, age-equivalent score. Normed on 540 children. Interrater reliability = 0.94. Construct validity = 0.87. Administration time: 7 min.
Test of Language Competence—Expanded Edition Wiig, E.G., & Secord, W. (1989). San Antontio, TX: Harcourt Assessment	Level 1: 5–9:11 yr Level 2: 9–8:11 yr	Metalinguistics, multiple meanings, inferences, figurative usage, conversational sentence production	Yields standard percentile for age, age-equivalent score. Has companion intervention program, which uses cognitive-linguistic approach. Administration time: 1 hr.
Test of Language Development—Primary (TOLD-P:3)/Intermediate (TOLD-I:3) Newcomer, P.L., & Hammill, D.D. (1997). Austin, TX: Pro-Ed	Primary: 4–8:11 yr Intermediate: 8:6 yr– 12:11 yr	Receptive and expressive semantics, syntax	Software available for scoring. Nationally standardized on more than 2436 children in 29 states, mostly white, urban; 50% white-collar. Item reliability = 0.93–0.99. Administration time: 40 min.
Test of Narrative Language (TNL) Gillam, R.B., & Pearson, N.A. (2004). Austin, TX: Pro-Ed	5–11:11 yr	Literal and inferential comprehension, use of language in narrative discourse	Normed on 1059 children from 20 states. High validity and reliability. Administration time: 15–20 min.
Test of Pragmatic Language Phelps-Terasaki, D., & Phelps-Gunn, T. (1992). Austin, TX: Pro-Ed	5–13:11 yr	Pragmatics	Can be used for adult remedial, English-as-a-Second Language, and aphasic populations. Yields standard, percentile scores. Internal consistency = 0.82. Reliability = 0.80. Standardized on 1016 children in 21 states. Administration time: 45 min.
Test of Problem Solving—Revised—Elementary Bowers, L., Barrett, M., Huisingh, R., Orman, J., & LoGiudice, C. (1994). East Moline, IL: LinguiSystems	6–11 yr	Explaining inferences, determining cause of events, answering negative and why questions, determining solutions, avoiding problems	Yields standard, percentile, age-equivalent scores. Standardized on 842 children. Administration time: 20 min.
Test of Relational Concepts—Revised Edmonston, N., & Thane, N.X. (1999). Washington, DC: Gallaudet University	3–7:11 yr	56 concepts: dimensional adjectives, spatial and temporal, quantitative, others	Yields standard, percentile score. Normed on 1000 children nationwide. Administration time: 10–15 min.
Test of Semantic Skills—Primary (TOSS-P) Bowers, L., Huisingh, R., LoGiudice, C., & Orman, J. (2002). East Moline, IL: LinguiSystems	4–8 yr	Receptive and expressive semantics: labels, categories, attributes, functions, definitions; has 6 themes: learning and playing, shopping, household, working, meals and health, and fitness	Yields standard, percentile, age-equivalent scores. Standardized on 1500 students nationwide. Administration time: 25–30 min. Previously called *Assessing Semantic Skills Through Everyday Themes (ASSET)*.

| TABLE 11-2 | A Sample of Language Assessment Tools for Grades K-5—cont'd |

TEST NAME (AUTHOR[S]/DATE/PUBLISHER)	AGE RANGE	AREAS ASSESSED	COMMENTS
Test of Word Finding—Second Edition German, D.J. (2000). Austin, TX: Pro-Ed	4:4–12:11 yr	Multisyllable and compound word retrieval, progressive and past tense verb forms	Yields standard, percentile, age- and grade-equivalent scores. Nationally standardized on 1836 students. Administration time: 20–30 min.
Test of Word Finding in Discourse German, D.J. (1991). Austin, TX: Pro-Ed	6:6–12:11 yr	Word retrieval in discourse	Provides word-finding behaviors index, productivity index. Yields standard scores, percentile ranks. Nationally standardized on 856 students. Administration time: 15–20 min.
Test of Word Knowledge Wiig, E.H., & Secord, W. (1992). San Antonio, TX: Harcourt Assessment	Level 1: 5–8 yr Level 2: 8–17 yr	Expressive and receptive semantics, definitions, antonyms, synonyms, multiple meanings	Yields standard, age-equivalent, percentile scores with confidence interval. Administration time: 30–60 min.
Test of Written Language-3 (TOWL-3) Hammill, D.D., & Larsen, S.C. (1996). Austin, TX: Pro-Ed	2nd–12th grade (7–17:11 yr)	Cognitive and linguistic components of language	Suggested use is to establish baseline. Can be given to individual or group. Two forms available so post-test results not confounded by memory. Software scoring system available. Yields standard, percentile, written language quotient scores. Standardized on more than 2000 students in 16 states. Administration time: 40 min.
Token Test for Children DiSimoni, F. (1978). Austin, TX: Pro-Ed	3–12 yr	Auditory comprehension, temporal and spatial concepts	Yields age- and grade-equivalent score. Standardized on 1300 children (urban and rural). Administration time: 10–15 min.
Utah Test of Language Development—4 Mecham, M.J. (2003). Austin, TX: Pro-Ed	3–9:11 yr	Receptive and expressive language, auditory comprehension	Yields standard scores and language quotient. Administration time: 30–45 min.
Wiig Assessment of Basic Concepts (WABC) Wiig, E. (2004). Greenville, SC: Super Duper Publications	2:6–7:11 yr	Receptive and expressive concept knowledge in 7 categories: color or shape; size, weight or volume; distance, time or speed; quantity or completeness; location or direction; condition or quality; sensation, emotion, or evaluation	Test is presented in interactive storybook format. Normed on 1200 children. Standard scores, percentile ranks, and age equivalents. Administration time: 10–15 min.
Wiig Criterion-Referenced Inventory of Language Wiig, E.H. (1990). San Antonio, TX: Harcourt Assessment	4–13 yr	Semantics, pragmatics, syntax, morphology	No norm-referenced scores; use as criterion-referenced procedure.
Woodcock Language Proficiency Battery—Revised Woodcock, R.W. (1991). Chicago, IL: Riverside Publishing	2–95 yr	Oral language, vocabulary, antonyms and synonyms, reading and writing	Compuscore software for scoring. Spanish form available. Yields standard, age- and grade-equivalent scores. Nationally standardized on 6300 students. Reliability coefficients = 0.95.

TABLE 11-2	**A Sample of Language Assessment Tools for Grades K-5—cont'd**		
TEST NAME (AUTHOR[S]/DATE/PUBLISHER)	**AGE RANGE**	**AREAS ASSESSED**	**COMMENTS**
The Word Test—2 (Elementary) Huisingh, R., Bowers, L., LoGiudice, C., & Orman, J. (2004). East Moline, IL: LinguiSystems	7–11 yr	Associations, synonyms and antonyms, semantic absurdities, definitions, multiple meanings	Yields standard, percentile, age-equivalent score. Standardized on more than 1282 students. Administration time: 30 min.

consultative or collaborative basis, in order to help build a language base for literacy for all the students in the class, as well as for those at risk.

PREASSESSMENT/REFERRAL

Traditionally, SLPs have only served those children with identified special educational needs. However, as we saw in Chapter 10, many school systems now make use of a preassessment process, often called "student success teams" (SST), to attempt to meet the needs of students within regular classes without identifying them as disabled. This is a general education process that attempts to help students who are having difficulties in school without the use of special education (Moore-Brown & Montgomery, 2001), but SLPs and other special educators, because of their expertise in helping children with difficulties, are often a part of these teams. The SST will meet to discuss students who seem to be having trouble, get a sense of the student's strengths and needs and brainstorm ways to help. This process has the advantage of helping schools avoid overidentifying students as "disabled," as is often the case for CLD children. Instead of saying there is something "wrong" with the child, SSTs attempt to make the classroom conform more closely to how the child needs to learn, rather than labeling him or her as disordered. If these accommodations are successful, they can avoid labeling a child who may be struggling not because of a disability but because of a lack of literacy experience, transient emotional problems, or cultural differences.

The SLP may work with the classroom teacher to observe learning problems the teacher suspects may be language-related and collaborate with the teacher to support the student so that she or he is able to succeed with only modest modifications of the classroom environment rather than special educational designation. Let's take Nick, from Chapter 10, as an example. Perhaps instead of referring him for an evaluation, his teacher might suggest that the school's SST take a look at him. The SLP might observe him in the classroom and note when he is having difficulty. She might do some dynamic assessment within the classroom setting and talk to the teacher about her findings. Perhaps there is another child in the class who is already on an IEP. The SLP might work collaboratively with the teacher on some study skills or metacognitive lessons in the classroom, pair Nick with the student on an IEP, and give them some

extra support as the teacher works with the rest of the class. They might decide Nick would benefit from some of the same supports the other student receives, such as simplified reading assignments, a peer to make sure they "get" classroom directions before beginning assignments, extra help from parents on spelling at home, a chance to listen to classroom novels on tape in addition to trying to read them independently. These accommodations could be instituted, without further assessment or the development of an IEP, and Nick's progress could be monitored. If these seem to help, and he is able to function in the classroom with them, a full assessment can be deferred, and reconsidered at a later time if problems arise.

USING STANDARDIZED TESTS IN THE L4L STAGE

Suppose we are very successful in our efforts to get teachers to refer students with LLD for oral language evaluation. What should we do with the students once we get them? As we've seen, many students who have trouble with academic work have at least marginally adequate oral language, particularly in the areas usually measured on standardized tests, such as syntax, morphology, and vocabulary. For this reason, informal, criterion-referenced procedures make up a large part of the assessment used to establish baseline function and set intervention goals for students with LLD. Are standardized tests necessary for these students?

School clinicians will probably find that some standardized testing is needed in the L4L stage. The reason can be summed up in one word: *eligibility*. Many states require that a student perform below a designated level on some standardized measure to qualify for special educational services, including the services of the SLP. States have differing criteria for eligibility for various kinds of speech-language services, but most include a requirement for some standardized testing. Moore-Brown and Montgomery (2001), for example, give examples of the variety of eligibility criteria used in various states within the United States. These include levels of performance on standardized tests, severity ratings, and general indicators of delay. At least one-third of the states reviewed require some form of standardized testing to establish eligibility. When a student has been referred by a teacher or identified as having language deficits as a result of a screening, a first step is often to establish the student's eligibility for services by means of standardized testing. Table 11-2 provides a sample of standardized tests developed for students in the L4L period.

If a pragmatically oriented checklist has been used as a referral tool, the clinician may not have much sense of what the student's performance in language form and content might be. To begin to get such a sense, a short conversational interaction, such as the one we talked about for assessing intelligibility for children with developing language in Chapter 8, can be used. By talking to the student informally for a brief time (say 5 minutes), an SLP can break the ice and give both participants a chance to get to know each other a little. The SLP also can get a feel for what the child's linguistic abilities and disabilities might be. This brief conversational sample can help point us toward the assessment instruments that will help establish the student's eligibility for services.

Screening for Language-Based Reading Disabilities Checklist

Child's name: _____ Birthday: _____

Date completed: _____ Age: _____

This checklist is designed to identify children who are at risk for language-based reading disabilities. It is intended for use with children at the end of kindergarten or beginning of first grade. Each of the descriptors that characterize the child's behavior/history should be checked. A child receiving a substantial number of checks should be consider at-risk for language disability.

Speech sound awareness

_____ Does not understand and enjoy rhymes

_____ Does not easily recognize that words may begin with the same sound

_____ Has difficulty counting the syllables in spoken words

_____ Has problems clapping hands or tapping feet in rhythm with songs and/or rhymes

_____ Demonstrates problems learning sound-letter correspondences

Written language awareness

_____ Does not orient book properly during book-looking

_____ Cannot identify words and letters in a picture book

Letter name knowledge

_____ Cannot recite the alphabet

_____ Cannot identify printed letters when named by teacher ("Where is the A?")

_____ Cannot name letters when asked

Word retrieval

_____ Has difficulty retrieving a specific word (e.g., calls a sheep a "goat" or says "you know, a woolly animal")

_____ Shows poor memory for classmates' names

FIGURE 11-3 ✦ Screening for language-based reading disabilities in kindergarten and first grade: A checklist. (Based on Catts, H. [1997]. The early identification of language-based reading disabilities. *Language, Speech, and Hearing Services in Schools, 28,* 88-89; and Justice, L., Invernizzi, M., & Meier, J. [2002]. Designing and implementing an early literacy screening protocol: Suggestions for the speech-language pathologist. *Language, Speech and Hearing Services in Schools, 33,* 84-101.)

_____ Speech is hesitant, filled with pauses or vocalizations (e.g., "um," "you know")

_____ Frequently uses words lacking specificity (e.g., "stuff," "thing," " what you call it")

Speech production/perception

_____ Has problems saying common words with difficult sound patterns (e.g., *animal, cinnamon, specific*)

_____ Mishears and subsequently mispronounces words or names

_____ Combines sound patterns of similar words (e.g., saying "escavator" for escalator)

_____ Shows frequent slips of the tongue (e.g., saying "brue blush" for blue brush)

Comprehension

_____ Only responds to part of a multiple-element request or instruction

_____ Requests multiple repetitions of instructions/directions with little improvement in comprehension

_____ Fails to understand age-appropriate stories

_____ Lacks understanding of spatial terms, such as left-right, front-back

Expressive language

_____ Talks in short sentences

_____ Makes errors in grammar (e.g., "he goed to the store," "me want that")

_____ Lacks variety in vocabulary (e.g., "uses "good" to mean happy, kind, polite)

_____ Has difficulty giving directions or explanations (e.g., may show multiple revisions or dead ends)

_____ Relates stories or events in a disorganized or incomplete manner

_____ May have much to say, but provides little specific detail

Literacy motivation

_____ Does not enjoy classroom story-time; wanders, fails to pay attention to stories read by teacher

_____ Shows little or no engagement in classroom literacy activities, such as writing, book-looking.

FIGURE 11-3 ✦—cont'd

If the clinician hears articulation errors, syntactic and morphological mistakes, or evidence of word-finding or vocabulary problems in the conversation, then tests that tap these areas can be used to establish eligibility. It may be, though, that the student's language form and content appear adequate to the "naked ear" or that the problems heard are not specific to one area but seem to involve a more generalized restriction of speech, conceptual content, organization, or pragmatic appropriateness. If this is the case, we will want to use a more broad-based approach to evaluation. Three types of standardized tests can be used to affect this approach: comprehensive language batteries, tests of pragmatics, and tests of learning-related language skills.

Comprehensive batteries are commonly used in the assessment of students with LLD. Most states allow children to qualify for services if they score below a certain level on some subtests of a standardized battery or if they score below criterion on one subtest of a similar area on two standardized batteries. California regulations provide this option, for example. So batteries that look at a broad spectrum of abilities will be most useful in identifying students, like many of our clients with LLD, who perform adequately in some aspects of language but have difficulty in a few areas that are interfering with their achievement in school. Some examples of test batteries that can be used in this way include *Clinical Evaluation of Language Fundamentals—4* (Semel, Wiig, & Secord, 2003; which also contains a checklist for assessing pragmatics), *Test of Language Development—3—Primary and Intermediate* (Newcomer & Hammill, 1997), and the *Utah Test of Language Development—4* (Mecham, 2003). These batteries can sample a range of oral language abilities, in the hope of identifying specific areas in which students are having problems that will qualify them for services, as well as pointing out areas of strength.

As we saw in Chapter 10, students with LLD commonly have pragmatic deficits, and some have their primary deficits in this area. Standardized tests of pragmatics, then, can be useful for establishing eligibility. As we discussed earlier, using a standardized test to assess pragmatic function is something like using a sound-level meter to assess the quality of a symphony. Since pragmatic function is the ability to use language appropriately in real conversation, its assessment in a formal setting is bound to be somewhat limited and artificial. Tests of pragmatics may not be a necessary part of the assessment battery for children at earlier language levels, who will have plenty of deficits in form and content. Still, these tests can be useful for documenting deficits at the L4L stage, when children have outgrown some of the more obvious form and content problems.

Standardized tests of pragmatics in students with LLD most likely will be used to establish eligibility for services. Some students with LLD will not score low enough on tests of language form and content to qualify for communication intervention. Using a test of pragmatics with these clients may provide information that substantiates our informal assessment of their deficits in pragmatic areas. In other words, we can use standardized tests of pragmatics for the basic purpose for which all standardized tests were designed: to show that a child is different from other children. A few examples of standardized tests in this area include the *Test of Pragmatic Language* (Phelps-Terasaki & Phelps-Gunn, 1992), the *Communication Abilities Diagnostic Test* (Johnston & Johnston, 1990), and *Test of Language Competence Expanded Edition* (Wiig & Secord, 1989). Recently, Young, Diehl, Morris, Hyman, and Bennetto (2005) showed that *Test of Pragmatic Language* was helpful in identifying pragmatic deficits in students with autism spectrum disorder.

The *Children's Communication Checklist* (Bishop & Baird, 2001) has also been shown to be useful for this purpose.

A third type of standardized test also can help assess students that the clinician believes need help with oral language foundations for the classroom. These tests look specifically at learning-related language skills. Some examples of these kinds of tests are the *Comprehensive Test of Phonological Processing* (Wagner, Torgenson, & Rashotte, 1999), the *Language Processing Test-Revised* (Richard & Hanner, 1985), the *Test of Awareness of Language Segments* (Sawyer, 1987), the *Test of Early Written Language—2* (Herron, Hresko, & Peak, 1996), the *Test of Relational Concepts-Revised* (Edmonston & Thane, 1999), the *Test of Word Finding in Discourse* (German, 1991), and the *Word Test—2—Revised* (Huisingh, Bowers, LoGuidice, & Orman, 2004). These tests specifically tap the language skills that are likely to be less developed in students with LLD. Tests such as these are likely to show that a student with LLD is significantly different from peers in areas of language skills that influence academic performance and can be used to help establish eligibility for services.

CRITERION-REFERENCED ASSESSMENT AND BEHAVIORAL OBSERVATION IN THE L4L STAGE

Once we have established a student's eligibility for services by means of a standardized test, we can go on to the other purposes of assessment: establishing baseline function and identifying targets for intervention. Let's look at the methods available for doing this in the various areas of oral language that we need to evaluate at the L4L stage.

PHONOLOGY

Most students with LLD who function at the L4L stage do not make a large number of phonological errors. Some distort a few sounds or retain one or two phonological simplification processes. When this is the case, procedures discussed for the developing language stage can be used to assess these problems. If obvious phonological errors are not evident, though, we may want to know how phonologically "robust" the child's system is. As we've discussed, researchers such as Catts (1986), Dollaghan and Campbell (1998), and Harris-Schmidt and Noell (1983) have shown that children with LLD often have trouble with phonologically demanding tasks, such as producing complex, unfamiliar words and phrases, even when their conversational speech is not full of errors. Such vulnerability may indicate problems with phonological awareness as well, as Webster and Plante (1992) suggested. Phonological awareness, as we've seen, is important for literacy acquisition. So part of the oral language assessment of a child with or at risk for LLD, particularly a child in the primary grades or one who is reading on a primary-grade level, should include some index of these higher-level phonological skills that serve as the foundation for learning to read.

There are several ways to approach this assessment. The first is to look at production skills in phonologically demanding contexts. Catts (1986) developed a series of words and phrases to be used to look at phonological production in complex tasks. These can be used with children in the second grade or older and can give an impression of the child's ability to deal with complex production demands. A short version of Catts's (1986) task is presented in Box 11-1. Any student who has significant difficulty pronouncing these words and phrases can be considered at risk for higher-level phonological deficits that can affect literacy acquisition. Since the Catts procedure is not a standardized test, there is no hard-and-fast failing score. However, a student who makes errors on more than 20% of the items and seems to struggle with the task can be seen as having higher-level phonological problems. Hodson's (1986) Multisyllabic Screening Protocol section of the *Assessment of Phonological Processes—Revised* and Dollaghan and Campbell's (1998) nonword repetition task, in which children are asked to repeat phonologically unfamiliar nonsense sequences, also can be used to measure this aspect of phonological skill. The stimuli for Dollaghan and Campbell's task are given in Box 11-2. Their research showed that children with language impairments scored significantly lower on the total percentage of phonemes correct (PCC) than did normally achieving peers on this task. This research suggests that children who score less than 75% PCC on this task can be considered at risk for LLD. Many standardized tests of phonological awareness also contain subtests that use nonword repetition tasks and provide standardized scores. The *Comprehensive Test of Phonological Processing* (Wagner, Torgeson, & Rashotte, 2000) and the *Children's Test of Nonword Repetition* (Gathercole

---

| **BOX 11-1** | **Complex Phonological Production Task** |

Naming Task

Have student name pictures of the following:
alligators
stethoscope
helicopter
submarine
kangaroo
buffalo
rhinoceros
vegetables
octopus
dinosaur
asparagus
hippopotamus
ornaments
broccoli
domino
gorilla
volcanos

| **BOX 11-1** | **Complex Phonological Production Task—cont'd** |

valentine
ambulances
aquarium

Word Repetition Task

Say each word, and have the student repeat it.
peculiar
Colorado
orchestra
animal
catalog
permanent
navigator
aluminum
cinnamon
symphony
specific
governor
pistachio
especially
probably
calendar
syllable
enemy
fudgesickle
pneumonia

Phrase Repetition Task

Say each phrase, and have the student repeat it.
Fly free in the Air Force.
A box of mixed biscuits.
Six slim sailors.
Have some fried flounder.
Shiny seashell necklace.
Big black bugs' blood.
Wash each dish twice.
He likes split pea soup.
He skied down the snow slope.
Tom threw Tim three thumbtacks.

Adapted from Catts, H. (1986). Speech production/phonological deficits in reading-disordered children. *Journal of Learning Disabilities, 19,* 504-508.

& Baddeley, 1996) are two examples. Table 11-3 presents a list of standardized tests of phonological awareness, indicating which contain nonword repetition subtests.

A second way to look at higher-level phonological skills in students with LLD is to examine phonological awareness directly. There are a variety of tests of phonological awareness currently

BOX 11-2	**Phonetic Transcriptions of Dollaghan and Campbell's (1998) Nonwords***

One Syllable	Two Syllable	Three Syllable	Four Syllable
/naɪb/	/teɪvak/	/tʃinɔɪtaʊb/	/veɪtatʃaɪdɪp/
/voʊp/	/tʃoʊvæg/	/naɪtʃoʊveɪp/	/dævoʊnɔɪtʃig/
/taʊʤ/	/vætʃaɪp/	/dɔɪtaʊvæb/	/naɪtʃɔɪtaʊvub/
/dɔɪf/	/nɔɪtaʊf/	/teɪvɔɪtʃaɪt/	/tævatʃinaɪg/

*These words were constructed to minimize familiarity and predictability in order to maximize differentiation between children with typical and impaired language at 6 to 10 years of age.

Reprinted with permission from Dollaghan, C., & Campbell, T. (1998). Nonword repetition and child language impairment. *Journal of Speech, Language, and Hearing Research, 41*, 1138.

on the market. Table 11-3 profiles some of these. The pitfall in using these tests, is that they can take a good deal of time to deliver a small amount of information; i.e., whether or not the child is at risk for literacy difficulty, that might be inferred as easily from a shorter assessment or more curriculum-based assessment.

A third approach to assessing higher-level phonological impairments was suggested by Swank (1994) and Catts, Fey, Zhang, and Tomblin (2002), who advocate assessment of *rapid automatized naming* (RAN). Bowers and Grieg (2003) and Wolf, O'Rourke, Gidney, Lovett, Cirino, and Morris, (2002) have reviewed evidence showing that RAN is also highly correlated with reading ability. In RAN tasks, students are asked to name common objects presented in a series as rapidly as they can. Children also can be asked to produce overlearned series such as days of the week or months of the year. Performance on tasks such as these has been shown to discriminate between good and poor readers. Some standardized tests, such as the *Clinical Evaluation of Language Fundamentals—4* (Semel, Wiig, & Secord, 2003), contain subtests that tap this ability.

Despite the importance of identifying risk for reading failure, and the known strong associations among nonword repetition, RAN, phonological awareness, and reading, the main goal of this assessment must always be kept in mind. That goal is to identify children in early primary grades who are *at risk* for reading failure and to provide early, preventive intervention to give them an opportunity to avert this failure. For older students already known to have reading deficits, phonological assessment is less important, and evaluation of other areas of oral language needed to support reading should be our focus. And even for younger children, shorter, informal methods of identifying risk, such as the checklists like the one in Figure 11-3 or suggested by Boudreau (2006), or simply working with kindergarten and first grade teachers to quickly identify children who are having trouble with standard classroom phonological awareness activities, as Justice and Kaderavek (2004a) have suggested, may be just as effective. And when we think about intervening for these problems, Catts (1999a) has reminded us that the aim of these interventions is to teach children to read and spell,

not to develop phonological awareness as a "splinter skill." Once basic phoneme segmentation, sound blending, and letter-sound correspondence has been mastered, we should move on to building other aspects of oral language skill to support reading development, rather than continuing to teach more and more advanced phonological awareness skills.

SEMANTICS

Receptive Vocabulary

Most general language batteries have a receptive vocabulary section, usually using a picture-pointing format. If the student scores below the normal range, a problem with receptive vocabulary can be identified. Further evaluation to probe for specific receptive vocabulary items to be targeted in the intervention program should focus on the words the student needs to succeed in the classroom. There are two ways we can accomplish this classroom-based vocabulary assessment.

Instructional Vocabulary. One way is for the clinician to observe in the student's class and note the kinds of spatial, temporal, logical, and directive vocabulary the teacher uses. These can form the basis for a criterion-referenced vocabulary assessment, in which the student is asked to follow directions containing these words, one target word per direction. For example, suppose the teacher typically tells the students, "Write your name in the upper right-hand corner of the paper, write the date below your name, and number your paper to 20 down the left side." The clinician might assess the student's understanding of the vocabulary in these directions by isolating each potential problem word and testing its comprehension in a game-like format, such as the one in Box 11-3. Any words the student has trouble comprehending that are common in the teacher's instructional language could be targeted as part of the intervention program. Alternatively, the teacher could be made aware of the student's difficulty, and consultation suggestions could be made to encourage the use of visual cues along with instructions, additional time for the student to process the instruction, and paraphrasing the instruction to give the student an extra chance to understand it.

TABLE 11-3 **Tests of Phonological Awareness**

TESTS	RAPID NAMING	WORD DISCRIMINATION	RHYMING	SEGMENTATION	ISOLATION	DELETION	SUBSTITUTION	BLENDING	GRAPHEMES	NON-WORD REPETITION
Children's Test of Nonword Repetition										X
Comprehensive Test of Phonological Processing (CTOPP) Tests of phonological awareness, memory, and rapid naming.	X			X		X		X		X
Goldman-Fristoe-Woodcock Auditory Skills Test Battery (GFW) Listening to taped words and pointing to a matching picture, repeating specified sounds in taped words, reading and spelling nonsense words, other auditory tasks.		X			X			X	X	X
Lindamood Auditory Conceptualization Test (LAC) Using colored blocks to represent differences or changes in sequences of speech-sounds.							X			

TABLE 11-3	Tests of Phonological Awareness—cont'd									
TESTS	RAPID NAMING	WORD DISCRIMINATION	RHYMING	SEGMENTATION	ISOLATION	DELETION	SUBSTITUTION	BLENDING	GRAPHEMES	NON-WORD REPETITION
NEPSY A developmental neuropsychological assessment	X									X
Phonological Abilities Test (PAT) by Muter, Hulme, & Snowling			X			X			X	
Rosner Test of Auditory Analysis Skills (TAAS) Say "cowboy" without the "cow." Say "picnic" without the "pic." Say "cart" without the "/t/." Say "blend" without the "/bl/."						X				
Roswell-Chall Auditory Blending Test Blending sequences of sounds spoken by the examiner.								X		
Test of Auditory-Perceptual Skills–Revised (TAPS-R): Auditory Word Discrimination Subtest Identifying whether two words spoken by examiner are SAME or DIFFERENT		X								

TABLE 11-3 **Tests of Phonological Awareness—cont'd**

TESTS	RAPID NAMING	WORD DISCRIMINATION	RHYMING	SEGMENTATION	ISOLATION	DELETION	SUBSTITUTION	BLENDING	GRAPHEMES	NON-WORD REPETITION
Test of Phonological Awareness (TOPA) Marking pictures of orally presented words that are distinguished by the same or different sound in the word-final position.					X					
The Phonological Awareness Test (TPAT) by Robertson & Salter			X	X	X	X	X	X	X	
Woodcock-Johnson III (WJ III) Incomplete Words, Sound Blending, Auditory Attention, Auditory Working Memory, Rapid Picture Naming, Word Attack, Spelling of Sounds, Sound Awareness.	X	X	X	X	X	X	X	X	X	

BOX 11-3 **Criterion-Referenced Assessment of Classroom Direction Vocabulary**

Clinician: Let's pretend you're a soldier. You're a good soldier. You always do what the sergeant says. Here's some paperwork the sergeant wants you to take care of. I'll be the sergeant and give some orders. You follow the sergeant's orders and write what the sergeant says to write on this paper. Listen carefully, now! Here we go!

1. OK, Private, draw a star in an *upper corner* of the paper.
2. Now, Private, draw a tank on the *right-hand side* of the paper.
3. Write today's *date*, Private.
4. Number your paper from 1 to 10.
5. Alright, Private, draw a line down the *left side* of the paper.
6. Now put a square in the *upper left-hand corner*.

Textbook Vocabulary. A second source of potentially problematic vocabulary is the student's classroom texts. If a student has receptive vocabulary deficits identified in the standardized portion of the assessment, we can probe for words in the texts that might be causing problems. We could then focus on expanding the understanding of these words as part of the intervention program.

There are a variety of ways to obtain lists of words from classroom texts to use as vocabulary probes. Many textbooks have glossaries at the end of each chapter or of the book that list words that would be new to most of the book's readers. These can be one source of words to probe for comprehension. Teachers sometimes base spelling lists or other classroom vocabulary work on words drawn from the texts used in class. These lists can be obtained from the teacher and used as the basis for the vocabulary assessment. The clinician also can review the student's homework with an eye toward seeing which words seem to be poorly understood.

We should remember when working with students with LLD that it is not only the technical, content vocabulary of the texts that might cause these students difficulty. More common spatial terms (*above, north*); temporal terms (*after, following*); and connectives (*however, consequently*) also may cause problems. We may want to read through some of the student's textbooks with an eye for terms such as these and generate our own list to be used as probes for vocabulary assessment.

Once we have found a list of words in the texts to probe, we need to decide how to assess whether the student understands them. Providing a definition is a metalinguistic skill that many students with LLD cannot do very well, even when they do know

generally what a word means. We could just ask the student whether he or she knows a particular word, but comprehension monitoring deficits may cause problems here. For some nouns, we may be able to ask the student to identify pictures referring to the words in question in the textbook. Words such as *planet, solar system*, etc., could be assessed this way. So could geographical terms such as *mountain, plateau*, and *piedmont*, which are used in maps or diagrams in social studies texts.

Many of the words we'll want to assess are not easily depicted, though. In such cases, we could try to get the student to act out or indicate the meaning of the word in some nonverbal way. We might, for example, ask the student to "Show me orbit" with two tennis balls or to "Show me division" with some raisins. For more general assessment, language batteries that include subtests of words that are often difficult for students with LLD can be used. The *Clinical Evaluation of Language Fundamentals—4* (Semel, Wiig, & Secord, 2003) and the *Detroit Tests of Learning Aptitude–Fourth Edition* (Hammill, 1998) are two examples. When students score below the normal range on these subtests, an item analysis can be done as an informal assessment of the specific vocabulary items that are hard for the student to understand. For some of the spatial, temporal, and connective words we are concerned about, we can ask the student to act out several versions of the same sentence that differ only by words in the category being tested. Examples of such sentences for informal assessment are given in Box 11-4.

Expressive Vocabulary

We talked in Chapter 8 about the relations between receptive and expressive vocabulary. We know receptive vocabulary is larger than expressive vocabulary in people of all ages. Fast mapping, though, can allow children to know just enough about a word to use it without understanding its fully elaborated meaning. Children may be using words that they only understand partially, and they may understand lots of words that they have very little occasion to use. The relationship between expressive and receptive vocabulary is likely to be complicated, so we may want to examine each one somewhat independently. In looking at expressive vocabulary skills, we would like to examine two basic components: lexical diversity and word retrieval.

Lexical Diversity. The ability to use a flexible, precise vocabulary contributes a great deal to the efficiency of our communication. The Type-Token Ratio (TTR; Templin, 1957) is a measure that has been used traditionally to assess lexical diversity. It involves counting the total number of words (tokens) in a 50-utterance speech sample and dividing this number into the number of different words (types) in the sample. Owen and Leonard (2002) showed that children with SLI did not generally differ from same-age peers on this measure. Watkins, Kelly, Harbers, and Hollis (1995) compared the ability of the TTR as opposed to the Number of Different Words (NDW) and Number of Total Words (NTW) in a speech sample to differentiate children with normal and impaired language development. They found that in speech samples of various sizes, the NDW and NTW measures were more sensitive esti-

BOX 11-4

BOX 11-4 | Informal Assessment of Spatial, Temporal, and Connective Terms

Spatial Terms

Materials: a paper with a sticker stuck in the middle, a pencil, a sheet with the directions written on it for the clinician to score as the student makes the dots.

Make dots *above* the sticker.
Make dots *below* the sticker.
Make dots *around* the sticker.
Make dots to the *right* of the sticker.
Make dots *beside* the sticker.
Make dots on the *left-hand side* of the sticker.

Temporal Terms

Materials: a whistle, bell, or other noisemaker; a sheet with the directions written on it for the clinician to score as the student uses the noisemaker.

Make a noise *after* I say "Go." (Clinician says "Go" after a pause.)
Make a noise *before* I say "Go." (Clinician says "Go" after a pause.)
Make a noise *while* I say "Go." (Clinician says "Go.")
Make a noise *as* I say "Go." (Clinician says "Go.")
Make a noise *when* I say "Go." (Clinician says "Go.")

Connective Terms

Materials: a whistle, bell, or other noisemaker; a sheet with the directions written on it for the clinician to score as the student uses the noisemaker.

Make a noise *if* I say "Go." (Clinician says "Go.")
Make a noise *although* I say "Go." (Clinician says "Go.")
Make a noise *unless* I say "Go." (Clinician says "Go.")
Make a noise *until* I say "Go." (Clinician says "Go" after a pause.)

mates of children's lexical diversity than the TTR. Klee (1992) also reported that NDW and NTW showed both developmental and diagnostic characteristics (that is, both increased significantly with age and both differentiated children with normal and impaired language). NDW and NTW produced in a conversational speech sample may, then, be the best means we have available to evaluate children's lexical diversity. These measures can be calculated automatically by computer-assisted speech sample analyses programs such as the *Systematic Analysis of Language Transcripts (SALT)* (Miller & Chapman, 1993). Leadholm and Miller (1992) presented data on NDW and NTW in the 100-utterance conversational speech samples of 27 typical school children in the Madison, Wisconsin, Reference Data Base. These data are summarized in Table 11-4. If NDW and NTW measures are collected from conversational samples of clients' speech and the values computed fall below the normal ranges given in Table 11-4, a deficit in lexical diversity could be diagnosed. Intervention could focus on increasing expressive vocabulary by focusing on words necessary for success in the curriculum. Miller (2006) also discusses methods of investigating vocabulary diversity in narrative language samples.

Word Retrieval. Another aspect of expressive vocabulary that is important to assess in the L4L stage is word retrieval. Word-finding difficulties are very common in students with LLD, as we've discussed. One clue to the presence of a word-retrieval problem would be a much higher score on a receptive vocabulary test, such as the *Peabody Picture Vocabulary Test—4* (Dunn & Dunn, 2006), than on an expressive vocabulary test, such as the *Expressive Vocabulary Test* (Williams, 1997). Another would be a teacher report of word-finding problems on one of our referral checklists, like the one in Figure 11-1. We also might hear some word-finding problems in our short conversational interaction, with which we began the assessment session.

If we think word retrieval might be a problem, we generally want to establish the fact of the difficulty with a standardized test or a portion of a test that investigates word finding specifically. It is a good idea to document a word-retrieval problem by means of a score on a norm-referenced assessment, rather than making a subjective judgment. Several tests listed in Table

TABLE 11-4 | Normal Range of Number of Different Words and Number of Total Words in 100-Utterance Speech Samples of Children between 5–11 Years

	NDW		NTW	
AGE	1 SD–	1 SD+	1 SD–	1 SD+
5-year-olds	156	206	439	602
7-year-olds	173	212	457	622
9-year-olds	183	235	496	687
11-year-olds	191	267	518	868

Normal range = (±1 standard deviation from group mean).

NDW = number of different words; NTW = number of total words.

Adapted from Leadholm, B., & Miller, J. (1992). *Language sample analysis: The Wisconsin guide.* Madison, WI: Wisconsin Department of Public Instruction.

11-2, including the *Test of Word Finding in Discourse* (German, 1991), assess word-retrieval skill. Several others, including the *Clinical Evaluation of Language Fundamentals—4* (Semel, Wiig, & Secord, 2003), the *Test of Semantic Skills—Primary* (Bowers, LoGiudice, Orman, & Huisingh, 2002), and the *Language Processing Test—Revised* (Richard & Hanner, 1995), also have subtests that assess word finding, on which item analyses can be done for criterion-referenced assessment. If a word-finding deficit is identified, we want to try to teach some word-finding strategies as part of our intervention program and build up the student's overall vocabulary abilities—both receptive and expressive—to provide a stronger semantic network that can help ameliorate word-retrieval problems.

Other Semantic Skills

Brackenbury and Pye (2005) discuss the importance of looking beyond vocabulary when assessing semantic skills. Several other aspects of semantic development that can be considered for assessment are discussed below.

Quick Incidental Learning (Fast Mapping). The ability to acquire new words quickly, with limited meanings, from very abbreviated exposure, is one of the ways in which children's vocabularies are able to grow so rapidly. Often called Quick Incidental Learning, or QUIL, this capacity has been shown to be present, but less well developed in children with language disorders (Dollaghan, 1987; Eyer, Leonard, Bedore, McGregor, Anderson, & Viescas, 2002). Many studies of QUIL use nonsense words to determine a child's ability to learn a new word from naturalistic interactions, and this ability to learn new words is often considered a good way to assess a child's intrinsic language skill, especially in children who are not native speakers of English or who may have impoverished language experience (Branckenbury & Pye, 2005). One way to assess QUIL clinically is to use the Diagnostic Evaluation of Language Variation (DELV; Seymour, Roeper, & Devilliers, 2003), which contains a QUIL subtest.

Semantic Relations between Clauses. One of the major changes in children's language in the school years is an increase in the use of sentences that contain more than one proposition or main idea. We examine these kinds of expressions when we look at complex sentence development in our assessment of productive syntax. We also can look at how students attempt to convey semantic relations between propositions, even when they are not using syntactically correct forms to do so. A student who is trying to express a variety of semantic relations between propositions, even with primitive syntactic forms, is showing a readiness to learn complex syntax. A student who is not doing this may need to work on more basic sentence forms and to hear more language in which propositions are conjoined syntactically before making production of complex syntax a goal.

Suppose we do our complex sentence analysis of a speech sample (which we'll discuss in the next section) and find very little use of any syntactically complex forms. We can then look at the sample for evidence of presyntactic expression of semantic relations between propositions. In normal development, children first express these relations by merely juxtaposing two clauses ("Mommy here, Daddy gone"). Later they conjoin with nonspecific conjunctions, primarily *and*. Students with LLD may show this kind of immature attempt at relating ideas. The kinds of relations we would expect to see emerging (Lahey, 1988) include the following:

1. Temporal ("Eat dinner and go to sleep")
2. Causal ("Go to store and buy shoes")
3. Conditional ("Eat dinner, go outside")
4. Epistemic ("I think draw pink")
5. Notice-perception ("Show me how do a somersault")
6. Specification ("I have a dog and it's brown")
7. Adversative ("The girls sit here and the boys sit there")

If students do not use complex syntax, we can look for presyntactic expression of these semantic relations between propositions in the speech sample. When they are present, they suggest that we teach syntactically correct forms for expressing these same relations. If neither the complex syntax nor the presyntactic expression of semantic relations between clauses is found, we may want to spend time exposing the student to literate language styles that contain complex syntax and provide opportunities for the student to paraphrase the language heard in these sessions. Such exposure may help the student see how ideas are related in language.

SYNTAX AND MORPHOLOGY

A Strategy for Assessing Receptive Syntax and Morphology

We've talked before about the need to assess syntax and morphology in the receptive and expressive modalities. We discussed why this is important: the fact that children frequently produce sentence forms even when they fail to perform correctly on comprehension tests of these same forms in settings where nonlinguistic cues have been removed (Chapman, 1978; Miller & Paul, 1995). So knowing that a child produces a sentence type does not necessarily mean that the child will fully comprehend the same sentence if it is heard in a decontextualized format.

We've also talked about the importance of assessing comprehension strategies. Paul (2000b) discussed the fact that children with LLD are likely to persist much longer than normally speaking peers in using several types of these strategies, particularly when confronted with complex sentences. Some of the difficulties that students with LLD have in understanding complex language can be traced to this protracted reliance on information other than that contained in the syntax of the sentence. If students at this stage persist in using strategies, they need to be taught how to get beyond their dependence on these processing shortcuts and to extract the appropriate information from syntactic forms. Sentences particularly vulnerable to this type of misinterpretation by students with LLD include passives ("A student is seen by a teacher" misinterpreted as "student sees teacher"); sentences with relative clauses embedded in the center between the subject-noun phrase and the main verb ("The boy who hit the girl ran away" misinterpreted as "girl ran away"); and sentences that certain adverbial conjunctions

("Before you eat your dessert, turn off the TV" misinterpreted as "eat dessert then turn off TV").

We've also talked about the need to assess both contextualized and decontextualized formats when we look at comprehension skills. We look at the decontextualized formats to determine how much *linguistic* comprehension a child displays and as a way to identify linguistic forms that can cause problems when few other cues are available. We also can look at comprehension in contextualized situations to find out whether a child can take advantage of the nonlinguistic cues in the environment.

The general strategy for assessing syntactic and morphological comprehension we discussed in Chapter 8 will differ somewhat for children in the L4L period, because standardized tests may not identify all the comprehension deficits that can give students problems in the classroom. So I'll give you a version of the general strategy for assessing grammatical comprehension that can be used in the L4L stage:

1. Use a standardized test of receptive syntax and morphology to determine deficits in this area.

   ▶ If the client performs below the normal range, use criterion-referenced decontextualized procedures, such as judgment tasks, to probe forms that appear to be causing trouble on the standardized measure. Look for use of comprehension strategies in responses to these tasks.

   ▶ If the client scores within the normal range but teacher referral indicates problems in classroom comprehension, observe teacher language in the classroom and textbook language (as outlined in the vocabulary section earlier in the chapter). Identify syntactic structures that may be causing difficulty. Some likely candidates include complex sentences with adverbial conjunctions (*because, so, after, although, unless,* etc.); sentences with relative clauses; passive sentences; and other sentences with unusual word order, such as pseudoclefts ("The one who lost the wallet was Maria") (Wallach & Miller, 1988). Probe comprehension of these structures with criterion-referenced, decontextualized procedures, such as judgment tasks (see Miller & Paul, 1995, for suggestions). Again, look for operation of strategies.

2. If the client performs poorly on the decontextualized criterion-referenced assessments, test the same forms in a contextualized format, providing familiar scripts and nonlinguistic contexts; facial, gestural, and intonational cues; language closely tied to objects in the immediate environment; and expected instructions.

3. If the child does better in this contextualized format, uses typical strategies, or both, then compare performance on comprehension to production. Target forms and structures the child comprehends well but does not produce as initial targets for a production approach. Target structures the child does not comprehend well for focused stimulation or verbal script approaches to work on comprehension and production in tandem.

4. If the child does not do better in the contextualized format and does not use strategies, provide structured input with complexity controlled, using more hybrid and clinician-directed activities for both comprehension and production.

Criterion-Referenced Methods for Assessing Receptive Syntax and Morphology

Now that we've outlined the basic strategy for receptive language assessment in the L4L stage, let's look at some of the methods available for doing both decontextualized and contextualized assessment.

Decontextualized Methods. In Chapter 2, we talked about several basic means for evaluating comprehension in decontextualized settings. These included picture pointing, behavioral compliance, object manipulation, and judgment. We've talked already in Chapter 8 about ways of using some of these methods. These methods will continue to be appropriate for use with students with LLD. In the L4L period, we can add judgment tasks to our repertoire, since school-age children are developmentally ready to make judgments of grammaticality. Judgment tasks are very convenient for assessment, because they don't require picturing or acting out linguistic stimuli. We can simply present a set of sentences and ask the client to judge whether they are in some sense "OK." We can use judgment tasks in a variety of ways to assess several areas of language competence. For the moment, though, let's look at two ways that are well-suited to assessing syntactic comprehension: judgment of semantic acceptability and judgment of appropriate interpretation.

Judgment of Semantic Acceptability. This method involves presenting a series of sentences and having the student tell whether each is "OK" or "silly." Alternatively, we can tell the student that we have two people, one who always says normal things and the other who always says ridiculous things. The "OK" picture can be of an ordinary-looking chap, such as the one in Figure 11-4. The "silly" picture can be a clownlike, silly person, as in Figure 11-5. We can display the pictures and give examples of OK and silly things each might say. We can then ask the student to point to the picture of the character who would say each sentence. We can then test grammatical forms that require the student to understand a transformation or grammatical rule to decide whether a sentence is OK or silly. Passive sentences, for example, like those listed in Box 11-5, can be probed this way.

Judgment of Appropriate Interpretation. A second way to use judgment tasks to assess comprehension in the L4L stage is to offer students two interpretations of a sentence and ask them to judge which is correct or to offer one interpretation and ask students to judge whether it is correct. If we are assessing understanding of sentences with adverbial clauses, for example, we can say, "The boy brushed his teeth after he ate his sandwich." We can then mime the two actions in correct order (eat sandwich, brush teeth) and ask, "Did I do it right?" We can then present other similar sentences and offer both correct and incorrect interpretations for the student to judge. Table 11-5 presents an example of this type of assessment for center-embedded relative clause sentences.

Assessing Use of Comprehension Strategies. If students respond incorrectly to these decontextualized comprehension activities, we can look for the use of strategies in their responses.

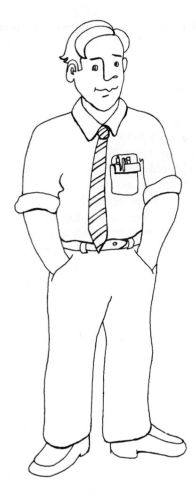

FIGURE 11-4 ✦ Norman Normal.

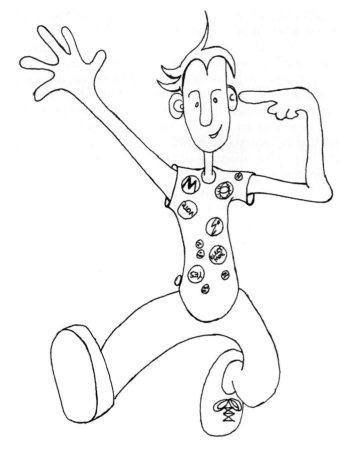

FIGURE 11-5 ✦ Chris Crazy.

The two types most likely to be used in the L4L period are *probable-event* or *probable-order-of-event strategies* and *word-order* or *order-of-mention strategies*. Evans and MacWhinney (1999) found evidence for the use of both these strategies in school-aged children with language impairments. Probable-event and probable-order-of-event strategies involve interpreting sentences to mean what we usually expect to happen. This strategy is similar to that used by preschoolers to interpret passive sentences. Preschoolers may correctly interpret "The dog was fed by the boy," for example. They can do this not because they understand passive sentences, but because they rely more on their knowledge of how things usually happen than on syntactic form.

Some students with LLD may continue to use this strategy for comprehending passives, even though normally developing children move beyond it by 4 or 5 years of age. Students with LLD also may misunderstand a sentence such as, "Before you wash your hair, dry your face" for the same reason. Ordinarily we would wash our hair before drying our face, but this sentence tells the listener to do something out of the ordinary. The student with LLD may mistakenly depend more on knowledge of the order in which things usually happen than on linguistic form. If a student seems to be having trouble with sentences with adverbial clauses, we can assess use of this strategy by giving several sentences for the student to mime that contain unusual orders of events. For passives, we can use the assessment in Box 11-5 and note whether the student does more poorly on the improbable-event sentences than the probable-event ones. If so, the probable-event strategy can be seen to operate.

The second kind of strategy we are likely to find in children with LLD is the word-order or order-of-mention strategy. Paul (1990) and Evans and MacWhinney (1999) reported that children with expressive language disorders are especially likely to use this strategy. Normally speaking children move beyond it by about age 7, but students with LLD may still use it into adolescence. We can see this strategy operating in assessments such as those in Table 11-5 and Box 11-5. Students with LLD may consistently misinterpret these sentences. For passives, they may interpret the first noun as the agent of the action, rather than the object, as the passive sentence form requires. "A hot dog is cooked by a girl," for example, will be understood as "hot dog cooks girl." For center-embedded relatives, the last noun-verb-noun sequence may be interpreted as the agent-action-object message of the sentence. So, for instance, "The cow that bit the goat was called Sadie" will be interpreted as "the goat was called Sadie."

If we find students with LLD persisting in using these strategies, we should address them in the intervention program. We

<table>
<tr><td>**BOX 11-5**</td><td>**A Judgment Task for Criterion-Referenced Assessment of Comprehension of Passive Sentences**</td></tr>
</table>

Here are pictures of two guys: Norman Normal and Chris Crazy. Norman Normal always says normal things like, "I like apples" and "He sees the rain." Chris Crazy always says silly things, like, "Apples like me" and "The rain sees him." I'm going to say some sentences. After each one, you tell me if you think it was said by Norman Normal or Chris Crazy. If it's a normal, OK sentence, you'll say Norman Normal said it. If it's silly, you'll say it was Chris Crazy that said it. Try this one.

A boy catches a ball.
A boy is carried by a flower.
A hot dog is cooked by a girl.
A bank is robbed by a man.
A girl is painted by a store.
An orange is picked by a boy.
A boy is lifted by a box.
A car is washed by a girl.
A cake is carried by a boy.
A cake is baked by a lady.
A car is started by a man.
A man is planted by a flower.
A ball is kicked by a girl.
A key is turned by a woman.
A man is climbed by a fence.
A ball is dropped by a woman.
A box is opened by a girl.
A man is cooked by an egg.

need to help the students get past these less mature heuristics for making sense of the language they hear. We want to provide ways for them to learn to attend to and derive meaning from the linguistic structures they encounter in the classroom and its reading materials. Techniques for providing this intervention will be given in the next chapter.

Assessing Comprehension in Contextualized Settings. We've talked about using nonstandardized assessment both to probe comprehension of specific forms and to look at strategies for comprehending difficult input. For both these purposes we are looking at comprehension in somewhat contrived situations. If we want to know more about how a child responds to language in a more naturalistic setting, we can set up some communicative situations and observe the child's responses. The reason for doing so, again, is as a contrast to the performance on the decontextualized situations. If a child does just fine on a standardized comprehension test or in decontextualized probes, there is no need to assess comprehension further in a naturalistic setting. But if the child is not so good at responding to language in formal contexts, it would be nice to know whether performance is better in more natural situations.

We know that many of our students with LLD have trouble with comprehension in one more-or-less natural setting: the classroom. Many of them will have found their way to us because of this trouble. We can observe the child in other, less-demanding communicative situations, though. We might ask the child to work with a peer and some materials. We might have the peer give instructions on how to play a board game we provide or complete a craft project with materials we supply. We can observe to determine how well the client comprehends messages in this setting. This kind of interaction can be a rich source of data on several other aspects of the client's communicative skills, including comprehension monitoring, requests for clarification, and use of other pragmatic skills. We can use the assessment of contextualized comprehension to look for errors or difficulties in understanding spoken language. We can note how frequently they occur and in response to what kinds

<table>
<tr><td>**TABLE 11-5**</td><td>**Example of a Judgment of Appropriate Interpretation Activity for Decontextualized, Criterion-Referenced Assessment of Center-Embedded Relative Clauses**</td></tr>
</table>

Present each sentence, and ask student to answer each question.

STIMULUS SENTENCE	QUESTION	CORRECT ANSWER
The boy who chased the cow was wearing a hat.	Was the cow wearing a hat?	No
The girl who rode the pony was named Sally.	Was the pony named Sally?	No
The crook who ran from the police officer was carrying a bag.	Was the crook carrying a bag?	Yes
The woman who lost her dog was wearing a sweater.	Was the dog wearing a sweater?	No
The cat that chased the dog was brown.	Was the dog brown?	No
The cow that bit the goat was called Sadie.	Was the cow called Sadie?	Yes

of linguistic input. These data can be used for comparison with the other comprehension information we've gathered, as the strategy we outlined earlier suggests.

Expressive Syntax

Deficits in productive syntax and morphology can be identified by means of standardized testing, just as they can in the developing language period. When they are, we need to remember that standardized tests are not ecologically valid assessments. Although they reliably tell when children are different from other children, they do not necessarily tell us what kinds of errors children make in spontaneous speech. For this reason, when a problem in expressive syntax has been documented by a standardized test, we want to obtain and analyze a sample of spontaneous speech.

We also may want to look at a sample of spontaneous speech even if the child does not score below the normal range on a standardized test of expressive syntax. The reason is that many of our students with LLD will not make gross errors in syntax and morphology, but their speech may be simpler and less elaborated than that of their peers. Alternatively, it may be more rambling and disorganized. Either type of deficit can cause problems by providing an insufficient base both for the understanding of literate language and for age-appropriate writing skills. For this reason, assessment of expressive syntax

in the speech of students with LLD may be part of the assessment even when the child does not score below the normal range on a test of syntax and morphology.

Collecting a Spontaneous Speech Sample. Evans and Craig (1992) showed that an interview format is a valid, reliable speech-sampling context for students with LLD. It requires no props, and in Evans and Craig's study it elicited more advanced language behaviors than did free-play interactions with toys for the 7- to 12-year age group. Evans and Craig suggested using an interview protocol following the format given in Box 11-6 to obtain a conversational sample from children with LLD. Nelson (1998) suggested supplementing the interview with "leading questions" designed to elicit an animated, emotional response. Examples of these kinds of questions have been added to the protocol in Box 11-6. Hadley (1998) also presented some alternative protocols for eliciting interview samples from school-age children.

Narrative samples are another way to gather information about a student's expressive abilities. Wagner, Nettelbladt, Sahlen, and Nilholm (2000) reported that narrative samples elicited more expanded phrases and grammatical morphemes than conversational samples in young children. Southwood and Russell (2004) found that free-play speech samples elicited more talk but less complex language than conversation or narrative, while narratives elicited the longest utterances. These studies suggest

---

| **BOX 11-6** | **Interview Protocol for Eliciting a Conversational Sample from Students with LLD** |

Introduction

"Let's talk a little."

Question 1 (5 minutes)

"What can you tell me about your family?"
  (Adult responds to the student with rephrasing of the student's comments or "Really! Tell me more about that.")
  Leading question (to be asked after the student has talked about question 1 for a few minutes):
  "Do you have any brothers and sisters? Do they ever bother your stuff?"

Question 2 (5 minutes)

"Are you in school? Tell me about it."
  (Adult responds same as above.)
  Leading question (to be asked after the student has talked about question 2 for a few minutes):
  "Did your teacher ever do anything that really bugged you?"

Question 3 (5 minutes)

"What do you do when you're not in school?"
  (Adult responds same as above.)
  Leading questions (to be asked after the student has talked about question 3 for a few minutes):
  "Did you ever get into an argument with a friend?"
  "Do you have a favorite sports team? Tell me about your favorite player."

Adapted from Evans, J., & Craig, H. (1992). Language sample collection and analysis: Interview compared to free play assessment contexts. *Journal of Speech and Hearing Research, 35,* 343-353; leading questions based on Nelson, N. (1998). *Childhood language disorders in context: Infancy through adolescence.* Columbus, OH: Merrill.

that in order to see the more complex end of the student's language abilities, conversation and narrative are appropriate contexts for eliciting language samples from school-aged students.

Transcribing the Speech Sample. We can use many of the transcription conventions that we discussed for the developing language period when recording a speech sample from a child in the L4L stage. One change we want to make, though, is in the way we segment our sample into utterances. In the developing language phase, we followed Lund and Duchan's (1993) guidelines. However, Reed, MacMillan, and McLeod (2001) examined the effects of varying rules for utterance segmentation from language samples of school-aged children and found that the type of segmentation used on a speech sample did lead to differences in findings, so choosing a segmentation method is important, particularly if we are following children's language growth over time. For students in the L4L stage, we may want to use a somewhat different approach to avoid skewing the mean length of utterance (MLU) or other analyses by long, run-on sentences strung together with *and*. To get around this problem, we can use the T-unit segmentation method developed by Hunt (1965). A *T-unit* is one main clause with all the subordinate clauses and nonclausal phrases attached to or embedded in it. All coordinated clauses are separated into separate T-units, unless they contain a co-referential subject deletion in the second clause ("He goes and loses it"). Clauses that begin with coordinating conjunctions *and*, *but*, or *or* would be considered to make up a new T-unit.

Suppose a client produced the following response to leading question No. 1 in Box 11-6:

> Yeah, my little brother, he's a real pain in the neck and he's always taking my stuff and he never asks first and then he goes and loses it or breaks it and so my mom yells at me when I slug him for it, but sometimes he's not so bad.

Here's how we'd segment this utterance into T-units:

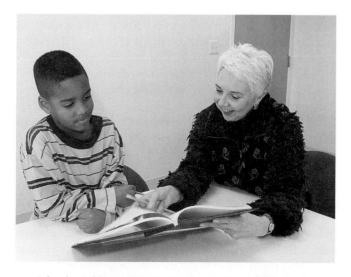

School-aged language samples can involve retelling stories from classroom literature selections.

T1: Yeah, my little brother, he's a real pain in the neck.
T2: (and) he's always taking my stuff.
T3: (and) he never asks first.
T4: (and) then he goes and loses it or breaks it [co-referential subjects deleted from second and third clauses].
T5: (and so) my mom yells at me when I slug him.
T6: (but) sometimes he's not so bad.

Using T-unit segmentation provides a more realistic picture of syntactic units in the L4L phase than does the method we would use for children in the developing language period.

Analyzing the Speech Sample

Analyzing Average T-Unit Length. We can look at MLU per T-unit in children with LLD, just as we looked at MLU per utterance for children with developing language, by counting the number of morphemes in the sample and dividing by the number of T-units. Again, it may not be necessary to compute MLU for every sample we examine. We may decide that MLU is going to be a useful measure, though, perhaps as a way to track progress over a course of intervention. When this is the case, using MLU per T-unit rather than per sentence will provide a more valid assessment of utterance length. Scott (1988) and Nippold (1998) showed that MLU per T-unit increases throughout the school years, but the changes are slow. In spoken language, MLU per T-unit increases from about 7.6 in third grade to about 8.8 in fifth. More changes in MLU per T-unit are seen in writing than in speech during this age range. We should not, then, expect to see dramatic changes, even as a result of intervention, in MLU per T-unit in the spoken language of children in the L4L stage.

A question that arises for samples from school-aged children concerns the unit of analysis for MLU: morpheme or word? Gutierrez-Clennen, Restrepo, Bedore, Pena, and Anderson (2000) report that MLU in words (MLU-w or sometimes called Mean Length of Response, MLR) is highly related to morphosyntactic production in both English and Spanish-speaking children. Moreover, MLU-w has been used in previous research on changes in sentence length during the school years (Hunt, 1965). For this reason, MLU is usually calculated for words rather than morphemes in children in the L4L stage.

Analyzing Syntactic Forms. When looking at conversational speech in students with LLD, we probably do *not* need to look at the broad range of structures that we examine in the developing language phase. If a student's MLU is less than 4.5 or if we hear omissions of grammatical morphemes, verb markers and auxiliaries, pronoun errors, or problems with negative or interrogative sentences, we can do the same kinds of speech-sample analyses we discussed in Chapter 8. But for many students with LLD, MLU is beyond Brown's stage V, basic sentence structures have been acquired, and obvious errors occur only rarely. In these cases, we want to look at just three aspects of the child's syntactic production: (1) analysis of errors in morphological and syntactic form, (2) use of complex syntax, and (3) disruptions.

Error Analysis. Scott & Windsor (2000) showed that production of grammatical errors was the measure that was best at distinguishing children with LLD from typical peers in naturalistic language sampling. Especially at the school-age level, the persistence of grammatical errors is an important index of impairment. If we transcribe the sample or use a computer-assisted format, we can do an error analysis by noting each grammatical error that occurs and making a list of those we find. We also might note whether these errors are consistently used at every opportunity or in every obligatory context or whether there is some correct usage. If we don't transcribe the sample but simply listen to an audiorecording of it some time later, we can make the same kind of list as we listen. An experienced clinician can even make a list of errors in real time during the collection of the interview sample, provided the errors are not too frequent. For beginning clinicians, though, it is better to work from a transcribed or audiorecorded sample. Forms that are in error in the sample can be targeted for intervention. Table 11-6 provides a sample worksheet to be used in this kind of error analysis, with some of the typical errors that may be seen in students with LLD. Clinicians using the form can add any additional error types that appear in a client's speech sample. Paul, McNamara, Reuler, Roy, and Peterson (2001), Restrepo (1998), as well as Scott and Windsor (2000) reported that number of grammatical errors in speech samples reliably discriminated between language normal and language delayed children whether they were English or Spanish speakers. Paul et al. (2001) showed that no English-speaking five year olds with typical language development produced more than 6 grammatical errors within a 50 utterance spontaneous speech sample, whereas all the children clinically classified as language delayed produced more than 6 errors.

Complex Sentence Analysis. Most students in the L4L stage will have acquired basic sentence forms. Forms that are just emerging or still lacking in their speech are likely to be in the category of complex sentences. Complex sentences are those that contain more than one verb phrase (Paul, 1981) in embedded or conjoined multiclause utterances. They are used to express specific semantic relations between clauses, such as those we discussed in the semantics section. Their use increases significantly throughout the school years and continues to do so through adolescence, particularly in the context of written language (Loban, 1976). Children who are unable to use syntactic means to combine propositions in speech consequently are at a distinct disadvantage in writing about the abstract, decontextualized content of the classroom.

Paul (1981) has presented a system for analyzing three aspects of complex sentence use that can be used with children in the L4L period. For many students in the L4L stage who do not make obvious errors of syntactic form, the complex sentence analysis may be the only evaluation of grammatical production we need to do. To perform this analysis, we first identify each sentence produced by the client that can be considered complex. If this is the only analysis we are doing of the transcript, we do not need to transcribe the entire sample. Instead we can listen to an audiorecording and write down just the sentences we intend to consider in the complex sentence analysis. If the *SALT* (Miller & Chapman, 1993) computer-assisted analysis procedure is used, it can identify complex sentences by means of the conjunctions contained within them and provide a list of all sentences with examples of these conjunctions. Either way, we want to generate a list of complex sentences that appear in the speech sample.

The first aspect of complex sentence use we can examine is the **proportion of complex to simple sentences** in the sample. Paul (1981) reported that by the time normally developing children's MLUs reach 5 (at an average age of 4 to 5 years), 20% of the sentences they use in spontaneous speech contain embedded or conjoined clauses. This suggests that one criterion for determining the maturity of a speech sample is to look at the proportion of the sentences that are complex. If we transcribe the entire sample, we can easily compute the percentage of complex sentences that appear. But if we are trying to increase our efficiency in language sampling and are using a "shortcut" of only transcribing the complex utterances, we can estimate this percentage.

One way to perform this estimation is to make a note or hash mark for each T-unit we hear as we listen to the tape of our sample. During the same pass, we can stop the tape to transcribe each complex sentence the sample contains. We can then get an estimate of the total number of T-units in the sample (by adding the number of complex sentences transcribed to the number of hash marks recorded). Then we can divide the number of complex sentences by the total number of T-units to get a percentage. If the percentage for any child in the L4L stage is substantially less than 20%, we can infer that this client is using fewer complex sentences than normally speaking peers and could benefit from intervention to increase speech complexity. If more than 20% of the sample is complex, we will not need to analyze any further. We can conclude that this client is progressing adequately in complex sentence use.

A second aspect of complex sentence analysis concerns the **types of complex sentences** that appear. This analysis can be done for clients who produce a smaller-than-normal proportion (less than 20%) of complex utterances. Paul (1981) assigned each complex sentence type that appeared in transcripts of normally developing children's speech to one of Brown's stages, according to the stage at which a majority of normally developing children produced each form. This stage assignment can be simplified for assessment purposes by dividing the complex types into two general groups: those that appear early in development (when MLUs are between 3 and 4) and those that appear later (when MLUs are between 4 and 5). Table 11-7 describes and gives examples of each sentence type in the early and late groups.

Before initiating intervention for use of a particular complex sentence type, though, we will probably want to use elicited production activities to probe for forms that are absent in spontaneous speech. Remember that a speech sample is just that—a *sample* of speech, not necessarily containing all the forms a client can use. Complex sentence forms can be elicited with cloze procedures, in which the clinician produces one clause and asks that client to "finish the sentence or thought" (e.g., "I think . . . ," "Mary wants to . . . ," "I know where. . . ."). An

TABLE 11-6	Example of a Worksheet for Error Analysis in Conversational Speech Gathered from a Student in the L4L Stage	

ERROR TYPE	NO. OF ERROR OCCURRENCES	NO. OF OPPORTUNITIES FOR ERROR
Pronoun usage me/I	I I I I	I I I I I I
Bound morphemes on nouns absent comparative marker	I I	I I I I I I I
Inflections on verbs absent past-tense marking	I I	I I I I
Errors on copula *be* VERBS is/are	I I I	I I I I I I
Subject/verb agreement errors absent third-person singular marker	I I	I I I I I
Auxiliary verb errors don't/doesn't	I I I	I I I
Errors in negation nobody/anybody	I I	I I
Errors in questions absent auxiliary inversion	I	I I I

alternative procedure is to ask the client to make up a sentence with *that* or *if*, or *when*, and so on, to probe conjunction use or to make up a sentence with *know, need to, know what to, wants me to,* or a similar construction to probe use of various complex sentence types.

If a genuine deficit in the use of certain complex sentence types is seen in spontaneous speech and confirmed through elicited production procedures, we can examine speech samples to see what kinds of complex sentences are in evidence. If the student is using only forms that are in the Early group in Table

TABLE 11-7   Complex Sentence Types Divided into Early and Late-Appearing Groups

SENTENCE TYPE	DESCRIPTION	EXAMPLE
Early Group (first appear in normal development when MLU is between 3 and 4)		
Simple infinitive	*Not* an early developing catenative such as *gonna, wanna, gotta, sposta, hafta, let's,* or *lemme; to* is present; subject is the same as main sentence, so it is deleted.	"He has to move." "She wants to get out."
Full propositional complements	Headed by "cognitive" verbs, such as *think, guess, wish, know, hope, wonder;* may or may not contain the conjunction *that.*	"I think that we have some." "Pretend you said it."
Simple *wh-* clause	Marked by conjunctions *what, who, where, when, why, how;* do *not* contain an infinitive *to* marker.	"I know what we could do." "Look how big I am."
Simple conjoinings	Two clauses joined by a conjunction, either coordinating (*and, but, so,* etc.) or subordinating (*because, after,* etc.)	"Close the gate so he can't get out." "I eat ice cream 'cause I like it."
Multiple embeddings	Sentences containing more than one embedded clause; one may include a catenative.	"It's gonna start to fall." "I think we gotta pour some water on it."
Embedded and conjoined	Sentences containing both an embedded and a conjoined clause; the embedding may be a catenative.	"It's not a bulldozer 'cause it doesn't have a scooper thing to scoop with." "He wants to stay at home and I don't know why."
Later Group (first appear in normal development when MLU is between 4 and 5)		
Infinitive clauses with different subjects	The embedded clause has a subject different from the main clause, so it is expressed.	"I want it to go chug." "Dad made this for me to drive."
Relative clauses	Function as adjectives; specify nouns; may or may not be marked with *which* or *that.*	"That's not the kind that I like." "They're boys that I know."
Gerunds	*-ing* forms used as noun clauses.	"I felt like turning it." "They can hear us talking on the tape."
wh- infinitives	Marked by conjunctions *what, who, where, when,* and *to.*	"I know what to do." "You know how to make one."
Unmarked infinitives	Headed by *make, help, watch,* or *let* with no *to* marker.	"Watch me jump." "Help me pick these up."

Adapted from Paul, R. (1981). Analyzing complex sentence development. In J.F. Miller (Ed.), *Assessing language production in children: Experimental procedures* (pp. 36-40). Needham Heights, MA: Allyn and Bacon.

11-7, we can develop intervention that attempts to elicit some of the more advanced forms. We can provide intensified input by means of literature-based script therapy that gives examples of the use of some of these forms. If the student is using a few forms from both the Early and Later groups, we may want to work on eliciting new forms in the Early group first. We can again target production as well as provide input in script-based formats to help the student to understand and use these structures. We'll talk about some specific methods for targeting complex sentences in our next chapter.

If a student is using hardly any syntactically well-formed versions of complex sentences, we can do the analysis of semantic relations between clauses that we talked about earlier. This analysis can be used to identify the relations the student is already expressing in less mature ways. Syntactic forms for expressing these same relations can then be incorporated into the intervention program.

The third area of complex sentence production we may want to look at concerns the **use of conjunctions**. By the end of the preschool period, normally developing children are using an average of six to eight different conjunctions in a 15-minute speech sample, including *and, if, because, when,* and *so* (Paul, 1981). If we find, in looking at the complex sentences of children in the L4L stage, that fewer than six different conjunctions appear in samples of this size, we can again probe for conjunction use with elicited production procedures. If the deficit is confirmed, we can target these early developing conjunctions that are not found in the transcript as part of the intervention program. If the semantic relational analysis shows that students are juxtaposing clauses without any explicit conjunctions, we can provide intervention to elicit use of these early developing conjunctions for expressing the semantic relations between clauses that the students are already encoding presyntactically.

Box 11-7 presents a portion of a speech sample from a 9-year-old student. Try practicing an analysis of complex sentences on this sample and determine whether a deficit in complex sentence use is seen. My analysis of the sample appears in Appendix 11-1.

Disruptions. Dollaghan and Campbell (1992) pointed out that many descriptions of children with LLD refer to their *disruptions in speech,* or "getting tangled up" when they try to talk. Frequent suggestions have been made in the LLD literature that these speakers are particularly prone to "mazes," or verbalized disruptions, false starts, and excessive revisions in their spontaneous speech. In some cases these disruptions are the most prominent feature of a student's expressive language disorder. Dollaghan and Campbell suggested looking in detail at speech disruptions as a way to quantify otherwise vague impressions of "tangled speech." They suggested further that

---

BOX 11-7	**Portion of a Speech Sample Derived from an Interview of a 9-Year-Old Student**

T1. I got two brothers
T2. (and) one of them, Marco, is a real pain.
T3. He never lets me play his video games,
T4. (and) he never wants to play two players, and just keeps playing and playing
T5. (and) he never dies or anything!
T6. I can get onto the eighth level when I get to play for long enough.
T7. I hardly ever do, because my dumb big brother always hogs it when I want to play.
T8. He knows why to be nice sometimes, because he always gives me his basketball cards when he gets doubles
T9. (and) I think I know why he does it.
T10. He wants to get Mom to take us to the card store.
T11. She'll only go when I ask her.
T12. See, this card store has all kinds of stuff that's real expensive
T13. (and) she hates it when we take all our money and spend it there
T14. She'll go when I ask because I never have as much money as Marco
T15. (and) she doesn't think it'll be too bad
T16. (and then) Marco says he wants to come, too,
T17. (and) she can't say "no" because she already said she'd take me!
T18. See, sharing the cards that he has doubles of with me means he can get to the store more often.

---

we use the analysis of disruptions only for those clients whose perceived deficits in expressive language cannot be reduced to semantic, syntactic, or phonological difficulties. For these clients, whose production problems are otherwise difficult to quantify, a detailed analysis of speech disruptions can help both to make deficits more explicit and to identify strategies for intervention. Dollaghan and Campbell found that the average number of disruptions, including both mazes and pauses of various types, in the spontaneous speech of typical students in 100-word speech samples (from which mazed words were excluded) was 5.31 (with a standard deviation of 1.82). These findings suggest that students who produce *more than eight* disruptions in speech samples of this size are producing speech that is significantly "tangled." Intervention for students with frequent speech disruptions can include using self-monitoring strategies to help students become aware of their own disruptions, metacognitive strategies to help them plan speech before they begin talking, and teaching them to use "editing expressions"—such as "Let me try that again"—when they get tangled. An adaptation of Dollaghan and Campbell's system for analyzing speech disruptions appears in Box 11-8.

PRAGMATICS

Remember that pragmatics is the area in which we are likely to find many of the communication problems of students with LLD. For students at the L4L stage, we want to assess pragmatic skills in two of the major discourse types we identified in Chapter 10: conversation and narrative. We'll expand our discussion to include expository and persuasive texts when we discuss advanced language in Chapters 13 and 14.

Pragmatics in Conversation

When we examine a student's skill in using conversational language, there are three major areas to think about.

1. An appropriately broad range of *communicative intentions,* or functions of communication.
2. Whether the student can *modify communicative style,* or register, for different interactive situations.
3. How the student can *manage discourse* turns, topics, and breakdowns.

We can use some of the assessments we discussed for the developing language period to get a general overview. For example, Prutting and Kirchner's *Pragmatic Protocol* (1983), in Figure 8-17 is a good assessment tool to use at the L4L stage as well as at earlier levels. Damaico's *Systematic Observation of Communicative Interaction* (SOCI; Damico, Oller, & Tetnowski, 1999) is another tool that may be used. Let's look at some additional methods for assessing each of these areas of pragmatic skill.

Communicative Intentions. One important question to ask concerns the range and maturity of communicative functions expressed by students with LLD. Tough (1977) examined the kinds of communicative functions expressed by typical children between 5 and 7 years old. These functions, according to Chapman (1981), reflect the cognitive changes going on during

| **BOX 11-8** | **System for Analyzing Speech Disruptions** |

1. Collect a speech sample, using a question or interview format.
2. Segment the sample into T-units.
3. Transcribe all words, portions of words, unglossable speechlike sounds, and silent pauses of more than 2 seconds in length.
4. Identify verbal mazes (false starts, repetitions, and revisions). Count the number of words *not* within mazes in the transcript. This is the "number of unmazed words" to be used to compute the percentage of disruptions in Step 6.
5. Identify each disruption in the transcript and count the frequency of each type of disruption and the total number of disruptions.

Disruption Types

Pauses
Filled: Nonlexical, one-syllable filler vocalizations, such as *um* or *er*
Silent: Silent intervals of 2 or more seconds in length
Pause strings: More than one silent or filled pause in succession ("He *(um)* [pause] said I could go")

Repetitions
Forward: Speaker repeats an incomplete linguistic unit and goes on to complete it following the repetition ("She she said I can go")
Exact: Speaker repeats a linguistic unit that has already been completed ("She said I can go I can go")
Backward: Speaker inserts an additional word or words before the repeated unit without changing the unit itself ("She said I think she said I can go")

Revisions
Recognizable modifications of a linguistic unit already produced by the speaker. They can be used to correct overt errors, add information, delete information, or for unknown reasons. They may involve lexical, grammatical, or phonological changes or some combination of these. *Examples:*
   "I have two sipter, sisters."
   "My older brother, my brother likes baseball."
   "My brother, I mean my sister is here."
   "I have a brother, two brothers."

Orphans
Linguistic units with no identifiable relationship to other units. *Examples* (in square brackets):
   "I saved up [in] all my allowance."
   "And [in] that was my car."
   "And [spuh, in] that's her date."

6. Divide the frequency of disruptions by the number of unmazed words in the sample (from step 4). Multiply by 100 to get the percentage of occurrence of disruptions per 100 unmazed words.
7. Determine whether there are more than seven or eight disruptions per 100 unmazed words to decide whether the student's speech is significantly "tangled."
8. Look for unusual types of disruptions. Also, inspect for patterns with respect to where disruptions occur. For example: (a) Do revisions seem to cluster in utterances that are longer than the speaker's average T-unit length or in complex sentences? If so, work on improving skills in complex syntax may be warranted. Part of the intervention monitoring could include analysis of speech to determine whether disruptions in targeted forms decrease as forms become well-learned. (b) Do most revisions seem to result from a need to correct errors or add or delete information? In this case, metacognitive strategies to improve planning skills may be useful. (c) Are revisions primarily phonological? This may indicate word-retrieval problems. Intervention might focus on developing word-finding strategies, using both semantic and phonological retrieval strategies.

Adapted from Dollaghan, C., & Campbell, T. (1992). A procedure for classifying disruptions in spontaneous language samples. *Topics in Language Disorders, 12,* 56-68.

the early school years. Such changes include an increased ability to monitor one's own behavior, to reason, to relate events and ideas to each other, and to engage in complex imaginative play. Students at the L4L stage should be showing evidence of at least some of these intentions, in addition to the basic assertive and responsive intentions in Fey's scheme. These advanced intentions can be observed in an interview, free play, or a peer interactional sample and can be coded in real time or from an audiorecording. The intentions identified by Tough appear in Table 11-8. When there is a dearth of these advanced intentions in the communication of a student with LLD, new forms and meanings taught in intervention should be modeled for the student in these kinds of intentions. Role-playing and other contexts that provide opportunities for students to use both pre-existing and newly learned language forms to serve these communicative functions also can be included in the intervention program.

Contextual Variation. Part of pragmatic skill is the ability to use the context of the communicative situation to decide how to say what we want to say. We use information about our listeners when we make these decisions, as well as information about the nonlinguistic context. Children talk differently to their teachers than they do to their peers and differently yet to their younger siblings, reflecting knowledge of the different age, status, and communicative competencies of these various listeners. We also talk differently depending on who has more rights in the

TABLE 11-8		Cognitive Uses of Language of Young School-Age Children	
MAJOR FUNCTION		**USE**	**EXAMPLES**
Directive	Self-directing	Monitoring actions	Child accompanies actions with words.
		Focusing control	"It won't turn. I need help."
		Forward planning	"I'm gonna cut this clay into two, then I'll flatten it."
	Other-directing	Demonstrating	"Put yours here, like this."
		Instructing	"Be careful, don't push it."
		Forward planning	"You'll need another block to finish it."
		Anticipating collaboration	"We're gonna have a crash! Make yours go fast so they can crash good!"
Interpretive	Reporting on present or past events	Labeling	"That's a cowboy; that's a sheriff."
		Elaborating	"We went to the beach, and it was too cold to go swimming, so we picked up stones and seashells."
		Associating	"I got one, but it's not like that one."
		Recognizing incongruity	"That house is too small for this doll."
		Awareness of sequence	"We went on vacation, and I got chicken pox, then Bob got them."
	Reasoning	Recognizing cause	"The ice cream got soft 'cause we forgot to put it in the fridge."
		Recognizing principles	"People don't like it if you take their stuff."
Projective	Predicting	Forecasting events	"My dad's gonna build me a playhouse."
		Anticipating consequences	"My mom'll be mad if I get home late."
		Surveying alternatives	"We could take a train or a car to my Grandma's."
		Forecasting possibilities	"If my thermos is broken, the milk'll leak all over my lunch."
		Recognizing problems and predicting solutions	"My zipper's broke; maybe my dad can fix it with a wrench."
	Empathetic	Projecting into others' feelings and experiences	"She doesn't like his teasing, and she's crying 'cause she didn't like it."
		Anticipating reactions of others	"She won't like that!"
	Imagining	Renaming	"This'll be the house."
		Commentary on play	On toy phone: "Doctor, my baby's sick!"
		Building scene	"This is such a big hospital. Will my baby be OK?"
		Role-playing	Playing doctor: "Now, now, Mrs. Jones, I'll take good care of your baby."
Relational	Self-maintaining	Express need	"Watch me! I can do it!"
		Protect self-interest	"That's mine! Give it back!"
		Justify	"I want red so I can draw a fire engine."
		Criticize	"I don't like your picture."
		Threaten	"Give me that or I'll hit you!"
	Interactional	Self-emphasize	"I'm the one that's the mommy."
		Other-recognizing	"Please give me my car back now."

List presented by Tough, J. (1977). *The development of meaning.* New York: Halsted Press; cited in Chapman, R. (1981). Exploring children's communicative intents. In J. Miller (Ed.), *Assessing language production in children.* Needham Heights, MA: Allyn and Bacon.

context. We ask for a pencil differently, for example, depending on whether the pencil belongs to us and we want it returned or it belongs to the listener and we want to borrow it. And we talk differently in different nonlinguistic contexts, depending on how formal we perceive them to be. I might talk to my students one way in the classroom and another way if I meet them in the ladies' room. These kinds of changes are called *register variation*.

Other changes involve knowledge of what our listeners know and don't know. We would describe a baseball game differently to someone who knew a lot about baseball than to someone (like me) who didn't. Similarly, you would describe your master's thesis on alaryngeal speech differently to your parents than to an otolaryngologist. These kinds of contextual variation depend on our assessment of our audience's state of background knowledge or *presupposition*. Skills in register variation and presupposition constitute one aspect of our communicative competence.

Assessing Register Variation. We can assess register variation by setting up role-playing situations in which we ask students to express the same basic communicative intent in several different contexts. We also can assess their understanding of register changes in the same activity, by displaying several different ways to convey an intention and seeing whether they can match each with an appropriate context. It is especially helpful in our remedial planning if we choose contexts that relate to the child's performance in school. Although we know normally developing children use a different register in talking to younger children, for example (as do most children with language impairments [Fey & Leonard, 1984]), this type of variation may not be very important for success in school. The kinds of variations needed for school success are more likely to include politeness variations and variations based on rights, social status, and degree of formality. Figure 11-6 gives some example role-playing activities that can be used to assess register variation in students with LLD.

If an assessment like this indicates that the student has difficulty making and understanding changes in speech style for different situations, remedial activities that target newly learned forms and meanings in a variety of situational contexts can be included in the remedial program. The clinician can model the appropriate use of these forms in various contexts and can work with the student to identify and practice use of these forms and meanings in a variety of contexts important in the client's social environment.

Assessing Presuppositional Skill. Many of the assessment activities proposed by Roth and Spekman (1984a, b) and summarized in Table 8-13 also will be useful for assessing presuppositional skills in students in the L4L stage. As outlined in the table, one activity is to have clients describe a sequence of pictures, each of which changes by one detail. We can note whether they use *ellipsis*, that is, whether they delete redundant information ("In this picture a boy is riding a bike; in this one he's not" ["riding a bike" is deleted since it is redundant]). We also can note whether clients use pronouns for nouns in subsequent pictures ("In this picture a girl is riding a bike; in this one *she's* walking"). And we can look to see whether they use indefinite

articles (*a, an*) first and definite articles (*the*) to describe the same picture later in the sequence. ("In this picture a dog is running; in the next one *the* dog's sitting"). The peer interaction we discussed earlier, in which one student instructs another in a game or project, also can yield useful information. For looking at presuppositional skill, we would want to ask the student with LLD to explain something to the normally developing peer.

Barrier games also are useful contexts for assessing the ability to tell a listener what he or she needs to know in a situation. This type of assessment is called a *referential communication task*. Referential communication might involve choosing a large blue circle from an array of blocks of various colors, sizes, and shapes. If the student told the listener to find a circle or a "blue one," and other round or blue blocks were available, an error in presuppositional encoding could be identified. If the student made these kinds of errors consistently, a presuppositional deficit could be inferred. Lloyd (1994) provided additional suggestions for assessing referential communication skills.

Many barrier game sets are available commercially, including *Barrier Games for Better Communication* (Deal & Hanuscin, 1999) and *Barrier Games with Unisets* (Marquis & Blog, 1993). They also can easily be assembled by the clinician, by gathering matching sets of objects or pictures. Barrier games also are useful for looking at the ways in which the client can improve unclear messages in response to requests for clarification from the clinician and at whether the client can request clarification in response to purposefully unclear messages from the clinician.

Discourse Management. The ability to orchestrate turns and topics and to repair breakdowns in conversation constitutes the realm of discourse management. The peer interaction we discussed before is a good context for looking at a student's ability to initiate a topic, begin a conversation, maintain a topic, and respond to requests for clarification. Again, having the student with LLD do the explaining is the best way to gather these kinds of data on discourse management. Brinton and Fujiki (1989, 1994) and Gruenewald and Pollack (1990) also provided methods that can be used in assessing discourse skills in school-aged children.

Although we are interested in all aspects of a client's discourse-management skill, the special discourse requirements of the classroom are particularly important. We talked in detail in the last chapter about what these requirements are. Let's look now at some methods we might use to assess a student's competence with them.

Figure 11-7 presents a checklist developed by Bedrosian (1985) to look at a client's skill in discourse management. The clinician can use the checklist to rate an observation of either conversational or classroom discourse. Ideally, the clinician would use the checklist to observe several different interactional situations, including clinician-client, client-peer, and client-teacher in a one-to-one setting, as well as observing the client in classroom discussion. The clinician can then look across these contexts to identify problems or areas of strength. When difficulties in discourse management are identified, the particular contexts

Expressive Activities

Have the student role-play producing each speech act in each context. Record the student's utterance, and make a judgment as to whether it is appropriate for each context.

Speech act	Context	Student utterance	Appropriate?
Request ice cream	1. Mother 2. Friend who has money to spend on the way home from school 3. Brother who took cone for a taste and won't give it back		
Greet	1. Principal 2. Friend 3. Grandparent		
Persuade	1. Father to give advance on allowance 2. Friend to lend a favorite sweater 3. Teacher to postpone a quiz		
Request information	1. From a teacher about a homework assignment 2. From a librarian at the town library 3. From a friend about a baseball game		

Receptive Activities

Ask the student to judge each speech act you produce according to whether it is appropriate in each context. If the student judges the act to be inappropriate, ask him or her to produce a better version.

Context	Speech act	Student judgment of appropriateness
Student requests a baseball from a friend	"Hey, dude, can I borrow your ball?"	
Teacher requests a pencil from a student	"May I please use your pencil?"	
Student requests a cookie in the cafeteria	"Give me that cookie right away!"	
Student greets a teacher	"How do you do, Ms. Hernandez?"	
Principal greets a student	"Good morning, James. How are you today?"	
Student greets a friend	"Hey, man, how's it going?"	
Student tries to get a teacher to lend a book from the class library	"Please, Ms. Jansen, I'll be especially careful with it. I'll bring it right back tomorrow!"	
Student tries to get a friend to give him a ride on the back of his bike	"You better let me ride on the back. I'm telling you, you better or else!"	
Student tries to get parent to increase allowance	"I want more money! I need it! I have to have it."	
Student asks teacher to repeat page numbers of math assignment	"I'm sorry. I didn't hear you. Could you say it again?"	
Student asks librarian to help find a book	"So where is it? Is it over here?"	
Student asks friend for the time	"Excuse me, Kim, but might I trouble you to ask the time, please?"	

FIGURE 11-6 ✦ An example worksheet for use with role-playing activities to assess register variation skills in students with LLD.

that are problematic can be incorporated into the intervention program. If classroom discourse is affected, the clinician can work with the teacher to find ways to make the "hidden curriculum" more explicit to the student and to facilitate more successful classroom interaction skills.

Silliman and Wilkinson (1991) proposed a strategy for assessing classroom discourse that uses a sequence of assessment tools, each focused on progressively narrower and more closely defined areas of performance. They suggested starting with a teacher referral checklist, such as the one in Figure 11-1,

to identify a problem. Next the clinician can use a checklist, such as the one in Figure 11-2, to guide a direct observation of several interactions. The subsequent step in their system involves a more focused observation of a single classroom discourse situation. Silliman and Wilkinson provided a variety of techniques for accomplishing this goal. One technique that may be particularly useful to the SLP is the *running record*. A running record is a slice of classroom life. In it, the clinician records in a narrative style everything that happens in sequence over the course of a 10- to 15-minute classroom interaction. The running

Name of client: _____

Date of interaction: _____

Type of participant interaction: _____

Type of setting: _____

Length of interaction: _____

Instructions: Check the appropriate skill descriptor that follows:

	Yes	No	Sometimes	NA
I. Topic initiations				
A. Frequency of client's topic initiations in comparison to the other participant(s) (check one).				
1. None				
2. Less than				
3. Approximately equal to				
4. More than				
B. Subject matter of topic initiations:				
1. Able to get attention of listener				
2. Repeats old topics on a daily basis				
3. Initiates new topics on a daily basis				
4. Able to greet others				
5. Able to express departures when leaving				
6. Able to make introductions				
7. Able to initiate needs				
8. Able to initiate questions:				
a. Requests for information				
b. Requests for repetition or clarification				
c. Requests for action				
d. Requests for permission				
9. Talks mostly about self				
10. Talks about the other, as well as self				
11. Talks about referents in the past				
12. Talks about referents in the future				
13. Talks about referents in the present				
14. Talks about fantasy-related referents				
15. Uses people's names appropriately				
16. Uses noise or sound-word play in appropriate situations				

FIGURE 11-7 ✦ Discourse skills checklist: molar analysis. (Used with permission from Bedrosian, J. [1985]. An approach to developing conversational competence. In D. Ripich and F. Spinelli [Eds.], *School discourse problem* [p. 239]. San Diego, CA: College-Hill Press.)

	Yes	No	Sometimes	NA
II. MAINTAINING TOPICS				
A. Able to keep a topic going				
1. Responds to questions				
2. Acknowledges topic (e.g., "Uh-huh")				
3. Offers new information that is related				
4. Requests more information about a topic				
5. Able to request repetition or clarification if message is not clear				
6. Able to repeat or answer questions about what another has talked about				
7. Agrees with others				
8. Disagrees with others				
B. Not able to keep a topic going				
1. Intentionally evades or ignores a question				
2. Initiates a topic immediately following a topic initiation by a prior speaker				
3. Engages in monologues when in a group				
III. USE OF EYE CONTACT				
A. Able to use eye contact to designate a listener in a group when initiating a topic				
B. Uses eye contact while listening				
IV. TURN-TAKING				
A. Is easily interrupted				
B. Interrupts others				
C. Answers questions for others				
D. Has long speaking turns				
E. Designates turns for others in a group				
F. Sensitive to listener cues (e.g., can tell if listener is interested or bored)				
G. Excuses self when interrupting				
V. POLITENESS				
A. Able to make indirect requests				
B. Uses commands				
C. Uses politeness markers of "Please," "Thank you," "Excuse me"				
VI. OBSERVATION OF NONVERBAL BEHAVIORS				
A. Stands or sits too close to people when talking				
B. Stands or sits too far away from people when talking				
C. Stands or sits at appropriate social distances when talking				
D. Uses nonverbal head nods to acknowledge				
E. Uses nonverbal means of getting attention to initiate a topic (e.g., taps on shoulder, points)				

FIGURE 11-7 ✦—cont'd

record can be examined with the teacher to identify the student's conflicts and sources of difficulty in the classroom and to check teacher perceptions and expectations to see where any mismatches may be occurring. Box 11-9 gives an example of a running record of classroom discourse, drawn from Silliman and Wilkinson.

After the running record has been discussed with the teacher, he or she and the clinician may collaborate to develop strategies, including making the "hidden curriculum" explicit or using peer tutoring, role-playing, and coaching by the clinician, to facilitate more successful client communication. They also may decide to carry the assessment one step further and produce a *critical incident report*. This is used to gather information to address a specific question. The question might be, "Does the client tune out teacher instructions?" or "Do cultural differences in rules for responding to questions make the client unwilling to answer the teacher?" If the teacher and clinician feel the need for more information to answer such specific questions, observations of incidents relevant to these questions can be made by the clinician, using the running record format, and subsequently discussed by the assessment team. Again, specific problems identified can be addressed by collaborative planning.

In the case of some critical incidents, a Systems model might be applied to the problem (that is, the difficulty may not only reside in the child but also in the interaction between the child and the environment). Cultural differences in language use would be a prime example of a situation in which a Systems model would be appropriate. If mismatches in communication style are identified, they could be worked from both ends. The clinician might work with the client to make the "hidden curriculum" explicit, explaining the classroom rules and asking the client to talk about how they differ from the rules of conversation at home. The client could be encouraged to learn and "play by" the classroom rules when in school, while preserving the pragmatics of the home culture in other settings. At the same time, the clinician could work with the teacher to understand the client's cultural differences and to make some accommodation for them in the classroom.

Pragmatics of Narrative

We talked in the last chapter about the importance of narrative skills in the acquisition of literacy and for success in school generally. Narrative skills are another area of discourse we want to address in the student with LLD in the L4L period. We can examine both comprehension and production of narrative discourse.

Comprehension and Inferencing. Understanding stories involves having expectations, or scripts, for how they will proceed. In other words, understanding and processing stories requires some knowledge of *story grammar*. But it also involves something more. Not everything that happens in stories is stated explicitly. Part of understanding a story is being able to infer some of this implicit information. In assessing how students make sense of stories, we need to look at both literal and inferential comprehension.

Literal story comprehension can be assessed by adapting a variety of materials designed to evaluate reading comprehension. The *Gray Silent Reading Tests—4th Edition* (Wiederholt & Bryant, 2000), and the *Woodcock Reading Mastery Tests— Normative Update* (Woodcock, 1998) are just two examples. Many such materials can be obtained from the school reading specialist. Alternatively, classroom reading material can be used. Either way, we can assess narrative comprehension by reading a story or passage to the client. Using commercial or clinician-created comprehension probes, we can have the student respond to orally presented questions about the setting, names and roles of characters, sequence of events, outcome, and resolution of the story.

Inferential comprehension can be assessed by asking students to explain why characters behaved as they did, to state what the character's goals and motivations were, and to talk about how characters felt at different points in the story. Some commercial reading tests include questions on inferential comprehension. Examples include *The Test of Narrative Language* (Gillam & Pearson, 2004), *The Qualitative Reading Inventory—3* (Leslie & Caldwell, 2001) and the *Flynt-Cooter Reading Inventory for the Classroom* (Flynt & Cooter, 2004). Westby (2005) suggested using "trickster tales," in which characters attempt to deceive others, as a good way to get at inferencing ability in children in later elementary grades. Some examples of trickster tales include *Miss Nelson Is Missing* (Allard & Marshall, 1977), *Stone Soup* (Brown, 1947), and folktales such as Uncle Remus or Anansi the Spider stories. Another way to

---

BOX 11-9	**Example of a Running Record of Classroom Discourse**

At the end of the count of 10 when the whole class is supposed to be sitting on the floor, D is not there. Instead he goes out the door of the class. One of the children calls the teacher's attention to this and she says, "D is being stubborn." She then engages the class in a conversation about being stubborn, asking them if they know what it means to be stubborn. Someone suggests that it means to be sad. Someone else says it means bad. The teacher says that you are stubborn if someone asks you to do something and you say (demonstrating) "No, I won't do it!" At this point one of the children says, "Yes. They ask you and you no like." (p. 304)

From Boggs, S. (1972). The meaning of questions and narratives to Hawaiian children. In C.B. Cazden, V.P. John, & D. Hymes (Eds.), *Functions of language in the classroom* (pp. 299–330). NY: Teacher's College Press; quoted in Silliman, E., & Wilkinson, L. (1991). *Communicating for learning: Classroom observations and collaboration.* Gaithersburg, MD: Aspen Publishers.

assess inferential comprehension is to stop the story at several points and ask the student to tell what will happen next. Norbury and Bishop (2003) found that students with a variety of communication disorders could make inferences in stories, but these were not always relevant to the story context, and Cain, Oakhill, and Elbro (2003) report that children with LLD were impaired in their ability to integrate information within a text in order to infer meaning of novel words. Wallach and Miller (1988) pointed out that children with LLD are capable of making inferences in story comprehension tasks, but they do not always marshal these abilities spontaneously. If inferential skills seem lacking, some dynamic assessment techniques can be used. These would involve actively coaching students to take pieces of information in the story and put them together to draw a conclusion. If the student does better with this kind of coaching, it can be expanded and intensified in the intervention program.

Narrative Production. Fey, Catts, Proctor-Williams, Tomblin, and Zhang (2004) reported in a large study of narrative production in school-aged children that story production tasks were found to be highly educationally relevant and should play a significant role in the evaluation of children with developmental LLD. Studies have shown narrative assessment to be sensitive to both pragmatic (Botting, 2002) and structural aspects of children's language abilities (Norbury & Bishop, 2003), and to show areas of deficit even when standardized tests do not (Manhardt & Rescorla, 2002). Hadley (1998) showed that students are more likely to show maze behaviors and to make errors in morphological marking in narrative contexts than they are in conversation. Guiterrez-Clennen and DeCurtis (2001) report that narratives collected in the native language can be used to identify disorders in children who do not speak English, although it is important to be aware of the ways in which narratives in different cultures vary (McCabe & Bliss, 2003). Narrative tasks, then, tend to be better at revealing the linguistic vulnerabilities in children with LLD than simpler conversational activities. That's one reason why assessing narrative production is an important part of the evaluation of school-age clients. There are a variety of ways to elicit narrative samples from students. Hughes, McGillivray, and Schmidek (1997) identified three types of narratives that are appropriate as assessment contexts for children in the L4L stage:

▶ *Personal narratives.* These involve asking the child to recount a salient personal experience. Suggestions for eliciting these include asking students to tell about a time when they were hurt, scared, or solved a problem.

▶ *Script narratives.* These require students to relate a routine series of events. Often it helps to give the student a reason for producing the script. For example, we can ask students to pretend they are explaining to a new student what happens in gym class or to a foreign visitor how to order food in a fast food restaurant.

▶ *Fictional narratives.* Children can be asked to generate a story, such as "Goldilocks and the Three Bears" or describe the plot of a TV show or movie they've watched. Alternatively, the clinician can tell a story, with or without pictorial support, and ask the student to retell it. Story generation is usually more difficult, but it is considered more representative. In either the generation or retelling task, visual stimuli in the form of single pictures, series of pictures, film strips or videos can be used. Providing visual support generally makes either type of fictional narrative task easier. Westby (1989b) advocated having students provide the narration for a wordless picture book, such as *A Boy, a Dog, and a Frog* (Mayer, 1967) or from a short video, such as one of the Max the Mouse series (Society for Visual Education, 1989).

Hughes, McGillivray, and Schmidek (1997) provide extensive guidance in eliciting, transcribing, segmenting, and analyzing language samples. They also provide numerous practice exercises to help clinicians refine their skills in narrative assessment. Gillam and Pearson's (2004) *Test of Narrative Language* employs stories with a variety of formats, such as those listed above.

Paul, Hernandez, Taylor, and Johnson (1996) found in their research on children's narratives that three characteristics distinguished the narratives of children with language disorders from those of their normally speaking peers:

1. Overall maturity of narrative, sometimes referred to as *story macrostructure*, as indexed by the degree of organization and number and type of story grammar elements included in the story.

2. Clear and appropriate use of linguistic markers such as pronouns, prepositions, and articles to provide cohesive ties throughout the story.

3. Use of precise and diverse vocabulary, a literate language style, advanced episodic structure and linguistic highlighting of the crux, or *high point* of the story, to create a comprehensible and interesting tale. Peterson and McCabe (1983) referred to this aspect as "sparkle" in children's stories.

Let's see how we might assess each of these areas to learn more about a client's narrative ability.

Narrative Macrostructure. There are a variety of means of assessing overall level of narrative maturity in the transcriptions of story samples we collect from students with LLD. We've already discussed Applebee's (1978) system. *The Strong Narrative Assessment Procedure* (SNAP; Strong, 1998) and the *Test of Narrative Language* (TNL; Gillam & Pearson, 2004) are commercially available materials that include detailed instructions for administration and scoring, as well as norm-referenced scores. Lahey's scheme for analyzing story macrostructure appears in Box 11-10. Hughes, McGillivray, and Schmidek (1997), Johnston (1982), McCabe and Rollins (1994), and Peterson and McCabe (1983) provided additional examples. Westby (2005) proposed a decision-tree structure for assessing the maturity of narrative organization and provided detailed instructions for assigning narrative stage using this method. Her decision tree appears in Figure 11-8. We also looked at the scheme based on Klecan-Aker and Kelty (1990) and Paul, Laszlo, and McFarland's (1992) adaptation of Applebee's (1978) narrative stages in Box 10-3. This method can also be used to rate the maturity of narrative organization. A modification of the simplified method of story macrostructure assessment, developed specifically for use with Mayer's Frog stories was used in a study by Norbury and Bishop (2003) and appears in Figure 11-9.

BOX 11-10 **Levels of Narrative Development**

Additive Chain

Propositions in the text are essentially independent so that they can be moved around within the text without changing the meaning. For narratives at this level, the following questions can be asked:

Was there more than a listing?
Were there any actions?
Was there a theme such as a repetition of an action, person, or setting?
Did some of the propositions describe a person or place?

Temporal Chain

Some of the propositions are sequentially related, so rearranging them would change the order of events in the story, but there is no cause-effect relation among them.

Causal Chain

A problem is described to which other propositions are causally related by enabling or causing other states or events. There is only one such unit in the story. For narratives at this level, the following questions should be asked:

Was the story a statement of a problem and some aspect of consequence with much information omitted, such as plans, goals, and resolution?
Was the causal chain automatic and not related to goals or plans?
Was the causal chain free of an obstacle between the problem and resolution?
Did an obstacle intervene in the process of trying to reach a goal?

Multiple Causal Chain

The story includes more than one causal chain or episode. For narratives at this level, the following questions should be asked:

Were the episodes related in an additive or temporal fashion, but not causally linked?
Did any of the episodes provide the cause, effect, or motivation for another episode?

For Stories at the Causal Chain Level or Above, Note Subcategories Contained in the Story

Initiating event or complication
Setting
Reaction (plans, goals of characters)
Internal response (changes of state or thought of characters)
Attempt (to solve the problem posed in the initiating event)
Consequence or resolution (achievement of characters' goals)

Adapted from Lahey, M. (1988). *Language disorders and language development*. New York: Macmillan Publishing.

McFadden and Gillam (1996) also provide a scheme for measuring overall narrative quality, using a set of rubrics and anchor stories. They reported that this scheme correlated moderately well with other text-level measures of narrative maturity. Their rubrics appear in Box 11-11. Hughes, McGillivray, and Schmidek (1997) suggest developing local anchor stories by collecting narratives from children with a range of abilities and grade levels in a particular school. The clinician can then meet with teachers to rate sets of stories and identify weak, adequate, good, and strong stories for each grade level. These collaboratively established anchor stories can serve as a basis for narrative assessment.

Regardless of which scheme we use, the assessment of narrative macrostructure is intended to tell us whether a student can produce narratives that include the major elements of a story grammar, all of which would be expected in stories of children of school age. When assessment indicates that story macrostructures are less than complete, we want to include narrative structure development as part of the intervention program. Westby (2005) advocated addressing this area by using stories that exemplify macrostructures at the level above the client's current story structure level. We'll look at the kinds of intervention activities this might entail in the next chapter.

Cohesion in Narrative. Cohesive ties are linguistic markers that bind sentences together to make them an integrated discourse unit rather than a series of unrelated utterances. Markers used for this purpose include pronouns; conjunctions; conjunctive adverbs (*nevertheless, on the other hand*); ellipsis (deleting redundant information); and the definite article *the.* Cain (2003) found there were significant differences in cohesion abilities

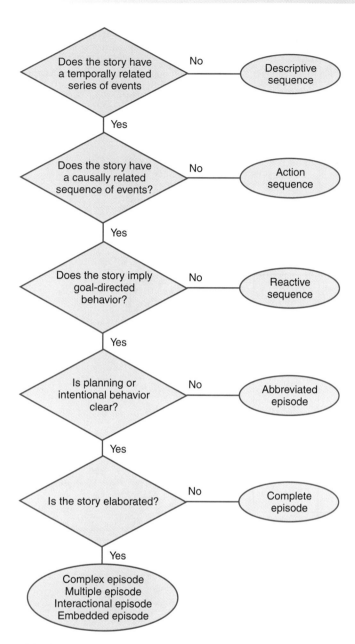

FIGURE 11-8 ✦ Story grammar decision tree. (Used with permission from Westby, C. [2005]. Assessing and remediating text comprehension problems [pp. 157-232]. In H. Catts and A. Kamhi (Eds.). *Language and Reading Disabilities, 2nd Edition*. Boston: Allyn & Bacon [p. 181].)

between students with LLD and those with normal achievement. Liles (1985) provided a detailed system for scoring cohesion in narrative samples, based on Halliday and Hasan's (1976) taxonomy. She defined cohesive markers as linguistic forms whose meanings cannot be interpreted without reference to information outside the sentence or clause in which the marker occurs. Cohesive markers signal listeners to "search" outside the sentence to complete its meaning. For clinical purposes, her system can be adapted, using the guidelines in Box 11-12. Beliavsky (2003) reported that kindergarten children showed up to 40% inappropriate or ambiguous use of cohesion in stories, but by first grade these levels had dropped to below 15%, and remained similar through the fourth grade. These findings, in conjunction with those reported by Paul, Hernandez, Taylor, and Johnson (1996) suggest that grade school children who produce narratives with fewer than 70% complete cohesive ties could be considered as having difficulty in producing a cohesive text. Remedial activities that focus on linking propositions in discourse with complete cohesive markers would be a way to address this deficit.

Story "Sparkle". What if an older elementary school student with LLD produces stories with adequate macrostructure and cohesion, yet we still get the feeling that the stories are not quite all they should be? Good stories contain more than just complete episodes and cohesive ties; they have what Peterson and McCabe (1983) call "sparkle." Several elements contribute to the degree to which a narrative has "sparkle": the richness of the vocabulary, the complexity of the episodes in the story, the creation of a "high point" to stress the story's climax, and the use of a literate language style. We only want to assess these aspects if narrative macrostructure and cohesion are found to be adequate, yet the older client's stories still seem lacking in some way. If deficits in macrostructure and cohesion are identified, it will not be necessary to carry the assessment further, since these more basic elements of story generation need to be addressed before we make any attempt to add "sparkle" to the student's stories.

Greenhalgh and Strong (2001) reported that simply counting the number of different words in a child's narrative did not provide a valid measure of lexical richness. This trait can be measured, however, by looking at the number of *unusual* words a child produces within a sample. Paul, Hernandez, Taylor, and Johnson, (1996) used the number of words not found on the Wepman and Hass (1969) list of the 500 most common words in the speech of 6-year-olds as a measure of lexical richness. This list appears in Appendix 11-2. To compute lexical richness, the clinician merely checks the words in the client's story against the words on the list. Any word that does not appear on the list in Appendix 11-2 is noted, and the number of words not on the list in the child's narrative production is counted. Paul, Laszlo, and McFarland (1992) used this measure to assess the lexical diversity of the stories of primary-grade children with normal and delayed language development and found the measure to reliably distinguish between the two groups. They reported that stories of kindergarten students with normal language abilities contained an average of 15 (±6) words not on the Wepman and Hass list. Students who use fewer than nine words not on the list, then, could be seen to be displaying a less-than-normally diverse vocabulary in storytelling. Miller (2006) developed a measure of vocabulary richness specifically for Mayer's *Frog* stories that can be computed using the SALT program for stories told in either English or Spanish. A reference database specific to this analysis is also available from the SALT program (http://www.languageanalysislab.com/).

Although we know that children begin using true narratives at 5 to 7 years of age, narrative development is by no means

	Definition	Example	Potential points	Normal range for 8 to 10 year old with typical development	Points earned
Global structure Initiating event	Problem that provides motivation for story	Boy wants to catch frog	1 for mention of characters 1 for problem	1.7-1.9	
Attempts	Things characters do to solve the initial problem	Boy attempts to catch frog with net; catches his dog by mistake	1 for each attempt reported	1.6-1.8	
Resolution	Satisfactory end to story that resolves initial problem	Frog follows boy home; he's happy when they're together	1 for mention of intention of action 1 for feelings of character	1.2-1.4	
Local structure Length	Total number of sentences in child's story	The boy went to the pond.	One point for each sentence	25-48	
Syntax	1. Number of complex sentences in story	Subordinate clauses (*When the boy saw the frog, he ran toward it.*) Complement clauses (*The boy wished he could catch the frog.*) Verb complements (*The boy was trying to catch the frog*). Full passive sentences (*The dog was caught by the net.*)	One point for each complex sentence	2.3-8.8	
	2. Number of tense marking errors	He look_in the water	One point for each error	0-1	
Semantics	Number of pieces of relevant information provided	1. Boys goes to pond 2. Boy's dog goes along	One point for each proposition	40-55	
Cohesion	Use of ambiguous pronouns	The boy and the frog looked at each other. *He* was mad.	One point for each ambiguous pronoun	0-3	
Mental state verbs	Use of verbs to describe thinking or talking	*Think, know, remember, forget, say, tell*	One point per mental verb	4.3-15.4	
Emotional terms	Use of words to describe emotions or internal states	The boy was sad.	One point per emotion term	0-3.6	

FIGURE 11-9 ✦ Narrative assessment scoresheet adapted from Norbury and Bishop (2003), using Mayer's (1967) *A Boy, a Dog, and a Frog.* (Adapted from Norbury and Bishop, 2003.)

complete at this age. There are two ways in which narratives change during these years. The first has to do with the complexity of the episodes within the story. Hughes, McGillivray, and Schmidek (1997) identified the following four levels of episode complexity beyond the basic true narrative (Table 11-9):

▶ *Multiple episodes.* More than one complete episode, each of which contains an initiating event, action, consequence, and reaction, is included in the story. For example, a child might tell a story about a trip to the doctor, which is preceded by a story of how he got sick.

▶ *Complex episodes.* These contain obstacles that complicate the solution or the main character's ability to carry out the plan developed in the story. For example, a girl might tell a story about how she wanted to get a horse, made a plan to earn the necessary money, met with opposition from her parents, but managed to overcome the opposition and achieve her goal.

▶ *Embedded episodes.* One episode occurs within another in the story. For example, a story about how a bride found her ideal wedding dress might have the story of how she met her groom embedded within it.

▶ *Interactive episodes.* The narrative tells the story from two different points of view. For example, the story of how the bride and groom met is told separately from each participant's perspective.

▶ The second change in narrative structure involves the inclusion of an increasingly elaborated high point, or climax to the story. McCabe (1995) suggested using high point analysis to look at these higher-level elaborations in the stories of school-age children. Table 11-10 defines several aspects of high point analysis.

The final aspect of story sparkle refers to the sophistication of linguistic forms used to tell the story. Westby (2005) identified four elements that provide an index of literary language

BOX 11-11   Scoring Rubrics for Narratives

Weak: Narrative consists of descriptions and poorly organized, uninteresting stories.

Adequate: Stories take one of four forms:

An account of events without a high point or climax.

A minimal narrative without elaboration.

A story without a resolution.

A confusing narrative with some strong descriptive elements.

Good: Narratives are captivating stories that contain problems and resolutions, but they may contain organizational weaknesses.

Strong: Narratives are easily understood and contain clear, integrated story lines; elaboration; interesting word choices; and some captivating features, such as a climax or plot twist or compelling personal voice.

Adapted from McFadden, T., & Gillam, R. (1996). An examination of the quality of narratives produced by children with language disorders. *Language, Speech, and Hearing Services in Schools, 27,* 48-56.

---

style in narratives. These are given in Box 11-13. Each element that appears in the story sample can be counted, and any of the four that appear rarely or not at all can be targeted for attention in the intervention program. Greenhalg and Strong (2001) found that measures of conjunctions and elaborated noun phrases differentiated children with LI from those with typical language. The values for literate language items seen in the narratives of typically developing children between 7 and 10 years of age appear in Table 11-11. These values suggest that students who produce fewer than the lower limit of these ranges should be considered to be using few literate language markers. It is important to note, though, that in elementary students some of these markers are used relatively rarely.

Why not try your hand at some narrative analysis? Use the narrative sample in Box 11-14, which was collected from a first grader, using Renfrew's (1991) story retelling task. Use the criteria in Box 10-3, Box 11-1, or Figure 11-8 to assess narrative macrostructure. Use Box 11-12 to guide a cohesion assessment. Assess "sparkle" by listing and counting the number of words in the story that are not on the Wepman-Hass list of the 500 most common words in children's speech (listed in Appendix 11-2). Also look for literary language style devices by counting the number of features listed in Box 11-13. Evaluate each aspect of this client's narrative and decide whether you would include

BOX 11-12   A Procedure for Scoring Cohesive Adequacy in Narrative Samples

1. Transcribe the narrative sample.
2. Read through the transcript once.
3. Read the transcript again. This time, underline each pronoun, conjunction, conjunctive adverb, elliptical utterance, or article that refers to information *outside* the sentence or clause in which it is used.

Examples

Pronoun: "There's a frog. *He* jumps off the lily pad."

Conjunction: "The frog wants to follow the boy, *but* the boy goes too fast."

Conjunctive adverb: "The frog was lonesome. *Still,* he wouldn't let the boy catch him."

Elliptical utterance: "The boy tried to catch the frog, but he couldn't" ("*catch the frog*" is deleted).

Article: "A frog was in the pond. And a boy wanted to catch *the* frog."

4. For each tie, make a judgment as to whether it is complete.

Complete ties are those that refer to information outside the sentence or clause that is easily found and is unambiguous.

Example

"The frog wanted to go with the boy and his dog. So *he* followed *them*."

Incomplete ties are those that refer to information that is not provided or missing from the text, or to information that is ambiguous.

Examples

Missing: "The frog was hopping. Then he tripped over *it*."

Ambiguous: "The boy was chasing the dog and the dog was chasing the frog. And *he* caught *him*."

5. Count the total number of cohesive markers in the sample. Then count the number of complete ties. Divide the number of complete ties by the total number of cohesive markers. If this proportion is less than 70%, a cohesive deficit can be inferred.

Adapted from Liles, B. (1985). Cohesion in the narratives of normal and language-disordered children. *Journal of Speech and Hearing Research, 28,* 123-133.

TABLE 11-9	A Summary of Later Stages of Narrative Development

DEVELOPMENTAL LEVEL (YR)	HIGH POINT ANALYSIS LEVEL	NARRATIVE LEVEL	STORY STRUCTURE
6	Beginning use of high point resolutions	True narrative	Mostly abbreviated episodes
7–8	Use of introducers and codas		Mostly complete episodes, including goals, internal motivations, and reactions
11		Complex narratives	Multiple episodes Complex episodes
13	Stories have elaborated high points, including several high point elements		Embedded episodes Interactive episodes

Adapted from Hughes, D., McGillivray, L., & Schmidek, M. (1997). *Guide to narrative language.* Eau Claire, WI: Thinking Publications.

TABLE 11-10	Group Mean and Standard Deviation Values for Literate Language Use by 7- to 10-Year-Olds with Typical Development

LITERATE LANGUAGE FORM	MEAN (AND SD) PER T-UNIT	NO. TO BE EXPECTED/50 T-UNIT SAMPLE*
Conjunctions	0.24 (0.2)	2–22
Elaborated noun phrases	0.17 (0.1)	3–13
Mental and linguistic verbs	0.11 (0.10)	1–10
Adverbs	0.008 (0.02)	0–2

*Based on multiplying ± 1 SD from mean values $\times$ 50 T-units.
Adapted from Greenhalgh, K., & Strong, C. (2001). Literate language features in spoken narratives of children with typical language and children with language impairments. *Language, Speech and Hearing Services in Schools, 32,* 114-135.

narrative activities in your intervention program. You'll find my evaluation of the story in Appendix 11-3. Some additional sources for narrative assessment ideas include Gillam, McFadden, and van Kleeck (1995), Strong (1998), Naremore, Densmore, and Harman (1995), and Scott and Windsor (2000).

Assessing the "Metas"

Metalinguistic Awareness

We've talked at length about the importance of metalinguistic awareness in both classroom discourse and the acquisition of literacy. Schuele and van Kleeck (1987) discussed several aspects of metalinguistic awareness that contribute to school success. These include consciousness of words, ability to segment words into sentences, and phonological awareness. Kamhi (1987) pointed out some additional metalinguistic skills of the L4L period. These are making judgments about language form and content (as in editing), analyzing language into linguistic units (such as analyzing words into syllables), manipulating these units (as in producing pig Latin), and understanding and producing language play (such as riddles, puns, and rhymes). Wallach and Miller (1988) and Nelson (1998) discussed the role of metapragmatic abilities: the ability to talk about appropriate uses of language in social situations.

We've already looked at some methods of assessing phonological awareness. These skills will be important to assess, particularly in children who are having trouble learning to read. Other aspects of metalinguistic awareness can be assessed simply by asking questions such as those in Box 11-15, drawn from Westby (2005).

Curriculum-based assessment (Nelson, 1998) can be particularly useful for assessing metalinguistic skills in the context of editing. The clinician can work with a client in the classroom to edit a writing assignment. Metalinguistic abilities to recognize and correct errors in the student's own writing can be clearly seen in this context. Deficits identified can be addressed in intervention activities that focus on editing activities.

Metapragmatic skills can be assessed in conversation with the client about rules for various discourse contexts. We might ask the student how the rules for asking for something politely differ from the rules for asking for something during an argument. It may be especially important to assess a student's awareness of the interactional expectations of the classroom. Difficulty with this kind of activity may suggest a need for the clinician to exert extra effort to make the "hidden curriculum" explicit for the client and to talk explicitly about how classroom discourse differs from that in other settings. Creaghead and Tattershall (1991) suggested questions such as those in Box 11-16 to assess metapragmatic knowledge of classroom discourse rules.

BOX 11-13	**Elements of Literary Language Style**

Conjunctions. *And* and *then* are excluded. Other conjunctions, such as (but not limited to) *when, since, so, as a result, if, until, however, before, after, while, because, therefore, however, although,* etc., are counted.

Elaborated noun phrases. Count noun phrases with more than two modifiers preceding the noun *(the two big dogs)* or with qualifiers such as prepositional phrases and relative clauses following the noun *(the big dog in the pet store; the boy who has a fishnet).*

Mental and linguistic verbs. Count verbs that denote cognitive *(think, wish, know, forget)* or linguistic *(say, promise, report, exclaim)* processes.

Adverbs. Count all adverbs, but note especially those that code aspects of tone, attitude, and manner that would be conveyed by stress and intonation in conversation *(angrily, hotly, ominously, threateningly).*

Adapted from Westby, C. (1998). Communicative refinement in school age and adolescence. In W. Hayes & B. Shulman (Eds.). *Communication development: Foundations, processes, and clinical applications* (pp. 311-360). Baltimore, MD: Williams & Wilkins.

If a student in the L4L stage has difficulty with these kinds of metalinguistic activities, a metalinguistic component should be a strong part of the intervention program. Metalinguistic activities are useful, though, for all students in the L4L stage. Metalinguistic skill is learned, remember, primarily through interactions that focus on communication itself and that use literate language styles. Many children with normal basic language skills have limited experience with metalinguistic awareness, so even children without identified language disorders can learn from these activities. Metalinguistic activities make especially good classroom collaborative lessons, because students with and without basic language deficits can benefit from them. We'll discuss some ideas for metalinguistic intervention activities in the next chapter.

Metacognitive Skills. Westby (2005) identified two aspects of metacognitive skills:

▶ *Self-regulation*: the ability to plan, organize and execute actions efficiently using consciously selected strategies.

▶ *Self-assessment*: understanding of the thinking process and the ability to consciously consider and reflect on knowledge and understanding of one's self and others.

Both of these abilities represent great stumbling blocks for many students with LLD, and they represent an area in which to consider assessment and intervention activities for students with LLD. Informal assessment of these abilities can often be accomplished in curriculum - based activities, which we will discuss shortly. Another method of assessing these skills is through activities like those used in Theory of Mind research (Baron-Cohen, 2000; Wellman, 1985). Activities based on this

TABLE 11-11	**Aspects of High Point Analysis**

HIGH POINT ELEMENT	DESCRIPTION	EXAMPLE
Introducer	Occurs at beginning; gives an overview of the story; serves to get listener's attention.	"You'll never guess what happened on my block last night!"
Orientation	Gives background and setting information.	"My buddy Malcolm, him and me were sittin' around on the stoop after dinner."
Complicating action	Shows how action proceeds to the high point.	"We didn't know it, but something had scared his dog, and it came rushing up to where we were and started barking like crazy at me."
Evaluation	Gives an assessment or emotional comment about the high point.	"I was really scared because he looked like he might not stop. He was growling and coming closer. Malcolm yelled for me to take off my red cap. I did, and all of a sudden he got quiet."
Resolution	Finishes off the event, and resolves any complications.	"He got the dog calmed down and explained that when the dog was upset, he went crazy if he saw someone wearing something red, because once a man in a red uniform had hit him with a stick."
Coda	Closes the story and connects the ending to the present context.	"I was real glad I'd gotten my cap off in time."

Adapted from McCabe, A. (1995). Evaluating narrative discourse skills. In K. Cole, P. Dale, & D. Thal (Eds.). *Assessment of communication and language* (pp. 121-141). Baltimore, MD: Paul H. Brookes; Hughes, D., McGillivray, L., & Schmidek, M. (1997). *Guide to narrative language.* Eau Claire, WI: Thinking Publications.

BOX 11-14	Narrative Sample from Story Retelling Task from a First Grader

T1: Once there was a man who was driving a bus.

T2: And the bus ran away.

T3: And the bus went on to the grass.

T4: But the bus and the train made faces at each other.

T5: And they couldn't because the train went in a tunnel and into a town.

T6: And then they went into the country and jumped over a fence and went up a hill.

T7: And it couldn't find its brakes because it didn't know how to.

T8: And it fell into the water.

T9: And then the owner came and called a crane to pull it out.

T10: And then they drove away.

Adapted from Renfrew, C. (1991). *The bus story: A test of continuous speech* (ed. 2) Old Headington, Oxford, England: C. Renfrew.

BOX 11-15	Sample Questions for Assessing Metalinguistic Skills

Do you know what a word is? Tell me three words.

I'm going to say a sentence. You tell me how many words are in it.

I've written a sentence on this paper. Can you circle the first word in it? The last word? How many words are in this sentence?

Max hates grapes, but he hates apples. Does that make sense? Why not?

How many syllables are in these words? Clap once for each syllable.

I'm going to say some things, and I want you to tell me whether each is a word or not:

    car

    cag

    if

    bune

    this

    girl

    an

    yours

    trup

I'm going to say some words, and I want you to tell me if they are long words or short words, and tell me why:

    Alligator (long word, long referent)

    Spaghetti (long word, long referent)

    Train (short word, long referent)

    Banana (long word, long referent)

    Hose (short word, long referent)

    Toe (short word, short referent)

    Fly (short word, short referent)

Do you know any jokes? Tell me one. I don't get it. Why is that funny?

What does *run* mean? Can it mean anything else?

Adapted from Westby, C. (1998a). Communicative refinement in school age and adolescence. In W. Hayes & B. Shulman (Eds.). *Communication development: Foundations, processes, and clinical applications* (pp. 311-360). Baltimore, MD: Williams & Wilkins; Westby, C. (2005). Assessing and facilitating text comprehension problems. In H. Catts & A. Kahmi (Eds.) *Language and reading disabilities* (2nd ed., pp. 157-232). Boston: Allyn & Bacon.

research are provided in Table 11-12, which are passed by 80% of typically developing children at age 7. The Developmental Evaluation of Language Variation (DELV; Seymour et al., 2003) also has a theory of mind narrative task as part of its Pragmatics subtest.

Barrier games can be used to assess self-appraisal of comprehension, as discussed earlier. The clinician can give purposefully unclear messages or can mumble essential parts of the message to see whether the student asks for clarification. The peer interaction activity, with the normally developing peer providing instructions for playing a game or doing a project, also can give us a glimpse at the ability of a client to monitor his understanding and ability to complete a task. Teacher interviews also can supply information on a student's metacognitive abilities. We can ask the teacher whether students ask appropriate questions about assignments, whether they give a signal when they have difficulty understanding, and how the teacher knows that students do not understand a direction or discussion. Think-aloud protocols are another way to get a window on the child's cognitive process. Here we present a children with a task and ask them to "think out loud" for us as they complete it, saying aloud each step in the completion of the task. We will discuss think-aloud methods more fully under dynamic and curriculum-based assessment. We'll discuss intervention techniques for these abilities in the next chapter.

CURRICULUM-BASED LANGUAGE ASSESSMENT

Nelson and Van Meter (2002) and Norris and Hoffman (1993) advocated using curriculum-based language assessment to observe how the student uses language in learning the curriculum of the classroom. Many of the criterion-referenced assessment techniques discussed in this chapter can be done in the context of curriculum-based assessment. The tools of this type of assessment include artifact analysis, onlooker observation, and dynamic assessment.

BOX 11-16	Suggestions for Assessing Metapragmatic Knowledge of Classroom Discourse Rules

"What is the most important thing you should always say in class?"

"How do you know when it's time for recess?"

"When is it OK to talk aloud without raising your hand in class?"

"When is it all right to ask the teacher a question?"

"What does your teacher say when she's angry?"

"What does your teacher do when it's time for a lesson to start?"

"What's the first thing you're supposed to do when school starts?"

"How do you know when your teacher is saying something really important?"

"How do you know when your teacher is making a joke?"

"What's the most important thing you should always do in school? What should you never do?"

"What's the last thing you should do at the end of the day before you leave school?"

Adapted from Creaghead, N., & Tattershall, S. (1991). Observation and assessment of classroom discourse skills. In C. Simon (Ed.), *Communication skills and classroom success* (pp. 105-134). San Diego, CA: College-Hill Press.

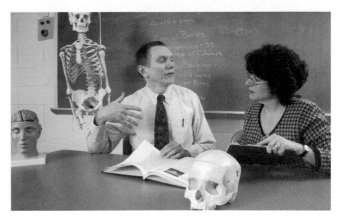

Collaborative intervention involves learning about the demands of the curriculum.

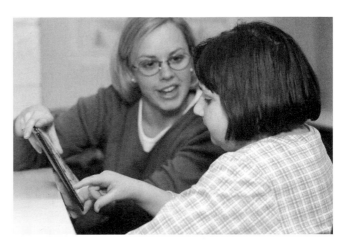

Assessment of school-age children includes curricular materials.

Artifact analysis examines products of the student's regular curricular activities, such as homework assignments, written work done in class, or projects completed independently or in cooperative learning groups. The clinician can look at these materials for evidence of various communicative skills, such as level of narrative development, literate language style, and use of cohesion. This analysis also can be used to document change in an intervention program. The advantage of this type of assessment is that it provides a means of *functional assessment*—a way to look at how the student uses communication in real,

TABLE 11-12	Theory of Mind Assessments for Metacognitive Skills

TASK	PROCEDURE
Know-remember	Child sees item hidden in one of two containers; after brief delay child is asked to find item, and is asked, "Did you know where it was? Did you guess where it was? Did you remember where it was?"
Guess	Child does not see where item is hidden, but must make a choice between two containers to find it. Child is asked, "Did you know where it was? Did you guess where it was? Did you remember where it was?"
Forget	Child watches toy who sees his coat put in one of two closets and is asked, "Does he know were his coat is? Why do you say he knows?" Later the character comes back to get his coat and looks in the wrong closet. Child is asked, "Did he know where his coat was? Did he remember? Did he forget? Why do you say he forgot?"

Adapted from Baron-Cohen, S. (2000). Theory of mind and autism: A fifteen year review. In S. Baron-Cohen, H. Tager-Flusberg, & D. J. Cohen (Eds.). *Understanding other minds: Perspectives from developmental cognitive neuroscience* (pp. 1-20). Oxford University Press: Wellman, H. (1985). The origins of metacognition. In D. Forrest-Pressley, G. MacKinnon, & T. Waller (Eds.). *Metacognition, cognition and human performance* (pp. 1-31). Orlando: Academic Press.

relevant situations. Artifact analysis done for this purpose is often referred to as *portfolio assessment*. Kratcoski (1998) discussed several ways we can use portfolio assessment as a tool for examining functional communication in school settings. She suggested collecting the following artifacts to include in a student's portfolio:

▶ Initial referral forms
▶ Language samples
▶ Narrative samples
▶ Observation notes
▶ Samples of student work that address questions such as:
  ▶ What are the language demands of this assignment?
  ▶ How did the student meet these demands?
  ▶ What are the strengths/needs demonstrated in the assignment?
  ▶ What strategies are evident in the student's approach to the task?
  ▶ Teacher interviews
  ▶ Student interviews
  ▶ Parent interviews
  ▶ Test results

Often, students are encouraged to make their own choices of their best samples to be included in the portfolio. The student and teacher or clinician evaluate the collected work together, using it to document changes in the student's work over the course of the intervention period. The artifacts are evaluated to identify areas in which goals have been met or work has substantially improved and to look at areas that need additional attention in the next cycle of intervention.

Onlooker observation involves watching, from a distance, as the student participates in classroom activities. Onlooker observation is valuable, for example, for assessing adherence to classroom discourse rules or use of communicative intentions. The running record is one type of onlooker observation.

Norris and Hoffman (1993) suggested using onlooker obser-vation not only to assess the student's performance in the class-room, but also to evaluate the demands that the classroom situa-tion places on the student. In doing this kind of evaluation, we can apply a Systems model (that is, the assessment could address changing both the student and the classroom environment). It may result in working to improve the student's participation in the classroom discourse and working with the teacher to modify the style of the discourse to make it more accessible to the student with LLD. Norris and Hoffman suggested a series of questions to use in guiding this onlooker assessment of classroom discourse. An adaptation of their scheme appears in Box 11-17.

DYNAMIC ASSESSMENT

In the context of curriculum-based assessment, this involves the clinician's working side by side with a student, using scaffolding techniques to facilitate the student's participation in a classroom activity. While doing so, the clinician observes whether the student succeeds more fully with the scaffolding than without it. If the student does better with a little help from the clinician, then the skill being facilitated would be seen as within the student's zone of proximal development, one that the student is ready to learn in an intervention program. Elliot (2003) argued that the primary purpose of dynamic assessment should be the identification of strategies that will help the child to succeed in the curriculum. Peña (1996) discussed a variety of dynamic language assessment methods that can be adapted for participant observation in the classroom. These include the following:

▶ *Diagnostic teaching.* A child is given a difficult task, then the clinician gives contextual support and cues. The clinician observes how the child responds to the cues; how much support, context, or prompting is needed to elicit the desired response. This information is used to develop a remedial plan.

BOX 11-17	**Questions for Guiding an Onlooker Assessment of Classroom Discourse for Students with LLD**

Are the objects and events discussed present (contextualized) or absent (decontextualized)?
How well does the student use the contextual support that is present?
Does the teacher provide more contextual support when the student fails to respond correctly?
Does the teacher associate information presented with the student's own experiences if the student fails to respond correctly?
How much social support is given to the student within the class?
How familiar are topics discussed in class?
How much abstraction is demanded of students in class discussions?
Is there a discrepancy between the level of abstraction of teacher's questions (e.g., "What are the three stages in the life cycle of an insect?" Question requires answer at an abstract level.) and the student's remarks (e.g., "I caught a bug once and it died." Comment limited to personal experience.).
What kinds and how much assistance are needed to increase the level of sophistication of the student's response?
Do the student's responses show disruptions (hesitations, pauses, false starts, word-finding problems) that indicate difficulty in responding at the level required?

Adapted from Norris, J., & Hoffman, P. (1993). *Whole-language intervention for school-age children.* San Diego, CA: Singular.

For example, we might give the child a writing task. Once the student does it without help, we see how providing a picture cue helps or how using another student's work as an example improves performance. After trying several such supports, we would choose the most effective for our continued intervention with the student.

▶ *Successive cuing.* Several levels of cues are provided, and the clinician observes which is most effective. For example, in helping a student with word-finding difficulties acquire new words from the classroom curriculum, we might give the student a list to learn, then ask the student to produce the words in a cloze activity. When the student gets stuck, we could sometimes offer a semantic cue, sometimes a phonological one, sometimes both. We could then assess what cues helped most. The intervention program would then develop self-cuing strategies for these supports.

▶ *Mediated learning experience.* This approach involves helping the student invoke metacognitive strategies. Students are given a task, such as finding synonyms for words. They are given mediation that explains the goal of the task (e.g., "We want to be able to have lots of different words to use for describing objects, events, and feelings."). Students are given strategies for finding synonyms, such as categorization, and comparing words and their meanings. They then are asked to find synonyms independently for a new set of words. The clinician observes whether the student independently invokes the strategies taught in completing the task with the new words. An example of a think-aloud protocol that might be used in this way appears in Table 11-13.

CONSIDERATIONS FOR THE OLDER CLIENT AT THE L4L STAGE

Some adolescents and young adults with moderate to severe LLD may function at the L4L stage, with oral language commensurate with the early elementary grade levels and minimal reading or writing skills. For these students, assessment concerns are similar to those for younger students with LLD, but a few special considerations may be necessary. These students may not be participating in a regular curriculum and may be engaged in primarily vocational or independent-living programs. These students will probably already be identified as eligible for services,

---

TABLE 11-13	**An Example of Dynamic Assessment of Metacognition with a Think-Aloud Protocol**

Present student with task, such as reading a section of the classroom social studies textbook and answering the questions at the end.

PRESENT PROMPTS	OBSERVE STRATEGIES
What do you think this section will be about? How do you know?	Scans text. Looks at title, headings. Looks at pictures. Identifies words.
After student reads a portion, stop him and ask, Why did X (event) happen? Why do you think that? How could you find out if you don't know?	Prediction based on prior knowledge Prediction based on cues in text Rereads to find answer Looks ahead to find answer in text
Choose a word that is likely to be unfamiliar to student. What do you think *mesa* means here? How could you tell?	Uses contextual cues Suggests using dictionary Suggests teacher or other resource Relates to personal experience
Select a point that is not stated explicitly. Why do you think the soldiers retreated to the mesa? Why did you decide that?	Infers based on text cues Infers based on prior knowledge Relates personal experience Draws analogy Rereads
Direct student to answer questions about section. What is your plan for answering the questions? What will you do if you don't know an answer? Do you think all the answers will be found in what you read?	Provides a sequence of actions Attempts to integrate information from text, illustrations, etc. Refers to differences between fact and opinion Refers to prior knowledge

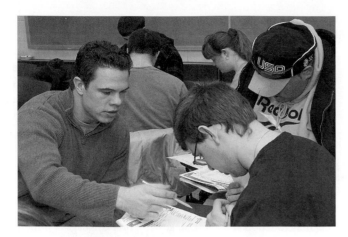

Curriculum-based assessment is appropriate for adolescents at the L4L stage.

so very little if any standardized testing is needed. Most assessment methods will be observational or criterion-referenced.

For these older clients, using chronological age-appropriate materials and evaluating functional communicative needs are the paramount assessment concerns, just as they were for adolescents with developing language. When we do criterion-referenced or observational assessments for the older, moderately to severely impaired client, we want to use situations and props that are fitting for a person of this age, such as materials from the client's occupational training program or objects from self-care and daily living activities that the client is learning to perform independently, or from leisure activities in which the client likes to engage.

There also may be some "fine points" of the language system, such as complex sentences or mature narratives that the young adult with moderate to severe impairment will never master. When this is the case, we would not want to withhold teaching other important skills that are usually thought of as more advanced than these, just as we would not do so for clients with developing language. McCormick (1997a) reminds us that the premises of ecological assessment include the following:

▶ There are no minimal criteria or prerequisites for communication intervention. Any student with difficulty communicating can benefit from instruction and should have the opportunity to participate in classroom and social interactions. This is true regardless of whether the student's IQ is within or below the normal range.

▶ The focus of intervention should be providing whatever supports students need to participate in school and other important environments.

Ecological inventories such as those used for adolescents with developing language can also help us with older clients at the L4L stage to determine what communicative skills are needed to succeed in the client's daily environments. For some children, these environments will be regular classrooms, in which they are included for some or all of their instruction. Elksnin and Elksnin (2001) discussed several elements that should be used in ecological assessment:

▶ *Observation*: The student is observed in relevant environments. These might include the inclusion classroom, vocational training setting, leisure settings, etc. Observation is used to identify the essential communication skills for the environments in which the student will need to function. Elksnin and Elksnin (2001), for example, found that for one of their students to succeed in a work setting, he needed to be able to carry on friendly conversations with co-workers in the break room. Goals identified this way become part of the student's communication program.

▶ *Interviews*: Teachers, aides, parents, counselors, and potential employers can be interviewed to identify the communication skills necessary for particular settings, and to determine gaps between the student's current communication level and the needs of the settings in which he will function. As always, an interview should be planned in advance, with a recording form constructed by the clinician to record information. Elksnin and Elksnin (2001) also suggest doing "social autopsies," by interviewing the student after social encounters in order to analyze events and determine assistance they may need to be more successful in the future.

▶ *Role play*: Students can be asked to act out a series of communication situations to determine how they might behave in settings that may be hard to observe (such as disputes) or on communication problems they have been working on in intervention. Before performing the role play, it is helpful to ask the student to rehearse the steps verbally.

McCormick (2003) outlined the steps we can use in the process of creating an ecological assessment, both for inclusion in regular educational settings, as well as for more community-referenced environments. These are summarized in Table 11-14.

For clients with very few reading and writing skills, for example, we might use an ecological inventory to determine what their literacy needs are in school, work, or independent living. These skills could be targeted even if reading and writing skills in general are at very low levels. Similarly, an ecological inventory of the client's school or work setting could be done to determine the discourse situations and rules the client must deal with on a day-to-day basis. These particular discourse needs could be addressed in the intervention program.

For students using augmentative or alternative communication (AAC) devices, the development of literacy continues to be an especially important goal, since AAC devices that use some form of the printed word provide the most viable means of communication for these students. Fallon, Light, McNaughton, Drager, and Hammer (2004) have shown that these students can acquire literacy skills, and such skills make an important contribution to their ability to communicate with the broadest range of interlocutors. Light and McNaughton (1993) have suggested that there are two crucial pieces to literacy programs for AAC students at the L4L level: developing appropriate expectations and fostering functional literacy.

Light and McNaughton argued that expectations for literacy in this group should be positive but realistic. Both parents and teachers should be given information on emerging literacy and the importance of reading and writing for these students.

TABLE 11-14	**Steps in the Process of Ecological Assessment**

STEP	PROCEDURES	OUTCOME
1. Get to know the child.	Interview parents to learn about case history, their fears and dreams, the student's strengths and needs; observe student in classroom and other relevant settings.	Picture of student's strengths, needs, and preferences; a vision statement
2. List activities and routines in a typical day in this setting.	Compile the student's weekly schedule, observe the client in several environments, determine demands of each.	Schedule of weekly activities; a prioritized list of environments and their requirements
3. State goals, and list key activities/routines and set priorities among them.	Identify broad goals; then list 3 or 4 activities or routines that need to be mastered in order to accomplish each goal.	List of broad goals for 3–5 priority activities
4. Observe and record behaviors of typical participants or conduct interviews to determine the expectations of each activity.	Do observations and interviews to determine component skills and concepts for each activity.	List of what typical students do to accomplish each activity
5. Observe the student in each activity.	Record observations and describe what the client currently does in the activity—the degree to which he or she shows the skills necessary for participation.	Description of student's present level of performance
6. Compare the student's behavior to expectations. Note discrepancies.	Compare client's performance in each activity to expectations/desired performance.	Description of the behaviors/skills student needs to learn to participate in each priority activity
7. Identify the language/communication skills needed to achieve expectations.	Identify reasons why activities are not successfully performed (e.g., lack of skills, knowledge, strategies; interfering behaviors; instructional problem; environmental obstacles).	List of the language/communication skills student needs to learn and what may be interfering with current performance
8. Identify communication skills not currently demonstrated.	Give behavioral objectives for each activity.	List of instructional objectives for each goal above
9. Outline communication goals for each activity.	Identify physical and instructional modifications, adaptations, and supports needed. Determine an instructional focus for each objective.	List of needed modifications, adaptations, supports, and instructional objectives for each goal
10. Develop an IEP for these goals.	Plan who, when, and how each objective will be achieved.	List of environmental adaptations, resources, supports, and instructional priorities for each goal

Adapted from McCormick, L. (2003). Ecological assessment and planning. In L. McCormick, D. Loeb, & R. Schiefelbusch (Eds.). *Supporting children with communication difficulties in inclusive settings* (pp. 235-258). Boston: Allyn & Bacon.

Enlisting parents' help by providing emerging literacy activities to do at home is an important first step. Parents can be asked to read appropriate stories, newspaper articles, shopping lists, and so forth to clients. They can be urged to talk with clients about letters, words, writing, and the purpose of print. Teachers can be encouraged to label objects in the classroom with word cards, to display print in the classroom, and to talk about the functions of reading and writing with students. Both parents and teachers should be on the lookout for signs of interest and readiness on the part of clients for more formal, focused instruction in reading and writing. When students send signals that this interest is present—such as "reading" labels placed by teachers around the environment, attempting to write notes or lists, taking an interest in naming letters or words, asking questions about what signs say, or recognizing environmental print such as product labels or stop signs—more formal instruction can be initiated. The research of Fallon et al. (2004) and Blischak, Shah, Lombardino, and Chiarella (2004) suggests that traditional direct instruction that includes work on both oral language bases in vocabulary knowledge, as well as work on phonological awareness and guided practice in single word reading is effective with these students, as it is with typical children. Paul (1998) has reviewed literature showing that literacy development in children who use AAC benefits from the use of communication devices with voice output. Erickson, Koppenhaver, Yoder, and Nance (1997) report that voice output devices can benefit both literacy and general communication in these children. It is thought that these devices help their users match auditory images to intended meanings and improve their phonological awareness. This, as we know, is an important foundation for reading. If children have not yet had the opportunity to use voice output AAC devices when literacy emergence seems near, these opportunities should be provided, if at all possible. Procedures for fostering functional literacy in these students are discussed in more detail in Chapter 12.

■ Conclusions

Nick and Maria are just two of the kinds of students with LLD that you may encounter in the elementary school. They express their language and learning deficits somewhat differently, and they react emotionally or behaviorally to their difficulties in different ways. Assessing their needs and those of other students at the L4L stage is a somewhat different problem than it was for children at earlier language levels. With younger children, we were looking primarily at deficits in language form and meaning. With students in the L4L stage, we need to investigate how they process and use language in an important but unique communicative environment: that of the classroom. This means that assessment must, to a great extent, focus on that environment. It must attempt to discover errors and gaps in the child's language competence and also to look at mismatches and misperceptions reflected in the student's language performance in this environment. Finally, the clinician needs to look at how a student's oral-language processing and use may be affecting the ability to move beyond oral language to the new modalities so necessary for success in school: the acquisition of literacy and literate language.

Let's take Maria as our example this time and see how her clinician might develop an assessment plan to begin to answer these questions and move toward developing an intervention program.

When Mr. McMahon, the school's SLP, circulated a teacher referral form to all the third-, fourth-, and fifth-grade teachers, the third-grade teacher was eager to fill one out for Maria. Mr. McMahon reviewed the form and talked with Maria's teacher and parents to place Maria on the Student Success Team list, so accommodations might be made for her in class. He observed her during academic subjects, and noted that she did not actively contribute to group activities, and seemed to be lost on many of her assignments. He suggested the teacher try pairing her with a higher achieving classmate who would help her organize her work and make sure she understood the directions, as well as giving her extra time to complete assignments and respond to questions. After a month, Maria was continuing to have difficulty and to complain of stomachaches and so on. It was decided a full evaluation was necessary.

The school learning disability and reading specialists were part of the assessment team. They arranged a pre-assessment conference with the teacher and parents to discuss concerns and plan the assessment program. In addition, Mr. McMahon had a talk with Maria. He asked her how she was getting on in school and whether she had any trouble there. He explained that he would like to help her do better and have an easier time in school. At first she was resistant and sullen, but she warmed up after a while and agreed she would like to do better. Mr. McMahon told her about some of the things he would be doing with her and asked if she would agree to help him help her. She said she would, and they made a date to begin the assessment the following week.

Mr. McMahon developed the following plan for Maria's language evaluation:

▶ Review Medical and Educational History: Obtain the records from Maria's hospital stay following her accident. Note the nature and extent of her injuries, the length of her coma, and her rate of recovery. Study school records from before and after the accident. (She had had standardized achievement testing done in second grade before the accident and again after the accident when she repeated the grade.) This information can show where she had started out academically and what kind of regression, if any, took place.

▶ Standardized Testing to Establish Eligibility: *Clinical Evaluation of Language Fundamentals—4 (CELF—4)* (if Maria scores within normal range in all areas, give *Test of Problem Solving* or *Test of Word Finding*)

▶ Criterion-Referenced Assessments and Behavioral Observations to Establish Baseline Function and Identify Intervention Targets (to be done in the context of regular sessions once eligibility has been established and the student has begun an intervention program): 5-minute conversational speech sample to assess intelligibility, syntactic, errors, and word-finding problems

▶ Assess Phonological Awareness: *Lindamood Auditory Conceptualization Test—3*

▶ If results of the receptive-language sections on the CELF—4 indicate problems, use curriculum-based onlooker assessment of the student's receptive vocabulary and syntax during a time when the teacher is giving instructions to the class. If classroom problems are evident, look for any signs that Maria can monitor her comprehension. Probe further in criterion-referenced assessments, using vocabulary and sentences drawn from teacher's instructional language and textbook material. Again, look for metacognitive as well as comprehension problems. Use both decontextualized (e.g., judgment tasks) and contextualized probes, and look for use of comprehension strategies in the decontextualized examples. Because of history of traumatic brain injury (TBI), expect delayed responses and inconsistent performance. Give extra time to respond, and give items several times if responded to incorrectly at first. Because Maria may do better in the less-distracting atmosphere of an individual assessment, contrast performance observed in the classroom-based onlooker assessment with performance in the individual settings.

▶ Audiorecord a sample of speech using an interview format. Evaluate the sample for syntactic and morphological errors and complex sentence use. If complex sentences are few, probe for complex forms and conjunctions that don't appear in the sample, using elicited production techniques. Also check for presyntactic semantic relations expressed in the sample. Because of history of TBI, consider analyzing speech disruptions as well.

▶ Do another curriculum-based onlooker assessment in the classroom, during a class project or discussion. Keep a running record, and note Maria's use of advanced communicative intentions and adherence to classroom discourse rules. Because of TBI history, look carefully for difficulty in reading others' nonverbal cues, difficulty in integrating information received, difficulty knowing what aspect of a question needs to be answered, apparent lack of responsiveness that may result from information overload, difficulty in processing a series of directions, and reduced ability to use abstract language. If problems are evident, probe register variation in role-playing situations and presuppositional skills in barrier games. Use this information and that derived from the classroom observation to work with the teacher to develop a pragmatic intervention program to address classroom discourse problems.

▶ Collect a narrative sample by asking Maria to tell a story from a wordless picture book. Assess level of narrative macrostructure. If structure is immature, assess cohesion. If both areas are weak, address narrative skills in the intervention program.

▶ Assess metalinguistic skills using curriculum-based artifact assessment. Have Maria bring in a writing sample from class. Go over it together to edit it. Assess whether and how well Maria can attend to metalinguistics in editing. Assess metacognitive skills using dynamic participant observation in the classroom. This area may be of particular importance because of the history of traumatic injury.

▶ Mr. McMahon was able to establish Maria's eligibility for services based on her performance on the CELF—4 as well as her medical history. The family agreed to an IEP that involved direct services by Mr. McMahon and the reading specialist, with consultation from the learning disabilities teacher. Mr. McMahon spent the first 2 weeks of his program completing the assessment plan. When he had accomplished all the assessments, he felt he knew a good deal about Maria and her strengths and needs and also about what her teacher expected from her in the classroom. He felt in a good position to design an intervention program that would address her needs and help her to succeed in the academic environment.

STUDY GUIDE

I. Child and Family in the Assessment Process
   A. Discuss family-centered practice as it relates to the school-age child.
   B. What role should the client have in the assessment process?
   C. What is the role of a case manager in an assessment of a school-age child?

II. Identifying Students for Communication Assessment
   A. Discuss kindergarten screening. How is it best accomplished? What are its advantages and disadvantages?
   B. Discuss criteria for choosing a screening instrument for school-age children.
   C. Describe several methods of case finding for the SLP in an elementary school setting.

III. Using Standardized Tests in the L4L Stage
   A. For what purpose are standardized tests used in the L4L stage?
   B. Why can establishing eligibility sometimes be a problem for children at this stage?
   C. When should standardized tests of pragmatics be used?

IV. Criterion-Referenced Assessment and Behavioral Observation in the L4L Stage
   A. What aspects of phonology are part of the assessment of a child in the L4L stage?
   B. Discuss two methods of assessing phonological awareness.
   C. How can we assess receptive vocabulary using curriculum-based methods? Using other informal methods?
   D. Discuss some aspects of expressive vocabulary that can be assessed with criterion-referenced procedures.
   E. Outline a general strategy for assessing receptive syntax and morphology in the L4L stage.
   F. Discuss some decontextualized methods of criterion-referenced comprehension assessment that are appropriate for children with LLD.
   G. How can we assess comprehension strategies in the L4L period?
   H. Discuss contextualized comprehension assessment techniques.
   I. Outline a strategy for assessing expressive syntax and morphology from a speech sample in children with LLD.
   J. Describe how to assess speech disruptions in a spontaneous speech sample. Under what conditions would you do this analysis?
   K. Describe the areas of conversational speech that can be assessed in a pragmatic evaluation of students with LLD. Give methods for assessing each.
   L. What are some methods for eliciting narrative samples in students with LLD?
   M. What aspects of narrative can be assessed in children in the L4L period? Discuss procedures for assessing each.
   N. What contributes to "sparkle" in children's stories?
   O. Why and how would you assess metalinguistic awareness in students with LLD?
   P. How can metapragmatic awareness be assessed? Why would you want to assess it?
   Q. Discuss reasons and methods of assessing comprehension monitoring.
   R. What are the three types of curriculum-based assessment? Describe how you might use each one as one aspect of the assessment of a student with LLD.

V. Considerations for the Older Client at the L4L Stage
   A. Discuss issues and procedures for assessing communication in a young adult who functions at the L4L stage.
   B. How can ecological inventories be used for students at the L4L stage?
   C. Outline the steps in developing an ecological inventory for a student at the L4L stage.
   D. What are some important considerations for developing literacy in older students at the L4L stage who use AAC systems?

Percentage Complex Sentences

15/18 = 83.3%

Complex Sentence Types

Early Developing

Simple infinitive: T4, T6, T7, T10, T16

Full propositional clause: T9, T15, T16, T17, T18

Simple *wh-* clause: T9

Simple or multiple conjoining: T4, T7, T8, T11, T13, T14

Multiple embedding: T9, T10, T16, T18

Embedding and conjoining in one sentence: T4, T6, T7, T8, T17

Later Developing

Infinitive clause with subject different from main sentence: T10

Relative clause: T12, T18

Gerund clause: T4, T18

wh- infinitive clause: T8

Unmarked infinitive clause: T3

Conjunctions Used

and, when, because, why, that

Evaluation

Adequate use of complex sentence constructions; small repertoire of conjunctions.

Plan

Probe conjunction use with elicited production tasks (e.g., ask student to "make up a sentence with *if . . .*"). If difficulties appear in elicited as well as spontaneous production, develop intervention activities to facilitate production of sentences with early developing conjunctions that are missing from the repertoire, such as *if, so, but,* and *how.* Target more advanced conjunctions (e.g., *unless, until, before, after, although,* etc.) when earlier-developing ones are used spontaneously.

A	Better	Chair	Eat
About	Big	Child	Else
Across	Bird	Children	End
After	Bit	Chop	Even
Again	Black	Clean	Ever
Against	Blank	Climb	Every
All	Boat	Close	Everybody
Almost	Book	Clothes	Everyone
Along	Both	Coal	Everything
Already	Bought	Coat	Except
Always	Box	Cold	Eye
Am	Boy	Come	Face
An	Brick	Corn	Faint
And	Bridge	Couch	Fall
Animal	Bring	Could	Farm
Another	Broke	Country	Fast
Ant	Broken	Couple	Father
Anybody	Brother	Cross	Feel
Anything	Brought	Cry	Fell
Are	Bug	Cut	Field
Arm	Bump	Dad	Fight
Army	Burglar	Dance	Find
Around	Burn	Dark	Finish
As	Bury	Daughter	Fire
Ask	But	Day	First
Asleep	Buy	Dead	Fish
At	By	Dear	Five
Ate	Cabin	Decide	Fix
Away	Call	Did	Floor
Baby	Came	Die	Flower
Back	Can	Dinosaur	Food
Bad	Car	Do	For
Bag	Card	Doctor	Forest
Barn	Care	Does	Forget
Be	Carry	Dog	Forgot
Because	Castle	Doll	Found
Bed	Cat	Done	Four
Bedroom	Catch	Door	Friend
Been	Caught	Down	From
Before	Cause	Dry	Funny
Behind	Cave	Each	Game
Below	Cemetery	Early	Garden

Gave	If	More	Pull
Get	In	Morning	Put
Girl	Inside	Mother	Rain
Give	Instrument	Mountain	Ran
Go	Into	Move	Read
Gone	Is	Much	Ready
Good	It	Must	Real
Got	Its	Mustache	Really
Grandfather	Jump	My	Rest
Grandma	Just	Name	Ride
Grandmother	Keep	Near	Right
Grass	Kept	Never	River
Grave	Kid	New	Robber
Great	Kill	Next	Rock
Ground	Kind	Nice	Room
Grow	Kind-of (kinda)	Night	Rope
Guess	Kiss	No	Run
Guitar	Knife	Not	Sad
Gun	Knock	Nothing	Said
Guy	Know	Now	Sail
Had	Lady	Of	Same
Hair	Lake	Off	Saw
Hand	Lamp	Oh	Say
Happen	Land	OK	School
Happily	Lay	Old	Sea
Happy	Leaf	On	See
Hard	Left	Once	Seed
Hardly	Lesson	One	Sent
Has	Let	Only	She
Hat	Light	Open	Shine
Have	Like	Or	Shoe
Hay	Line	Other	Shot
He	Listen	Out	Should
Head	Little	Outside	Shut
Heard	Live	Over	Sick
Help	Log	Own	Side
Her	Long	Paint	Sister
Here	Look	Painting	Sit
Herself	Lot	Paper	Six
High	Love	Part	Sky
Hill	Lunch	Pay	Sleep
Him	Mad	People	Snake
Himself	Made	Pet	Snow
His	Make	Pick	Snowy
Hold	Man	Picture	So
Hole	Marry	Piece	Some
Home	May	Place	Somebody
Horse	Maybe	Plant	Someone
Hospital	Me	Play	Someplace
Hot	Mean	Plow	Something
House	Men	Police	Sometimes
How	Might	Pond	Somewhere
Hundred	Minute	Practice	Soon
Hurt	Mom	Pray	Sort-of (sorta)
Husband	Money	Pretty	Stair
I	Monster	Probably	Stand

Star	These	Two	Where
Start	They	Under	While
Statue	Thing	Until	White
Stay	Think	Up	Who
Step	This	Upon	Why
Stick	Those	Us	Wife
Stone	Thought	Use	Will
Stop	Thousand	Very	Window
Store	Three	Violin	Winter
Storm	Through	Wait	With
Story	Tie	Wake	Woke
Stuff	Till	Walk	Wolf
Summer	Time	Wall	Woman
Sun	Tired	Want	Won
Swim	To	War	Wonder
Table	Together	Was	Wood
Take	Told	Watch	Work
Talk	Too	Water	Would
Teach	Took	Way	Wreck
Tell	Top	We	Wrong
Ten	Tornado	Wear	Yeah
That	Tree	Well	Year
The	Try	Went	Yes
Their	Tune	What	Yet
Them	Turn	Whatever	You
Then	Turtle	When	Your
There	TV		

From Wepman, J., & Hass, W. (1969). *A spoken word count*. Chicago, IL: Language Resource Association.

Narrative Macrostructure

T1 = setting

T2 = initiating event

T3-6 = description of characters' actions without much sense of plot, plan, or motivation

T7 = attempt (use of verb *know* indicates some internal response)

T8 = consequence

T9 = reaction (does not include character motivation; physical reaction only; contains temporal element then)

T10 = abrupt end

Narrative stage using scheme in Box 10-3: 4 (Chain)

Narrative stage using scheme in Box 11-10: Temporal Chain

Narrative stage using scheme in Figure 11-8: Action Sequence

Cohesion Analysis Based on Scheme in Box 11-12:

Cohesive Marker T-Unit No./Item	Cohesive Adequacy Analysis Tied to Information in T-unit No./Item	Marker Judgment*
2/the bus	1/a bus	C
3/the bus	1/a bus	C
4/the bus	1/a bus	C
4/the train	—	I
4/but	conj.	I
5/they	4/bus and train	C
5/couldn't	ellipsis	I
5/the train	4/bus and train	C
5/because	conj.	I
6/then	conj.	C
6/they	4/bus and train	C
7/it	—	I
7/its	—	I
7/because	conj.	C
7/it	—	I
7/know how to	ellipsis	I
8/it	—	I
9/then	conj.	C
9/the owner	1/a man	C
9/it	—	I
10/then	conj.	C
10/they	—	I

*C = Complete tie; I = incomplete tie.

11/22 = 50% complete ties.

Lexical Richness

Nine words not in Wepman-Hass list (Appendix 11-2): *brakes, bus, crane, driving/drove, fence, owner, town, train, tunnel*

Literary Language Style (Box 11-13)

1. Conjunctions: *but, because, who, then*
2. Elaborated noun phrases: T1—"who was driving . . ."

3. Mental and lingusitic verbs: T7—*know*
4. Adverbs: none

Evaluation

Little evidence of literary language style, poor use of cohesion, immature macrostructure, marginal lexical richness. Include narrative goals, focusing first on macrostructure and cohesion, within intervention program.

INTERVENING AT THE LANGUAGE-FOR-LEARNING STAGE

CHAPTER OBJECTIVES

Readers of this chapter will be able to do the following:
- List the elements needed in a plan for communication intervention at the elementary school level.
- Name the required elements in an Individualized Educational Plan.
- Define and describe appropriate intervention goals at the elementary school level.
- List a variety of intervention activities at the elementary school level.

- Describe several service delivery models at the elementary school level.
- Discuss the role of various intervention agents at the elementary school level and the ways in which they structure collaboration.
- Carry out language analysis procedures for conversation and narratives.
- Apply concepts discussed to the education of students with severe disabilities in elementary schools.

Willie had been late to begin talking when he was a toddler. His parents were concerned about him and asked their pediatrician about it. The pediatrician had Willie's hearing tested and found that he had a mild sensorineural loss in the right ear and a moderate loss in the left. He began wearing hearing aids and was enrolled in an early intervention program. His oral language skills began to improve, and by the time he reached kindergarten, he was able to pass a screening for entrance into a mainstream program. The regular kindergarten teacher referred him for additional speech and language intervention midway through the year, though, because of some mild problems with the intelligibility of his speech and a concern about "immature language." He worked with a speech-language pathologist (SLP), Ms. Johnson, during kindergarten and first grade on basic oral language skills, including increasing intelligibility, use of auxiliary verbs and verb marking, increasing vocabulary, and other skills at the developing language level. Ms. Johnson helped his teachers set up and use a classroom amplification system to improve Willie's reception of the teacher's language input. By the end of first grade he had mastered most of the basic oral language skills his clinician had targeted. Language analysis showed he was functioning at or above Brown's stage V in most areas of productive language. He scored within the normal range, although at the low end, on receptive language and vocabulary assessments. Ms. Johnson put Willie on monitoring status at the end of first grade, and Willie went on to second grade.

Toward the end of his second-grade year, Ms. Johnson received another referral for Willie. His second-grade teacher reported that Willie was "not listening" in class; was having trouble with reading and writing; couldn't organize his materials or complete independent work; and was "acting like a clown," getting attention by being silly and boisterous. Generally, he seemed unable to keep up with the other second-graders in "getting" the information being studied in the subject areas. The second-grade teacher felt he could not function in a mainstream classroom and needed a special program for children with hearing impairments.

Willie was seen by the Student Success Team. They made modifications in his assistive listening system, moved his seat to the front of the room, and advised the teacher to look directly at him when she spoke to him. However, when another marking period went by without much improvement in his classroom performance, it was decided that he needed special help. After an intensive evaluation including both standardized and criterion-referenced assessments in collaboration with the audiologist and learning-disability and reading specialists on the school assessment team, as well as two classroom observations for some curriculum-based evaluation, Ms. Johnson concluded that Willie could benefit from speech/language services. This time, though, his needs were different. They were not in the area of basic oral language skills, but concerned his ability to use and understand language to participate fully in the life of the classroom and to move beyond basic oral language to higher-level linguistic functions, including reading, writing, and the complex discourse demands of the classroom. Still, Ms. Johnson felt that Willie had enough language skill to continue in a mainstream classroom if he received the appropriate support. Ms. Johnson began to work with Willie's family and with the reading and learning-disability specialists and audiologist to design a program for Willie's third-grade year that would meet his needs and help him succeed in the mainstream setting.

Although Willie's hearing impairment figures in his difficulties in school, the pattern of his development is in some ways typical of many children with problems at the language-for-learning (L4L) level. They may start out with a primary problem in oral language, grow out of that (with some help from the SLP), and grow into a different kind of problem, one with managing in school. Let's talk about how to plan and deliver intervention for children whose language skills lead to difficulty in meeting the demands of the school curriculum.

PLANNING INTERVENTION IN THE L4L STAGE

Students being seen for language intervention in the L4L period usually require *transdisciplinary planning*, which, you'll remember, means that specialists and teachers work together, not just within but across their disciplines, to design an effective intervention program. Services need to be coordinated among the specialists, in consultation with the regular or special-education teacher, to ensure that the student's program is coherent and addresses all aspects of the student's needs and includes the family's perspective (Prelock, Beatson, Contompasis, & Kirk, 1999).

The Individualized Educational Plan (IEP) meeting provides an excellent opportunity to engage in this kind of collaborative planning. Since the IEP meeting is required by law, everyone involved in the student's program will be present. Parents will be there, too, so their input can be incorporated. If the SLP serves as service coordinator, she or he can initiate a discussion among the team as to who will do what and when and how to be sure the program flows smoothly and makes sense for the student. To make the intervention truly transdisciplinary, the SLP needs to work with the other educators to outline the client's needs and figure out how each can best be served. Take Willie, for example. His hearing impairment needs to be carefully monitored and his aids and assistive listening devices managed. He needs to work on basic reading and writing skills. He also needs to learn to communicate more effectively in the classroom, be more organized in his work habits, and improve his use of the hearing he has in classroom situations. And he needs help learning the material being presented in the classroom. Who helps him with what?

In transdisciplinary intervention, specialists don't work independently on separate intervention agendas. Instead they decide with the classroom teacher what Willie's most immediate needs are and divide up the responsibilities according to the strengths of each professional. Monitoring his hearing and managing his audiometric equipment would fall to the audiologist. Work on basic reading and writing skills would obviously be under the direction of the reading specialist. The learning-disability teacher might work with Willie or in consultation with the classroom teacher to develop better organizational and study skills and help with mastering classroom content. The SLP might work with the classroom teacher to give Willie some listening strategies in the classroom and might help the teacher to modify some of the classroom procedures to make it easier for Willie to succeed. The language pathologist also might consult with the full team about some of the higher-level oral language skills that Willie needs to work on to succeed in the other areas of the curriculum. The SLP could address these skills in oral language activities, developing comprehension-monitoring and metacognitive strategies for Willie to use in focusing on these higher-level targets. The SLP might share these strategies with the classroom teacher, who would encourage Willie to use them in the classroom. The reading and LD specialist also might encourage Willie to use the same comprehension monitoring and metacognitive strategies in their work with him. In this way, a focused and coherent program might be developed in which the work of each specialist would contribute interactively to fostering Willie's development (Silliman, Ford, Beasman, & Evans, 1999).

PLANNING INTERVENTION WITH THE IEP

The IEP for a school-age child differs somewhat from the IFSP the infants and toddlers, as we have discussed. It requires, participation and signature of all parties, from both the family and the school, at the IEP meeting. Since the law emphasizes including children with disabilities in the regular curriculum, the regular education teacher must be part of the team. The IEP also includes a statement of the student's present levels of educational performance, a statement of annual goals and objectives with criteria for determining whether each has been achieved, a summary of all special-educational services and related services (such as transportation) to be provided, a statement of the extent of participation in the regular education program, a justification of the student's placement in the least-restrictive setting for that pupil, a statement of modifications needed in the regular classroom program to accommodate the student, the projected dates for initiating services, the duration of services, and the proposed date of review.

IEP goals at the L4L stage may include targets in traditional oral language areas, such as increasing sentence length, expanding vocabulary, and increasing use of appropriate request forms. They also can include goals directed at improving classroom performance and integrating oral language and literacy. Sample IEP goals for these kinds of targets might include following classroom directions, demonstrating comprehension of classroom textbooks, producing a cohesive story, or explaining the meaning of technical terms in the curriculum. Simon (1999) provided some examples of ways to design curriculum-based goals for the IEP. She suggested, for example, that objectives be embedded into larger goals based on the curriculum.

For example, an IEP goal might state "Willie will be able to define target vocabulary with 80% accuracy *when discussing key vocabulary items from classroom lessons.*" Farber, Denenberg, Klyman, and Lachman (1992), Nelson (1988), and Prelock, Miller and Reed (1993) also provided extensive examples of IEP goals that can be written to address classroom performance and literacy development in students with language learning disabilities (LLD).

Procedures for modifying the classroom environment so that the child with special needs can participate are an especially important aspect of the IEP for a child at the elementary school level. These modifications might include providing auditory training equipment for a child like Willie or modifying grading so that a child with a developmental disability can be graded on a pass/fail basis. Other modifications might involve providing an aide to help a student with autism participate in classroom activities or a Sign or oral interpreter to translate classroom language for a hearing-impaired or deaf-blind student. Tests might have to be modified for a student with attention-deficit hyperactivity disorder (ADHD), so that there were only a few questions per page. Written texts might need to be read to a blind student or to one with a severe reading disorder. Any such modification would have to be stated on the IEP.

Justifying a placement as least restrictive also is important in this age range. Any placement that moves the student away from the regular classroom or neighborhood school must be justified on the basis of an inability to provide appropriate education in the mainstream setting. Particularly for students with mild to moderate disabilities, the Individuals with Disabilities Education Act (IDEA) gives strong support for *inclusion*, or integrated education within the general classroom. Silliman, Ford, Beasman, and Evans (1999) provide one model for achieving this inclusion for students with LLD. Appendix 12-1 provides a model of what an IEP form might look like. Each educational agency must develop its own form, so the one your school uses may not look just like this. Although there are no mandatory forms for use in creating IEPs, the 2004 reauthorization of the IDEA provides for the development of model IEP forms. However, as of this writing, these models have not yet been disseminated. Whatever form is used, however, it must contain the components we've discussed.

SECTION 504 OF THE REHABILITATION ACT OF 1973

One other area of federal legislation affects intervention planning for school-age children. Section 504 of the Rehabilitation Act of 1973 prohibits agencies that receive federal monies from discriminating against people on the basis of their disabilities. This legislation actually laid the basis for IDEA, since it meant, in practice, that schools could not exclude children because they had a disability (as they had up until that time). Some children have "504 plans" rather than IEPs in schools because they may not qualify for services under the special education eligibility laws of their states. For example, children with ADD who do not have other learning disabilities may not qualify for

special education. Many of these students will have accommodation plans under Section 504.

FAMILY-CENTERED INTERVENTION FOR THE SCHOOL-AGE CHILD

The IDEA requires that families participate in the IEP meeting and in designing the educational program for a student with special needs. What does this mean for a school-age child, for whom intervention will take place primarily in the educational setting, often without direct involvement of parents in the day-to-day program? For us as SLPs it means keeping the family in mind and informed throughout the assessment and intervention processes, not just at the IEP meeting. Parents usually appreciate weekly notes or newsletters sent home with students. A regular telephone call every few months (not just when problems come up) to discuss progress and get input and feedback from parents also can be helpful. Again, the key to family-centered practice in the L4L stage, just as for younger clients, is an attitude of openness, respect, and concern for the family as well as for the client. Using the communication strategies outlined in Table 6-1 can be helpful in working with families of school-age children as well as those of younger children. Prelock et al. (1999) also provide guidance on including families in programs for our students.

Students in the L4L stage are old enough to have their own perspectives considered in planning the intervention program, as well as those of their parents. Enlisting clients in identifying their own areas of strengths and weaknesses and in setting priorities for working on goals identified in the assessment can help to ensure cooperation and make clients feel that the intervention is really for them. A short questionnaire such as that in Figure 12-1 can be used as a basis for an interview with the client in the beginning of an intervention program. The clinician can ask these questions; record the clients' responses; and discuss the intervention program with the student, pointing out how the activities will address the needs and preferences the client expressed. This kind of collaborative planning with school-age children not only helps them to take responsibility

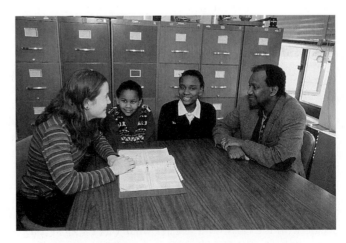

Students and their families can participate in planning intervention at the L4L stage.

Name _____

Date _____

Teacher _____

Grade _____

Please answer the following questions to help me figure out ways to make school more interesting and fun for you.

What's your best subject in school? Why is that your favorite?

What part of school is hardest for you? Why is it hard?

What would you like to read more about?

_____ Famous people   _____ Adventures

_____ Space or science fiction   _____ Sports

_____ Hobbies   _____ History

_____ Other? _____

What kinds of things do you like to read?

_____ Books   _____ Comics

_____ Newspapers   _____ Magazines

_____ Poems   _____ Plays

_____ Other? _____

What do you like to write?

_____ Letters   _____ Crossword puzzles

_____ Poems   _____ Stories

_____ Reports   _____ Diaries

_____ Other? _____

How do you learn best?

_____ Large group, when the teacher explains something to everyone

_____ Small group   _____ Working with one other student

_____ Working alone with the teacher   _____ By yourself

_____ Watching films   _____ Listening to tapes

_____ Doing "hands on" experiments   _____ Working on a computer

_____ Other? _____

What would you like to do better on in school?

What do you think we could do together to help you do better?

What do you wish your teacher did that would make it easier for you to do well in school?

Tests are hard for everyone, but what would help you do better on tests?

_____ Having extra time to finish   _____ Having fewer questions on each page

_____ Having someone read you the questions _____ Having the questions on tape to listen to

_____ Being able to tell someone your answers instead of writing them down

What would you like to change about the way you work in school?

FIGURE 12-1 ✦ A sample questionnaire for including school-aged clients in intervention planning. (Adapted from Waldron, K. [1992]. *Teaching students with learning disabilities.* San Diego, CA: Singular Publishing Group.)

for their own learning, but maximizes the chances for their complete cooperation in the intervention program.

BEHAVIORAL ISSUES IN INTERVENTION PLANNING

We've talked before about the fact that students with LLD frequently have attentional and behavioral problems that inter-

fere with their ability to take advantage of instruction, both in the classroom and in the intervention setting. This is a fact of life in working with children with special needs, one that unfortunately will not go away. Our best approach is to be prepared to deal with behavior problems, to expect them, and to have some strategies in place for addressing them. Most specialists in the management of problem behaviors today advocate the use of *positive behavior support* (PBS) (e.g., Bopp, Brown, &

Mirenda, 2004; Peck & Scarpati, 2004). PBS represents a movement away from punishment-based approaches that emphasize obedience and compliance and toward instruction that emphasizes functional skill development. In addition, PBS includes engineering environments that make problem behavior less likely to occur (Carr et al., 2002; Gunlap, 2005; Renzaglia, Karvonen, Drasgow, & Stoxen, 2003). PBS consists of two procedures: conducting a functional behavior assessment (FBA) and implementing comprehensive intervention.

FBA is a procedure used to identify why problem behavior occurs and what purpose it serves. Functional assessment procedures usually consist of collecting information about the maladaptive behavior through checklists, interviews, and direct observation of the problem behavior, recording important aspects of the situation in which it occurs. O'Neill et al. (1997) provide detailed instructions for conducting FBA. Typically, FBA is performed by the school psychologist or behavior specialist, although the SLP may be one of the professionals who responds to the questionnaires or checklists.

The second procedure of positive behavior support is developing and implementing comprehensive interventions that address the functions of the behavior, as determined by the functional assessment. The program is implemented throughout the day across settings by means of multiple intervention strategies developed by the team. Although FBA may be conducted by the psychologist, the delivery of PBS intervention requires the collaboration of everyone on the student's educational team. The SLP's role is often to deliver *functional communication training* (FCT), in which we teach students to replace socially unacceptable behavior with a more adaptive communicative act (Bopp et al., 2004). Buschbacher and Fox (2003) discuss the components of a comprehensive intervention plan, which include the following:

▶ *Behavior hypotheses*: statements of the most probable antecedents, maintaining factors and communicative functions of the problem behavior, as suggested by the FBA. For example, the team might hypothesize that Willie is clowning because he does not understand the directions for particular class activities.

▶ *Long-term supports*: strategies to assist the student's overall development and interactions to create the optimum quality of life for the student. These might include, for example, having the school nurse check Willie's hearing aid batteries each morning to be sure he is hearing optimally.

▶ *Prevention strategies*: changes in the environment that will minimize the likelihood that the problem behavior will occur. These will be inferred from the FBA, but must fit into the natural routines of the classroom. For example, the teacher might provide written or pictured directions on the blackboard as she explains them, and assign Willie a "buddy" to work with in case he still has trouble understanding what to do.

▶ *Replacement social and communication skills (FCT)*: Adaptive and conventional communication skills are taught that can replace maladaptive behaviors. For example, Willie might be instructed to address questions about classroom instructions to his buddy, rather than acting out. Replacement

behaviors should be functionally equivalent to the problem behavior, and should result in faster and more consistent achievement of the behavior's goal.

▶ *Consequential strategies*: These outline how the team responds to both the replacement skills and the maladaptive behavior. It is important to ensure that rewards for the replacement should exceed those for the problem behavior. In Willie's example, the teacher might assiduously ignore any clowning, but provide rapid and lavish praise, perhaps combined with tokens that can be accumulated for a prize or special privilege, when Willie works quietly with his buddy to complete an assignment.

A related strategy was suggested by LaVigna (1987): *differential reinforcement of other (DRO)* behavior. In this method, the student is reinforced after a specified period in which an undesirable behavior has *not* occurred. Reinforcement is not dependent on the production of any specific behavior, only on some target behavior's being omitted. Suppose Willie is constantly getting up out of his seat and wandering around the room and talking to other students, when he should be working on a written assignment. Using DRO, the teacher or clinician would provide reinforcement for every 3 minutes in which he did *not* wander around and bother others. He would not have to be completing his own work to receive the reinforcement; he would only have to *not* engage in the disruptive behavior. Once some success was achieved, the intervals between reinforcements would be lengthened. Eventually, behavior that substitutes for the undesired one can be shaped into the behavior in which we really want the student to engage. If Willie is first reinforced for not bothering others, eventually we can up the ante, requiring him to stay in his own seat to get the reinforcement. When that has been accomplished, reinforcement can become contingent on his completing his own work.

Another strategy that appears useful for managing problem behavior is the Social Story (Gray, 1995a). These stories were developed to assist children with autism to manage their behavior in social settings, but can be used with any child who needs positive behavioral support. Kuoch and Mirenda (2003) showed that using these stories provided long-lasting replacement of appropriate behaviors for maladaptive ones. Social Stories can be written individually for children, or taken from commercial materials that present a range of social stories for common situations (Gray, 2000). The Social Story contains three basic elements:

▶ Descriptive sentences: identify a social setting the child finds problematic and describe it (The bell rings when recess is over. Everyone gets in line.)

▶ Directive sentences: tell what the child should do to be successful in the target situation (When the bell rings I stop playing. I get in line. I wait for the teacher.)

▶ Perspective sentences: describe internal states of others during the target situation (My teacher will feel happy when everyone is in line. I will feel good that I followed the rules.)

For children identified as having special educational needs, IDEA provides protections against penalties for behavior that is part of their disability. Although many schools, in the wake of recent episodes of violence on school premises, have adopted "zero tolerance" policies for certain behavior such that the first infraction leads to automatic suspension or expulsion, children with disabilities cannot be punished this way if the infraction was related to their disorder. For example, a school may have a "zero tolerance" policy for wearing a hat in school (as part of regulations against "gang paraphernalia"), but if a child with autism insists on wearing a hat because he has a need for sameness and removing his hat would cause him inordinate disorganization and distress, he cannot be punished for breaking this rule. However, the team certainly can work with him to help him overcome his need for the hat, or to replace it with an alternative more acceptable to school administrators.

Managing behavior is an unavoidable part of the work of any clinician who deals with children. Clinicians who want to engage in transdisciplinary and collaborative intervention need to be especially aware of discipline issues and to work with the team to establish consistent strategies. The best offense here is a good defense. Being prepared for discipline problems before they happen, with plans and strategies for addressing them as a team effort, keeps them to a manageable minimum.

INTERVENTION PRODUCTS IN THE L4L PERIOD

Many of the language difficulties we discussed in Chapter 10 and assessed in Chapter 11 will be important objectives of the intervention programs we design for children in the L4L stage. We want to address the language forms that appear in normal development during this period. These include use of advanced morphological markers, complex sentences, abstract vocabulary, adverbial marking, precise conjunctions, linguistic cohesion markers, and elaboration of noun phrases. We also want to help students with LLD to make better use of the language they have. This goal would include reducing word-finding problems, and increasing the flexibility and sensitivity of use of language forms employed to accomplish a range of pragmatic goals, such as politeness, persuasiveness, explicitness, and clarification. Developing use of more varied discourse structures, such as the classroom discourse and narrative structures we outlined in Chapter 10, will also be important. As we saw in Chapter 10, though, language intervention in the L4L period entails more than targeting specific oral language objectives. It also means finding ways to help the student learn the language needed and use the language learned to succeed in the classroom. Let's think about how this basic goal influences intervention planning in the L4L period.

We've been referring to the period of language development that normally takes place between 5 and 12 years of age as the "language for learning" stage. Westby (1991) suggested that during the elementary school years, children move from learning to talk, which was the prime accomplishment of the preschool period, to "talking to learn." In talking to learn, children acquire, among other things, a new style or register of language. Westby called this the *literate language* style. We discussed

aspects of this style and contrasted it to oral language use in Table 10-3.

One important goal of intervention in the L4L period is to develop a literate language style. Access to this "language for learning" register enables a student to engage in "talking to learn," as well as to understand written forms of communication, which generally have a literate language format. One of the reasons narrative skills are so important in the L4L stage is that they form a bridge, or middle ground, between the familiar, contextualized language of conversation and the abstract, decontextualized style of literate language (Westby, 2005). In helping students develop a literate language style, improving oral narrative skill is often a useful first step. What else is needed? Let's look at four principles that can guide intervention in the L4L period. Using these principles to help us choose intervention targets and procedures can ensure that our intervention not only addresses oral language skills but also works toward developing a literate language register.

GUIDING PRINCIPLES OF INTERVENTION AT THE L4L STAGE

Curriculum-Based Instruction

The first principle was articulated by Wallach (1989) and is reinforced by regulations in IDEA. SLPs working with clients at school-age levels should refrain from having their own independent intervention agenda. Instead, they should target goals that are curriculum based (Ehren, 2000b). Let's take Willie as our example again. Suppose that we find as a result of our assessment that Willie has very limited complex sentence production. Following the principle of curriculum-based instruction, we would use onlooker assessment procedures to find out what aspects of Willie's participation in the curriculum require complex sentence use. We would then work on his complex productions within those curricular contexts. Perhaps he needs to be able to answer content questions more concisely in class. We could work on using complex sentences to answer questions modeled after teacher questions drawn from a classroom observation. Maybe he needs to report on past events more precisely, using appropriate temporal conjunctions. If so, we could have him "practice" for sharing times or group discussions by "prepping" him to organize his contribution with complex sentences and conjunctions. The point is to avoid work on a language agenda isolated from the ways the language will be used to participate in the curriculum. Instead we want to integrate our language intervention with the demands our students face in the classroom every day.

Integrate Oral and Written Language

The second principle that should guide intervention in the L4L period was suggested by Gerber (1993) and Berninger (2000). They advocated another type of integration: the integration of oral and written language. This means that we want to provide both oral and written opportunities for students to practice the forms and functions targeted in the intervention.

For students functioning at primary-grade levels, we want to address skills that contribute to both oral and written language development. In addition to basic oral language approaches, then, we want to include literacy socialization, metalinguistic and phonological awareness, as well as narrative activities. We might work on comprehension and use of abstract vocabulary, for example, not just in oral exercises but also in activities that involve printed forms. Vocabulary sessions might include literacy socialization activities such as book reading and discussion of the words in the text. We might ask students to identify target words in the book we've discussed. In a similar vein, we could include phonological awareness (PA) activities in the vocabulary program. We could have students decide whether a word we were working on was a "long" or "short" word, how many syllables it had, what words rhyme with it, what sounds it begins and ends with, how many sounds are heard in the word, what letters might be used to represent those sounds, and so on.

For students functioning at the intermediate-grade levels, integrating oral and written language remains important. Even if these students are seeing the reading or learning disability specialist, we need to encourage them to "pull together" the oral language skills we are helping them develop. The best way to attain this goal is to provide a variety of language experiences addressing each objective. Experiences early in the program might be primarily oral and highly contextualized, such as face-to-face conversation. But as we continue to work on a goal, it can be addressed in increasingly literate, decontextualized activities, such as oral narrative contexts, and eventually in reading comprehension activities.

Go Meta

The third principle guiding intervention in the L4L stage was presented by Wallach and Miller (1988). In their words, intervention in the L4L period should focus on the "metas," activities that direct conscious attention to the language and cognitive skills a student uses in the curriculum. "Meta" skills include talking about talking and thinking about thinking. All the activities we do around any of our language objectives ought to be done on two levels. On the first level, we demonstrate through models and practice how particular forms and functions of language work, just as we would for a child at an earlier language stage. On the second, or "meta," level, the client and clinician talk about the language forms and functions being used and state rules and principles explicitly, focusing attention on the structure of language.

"Going meta" can involve a variety of activities aimed at bringing the clients' language use and comprehension to a higher level of awareness. Basic comprehension activities for vocabulary and syntax can be supplemented by comprehension monitoring instruction. Activities aimed at production of language forms, such as advanced morphemes, complex sentences, and adverbial usage, can be introduced with basic-level activities and expanded with metalinguistic discussions. In these, the client can state when and why these forms are used, tell what meaning they encode, explain how to use linguistic or nonlinguistic

context to decide what form is appropriate, and so on. Work on improving classroom discourse skills, such as listening, making relevant contributions, knowing when to talk and when not to, what to talk about and what not to—all the aspects of the "hidden curriculum"—are ideal contexts for metapragmatic activities. The clinician can get students to state classroom rules explicitly, role-play appropriate and inappropriate language use, role-play the teacher as the clinician role-plays the student making various classroom discourse errors, discuss why things go wrong for the client in the classroom, and brainstorm alternative language strategies.

Preventive Intervention

The fourth principle to consider in working with primary school clients is the notion of preventive intervention. We've talked before about preventive intervention as a means of delaying or circumventing the occurrence of symptoms. Preventive intervention can apply to our work with children who have a history of language disorders as preschoolers or who have language deficits and continue to function at developing language levels in the primary grades. These students may not yet be diagnosed as LLD, but everything we know about LLD suggests that these clients have a good chance of eventually graduating to that diagnosis. Why wait for it to happen?

We can apply the other three principles already discussed to our work with these children. If they are already involved in intervention at the developing language level, we can supplement the oral language program. We can work on semantic and syntactic targets in curriculum-based activities. We can integrate oral and written language approaches by focusing on emerging literacy skills through literature-based script activities and on PA. If the client is working on phonological production targets, these would be an ideal setting for developing PA skills at the same time. We can also "go meta," even while working on preschool-level language goals. We can point out written versions of the words and sentence types we are working on, state explicitly the rules we are teaching, ask students to judge the appropriateness of discourse that contains the targets, and have students talk about the rules and when they apply.

We can use screening protocols for late kindergartners and early first-graders, such as those we discussed in Chapter 11 (Catts, 1986; Gilbertson & Bramlett, 1998; Justice, Invernizzi, & Meier, 2002), to identify children with weak PA skills. These children, who are known to be at risk for reading difficulty, can receive preventive intervention in the form of specific PA training.

We also can provide this kind of preventive work even for students who are not receiving direct intervention. We accomplish this through collaborative instruction in the classrooms of children who are identified as having language disorders. If we work in primary classrooms, providing language activities that foster emerging literacy, PA, and metalinguistic skill, we are exerting a preventive influence on other children in the class. These children, who may be at risk for LLD because of a history of language delay, poor literacy socialization, or cultural differences, would not receive any direct services until they started to fail in school. A preventive approach through collaborative intervention at the primary grade level can have far-reaching effects on these vulnerable children, as well as on the identified clients in the class.

Summary

We might say, then, that in addition to the basic language goals we've outlined for the L4L stage, four additional considerations should guide our intervention planning. These are (1) making intervention curriculum-based, rather than independent and isolated; (2) integrating oral and written forms of expression in addressing language goals, moving from oral to literate formats for communication as we work on language objectives; (3) "going meta," attempting to bring all the language we work on to a higher level of awareness; and (4) using preventive intervention in primary grades to attempt to ward off LLDs in vulnerable children. Let's see how we might use these principles to design intervention activities.

INTERVENTION PROCESSES IN THE L4L PERIOD

Remember that we've been discussing intervention procedures under three basic categories: clinician directed (CD), child centered (CC), and hybrid. Let's take a look at some of the kinds of activities at the L4L level that might fall in each category.

CLINICIAN-DIRECTED INTERVENTION IN THE L4L STAGE

CD activities, using drill play contexts, can be used for a variety of goals at the L4L stage. PA is often targeted in a drill play format, for example. Students are given a set of tokens, nickels for vowels and pennies for consonants, perhaps. The clinician demonstrates segmenting a vowel-consonnat (VC) word, such as *oat* (/ot/), by moving the nickel as /o/ is pronounced and the penny as the /t/ is produced. The students are then instructed to follow the clinician's model and move their coins as the sounds are pronounced. When students can accomplish this kind of phonological segmentation, CVC (*coat*) words can be introduced. Eventually, CCV (*blue*), CCVC (*stone*), CVCC (*taps*), and CCVCC (*blast*) words can be incorporated into the activity. Many of the PA programs used in research demonstrating the efficacy of PA training on literacy (e.g., Ehri, et al., 2001; Gillon, 2000) make use of this format.

CD activities can, of course, be used to target morphological markers, vocabulary, and sentence structures at the L4L stage, just as they can at the developing language period. In using CD activities for these targets, though, we want to be sure *not* to be operating on an independent agenda, targeting forms just because they are identified as deficits in the assessment. The principles we discussed earlier still apply. We can address goals with drill and operant procedures, but we want to be sure that the drills focus on using these forms in ways that are relevant to the curriculum.

We might decide, for example, that a first-grader with deficits in advanced morphological markers really needed to develop proficiency with *-er* and *-est* because these were used frequently in the math curriculum ("Find the larger number," "Find the smallest number"). In this case we would develop *-er* and *-est* drills in number-related contexts. The student might be asked to repeat, and demonstrate with chips or counters, a list of number statements containing *larger*: "Two is *larger* than one, three is *larger* than two," and so on. The student could then be asked to complete a series of cloze statements, such as "Of 10 and 9, 10 is _____." The same process could be repeated with *smaller*. The next step would be to use cloze statements in which the student had to decide, with the help of chips or counters, whether *smaller* or *larger* were appropriate ("Of 6 and 7, 6 is _____; of 5 and 4, 5 is _____", and so on). The same process could be followed for *largest*, then for *smallest*, then for the two combined in cloze drills ("Of 6, 7, and 8, 8 is _____; of 9, 10, and 11, 9 is _____"; and so on). Eventually all four terms would be included in an activity. The point to remember about CD activities at the L4L stage is that they are appropriate methods for addressing goals, so long as the goals themselves conform to the four principles we discussed earlier. We want to avoid isolated CD drills that do not relate in any way to the classroom curriculum.

Another application of CD techniques is what Marshall (1991) and Silliman (1987) referred to as cognitive behavior modification (CBM). CBM is a CD approach to developing comprehension-monitoring and metacognitive strategies for increasing learning skills. It is, essentially, an operant way to "go meta." CBM involves three basic steps:

1. The clinician tells the client explicitly what strategy will be developed, why it is important, and what procedures will be used to attain the strategy. The clinician might, for example, tell clients that they were going to work on deciding whether they had understood all the information in a paragraph read by the clinician. The clinician might explain that it is important to know when we don't understand something so that we can ask questions, ask for repetition, or seek further information. The clinician would then explain that she will model how to talk through the process of deciding whether the paragraph was understood and will have the clients follow this model.

2. The clinician "thinks out loud" to demonstrate how the strategy is accomplished. She might read a paragraph out loud, then ask herself, "Now, do I understand what it was about? Let's see, it was about X. OK, do I remember the details about X? Well, there was A, B, and I think there was another one, but I can't remember it. I'll have to ask about that one. Did I understand all the words? There was one word I didn't know. I think it was 'magna' or something like that. I'll have to ask the teacher or look that up in the dictionary." The clinician could write each question she asked herself as she asked it and make a note as to the answer she gave herself after each question.

3. The clinician has each client model this thinking out-loud process in turn. For our comprehension-monitoring example, the clinician would read the paragraph again and ask a student to talk through the list of questions that she generated.

In this example she would have the students ask themselves "Did I understand what it was about? Did I remember the details? Did I understand all the words?" Students would then note their own answers to each question and take the actions needed, such as looking up one of the words in the dictionary.

This process would be repeated numerous times, until clients were able to generate self-monitoring questions spontaneously. Then more advanced material, such as longer passages or text the clients read themselves, would be used, with the same procedures. CBM is another way we can use explicit, CD procedures to find ways to help students with LLD succeed in the classroom.

CHILD-CENTERED INTERVENTION IN THE L4L STAGE

Scaffolding

The most common CC techniques at the school age level involve *scaffolding*. Scaffolding involves identifying the student's zone of proximal development (ZPD) in curricular language skills, and devising activities that scaffold his current level of function into the ZPD by means of clinician support. These techniques can be used by the clinician in interactions with students with LLD and also can be provided to classroom teachers in consultative formats. When we give teachers very specific techniques to use, our chances of influencing their interactions with the students with LLD in their classrooms are greatly enhanced, and the chances for success of our consultative efforts in general increase. Gerber (1993) described three forms of scaffolding that can be used in working with students with LLD.

Creation of Optimal Task Conditions. This form of scaffolding involves reducing the amount of stress and undue effort a student uses to complete a curricular task. In practice, it means working with the classroom teacher to reduce the amount of material a student has to process and to present the material in smaller units with extra time allowed for task completion. Suppose Willie is required to write one book report a month on a book he reads independently. The clinician can discuss modifying this requirement with the classroom teacher. The clinician might suggest that instead of letting Willie choose any book from the class library, as the mainstream children do, he be given his own "shelf" in the library with books that are written at his level of reading or narrative development. For example, when a book report is assigned, the clinician can provide several books for Willie's "private shelf" in the classroom library that are at the level of narrative development just above his current level, as identified by assessment. After reading or listening to these books and preparing appropriate book reports, Willie can be reassessed. If narrative stage has improved, the shelf can be stocked with books at the next, higher level. Box 12-1 contains examples of well-known books at a range of narrative complexity levels, compiled from suggestions of Wallach (1989) and Westby (2005).

In addition to providing scaffolding in terms of narrative structure, the clinician can also create optimal task demands by structuring the written work the student is required to produce. Take our book report example again. The clinician might suggest to the teacher that instead of being asked to produce a free-form book report, Willie be given a form to complete. The clinician might give the teacher a series of increasingly complex forms to use, suggesting that when the student becomes adept at writing reports using one form, the next in the sequence can be required for subsequent reports. Westby (2005) provided such a series of book report formats that can be used to scaffold a client's performance. An adaptation of her series appears in Box 12-2. An example book report form can be found in Figure 12-2.

Guidance of Selective Attention. This form of scaffolding involves highlighting important information by using visual, verbal, and intonational cues. Using this device, a clinician can, for example, use a highlighting marker to call attention to potentially difficult words in a photocopied passage from a textbook. Before students read, or watch as the clinician reads the passage to them, they can be told to look for these words, try to guess what they mean, or to let the clinician know whether they need to look them up in the dictionary. Similarly, the clinician can read the passage with heavy intonational stress on the same words, telling the students beforehand to listen for them because they may be tricky and to decide whether they can guess their meaning or need to look up their definitions.

Provision of External Support. The clinician can "prime" students to succeed in classroom activities. This can be done especially effectively in service delivery systems that combine collaborative intervention with some clinical sessions. Suppose the clinician is doing a collaborative lesson on listening skills in a client's classroom. She can "prep" clients for the lesson in a pull-out session, previewing what she will be covering and some of the questions she will be asking. She might tell the clients ahead of time that she will be asking the class to think about and make a list of "good listening behaviors." She could preview the activity with the clients, helping them to generate their own list. When she gives the lesson in the classroom, the clients already know the right answers! Allowing them to demonstrate their knowledge to the mainstream students not only reviews and reinforces the information for the clients, but also allows them to "look smart" before the other students. Such an opportunity can give a real boost in self-esteem to clients who often find themselves trailing behind the rest of the class.

HYBRID INTERVENTION IN THE L4L STAGE

A great number of the intervention methods we use with students at the L4L stage are of the hybrid variety, with some degree of direction by the clinician but less structure than traditional operant procedures. We'll look at examples of hybrid procedures that might be used to address some of the major goals of the L4L period, but these examples are by no means exhaustive. Additional sources of ideas include DeKemel (2003), Dodge (1998), Falk-Ross (2002), Gerber (1993), Haynes, Moran,

BOX 12-1 | **Suggestions for Books at Various Stages of Narrative Macrostructure Development**

1. For students currently producing narratives at the Heap stage, provide books at the Sequence level, in which there is a recurring theme but the order of events doesn't matter:
   Abuela's Weave by Omar Castenada
   Charlie Needs a Cloak by Tommie DePaola
   King Bidgood's in the Bathtub by Audrey & Don Wood
   The Gingerbread Boy by Paul Galdone
   The Goat and the Rug by Charles L. Blood, Martin Link, & Nancy Winslow Parker
   The House that Jack Built by Paul Galdone
   The Snowy Day by Ezra Jack Keats
   The Very Hungry Caterpillar by Eric Carle

2. For students currently producing narratives at the Sequence stage, provide books at the Primitive Narrative level, which have a main theme and involve some understanding of attempts and actions and ability to interpret events:
   Alexander and the Terrible, Horrible, No Good, Very Bad Day by Judith Viorst
   Alice Gets Ready for School by Cynthia Jabar
   George and Martha by James Marshall
   Kevin's Grandmother by Barbara Williams
   Mr. Happy; Mr. Fussy; Mr. Bounce; Mr. Worry; etc. by Roger Hargraves
   Rotten Ralph by Jack Gentos
   Round Robin by Jack Kent

3. For students currently producing narratives at the Primitive Narrative stage, provide books at the Chain level, which involve some understanding of cause-effect and character motivation:
   Drummer Hoff by Ed Emberley
   Feelings by Aliki
   If I Had by Mercer Mayer
   If You Give a Mouse a Cookie; If You Give a Moose a Muffin by L. Numeroff
   Just for You by Mercer Mayer
   Keep Your Mouth Closed, Dear by Aliki
   The King's Tea by T.H. Nonle
   The Little Red Hen by Paul Galdone
   Tingo, Tango, Mango Tree by Marcia K. Vaughan & Yvonne Buchanan
   Today I Feel Silly by Jamie Lee Curtis
   What are YOU so Grumpy About? by Tom Lichtenheld
   Why Mosquitoes Buzz in People's Ears by Vernal Aardema & Leo and Diane Dillon
   Why the Sun and the Moon Live in the Sky by Elphinstone Dayrell

4. For students functioning at the Chain level, provide books with a simple True Narrative structure, plots that have character development, sequences of actions motivated by characters' goals and plans, and a resolution of the story's problem:
   Bread and Jam for Francis by Russell Hoban
   Elbert's Bad Word by Audrey & Don Wood
   Fantastic Mr. Fox by Roald Dahl
   Franklin in the Dark by Paulette Bourgeois & Brenda Clark
   Hetty and Harriet by Graham Oakley
   Ira Sleeps Over by B. Waber
   Owl at Home by Arnold Lobel
   The Three Little Pigs by Paul Galdone

Adapted from Wallach, G. (speaker). (1989). *Children's reading and writing disorders: The role of the speech language pathologist* (ASHA Teleconference Tape Series). Rockville, MD: American Speech-Language-Hearing Association; and Westby, C. (2005). Assessing and remediating text comprehension problems. In H. Catts & A. Kamhi (Eds.). *Language and reading disabilities—2nd Ed.* (pp. 157-232). Boston: Allyn & Bacon.

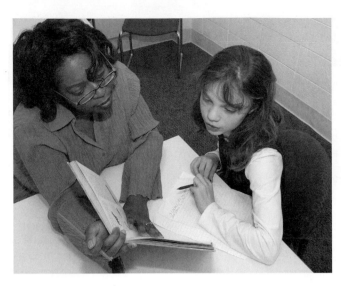

Intervention for children with LLD often includes scaffolding and guidance of selective attention in classroom materials.

and Pindzola (1999), Kuder (1997), Paul (1992b), Secord (1990), Simon (1991a), Wallach and Butler (1994), Wallach and Miller (1988), Westby (2005), and Wiig and Semel (1984). The suggestions here are meant only to start you thinking about how hybrid intervention activities for this developmental period might be designed. The rest is up to your own creativity. Remember, too, that when we talk about hybrid activities that can be used to address specific intervention targets, the targets themselves should always be selected with our four guiding principles of intervention at the L4L stage in mind.

Semantics

Vocabulary. Research (Biemiller, 2003; Dole, Sloan, & Trathen, 1995) has shown that students with more extensive vocabularies do better in reading comprehension as well as in oral language activities. But these studies also demonstrate that having students look words up in a dictionary does not transfer word knowledge very effectively to reading comprehension tasks. Something more is needed to develop the kind of understanding that improves reading skills. Blanchowicz (1986) outlined the following five-step program that can be used to deepen both receptive and expressive lexical skills:

BOX 12-2 | **Book Report Sequence**

Book Report 1: Description

Identify title.
Identify author.
Draw a picture of a favorite part of the story.
Describe the pictures in the book.

Book Report 2: Sequence 1

Identify title.
Identify author.
Name the major characters.
Tell the first thing that happened in the story.
Tell how the story ends.

Book Report 3: Sequence 2

Identify title.
Identify author.
Name the major characters.
Tell three things, in sequence, that happened in the story.
Retell the story with pictures.

Book Report 4: Primitive Narrative

Identify title.
Identify author.
Respond to a 'why' question about a physical cause (Why did the first little pig's house fall down?)
Tell three things, in sequence, that happened in the story.
Retell the story with pictures.

BOX 12-2 | **Book Report Sequence—cont'd**

Book Report 5: Chain Narrative

Identify title.
Identify author.
Tell what a character in the story wants.
Identify a feeling experienced by a main character.
Explain how you know the character feels this way.
Retell the story with pictures.

Book Report 6: True Narrative-Abbreviated Episode

Identify title.
Identify author.
Tell what a character wants.
Explain why the character feels this way.
Retell the story without pictures.

Book Report 7: True Narrative

Identify title.
Identify author.
Tell the problem in the story.
Tell how the characters solved the problem.
Retell the story in your own words.

Adapted from Westby, C. (2005). Assessing and remediating text comprehension problems. In H. Catts & A. Kamhi (Eds.). *Language and reading disabilities–2nd Ed.* (pp. 157-232). Boston: Allyn & Bacon.

Title: _____

Author: _____

Characters: _____
_____
_____
_____

Three things that happened:

1. _____

2. _____

3. _____

Retell the story with pictures:

FIGURE 12-2 ✦ Sample book report form for book report. (Adapted from Westby, C. [2005]. Assessing and remediating text comprehension problems. In H. Catts & A. Kamhi (Eds.). _Language and reading disabilities—3rd Ed._ [pp. 157-232]. Boston, MA: Allyn & Bacon.)

1. _Activate what students already know._ To accomplish this, Blanchowicz suggested _exclusive brainstorming._ A topic from the curriculum, such as a content unit or work of literature being read in the classroom, is chosen. The clinician selects a set of words from it that may give the clients trouble or asks the students to make a list of words they found hard in the text. The clinician also selects a list of words from a different classroom unit. The clinician presents the words to the students in oral and written form. The students discuss the words and decide which ones go with their topic for the day and which don't. To make this decision, students are encouraged to use a knowledge rating checklist like the one in Table 12-1 to foreground whatever knowledge they have about the words.

2. _Make connections among words and topics._ The clinician gives students a list of words from a textbook or literature selection and asks them to guess the topic of the selection. A "Predict-O-Gram," like the one in Box 12-3, can be used to help students predict how the words will be used in the selection. In this example, a story grammar format is used to guide the predictions. In this way, work on story macrostructure can accompany vocabulary development. Another way to foster connections among words is to use "word maps" (Westby, 2005). Figure 12-3 shows one type of map, relating words around a theme. Figure 12-4 shows a map relating synonyms by their level of intensity.

3. _Use both spoken and written contexts._ Here the goal is to expose the students to the words in a variety of language experiences. Using a science lesson as an example, the clinician could first read the science passage to the students, asking them to raise their hand when they hear one of the words on their word list from (1). The students could then write a list of the words and discuss what they know about each one. They might then be asked to do the knowledge rating checklist again, to list the words they now feel they can define and read their list to the group. The group could together generate definitions for each word, then compile a group glossary, by writing down the definition they gave orally for each word.

4. _Refine and reformulate meanings._ Here, again, we need to expose the student to the words in varying contexts. The

TABLE 12-1	A Knowledge Rating Checklist for Words that Do and Do Not Pertain to the Topic "Solar System"

HOW MUCH DO WE KNOW ABOUT THESE WORDS?

WORD	CAN DEFINE	HAVE SEEN/HEARD	BEATS ME!
Asteroid		X	
Orbit	X		
Nebula			X
Lunar		X	
Interstellar		X	
Volcanic	X		
Axis		X	
Rotation		X	
Magma			X

Adapted from Blanchowicz, C. (1986). Making connections: Alternatives to the vocabulary notebook. _Journal of Reading, 29,_ 643-649.

| **BOX 12-3** | **A Predict-O-Gram for Vocabulary Chosen from a Literature Selection** |

Predict in what part of the story the author will use these words: *boa, butler, croquet mallet, cure, disappear, elegant, gazebo, relief, shocked, shriveled, snickering, wizard*

The setting	**The characters**	**The problem**	**The action**	**The resolution**
elegant	*butler*	*croquet mallet*	*snickering*	*cure*
gazebo	*wizard*	*boa*	*shocked*	*relief*
			shriveled	*disappear*

Adapted from Blanchowicz, C. (1986). Making connections: Alternatives to the vocabulary notebook. *Journal of Reading, 29,* 643-649; literature selection; Wood, A. (1988). *Elbert's Bad Word.* San Diego, CA: Harcourt, Brace, Jovanovich.

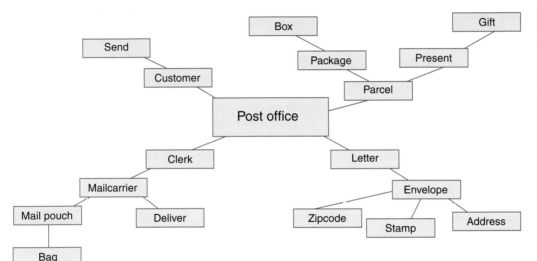

FIGURE 12-3 ✦ Visual map for the "visiting the post office" script used in working on word retrieval in primary grades. (Adapted from Yoshingaga-Itano, C., & Downey, D. [1986]. A hearing-impaired child's acquisition of schemata: Something's missing. *Topics in Language Disorders, 7,* 45-57; and Wallach, G., & Miller, L. [1988]. *Language intervention and academic success.* Boston, MA: College Hill.)

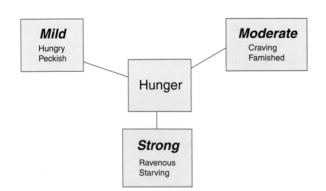

FIGURE 12-4 ✦ Word map for *hunger* by synonym intensity.

students could be asked to tell as much as they know about each word and name the words they still have trouble understanding. The teacher could help the students look these words up in the dictionary and discuss their meanings further. The clinician might read the students the passage containing the words from their science text and from a library book on the same topic. The students could talk about how the words are used in each selection. They might comment on which selection helped them learn more about what the words

mean, if any have parts in common with other words they know, which was easier to understand, and which they liked better and why.

5. *Use the words for writing and additional reading.* The clinician might have students write a science fiction story about the solar system, using words from the list. The clinician could ask students to listen to each other read their stories. Finally, they can write a group story using their favorite parts from each of the individual stories, with the stipulation that the group story must contain all the words on the list.

The main thrust of this approach is that vocabulary development should be an in-depth procedure. I like to call this approach *elaborated exposure.* For students with LLD, listing and defining words is just not enough to get the words firmly implanted in their lexicon. They need to engage, both receptively and expressively, in a variety of experiences with words that intensify and expand their knowledge of meanings. Such elaborated exposure helps to ensure that the words learned are retained and accessible.

A second approach to vocabulary development was suggested by Dole, Sloan, and Trathen (1995). This is a somewhat metacognitive approach, which attempts to teach students strategies for learning new words, rather than a particular set of new words themselves (we'll talk more about learning strategies approaches to intervention in Chapter 14). Students in this program are taught first to use three criteria to select important unknown words from their classroom reading sections:

1. They must not know what the word means.
2. The word must be used in the assigned selection.
3. The word must be key to describing a character, event, or idea in the selection.

Students must justify their choice of each word on these grounds. Teachers first model this procedure, then students select their own words and write them in a list. After each word, they write a guess as to what it might mean, based on their review of the context in which they encountered it. They then look up the word in the dictionary and write down the one meaning most appropriate for this context. Next the students reread the words aloud in context and read the definition they found most appropriate. They talk about how each word's meaning relates to the plot or main point of the selection and why each word might have been chosen by the author to convey this meaning. Sloan et al. report significant improvement in students' understanding of word meaning when they are taught this strategy, as opposed to a more traditional program in which students simply look up words the teacher gives them, without contextual discussion.

DeKemel (2003) stresses that although building curricular-related vocabulary through elaborated exposure is an important aspect of language instruction for students with LLD, we cannot ignore the fact that children will encounter words they do not know, and will need to develop dictionary skills to understand such words. She advocates combining elaborated exposure with specific instruction in the use of the dictionary and thesaurus, using the following methods:

▶ Keep a dictionary and thesaurus available in each classroom and therapy room.
▶ Teach skills for alphabetizing and using the alphabetic system to find words in reference books.
▶ Explicitly teach the various parts of dictionary entries, including pronunciation key, etymology, and the meaning of the order of definitions.
▶ Focus on word study; pointing out parts of words (roots and affixes) and the concept of identifying roots they know within new words.
▶ Explain the meaning of abbreviations used, such as *n.* for *noun.*
▶ Point out the use of sentences in the dictionary to help illustrate meaning and usage.
▶ Once a definition is found, use the thesaurus to identify words related in meaning.
▶ Teach how to use synonyms to eliminate redundancy, create more precise expression.
▶ Always take newly defined words back to usage contexts, such as curricular themes and texts.

Biemiller (2003) reports that research supports the use of an oral reading context for introducing new words. His studies suggest that reading texts to children, picking out words likely to be unfamiliar and explaining them within the context of the story or passage is sufficient for typical students to acquire two or three new words per session. Students with LLD will need additional exposure, but consulting with teachers to provide this kind of direct instruction and then providing more elaborated exposure in therapy sessions can help our students' vocabulary keep up with their peers. Biemiller also advocates for teaching all students explicitly to ask the teacher or SLP about words they do not know.

The *Word Study* approach lends itself to the development not only of vocabulary, but of morphology and spelling, as well. Bloodgood and Pacifici (2004) suggested several activities that can be used in a word study approach to vocabulary development. These are outlined in Table 12-2. Box 12-4 lists children's books suggested by Bloodgood and Pacifici that can be used in a word study approach.

Whatever specific approach is used, recent research (Throneburg, Calvert, Sturm, Paramboukas, & Paul, 2000) suggests that an in-class, collaborative model is more effective for teaching curricular vocabulary to students who qualified for speech or language services than a traditional pull-out model. So, however we decide to teach new vocabulary to students with IEPs, incorporating a collaborative approach will be advantageous. And explicitly linking word study to spelling can also be helpful for students struggling with this aspect of literacy, as well (Bauman et al., 2002).

Word Finding. In Chapter 10 we talked about the fact that word-finding problems are frequently observed in students with LLD. We said they may be caused by semantic or phonological problems or some combination of the two (German & Newman, 2004). Therefore, to address word-finding problems, we need to work on several levels. One way to address the semantic side of word-retrieval difficulties is to do the kind of elaborated exposure work on vocabulary that we just discussed. By expanding and deepening students' knowledge of word meaning, we increase the connections among words in the students' semantic network. These stronger links and more elaborated understanding will, in themselves, decrease word-retrieval problems.

Wallach and Miller (1988) suggested using visual maps to help increase the semantic associations among words around a specific curriculum topic. For students in primary grades, topics with which students have some direct experience may be used. Yoshinaga-Itano and Downey (1986) suggested using familiar scripts, such as going to the doctor or visiting the post office, as bases for visual mapping. Figure 12-3 gives an example of a visual map for a "going to the post office" script that might be used in conjunction with a "community helpers" unit with primary students who show word-finding difficulties. Visual mapping helps students use semantic strategies to overcome word-finding problems.

Massed practice can help increase speed of retrieval. Here students time themselves as they produce a list of vocabulary words associated with a curriculum-based unit. Students in intermediate grades could, for example, name all the layers of the rain forest that they have studied or all the parts of the food

| TABLE 12-2 | Activities for Supporting Vocabulary, Morphology, and Spelling through Word Study | | |

ACTIVITY	GRADE LEVEL	ACTIVITY	RESOURCES
Root of the day	3–6	Teacher/SLP writes a Greek or Latin root on the board at the beginning of the week (e.g., *tele*). Students add words they think are related (e.g., telephone, telegraph, television). Later, students discuss what the root might mean based on the words in their list. Volunteers check meaning in the dictionary; students add these to notebooks or cards.	*Word Journeys* (Ganske, 2000) *Words Their Way* (Bear et al., 2000)
Roots and branches	4–6	Teacher/SLP places a root word in the center of a tree trunk drawn on chart paper. Students in groups record derived words on branches in one color. Volunteers find the meanings in the dictionary and record them on the branches in a second color.	Greek mythology, *American Heritage Dictionary of Indo-European Roots* (Watkins, 1985)
Word sorting	3–6	Teacher/SLP introduces two related sound patterns (e.g., short *i*, long *i*), and a list of words for each (stick, time, find, guide, miss, wild, blimp); students sort the words into the two patterns (short: miss, blimp, stick; long: time, find, guide). They then attempt to find spelling patterns (e.g., what determines whether the *i* is long or short).	*Explorations in Developmental Spelling* (Bear & Templeton, 1998)
Homophone rummy	4–6	After introducing the concept of homophones (words that sound the same but are spelled differently), homophone pairs are written on cards, and various matching games (Rummy, Concentration, Uno, etc.) are played with them. To make a pair, however, students must give correct definitions for each word. Challenges are resolved by looking the words up in the dictionary.	*Eight Ate: A Feast of Homonym Riddles* (Terban, 1982)
Homograph concentration	4–6	After introducing the concept of homographs (words that are spelled the same but pronounced differently), pairs of sentences containing homographs are written on card stock. Cards are placed face down, as for Concentration. Players turn over pairs of cards until a match is found. Players must read the two matching sentences aloud and give a description of the meaning of the homograph in each of the two sentences.	*The Dove Dove: Funny Homograph Riddles* (Terban, 1988)

Adapted from Bloodgood, J., & Pacifici, L. (2004). Bringing word study to intermediate classrooms: Here are four original word study units teachers can easily implement themselves. *The Reading Teacher, 58,* 250-264.

pyramid. Students at the primary level can be asked to name all the days of the week or months of the year. The listing would be timed and repeated until retrieval is rapid and effortless. Then new vocabulary could be introduced.

Research (German, 2002) has suggested, though, that approaches that incorporate phonological cues, may be especially effective. Vocabulary work can, then, be organized around phonological similarities. We might do a session on *bl* words, for example, using some of the words from a current classroom theme, work of literature, or classroom discourse activity. At the primary grades, such words might include *blue, black, blast,* and *blaze* during a classroom unit on colors or fire prevention. At the intermediate level, we might use words such as *blatant, blunder, blush,* and *blame* in conjunction with work on classroom discourse skills. Work on

meanings and uses of the words could be supplemented with cloze activities in which the clients supply the words in sentences constructed by the clinician. The clinician might write sentences such as the following for the intermediate-grade students:

> When I talk out of turn in class, the teacher gives me a dirty look and I _____.
> When someone gives the wrong answer, it's _____ly obvious because the teacher says, "Any other ideas?"
> Talking without raising your hand is a _____.

If students have trouble remembering the word needed to fill in the blank, the clinician can remind them, "Remember,

| **BOX 12-4** | **Children's Books Supporting Vocabulary, Morphology, and Spelling through Word Study** |

Children's Books for Word Play

Barrett, J. (1998). *Things That Are the Most in the World*. Illustrated by J. Nickle. New York: Simon & Schuster

Cleary, B.F. (2000). *A Mink, a Rink, a Skating Rink: What Is a Noun?* Illustrated by J. Prosmitsky. Minneapolis: Carolrhoda

Cleary, B.F. (2001). *Hairy, Scary, Ordinary: What Is an Adjective?* Illustrated by J. Prosmitsky. Minneapolis: Carolrhoda

Cleary, B.F. (2001). *To Root, to Toot, to Parachute: What Is a Verb?* Illustrated by J. Prosmitsky. Minneapolis: Carolrhoda

Cleary, B.F. (2002). *Under, over, by the Clover: What Is a Preposition?* Illustrated by B.F. Gable. Minneapolis: Carolrhoda

Cleary, B.F. (2003). *Dearly, Nearly, Insincerely: What Is an Adverb?* Illustrated by B.F. Gable. Minneapolis: Carolrhoda

Ernst, M. (1960). *In a Word*. Illustrated by J. Thurber. New York: Harper & Row

Ghigna, C. (1999). *See the Yak Yak*. Illustrated by B. Lies. New York: Random House

Gwynne, F. (1970). *The King Who Rained*. New York: Simon & Schuster

Gwynne, F. (1976). *A Chocolate Moose for Dinner*. New York: Simon & Schuster

Gwynne, F. (1988). *A Little Pigeon Toad*. New York: Simon & Schuster

Heller, R. (1987). *A Cache of Jewels and Other Collective Nouns*. New York: Putnam

Heller, R. (1988). *Kites Sail High: A Book about Verbs*. New York: Putnam

Heller, R. (1989). *Many Luscious Lollipops: A Book about Adjectives*. New York: Putnam

Helter, R. (1990). *Merry-Go-Round: A Book about Nouns*. New York: Putnam & Grosset

Heller, R. (1990). *Up, Up and Away: A Book about Adverbs*. New York: Putnam

Heller, R. (1995). *Behind the Mask: A Book about Prepositions*. New York: Putnam & Grosset

Heller, R. (1997). *Mine, All Mine: A Book about Pronouns*. New York: Putnam & Grosset

Heller, R. (1998). *Fantastic! Wow! And Unreal! A Book about Interjections and Conjunctions*. New York: Penguin Putnam

Hepworth, C. (1998). *Bug Off! A Swarm of Insect Words*. New York: Penguin Putnam

Martin, J. (1991). *Carrot/parrot*. New York: Simon & Schuster

Martin, J. (1991). *Mitten/kitten*. New York: Simon & Schuster

McMillan. B. (1990). *One Sun: A Book of Terse Verse*. New York: Holiday House

Steig, W. (1968). *C D B!* New York: Simon & Schuster

Steig, W. (1984). *C D C?* New York: Farrar Straus Giroux

Strauss, B., & Friedland, H. (1987). *See You Later Alligator … A First Book of Rhyming Word-Play*. Illustrated by T. d'Elgin. Los Angeles: Price Stern Sloan

Terban, M. (1982). *Eight Ate: A Feast of Homonym Riddles*. Illustrated by G. Maestro. New York: Houghton Mifflin

Terban, M. (1983). *In a Pickle, and Other Funny Idioms*. Illustrated by G. Maestro. New York: Clarion

Terban, M. (1984). *I Think I Thought, and Other Tricky Verbs*. Illustrated by G. Maestro. New York: Clarion

Terban, M. (1987). *Mad as a Wet Hen/And Other Funny Idioms*. Illustrated by G. Maestro. New York: Clarion

Terban, M. (1988). *The Dove Dove: Funny Homograph Riddles*. Illustrated by T. Huffman. New York: Clarion

Terban, M. (1988). *Guppies in Tuxedos: Funny Eponyms*. Illustrated by G. Maestro. New York: Clarion

Terban, M. (1989). *Superdupers/Really Funny Real Words*. Illustrated by G. Maestro. New York: Clarion

Terban, M. (1990). *Punching the Clock: Funny Action Idioms*. Illustrated by T. Huffman. New York: Clarion

Terban, M. (1991). *Hey, Hay! A Wagonful of Funny Homonym Riddles*. Illustrated by K. Hawkes. New York: Clarion

Terban, M. (1993). *It Figures/Fun Figures of Speech*. Illustrated by G. Maestro. New York: Clarion

Terban, M. (1996). *Scholastic Dictionary of Idioms*. New York: Scholastic

Terban, M. (2000). *Punctuation Power/Punctuation and How to Use It*. New York: Scholastic

Walton, R. (1998). *Why the Banana Split*. Illustrated by J. Holder. Layton, UT: Gibbs Smith

Wood, A. (1982). *Quick as a Cricket*. Illustrated by D. Wood. Swindon, UK: Child's Play

Wood, A. (1988). *Elbert's Bad Word*. Illustrated by A. & D. Wood. Orlando, FL: Harcourt Brace, Jovanovich

Booklist from Bloodgood, J.W., & Pacifici, L.C. (2004, November). Bringing word study to intermediate classrooms. *The Reading Teacher, 58,* 250-263. Reprinted with permission of the International Reading Association.

all the words we've been working on begin with *bl*. Try to remember the word by saying the beginning to yourself, and see whether that helps you remember the rest. When the teacher gives you a look, you /bl/. . . ?" Later, a second set of words with a different phonological pattern can be introduced and the two patterns can be used in the cloze procedure, with the clinician encouraging the students to try to remember which of the two beginnings start the word.

Gerber (1993) suggested further work to focus students' attention on the phonological properties of words. Students can be given phonological cues in games in which they guess a word after a clinician's clue. Again, the words can be drawn from classroom themes. The clinician might say:

> Here are pictures of five people in our school. I'm thinking of one whose job has four syllables. (secretary)
> Here are pictures of six foods. I'm thinking of one that rhymes with *seen*. (bean)
> Here are maps of three countries we've studied. I'm thinking of one that starts with /s/. (Spain)

Another application of phonological retrieval strategies combines work on vocabulary and spelling. Fulk and Stormont-Spurgin (1995) emphasized the importance of teaching spelling through analogy by pointing out, for example, that when two words rhyme, the last part of each word is often spelled the same. We can use these spelling analogies to highlight a variety of phonological similarities among words (for example, same ending, same beginning sound, same sound in the middle represented by double letters, same short vowel sound). By focusing on the structural similarity among words and pairing these sound similarities with written forms, we provide students with both auditory and visual images of the word for storage, again deepening and elaborating knowledge of words. In this way, we not only build vocabulary strength, but adhere to our principle of integrating oral and written instruction and provide a good foundation for increasing knowledge of words' written representation—their spelling—as well.

German (2002) investigated a word retrieval program that made use of words drawn from the curriculum and included three elements: metalinguistic reinforcement, phonemic neighbor cues, and rehearsal. These strategies are summarized in Box 12-5. German reported that these strategies were effective in improving students' access to words trained, but not to untrained words.

Helping students learn to use both semantic and phonological cues to aid in word finding provides the students with a broad-based strategy for improving their word-retrieval skills. There also are commercially available programs that target word finding, such as German's (2005) *Word Finding Intervention Program*.

Semantic Integration and Inferencing. As we have seen, students with LLD appear to have difficulties in spontaneously putting information together and drawing inferences from language they hear or read (DeKemel, 2003; Letts & Leinionen, 2001), although they do better in listening contexts than when reading (Wright & Newhoff, 2001). This suggests work on this area should begin with material the clinician tells or reads to the student before working on inferencing in material the student reads himself. Literature-based activities are an excellent frame-

---

BOX 12-5	**Word Retrieval Strategies**

1. **Metalinguistic Reinforcement:** Make student aware of syllable structure of target word. Present a grid of cells representing the number of syllables for the target word:

Segment the word into syllables for the student, and have student write each syllable in one of the boxes:

Hip	po	po	ta	mus

The student is then asked to say each syllable while touching its box, and to pronounce each syllable along with a clap.

2. **Phonemic Neighbor Cue:** The student is given a prompt word that is a 'phonemic neighbor,' or shares some phonemic properties of the target word. Examples include *hip* for hippopotamus, *try* and *angle* for triangle, *help* and *mitt* for helmet, *card* for cardinal. Students are taught to link each cue to the target word and to think of the prompt word but not say it (so the prompt will not interfere with access to the target: "Think *card*, say cardinal").

3. **Rehearsal:** Massed practice, in response to picture or written cues is used, but the requirement also to use each target word in a sentence is added.

From German, D.J. (2002). A phonologically based strategy to improve word-finding abilities in children. *Communiation Disorder Quarterly, 23,* 179-192.

work for developing semantic integration skills—the ability to synthesize ideas from several linguistic units. Inferencing activities take advantage of this ability. McGee and Johnson (2003) showed that specific training in drawing inferences resulted in significant improvement in primary aged children with LLD. One way to develop inferencing and semantic integration is to use prediction activities. Students can be read part of a short story or picture book from the classroom literature selection and asked to predict what they think will happen next and why. They can be asked to draw a picture of what they think the next part of the story will look like and to label or describe the picture in writing. Commercial materials also are available, such as Matthews' (1995) *Jump to a Conclusion!*

Students also can write their own stories around classroom themes or curricular content, individually or in small groups. They can be told to leave off the ending or to write the ending on a separate sheet of paper. For the second part of the lesson, the stories (without the endings) can then be passed to another student or group for a meaningful ending to be added. The completed stories might then be read aloud and the reasons for the chosen endings discussed and evaluated. If the original authors wrote the endings on a separate sheet of paper, these can be shared and compared with those produced in the second part of the activity. The students could evaluate which ending was better and why. Book series such as the TwistAPlot (Scholastic) and Choose Your Own Adventure series (Bantam Books), which are designed to allow readers to select among endings, also can be used in these activities. If necessary, the clinician can read the text to the students.

Interactive computer games also are very useful for this purpose. Many computer games used in schools allow students to select what comes next in a story or simulation activity. These programs, if available, can be used with students with LLD, with clinician assistance, if necessary, in reading the text on the screen. When working with computer games with students, we need to provide a lot of contextual and metalinguistic support. We want to be sure that the students are really attending to the semantic integration of the information and not getting so involved in the game that they are not focusing on the goal of the activity. Reminding students to remember the information in the story that they already know, think about what might happen next, and guess about the consequences of characters' actions can help to keep their inferencing at an awareness level.

Wallach and Miller (1988) also discussed some semantic integration and inferencing activities that can be done around smaller pieces of text. They cited Johnson and von Hoff Johnson's (1986) suggestion to present students with various sentences, following each one with a question that requires an inference. The sentences can relate to a curricular unit or be drawn from a classroom literature selection or theme-based unit. For example, if the class is reading *The Fox Went Out on a Chilly Night* (Spier, 1961), the following sentences and inferential questions might be presented:

---

1. The fox went out on a chilly night.
   What season of the year was it?
2. Then old mother Giggle-gaggle jumped out of bed.
   What was she doing before she heard the fox?
3. She cried, "John, John, the gray goose is gone and the fox is on the town."
   Who is John?
4. There were the little ones 8-9-10. They said, "Daddy, better go back there again, 'cuz it must be a wonderful town.
   Who are the little ones? Have they ever been to town before?

Inferencing activities also can be done around classroom themes. For example, if students are studying Mexico in geography or social studies, they can be presented with a selection such as the following:

Señora Rodriguez got out her cornmeal. She mixed it carefully with a small amount of water, then rolled the dough into a very thin circle. She filled it with some beans she'd fried, then put it in the oven. What was she doing?

Wallach and Miller also suggested helping students become more conscious of inferencing by producing "sentence bridges" to make inferred information explicit. For example, students working on a weather unit in science might be presented with the following two sentences:

Sam and Dave looked up at the dark and cloudy summer sky. They decided to listen to the game on the radio.

Students could be asked to explain how the second sentence might follow from the first. They could then be asked to fill in the middle with the clinician's guidance, after discussing why cloudy weather might lead to listening to a ball game on the radio. They might generate sentence bridges such as:

It looked as if it would rain.
They didn't want to drive all the way to the city in bad weather and sit in the rain all day.
It would be more fun to stay home and be warm and dry.

Syntax

Integrating Expression and Comprehension in Intervention. We talked in Chapter 3 about the principle of focusing on production in intervention, even when deficits in comprehension are identified in the assessment. Assessment data on comprehension and comprehension strategies can be used, as in the developing language period, to help select methods of intervention. If, for example, a student has trouble both understanding and producing passive sentences, work on producing passive sentences can take place in contexts such as literature-based script approaches and focused stimulation activities that provide opportunities for both comprehension and production of target forms. If comprehension is adequate and only production is limited, activities that integrate oral and written expression can be used, with less emphasis on providing input for comprehension development.

What if the assessment data tell us that the student uses comprehension strategies to process sentences that we are targeting for expressive work? Here an approach that includes both an expressive and receptive focus at a metalinguistic level will be helpful. If, again, passive sentences were the target, we might give the student pairs of sentences taken from classroom content. We might use the following sentences if *Gentle Ben* (Morey, 1965) were being read in class:

> Fog Benson always kept Ben chained.
> Ben was always kept chained by Fog Benson.

Students would be asked to discuss the characters in the story, to recall that Fog was the man who owned the bear, Ben. They could then be asked to draw a picture to illustrate the first sentence, decide whether the first and second sentences meant the same or different things, and tell why they knew ("Ben couldn't keep Fog chained, since Fog was the owner"). The clinician could then focus metalinguistically on the structure of the sentence, discuss what the *was* and *by* signaled, and give other examples of passive sentences. Students could be asked to generate more sentences about what characters in the story did to someone ("Mark's mother protected him, Mark's father frightened him, Fog shot Ben in Mark's dream"). The clinician could write the sentences down, give a passive equivalent for some, then ask students to generate the passive equivalents. At the end of the activity, the structures that signal the passive could be discussed again. Subsequent activities could use the same procedures applied to different classroom material. A similar approach could be used for other sentence forms on which assessment data indicate strategies are operating. These forms might include sentences with *before* and *after*; those with center-embedded relative clauses ("The man who owned the bear was named Fog Benson."); and other sentences, such as clefts, with unusual word order ("It was Fog Benson who owned the bear.").

In choosing syntactic forms to target at the L4L period, again, we want to remember to take into account data from *both* the assessment of a student's syntactic abilities *and* from assessment and understanding of the demands of classroom discourse as well as the literary language requirements of the curriculum. It also may be possible to do some preventive intervention by addressing forms we know are important for these contexts. The following sections contain some examples of these kinds of forms that contribute to classroom success and move language toward the literate end of the oral-literate continuum.

Advanced Morphology. Windsor, Scott, and Street (2000) showed that although children with LLD showed relatively high levels of correct morphological production in speech after age 7, they had significantly more errors in writing. When we work

with students with LLD on morphology, then, it is important to practice both saying and writing the markers in appropriate contexts. Gerber (1993) suggested that one way to address advanced morphological usage is to develop an understanding of the relationships between root words and derivations. Students can play matching or "Concentration" games with pairs of cards. Each pair would contain two words that share a common root. One of the words in each pair can be drawn from classroom activities. Students would be required to match the related words, for example:

social	**monster**	**clinic**
society	monstrous	clinician
school	**order**	**medicine**
scholastic	disorder	medical
danger	**muscle**	
dangerous	muscular	

In discussing how the words are related in meaning, we also can point out the relations in spelling, following the suggestion of Chomsky (1980). For example, we might show students that *muscle* and *muscular* both have a *c* in them, although the *c* is pronounced only in *muscular*. Students can be told that if they have trouble remembering how to spell *muscle*, they can remind themselves of the word *muscular*, in which the sound of the letter *c* is clearly heard. The same approach can be used to discuss the spelling of *medicine*. If the students can't remember whether to spell the /s/ sound in *medicine* with an *s* or a *c*, they can remind themselves of *medical*, in which a *c* is clearly the spelling. Similar reasoning can be used to discuss *social* and *society*, and many other terms. In fact, the students can be told that one of the reasons spelling in English has so many irregularities is that our writing system often preserves these connections among related words by retaining similar spelling patterns even when pronunciation changes over time (Chomsky & Halle, 1968). Frequently reminding students of these connections in succeeding work on morphology and vocabulary can help to build not only oral language skills but spelling ability. Evidence (Bhattacharya & Ehri, 2004) suggests that analytic approaches such as these help struggling readers both to recognize and spell new words more effectively.

Complex Sentences. Literature-based script approaches are great for developing complex sentence use, as they are for so many other language goals. Some examples of books for complex sentence development were provided in Appendix 9-1. Just one additional example that is especially appropriate for school-age children is *When I Was Young in the Mountains* (Rylant, 1982). This book has more mature content than most of those listed in Chapter 9 and can be used to encourage use of temporal conjunctions, among other things.

Other approaches to the development of complex syntax were suggested by Wallach and Miller (1988). They have students analyze complex sentences taken from classroom content or newspaper stories on topics of interest. The students first identify propositions included within the meaning of a complex sentence. Then they write out the propositions. For example, the clinician might choose a sentence from a classroom literature selection like *Charlotte's Web* (White, 1952):

> Every afternoon, when the school bus stopped in front of her house, [Fern] jumped out and ran to the kitchen to fix another bottle for [Wilbur].

Students might identify which of the following sentences' meaning were contained in the complex one:

> The school bus stopped at Fern's house every afternoon.
> Fern ran to the kitchen as soon as she got home from school.
> Wilbur's bottles were kept in the kitchen.
> Fern jumped in the kitchen.

The activity can then be reversed by supplying students with several sentences and asking them to find ways to combine them into one. This task can be done either orally or in writing, or on word-processing equipment. Using *Charlotte's Web* as our literature base again, we might ask students to combine the following sentences into one:

> Wilbur climbed up on top of the manure pile.
> Wilbur was full of energy and hope.
> The rat and the spider were watching Wilbur climb.

Paraphrasing is another way to develop complex sentence skills. Paul (1992b) suggested giving students sentences in two different forms, such as:

> Charlotte wove some words in the web.
> Some words were woven in the web by Charlotte.

Students can discuss whether the sentences mean the same thing and why they might choose one over the other. The clinician might ask, "Which one would you say to a friend? Which one would you use if you were writing a book?" and other questions. Students can then be given sentences to paraphrase (or "say a different way") on their own or in groups.

Wallach and Miller (1988) used picture sequences to discuss clause order in complex sentences. Students can be given pictures to place in correct order corresponding to a spoken or written sentence. Alternatively, the students can draw the pictures themselves, based on a literature selection. For example, they can draw a picture of Fern holding Wilbur on her lap and another of Fern feeding Wilbur a bottle. The clinician can present the following sentences and ask the students to arrange the pictures according to what the sentences say:

> Fern held Wilbur before she fed him.
> Fern held Wilbur after she fed him.
> After she fed Wilbur, Fern held him.
> Before she fed Wilbur, Fern held him.

As always, we would follow up such activities with metalinguistic discussions about how the different sentences convey different meanings, which pairs mean the same, in what situations each sentence would be most appropriate, and so on.

Preventive Intervention: Developing the Syntax of Literate Language. We can help students learn to use forms that build toward a more complex, literate language style, even without having extensive assessment data on this aspect of syntax. This type of work would be considered preventive intervention. It can help to minimize or head off later problems with literary language genres. Since we know these forms are needed for a literate language style, they can be included in the intervention program even if they were not addressed specifically in the assessment process. In the case of work on literate language style markers in both noun phrase and verb phrase elaboration, we would want to include these activities as supplements to the work on syntactic forms in which the client had identified deficits. We saw in Chapter 11 that the use of elaborated noun phrases is one aspect of the literate language style. We can encourage students to move from simple, unelaborated forms to providing more detail and modulation in their sentences. Elaboration of the verb phrase through adverbial and auxiliary marking is another aspect of the literate language style that can be addressed in preventive intervention. Again, literature-based approaches are very helpful here. It is also important to remember that, as Gummersall and Strong (1999) showed, repeated modeling and opportunities to practice are necessary for children with LLD to acquire these new forms.

Noun Phrase Elaboration. To encourage use of *multiple modifiers* and *prepositional phrases* to elaborate noun phrases, the clinician might write modifiers, prepositional phrases, or both, taken from the classroom literature selection or from a theme-based unit, on cards given to each student or group. Several nouns from the selection would be displayed on similar cards. Students would be asked to choose noun cards that could be elaborated with the modifiers and phrases they have. After discussing how the modifiers and phrases give more information about the nouns, students could be asked to put the noun phrases they've developed into sentences relating to the story or theme. They could then be asked to generate other modifiers or prepositional phrases that could modify the same nouns and to talk about how the meanings of the noun phrases would change accordingly. They might then write sentences with these new elaborated noun phrases. Eventually, new nouns could be introduced for which the students can generate modifiers and prepositional phrases, based on the ones with which they have become familiar in the earlier exercises.

To increase noun phrase elaboration with *relative clauses*, the clinician might use a story such as "The House that Jack Built." Gerber (1993) suggested writing each clause in the story on a strip of oak tag and allowing students to add their strip to the story as it is read. Students can then write their own version of the story, such as "This Is the House that Miguel Built," using different clauses to elaborate the tale.

To work on relative clause development at a higher level, Gerber (1993) suggested another activity. Each student or group is given a relative clause relating to a classroom theme (for example, *who study the earth's atmosphere*), written on an oak tag strip. The strip can be color coded so it can be referred to as "the red one" instead of as "the relative clause." Each student also receives a different-colored strip containing a subject noun phrase (for example, *The astronauts*) and one with a verb phrase (for example, *gather information for scientists*). The students see how many different, meaningful sentences they can form with their strips, writing each sentence down as they form it. The groups can compare their sentences and talk about how placing the relative clause (or red strip) in different places changes the meaning of the sentence.

Verb Phrase Elaboration. Nippold (1998) suggested working on the relative magnitude of adverbs. Students can be given cards with words such as *slightly*, *somewhat*, *quite*, *unusually*, and *extremely*. They can be asked to use the adverbs (or "words on blue cards") to fill in blanks in a passage relating to curricular content. For example, the clinician might write the following:

> Scientists worry that global warming is increasing average temperatures. Weather in some parts of the county has been _____ hot.

Students could decide which of their words best completes the sentence. Alternatively, the clinician could write three versions of the second sentence and ask students to discuss the meaning of each and talk about why they might choose one over the other as the best follow-up to the first sentence:

> Weather in some parts of the county has been slightly hot.
> Weather in some parts of the county has been unusually hot.
> Weather in some parts of the county has been quite hot.

Another way to encourage adverbial use is to present a list of adverbs relating to emotions. This can be combined with "intensity maps" like the one in Figure 12-4. Dialogue can be drawn from a classroom literature selection and students can be asked to choose the adverb (or "blue card") that could be used to show how the character would say that part of the story. Suppose students are reading *Curious George Rides a Bike* (Rey, 1952) in class. The children could be given the adverbs *sadly*, *angrily*, *curiously*, and *excitedly*. Then they could be asked to choose which one could be used to describe the way characters might speak in the following parts of the story:

> "I wonder what the river is like further on," said George
> _____.
> "We cannot use little monkeys who don't do as they are told!" said the director _____.
> "I won't be able to play the trumpet in the show now," George said _____.
> "There's George!" said the Man in the Yellow Hat
> _____.

Auxiliary Verb Marking. As DeKemel (2003) noted, children with specific language disorders typically have inordinate trouble learning the verb system of English. Using varied and combined auxiliaries to modulate the meaning of verbs in sentences is an important aspect of elaborating meaning, and provides opportunities to discuss roots and affixes in a metalinguistic, word study format. Literature-based script approaches can be used here, too. Texts familiar to students can be modified to include repeated instances of present perfect tense (*have arrived*), past perfect tense (*had arrived*), and auxiliary combinations (*could have arrived, could have been delayed*). These "homemade books" can be read repeatedly to children, following the procedures developed by Kirchner (1991) and outlined in Chapter 9. For example, if *Mr. Brown Can Moo, Can You?* (Seuss, 1970) is being read in the clients' classroom, the clinician can make a photocopy of each of its pages and paste over the usual text with versions that contain target forms. The book might be made to read, "Mr. Brown has mooed, have you?" and so on. As just one more example, the texts of Joslin's books on manners in silly situations, *What Do You Do, Dear?* (Joslin, 1961) and *What Do You Say, Dear?* (Joslin, 1986), could be modified to be read as "What could you have done, dear?" and "What could you have said, dear?"

Fey (1986) suggested that advanced auxiliary marking also can be taught by setting up a discourse context in which such forms are required. For example, the clinician might retell a story the students are reading in class, asking questions that create a context for the use of the past perfect tense. After reading the students the story, the clinician might say the following:

> A little old woman decided to bake a gingerbread boy. She had made the dough and put it in the oven, but when she opened the door, the oven was empty. What had happened?
> (The gingerbread boy had run away.)
> The woman yelled for him to stop, but the gingerbread boy ran on. The gingerbread boy ran past a little old man, who had stopped his work. What had happened to make him stop?
> (He had heard the little old woman yelling.)

Pragmatics

Conversational Discourse. We've talked about some of the conversational difficulties of our students with LLD. When assessing conversational discourse, we looked at the range of advanced intentions expressed; the way the client can modify the message depending on the context; and the management of discourse turns, topics, and breakdowns. We can address each of these areas in intervention.

A variety of conversational pragmatic programs are available commercially, many geared toward working with students with autism spectrum disorders. Some examples of these appear in Table 12-3.

As just one example, Dodge (1998) presented a program on general communication skills for elementary students that can be presented in classrooms for both mainstream and LLD

TABLE 12-3	**Examples of Commercially Available Programs for Addressing Conversational Pragmatics**	
TITLE	**AUTHOR**	**PUBLISHER**
"Ask and Answer" Social Skills Games	K. Spieloogle, M. Cullough, & M. DeShang	SuperDuper
Let's Be Better Friends: The Peer Integration Program	M.B. DeLaney, N. Griffin, & K. Fox	Janelle Publications
Maxwell's Manor: A Social Language Game	C. LoGiudice & N. McConnell	LinguiSystems
Positive Pragmatic Games	K. Gill & J. DeNinno	SuperDuper
Promoting Social Communication: Children with Developmental Disabilities from Birth to Adolescence	H. Goldstein, L.A. Kaczmarek, & K.M. English	Alimed Inc.
Ready-to-Use Social Skills Lessons & Activities for Grades PreK–K	R. Weltmann Begun, editor	Jossey-Bass
Ready-to-Use Social Skills Lessons & Activities for Grades 1–3	R. Weltmann Begun, editor	Jossey-Bass
Ready-to-Use Social Skills Lessons & Activities for Grades 4–6	R. Weltmann Begun, editor	Jossey-Bass
Room 14: A Social Language Program	C. Wilson	LinguiSystems
Scripting Junior: Social Skill Role-Plays	L. Miller	Thinking Publications
Social Communication Skills for Children	W. McGam & G. Werven	Pro-Ed Inc.
Social Skill Builder Software		Academic Communication Associates
Social Star	N. Gajewski, P. Hirn, & P. Mayo	Thinking Publications
Talk About Activities: Developing Social Communication Skills	A. Kelly	Pro-Ed Inc
Talk About: A Social Communication Skills Package	A. Kelly	Pro-Ed Inc
Talk! Talk! Talk! Tools to Facilitate Language	N. Muir, S. McCaig, K. Gerylo, M. Gompf, T. Burke, & P. Lumsden	Thinking Publications
The Socially Speaking Game	A. Schroeder	SuperDuper

students. In addition, incidental teaching contexts, such as those discussed for children in the developing language phase, can be modified to provide opportunities for students to use advanced communicative intentions. Suppose you found that a client expressed few advanced intentions, such as using language to reason and report. You might set up an activity in which students had to solve a problem, such as how to make a spider web out of black yarn (continuing our *Charlotte's Web* theme). After letting students try on their own, you might report their success to them ("You figured out how to start the web. You wound the yarn around your hand. Then you put the yarn on the desk, cut off a piece, and lay a bigger circle of yarn around it"). You might then "think out loud" about how to proceed with the next step. When the project was completed, you could ask the students to think about how they might tell another student how to do the task. You might ask them to reason about why they had trouble at first, or about other ways to approach it. As they do this, you can provide additional models of reporting and reasoning as expansions or extensions of the clients' comments.

Contextual variation can be practiced through role-playing. Variations can be made for the following purposes:

1. Politeness ("Let's pretend you're a mom asking her son to get her a pencil. Now pretend you're a teacher asking a student. Now be a teenager asking his friend. Now be a boy asking his sister for the pencil she borrowed.")
2. Tact ("Pretend you're a doctor telling a patient she needs an operation. Pretend you're telling a friend you already have the book she gave you for your birthday.")
3. Assertiveness ("Pretend you want to tell your friend something, but she's not listening. Pretend your sister is hurt and you need to tell your mother, who is talking on the telephone.")

Bedrosian (1985), Brinton and Fujiki (1989;1995), Brinton, Robinson, and Fujiki (2004), Mentis (1994), Naremore, Densmore, and Harman (1995), and Paul and Sutherland (2003) presented many suggestions for activities that can be used to address a variety of discourse management skills. As one example of a topic-maintenance activity, Brinton and Fujiki (1989) suggested engaging the client in a conversation about a topic of the child's interest. The clinician provides scaffolding to remain on the topic. If the child begins to wander from the topic of how he liked the basketball game he saw over the weekend, the clinician might comment, "That sounded like a great game you saw. Tell me about the most exciting play." Gradually, the scaffolding should be reduced, so that only cues are provided (for example, "Is that what we're talking about?" can be used at first and then later just a tap on the wrist). The client can then be asked to have a similar conversation with a peer. The clinician can sit beside the client and give the cue (a tap on the wrist) if the client strays from the topic, whispering a verbal cue or a prompt for an appropriate comment in the client's ear, if necessary.

Paul and Sutherland (2003) suggested activities such as conversational mapping, in which children make a "scrapbook" containing one page for each friend. Each page contains a picture or drawing of a child the client would like to talk with, along with pictures of things the client knows each "friend" likes or is interested in. They role-play talking to each "friend" with the clinician, by asking one question about what the "friend" likes, and saying two things about that topic before introducing a new topic. After role-playing, they try approaching the new "friend" in a similar way, and report back to the clinician on how it went.

Brinton et al. (2004) presented a case study of a conversational treatment program, which is summarized in Box 12-6. It is important to note that their program lasted for 2 years, suggesting that in order to make significant changes in a client's conversational style, extensive intervention will often be required.

We talked about the use of barrier games, or referential communication activities, for assessment of presuppositional skills and of the ability to clarify and request clarification. Barrier games also can be used in intervention for discourse management. The clinician, as speaker, can model appropriate presuppositional behavior, pointing out to the client how the clinician's message was effective because it contained appropriate information. Again, vocabulary and sentence structures being targeted in intervention can be used in these barrier games, to help the student learn to use new forms and meanings in presuppositionally appropriate ways.

For work on clarification and communicative repair, the client can be given a turn as speaker in a barrier game, with the clinician requesting clarification as frequently as possible during the exchange. Discussion about the interaction can follow, with the clinician pointing out how important it is to ask when we don't understand something. Roles can then be reversed. This time the clinician can give purposefully unclear messages. Nonsense words can be inserted in the message, or part of it can be mumbled. If the student fails to request clarification, the clinician can allow the task to be completed. Then

---

| **BOX 12-6** | **Elements of Conversational Treatment Study of Brinton, Robinson, and Fujiki (2004)** |

1. Watch short film clips from movies client had seen and role-play scenarios in them to increase awareness of the social, emotional, and contextual information needed to function appropriately in conversation.
2. Have client consider and comment on the exchange of messages between conversational partners.
3. Review videotapes depicting clinic personnel role-playing events and interactions similar to those client had experienced at school, portraying difficult, isolating, or harassing incidents (e.g., peers ridiculing a student who was standing alone) and have client describe how various characters felt and what their intent was at different points in the interaction.
4. Generate possible conversation topics, write them on slips of paper, place them in a can; pick one at random.
5. Clinician models steps for the "conversation game": read the paper and take a moment to think about the topic, then make one comment on the topic, ask a question, and listen to the response.
6. Increase complexity of "rules" for the "conversation game" as client masters previous level:
   Make two comments on the topic, ask a question, and listen to the response.
   Make two comments on the topic, ask a question, listen to the response, and comment on that response.
   Make two comments on the topic, ask a question, listen to the response, comment on that response, ask a related question, and listen to the response.
   Make several comments on the topic, ask a question, listen to the response, make some comments on that response, ask a related question, and listen to the response.
7. Additional strategies initiated at later points in the program include:
   Ask for your partner's opinion.
   Talk approximately the same amount of time as your partner does (balance the conversation).
   Determine what interests your partner.
   Draw your listener(s) into the conversation.
   Respond to your listener's needs.
8. Later sessions provide cues to client's failure to adhere to appropriate conversational give and take. Each cue is demonstrated, then given in context if client begins dominating the conversation or ignoring listener needs:
   Yawn
   Look at watch
   Look away from client
   Client is taught first to recognize these cues, then to develop appropriate responses to them.

errors in completion can be discussed and the clinician can point out that some of the message was unclear, ask the client whether he or she detected the miscommunication, and ask what he or she might have done. The interaction can then be replayed, with the client coached to request clarification at appropriate points. Additional activities can provide opportunities for the client to experience such unclear messages and respond to them. As we saw in Chapter 11, many commercial materials, such as *Make-It Yourself Barrier Activities* (McKinley & Schwartz, 1987), *Barrier Games for Better Communication* (Deal & Hanuscin, 1999), and *Creatures & Critters* (Marquis, 2004), are available for use in barrier games.

Classroom Discourse Skill. We talked in the last chapter about using classroom observation methods to identify any difficulties a student might be having with the "hidden curriculum" of classroom discourse (Christie, 2003; DeKemel, 2003). Some of the work to improve classroom discourse performance involves working with the teacher in a consulting role to modify the demands of the classroom. We'll talk about this role a bit later. We also can work with the child, though, to improve some classroom discourse skills.

Ripich and Spinelli (1985) suggested using the intervention setting to construct a "miniclassroom." In this setting, "hidden curriculum" rules are first discussed and made explicit, then practiced. Each miniclass session begins with a discussion of a school event or routine. Creaghead (1990) provided a variety of classroom routines or scripts that serve as a basis for these discussions. These are listed in Table 12-4.

After discussing the hidden rules and structure of each script, the students do an activity involving the script, with some taking roles of students and one taking the role of the teacher. The miniclass might, for example, role-play coming to class and doing a show-and-tell or sharing time. The student playing the teacher role would be encouraged to provide specific correction to students who fail to adhere to the rules the group generated to describe the hidden curriculum of the activity. When the clinician plays the role of teacher, he or she can purposefully give unclear directions or violate the rules of the script to encourage students to ask for clarification and assert themselves in a group setting.

Narrative Skill. We've already discussed some ways to develop inferencing in narrative and to scaffold narrative macrostructure. Let's look at a few more examples of activities that can be used to increase narrative comprehension and production to fortify this important bridge from oral to literate language.

Comprehending Narratives. Norris and Hoffman (1993) advocated developing a *preparatory set* with students before they read a story to activate their background knowledge about the story's topic and to get them ready to take in the new information the story will provide. Hoggan and Strong (1994) suggested using the story's title to establish a preparatory set by asking students to talk about what they know about specific words in the title and to identify words or concepts with which the students are unfamiliar. Unknown words can be discussed, and students can act out meanings of words. However, Stahl (2004) pointed out that the discussion of background knowledge must be carefully constrained by the teacher, or it is likely to lead away from the text to personal experiences of students that may not be relevant. She advocates targeted discussions of background knowledge, guided by the teacher with focused discussion of what students know about teacher-selected, relevant topics before reading or listening to a text, and open-ended questions evoking background knowledge relevant to specific events during the story.

Nessel (1989) and Stahl (2004) suggest using *directed reading-thinking activities* to establish preparatory sets. Here students are shown the book to be read and told the title, but not told the story's topic. Students are asked to make predictions about the topic of the story and to give support for their opinions. Predictions are listed, so they can be compared to the events in the story after it is read in its entirety. Students then hear the first few paragraphs and are asked whether they want to change their predictions. After reading the whole story, students are asked to compare their predictions to what happened in the story, identify predictions that were correct, and contrast those

TABLE 12-4	**Scripts Used in Classroom Discourse**	
EVENT SCRIPTS	**ORAL SCRIPTS**	**WRITTEN SCRIPTS**
Coming to class	Getting help from teacher	Writing about personal experiences
Following directions	Sharing information	Writing book reports
Completing worksheets or workbooks	Talking with peers	Writing about current events
Listening in a group	Reading aloud	Writing reports in subject areas
Taking tests	Explaining or defending behavior	Creative writing
Taking home and turning in homework	Giving oral reports	Writing messages
Lunch or recess	Show-and-tell or sharing time	Journal writing
Dismissal	Requesting clarification	

Adapted from Creaghead, N. (1990). Mutual empowerment through collaboration: A new script for an old problem. In W. Secord (Ed.). *Best practices in school speech-language pathology* (vol. 1) (pp. 106-116). San Antonio, TX: Psychological Corp., Harcourt Brace Jovanovich. Reproduced by permission.

that did not turn out to be true. Students can explain what events in the story led to different conclusions than the ones they predicted.

Literature webbing is another prediction technique reported to have significant effects on young readers' ability to predict and retell story events (Stahl, 2004). The teacher or SLP writes key events from a story on cards, and gives each group of students a set of these cards in random order before hearing a story. Each group organizes the cards into the order they predict will occur in the story. They then hear or read the story, check their predicted order, and discuss any changes they need to make and why.

Westby (2005) suggested that another way to enhance understanding of narrative is through repeated, scaffolded exposure. In addition to the scaffolding techniques we've already discussed, we also can work with the texts we provide to students to identify story grammar elements. After reading the story, we can ask a series of questions, such as the following:

▸ Where did the story happen?

▸ Who were the important people in it?

▸ What problem got the story going?

▸ How did the people try to solve the problem?

▸ How did it end?

The questions chosen would depend on the student's current level of narrative functioning. If, for example, we were working with students at a Primitive Narrative level, using a story like *Just for You* (Mayer, 1975), which is at a Chain level, we would ask questions to elicit Chain-level responses. These would include the following:

▸ Who were the important characters (after explaining that a character is a person or animal in a story)?

▸ What problem is the little bunny trying to solve on this page? (He wants to do something nice for his mom.)

▸ How did he try to solve the problem? (He tries to make her breakfast.)

▸ What happens? (He spills the eggs on the floor.)

After working orally on asking questions related to the story grammar, we might list all the story grammar elements for the level of narrative at which the students are working, discussing and explaining the vocabulary as we do so. We might then read another story at the same level and ask the students to pose the story-grammar-element questions to each other. The next step would be to write a group book report, using one of Westby's book report forms from Box 12-2. Later, students can be asked to write individual book reports, again using a form, after a group discussion of the story grammar elements in another story at the same level. When students can comfortably comprehend stories at this level, stories at a higher level of narrative can be introduced. Dimino, Taylor, and Gersten (1995) reviewed research demonstrating that story grammar instruction promoted comprehension of narrative texts in students with LLD as well as in those at risk. A related technique uses teacher "think-alouds" to model processing of the story during oral reading. The teacher/SLP voices all the things she notices, does, visualizes, feels, and asks herself during the reading of a text. Wilhelm (2001) showed that this strategy also improved comprehension.

Hoggan and Strong (1994) suggested supplementing these kinds of activities with visual aids. A story flow chart (Ollman, 1989) can be used to help students visualize the relations among events in the story. After reading, the clinician can ask students to call out the major events they remember from the story. The students' ideas are listed on the board. The clinician then draws the chart and has the students place the events they listed in the appropriate place on the chart. Figure 12-5 illustrates a flow chart developed from A.A. Milne's (1926) "In which Pooh Goes Visiting and Gets into a Tight Place." Garner and Bochna (2004) showed that instruction like this in narrative text structure provided persistent improvements in typical first graders' reading comprehension. Boyle (1996) demonstrated that this kind of mapping resulted in LLD students showing substantial gains in both literal and inferential comprehension. Stahl (2004) also suggests using visual imagery to improve story comprehension. Teachers demonstrate how to "paint a picture in your mind" first of several displayed objects, then of events heard or read in stories. Think-aloud protocols can be used to model the visualization process. Stahl reports that visualization training increased both comprehension and retelling in primary grade children.

For students at True Narrative levels of development, Westby (1991) suggested using stories that highlight aspects of the story grammar that are most likely to be difficult for students with LLD. She advocated helping students become aware of character traits by reading several books about one set of characters and having students discuss and list the character's attributes. This procedure lends itself well to having students write their own stories about the characters they have been discussing, being sure to maintain the personalities they have described. Series popular with children, such as Harry Potter (Rowling [Scholastic]), Animorphs and Megamorphs (K.A. Applegate [Scholastic Books]), Nancy Drew (C. Keene [Simon & Schuster]), the Hardy Boys (D.W. Dixon [Simon & Schuster]), or the Moomintroll books (T. Jansson [Farrar, Straus, and Giroux]) can be helpful here.

Students with LLD also are likely to have trouble understanding how feelings can motivate actions in stories. Westby (2005) suggested using wordless picture books, such as Mayer's "boy and frog" series (Dial Books) or *What Whiskers Did* (Carroll, 1965), for this purpose. Students can be encouraged to talk about the feelings portrayed by characters in the pictures, to give words for the feelings, and to talk about how the feelings drive the action of the story. Students can then make posters by cutting out or drawing pictures of people who exemplify emotions they discussed in the story. The "angry" poster might then serve as the basis for writing a group story about what made all the people on it angry. The "sad" poster could be used to generate another story, and so on. Alternatively, Hoggan and Strong suggested making an "Internal States Chart." Each character in a story is listed, and students are encouraged to talk about how that character felt at different points in the story. An example of an Internal States Chart, based on the story of "Androcles and the Lion" (Baldwin, 1955), is given in Table 12-5.

Student Ideas

Pooh wants to visit Rabbit in Rabbit's hole.	Rabbit tries to help.
Rabbit is worried.	Rabbit gets Christopher Robin.
Pooh eats all Rabbit's food.	Christopher Robin says Pooh has to wait to get thin.
Pooh tries to get out.	He reads to Pooh.
He gets stuck.	

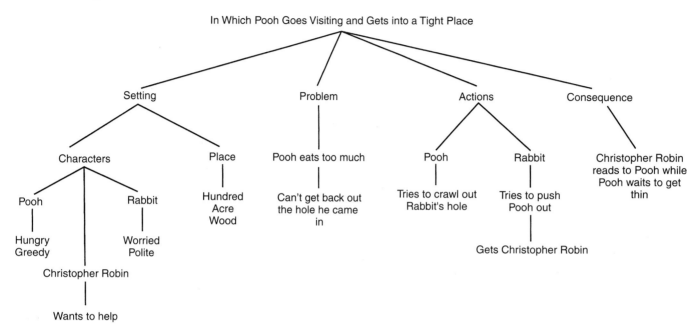

FIGURE 12-5 ✦ Flow chart of A.A. Milne's (1926) "In which Pooh Goes Visiting and Gets into a Tight Place." (Adapted from Hoggan, K., & Strong, C. [1994]. The magic of "once upon a time": Narrative teaching strategies. *Language, Speech, and Hearing Services in Schools, 25,* 76-89; and Ollman, H. [1989]. Cause and effect in the real world. *Journal of Reading, 33,* 224-225.)

TABLE 12-5	An Internal States Chart for the Story "Androcles and the Lion"

CHARACTER	FEELING	EVENT	MOTIVE
Androcles	Fear	Meets lion	Lion may eat him
Lion	Pain	Roars and frightens Androcles	Thorn in foot
People who watch Androcles and Lion in arena	Surprise	Lion will not eat Androcles	They expected lion to be fierce

Adapted from Hoggan, K., & Strong, C. (1994). The magic of "once upon a time": Narrative teaching strategies. *Language, Speech, and Hearing Services in Schools, 25,* 76-89; and Baldwin, J. (1955). Androcles and the lion. In *Favorite tales of long ago.* New York: J.P. Dutton.

Students with LLD often have trouble recognizing how characters' plans and intentions affect events in the story. Here Westby (2005) suggested using "trickster tales," in which a character achieves goals through deceit. Some examples include *Miss Nelson Is Missing* (Allard & Marshall, 1977), *Tales of an Ashanti Father* (Appiah, 1989), *Stone Soup* (Brown, 1947), *Iktomi and the Boulder: A Plains Indian Story* (Goble, 1988), *Anansi and the Moss-Covered Rock* (Kimmel, 1990), *How Rooster Saved the Day* (Lobel, 1977), and *Raven the Trickster: Legends of the North American Indians* (Robinson, 1982). Jarvey and McKeough (2003) found that using character webs to help students map out the strengths, weaknesses, desires, and fears of characters in trickster tales was particularly helpful in understanding these story forms (Figure 12-6). Students can discuss how the character tricked others in the story, how their actions did not match their intentions, and whether the characters were right to deceive as they did. For follow-up, older students can write a story about a time, real or imagined, that someone tricked them and how they felt when they realized what happened.

Other procedures for working on story comprehension can be adapted from material designed for reading comprehension activities. The clinician can adapt these materials by reading the text to the students, reading the students the comprehension questions, allowing the students to work on answering the

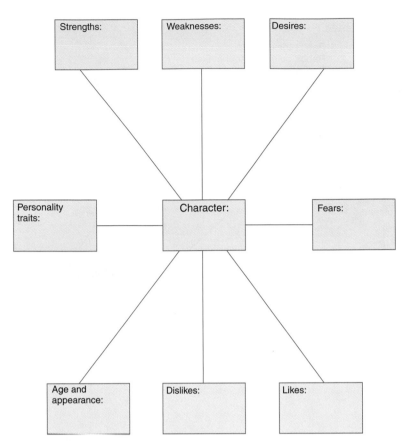

Strengths:

Weaknesses:

Desires:

Personality traits:

Character:

Fears:

Age and appearance:

Dislikes:

Likes:

FIGURE 12-6 ✦ Character web for use with trickster tales.

questions in cooperative learning groups, and having the students generate their own comprehension questions to follow up the texts provided in the materials. It is important, though, to avoid too-heavy reliance on these traditional kinds of comprehension materials that focus on the details, sequences, facts, and literal interpretations necessary but not sufficient for authentic comprehension of texts. Kamhi (1997) and Westby (2005) argued that these basic comprehension activities should be supplemented by those that involve the reader in a more elaborated and personal response to the story. These activities include relating personal experiences to the story; finding similarities between the story and others the students have read or heard; and talking about not only what characters do but about how they feel and what their plans, goals, and motivations for action are.

One way to approach this more elaborated level of comprehension was proposed by Hoggan and Strong (1994). They described the Question-Answer Relationship Techniques (QART) developed by Raphael (1984) to deepen students' understanding of narrative texts. Here, a clinician would first introduce four types of questions most frequently asked about stories. The clinician would ask example questions of each type about a story the group had read or heard. Students would then be encouraged to find the answers, using information from both the text and their own background knowledge. Examples of the four question types used in this technique, using *Three Billy Goats Gruff* (Rudin, 1982) as the sample text, can be found

in Box 12-7. Mastropieri and Scruggs (1997) have shown that teacher-led questions such as these are an especially effective technique for improving text comprehension in students with LLD, particularly if the activity is followed by instruction that leads students to use self-questioning strategies in their independent reading.

Whatever techniques are used to enhance story comprehension, recent research (Adams, 1997; Pressley, 1998; Pressley Wharton-McDonald, 1997; Stahl, 2004) has demonstrated that comprehension skills must be addressed with direct instruction that teaches children explicit strategies for getting meaning from what they read or hear, and this is even more true for students with LLD (Gleason, 1995; Nation, Clarke, Marshall, & Durand, 2004; Rabren, Darch, & Eaves, 1999). Activities such as the ones outlined in this section, then, make excellent collaborative teaching lessons, as well as direct service activities. All the students in the classroom, as well as those with special needs, benefit from this kind of direct comprehension instruction.

Composing Narratives. Narrative production provides an excellent context for implementing our intervention principle of integrating oral and written language in intervention. Norris and Hoffman (1993) suggested some ways to start the process of producing stories with students at low levels of writing ability. Beginning writers can be given a photocopy of a page or pages from a favorite story and some typewriter correction fluid. They can be asked to change as many elements of the story

| **BOX 12-7** | **Question Types Used in the QART Technique** |

Question Type 1: Right There

The answer can be found easily in the story. The words for the question and the words for the answer can be found in the same sentence.

> Q1: Why did the littlest billy goat decide to cross the bridge?
> A: He couldn't wait any longer to eat the sweet grass on the other side.

Question Type 2: Think and Search

The answer can be found in the story but requires information from more than one sentence or paragraph.

> Q2: Why were the billy goats afraid to cross the bridge?
> A: A mean troll lived under the bridge, and he threatened to eat anyone who tried to cross.

Question Type 3: Author and You

The answer is not in the story. Students need to think about what they already know about the topic and combine that knowledge with what the author provides in the story to infer the answer to the question.

> Q3: Why did the troll let the littlest billy goat go by without eating him?
> A: He was greedy and thought that he could get more to eat by waiting for the bigger brother.

Question Type 4: On My Own

An inferential question that encourages students to search their knowledge base. The answer to the question is relevant to the text but does not appear in it.

> Q4: What would you do if a bully like the troll in the story was keeping you and your friends from going somewhere?

Adapted from Hoggan, K., & Strong, C. (1994). The magic of "once upon a time": Narrative teaching strategies. *Language, Speech, and Hearing Services in Schools, 25,* 76-89; and Raphael, T. (1984). Teaching learners about sources of information for answering comprehension questions. *Journal of Reading, 27,* 303-311.

---

as they like by "whiting out" a word or words and supplying their own replacement words. Later, specific kinds of alterations can be used, such as asking the student to add to the text by putting in adjectives, prepositional phrases, or new clauses.

Ukrainetz (1998) suggests another strategy for this level of story production. She uses "stickwriting" to help children at early narrative levels preserve the stories they produce. This technique encourages students to plan and record stories using simple pictographs in order to give developmentally younger students a quick and easy method for representing characters, settings, and sequences of actions, while avoiding the frustration often involved in writing at this level. She suggests using "stickwriting" to help students plan and represent time sequences in their stories. She uses the technique, along with verbal prompting, to help students to sequence events in their stories ("What happened first. Draw a quick picture of that. Then what? Draw that next. Remember to keep the drawing quick and easy."). After the stickwriting is completed, the student "reads" the story back to the clinician with support from the pictographic cues. Research on this technique demonstrates its benefits for increasing length and quality of early narratives and for allowing a greater focus on content, rather than the mechanics of writing. After stories are initially represented this way, they can be translated into more conventional written

form. Figure 12-7 presents two examples of students' "stick-writing" stories.

For students with some facility in the mechanics of writing, who are ready to do more independent narrative production, Stewart (1991) suggested introducing and discussing the parts of the story grammar, as we did in the comprehension activities, and using these as a basis for students to produce their own stories. This can be done whenever students reach a True Narrative stage of story development. Posting the story grammar elements on a wall chart can serve as a guide to the composition, which may be spoken, dictated, written, or typed, depending on the students' abilities. Other visual aids, such as the Story Grammar Marker (Moreau & Fidrych, 1998), also can be useful.

Story maps or webs also can be used to guide students' composition of stories, using formats like the one in Figure 12-5 and leaving the nodes blank for students to fill in and use later to structure their written productions. Zipprich (1995) showed that these techniques were effective in increasing planning time and improving quality of story writing in children with LLD.

Students also can be asked to generate group stories by modifying stories they have read or heard. They might listen to the clinician tell "Goldilocks and the Three Bears," for example, and then read James Marshall's (1988) humorous version of the

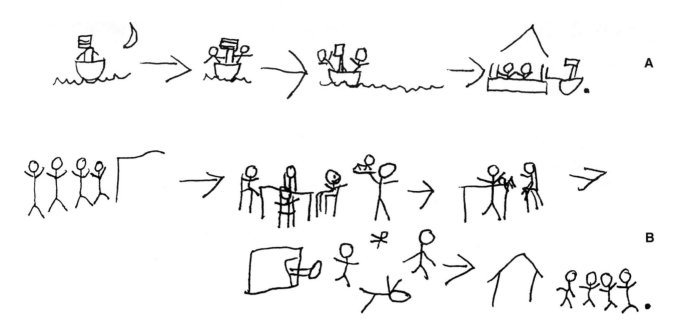

FIGURE 12-7 ✦ Two examples of a pictogram from (*A*) a fourth-grade student with language impairment showing a boat rescue story and (*B*) a typical second-grade student showing a frog escaping from a restaurant.
(Reprinted with permission from T. Ukrainetz [1998]. Stickwriting stories: A quick and easy narrative representational strategy. *Language, Speech, and Hearing Services in Schools, 29,* 200.)

tale. Another possibility is to listen to "Little Red Riding Hood," then read the Chinese version, *Lon Po Po* (Young, 1989). They could then be asked to write their own version. The resulting story can be illustrated and read to the rest of the class or to younger students. Later activities can include generating stories about students' own experiences as they relate to a literature selection they hear. If students are reading *Little House in the Big Woods* (Wilder, 1932) in class, for example, they might write stories about a time they helped their parents make or do something at home. Students can be reminded to refer to the story grammar visual aid to guide their compositions. Many additional ideas for facilitating narrative skills can be found in Apel and Masterson (2005), DeKemel (2003), Falk-Ross (2002), Merritt, Culatta, and Trostle (1998), and Roth (2000).

Word-processing computer programs also can be used in these kinds of activities. Software programs, such as *Kidspiration* (Inspiration Software, Portland, OR), *Kidwriter* (Spinnaker Software, Cambridge, Mass.), *Explore-a-Story* (D.C. Health, Cambridge, Mass.), and *Logowriter* (Log Computer Systems, New York), allow students to produce text and select graphics to illustrate stories and to rearrange elements of classic stories to create new versions. Cochran and Bull (1991) discussed additional ways to integrate word processing in language instruction at the L4L stage. Roth (2000) summarized a range of strategies, in addition to those already mentioned that can be used to improve narrative production in students with LLD. These are summarized in Box 12-8. Many of these approaches will be discussed in more detail later in this chapter and in Chapter 14.

Cohesion. Although cohesive markers such as pronouns, conjunctions, and articles (*a/an/the*) are used in a variety of texts in addition to narratives, stories rely especially on

cohesion as an important element in their structure, and they are excellent contexts for developing cohesion skills. Let's look at some ideas for developing awareness and use of cohesive markers in narratives. As usual, we want to choose narratives that come from classroom literature selections or coordinate with curriculum themes.

Wallach and Miller (1988) provided a variety of activities for developing cohesive skills. They suggested working on pronouns by taking sentences that contain a referent and a pronoun from a literature selection. If we use the example of *Little House in the Big Woods* again, we might choose the following sentences:

> Every evening before he began to tell stories, Pa made bullets for his next day's hunting. Laura and Mary helped him.

The clinician can help the students to identify pronouns and referents in the sentences. A pronoun chart like the one in Table 12-6 can be a useful adjunct to this discussion.

The students can look for additional examples of pronouns and their referents in the text and generate their own sentences with pronouns about the characters in the story. The clinician can then present sentences with ambiguous referents, like the following:

> He told them a great story.

Students can be asked to guess what characters from the story might go with the pronouns. They can then write more text around the sentence to remove the ambiguity. Other activities

---

BOX 12-8   **Procedures for Improving Narrative Production**

Prewriting: Drawing by hand or with computer programs such as *The Amazing Writing Machine* (Broderbund, 1999), The *Ultimate Writing and Creativity Center* (The Learning Company, 1996), and *Curious George Paint and Print Studio* (Pearson Software, 2000).

Story web: A graphic organizer in which each element of story grammar is represented as a node on a web.

Schematic story structure: Each story grammar component is sequentially introduced and defined. Students identify these elements in stories, and build their own stories using the following:

   Story frames: written starters for each story grammar element are provided in a cloze task.

   Scrambled stories: a written story is presented with one element out of sequence; students recognize it and restructure.

   Story grammar facilitation: students are given cards with story grammar elements written on them, which they use to organize their story.

   Story grammar cue cards: students are given a check list containing the story grammar elements that they check off as they include each element in their story.

   Story prompts: a set of questions or prompts the student answers to produce each story grammar element.

   Acronyms: SPACE (Setting, Problem, Action, Consequence, End), for example, are used to help students remember to include all story parts in order.

   Self-regulated strategy development (SRSD): This approach involves teaching the planning, production, and revision processes. It can make use of "think sheets" that serve as cues for student to carry out specific activities within each of these phases.

Adapted from Roth, F. (2000). Narrative writing: Development and teaching with children with writing difficulties. *Topics in Language Disorders, 20(4),* 15-28.

TABLE 12-6   **Words that Stand for People: A Pronoun Cohesion Chart**

	BOYS AND GIRLS	ONLY GIRLS	ONLY BOYS
One person	I, me, my, mine, myself	She, her, hers, herself	He, him, his, himself
One or more people	You, your, yours, yourself, yourselves		
More than one person	We, us, our, ours, ourselves, they, them, their, theirs, themselves		

Adapted from Wallach, G., & Miller, L. (1988). *Language intervention and academic success.* Boston, MA: College-Hill Press; and Bauman, J. (1986). Teaching third-grade students to comprehend anaphoric relationships: The application of a direct instruction model. *Reading Research Quarterly, 21,* 70-90.

---

might involve substituting pronouns for some of the nouns in the text to see whether it can still be understood; substituting nouns for some of the pronouns; and writing summaries of individual chapters in the book, using pronouns carefully to provide cohesion. As always, metalinguistic discussion should accompany each phase of the activity, to give the students opportunities to evaluate the effect of using and changing pronouns on the cohesion of the text (or on "how the story hangs together and is easy to follow").

Work on the development of cohesion through conjunction use is particularly helpful because complex sentences that encode various semantic relations between propositions can be used in the process. These sentences and relations are frequently identified as intervention targets in our assessment of students with LLD. Working on complex sentence forms and on combining semantic relations between propositions in the context of narrative is another way to adhere to one of our guiding principles for intervention in the L4L period; that is, to integrate intervention targets identified in the assessment with work toward a literate language style. Let's look at some ideas for doing this.

Wallach and Miller (1988) suggested taking propositions from classroom literature selections and working on combining them using appropriate conjunctions and relations. Following Lahey's (1988) sequence as discussed earlier, we would work on relations and conjunctions in the following order:

1. Temporal relations with conjunctions *then, when, before, after,* etc.
2. Causal relations with conjunctions *because, so,* etc.
3. Conditional relations with conjunctions *if-then*
4. Epistemic relations with conjunction *that*
5. Notice-perception relations with *wh-* conjunctions such as *what, where, how,* etc.
6. Specification relations with conjunctions *that, which*
7. Adversative relations with conjunctions *but, though, although,* etc.

Let's use *Little House in the Big Woods* as our example again. Suppose you were working at early stages with third-graders. You might ask students to combine the following propositions from the story:

> Laura touched the shiny, hot bullet.
> Laura burned her finger.

For later stages of development, with fifth-graders say, you might choose the following propositions:

> The bullet was too hot to touch.
> The bullet shone so brightly that Laura couldn't help touching it.

Either way, you would encourage the students to think about how the two ideas might go together and discuss possibilities for how they might be combined in one sentence. Students could then generate a sentence, with the clinician's help at first, which combined the two ideas with a conjunction or "hooking-up word." Again, a wall chart listing conjunctions, each with a hook drawn from it to symbolize its linking function, could serve as a reference. Students might be asked to generate, orally or in writing, other ideas in the story that could be "hooked up" with the same conjunction. Students might then write their own story, with the stipulation that the target conjunction appear three times in it. When other conjunctions have been addressed, stories can be required to contain one instance of each of the conjunctions the students have been learning. As always, stories should be discussed when completed, to allow students to evaluate how well they have used the target conjunctions to "hook up" ideas in the story.

Naremore, Densmore, and Harman (1995) suggested a strategy-based approach for helping children produce cohesive narratives. They begin by having students first identify the main idea in a story read to them and then in a story they intend to produce. They are then instructed to find a way to tie each sentence to the main idea by using one of the four following devices:

1. Pronouns
2. Repetition of key words
3. Substitutions for key words
4. Lists of items relating to the main idea

Students are first given examples of stories that omit these cohesive ties and are asked to change them to improve their cohesion. They then develop their own versions, using appropriate cohesive markers. Paul (1992b) provided some additional activities for developing conjunctions and semantic relations between propositions in stories.

The Metas

Many of the activities we've been discussing in this chapter have metalinguistic components. We want to provide students with the opportunity to talk about and evaluate all the language they use in our intervention program, to bring it to a higher level of awareness. The following activities provide some additional suggestions for helping students attend to, think about, and use "meta" skills.

Phonological Awareness. We've already talked at length about the importance of PA in the process of learning to read and about the need to integrate PA with other approaches to reading instruction. PA may be part of the intervention program for primary grade children with higher-level phonological difficulties that were identified during assessment that makes use of phonological production, with tasks or the checklists we discussed in Chapter 11, or with classroom-based methods like those suggested by Justice et al. (2002). Even students in intermediate grades who are having reading difficulty can benefit from explicit PA instruction with the SLP, in conjunction with remedial reading help from the reading or LD specialist. Remember, though, that we don't want to develop PA as an isolated skill. We only want to address it to the extent that it helps students decode words for reading and encode for spelling. For older students, PA activities should be used only until students can accurately segment words into sounds, represent sounds with appropriate letters, and synthesize letter sounds to decode words. At that point, more targeted reading and spelling instruction should be implemented (Catts, 1999a; Torgesen, Otaiba, & Grek, 2005).

PA work also makes sense as a target of preventive intervention. Primary-grade students with a history of language problems or unintelligible speech and those who are still functioning at developing language levels are particularly vulnerable to problems in learning to read. Similarly, students from low-income or culturally different backgrounds who have little literacy socialization experience when they come to school are prone to reading problems. All these students would be considered at risk for reading failure. Foorman and Torgesen (2001) reviewed a broad range of literature on promoting literacy and identified the following elements to be necessary for reading success for all children. These include explicit instruction in the following:

- Phonemic awareness and decoding
- Fluency in word recognition
- Comprehension strategies for processing texts and deriving meaning from them
- Vocabulary
- Spelling
- Writing

For students at risk for reading failure, Foorman and Torgesen's review indicates that these children do *not* need a different program of instruction; instead they need more of the same: more intensive provision of explicit and comprehensive instruction on the same elements we listed above, in individual and small group settings that provide high levels of both emotional support and cognitive scaffolding. Blachman et al. (2000) showed that the same applied to children in grades 2–3 with poor reading skills. And Wright and Jacobs (2003) demonstrated that combining PA instruction with direct teaching of metalinguistic concepts (such as letter, word, syllable, vowel, consonant) and metacognitive strategies (such as planning and self-monitoring) was even more advantageous for struggling readers. That's why it makes such good sense for SLPs to work with teachers in primary classrooms to deliver this explicit instruction to all children, and observe who has trouble with it, as Justice and Kaderavek (2004a) suggested. These children then can be picked up for more intensive instruction before they begin to fail. Research (Hadley, Simmerman, Long, & Luna, 2000) provides some evidence that an SLP/classroom teacher collaborative approach is more effective in preventing reading failure than is the traditional classroom teacher-alone model.

PA training can take place in a variety of intervention contexts. For preschoolers or students at developing language levels, it can be integrated with work on phonological production. Here, target words can be presented in both oral and written form. In addition to producing words with the target sounds, students can be encouraged to identify words that contain the target sounds, first at the beginning and later at the end of words. Students can go for "scavenger hunts" around the school or through magazines for objects or pictures that contain the target sound in initial or final position. The clinician can keep a list of words the student found, pointing out the spelling of the target sound in each word and reminding the student that it is how we spell the target sound. The same kinds of activities can be used for consonant blends if children are addressing cluster reduction, or for digraphs such as *sh*, *ch*, and *th* that represent frequently misarticulated fricative and affricate sounds.

PA activities like these also can be used with groups either in pull-out sessions or in collaborative classroom lessons. PA activities are especially beneficial classroom collaborative material. Many children, in addition to the identified clients, benefit from work on increasing awareness of the sound structure of words and its relation to the alphabetic writing system. Some materials for PA activities are commercially available, including Adams, Foorman, Lundberg, and Beeler's (1998) *Phonological Awareness in Young Children: A Classroom Curriculum*; Blachman, Ball, Black, and Tangel's (2000) *Road to Code*; Donnelly, Thomsen, Huber, and Schoemer's (1992) program; Gillon's (2000) *Phonological Awareness Training*; and Stone's (1992) *Animated Alphabet*. Van Kleeck (1990) discussed the sequence of acquisition of PA skills that can serve as a curriculum guide for developing a clinician-constructed PA program. This sequence is summarized in Box 12-9. We should recall, though, that recent research (Catts, 1999b; Gilbertson & Bramlett, 1998; Nation & Hulme, 1997) has shown that the PA skills most closely related to reading are phoneme segmentation (that is, being able to break a word into its component sounds [for example, segmenting *dog* into /d/, /a/, and /g/]), letter-sound correspondence (knowing that the letter B stands for the sound /b/) and blending (being able to combine sounds to form a word [for example, what do /d/ and /at/ make when you put them together? (*dot*)]). These are the skills, then, that we will want to focus on in providing intervention in this area.

We would start with rhyming for children with very low levels of PA. Using rhyming texts from classroom literature selections, we would encourage students to play with the rhymes in the stories, to substitute other words that rhyme, make up nonsense words that rhyme, and write alternate or additional verses for the rhymes in group story contexts. The focus in these activities is on awareness of sound patterns, not yet on spelling. But when two rhyming words that are spelled with the same final sequence of letters come up, we can take the opportunity to write them, pointing out that they not only sound the same, but use the same letters at the end.

BOX 12-9	A Summary of the Normal Sequence of Acquisition of Phonological Awareness Skills

Rhyming
Ability to segment words into syllables
Ability to identify words with the same beginning sound (alliteration)
Ability to identify words with the same final sound
Ability to count sounds in words and to segment CV, VC, and CVC words into phonemes
Ability to segment CCVC, CVCC, and CCVCC words into phonemes
Ability to manipulate sounds in words, i.e., say *fun* without the /f/, take the /t/ from the beginning of *ten* and put it at the end

Adapted from Van Kleeck, A. (1990). Emergent literacy: Learning about print before learning to read. *Topics in Language Disorders, 10,* 25-45.

After working on rhyming, we can progress to asking students to segment words into syllables. Rhythmic activities are fun here. Students can form a rhythm band and "play" the number of syllables in words taken from classroom literature or a theme-based unit. Paul (1992b) suggested "dances with words" in which students perform a different movement for each syllable in words from classroom reading selections.

Working on alliterative words is a common practice in primary classrooms, and Gilbertson and Bramlett (1998) have shown that this skill, too, is predictive of reading achievement. Students can make group or individual books with drawings or cut out pictures of words that have the same first sound. The books can be theme based to relate to classroom content. They might focus on foods that begin with /m/ in a nutrition unit or vehicles that begin with /t/ for a transportation unit. Letters also can be associated with the sounds, by writing the letter for the sound the words share on each page of the book. Students in phonological therapy can be encouraged to produce these theme-related picture albums using sounds from their intervention targets.

Yopp (1992) suggested using songs and rhymes in this type of activity. For example, a jingle can be sung to the tune of "Jimmy Crack Corn:"

Who has a word that begins with /s/?
Who has a word that begins with /s/?
Who has a word that begins with /s/?
It must begin with /s/!

The group sings the song together, then each student volunteers a word to be sung in the lyric:

Sun is a word that begins with /s/!
Sun is a word that begins with /s/!
Sun is a word that begins with /s/!
Sun starts with the /s/ sound!

Alternatively, students can be encouraged to identify initial sound similarities among words. Yopp (1992) suggested an activity using an "Old MacDonald" variation:

What is the sound that starts these words:
Toad, train, top (Wait for response from students.)
/t/ is the sound that starts these words:
Toad, train, top
With a /t/, /t/, here...

The same format can be used to help students identify words that share a common final (duck, cake, beak) or medial (leaf, deep, meat) sound.

Counting sounds and segmenting sounds in words is the next phase of the development of PA and is crucial to reading development. Several activities have been suggested in the literature to achieve this step. Yopp proposed using the tune of "Twinkle, Twinkle, Little Star" as a basis for sound counting:

Listen, listen to my word
And count all the sounds you heard. (spoken): top
/t/ is one sound
/a/ makes two sounds
/p/ makes three sounds
Top has three sounds, it's true
What a good listener that makes you!

Additional suggestions from Yopp and Yopp (2000) appear in Box 12-10.

Elkonin's (1973) sound-counting technique used small disks or coins to represent sounds. Children are presented with a picture of a CV (*me*), VC (*up*), or CVC (*sun*) word, with a small box drawn under the word for each sound it contains, as shown in Figure 12-8. The clinician says the word, prolonging the first sound while modeling moving one coin into the leftmost box. The next sound is pronounced as the clinician moves another coin into the next box. Students are then encouraged to try the same thing. Later words with CV, VC, and CVC shapes are provided for students to do independently. They can be asked to count how many coins they need for other words with these shapes. Eventually, more complex word shapes can be added. When students are proficient at this segmentation task, one type of coin can be provided for the consonants in the word and a different coin for the vowels. Eventually, students are given disks with the letters to represent each sound in the word they are segmenting, and the correspondence between the letter and the sound is highlighted during the activity. The words used in the activity can then be incorporated in stories or poems the students produce around classroom themes, with the students providing spellings for the words based on their segmentation activities. Torgesen et al. (2005) suggested additional activities along this line. Gillon's (2000) program, which demonstrated positive effects of PA training on reading, follows similar procedures.

Word sorts are another technique that has been shown to facilitate PA (Joseph, 2000). Here, each child in the group receives a set of chips and three cards, each with a word exemplifying a different word family. For example:

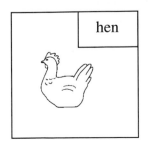

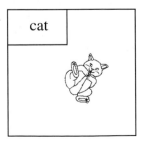

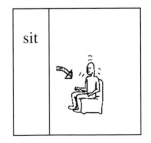

BOX 12-10	**Additional Suggestions for Phonological Awareness Activities**

Onset-Rime Awareness

Mail a Package: Use a large box or container with a lid to serve as a mailbox. Cut a slit in the lid through which cards can be deposited into the box or container. Give each child a picture card of an object and ask each child to show his or her card to the class and name the object. The objects should be single-syllable words such as *cup, ring, flag, street, rug, dog, cat, plum, brick*. The leader says the name of an object by segmenting it into its onset and rime components (c-up, r-ing, fl-ag, str-eet, and so on). The child who has the picture of the object named holds the card in the air, blends the sounds to say the word, and brings the card forward to mail as the group chants:

A package! A package! What can it be? A package! A package! I hope it's for me!

Sound Synthesis

Going on a Word Hunt: Read *We're Going on a Bear Hunt* by Michael Rosen. Then propose to go on a *word* hunt. Have children sit on the floor with their feet together and their knees bent up. Everyone slaps their toes, then slaps their knees with the beat of the chant. Keep the rhythm going throughout the chant. The teacher begins and the students echo.

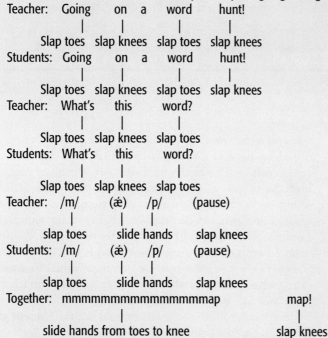

Teacher: Going   on   a   word   hunt!
            | | | |
         Slap toes slap knees slap toes slap knees
Students: Going   on   a   word   hunt!
            | | | |
         Slap toes slap knees slap toes slap knees
Teacher: What's   this   word?
            | | |
         Slap toes slap knees slap toes
Students: What's   this   word?
            | | |
         Slap toes slap knees slap toes
Teacher: /m/   (ǎ)   /p/   (pause)
            | | |
         slap toes   slide hands   slap knees
Students: /m/   (ǎ)   /p/   (pause)
            | | |
         slap toes   slide hands   slap knees
Together: mmmmmmmmmmmmmmmmap   map!
             | |
         slide hands from toes to knee   slap knees

Use single-syllable words that begin with continuant sounds so that they may be elongated as hands are sliding from the toes to the knees for the final part of the chant (as in mmmmmmap, above), such as *light, six, man, van, no, zoo, fist*.

Make a Word: Select rime units (such as *–at*) to focus upon. Have a card with the letters written on it. In a bag have letter cards that may serve as the onset for this family. A child draws a card from the bag. The class says the sound of the letter drawn, blends it with the *-at* and determines whether or not a real word is made. Students give a thumbs up or thumbs down. For instance, a student draws the card *b*. Students say /b/ and blend it with /at/, /b/–/at/: bat. Everyone indicates thumbs up because this is a real word. Someone else draws the letter *g*. Students say /g/–/at/: gat! Thumbs down for this one.

Phoneme Awareness

Find Your Partners: Using a set of picture cards with which the children are familiar, distribute the cards so that each child has one. Be sure that each card can be matched with another that begins or ends with the same sound or has the same sound in the medial position. For example, if you choose to focus on ending sounds, you should select cards such as dog and flag, and hat and nut. Then tell the children that once you give the signal, they are each to circulate and find a classmate whose card shares the same sound in the targeted position.

Bag Game: Have a large grocery bag or box that contains many small plastic bags that can be sealed so that objects do not fall out. In each of these smaller bags place one object and the number of interlocking cubes as there are sounds in the name of the object. For instance, one bag might contain a key and two cubes that are connected (representing the two sounds in key: /k/ and /i/). Another bag might contain a dime and three cubes that are connected for the three sounds in dime, etc. To begin the activity, ask a volunteer to draw a small bag from the large grocery bag. The child opens the small bag, pulls out the object and the cubes. He or she names the object and then says the sounds in the object, breaking apart the cubes as he or she speaks each sound.

Scavenger Hunt: Organize children into teams of about three. Give each team a bag or box that has on it a letter and picture of an object that begins with that letter. For instance, one team receives a bag with the letter M on it and a picture of a monkey; another team receives a bag with the letter S on it and a picture of a snake. Children then set off on a scavenger hunt to find objects in the classroom that begin with their target sound. Children with the B bag may locate a baby doll in the housekeeping center, a block in the building area, a brush in the painting area, and a book from the library corner. Children with the bag that has the letter P written on it may find a pencil, pen, and paper to put in their bag. Give the children enough time and support to be successful, then bring them together to state their target sound and share their objects. Then they may return their objects, trade bags, and repeat the activity.

Adapted from Yopp, H., & Yopp, R. (2000). Supporting phonemic awareness development in the classroom. *Reading Teacher, 54,* 130-143.

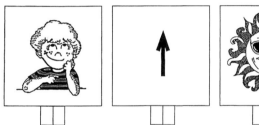
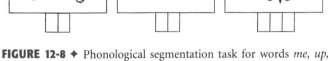

FIGURE 12-8 ✦ Phonological segmentation task for words *me, up,* and *sun.*
(Adapted from Elkonin, D. [1973]. U.S.S.R. In J. Downing [Ed.]. *Comparative reading.* New York: MacMillan.)

The clinician then reads a word from one of the families (e.g., *pen* [hen family]). The students put a chip in the box the new word belongs to; the clinician then gives each a card with the new word written on it to exchange for the chip. After a number of examples, the clinician gives each student a set of cards with words from the three families written on them for the students to sort visually, calling attention to the similarities in letters in the words among the family (hen: pen, ten, den; cat: hat, mat, sat; sit: hit, bit, lit).

Another thing we have learned from recent reading research is the importance of combining instruction on letter-sound correspondence and print concepts with PA (Blachman, 1997; Kaderavek & Justice, 2004a). Slingerland's (1971) method is another way of reinforcing letter-sound correspondence knowledge in a PA activity. It uses small letter squares, like Scrabble tiles, to allow children to "play" with sounds to segment and synthesize words. A small group of students can be given one vowel tile and several consonant tiles. The sounds associated with each letter can be discussed ("the *o* you have can spell the sound /a/. So you can make words that have the sound /a/ in them. Who knows what sound this letter *b* can spell?"). Students can be asked to see how many words they can form with the five or six letters they are given. Allowing them to synthesize nonsense words adds to the fun of the activity. They can then read one of their words to another group, who must guess what letters they used to form it. Later, more tiles can be introduced into the activity. Students can write stories around classroom themes with the words they form or write silly poems with the nonsense words. Segers and Verhoeven (2004) report that PA training, using activities similar to the ones we've discussed, but delivered via a computer game incorporating normal, unmanipulated speech, also benefited kindergarten age children at risk for reading difficulty.

One additional lesson of the recent literature (Gilbertson & Bramlett, 1998; O'Connor & Jenkins, 1995) is the usefulness of incorporating spelling activities in PA programs. O'Connor and Jenkins developed a series of steps in a combined PA/spelling program for kindergartners. Their sequence is presented in Box 12-11. They were able to demonstrate that kindergartners who practiced representing sounds in spoken words with letters developed more complete generalization of their phonological knowledge, which facilitated their acquisition of decoding and spelling skills. Joseph's (2000) program, for example, includes a third step in which children are given a piece of paper with the three word families they have been using for sorting activities written for them at the top:

BOX 12-11	Sequenced Tasks Used by O'Connor and Jenkins (1995) in a Combined Phonological Awareness/Spelling Program for Kindergartners at Risk for LLD

Lessons 1–2 (10 minutes each)

1. Show me the [magnetic] letter that makes this sound.
2. Write the letter that makes this sound.
3. Show me the [magnetic] letter that starts this word.
4. Write the letter that starts this word.
5. Show me the [magnetic] letter that ends this word.
6. Write the letter that ends this word.

Lessons 3–18 (10 minutes each)

1. Show me how you spell these words with your [magnetic] letters (6–7 words chosen from selections the children had read or heard in their literature program).
2. Write these words (same 6–7 words).

Corrective Feedback (if children had difficulty spelling a word)

1. Say the sound at the beginning of the word. (Model or correct, if necessary.)
2. Show me the letter for the first sound. (Model or correct, if necessary.)
3. Say the next sound in the word. (Model or correct, if necessary.)
4. Show me the letter for that sound. (Model or correct, if necessary.)
5. Say the last sound in this word. (Model or correct, if necessary.)
6. Show me the letter for the last sound. (Model or correct, if necessary.)
7. Now write the first sound, etc.

Hen	Cat	Sit

The clinician then says words they have worked with in the sorting activities (*hat, pen, lit, ten*), and the students spell each word beneath the word that shares its family.

Higher-level PA activities for older students who struggle with reading can involve additional word play and sound manipulation practice. One excellent sound manipulation technique is pig Latin. The word formation rules for pig Latin require taking the first sound (not letter) from a word, putting it at the end, and adding /e/. In pig Latin, *teacher* becomes "eacher-tay."

"*Shoe*" becomes "oo-shay." When students are proficient, they can create their own secret languages, specifying the rules, discussing exceptions, and writing out how the code works. Launer (1993) also suggested using the popular "oldie," "The Name Game," which specifies rules for changing the pronunciation of names ("Anna, Anna, bo-banna, banana-fanna," etc.). Again, when students have mastered the rules of this game, they can attempt making them explicit ("First you say the name twice, then say 'bo' and change the first sound in the name to /b/ . . .") as well as devise alternatives of their own. These kinds of activities help to bring the sound structure of words to a higher level of awareness and also provide students with important opportunities to talk about and manipulate the sounds of language. They fit in especially well with classroom science units on sound energy; social studies units on communication; and literature selections about spies, detectives, people who have trouble understanding each other, or children who form secret clubs. But always keep in mind Catts' (1999a) advice not to focus on PA to the exclusion of other literacy skills. Instead, use a limited amount of these activities to help focus students' attention on sound structure, then work with teachers and specialists to provide more focused instruction and practice in decoding, comprehension, and spelling. PA activities make excellent points of collaboration on spelling instruction, if the SLP works closely with the teacher to choose words for PA activities that are related to classroom spelling lists. And

Berninger et al. (2003) showed that combining PA and comprehension instruction resulted in higher gains in reading than PA instruction alone.

Wright and Jacobs (2003) demonstrated that instruction in metalinguistic and metacognitive strategies, in conjunction with PA instruction, also improved reading performance in elementary students with LLD significantly more than PA instruction alone. In addition to increasing PA skills, we want to help students with LLD become more aware of a variety of other aspects of language (metalinguistics) and become more conscious and able to plan their thinking processes (metacognition). Let's examine how we can achieve these goals with elementary school students.

Metalinguistics. Of course, we want to follow up all our activities at the L4L level with talk about the language in the activity. Here are a few additional ways to introduce metalinguistics to students with LLD. We can use classroom literature selections as material for metalinguistic awareness activities. Wallach and Miller (1988) suggested using paraphrasing activities for metalinguistic development. Students can be asked to rephrase a sentence or paragraph, simply finding another way to say the same thing. Later activities can include rewriting a textbook passage for a younger student, recasting a text selection as a picture or cartoon, and reworking material from textbooks as diagrams or maps. All these activities can help students focus on the form of communication.

Editing is an excellent activity to develop metalinguistic awareness. Students with LLD can edit their own and each others' classroom written work with input from the SLP, either in small groups or in metalinguistic activities taught collaboratively with the whole class. The clinician can begin by offering a sample, in which some intentional mistakes have been inserted. Errors of syntax ("We took bus a on a field trip"), morphological marking ("Our class visit a museum yesterday"), word use ("Everything in it was modern, at least a hundred years old"), conjunction choice ("We were late so the bus had a flat tire"), spelling ("We were glad to have a day away from skool"), capitalization and punctuation ("the bus ride was long?"), and logic ("We knew we'd get back in time for lunch, so we ate at the museum") can be included, depending on the students' levels and the activity's goals. In initial editing work, one type of error at a time should be included. Later, errors of different types can be interspersed in the selection. As the students identify the clinician's errors, discussion about what the error is, why it is wrong, and what should be done to change it can occur. Books that encourage metalinguistic awareness, like those in Box 12-4 can also provide opportunities for metalinguistic discussion.

Students can then be asked to write a related sample, intentionally including errors of the type they just discussed. Work can be exchanged so that students can discover these intentionally inserted errors. This introduction helps students to feel that errors are Okay and that working with errors is what editing is all about. No one produces perfect work the first time. What is important is to be able to evaluate our own writing and recognize and correct errors when they appear. As

a final step, students' classroom assignments can be exchanged for editing. Pretending to be newspaper editors working on each other's copy (even wearing green eye shades or using a blue pencil, like old-time editors) can add extra interest to this activity. Using the edited writing to compile a class newspaper or magazine that is distributed to other students or parents can provide a meaningful outcome.

Spelling activities are another excellent context for metalinguistic discussion. Using word study approaches to spelling, like those discussed earlier, sets the stage for focusing attention on the sound structure and meaning relations among words. Apel and Masterson (2001) and Scott (2000) provide additional ideas for metalinguistic spelling instruction.

Metacognition. We've talked about the importance of helping our students with LLD become more aware of the processes needed for successful participation in school. Developing skills for organizing and evaluating a variety of thinking processes involves *metacognition*—the ability to assess our own cognitive processes. Although the development of metacognitive skills is a dominant theme in our work with adolescents with LLD, we can begin to build these skills at the L4L level. Moreover, work on metacognition is an additional source of material for classroom collaborative lessons. What teacher wouldn't want a specialist to help her whole class improve organization and study skills? In this chapter, we'll look at some beginning metacognitive activities and examine some more advanced ones in Chapter 14.

Comprehension Monitoring. Dollaghan (1987) presented a series of activities that has been successful in helping elementary students learn to monitor and assess their comprehension. Using this method, children are first taught to recognize inadequacies in the acoustic signal and to react to them. The clinician gives the students a series of directions, some of which are adequate and some of which are difficult to understand. In the inadequate directions, the clinician tells the student to do something in a voice that is too soft to be heard, spoken too fast to be understood, or spoken with competing noise (knocking on the table with a wooden block). Before hearing each direction, students are told to ask if they don't understand the message. To follow our principle of making intervention relevant to the classroom, we can use directions like those the teacher typically gives. We might whisper a direction such as "Put your name in the upper right-hand corner of your paper" in a voice so soft the student cannot hear it. We might say, "Number your paper from 1 to 20, skipping a line between each," as quickly as we can, so it will be hard for students to understand. We might tell the students to spell the words *rock*, *sleep*, and *ride* as we bang a block loudly on the table.

When students have experienced several sessions of this training and consistently request clarification for the inadequate messages, more complex inadequacies are introduced. At this next level, adequate directions are interspersed with those that are inexplicit or ambiguous, contain unknown words, or are inordinately complex. Students might be told, for example, to "Write an *epistle* to your mother" (unknown word), "Put your name here" (no gestural cue; inexplicit), or "If you have ever been to California and have never been to Arizona, then put your name in the lower left-hand corner of the paper" (overly complex). Again, each direction is preceded by an instruction to ask if the message is not clear. Dollaghan (1987) reported that 10 sessions of this type of training over 4 to 5 weeks was effective in increasing comprehension monitoring in students with LLD, even after the intervention had ended. She advocated comprehension-monitoring instruction as a beneficial supplement to other activities to increase classroom comprehension skills in these students.

Organizational and Learning Strategies. These strategies involve teaching students to actively control, coordinate, and monitor their learning activities and processes. Several kinds of strategies are available, such as the following:

▸ *Creating inferential sets* by invoking all the background information and prior knowledge we have about a topic when attempting to learn new information about it and asking ourselves a set of prereading questions, such as "What do I already know about this topic? What questions can I ask about it?" These questions help students foreground their prior knowledge and look for relevant information in the text. Heller (1986) proposed using a "What I Know" chart to follow up the reading. On the chart, students fill in what they knew before reading, what they learned from the reading, and what they still need to know. An example of a "What I Know" chart appears in Figure 12-9.

▸ *Self-questioning.* After creating an inferential set, students are taught to stop during an assignment and ask themselves questions, such as those that could fill in their "What I Know" chart. In addition, students are taught to ask themselves a series of self-guiding questions as they work through a classroom assignment, individually or in cooperative learning groups. After the clinician models and has the students practice asking themselves the questions, they can be posted prominently on a poster in the class or intervention room. Students can make the poster themselves, as one of the activities that use the self-guiding questions. Questions appropriate for students in the L4L period can be posted and students can be referred to them:

▸ What is my job; what am I supposed to do?
▸ What is my plan; how can I do it?
▸ Am I using my plan?
▸ How did I do?

▸ *Think alouds.* The clinician models the thought processes that go into the completion of a literacy-based task by voicing each step. For example, you might model writing a book report for students by saying, "OK, I need to tell who the characters in this book are. Well, I remember a character is someone who is important in the story. In this story, the important characters are Fantastic Mr. Fox, and…. Then I want to talk about where the story happened. I remember a lot of what happened in this story is in the Fox's den and the Farmers' cellar, so I'll put that in the book report…"

▸ *Reciprocal teaching and buddy programs* involve grouping or pairing students to accomplish a task, and having students cue each other to use the following while completing their assignment:

▸ Predict
▸ Generate questions
▸ Summarize
▸ Clarify

▸ *Using graphic organizers and sensory imaging.* Students are taught to draw, map, or visualize material to help them comprehend and recall it.

Metacognitive strategies like these can be introduced by the clinician in pull-out sessions or in classroom collaborative lessons. Follow-up can be provided by the classroom teacher in consultation with the SLP.

Topic: Solar system		
What I need to learn: How do the parts of the solar system move?		
What I knew before reading	**What I know now**	**What I don't know yet**
Earth goes around sun	Moon goes around earth	Why isn't moon always full?
Earth turns to make day and night	Axis	Why is there midnight sun in Alaska?
Other planets are in solar system	Mars is near Earth	Names of all planets

FIGURE 12-9 ✦ "What I Know" chart.
(Adapted from Heller, M. [1986]. How do you know what you know? Metacognitive modeling in the content areas. *Journal of Reading, 29,* 415-422; and Wallach, G., & Miller, L. [1988]. *Language intervention and academic success.* Boston, MA: College-Hill Press.)

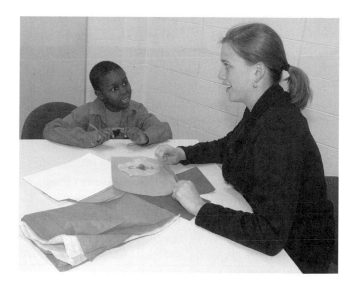

Intervention for students with LLD can involve using language for planning and problem-solving.

INTERVENTION CONTEXTS IN THE L4L PERIOD

SCHEDULING

One problem that often comes up in choosing contexts for intervention in school settings is the scheduling difficulties attendant on providing services in more than one school building. Traveling from one school to another often makes it difficult for an SLP to engage in collaborative work or to provide curriculum-based instruction because there is little time for working with teachers and other school personnel. Besides limiting the SLP's ability to provide innovative service, this situation often leaves SLPs feeling isolated and not really a member of the community of any of the schools served.

Taylor (1992) suggested a solution to this problem: intensive cycle scheduling. Instead of seeing students for 30 to 45 minutes once or twice weekly over the course of a school year, students are seen in more concentrated time periods, perhaps four times a week for 6 to 10 weeks, then "furloughed" to be picked up during another cycle later in the year. This schedule allows SLPs to spend longer periods in each school, get to know the faculty, have time to do classroom observations and curriculum-based assessments, coordinate with teachers to provide collaborative instruction, and meet with parents. It is especially helpful for SLPs in rural districts, where schools may be far apart. Here intensive cycle scheduling can eliminate the need to spend large amounts of the day traveling between sites instead of delivering service. IEPs can easily be written to stipulate a total number of hours of service to be provided over the course of the school year, rather than a number of hours per week. This type of intervention planning gives the SLP flexibility to develop the scheduling model that serves students best.

Soliday (2004) described another alternative, the 3:1 model. Here, traditional, direct intervention to students is delivered for three consecutive weeks, followed by a week of consultative services. Here, intervention time is planned on the IEP by the month, rather than the week. Activities during the consultative week include the following:

- Consultation with teachers, paraprofessionals, parents, other specialists
- Student evaluations
- Completion of third party medical billing
- Participation in special education meetings
- Participation in small group workshop/instruction

Soliday reports that this model allowed for greater planning opportunities with classroom teachers, in order to bring therapy goals into line with the general curriculum and also resulted in high levels of satisfaction among clinicians, teachers, and parents.

These examples demonstrate that a creative clinician has a variety of options for planning and delivering services "outside the box" of traditional intervention where all students are seen only in direct therapy settings on the same schedule every week.

AGENTS OF INTERVENTION

We talked in Chapter 9 about using paraprofessionals and peers as agents of intervention. The National Joint Committee on Learning Disabilities (1999) emphasizes that the main purpose of paraprofessionals in schools is to increase the frequency, intensity, efficiency, and availability of instructional help and to assist with generalization of newly learned skills to multiple settings. Blosser and Neidecker (2002) review the guidelines for permitted and non-permitted activities for SLP assistants under the supervision of SLPs in schools. These appear in Table 12-7.

Paraprofessionals can deliver structured CD or hybrid intervention to individuals or small groups, under the direction of the clinician, who decides on intervention goals and procedures. The clinician designs a lesson plan in detail, including the

TABLE 12-7	**Examples of Permitted and Nonpermitted Activities for SLP Assistants**

PERMITTED ACTIVITIES	NONPERMITTED ACTIVITIES
Conduct speech, language, and hearing screenings.	Conduct standardized testing or diagnostic assessment.
Follow documented treatment plans.	Interpret test or assessment results.
Document client progress in therapy and mainstream settings.	Provide counseling.
Assist during assessment.	Write IEPs.
Prepare clinic materials and perform clerical duties (filing, etc.).	Implement treatment without supervision.
Program AAC devices.	Select or discharge students from intervention.
Prepare schedules.	Make referrals.
Display data on charts, graphs, etc.	Share clinical information with anyone or communicate with family or staff without SLP direction.
Check and maintain equipment	Represent self as SLP.

Adapted from Blosser, J., & Neidercker, E. (2002). *School programs in speech-language pathology: Organization and service delivery*—4th Ed. Boston: Allyn & Bacon.

linguistic stimuli to be used; materials and activities to be employed; targeted responses; and reinforcement or corrective feedback to be given; and gives the plan to the paraprofessional to administer. Alternatively, the clinician might provide a commercially available lesson. Either way, responsibility for assessment, IEP development, intervention planning, ongoing evaluation, and parent-teacher communication remains with the clinician.

Another potential agent of intervention for the school-age client is an older or same-age peer. Wilkinson, Milosky, and Genishi (1986) reported that when students with mixed abilities are placed in small-group settings, those with higher achievement tended to model effective speaking styles. Paul (2003) reviewed a range of research on social skills training and found the research to suggest that peer-mediated approaches were consistently more effective interventions for children with a variety of disabilities at a range of age levels than were adult-directed social skills programs. A higher-achieving student can first be designated "group leader" and asked to guide the others in the group in carrying out a classroom task. The student with LLD can be assigned to be leader in the next session, reminded to use effective language as the peer did, and then conduct the group. If the clinician audiorecords the session, the students can listen to it later and evaluate the effectiveness of the communication. Together they can develop lists of rules for "good communicating." After several experiences like this, the student with LLD can serve as a tutor for a younger student. The clinician can remind the tutor to use the effective communication styles learned in the peer situation.

Cooperative learning groups are another excellent opportunity for peer interaction and instruction. In these groups, a problem or assignment must be completed by the group as a whole, who work together to devise a solution that involves

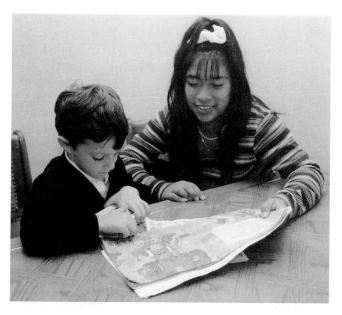

Students with LLD can tutor younger peers to practice communication strategies.

the entire group. For example, each group can be assigned to write a story about a classroom topic, with at least one sentence contributed by each group member. The students can help each other edit their sentences, but each member must provide an original contribution. In activities like these, peers can share their skills, and students with LLD can see competent skills modeled. Using cooperative learning groups in collaborative classroom work requires careful placement of students in groups, so that students on IEPs get exposure to more linguistically advanced peers. It's also a good idea to include a task in some part of the activity that the students with LLD are good at, so they can feel competent, too. If one student with LLD is a good artist, build drawing into the assignment. If another is a sports expert, require knowledge of sports trivia as part of the activity. Kuder (1997), McCormick (1997a), and Paul (2003) presented guidelines for facilitating interactions between students with disabilities and their typical peers in learning groups. These are summarized in Box 12-12.

SERVICE DELIVERY MODELS

We've talked before about the major contexts for intervention: the clinical model, the language-based classroom, and the collaborative and consultant models. For clinicians working in school settings, all these models will be relevant, particularly because just about every type of communication disorder will be seen in these settings. That's because IDEA legislation mandates "that removal of children with disabilities from the regular education environment occurs only when the nature or severity of the disability is such that education in regular classes with the use of supplementary aids and services cannot be achieved satisfactorily" (Section 612 [5], Part B).

The spirit behind this language is that children should in every case possible be placed in the general education class that they would attend if they did not have a disability. This placement option is referred to as *inclusion*. Inclusion should be about restructuring classrooms and schools to support and provide for the special needs of children with disabilities (McCormick, 1997b), not just having them passively "sit in." Although this ideal is not always met in practice, it does mean that children with all types and degrees of communication disorders will be found in public school settings, because IDEA says that, generally, they belong there and not in segregated special placements. Although we have concentrated in Chapters 11 and 12 on the assessment and intervention needs of children with LLD who function close to the same level as their chronological age peers, we should remember that school SLPs will find on their caseloads children functioning at all levels of development. If schools adhere to the spirit of IDEA, many of these lower-functioning students will be served, at least part of the time, in general education classrooms. McCormick, Loeb, and Schiefelbusch (2003) provide extensive guidance to clinicians working in inclusive settings for meeting the wide range of educational and communicative needs these children present. Like everything else in our field, though, inclusion is not universally accepted as the optimal approach for all students.

BOX 12-12 | **Guidelines for Facilitating Interactions between Typical Students and those with Disabilities in Learning Groups**

Provide service in the least-restrictive environment, as required by law.

Students with LLD can tutor younger peers to practice communication strategies.

Increase the clients' opportunities for interacting with the mainstream teacher and peers, decreasing the amount of classroom content "missed" because of being pulled out, and making the students' day more cohesive and integrated.

Target success in the natural environment with relevant tasks that encourage participation in both the overt and the hidden curricula.

Make students and teachers see language intervention as more meaningful because they perceive its relation to their daily work in school.

Provide greater opportunities for generalization across curriculum areas.

Provide beneficial input or modification of classroom instruction that helps not only the identified client but other students in the class.

Encourage teamwork and transdisciplinary practice among teachers, special educators, and SLPs, making SLPs a more integral part of the school community.

Provide peers with concrete strategies to use in interaction, such as prompting the student with a disability to produce a particular behavior (you make a list of all the cities in the state we need to study), and praising completed work.

Adapted from Kuder, S. (1997). *Teaching students with language and communication disabilities.* Boston, MA: Allyn & Bacon; McCormick, L. (1997a). Ecological assessment and planning. In L. McCormick, D. Loeb, & R. Shiefelbusch (Edds.). *Supporting children with communication difficulties in inclusive settings*—Second edition (pp. 235-258). Boston: Allyn & Bacon; Paul, R. (2003a). Enhancing social communication in high functioning individuals with autistic spectrum disorders. *Child and Adolescent Psychiatric Clinics of North America, 12,* 87-106.

Simon (1998), for example, raised questions about whether students with moderate to severe disabilities can receive sufficiently intense language intervention in a full inclusion setting. And ASHA (2000) reminds us that inclusive practices consist of a range of service-delivery options and recommends that an array of models be used to implement services to students with communication disorders. One size doesn't fit all, and some students can benefit from specialized services, at least some of the time.

With such variation in the level of functioning and extent of the needs of their students, school SLPs have a big job to do! Unfortunately, the scope of our responsibilities does not always limit the size of our caseload as it should. O'Connell (1997) reported that the national caseload average is 52, and some school SLPs have caseloads in the 70s, 80s, or even 90s! Although ASHA (2000) does not recommend a caseload maximum, it does argue that the caseload should be compatible with appropriate and effective intervention. Moreover, it advocates using the concept of *workload*, which subsumes all the activities in which the SLP participates. Workload takes into account not only the number of students an SLP serves, but also the paperwork, consultation, collaboration, conferencing, and supervision we provide. Clearly, we have some work to do in advocating for both caseloads and workloads that allow us to serve our varied client base in public schools with the level of service they require. That said, let's discuss the various service delivery models that are appropriate at the L4L level.

The Clinical Model

The traditional clinical or pull-out model of intervention is, of course, one aspect of service delivery in schools. Many children in the L4L period can benefit from the relatively quiet, less-distracting setting provided in the clinical model, as well as from the intensive attention and scaffolding that can be given in this setting. We also may want to consider, though, supplementing the clinical model with some other forms of service delivery. One possibility is the "pull-out/sit-in" approach. Here, part of the client's intervention time is spent in a clinical setting and part is spent in the classroom with participant observation-based intervention (Nelson, 1998) or with the clinician doing a collaborative lesson with the whole group.

The advantage of this approach is that the student with LLD can be "prepped" in the pull-out session. That is, the clinician can give the client a preview of a classroom lesson and prime the student to produce appropriate responses. Alternatively, the clinician can use pull-out sessions after classroom work to evaluate and "go meta" on some of the material introduced in the classroom. Using participant observation, the clinician can sit in with the student during a classroom activity, then talk about his or her performance and how to improve it in a pull-out session later.

O'Connell (1997) also suggested that clinical sessions are useful for developing basic skills that may not be relevant to the rest of the classroom, such as motor placement cues for sound production. She also advocates using clinical sessions to review recordings of the client's communication during classroom activities. This is a "sit-in/pull-out" rather than "pull-out/sit-in" approach, in which the clinician does work in the classroom, then encourages the client to monitor his or her own performance from the recording information.

The Language-Based Classroom

Feinberg (1981), McBride and Levy (1981), and Moore-Brown and Montgomery (2001) provided models of self-contained language stimulation classrooms at the primary-grade level. Generally, these classrooms will be designed to serve more severely impaired students with communication deficits that would make it difficult for them to participate in the mainstream class. In these programs, the SLP serves as the classroom teacher and creates a program focused on developing oral language skills and emergent literacy. Some SLPs especially like this model because it allows them to spend the whole day with a small group of students, getting to know them in a way they never could get to know a caseload of 40. Many of the activities we have discussed for addressing vocabulary, syntax, classroom discourse, and literate language styles are appropriate in these settings. Theme-based and naturalistic approaches are often incorporated in these programs, along with more structured activities focused on the development of listening, speaking, and reading and writing skills.

Some SLPs in schools may work as resource-room teachers in classrooms for children with LLD. The clinician may work closely with a special educator in these settings. Students generally spend part of their day in the resource room and part in the regular classroom. Often resource rooms focus on content mastery; that is, helping students to succeed in the curriculum being taught in the regular classroom. For this aspect of the resource-room curriculum, the SLP is especially well-equipped to provide metacognitive instruction that focuses on comprehension monitoring and learning strategies. In addition, the SLP can help provide curriculum-based assessment of the linguistic demands of the curriculum. Reviewing textbooks and observing in the mainstream class for teacher talk and hidden curriculum patterns can help the clinician provide focused intervention activities that address the specific requirements of the classrooms in which our clients must function.

A second function of the SLP in the resource-room setting is to provide instruction in general communication skills, especially in literate language style. The activities that we have discussed for developing more elaborated language, in conversation and classroom discourse and in work on narrative and other literate language materials, can all be used in the resource room, as well as in the clinical model. These activities help students to build the oral language foundation needed for success in school. Dodge (1998), Plourde (1985; 1989), and Bruder (2004) provided additional materials for developing a variety of communication skills at the elementary level that can be used effectively in the resource-room setting (see Table 12-3).

Consultation and Collaboration

Simon (1987) was one of the first to argue for the importance of moving SLPs out of the "broom closet" and into the mainstream of the school environment. This move has advantages for the client, the educational team, and students in the mainstream classroom who may be having difficulty but are not identified as eligible for services. Both consultation and collaboration offer SLPs ways to achieve the goal of fuller citizenship in the schools in which we work. And the 2004 reauthorization of IDEA puts the law behind the effort to bring SLPs into the classroom and our services to bear on success in the curriculum. Let's look at each of these service-delivery models and talk about how they can be implemented.

Consultation. When working in a consultative role, our goal is to help teachers find ways to increase the student's success in the classroom. It's much easier to achieve this goal if we have gathered some knowledge of the classroom environment through our curriculum-based assessments. This curriculum-based information is extremely helpful in working with teachers to identify obstacles that our students find difficult to overcome in the mainstream curriculum. Doing some classroom observation and curriculum-based assessment is fundamental to developing an effective consultation program.

Moore-Brown and Montgomery (2001) define *consultation* as helping another professional to assist a student. So one means of consultation is work with teachers to find ways to help our students succeed within the curriculum the teacher presents. Lasky (1991) provided some suggestions for working with teachers on modifying the presentation of information during instruction in the classroom. Box 12-13 lists some of Lasky's ideas that can be shared with teachers.

In working with teachers in a consultative role, it is important to remember that teachers are the experts on classroom issues. Our job is not to criticize or tell the teacher to teach differently. Instead, we want to work with the teacher to give the client the best chance for success. An effective approach to consultative sessions is to present the problems that we see our client having in the classroom and ask teachers how we can best help them to help the student succeed. Once areas of shared concern and ways in which the teacher is willing to modify the curriculum have been identified, concrete, specific suggestions like those in Box 12-13 can be presented. The SLP ought to be willing to do some of the modification for the teacher, if necessary, such as recopying tests with larger print and fewer questions per page or arranging for a volunteer to audiotape classroom readings for the student to use. This makes the modification a shared activity, not one imposed on the teacher by the SLP. Sharing responsibility for the student's success is what consultation should be all about.

O'Connell (1997) reminds us that serving in a consultant role does not need to mean being an "expert" who knows more about everything than the teacher. In many cases, in fact, we can learn a lot from teachers about managing classroom lessons, or choosing developmentally appropriate curricula and materials. What consultation does mean is using the special insight we have developed into the nature and structure of communication to help teachers sharpen their observation skills in these areas and perhaps think about their own and their textbooks' language more critically. For example, a teacher may tell us that a student "refuses" to complete social studies assignments. The consulting SLP might suggest that she and the teacher review the instructions in the textbook. While reviewing them, the SLP might exclaim, "Wow, look at this sentence! It's got three subordinate clauses. I wonder if that's why Maria

---

| **BOX 12-13** | **Consultation Suggestions for Modifying Classroom Presentation** |

Provide Contextual Cues

State the topic to be discussed.

Supply a prepared outline.

Use visual support, such as writing important information on the blackboard or using charts, pictures, or diagrams, etc. For example:

$$\left.\begin{array}{l}\text{plus}\\\text{and}\\\text{sum}\end{array}\right\} \text{ADD} \qquad \left.\begin{array}{l}\text{minus}\\\text{take away}\\\text{difference}\end{array}\right\} \text{SUBTRACT}$$

Present questions that review major points to focus student attention on these points.

Provide Redundancy

As instructions are given verbally, write them on the board at the same time.

Paraphrase information in the lesson, giving each main point several times with different wording each time.

Relate New Information to What Is Already Known

Help students establish an anticipatory set by asking what they know about the topic.

Ask students to talk about personal experiences with the topic.

Personalize information: talk about curriculum topics by using names of students in the class ("Suppose Jose wants to start a rock collection . . .").

Slow Down Presentation Rate

Talk in a slower-than-normal manner.

Pause for 2 seconds at the end of long sentences.

Decrease Distraction and Stress

Allow student to take tests or complete assignments with only a few problems per page.

Relax time limits for the client on timed assignments.

Allow clients alternate modes of presentation, such as listening to material on audiotape with headphones instead of reading it independently.

Allow clients alternate modes of response, such as tape recording homework rather than writing it or using a word processor instead of hand-writing assignments.

Give Preferential Seating

Have students with LLD work in a quiet part of the room

Provide a study "carrel" by placing three sides of a large cardboard box on the client's desk to screen out distractions.

Have clients sit near the teacher during instructional times.

Adapted from Lasky, E. (1991). Comprehending and processing of information in clinic and classroom. In C.S. Simon (Ed.). *Communication skills and classroom success* (pp. 113-134). San Diego, CA: College-Hill Press.

---

isn't doing her work. Maybe she can't understand what she's supposed to do. Is there anything we could do to simplify these directions for her?"

Another important function the SLP can serve in a consulting role concerns in-service education for teachers. Cirrin (1989) suggested three formats for in-service education that can help us to share information about the needs of our students and foster a sense of joint responsibility for their learning. In the *demonstration* format, specialists from several disciplines can demonstrate materials (such as Westby's [2005] book report forms), methods (such as CBM), or activities (such as PA) that

could be used in the classroom to foster success for clients as well as mainstream students. The *case-study* method provides an opportunity for specialists and regular educators to discuss a particular case in depth, so that principles and problems can be seen from a variety of points of view. Using a case from a previous year, for example (with names removed, of course), is a great way to practice transdisciplinary program planning. A *literature* session allows professionals to get together to talk about some readings they have selected. One or two disciplines might choose articles to provide to the participants, who would read them before the in-service. The in-service itself would give participants an opportunity to discuss their responses to the material. Another way to use the literature format is to provide the group with selected children's literature and work together to find ways to address oral and written language goals through the use of these selections. Prelock, Miller, and Reed (1995) also provided an outline of a series of in-service presentations to encourage collaboration between SLPs and classroom teachers. It appears in Box 12-14.

The point of these kinds of in-service presentations is to move away from the lecture format in which we present ourselves as experts and to move toward the development of transdisciplinary planning and practice by involving participants actively in the material being presented. Since we work hard at encouraging our clients to be active learners, doesn't it make sense to do the same for the colleagues with whom we want to work?

Collaboration. Providing collaborative intervention by "sitting in" or "guest teaching" in mainstream classrooms is another extension of our role as SLPs. While it may be challenging to those of us who consider our primary role to be clinician rather than teacher, collaborative intervention's advan-

---

| **BOX 12-14** | **In-Service Training for Teachers and SLPs Who Are Collaborating to Provide Services to Children with Communication Disabilities in the Regular Classroom** |

Training Course Outline

Session I: Language in the Classroom: Getting Perspective on Collaborating, Sharing Roles, and Teaming

Objectives
1. To share the perspectives of participants involved in collaborative service delivery on meeting the needs of at-risk students with communication disorders in the regular classroom.
2. To recognize those roles shared by teachers and speech-language pathologists as they assess and intervene with students.
3. To understand a transdisciplinary philosophy for teaming, including role exchange, role release, and role support.

Activity
Videotape viewing of collaborative planning meetings, classroom activities, and follow-up

Session II: Normal Communication Development and Communication Disorders in the Classroom

Objectives
1. To understand normal communication and language development in school-age children.
2. To recognize communication disorders common to the classroom.
3. To understand the pervasive nature of language deficits in children with handicaps.

Activity
Role playing an initial collaborative meeting

Session III: Identifying and Managing Classroom Language Demands: What Are the Scripts?

Objectives
1. To gain a broader understanding of the impact traditional classroom methods have on the student with communication disorders.
2. To identify scripts in the classroom.
3. To explain a process-based approach for managing classroom language demands.

Activity
Developing and implementing a communication skills "script" in the classroom

Session IV: Assessing Communication Problems in the Classroom: A Collaborative Approach

Objectives
1. To understand curriculum-based language assessment.
2. To provide a framework for collaborative assessment using language-based curriculum analysis, checklists, and observation logs.
3. To suggest ways of establishing collaborative data collection practices during classroom activities.

Activity
Practicing team assessment

| BOX 12-14 | **In-Service Training for Teachers and SLPs Who Are Collaborating to Provide Services to Children with Communication Disabilities in the Regular Classroom—cont'd** |

Session V: Strategies for Managing the Language of Math

Objectives
1. To recognize the language complexity in the math curriculum and in text materials.
2. To gain skills in adapting curriculum materials for elementary students with communication disorders.
3. To learn strategies for collaborating with students to enhance their performance in math application, computation, and problem solving.

Activity
Explaining math problems in third grade

Session VI: Using Literature in the Classroom

Objectives
1. To examine the development of oral and written language.
2. To learn strategies for implementing literature use in elementary classrooms.
3. To recognize and manage the reading difficulties of at-risk students and students with communication disorders.

Activity
Sharing a writing project

Session VII: Issues in Collaborative Service Delivery: Scheduling, IEP Development, and Conflict Resolution

Objectives
1. To explain a process for determining the type(s) of service delivery a student with communication disorders should receive.
2. To recognize the role of regular and special education teachers, parents, and students in developing IEPs for students with communication disorders.
3. To discuss barriers to effective communication when working with a team.

Activity
Conflict resolution through role-play

---

tages, such as the ones previously discussed, are powerful enough to warrant taking on this challenge. There have been a few studies, too, (Ellis, Schlaudecker, & Regimbal, 1995; Farber & Klein, 1999; Throneburg et al., 2000) that demonstrate the effectiveness of this approach, at least in early primary grades. Creaghead (1994) discussed the essential elements in successful collaboration. They include building administrative support, developing relationships with teachers, and creating effective collaborative lessons and curricular units. Let's see how we can accomplish each aspect of the development of these intervention programs.

Building Administrative Support. SLPs interested in collaborative intervention may need to do some groundwork with school administrators to convince them to provide the coordination time necessary. One important aspect of this support is the availability of time for coordination with other teachers. We need to talk with the teachers involved, not in the hall or during recess duty, but in regular, specified meetings. These

meetings are a crucial first step in establishing workable collaboration and consultation. Administrative support for the development of these service delivery models is essential for their success. DeKemel (2003), Moore-Brown and Montgomery (2001), and Prelock, Miller, and Reed (1995) discussed some methods of building this administrative support. Prelock et al. emphasized that one of the most important arguments concerns the way in which collaboration allows SLPs to support not only students on IEPs, but other at-risk students who may not qualify for direct services. By working alongside classroom teachers and modifying and enhancing the learning of students with a variety of difficulties, we help to ensure the success of all students. Other arguments we can make to administrators include stressing the increase in SLP productivity available with the model because both clients and other children in the class are affected; presenting the idea to administrators in a one-page written format that summarizes its strengths, with additional justification provided only when it is requested;

keeping administrators updated on successes with short monthly memos; providing building principals with a monthly calendar of SLP activities; inviting administrators to attend collaborative planning meetings; and offering to present information about the program at faculty meetings and "parents' nights." To facilitate the establishment of collaboration, weekly team meetings will need to be scheduled. Usually 30 to 45 minutes is needed in the early phases. Prelock et al. report, though, that after a few months, teams become more efficient and comfortable with each other, and the need for weekly planning decreases.

Using intensive cycle scheduling or the 3:1 model (Soliday, 2004) are additional ways to support collaboration for SLPs. By working consistently in one building for some time, scheduling collaborative or "pull-out/sit-in" service delivery models becomes less of a strategic nightmare. Keeping faculty and administrators aware of your schedule by posting it in the school office helps to increase your visibility and accountability.

Developing Collaborative Relations. Building relationships with teachers is the next step in successful collaboration. O'Connell (1997) and Blosser and Neidecker (2002) suggested that the best relationships are usually built one teacher at a time. SLPs frequently begin collaborative intervention with one teacher with whom they have a good personal relationship, work in that class for a few months, and let the word spread. Frequently other teachers express willingness to have collaborative lessons in their rooms as well, or at least are more amenable to the idea when they've seen it work well for a colleague. Prelock et al. (1995) suggest that SLPs attend curriculum and grade-level meetings to become familiar with classroom content and procedure. They also advocate offering teachers a "gift of time" by grading the papers of students on IEPs or decorating classroom bulletin boards. These activities not only delight the teacher, but allow the SLP to get to know clients' class work and support language goals within the classroom environment. Hosting breakfast meetings to explain collaboration and to recruit new teacher collaborationists and giving video demonstrations are also great ways to tell teachers about collaborative ventures. Peña and Quinn (2003) emphasize the importance of providing meaningful incentives to teachers for collaboration, particularly through recognition by administrators. And of course, in-service presentations are always a good opportunity to plug your program.

A variety of ways to implement collaboration in classrooms are discussed by Blosser and Neidecker (2002), DeKemel (2003), Moore-Brown and Montgomery (2001), and O'Connell (1997). These arrangements are displayed in graphic models, suggested by Friend and Bursuck (2000), in Figure 12-10.

It is probably unrealistic to expect that collaboration is possible with every teacher in a school. But after a successful year, you might approach a teacher with whom you work particularly well and ask whether he or she would be willing to cluster several of your clients in that class for the following year. If the teacher is willing, administrative support should also be sought. Clustering this way maximizes the efficiency of your intervention and ensures a receptive classroom for your clients.

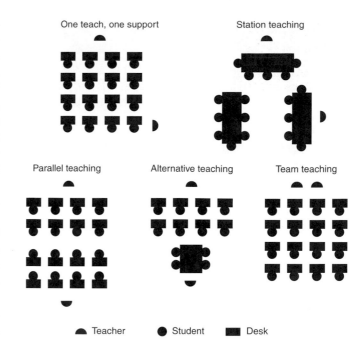

FIGURE 12-10 ✦ Co-teaching approaches.
(Reprinted with permission from Friend, M., & Bursuck, W.D. [2000]. *Including students with special needs: A practical guide for classroom teachers.* Boston, MA: Allyn & Bacon.)

Effective Lesson Planning. The third piece of the collaborative intervention program is the classroom lesson itself. Christensen and Luckett (1990) provided helpful guidelines on developing these lessons. It is a good idea for the SLP to take the lead, at least at first, in lesson development. This approach avoids the potential difficulty of the SLP being "used" as an aide in the classroom. It is important, though, to consult with the teacher about the lesson, to ensure that it is something he or she wants for the whole class, and to intertwine it with other activities and themes going on in the classroom. Christensen and Luckett suggested drawing the lesson content at first from commercial sources. Box 12-15 provides a list of possible sources that can be helpful in developing classroom collaborative lessons. Many of the activities we discussed in the sections on hybrid intervention techniques also can be adapted to the classroom setting. As you become more accustomed to classroom lesson planning, you will feel more confident in adapting and originating your own material.

In addition to the content of the lesson, the structure also is important. One way to structure the lesson is by means of cooperative learning groups. The SLP can present the lesson, break the class into groups, and supervise half of the groups directly while the classroom teacher supervises the other half. Usually the SLP arranges to have the clients with IEPs in the groups he or she supervises. A second way is to use what Waldron (1992) called "Academic Clubs." In this model, the SLP works in the classroom with part of the group on a lesson developed for those "club" members, while the teacher works on another lesson with the rest of the class. The "club" includes the students on IEPs but also includes others in the class. The "clubs" can

BOX 12-15	Some Sources for Collaborative Classroom Lessons

- *Classroom Listening and Speaking* (K, 1–2, 3–4, 5–6, by themes) by L. Plourde, Pro-Ed
- *Blooming Experiments/Holidays/Recipes/Arts and Crafts/Language Arts* series by Linguisystems
- *Classroom Language Intervention* by Children's Language Institute, Communication Skillbuilders
- *Collaborate! Celebrate!* series by Linguisystems
- *The Communication Lab (I and II)* by E.P. Dodge, Singular
- *Curriculum for Oral Language Development* by L. Mattes, Academic Communication Associates
- *Handbooks for Exercises of Language Processing* by A. Lazzari & P. Peters, Linguisystems
- *Jump to a Conclusion* by Tom Matthews, Academic Communication Associates
- *Language Lessons in the Classroom* by S. Diamond, Thinking Publications
- *Language Through Literature* by V. Rothstein & R. Termansen, Pro-Ed
- *Making Words* by P. Cunningham & J. Cunningham, *Reading Teacher, 46,* 106-113
- *The Magic of Stories* by C. Strong & K. North, Thinking Publications
- *More than Words* by K. Donnelly, S. Thomsen, L. Huber, & D. Schoemer, Communication Skillbuilders
- *Peabody Language Development Kits* by L. Dunn & J. Smith, American Guidance Service
- *Phonological Awareness in Young Children: A Classroom Curriculum* by M. Adams, B. Foorman, I. Lundberg, & T. Beeler, Paul H. Brookes Publishers
- *SCAMPER Strategies* by C. Esterreicher, Thinking Publications
- *The Story Grammar Marker* by M. Moreau & H. Fidrych, SGM, Inc.
- *Story Making* by R. Peura & C. DeBoer, Thinking Publications
- *Storybook-Centered Lesson Plans* by J. Norris & P. Hoffman, Communication Skillbuilders
- *Storybuilding* by P. Hudson-Nechkash, Thinking Publications
- *Thematic Unit on Listening* by M. Donahue, C. Nelson, & K. Czarnik, *Topics in Language Disorders,* 17(3), 51-61
- *Warm-up Exercises, Books 1 and 2* by R. Kisner & B. Knowles, Thinking Publications
- *What's the Story?* by M. Bernarding, Communication Skillbuilders
- *Why Didn't I Think of That?* Janelle Publications

Adapted from Christensen, S., & Luckett, C. (1990). Getting into the classroom and making it work! *Language, Speech, and Hearing Services in Schools, 21,* 110-113.

be organized around student interests. For example, the client and all other students in the class who are interested in basketball might join the "Dribblers' Club." The SLP can prepare lessons with a basketball theme that address the needs of the client as well as other class members. They might use statistics in the newspaper to write a report of a recent game, for example, then edit, rewrite, and "publish" the report. The "club" can last for several weeks, then another "club" can be formed with a different theme, involving different mainstream students. A "Secret Agents' Club," for example, might address higher-level PA skills for the client and others in the class whose reading might need improvement. Letting students in the club just because they want to learn secret agent techniques is fine, too!

Kuder (1997) suggested some techniques that can work well in these groups. He suggested that groups be given an assignment to complete with a set of materials from which they must choose. For example, if the collaborative lesson is on predicting story outcomes, students may be given four incomplete stories. Their job is to choose the group's favorite, then choose an ending for it together. Rewriting for varying audiences is another activity that can be useful. Each group in the class, for example, may be assigned to write their story's ending for a different audience. One might be assigned to a kindergarten audience,

another, an audience of science teachers, and so on. Once each group has written its story, they then can be asked to listen to the other groups' stories and then rewrite their ending for a different audience.

Christensen and Luckett (1990) also stressed the importance of providing a well-structured lesson plan, both for the teacher's benefit and for our own. If you are not too familiar with classroom intervention, you will probably feel more secure having a written-out plan to refer to in case nerves interfere with your memory! Christensen and Luckett provided a structured framework for classroom lessons, which appears in Box 12-16.

Christensen and Luckett reminded us to involve the teacher in the lesson by providing a lesson plan and specific activities to perform. In addition, it is crucial to maintain discipline during the lesson. Talking with the teacher before beginning the collaborative program about the discipline techniques to which the students are accustomed is often helpful. Working with the teacher to gear the lesson to classroom themes and content, being on time, and providing materials for follow-up also help to keep the collaboration going smoothly. It is a good idea to give the teacher some commercially prepared lesson plans to use as backup in case illness or emergency keeps you out of

BOX 12-16	A Framework for Collaborative Classroom Lesson Plans

Create an Anticipatory Set

Focus students' attention on the topic to be discussed. ("Today we'll talk about how characters in a story make plans to solve their problems.")

State the Objective

Tell the students what you expect them to learn as a result of the lesson. ("We'll learn to look for ways characters plan their actions in a story.")

Give the Purpose of the Lesson

Tell students how the learning will benefit them. ("It helps us understand stories better if we look for the ways characters make and carry out their plans.")

Provide an Input Model

Tell the students what to look for; provide an example, check for understanding, monitor and adjust the instruction if necessary. ("You read the story *Curious George Rides a Bike*. Remember that George wanted to make a boat. He used his newspapers and made a whole fleet. But then he had another problem! What was it? Can you tell how he tried to solve that problem?")

Provide Guided Practice

Have the students complete an activity under adult supervision and scaffolding. ("How did George try to solve this next problem? What was his plan? Can you think of another way he might have tried to solve it? Let's make a list.")

Close the Lesson

Review the objective and purpose and ask students to tell what they learned. ("Poor George got himself into trouble quite a few times in this story. Each time he came up with a plan to solve his problem. What was his first problem? How did he plan to solve it? What was the next . . . ? Each time George came up with a plan. The plan didn't always work out just the way he wanted, but he tried to solve his problems by planning his actions. That's what characters in stories often do. They try to plan a way to solve their problems.)

Provide Distributive Practice

Leave follow-up activities for the teacher to do so students can review and practice in a different setting what they learned in the lesson. ("Your teacher will be reading you another story this week. When I come back, I'd like each of you to have a list of some of the plans the character in your new story used to solve the problem in that story. Maybe you can act them out for me!")

Adapted from Christensen, S., & Luckett, C. (1990). Getting into the classroom and making it work! *Language, Speech, and Hearing Services in Schools, 21,* 110-113.

---

the classroom at the scheduled time. And it is smart to ask the classroom teacher for a critique of your lessons. This can provide helpful feedback and let teachers know that we are willing to learn from their expertise in the classroom.

Collaborative Curriculum Planning. As we've seen, IDEA legislation promotes including children with disabilities in the regular education curriculum. This means that one of our important roles will be finding ways to work with classroom teachers to design and modify the curriculum and provide appropriate accommodations so that our students learn what the other students in the class do. Freedman and Wiig (1995) developed a set of forms to aid in this collaborative planning process. The forms appear in Appendix 12-2. They can be used to help

structure our interactions with teachers and provide a means of thinking together about the prerequisites, content, and accommodations necessary to enable our students to get the most out of their participation in the classroom. Once team members have used forms like these a few times to plan curriculum units, the process becomes familiar and routine, so that planning can proceed quickly and efficiently.

CONSIDERATIONS FOR THE OLDER CLIENT AT THE L4L STAGE

For adolescents and young adults functioning at elementary grade levels of language and literacy, the main goal of intervention is to foster independence in vocational and living situations to as great an extent as possible. Having functional social discourse skills is very important in making this transition, as is having some functional literacy. Bedrosian (1985), Kilman and Negri-Schoultz (1987), and Paul (2003) presented examples of programs for developing social discourse skills in older clients with moderate to severe language disorders. Since these clients may not develop all the "fine points" of language, intervention targets must be chosen on the basis of providing a functional repertoire, whether spoken or employing AAC, for the environments in which the client must manage. Matching the client's language skills to the requirements of the social or vocational situation is vital.

Falvey, Grenot-Scheyer, and Luddy (1987) argued that curricula for these students should be *community referenced*. That means we should relate targets to the major domains in which the student must function. These domains would include domestic, recreational, and vocational settings. For each, ecological inventories can be used to assess what communication skills are needed. This often involves making contact with community settings to which the student will eventually transition and beginning to set up links before the student leaves school. Intervention can focus on providing the skills needed for these most crucial environments.

For all students with severe disabilities, teaching functional communication skills is essential (Sigafoos et al., 2004). Functional communication skills, as we've discussed before, are those that can be used to express basic wants and needs, and enable the speaker to obtain desired outcomes through the mediation of a listener. These will need to be matched to the environments in which the student will be involved, relying on ecological inventories and observations.

While these students are in school, every effort should be made to maximize literacy, using chronologically age-appropriate reading material, since the greater their reading skill, the more independent living options are available. Besides continuing to read and hear stories, the adolescent at the L4L stage should be given focused instruction in PA, letter-sound

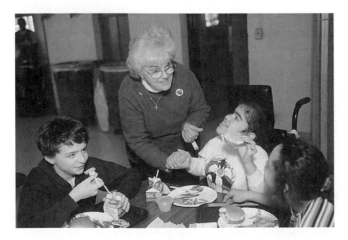

Intervention for older clients at the L4L stage
is community referenced.

correspondence, reading comprehension, writing, and spelling. Erickson, Koppenhaver, Yoder, and Nance (1997) found that the *Making Words Program* (Cunningham & Cunningham, 1992), which teaches children to systematically combine letters to form words, was easily adapted for use with a student with multiple disabilities. Basil and Reyes (2003) as well as Hetzroni and Schanin (2002) report that computer assisted programs that involve massed practice and scaffolding were successful in promoting literacy in students with severe disabilities. For older students at the L4L level, practice reading job applications, newspaper advertisements, and magazines on topics of interest should be part of the literacy program. Writing work should focus on filling out forms of various kinds, writing letters of inquiry about jobs and housing, and developing writing skills important for domestic independence, such as copying and organizing recipes, paying and filing bills, making shopping lists, and keeping household records. Clients also should be taught "meta" skills for deciding when they do not understand something they read, such as a contract or work agreement, so they know when they need to seek assistance to avoid being taken advantage of.

Ideally this literacy instruction should be integrated with other activities in the student's educational program (Blackstone, 1989). For example, reading vocabulary for ordering food from a restaurant menu can be taught in the context of a community living or recreation unit on going out to eat. Writing skills can be taught in conjunction with a unit on shopping and menu planning, as the student writes a shopping list and searches for the food on the list on the grocery shelves. Reading and writing should be integrated within the student's program systematically throughout the day, rather than in one short instructional session (Calculator & Jorgensen, 1991; Erickson, Koppenhaver, Yoder, & Nance, 1997).

■ CONCLUSIONS

Children like Willie—whose difficulties in school include not only basic oral language but also reading, writing, and functioning in the classroom—need help that goes beyond addressing vocabulary and syntactic skills. Work with these students must focus on the oral and written language skills needed for success in school and in life. To be fully successful, this kind of intervention involves more than a few sessions a week of isolated "speech therapy." It needs to be coordinated and integrated with the rest of his educational program. Let's see how we might design an intervention plan for a student like Willie to achieve this kind of integrated service delivery.

In May of Willie's second-grade year, Ms. Johnson met with the assessment team that had recently completed Willie's evaluation. The first order of business was to review Willie's audiometric data and design an assistive listening system that would increase his ability to receive auditory input from the teacher. It turned out that Willie's hearing aids needed adjustment and that the classroom amplification system had not been working properly. As a result, Willie had not been receiving optimal auditory input.

Ms. Johnson felt that this could be part of the reason for the deterioration in Willie's behavior. Ms. Johnson and the audiologist worked with the classroom teacher to show her how to "troubleshoot" Willie's auditory equipment each day and to report any malfunctions to them immediately. Willie also was taught to check the batteries on his hearing aid himself, to increase his independence and "ownership" of his hearing needs. The team agreed that Willie also needed help with basic reading comprehension. Ms. Johnson explained that although Willie's oral language sounded adequate to the naked ear, he needed to work on understanding and producing more complex language forms and meanings that are used in the literate language style. His classroom discourse skills, particularly in understanding teacher talk and textbook language, were poor. Ms. Johnson felt this might be a result of his not having heard very well throughout the year, and also might be the cause of some of his behavior problems. The team discussed behavioral issues and decided to see how the change in his aural rehabilitation devices and the work on reading and language skills would affect behavior before taking any further steps.

The team met with Willie's family to plan his third-grade program. Initially, the classroom teacher suggested that Willie spend half his day in a resource classroom to work on content mastery, behavioral issues, and language and reading skills. Willie's parents were opposed to this plan, however. They felt Ms. Johnson had worked with him before to good effect and thought that with her help as well as that of the other specialists, he could function in a regular classroom. After some discussion, the team decided that Willie would be placed in Ms. Dunthorpe's third-grade classroom for the first semester of the next school year. Ms. Dunthorpe had two other of Ms. Johnson's clients slotted to be in her class and had been working collaboratively with Ms. Johnson for 2 years now. Ms. Johnson thought that she and Ms. Dunthorpe could develop an appropriate program for Willie in the classroom, if the parents would agree to support all the behavioral interventions the team suggested, to manage his hearing aids carefully at home, and to learn along with Willie to troubleshoot the devices daily. They also were asked to agree to reassess the situation at the end of the first semester to see how it was working. The family agreed to this plan.

Ms. Johnson was using a 3:1 schedule that year. She arranged with Ms. Johnson to see Willie in a small group for curriculum-based language work 3 times a week during her direct service weeks and to present three collaborative lessons in the classroom for each of her collaboration weeks. During week 2 of the 3:1 schedule, Ms. Johnson and the reading specialist worked collaboratively to address comprehension of both oral and written language. The learning disability specialist worked on a consultative basis with Ms. Dunthorpe to keep on top of behavioral issues in the classroom and to help devise modifications of classroom instruction that would help Willie succeed. The audiologist worked with both Willie and Ms. Dunthorpe to make sure they understood how to test and troubleshoot his hearing aids and auditory-training device, and consulted monthly on how the troubleshooting was going. Ms. Johnson met monthly with the team—consisting of the teacher, reading specialist, LD specialist, audiologist, and herself—to monitor and provide input and consultation on Willie's classroom program. At the end of the third 3:1 cycle, Ms. Johnson "furloughed" Willie from direct speech and language

service, but continued to meet monthly on a consultative basis with his team, and to provide a monthly collaborative session in Willie's class on "listening skills." At the end of the first semester, Ms. Johnson did a classroom-based assessment. Willie was managing in class, and behavioral problems were significantly reduced. The parent-educator team met again, and everyone felt that Willie was progressing satisfactorily, although he still had some difficulties. Willie's mother was eager for Willie to receive some more direct service from Ms. Johnson, who agreed to pick him up again for once-a-week sessions during her direct service weeks.

STUDY GUIDE

I. Planning Intervention in the L4L Stage
   A. What is transdisciplinary intervention? How can it be incorporated into IEP development?
   B. What kinds of modifications of the classroom program might be included in an IEP for a school-age child?
   C. Discuss family involvement in the intervention program for a school-age child.
   D. How can the student be involved in intervention planning?
   E. Discuss behavior management techniques that can be used in classroom intervention for students in the L4L stage.

II. Intervention Products in the L4L Period
   A. What four principles should guide intervention at the L4L stage?
   B. What is *preventive intervention*?

III. Intervention Processes in the L4L Period
   A. What is the role of CD intervention in the L4L period?
   B. What kinds of goals are appropriately targeted with CD approaches at the L4L level?
   C. Discuss forms of scaffolding that can be helpful to students with LLD.
   D. Describe the basic principles and some activities for addressing vocabulary development in the L4L stage.
   E. Discuss approaches to word-retrieval problems.
   F. What are some ways to work on semantic integration and inferencing ability?
   G. Discuss using assessment data on comprehension skills and strategies to design a program for syntactic intervention.
   H. How can literature-based approaches be used to target syntactic skills?
   I. Discuss methods for addressing the development of advanced morphological markers. How can this work be used to work on spelling, too?
   J. Discuss the role of developing literate language syntax in a preventive intervention program.
   K. How can conversational discourse skills be targeted in an intervention program?
   L. Describe methods for working on classroom discourse skills.

M. What are some intervention approaches for developing narrative comprehension?

N. Describe a story-grammar approach to intervention for narrative production.

O. Discuss some methods for developing cohesive marking in stories.

P. Describe the sequence of development of phonological awareness and give some activities that can be used to develop each level.

Q. Discuss some curriculum- and literature-based metalinguistic awareness activities.

R. How can editing student writing be used as a metalinguistic activity?

S. Describe Dollaghan's comprehension-monitoring program.

T. Describe some organizational and learning strategies that can be taught at the L4L stage.

IV. Intervention Contexts in the L4L Period

A. Discuss some alternative forms of scheduling for the school SLP.

B. Discuss the role of SLP assistants in school settings. How should they interact with clients?

C. What are the advantages and disadvantages of a clinical or pull-out model of service delivery in schools?

D. Discuss the roles an SLP can play in a language-based or resource classroom.

E. Why is collaborative or consultative intervention an important adjunct to service delivery in schools?

F. Discuss how an SLP can maximize the effectiveness of a consultative program.

G. Describe three types of in-service presentations an SLP might give in a school setting.

H. What are some strategies for developing administrative support for a collaborative program?

I. Discuss positive behavioral support and the SLP's role in it.

J. Describe several different forms of implementation of collaborative teaching.

K. Describe the framework for an effective classroom lesson.

L. What are some ways we can involve teachers as we develop collaborative programming?

V. Considerations for the Older Client at the L4L Stage

A. What is the goal of intervention for an adolescent or young adult at the L4L stage of development?

B. What is a community-referenced curriculum, and how can it be implemented?

C. What are some ways to develop functional reading and writing skills for these students?

SAMPLE FORMAT FOR AN INDIVIDUALIZED EDUCATION PROGRAM

Student _____

Birthdate _____

Least Restrictive Environment Considered

1. Placement Options:
   ____ Regular class with support   ____ Full-time regular education
   ____ Other ____   ____ Full-time special education

   Provide reasons for rejecting other options _____

2. Location: ____ Neighborhood school   ____ Other school in district
               ____ Home-based instruction   ____ Other (specify) ____

   Provide reasons for rejecting other options _____

3. Opportunities for interaction with peers: ____ Lunch   ____ Recess
   ____ Class time   ____ Transportation   ____ Small group/tutoring
   ____ Other (specify) ____

4. Nonacademic and Extracurricular Involvement   ____ Sports
   ____ Intramurals   ____ Clubs   ____ Performing arts
   ____ Other (specify) ____
   If none, explain _____

	Estimated hrs/yr	Anticipated dates Start	End
Placement			
Regular classroom			
Special education			
Support services			
Speech and language			
Extended school year (ESY)			
____ Student qualifies for ESY			
____ Student does not qualify for ESY			
____ Decision deferred until May			
Vocational program			
____ Special designs			
Signatures of IEP participants			
Parent or surrogate parent ____			
Teacher or therapist ____			
District representative ____			
Other ____			
Other ____			
Physical Education			
____ Regular			
____ Special ed.			
____ P.E. requirement completed			
____ Regular education			

PARENTAL DECISION

My rights and responsibilities have been shared with me in writing in a manner which I fully understand. I have had the opportunity to participate in the development of the Individualized Education Program for my child and agree with its contents. I fully understand my child's present levels of performance and understand all programs and services which will be provided. I have participated in the development of the annual goals and objectives and I understand that the objectives which I have reviewed will be revised as progress is demonstrated towards the attainment of annual goals. I am aware that my participation and cooperation are needed if the Individualized Education Program is to be successful and I offer my support. I grant permission for my child/ward to participate in all aspects of this program. I understand that the program will be revised no later than one year from the date of my signature and that I will be notified if major changes in the program are necessary.

Parent or guardian (or adult student)	**APPROVAL**	Signature _____	Date _____
Parent or guardian	**REJECTION**	Signature _____	Date _____

Continued

Present Level of Performance

Academic:

Physical:

Adaptive:

Communication:

Related Services and Program Modifications

Transportation needs or restrictions:

_____ Regular bus

_____ Special education bus

_____ Wheelchair

_____ Carseat

_____ Special restraints

_____ Other _____

_____ Must have adult meet bus

_____ Child cannot walk to bus stop

_____ Child cannot cross in front of bus without assistance

_____ Child needs help on and off the bus

_____ Other _____

Program modifications:

_____ Pass/fail grading

_____ Classroom aide

_____ Auditory training equipment

_____ Preferential seating

_____ Modification of testing

_____ Written material presented orally

_____ Classroom interpreter

_____ Other _____

Parental Participation

Describe plans for parent participation in implementing the student's individualized education program.

Instructional Objectives

Student's Name _____

Service Provided _____

Annual Goal _____

School _____ Grade _____

Teacher/therapist _____

BENCHMARK	PROFICIENCY	MEASURED BY	PROJECTED BEGINNING	PROJECTED ENDING	ACTUAL COMPLETION

Parental Participation

Describe plans for parent participation in implementing the student's Instructional Objectives.

FORM FOR PLANNING CURRICULUM LESSONS AND UNITS

CURRICULUM – SPECIFIED GOALS OR OUTCOMES

- PRIORITIZE
- LOOK BEYOND THE OBVIOUS
- BE MEANS-END DIRECTED
- IF THEY LEARN NOTHING ELSE . . .
- WHAT IS MEANINGFUL . . .

ESSENTIAL EVERYONE MUST LEARN THIS

MOST SHOULD LEARN THIS

IF THEY CAN . . . I WANT SOME TO LEARN THIS

What prior knowledge or PRECONCEPTS must they have? What processes or skills must they know?

How can I probe for these preconcepts, processes? What questions can I ask? Will this be part of an orienting unit?

CORE VOCABULARY

Adapted from Freedman, E., & Wiig, E. (1995). Classroom management and instruction for adolescents with learning disabilities. *Seminars in Speech and Language, 16*, 62-64.

SEQUENCING THE UNIT

1. What will I do for students who do not have the necessary preconcepts, processes or skills – Preteach, use cooperative learning, design a preteaching unit for some and enriching activities for others, extend the orienting unit . . .

2. TEACHING THE CONCEPTS – (IN OUTLINE)
REMEMBER TO USE GUIDED QUESTIONING, MEDIATION, AND SCAFFOLDING.
How will I develop the VOCABULARY for the CONCEPT(S)?

MODIFICATIONS FOR STUDENTS WITH SPECIAL NEEDS

Continued

MODIFICATIONS FOR STUDENTS WITH SPECIAL NEEDS

What activities or aspects of the whole unit will ensure generalization and develop:

ORAL LANGUAGE	READING	WRITTEN LANGUAGE	SPECIAL SKILLS (e.g.,study skills research,etc.)

3. **EVALUATION**

- Did every student have equal access to the learning opportunity because I ensured that they all had the necessary preconcepts, vocabulary, skills, and modifications for special needs?
- Has every student learned something and how can I evaluate this range of learning?

CHAPTER 13

ASSESSING ADVANCED LANGUAGE

CHAPTER OBJECTIVES

Readers of this chapter will be able to do the following:
- Describe typical language development in adolescence.
- Discuss issues of student-centered assessment at the secondary school level.
- Discuss screening, case-finding, and eligibility for services for students in secondary schools.
- Describe the uses of standardized tests, criterion-referenced methods, and observational assessment at the secondary level.
- Outline methods of assessment of functional communication for adolescent students with severe disabilities.

Crystal had two younger brothers who were both diagnosed with fragile X syndrome when she was in third grade. At that time, Crystal was tested, too, and found to be positive for the syndrome. Before that, she'd been thought of by her teachers as something of a "slow learner," who had barely managed to stay at grade level. Once the diagnosis was established, she received a thorough assessment. She was found not to be eligible for services in third grade, since she was functioning within normal limits, although near the borderline. She was put on monitoring status and reevaluated 1 year later. By that time, her scores on a battery of oral language and reading tests had slipped below the cut-off and qualified her for services in language and reading. She received intervention throughout fourth and fifth grades and was able to function in regular classes. By the end of fifth grade she was making satisfactory progress, had age-appropriate oral language skills in most areas, and was reading on a fourth-grade level. It was decided to send her on to middle school with her class, to furlough her from direct intervention, and to monitor her progress.

Mr. Janis was the speech-language pathologist (SLP) at Crystal's middle school. He gave her the CELF-4 Screening Test (Semel, Wiig, & Secord, 2004) during her sixth-grade year and found her performance to be broadly within normal limits, although at the low end. In talking to her teachers, Mr. Janis gathered that Crystal was having a few problems but wasn't failing any courses and wasn't showing any behavioral difficulties, although they noted that she had some trouble paying attention. The teachers felt they could give her a little extra help in the classroom, and she would be able to get by. Mr. Janis

gave them some information about fragile X syndrome in girls, provided some tips for modifying classroom assignments and presentation, and asked them to let him know whether things changed. He placed Crystal on monitor status for another year. When he gave her the CELF-4 screening again in seventh grade, though, her score fell just short of passing. He talked to some of her teachers and found that she was beginning to have trouble with the lecture material presented in class, with completing independent assignments, and with keeping up with reading. They felt she sometimes seemed lost in the shuffle. Mr. Janis decided to do a full-scale assessment and find out what Crystal needed to help keep her on track.

Crystal is like many children who have language learning disorders (LLD) that stem from a variety of sources. She is one of what Launer (1993) called "the porpoise kids," whose deficits go below the surface at times and then leap up again at points when the demands of the curriculum increase. These points often occur in fourth and seventh grades, where, in each case, new and taxing changes in the curriculum and in teachers' expectations of students come into play. Crystal is typical of adolescents with LLD in another way, too. Most don't appear on the SLP's doorstep with no history. Almost always, unless they have recently suffered a traumatic injury, they have been assessed and have received services before, often during their elementary years. That means that they don't enter our caseloads as clean slates. A great deal of information about their language and learning history is available. The goal of assessment for this period of advanced language development is to use the data available in their files to select assessment questions and focus on the most relevant areas for in-depth appraisal.

LANGUAGE DEVELOPMENT IN ADOLESCENCE

What do we mean by *advanced language development*? In general, we mean the language normally learned when children are in the adolescent years, from age 12 through early adulthood, when they attend middle and high school. Of course, some students in secondary schools are functioning at lower levels of language development. Some are still in the language-for-learning (L4L) stage, with few literate language and literacy skills. Some with severe disorders are still at developing language levels. There may be students with profound disabilities who still function at emerging language or prelinguistic stages. For these students, the SLP uses assessment procedures appropriate for developmental level, of course. It is important, however, to do some functional assessment, such as ecological inventories, to determine these students' communicative needs in community-referenced environments, as we discussed previously.

Adolescents who are functioning at advanced language levels have not only mastered the basic skills of the developing language period but also achieved some of the goals outlined in Chapter 12. That is, they can produce and understand true narratives and some complex sentences, make some inferences, carry on marginally adequate conversations, engage in some metalinguistic discussions, and so on. While these abilities may be present in some aspects of their interactions, though, their skills are, in Nelson's (1998) words, "wobbly." Oral language facility can easily be disrupted by stress, when dealing with unfamiliar material or new vocabulary, or when faced with some new communicative goal (such as asking for a date) or cognitive function (such as formulating a scientific hypothesis). Word finding often continues to be a problem.

The new skills that normal adolescents are learning during the period of advanced language are primarily concerned with the development of language for more intensive social interactions, with language at the literate end of the oral-literate continuum, and with abilities related to critical thinking (Whitmore, 2000). Vocabulary acquisition involves literate language forms (Nippold, 1998; Westby, 2005) such as the following:

▶ Advanced adverbial conjuncts (*similarly, moreover, consequently, in contrast, rather, nonetheless*)
▶ Adverbs of likelihood (*definitely, possibly*) and magnitude (*extremely, considerably*)
▶ Precise and technical terms related to curricular content (*abscissa, bacteria, pollination, fascism*)
▶ Verbs with presuppositional (*regret*), metalinguistic (*predict, infer, imply*), and metacognitive (*hypothesize, observe*) components
▶ Words with multiple meanings (*strike* the ball, *strike* at the factory; *run* for office, *run* the office)
▶ Words with multiple functions (*hard* stone, *hard* water, *hard* feelings)

In addition, adolescents acquire more than just a larger vocabulary. They learn to elaborate and expand the meanings of known words (*cold* meaning temperature; *cold* meaning affect) and to understand connections among words related in various ways, such as by derivation (*clinic, clinician*) or by meaning, such as antonyms (for example, *reluctant* and *enthusiastic*); synonyms (for example, *huge* and *enormous*); or sound (homonyms [for example, *pair* and *pear*]) (Nippold, 1998). They also acquire more sophisticated abilities for defining words. Nippold, Hegel, Sohlberg, and Schwarz (1999) showed that between sixth and twelfth grades, students increased in their ability to provide the most advanced type of definition for abstract nouns, the *Aristotelian* type. This type of definition contains a superordinate term and a description with one or more characteristics (for example, *happiness* is a feeling [superordinate term] of pleasure of gladness resulting from a positive experience [description of characteristics]). Sixth-graders produced only one or two of 16 responses at this level, whereas twelfth-graders produced an average of six of 16.

New syntactic skills include growth both inside sentences (intrasentential) and between sentences (intersentential). Growth within sentences is seen in small but regular increases in sentence length throughout the school years. Longer sentences are used for particular purposes, though, including narrative, persuasion, and writing. Reed, Griffith, and Rasmussen (1998) reported that adolescents used morphosyntactic markers (verb marking, negative forms, etc.) more frequently than did younger children. Nippold, Ward-Lonergan, and Fanning (2005) showed that persuasive contexts elicited the most advanced syntactic forms in adolescents' writing. These results indicate that the use of increasing numbers of basic grammatical markers is one means by which sentences become longer during the adolescent years. Intrasentential growth, then, is seen both in the use of newly acquired forms, as well as in increased density of earlier-acquired forms within sentences. Intrasentential growth also is seen in the increasing use of subordinate and coordinate clauses, as well as in the use of low-frequency syntactic structures associated with literate language style.

Intersentential growth in the forms used to link sentences also is an important part of adolescent language development. The use of conjunctions and other forms of cohesive devices becomes more frequent and effective during the secondary school years (Nippold, 2000).

In addition to these new semantic and syntactic skills, typical adolescents develop a variety of new pragmatic abilities. They begin to use and understand language that has a figurative, rather than literal, function (Nippold & Haq, 1996; Nippold, Moran, & Swartz, 2001; Quals & O'Brien, 2003). They make puns, use sarcasm, and gradually learn to use and comprehend metaphors ("she's a whirlwind"), similes ("like a diamond in the sky"), proverbs ("a stitch in time saves nine"), and idioms ("raining cats and dogs"). Slang and in-group language become important, and the ability to discern the appropriate uses of this slang helps to determine group membership and peer acceptance (Nippold, 1998). Also, adolescents become significantly more proficient at using communication for purposes such as persuasion, negotiation, and establishing social dominance (Nippold, 1994). Moreover, unlike in earlier childhood when friendship revolved around shared activity, in adolescence, talk itself becomes the major medium of social interaction. It represents a new aspect of the teen's relation to the social world, where friendship is negotiated primarily by "just talking," sharing intimacies and experiences for the sake of communication alone (Raffaelli & Duckett, 1989).

School also plays a role in the normal adolescent's language development. New forms of discourse, such as class lectures and expository texts, are introduced in the curriculum, and students need to learn to process and produce them. Secondary school requires students to produce more extended written forms of communication than they did at the elementary grades. Students are required to produce not only stories, but expository and persuasive texts. The understanding of these texts undergoes a predictable sequence of development during the secondary school years (Scott, 2005). These written forms require a great deal of metacognitive and metalinguistic activity. Formal operational thought, the new cognitive development of the adolescent period, greatly extends the student's capacity to think about thinking processes and to entertain hypotheses, coordinate abstractions, and use logical operations. Formal operational thought emerges during this period in normal development (Kamhi & Lee, 1988; Nippold, 1998) and is elabo-

rated throughout the secondary school years. School work builds on formal thought capacities by teaching mathematics and science that make use of and provide practice in exercising these skills. Formal operational thinking also allows teens to develop a variety of verbal-reasoning and critical-thinking skills (Nippold, 1998). Analogical or inductive reasoning ("Apple is to fruit as potato is to vegetable") develops. Adolescents learn to use syllogisms or deductive reasoning, in problems such as "John is taller than Mary. Mary is taller than Pete. Who is tallest—John, Mary, or Pete?" These formal-operational and verbal-reasoning skills, in normal teens, also allow for a much greater range of metacognitive activities than are typical of elementary-age children. Again, the school curriculum both demands and provides forums for practicing these skills.

The kinds of demands that the middle and high school curriculum place on students were discussed by Montgomery and Levine (1995), Schumaker and Deshler (1984), and Whitmire (2000). These are summarized in Box 13-1. These demands draw on many of the abilities we've been discussing that normally evolve during the adolescent years. For adolescents with LLD, as we've seen, the oral language and literacy skills developed during the elementary years may still be "wobbly." These shaky skills can form a weak foundation for the advanced language required by the more intense demands of the secondary curriculum. It is likely that children who had difficulties acquiring

---

BOX 13-1   Curriculum Demands at Advanced Language Levels

- Deal with multiple teachers, with varied teaching styles and modes of communication, and follow classroom rules for each.
- Use already automatized skills (e.g., reading fluency) and increasing base of knowledge to gain information from material written at middle and high school reading levels.
- Be able to retrieve prior knowledge of several different procedures (e.g., writing a business letter; recalling technical names for parts of a business machine written about in letter; using writing conventions such as spelling, capitalization, punctuation) simultaneously in order to complete classroom assignments.
- Be able to increase the amount of work produced (e.g., write longer reports, more frequent written assignments), necessitating quicker, more efficient production, use of organizational strategies and problem solving skills for scheduling tasks, etc.
- Be able to use "working memory" to reason, process large chunks of material, follow multistep instructions.
- Be able to deal with the stress of using more focused and sustained attention for increasing periods of time.
- Use self- and comprehension-monitoring and metacognition to determine priority and saliency of classroom material.
- Work independently with little help from the teacher.
- Master increasingly decontextualized, abstract, symbolic material to participate in discussions and assignments about curricular material.
- Complete homework and other assignments independently.
- Gain information from lectures, films, and student reports.
- Take notes independently.
- Demonstrate knowledge by studying and recalling information or tests with various formats (essay, multiple choice, true/false).
- Express oneself in writing in various formats (essays, descriptions, narratives, and explanations).
- Use logical and critical thinking to evaluate information presented.

Adapted from Montgomery, J., & Levine, M. (1995). Developmental language impairments: Their transactions with other neurodevelopmental factors during the adolescent years. *Seminars in Speech and Language, 16,* 2; and Schumaker, J., & Deshler, D. (1984). Setting demand variables: A major factor in program planning for the LD adolescent. *Topics in Language Disorders, 4,* 22-40.

oral language and literacy at the L4L stage will continue to have problems with advanced language during the secondary school years. Let's talk about how we can assess these advanced language skills to identify ways to help our students with LLD manage in the secondary school environment.

STUDENT-CENTERED ASSESSMENT

We've talked often about the importance of the client's family in any successful program of assessment and intervention. We still want to keep families involved and informed in an adolescent's program, using some of the techniques we talked about in Chapters 11 and 12. However, one of the hallmarks of adolescence is the beginning of a movement away from the family of origin as the primary social unit, toward more independence and peer-group orientation. We need to think about this developmental shift in planning assessment for this age group. We can attempt to provide a *student*-centered program when working with clients at advanced language levels. Let's see how we might do it.

McKinley and Larsen (2003) discussed the importance of student motivation in assessing adolescents. They suggested, first, that the clinician have no "hidden agenda" in the assessment process. Larson and McKinley (1995) advocated telling the student what behaviors (listening, speaking, thinking, writing, etc.) are going to be assessed. Tests and other methods to be used in the assessment can be introduced to the client and the purpose of each explained. Other assessment methods to be used, such as speech, narrative, or writing sampling, also can be previewed, with an explanation of the uses to which the clinician will put each procedure. Teens also need to know why particular behaviors are being assessed. Clinicians can explain, for example, that it is important to know about the student's listening and understanding of words and sentences so that we can figure out how problems with listening might be getting in the way of succeeding in the classroom or interacting successfully with friends. It is important to emphasize to adolescents that the skills we are assessing are important not only for succeeding in school but also for interacting with peers and for developing vocational and independent-living skills.

The goal of such a student-centered approach to assessment is to establish a cooperative partnership between the teen and the clinician. Only through this partnership can we get the clearest picture of the adolescent's abilities. And, if we decide intervention is warranted, this partnership stands us in good stead for achieving the full cooperation of the client and eliciting the most highly motivated performance. One method that can be used to assist in this student-centered assessment is to ask the student to do some self-assessment. Grambau (1993) provided one example of such a self-assessment inventory; an adaptation is given in Figure 13-1. This form can be given to the student at the beginning of the evaluation. The student's self-assessment can be used to guide the process, focusing the clinician's attention on areas in which students perceive themselves to be having trouble. These areas can be investigated in depth as part of the assessment.

SCREENING, CASE FINDING, AND ESTABLISHING ELIGIBILITY WITH STANDARDIZED TESTS IN THE ADVANCED LANGUAGE STAGE

Larson and McKinley (1995) suggested that mass screening for language disorders in secondary schools is probably not an efficient use of the SLP's time. Instead, they proposed having any screening that does take place focus on at-risk populations. These would include adolescents placed in special classrooms, students receiving remedial reading assistance, those in danger of dropping out of school, and those having academic problems that aren't caused primarily by lack of motivation. Sanger, Moore-Brown, Magnuson, and Svoboda (2003) have reported an unusually high prevalence of unidentified language disorders among adolescent delinquents, so it is important to screen students who seem to be having behavioral or social difficulties, even if they have not been previously thought to have communication problems. Such students would be likely to have LLD and to benefit from assessment and intervention with the language pathologist. A sampling of screening tests available for use with students at advanced language levels appears in Table 13-1. These screening measures need to be used with some caution, though. Nelson (1998) pointed out that many screening tests developed for adolescents may not be sensitive to the problems that can occur at advanced language levels and have an impact on school and personal adjustment. If an at-risk student passes one of these screenings but the clinician has a "hunch" that the passing score is not a good reflection of the student's functional language ability, a talk with some of the student's teachers may be warranted. If the teachers confirm the clinician's hunch that language disabilities are getting in the student's way, some standardized testing in greater depth may be warranted to determine whether the student would be eligible for services on the basis of scores from more extensive testing.

Other sources of referral, in addition to screening populations like those identified by Larson and McKinley (1995), are most likely to be the teachers and counselors who work with students in the school. For these referral sources, it is especially important to provide practical criteria for making referral. Referrals are not likely to be made if teachers are frequently told that the students they refer fail to qualify for services. Using a pragmatically oriented checklist, like the ones in Figures 11-1 and 11-2, can be helpful for eliciting referrals from these sources. So can a referral checklist that focuses on skills like those in Box 13-1 that are required by the secondary curriculum. Figure 13-2 gives an example of a checklist that incorporates the pragmatic aspects of Figure 11-1 and adds some of the curricular demands of Box 13-1. A checklist like this can be given to teachers at in-service programs that discuss adolescent language and the needs of students with LLD at this level. Alternatively, it can be distributed to teachers with a short cover note explaining the clinician's interest in helping students to acquire language skills that will increase success in the classroom. Teachers can be asked to fill out the form for any student whom they suspect may have "wobbly" language abilities. Wiig

Learning skills	I'm good	I'm ok	I get by	I need some help	Aah! Help! Help!
Answering questions about my reading					
Asking questions when I don't understand					
Editing my writing					
Finding main ideas in textbooks					
Finding time to finish all my work					
Finishing assignments					
Following directions					
Interest in school work					
Organizing my thoughts					
Participating in class discussion					
Penmanship					
Reviewing and studying for tests					
Spelling and punctuation					
Taking notes					
Taking tests					
Understanding teachers' lectures					
Understanding what I read					
Using a dictionary or other reference books					
Vocabulary					
Writing papers					

FIGURE 13-1 ✦ A sample student self-assessment form for focusing evaluation in the advanced language stage. (Adapted from Grambau, M. [1993]. *Study smarter, not harder.* Kent, WA: Classic Printing.)

TABLE 13-1	A Sample of Language-Screening Instruments, Grades 6-12

TEST	AGE LEVEL	AREAS ASSESSED	COMMENTS
Adolescent Language Screening Test Morgan, D.L., & Guilford, A.M. (1984). Austin, TX: Pro-Ed	11–17 yr	Pragmatics, receptive and expressive vocabulary; concepts; sentence formation; morphology; phonology	Outlines dimensions needing further testing. Administration time: 15 min.
CELF-4 Screening Test Semel, E., Wiig, E.H., & Secord, W. (2004). San Antonio, TX: Harcourt Assessment	5–21 yr	Receptive, expressive, grammatical, and semantic skills	Correlates with CELF-4. Yields a criterion score. Administration time: 15 min.
Speech and Language Evaluation Scale Fressola, D.R., & Hoerchler, S.C. (1989). Columbia, MO: Hawthorne Educational Services	4:6–18+ yr	Articulation and voice, fluency, pragmatics, form	Has teacher rating scale plus speech and language scale. Normed on 4,501 students. Administration time: 20 min.

Student name _____

Grade/subject _____

Teacher _____

Date _____

To the teacher: Please mark any item below if it is of concern (+) or serious concern (++).

Reading

_____ Gains information from independent reading assignments at grade level

_____ Studies for tests effectively

_____ Identifies main ideas in reading

_____ Follows written directions without difficulty

_____ Uses references (dictionaries, Internet, atlases) effectively

Writing

_____ Expresses thoughts clearly in writing

_____ Uses forethought to plan writing assignments

_____ Has legible handwriting

_____ Uses adequate spelling

_____ Uses correct punctuation/capitalization

_____ Uses appropriate grammatical complexity

_____ Takes adequate notes

_____ Completes written assignments

_____ Applies adequate editing skills

_____ Can perform on short-answer tests

_____ Can perform on essay tests

Speaking

_____ Speaks with adequate pronunciation, fluency, and correct grammar

_____ Uses age-appropriate complexity

_____ Gives accurate information

_____ Can follow discussion agenda set by teacher

_____ Produces responses without long delays

_____ Discusses everyday topics appropriately

_____ Participates adequately in class discussions on curricular topics

_____ Uses appropriate specific vocabulary

_____ Organizes thoughts adequately when speaking

_____ Keeps to the point in speaking, without undue redundancy

_____ Asks questions when clarification is needed

_____ Follows classroom rules for speaking

_____ Uses and "gets" humor appropriately

_____ Is polite and tactful

_____ Can express opinions clearly

_____ Has no trouble finding words during speaking

Listening

_____ Follows oral direction the first time

_____ Can understand class lectures

_____ Understands idioms, proverbs, slang in context

_____ Can follow material presented in films, student reports, audiotapes, CD-ROM

_____ Can answer questions based on lecture and other orally presented material

_____ Can later recall and relate information from orally presented material

Organization

_____ Can work independently

_____ Organizes material in assignment books, planners, calendars, etc.

_____ Seems "with it" in class discussions

_____ Can think problems through, using reasoning skills and thinking out loud

FIGURE 13-2 ✦ A sample checklist for referral at the advanced language level.
(Adapted from Damico, J. [1985]. Clinical discourse analysis: A functional language assessment technique. In C.S. Simon [Ed.], *Communication skills and classroom success: Assessment of language-learning disabled students* (pp. 165-206). San Diego, CA: College-Hill Press; O'Connell, P. [1997]. *Speech, language and hearing programs in schools* [pp. 137-139]. Gaithersburg, MD: Aspen.)

(1995) pointed out that it is especially important to avoid jargon and confusing questions in these referral forms. Secondary teachers are often reluctant to complete clinician-generated checklists if they are in any way difficult or unclear. If teachers are unwilling to fill out the forms, the SLP might arrange a short meeting with the teacher and ask the teacher to think of any students who might be having trouble. The clinician can simply ask the questions on the form and record the answers for each student about whom the teacher has concerns.

Students who show significant problems on an inventory like the one in Figure 13-2 can be assessed for eligibility using standardized test batteries. A screening test would not be necessary, since the screening was done by the teacher by filling out the checklist. When choosing and interpreting standardized tests at advanced language levels, we need to bear in mind all the warnings we have discussed all along for standardized tests. Several are particularly germane in the advanced language period. The need to identify pragmatic as well as semantic and syntactic

areas of need is especially important, since pragmatics may be the area of greatest deficit in adolescents with LLD.

Like screening tests, standardized tests at advanced language levels may not be sufficiently sensitive to higher-level language skills to identify deficits in students with minimally adequate basic oral language abilities who are still having trouble with secondary school work. They also may fail to sample the extended discourse contexts, like narratives and textbook expository prose, that are necessary for success in school. Nelson (1998) suggested that the most appropriate uses of standardized tests of advanced language include identifying the dimensions of the language disorder—dimensions such as oral language, written expression, and comprehension of language forms in listening and reading. We can, then, select standardized tests for adolescents using a strategy similar to the one discussed for elementary students in Chapter 12. That is, we can use standardized tests that sample a broad spectrum of oral and written receptive and expressive abilities. If necessary, the assessment for eligibility can be supplemented with tests of pragmatics and tests of learning-related skills to establish eligibility, as we discussed in Chapter 11. At the advanced language level, some tests particularly helpful in this regard include the following:

▶ *Test of Word Knowledge* (Wiig & Secord, 1992a): assesses aspects of lexical skill including definitions, synonyms, antonyms, metalinguistics, and figurative language.

▶ *Test of Language Competence—Expanded* (Wiig & Secord, 1989): provides assessment of structural ambiguities, figurative language, and ability to draw inferences.

▶ *Test of Adolescent and Adult Language—3* (Hammill, Brown, Larsen, & Wiederholt, 1994): provides broad assessment of syntactic forms in the Listening Grammar, Speaking Grammar, Reading Grammar, and Writing Grammar subtests.

▶ *Clinical Evaluation of Language Fundamentals—4* (Semel, Wiig, & Secord, 2003): the Formulating Sentences, Recalling Sentences, and Sentence Assembly subtests tap various aspects of grammatical production.

▶ *Test of Language Development-Intermediate—3* (Hammill & Newcomer, 1997): the Sentence Combining and Word Ordering subtests have shown good correlations with production in spontaneous discourse (Scott & Stokes, 1995).

▶ *Test of Written Language—3* (Hammill & Larsen, 1996): measures structural elements in writing in students to age 17.

▶ *Comprehensive Assessment of Spoken Language* (Carrow-Woolfolk, 1999): measures semantic, syntactic, pragmatic, and supralinguistic aspects of language.

Table 13-2 provides a list of standardized tests that are appropriate for students at advanced language levels.

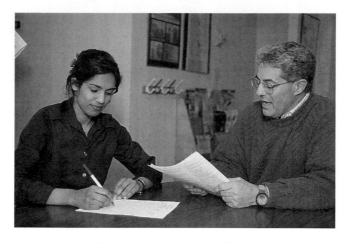
Standardized assessments of advanced language include written and spoken language.

A third source of referral at the secondary school level is the students themselves. Taylor (1992) suggested that we should "market" our services to adolescents directly, as well as to their teachers. Several components of a secondary-level communication program are necessary to attract student self-referrals. First, activity with the SLP must result in academic credit toward graduation (Larson, McKinley, & Boley, 1993). Students will not be willing to devote time voluntarily to activities for which they receive no credit. Larson and McKinley (2003b) also suggested taking care in naming programs, so that they sound like academic courses rather than therapy. *Communication Studies,*

TABLE 13-2	**A Sample of Language Assessment Tools, Grades 6-12**

TEST NAME, AUTHOR(S), DATE, PUBLISHER	AGE RANGE	AREAS ASSESSED	COMMENTS
Adapted Sequenced Inventory of Communication Development for Adolescents and Adults with Severe Handicaps McClennen, S.E. (1989). Melbourne, Australia: Psych Press	Adolescent–adult	Speaking, listening	For use with people with hearing loss, legal blindness, epilepsy, spastic quadriplegia, nonambulation. Similar to Sequenced Inventory of Communication Development. Yields age-equivalent scores.
Assessment of Classroom Communication and Study Skills (ACCSS) Simon, C.S. (1998). Eau Claire, WI: Thinking Publications	10–18 yr	Oral and written directions, inferences, math word problems	Group or individual administration. Administration time: 40–60 min.
Bader Reading and Language Inventory—5th Edition Bader, L. (2004). Upper Saddle River, NJ: Prentice Hall	7 yr–adult	Inventory of tests to assess reading and language abilities	Graded reading passages for all ages and skill levels. Preliteracy tests, including cloze tests to assess the knowledge of semantics and syntactic processing, phonics, and structural analysis. Interest and attitude tests for a more accurate diagnosis.

TABLE 13-2	A Sample of Language Assessment Tools, Grades 6-12—cont'd

TEST NAME, AUTHOR(S), DATE, PUBLISHER	AGE RANGE	AREAS ASSESSED	COMMENTS
Bilingual Syntax Measure II Burt, M.K., & Dulay, H.C. (1978); San Antonio, TX: Harcourt Assessment	Grades 3–12	Syntax mastery (expressive) Tests in English and Spanish	Yields criterion-referenced "levels of proficiency." Administration time: 10–15 min.
Clinical Evaluation of Language Fundamentals—4 Semel, E., Wiig, E.H., & Secord, W. (2003). San Antonio, TX: Harcourt Assessment	5–21 yr	Semantics, syntax, memory, receptive and expressive, composite	Software scoring package available (CELF-4 Clinical Assistant). Screening also available for ages 5–21. 11 subtests. Yields standard, percentile, age-equivalent scores. Normed on 2,400 students. Administration time: 30–60 min.
Comprehensive Assessment of Spoken Language Carrow-Woolfolk, E. (1999). Circle Pines, MN: AGS Publications	7–21 yr	Lexical, syntactic, pragmatic awareness of appropriate forms, complex comprehension	Software package for scoring available. Yields percentiles, stanines, standard scores, and age equivalents.
Expressive One-Word Picture Vocabulary Test—2000 Edition Brownell, R. (Ed.). (2000). Novato, CA: Academic Therapy Publications	2–18 yr	Naming	Spanish version available. Yields standard, percentile, age-equivalent scores. Administration time: 20 min.
Evaluating Communicative Competence Simon, C.S. (1994). Eau Claire, WI: Thinking Publications	10–18 yr	Language processing, metalinguistic skills, functional uses of language	Yields criterion-referenced information.
Fullerton Language Test for Adolescents, Second Edition Thorum, A.R. (1986). Austin, TX: Pro-Ed	11 yr–adult	Auditory synthesis, morphology, oral commands, convergent and divergent production, syllabification, grammar competency, idioms	Yields standard scores. Standardized on 762 adolescents. Administration time: 40 min.
Functional Communication Profile—Revised Kleiman, L.I. (2003). East Moline, IL: LinguiSystems	3 yr–adult	Functional communication profile in 11 areas: sensory, attentiveness, receptive language, expressive language, pragmatic/social, speech, voice, oral, fluency, non-oral communication	Targets practical skills that people encounter daily. Especially useful for clients diagnosed with autism, PDD, or severe disorders. Administration time: 45–90 min.
Language Assessment Scales-Reading and Writing (LAS R/W) Duncan, S., & DeAvila, E. (1994). Monterey, CA: CTB-McGraw-Hill	Grades 2–12	English proficiency	Administration time: 60–90 min. Measures English language reading and writing proficiency of students whose first language is not English.
Oral and Written Language Scales (OWLS): Written Expression Scale Carrow-Woolfolk, E. (1996). Circle Pines, MN: American Guidance Service	5–21 yr	Measures use of conventions, linguistic forms, and the ability to communicate meaningfully in writing	Administration time: 10–30 min.
Peabody Picture Vocabulary Test—4 Dunn, L.M., & Dunn, L.M. (2006). Circle Pines, MN: American Guidance Service	2:6 yr–adult	Receptive vocabulary	Spanish version available. Yields standard, percentile, age-equivalent scores, stanine. Provides standard error of measurement. Standardized on 4,012 subjects 2–18 yr old.

TABLE 13-2	A Sample of Language Assessment Tools, Grades 6-12—cont'd

TEST NAME, AUTHOR(S), DATE, PUBLISHER	AGE RANGE	AREAS ASSESSED	COMMENTS
Receptive One-Word Picture Vocabulary Test—2000 Edition Brownell, R. (Ed.). (2000). Novato, CA: Academic Therapy Publications	12–15:11 yr	Receptive vocabulary	Spanish version available. Yields standard, percentile, age-equivalent score. Similar to norming population for *Expressive One-Word Picture Vocabulary Test.* Administration time: 20 min.
Rhode Island Test of Language Structure Engen, E., & Engen, T. (1983). Austin, TX: Pro-Ed	3–20 yr	Receptive syntax	Designed for hearing impaired, but can be used for ESL populations or for students with LLD or developmental disorders. Yields criterion-referenced information. Standardized on 513 children with hearing impairments and 283 normal-hearing children. Administration time: 30 min.
Test of Adolescent and Adult Language—3 Hammill, D.D., Brown, V.L., Larsen, S.C., & Wiederholt, J.L. (1994). Austin, TX: Pro-Ed	12–24:11 yr	Receptive and expressive, vocabulary and grammar, reading and writing, auditory comprehension	Has software scoring program. Yields standard scores, means, and standard deviations for age. Normed on 3,000 students in 20 states plus 3 Canadian provinces.
Test of Adolescent/Adult Word Finding German, D.J. (1990). Austin, TX: Pro-Ed	12–80 yr	Naming, nouns, verbs, sentence completion, description, categories	Administration time: 45–60 min. Has 40-item brief test. Measures accuracy, speed, and secondary characteristics such as extra verbalization, gesturing, substitutions. Provides standard, percentile scores. Nationally standardized on 1,753 students. Has grade norms for grades 7–12; age norms for 12–80 yr.
Test of Language Competence—Expanded Edition Wiig, E.H., & Secord, W. (1989). San Antonio, TX: Harcourt Assessment	Level 2: 10–18:11 yr	Metalinguistics, multiple meanings, multiple inferences, figurative usage, conversational sentence production	Administration time: 20–30 min. Has companion intervention program, *Steps to Language Competence-Developing Metalinguistic Strategies* (Wiig); which uses cognitive-linguistic approach. Yields standard, percentile, age-equivalent score. Receptive and expressive composite scores. Administration time: 1 hr.
Test of Language Development—Intermediate Hammill, D., & Newcomer, P. (1997). Austin, TX: Pro-Ed	8–12:11 yr	Sentence combining, word ordering, and grammatical comprehension, and picture vocabulary	Administration time: 40 min.

TABLE 13-2	A Sample of Language Assessment Tools, Grades 6-12—cont'd

TEST NAME, AUTHOR(S), DATE, PUBLISHER	AGE RANGE	AREAS ASSESSED	COMMENTS
Test of Problem Solving—Adolescent Bowers, L., Barrett, M., Huisingh, M., Orman, J.L., & LoGuidice, C. (1991). East Moline, IL: LinguiSystems	12–17:11 yr	Fair-mindedness, oversimplification, analyzing, thinking independently, evaluating and clarifying, generating solutions	Yields standard, percentile, age-equivalent scores. Standardized on 1,000 students. Administration time: 20 min.
Test of Word Knowledge Wiig, E.H., & Secord, W. (1992). San Antonio, TX: Harcourt Assessment	Level 2: 8–17 yr	Expressive and receptive semantics, definitions, antonyms, synonyms, multiple meanings	Yields standard, percentile, age-equivalent scores. Provides confidence interval, receptive and expressive composite. Administration time: 1 hr.
Test of Written Expression McGhee, R., Bryant, B., Larson, S., & Rivera, D. (1995). Austin, TX: Pro-Ed	6:6–14:11 yr	Provides a comprehensive assessment of writing achievement	
Test of Written English (TWE) Anderson, V., & Thompson, S. (1988). Novato, CA: Academic Therapy Publications	6–11+ yr	Screens mastery of capitalization, punctuation, written expression, and paragraph writing	Administration time: less than 30 min.
Test of Written Language—3 (TOWL-3) Hammill, D.D., & Larsen, S.C. (1996). Austin, TX: Pro-Ed	Grades 2–12 (7:6–17:11 yr)	Cognitive and linguistic components of language	Can be given to individual or group. Yields standard score, written language quotient. Standardized on more than 2,000 students in 16 states.
Woodcock Language Proficiency Battery—Revised Woodcock, R.W. (1991). Chicago, IL: Riverside Publishing	2–95 yr	Oral language, vocabulary, antonyms and synonyms, reading and writing	Administration time: 40 min. Has Compuscore software. Yields standard, age- and grade-equivalent scores. Nationally standardized on 6,300 students.
The Word Test—2—Adolescent Bowers, L., Huisingh, R., Orman, J., & LoGiudice, C. (2005). East Moline, IL: LinguiSystems	12–17:11 yr	Brand names, synonyms, signs of the times, definitions	Administration time: 20–60 min. Yields standard, percentile, age-equivalent scores. Standardized on more than 1,500 students.
Writing Process Test Warden, M., & Hutchinson, T. (1992). Austin, TX: Pro-Ed	Grades 2–12	Writing, critical thinking	Provides normative data.
Written Language Assessment Grill, J., & Kirwin, K. (1990). Novato, CA: Academic Therapy Publications	8–18 yr	Assesses language with writing samples	

Effective Communication, and *Communication Laboratory* are some examples of likely titles. Third, the program should emphasize the interactions among speaking, listening, reading, and writing and their effects not only on academic but also on interpersonal and vocational success. Marketing to students, in the form of pamphlets, notices, and talks to classes, should focus on how improving language skills helps students succeed in both school and life.

Of course, students who refer themselves must qualify for services, just as students referred from other sources do. Using a self-assessment checklist like the one in Figure 13-1 can be an effective screening measure for adolescent self-referrals. If the student checks only a few of the areas on the form, the student's problem may not qualify him or her for intervention services. The clinician might talk briefly with such students to give them focused tips on study skills or peer communication or in whatever area they were feeling inadequate. Alternatively, the SLP might refer these students to the school counselor.

CRITERION-REFERENCED ASSESSMENT AND BEHAVIORAL OBSERVATION IN THE ADVANCED LANGUAGE STAGE

We've talked several times about the fact that standardized tests are needed to establish eligibility for services but are limited in their ability to serve as a basis for intervention planning. This principle still holds at the advanced language level. Criterion-referenced assessments and structured behavioral observations form the bulk of the assessment procedure at this stage. The errors and difficulties seen in the speech and writing samples we collect early in the assessment can point us toward the kinds of criterion-referenced evaluations we will want to complete. Let's look at the major areas of development of advanced language and give some ideas for criterion-referenced procedures to use to examine each one. Remember, though, that it probably won't be necessary to assess all areas for all students. Standardized testing, referral information, and the conversational and writing samples we collect can be used to focus the evaluation. And because our students at advanced language levels almost always have long histories of assessment and intervention, this information, too, is important in focusing on areas for assessment.

The first thing we need to do after establishing a student's eligibility for services is to decide whether the student is functioning in the advanced language stage or at a lower level. In the L4L stage, we used a short conversational sample to place the student in a general level of development to plan further assessments. This sample can be useful in the advanced language stage, too. A good supplement to the conversational sample, though, is a short sample of the student's writing. We can ask the student to come to the first assessment session with a sample of a homework assignment or an English composition recently completed. Examining these artifacts can help us to decide whether the student has achieved some of the basic skills of the L4L stage, such as the ability to write more-or-less grammatical sentences, to spell with some degree of accuracy, and to organize a sequence of thoughts and express them somewhat comprehensibly. We'll talk more about detailed analysis of writing skill later. It's important to remember, too, that adolescents referred for assessment still have significant difficulty with written expression, even when they are functioning at the advanced language stage. However, looking at a writing sample briefly as part of the preassessment decision-making can help to decide whether advanced language tasks are relevant for this student or whether the student is functioning more at an elementary level of oral and written language.

Students at an L4L level will probably make a few grammatical errors in speech and will display writing samples that are brief; contain short, simple sentences; show difficulty with the mechanics of spelling, capitalization, and punctuation; have little or no organization or macrostructure; and show sparse expression of ideas. In other words, their writing will be like that of a third- or fourth-grader rather than a secondary student. Students functioning at advanced language stages may display word-finding problems, limited vocabulary, and pragmatic errors in conversation, but will have mastered basic oral language rules. Their writing will be less mature and sophisticated than that of their peers but will display some competence with mechanics, some limited use of complex sentences, and some degree of organization and semantic content (Scott, 1999). For students appearing to function at L4L stages in the secondary school years, assessment can focus on areas outlined in Chapter 11, along with some assessment of functional skills needed to survive in the academic and vocational environments that students must face. For students who have basic oral and written language skills, assessment of areas of advanced language development can proceed. Let's look at some of the areas that can be a part of this assessment.

SEMANTICS

The Literate Lexicon

Nippold (1998) discussed the importance of the development in adolescence of a "literate lexicon," the words needed to understand and produce language near the literate end of the oral-literate continuum. One important aspect of the development of a literate lexicon is the ability to use "contextual abstraction" (Sternberg, 1987) to infer the meaning of a new word from the linguistic cues that accompany it. We can assess students' ability to do this by having them read (or listen to the clinician read) a passage that has some difficult, unfamiliar words. We can ask students to guess what the difficult words mean and to tell why they think so. Students who have trouble using context to infer meaning in these activities can be given practice in doing so as part of the intervention program.

Nippold (2000) identified several categories of words particularly important for the literate lexicon. These include nouns for technical and curriculum activities (*salutation, oppression, circumference, proton*). Words like these can be identified and assessed using curriculum-based methods such as those discussed in Chapter 12. Artifact analysis is a particularly useful format here. Students' written work can be analyzed to see which curricular vocabulary items are misused or avoided. These words can be focused on in the intervention program.

Another class of words in the literate lexicon is verbs used in discussions of spoken and written language interpretation and for talking about cognitive and logical processes (Nippold, 2000). They include verbs that refer to both metacognitive (*remember, doubt, infer, hypothesize, conclude, assume*) and metalinguistic (*assert, concede, imply, predict, report, interpret, confirm*) activities. Verbs with presuppositional aspects in their meaning also would be included in the category. Two types of verbs have presuppositional components: *factives* and *nonfactives*. Factive verbs presuppose or assume the truth of the following clause ("We *regret* that your application is denied.") They include examples such as *know, notice, forget*, and *regret*. With non-factive verbs, the truth of the following proposition is uncertain ("I *suppose* my application was denied.") They include verbs such as *think, believe, figure, say, suppose,* and *guess.*

Nippold (1998) reported that these verbs continue to develop and expand in meaning in the vocabularies of normally developing adolescents. There is good reason to believe, then, that they can cause difficulties for students with LLD. Assessment of vocabulary with standardized tests can be supplemented with informal assessment of verbs like these, since they are likely to cause problems and are necessary to establish competency with literate language. Here a metalinguistic approach to assessment can be used. The clinician can simply present a list of curriculum-related words gathered from classroom teachers and ask clients to tell what they know about them. A "Knowledge Rating Checklist" like the one in Figure 12-1 can be helpful. Students can fill out the chart for each word on the clinician's list, and the clinician can work with students on words whose meanings are shaky for them.

Word Retrieval

When we talked about word-finding difficulties for children in the L4L stage, we discussed the fact that a large discrepancy between scores on a receptive vocabulary test and an expressive vocabulary test is one signal of this problem. At the advanced language level, tests such as the *Receptive One-Word Picture Vocabulary Test–2000 Edition* (Brownell, 2000) and the *Expressive One-Word Picture Vocabulary Test—2000 Edition* (Brownell, 2000), as well as the *Peabody Picture Vocabulary Test—4* (Dunn & Dunn, 2006) and the *Expressive Vocabulary Test—2* (Williams, 2006), might be used for this purpose. Tests specifically designed to assess word retrieval include the *Rapid Automatized Naming Task* (Wolf & Denckla, 2005) and the *Test of Adolescent/Adult Word Finding* (German, 1990). Teacher report of word-finding problems or referral checklists would be another. A clinician-made form, like those we've discussed, or a commercially available one, like German and German's (1993) *Word-Finding Referral Checklist* can be used. We also might hear some word-finding problems in our short conversational interaction, with which we began the assessment session. In fact, Tingley, Kyte, Johnson, and Beitchman (2003) suggest that it is always important to supplement single-word testing with a conversational sample in assessing word-finding, since their research suggests only weak relationships between single-word tests and disruptions in conversational speech.

Word Definitions

We use the standard expressive and receptive vocabulary tests just discussed to give a general picture of vocabulary development. Crais (1990), however, emphasized the limitations of these tests in that they give a "yes or no" answer as to whether a particular word is "known," when in reality there are many levels of "knowing" involved in lexical acquisition. Having a partial representation of the meaning of a word is not adequate, for example, to produce a complete definition of the word.

Using word definition tasks to assess advanced language stages is appropriate, since the ability to define words is generally

acquired by the time normally developing children reach this stage (Nippold, 1995). Several tests of adolescent language have definition subtests that can be used as criterion-referenced assessments. These include *The Comprehensive Receptive and Expressive Vocabulary Test—2nd Edition* (Wallace & Hammill, 2002), *The Test of Word Knowledge* (Wiig & Secord, 1992a), and *The Word Test 2—Adolescent* (Huisingh et al., 2005). We also can simply ask students to give definitions for words derived from textbook or literature selections that they are studying in class. We can assess these informally elicited definitions using the following scoring rubric suggested by Nippold, Hegel, Sohlberg, and Schwarz (1999) and Pease, Gleason, and Pan (1993):

▶ **2 points:** contains an accurate superordinate term and describes the word with one or more accurate characteristics (X is a Y that Z; a robin is a bird that has a red breast)
▶ **1 point:** contains an accurate superordinate term but does not describe the word accurately (X is a Y; "happiness is a feeling"); describes the word with one or more accurate characteristics, but does not contain an accurate superordinate term (X is when Y; "happiness is when you're glad")
▶ **0 points:** attempts a response, but it does not contain an accurate superordinate term or accurate description/characteristic; no response

Nippold and Haq's results suggest that students in sixth grade should receive at least one point for more than half the words presented; those in ninth grade should receive at least one point for more than 75% of the words presented, and those in twelfth grade should receive 2 points for more than half the words presented.

If students have difficulty producing definitions, then we should work on enhancing their understanding of the meanings and uses of the words in question in the intervention program. We also should provide students with experience in word definition tasks as part of the program. These experiences include looking up, reading, reproducing, and eventually generating definitions for the words targeted in the treatment program.

Word Relations

To be competent with words, we need to know more than what the words mean. It also is necessary to know how words are related. Students at advanced language levels need to be able to consider that words may have more than one meaning. They have to be able to substitute words with similar meanings to avoid using the same word over and over again in their writing. They need to compare and contrast word meanings to choose the best word to express their idea. They also must choose correct spellings for words that are pronounced similarly (*their, there*) and use context to decide which meaning is being expressed by a spelling with more than one pronunciation ("I *read* the paper every day," "I *read* the paper yesterday").

Again, subtests of standardized instruments are available to use as criterion-referenced assessment for looking at these kinds of skills. *The Clinical Evaluation of Language Fundamentals—4* (Semel, Wiig, & Secord, 2003) has sections testing semantic relationships, as do the *Detroit Test of Learning Aptitude—4* (Hammill, 1998), the *Test of Language Competence—Expanded*

Edition (Wiig & Secord, 1989), the *Test of Language Development-Intermediate—III* (Hammill & Newcomer, 1997), the *Woodcock Language Proficiency Battery—Revised* (Woodcock, 1991), and *The Word Test 2—Adolescent* (Huisingh et al., 2005).

Understanding of multiple meanings can be assessed with definition tasks. We might give a student a word, such as *run* or *can*, that has several common meanings and ask the student to give a definition, and then give another one. We can observe whether students are able to generate alternative meanings without support. If they can't, some dynamic assessment can be tried, in which we give "clues," such as "Tell me what *run* means when you're talking about a race. What does it mean when you're talking about an election?" If these clues help students who were at first unable to generate multiple meanings, a learning-strategy approach might be used to help the student use self-questioning to determine whether multiple meanings of a word need to be invoked, to understand jokes, for example. If the "clues" don't help, more direct attention to words with multiple meanings might be provided in the intervention program.

Artifact analysis is another way to obtain criterion-referenced assessment of word-relation skills. Going over a student's writing to look for inability to substitute words with similar meaning, so that the same word recurs frequently, can clue us in to the need to work on synonyms and develop sets of synonymous words in the intervention program. Other usage errors in writing, such as writing *red* when the student means *read*, are also clues to the need for work in the area. So are misuses of words, such as using *assess* when *access* is meant.

Other curriculum-based forms of assessment also can be used. These would include reading a passage with a student, from a classroom literature selection, for example. The clinician could ask the student to substitute a synonym for several of the words, ask for antonyms for words, have the student compare and contrast the meanings of related pairs of words in the passage, and ask the student to generate other meanings for a word in the passage that could have more than one. For example, the clinician might present the following passage from *The Call of the Wild* (London, 1963, pp. 3-4):

> Buck did not read the newspapers, or he would have known that trouble was *brewing*, not alone for himself but for every tidewater dog…Because men, *groping* in the *Arctic* darkness, had found a yellow metal, and because steamship and *transportation* companies were *booming* the find, thousands of men were rushing to the Northland…These men wanted dogs…to *toil*…

You might ask the student to supply a word that could be substituted in this context for *brewing*, *groping*, or *booming*. You could ask what *brewing* means in this context and what else it could mean, what the opposite of *Arctic* or *toil* is (*tropical*, *play*), and how the words *Arctic* and *Northland* are related in meaning. All these activities, of course, require a good deal of metalinguistic skill. If the student cannot perform them, the failure may be a result of poor metalinguistic ability rather than a lack of lexical knowledge. Still, both levels of knowledge, lexical

and metalinguistic, are necessary to be fully competent with language at the literate end of the continuum. Assessing these skills with metalinguistic tasks will give us an idea whether students can handle the demands of the metalinguistics of word relations. If they can't, practice with such activities in a curriculum-based intervention program will improve both lexical and metalinguistic ability.

Figurative Language

As we've discussed, the ability to use language in nonliteral ways is one of the important developments of the advanced language period. Rinaldi (2000) has shown that students with LLD are less able than peers to use context to understand implied meanings and to rule out literal interpretations when they did not know the non-literal meaning of an expression. A few adolescent test batteries have figurative-language processing subtests. The *Test of Language Competence–Expanded* (Wiig & Secord, 1989) and the *Comprehensive Assessment of Spoken Language* (Carrow-Woolfolk, 2001) are two examples. We also can use curriculum-based assessment to document deficits in this area. Literature selections from the student's English class can be analyzed by the clinician for similes, metaphors, idioms, and proverbs. These figures can be presented in context to the student, who is asked to provide an interpretation. We can look at our *The Call of the Wild* (London, 1963, pp. 4–6) example again:

> Buck lived in a big house in the *sun-kissed* Santa Clara valley…And over this great domain Buck ruled…for *he was king*…He had a fine pride in himself, was ever a trifle egotistical *as a country gentleman*…

A clinician could ask the student to decide whether the sun really kissed the valley and whether Buck was really a king. The student could be asked to explain what these metaphors did mean and why the author might use them. A similar procedure could be used for the simile *egotistical as a country gentleman*. Again, these metalinguistic activities require more than basic comprehension of the figurative language forms. But these activities are the kind that will be demanded by the curriculum in which students must function. If assessment of figurative language in contexts like these indicates weakness on the part of the student, intervention that encourages work with figurative forms at a variety of levels can be instituted. In general, figures that refer to concrete objects ("The early bird catches the worm") are easier than those with abstract words only ("Two wrongs don't make a right"). Familiar sayings ("Too many cooks spoil the broth") are easier than unfamiliar ones ("Two captains will sink a ship"). However, Nippold and Taylor (2002) showed that there is a developmental progression in the understanding of idioms from childhood to adolescence so that the familiarity of the idiom becomes less important in determining its difficulty for older students, as they gain greater skill in using context to determine meaning. Qualls and O'Brien (2003) showed that context facilitates idiom comprehension, so that presenting idioms within a story setting aids students in determining their meaning. We can give students practice hearing, reading, interpreting, talking about, and creating figurative forms in a variety of contexts to increase both comprehension and metalinguistic awareness of these modes of expression.

Qualls and O'Brien (2003) selected a list of 24 idioms that represented a range of familiarity to speakers of English. These are presented in Table 13-3.

Students who have difficulty inferring and explaining the meaning of common figures in tasks such as these can benefit from exposure to and metalinguistic discussion about idioms in the intervention program that employs contexts in which the students are encouraged to infer the idiom's meaning.

Semantic Integration

We talked at length in Chapter 11 about assessing semantic integration in the L4L period. Many of the same procedures, using grade-appropriate material, can be used in the advanced language stage as well. The Inference subtest of the *California Test of Mental Maturity* (Sullivan, Clark, & Tiegs, 1961) and of the *Test of Language Competence—Expanded Edition* (Wiig & Secord, 1989) also can be used as a criterion-referenced procedure to assess this area. Kamhi and Johnston (1992) devised the Propositional Complexity Analysis, which looks at the semantic content of spontaneous speech samples. This procedure can provide an additional means of assessing how the client combines ideas in discourse.

Verbal Reasoning

The language of thinking, used to solve problems, to plan, organize, predict, speculate, and hypothesize, becomes a major function of communication in the advanced language stage. The ability to use language to extend thinking, reflect on thinking, and entertain several cognitive viewpoints at once are hallmarks of formal operational thought. Students who cannot engage in this kind of language use will be at a distinct disadvantage in many areas of the curriculum, including science, mathematics, and social studies topics such as history and geography. Several standardized tests assess verbal reasoning. These include the *Cornell Reasoning Tests* (Ennis et al., 1965), and the *Matrix Analogies Tests* (Naglieri, 1985). Subtests of some comprehen-

sive batteries also can provide helpful criterion-referenced information on a student's facility with verbal reasoning. The *Woodcock Language Proficiency Battery—Revised* (Woodcock, 1991), the *Illinois Test of Psycholinguistic Abilities—3rd Edition* (Hammill, Mather, & Roberts, 2001), *Wechsler Intelligence Scale for Children—4th Ed.* (Wechsler, 2005), *Differential Aptitude Test-—5th Ed.* (Bennett, Seashore, & Wesman, 1990), and the *Test of Problem Solving* have verbal reasoning sections. Students who have significant difficulties in these areas are helped by working on analogies, syllogisms, and using language to talk through logical problems in the intervention program.

SYNTAX AND MORPHOLOGY

Comprehension

Students at advanced language stages should be able to comprehend virtually all the sentence types in the language and should no longer use comprehension strategies for processing difficult sentences. Several language batteries for adolescents have receptive syntax subtests that can be used as criterion-referenced assessments. Some examples include the *Clinical Evaluation of Language Fundamentals—4* (Semel, Wiig, & Secord, 2003), the *Test of Adolescent and Adult Language—3* (Hammill, Brown, Larsen, & Wiederholt, 1997), and the *Test of Language Development—Intermediate—3* (Hammill & Newcomer, 1997). If deficits are identified on receptive syntactic testing or if comprehension strategy use is seen to persist on these measures, intervention should include an input component, as we've discussed for earlier stages of development. Activities aimed at eliciting production of advanced language forms should be supplemented with literature-based and curriculum-based script activities. These activities should provide intensive exposure in context to the forms for which comprehension is "wobbly," and metalinguistic discussion about their meaning to build the comprehension base for these structures.

Production

You probably are familiar by now with the arguments about using a language sample to assess syntactic production. Sampling how a student uses language to communicate in real interactive

---

TABLE 13-3	Common Idioms in English, at Three Levels of Familiarity	
LOW FAMILIARITY	**MODERATE FAMILIARITY**	**HIGH FAMILIARITY**
Take down a peg	Go into one's shell	Let off some steam
Vote with one's feet	Strike the right note	Go around in circles
Paper over the cracks	Keep up one's end	Put one's foot down
Hoe ones's own row	Cross swords with someone	Breathe down someone's neck
Talk through one's hat	Blow away the cobwebs	Put their heads together
Lead with one's chin	Make one's hair curl	Skate on thin ice
Rise to the bait	Throw to the wolves	Beat around the bush
Have a hollow ring	Go against the grain	Read between the lines

Adapted from Nippold, M., Taylor, C., & Baker, J. (1996). Idiom understanding in Australian youth. *Journal of Speech and Hearing Research, 39,* 442-447; Qualls, C., & O'Brien, R. (2003). Contextual variation, familiarity, academic literacy and rural adolescents' idiom knowledge. *Language, Speech and Hearing Services in Schools, 34,* 69-79.

situations provides the most ecologically valid assessment of productive syntax. But what kind of sample should we elicit from a student in the advanced language stage? The use of forms toward the literate end of the oral-literate continuum is the major area we are interested in assessing at this age range. Hadley (1998) suggested that contextual factors are especially important for selecting a sampling situation at this stage. Many interactive situations, such as peer conversations or even informal discourse with adults, do not elicit the advanced forms we are interested in sampling. So we want to select a context that gives us a good chance of observing some of these advanced language forms. This suggests that communication tasks near the literate end of the continuum may be a better source of information on these variables than conversation.

Many researchers looking at the syntax of advanced language have used narrative tasks (Blake, Quartaro, & Onorati, 1993; Hadley, 1998; Klecan-Aker & Hedrick, 1985; Morris & Crump; 1982, Nippold, 1998; O'Donnell, Griffin, & Norris, 1967; Scott & Stokes, 1995; Scott & Windsor, 2000). These sampling contexts have several advantages. First, much of the data on syntactic production in adolescents is based on these kinds of tasks. Using them in assessment, then, makes the client's sample more directly comparable to those in the literature. Second, narrative samples also can be analyzed for other aspects of advanced language, such as cohesion, use of literate lexical items, and narrative stage. Finally, narratives from children at this developmental level have been shown to contain more complex language forms than conversation does (Hadley, 1998). Narratives are, then, more likely to provide examples of the literate language that we hope to elicit. For these reasons, narratives probably make optimal speech sampling contexts for adolescents.

As we discussed when we talked about assessing narrative in younger children, there are several ways to elicit these samples. Weiss, Temperly, Stierwalt, and Robin (1993) suggested using cartoon strips from the newspaper, with the words "whited-out," to elicit narrative samples. Wordless picture books, such as *A Boy, a Dog, and a Frog* (Mayer, 1967), or films, filmstrips, or videos based on them (for example, *Frog, Where Are You?* [Osbourne & Templeton, 1994]) also can be used by asking the student to first look through the pictures and then to tell the story as if reading to a child for whom he or she is baby-sitting. Hadley (1998) suggested a two-step procedure. Students are first asked to retell an episode from a story after looking at pictures or a film of it. They then are asked to generate an ending for the story. This procedure provides an opportunity for clinicians to see whether students do better (as we would expect) when some visual support is provided, and how a student is able to organize and generate a story episode independently.

Because of the importance of written expression at the advanced language stage, it is wise to assess syntactic and morphological production in written as well as oral samples. Windsor, Scott, and Street (2000), for example, showed that middle schoolers with LLD were more likely to make morphological errors in their written than spoken language samples. Nippold et al. (2005) showed that persuasive writing contexts elicited students' most advanced level of syntactic production.

Artifact analysis (Nelson, 1998) can be used to assess compositions that students have prepared for English classes. Alternatively, written samples can be elicited in situations that parallel those used to elicit speech. Getting both a written and a spoken sample using the same sampling context—whether it be a personal narrative, retelling a film plot, or narrating a picture book or comic strip—can be valuable for looking at the ways in which oral and written skills compare.

Scott and Stokes (1995) suggested analyzing three aspects of syntactic and morphological production at the advanced language stage: T-unit length, use of subordination, and use of higher level structures. All three have been analyzed in the literature in both spoken and written language samples of students at advanced language levels (Scott, 2005). Let's see how we might apply these three analyses to samples of spoken and written language that we collect from our adolescent clients.

T-Unit Length. We talked in Chapter 11 about the use of T-units to analyze speech samples from children in the elementary years. We use this method to correct for long, run-on sentences that could bias scoring. A T-unit, remember, is one main clause with all the subordinate clauses and nonclausal phrases attached to or embedded in it. All coordinated clauses are separated out into separate T-units, unless they contain a co-referential subject deletion in the second clause ("She swings and misses"). Clauses that begin with the coordinating conjunctions *and, but,* or *or* would be considered to comprise a new T-unit.

Loban (1976) documented small but steady increases in T-unit length in words during adolescence, with bigger changes in writing than in speech. Table 13-4 gives the values Loban reported for T-unit lengths in words for oral and written samples from students from sixth through twelfth grades. Notice that T-units for adolescents in the literature have been calculated in words, not in morphemes. When we do T-unit analyses for adolescents and want to compare them to published norms, then, we need to remember to use words rather than morphemes as the unit of analysis. Scott and Windsor (2000) showed that T-unit lengths were significantly lower for children with LLD than for typical peers, whereas the number of grammatical errors was higher.

We should note another important feature of the information in Table 13-4. In early adolescence, in sixth and seventh grades, oral T-unit lengths are greater than those produced in written samples. In mid-adolescence, at eighth or ninth grade, the oral and written samples have about equal T-unit lengths. By late adolescence, in about tenth grade, though, written samples contain longer T-units than do oral ones, and this difference increases up through twelfth grade. Although Scott (2005) reports that T-unit lengths have not been found to differentiate students with LLD from those with typical development, it is useful to use T-unit length to document this important shift. When sampling oral and written expression at these age levels, it will be important, particularly for students in mid- to late adolescence, to determine whether T-unit length in written production is catching up to and eventually exceeding that of oral language. If it is not, we need to be sure to augment work on advanced oral language forms with activities aimed at increasing the complexity of written language as well.

TABLE 13-4	T-unit Lengths in Words for Spoken and Written Samples Collected from Adolescent Students	
GRADE	AVERAGE T-UNIT LENGTH IN WORDS PRODUCED IN SPOKEN SAMPLES	AVERAGE T-UNIT LENGTH IN WORDS PRODUCED IN WRITTEN SAMPLES
6	9.8	9.0
8	10.7	10.4
10	10.7	11.8
12	11.7	13.3

Adapted from Loban, W. (1976). *Language development: Kindergarten through grade twelve.* Urbana, IL: National Council of Teachers of English.

Box 13-2 contains a sample of an oral narrative describing a movie seen by an adolescent student, "Charlie." Why not try dividing it into T-units and computing average T-unit length in words for this sample? My analysis appears in Appendix 13-1. You may want to consider whether Charlie's T-unit length in spoken narrative is appropriate for a tenth-grader.

Clause Density. Scott and Stokes (1995) suggested another index of syntactic complexity that can be used to assess adolescent language samples: an index of the density of clauses within sentences, often referred to as the *subordination index.* They define clause density as "a ratio of the total number of clauses (main and subordinate) summed across [T-units], and divided by the number of [T-units] in a sample" (p. 310). In other words, if a T-unit contains just one main clause, it receives a clause count of 1. The T-unit from Charlie's sample, "*It was for monkeys and chimpanzees,*" contains just one main clause. A T-unit such as, "*Then after they graduated, they took them into this plane,*" would receive a clause count of 2: one for the main clause, "they took them into this plane," and one for the adverbial clause, "then after they graduated." The T-unit, "*There was a boy who was about 21 who stole a plane with a woman and champagne in the cockpit,*" would receive a clause count of 3: one for the main clause "there was a boy," one for the relative clause "who was about 21," one for the relative clause "who stole a plane with a woman and champagne in the cockpit."

The number of clauses for each T-unit in the sample would be summed, then divided by the number of T-units, to obtain the subordination index for the sample. Nippold (1998) reported values for Loban's (1976) study of subordination in speech and writing of secondary school students. These appear in Table 13-5. Note again that in early adolescence, the subordination index is higher in speech than in writing. In mid- to late adolescence, the values in written samples are similar to or slightly higher than those seen in speech. Note, too, that the increases in this score throughout adolescence are very small, suggesting that we should not expect to see big changes in this measure through the secondary school years. Nippold et al. (2005) and Scott (2005) remind us, too, that the use of subordination is highly dependent on the situation and audience. That's why it is especially important to choose a sampling context that falls near the literate end of the continuum if we are looking for

more advanced sentences. To interpret this analysis, a rule of thumb would be to see whether the subordination index is at least 1.3 in spoken samples for all adolescents and whether the index in written samples is at least equal to the index in a spoken sample for students in mid- to late adolescence. If we see subordination indices at these levels, we can conclude that the student's expressive language is of adequate complexity. If the subordination index is close to 1.0 or if the index in a written sample from a student in eighth grade or higher is noticeably less than that of the spoken sample, work on increasing use of subordination in formal speech and writing can be included in the intervention program. Why not try computing a subordination index for Charlie's sample in Box 13-2?

Use of High-Level Structures. Scott and Stokes (1995) discussed a variety of syntactic structures that appear with relatively low frequency but serve as markers of an advanced, literate language style. Table 13-6 lists these structures. We can examine the oral and written narrative samples collected from adolescents for the presence of the forms listed in Table 13-6 as one aspect of our assessment. Students who provide several instances of several categories of these markers in a short narrative or written sample can be considered to be producing adequately complex forms of expression.

Two caveats need to be kept in mind when looking for these higher level structures. First, context is very important in eliciting these forms. They only appear in relatively formal situations (Eckert, 1990), and their use is never obligatory. It is always a matter of making an appropriate choice of form for a particular audience or genre. Scott and Stokes suggest choosing contexts that involve cognitive planning in order to elicit these forms. Again, narrative is a good example of this kind of planned discourse. To increase the chances of finding some in our narrative samples, we can ask students to "tell me the story of a movie you saw recently. I haven't seen it, so try to tell the story as clearly as you can. Tell it the way it would sound if I read about it in a magazine." For written samples, we can ask students to "write the story of the movie as if you were writing a book or magazine article about the movie."

The second warning we need to bear in mind is that these are low-frequency forms. It is not likely that we will find more than a few instances of any of these forms in one short sample.

| BOX 13-2 | Oral Narrative Sample: Retelling of a Movie Plot Produced by "Charlie," A Tenth-Grade Student |

There was a boy who was about 21 who stole a plane with a woman and champagne in the cockpit, and then he got court-martialed for that and then they sent him to a research study. It was for monkeys and chimpanzees. They taught them how to fly, and then what they would do is to have three classes. White would be a freshman, blue a junior, and red a senior and they would teach them how to fly. Then after they graduated, they took them into this plane. There's this one area, called the radiation area and they put them in a simulator and exposed them to radiation treatment and they wanted to see how long they would fly until they would die and so they could see how long humans could fly if they could pilot their missions if the Russians had an attack on us and then what the boy did is he had a friend, a chimpanzee that knew sign language and he talked to him and he taught the other apes and they were going to kill his friend with the radiation thing. There were these people from the Air Force Patrol and they were watching the studies and he didn't want them to kill his monkey and so what he did was he called the lady who taught him sign language and she came and they stole a plane with the monkeys in it and they finally escaped.

| TABLE 13-5 | Subordination Index Figures in Spoken and Written Samples from Secondary School Students |

GRADE	AVERAGE SUBORDINATION INDEX PRODUCED IN SPOKEN SAMPLES	AVERAGE SUBORDINATION INDEX PRODUCED IN WRITTEN SAMPLES
6	1.4	1.3
8	1.4	1.5
10	1.5	1.5
12	1.6	1.6

Adapted from Scott, C. (1989). Spoken and written syntax. In M. Nippold (Ed.). *Later language development* (pp. 49-96). Boston, MA: College-Hill Press; and Loban, W. (1976). *Language development: Kindergarten through grade twelve.* Urbana, IL: National Council of Teachers of English.

Nippold et al. (2005) reported that 15% to 20% of adolescents' utterances included relative and adverbial clauses, for example, and this result was in the context of persuasive discourse, which tends to elicit higher-than-normal levels of these forms. Further, a given sample will not contain instances of all the types listed. In this analysis, we are not really looking for the appearance of any one particular structure, but only at whether several examples of these kinds of structures appear. If they do, and findings on T-unit length and subordination index confirm the finding, we can conclude that the student has some command of literate syntax. If they do not, and findings on T-unit length and subordination yield corresponding information, we can identify a deficit in advanced syntax. If such a deficit is identified, intervention would focus on developing a range of literate syntax forms. Exposing the student to literate language forms in reading material (read to the student if necessary) will be part of this intervention.

Take a look at Charlie's sample in Box 13-2. Try making a list of the high level structures from Scott and Stokes' list in Table 13-6 that appear in the sample. What would your assessment of Charlie's use of high level structures in this sample be? My list is in Appendix 13-1. Looking across the three measures of expression computed for this sample, how would you rate Charlie's syntactic complexity? My computation and evaluation are given in Appendix 13-1. Figure 13-3 presents a sample of Charlie's written expression. Try doing these three measures on the written sample and compare them to the spoken one. What would your conclusion about his expressive syntactic skill be on the basis of this comparison? My assessment of the written sample appears in Appendix 13-2.

PRAGMATICS

Pragmatic skills acquired in adolescence, like those children learn in the L4L stage, function to allow the student to operate in wider social circles and in a greater variety of discourse genres. While the changes that take place in semantic and syntactic development in adolescence are often subtle and need special contexts to be observed, the pragmatic changes that take place at this time are major and often painfully obvious to the adults who deal with young people in this stage of development. (Sarcasm, for example, is one of the new functions of language that emerges in teenagers, often to their elders' dismay.) We can look at two areas of pragmatic development that undergo these significant changes in adolescence: *conversational skills* and the expansion of competence in several *discourse genres.*

| TABLE 13-6 | **High-Level, Low-Frequency Structural Markers of Advanced Syntax** |

SYNTACTIC CATEGORY	STRUCTURE	EXAMPLES
Morphology	Prefixes and suffixes	*Unplanned, replay, helpless, requirement*
	Nominalization (noun forms of verbs)	*Adaptation, establishment*
	Use of past and present participle forms of verbs as adjectives	Her *broken* CD player; *a growing* plant
	Later developing conjunctions	*Otherwise, instead, after all, only, still, though, anyway, in all, finally, when, because*
	Adverbial sentence connectives (conjuncts)	*Nevertheless, furthermore, therefore, for example, in addition*
Noun phrase (NP) elaboration	NP pre-modification with two or more adjectives	Her *cute, black* puppy
	NP post-modification with:	
	Past participles	A tree *called the willow*
	Present participles	A machine *controlling his brain*
	Infinitives	A good way *to fish*
	Appositives	Mr. Smith, *the mail carrier*
	Relative clauses	A woman *who lives nearby*
	Elaboration	Dogs such *as Collies, Spaniels, and German Shepherds*
	Prepositional phrases	The cyclist *in the lead position*
Verb phrase (VP) elaboration	Multiple auxiliaries	We *could have* missed it
	Perfect aspect	We *had been studying* all night
	Passive voice	The house *was designed by a* famous architect
Adverbial use	With adjectives	*extremely* large
	Adverbial phrases	*Awfully quickly*
Complex sentence types	More than one clause type in a sentence	He wants to pass, but he doesn't know how to study
	"Left-branching" clauses (clauses that appear near the beginning of the sentence):	*Getting into college* won't be hard for Amy to do
	Preposed adverbial clauses	*After we study,* we'll go for pizza
	Center-embedded relative clauses	The boy *who sits behind me* in English is cute
	Noun clauses as subjects	*Passing Mr. Haywood's class* is tough
		To get a C in biology is an accomplishment
	Sentences using word order variations for theme and focus, such as cleft sentences	*It was our team* that won the game
		The one who got there first was the winner
		What I really want is a different English teacher

Adapted from Nippold, M. (1998). *Later language development: The school-age and adolescent years.* Austin, TX: Pro-Ed; and Scott, C., & Stokes, S. (1995). Measures of syntax in school-age children and adolescents. *Language, Speech, and Hearing Services in Schools, 26,* 309-317.

Conversational Pragmatics

Lapadat (1991) showed that adolescents with LLD performed like younger normally developing children in terms of their pragmatic skills. This work suggested that the flexible use of language finely tuned to interpersonal nuances, which is normally acquired during the teen years, may be lacking for our clients, even when basic semantic and syntactic skills are present. Adams (2002) reviewed data that suggests pragmatic problems to be common in many students with a variety of communication and language-learning disorders. Adams (2002) suggested organizing conversational analysis around four major areas:

▶ Initiation and responsiveness
▶ Turn-taking and repair
▶ Topic structure
▶ Cohesion/coherence

These major aspects of conversation can serve as a starting point for developing a conversational analysis method. However, Reed, Bradfield, and McAllister (1998) reported that although SLPs believed that discourse management skills were the most important pragmatic areas to address with adolescents, the youngsters themselves believed that language used for empathy and affiliation was more crucial for positive peer relationships. Turstra, Ciccia, and Seaton (2003) examined conversational behaviors in typically developing adolescents engaged in 3-minute interactions with peers and found that behaviors occurring at the highest rates were looking at the

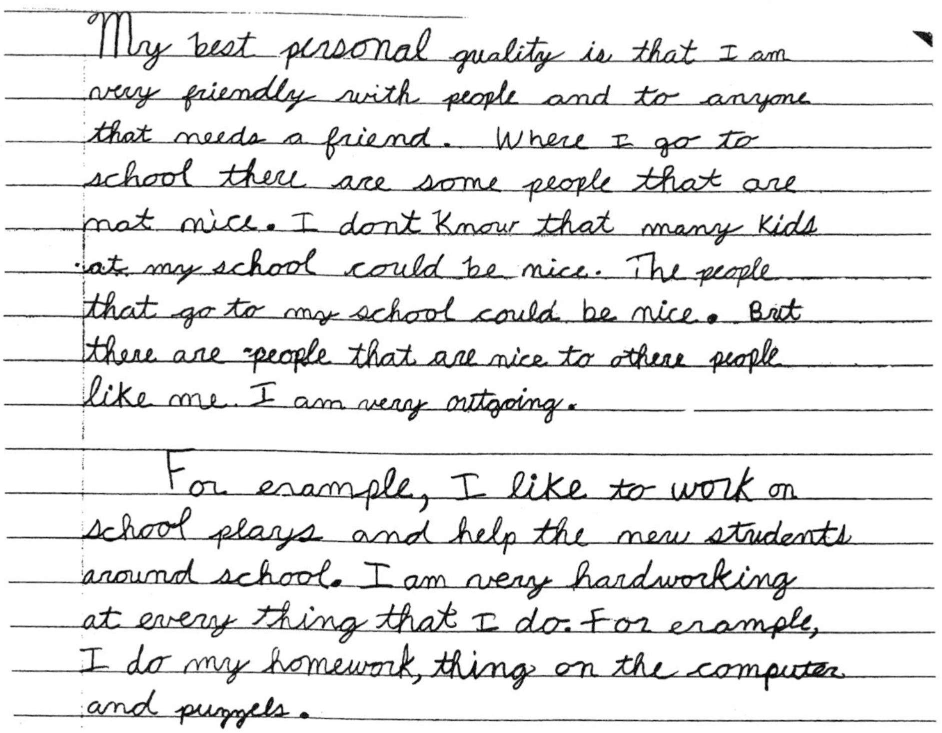

My best personal quality is that I am very friendly with people and to anyone that needs a friend. Where I go to school there are some people that are not nice. I dont Know that many Kids at my school could be nice. The people that go to my school could be nice. But there are people that are nice to othere people like me. I am very outgoing.

For example, I like to work on school plays and help the new students around school. I am very hardworking at every thing that I do. For example, I do my homework, thing on the computer and puzzels.

FIGURE 13-3 ✦ Charlie's written language sample (tenth grade).

partner (especially during listening), nodding and showing positive facial expressions, using back-channel responses indicating understanding and agreement (such as "uh-huh" or "yeah"), and giving contingent responses. Behaviors that occurred with very low frequency included negative emotions, turning away, asking for clarification, and failing to answer questions. These findings suggest that we need to be careful about choosing pragmatic targets in this age range. That is, while focusing on discourse structure and content aspects of conversation are important, these areas should be supplemented by a look at the use of appropriate paralinguistic behaviors in peer interactions. Moreover, we need to help teens find ways to express empathy and establish affiliation through conversation. Again, involving the student in the assessment process is a good way to keep priorities on track. And observing a peer-to-peer conversation, even a short one, such as Turstra used, can provide especially useful information, since Turstra (2001) showed that there were significant differences in conversational behaviors of students with LLD when talking to adults as opposed to peers.

Using a general pragmatic assessment, such as Prutting and Kirchner's (1983) *Pragmatic Protocol* (Figure 8-17), Damico's *Systematic Observation of Communicative Interaction* (1992), Bedrosian's (1985) *Discourse Skills Checklist* (Figure 11-7), or Bishop's *Children's Communication Checklist* (2003) may point to some areas of difficulty for students with LLD. But the specific deficits most likely to cause problems for this age group are often not represented on more global scales designed for younger children.

Larson and McKinley (2003a) designed a conversational assessment specifically for clients in the advanced language stage. Their *Adolescent Conversational Analysis* looks at linguistic and paralinguistic features and examines use of communicative functions and conversational rules. Figure 13-4 provides an abbreviated version of Larson and McKinley's procedure, which can be used to analyze an unstructured conversation between the adolescent and a familiar partner. Larson and McKinley suggested looking at several samples of the client interacting with different partners in various settings to get a complete picture of conversational competence.

Another method that can be considered for assessing conversational skill is Landa et al.'s (1992) *Pragmatic Rating Scale* (PRS). This measure was designed for use in a conversational context with adult family members of children with autism and related conditions. Paul and Sutherland (2005) reports that PRS scores from adolescents with typical development differ significantly from those of high functioning teens with autism spectrum disorders. Subjects in the typical group uniformly scored 5 or lower on this measure. These data suggest that scores above 6 on the PRS are likely to be indicative of a deficit in pragmatic ability. A rating form for the PRS appears in Figure 13-5. Additional assessments that can be considered include Bishop et al.'s *Assessment of Language Impaired Children's Conversation* and Rinaldi's (2001) *Social Use of Language Programme.*

Looking at conversational skill in free speech interactions can yield very valuable information. This method is, however, extremely time consuming and labor intensive. When doing initial evaluations to determine whether conversational pragmatics needs to be targeted in the intervention program, there are some shortcuts to conversational analysis that can give us useful information. These include norm-referenced instruments, structured behavioral observations, and nonstandardized role-playing procedures.

	Appropriate	Inappropriate	No opportunity to observe	Comments
Listener role				
Vocabulary				
Syntax				
Main ideas				
Cooperative manner				
Gives feedback				
Speaker role: language features				
Syntax				
Questions				
Figurative language				
Nonspecific language				
Precise vocabulary				
Word retrieval				
Mazes and dysfluencies				
Speaker role: paralinguistic features				
Suprasegmental features				
Fluency				
Intelligibility				
Speaker role: communicative functions				
Give information				
Receive information				
Describe				
Persuade				
Express opinion/belief				
Indicate readiness				
Solve problems verbally				
Entertain				
Conversational rules				
Verbal turns/topics				
Initiation				
Topic choice				
Topic maintenance				
Topic switch				
Turn-taking				
Repair/revision				
Interruption				
Verbal politeness				
Quantity				
Sincerity				
Relevance				
Clarity				
Tact				
Nonverbal				
Gestures				
Facial expressions				
Eye contact				
Proxemics				

FIGURE 13-4 ✦ Adolescent conversational analysis. Adapted from Larson, V., and McKinley, N. (2003a). *Communication solutions for older students: Assessment and intervention strategies.* Eau Claire, WI: Thinking Publications.

Norm-Referenced Conversational Assessments. Several norm-referenced instruments are available for probing pragmatic skills at the adolescent level. These include the *Test of Language Competence—Expanded Edition* (Wiig & Secord, 1989), the *Pragmatic Checklist from the CELF-4* (Semel, Wiig, & Secord, 2004), and Bishop's *Children's Communication Checklist* (2003). These norm-referenced measures can be helpful for establishing eligibility for students at advanced language stages, who may perform adequately on tests focusing on semantics and syntax. They also can identify areas that we may want to

	0	1	2
Inappropriate or absent greeting	—	—	—
Strikingly candid	—	—	—
Overly direct or blunt	—	—	—
Inappropriately formal	—	—	—
Inappropriately informal	—	—	—
Overly talkative	—	—	—
Irrelevant or inappropriate detail	—	—	—
Content 'out of sync' with interlocutor	—	—	—
Confusing accounts	—	—	—
Topic preoccupation/perseveration	—	—	—
Unresponsive to cues	—	—	—
Little reciprocal to-and-fro exchange	—	—	—
Terse	—	—	—
Odd humor	—	—	—
Insufficient background information	—	—	—
Failure to reference pronouns or other terms	—	—	—
Inadequate clarification	—	—	—
Vague accounts	—	—	—
Scripted, stereotyped discourse	—	—	—
Awkward expression of ideas	—	—	—
Indistinct or mispronounced speech	—	—	—
Inappropriate rate of speech	—	—	—
Inappropriate intonation	—	—	—
Inappropriate volume	—	—	—
Excessive pauses, reformulations	—	—	—
Unusual rhythm, fluency	—	—	—
Inappropriate physical distance	—	—	—
Inappropriate gestures	—	—	—
Inappropriate facial expression	—	—	—
Inappropriate use of gaze	—	—	—

Subject's total score: _____

0, Normal; 1, Moderately inappropriate; 2, Absent or highly inappropriate.
Total scores of 6 or above are indicative of pragmatic disorders.

FIGURE 13-5 ✦ Score form based on Landa et al.'s (1992) *Pragmatic Rating Scale.*

examine in structured observations to determine whether intervention in these areas would be of use to the student.

Structured Observations. Adams (2002) suggested that, while natural conversational sampling is the most ecologically valid method, there may be some critical behaviors that simply fail to appear in natural interactions. We must not assume these behaviors are absent from the child's repertoire, simply because they don't appear in a short sample. Brinton and Fujiki

(1992) suggested using probes within the interaction to solve this problem. That is, instead of, or in addition to observing an unstructured peer-to-peer conversation with the client, the clinician can provide stimuli to examine critical aspects of conversational behavior within the interaction and evaluate the client's response to each probe. Table 13-7 presents the probes Brinton and Fujiki suggested. If using probes as a screening measure, students who are unable to respond to these probes appropriately can be given more intensive assessment, using a procedure like Larson and McKinley's (2003a) or Bishop et al.'s to examine a broad range of conversational skills.

Several authors have designed methods of structured observation that can be used to look at conversational pragmatics in the adolescent years. Simon's (1994) *Evaluating Communicative Competence* provides activities for looking at conversational skill in adolescents. Brown, Anderson, Shillock, and Yule (1984) supplied procedures for examining presuppositional abilities. Adams and Bishop (1990) also provided a framework for looking at conversational exchanges in adolescents. They used pictures of common situations, such as a doctor examining a sick child, a girl having a birthday party, and a couple with a broken-down car, and asked students to describe experiences *of their own* that were similar to those in the pictures.

Role-Playing. Role-playing is a third method that can be used to assess adolescent conversational skill. Nippold (1998) discussed the development of two specific skills that contribute to conversational competence in adolescence: interpersonal negotiation strategies and the use of special speech registers for a variety of specific interactional contexts. Both these skills can be examined by creating hypothetical situations for students to act out in role-playing activities.

Negotiation Strategies. The ability to use language effectively to persuade others, to present our point of view, and to resolve conflicts has a great effect on self-esteem, popularity, and successful adjustment in adolescence and adulthood. These skills develop considerably during the secondary school years (Nippold et al., 2005; Selman et al., 1986; Whitmire, 2000) and represent areas in which adolescents with LLD can be expected to have difficulty.

We can use role-playing and hypothetical situations to get a sense of a student's ability to use linguistic negotiation strategies. Selman, Beardslee, Schultz, Krupa, and Podorefsky (1986) and McDonald and Turkstra (1998) presented adolescents with hypothetical situations such as the following to determine the kinds of negotiation skills present in secondary school students:

 Dan and his girlfriend are out on a date together. Dan wants to start going out with other girls, but he doesn't think his girlfriend will like that. What should he say?

John works in a grocery store after school. He is only supposed to work for 10 hours a week, but his boss keeps asking him at the last minute to work really late on Friday nights. Even though his boss pays him for his extra time, John doesn't like to be asked to work at the last minute. What should he say?

Caitlin wants to go camping for the weekend with her friend Josie, but she knows her parents don't like Josie much. What should she say to them to convince them to let her and Josie go?

We can ask our clients to tell us, for each hypothetical situation, "What should he or she say?" We also can ask clients to describe the potential conflict, say why they chose the language they did, and talk about what feelings might come up in such a situation. In analyzing the student's response to situations like these, we can look at the degree to which the student can talk about feelings and long-term consequences of the protagonist's actions and determine whether the student attempted to find a solution that would preserve the two characters' relationship using compromise and mutual agreement. Less mature

TABLE 13-7	**Probes for Eliciting Conversational Behavior in Adolescents**		

CLINICIAN'S PROBE	EXAMPLE	TARGET ELICITED BEHAVIOR	EXAMPLE
Topic initiation	"By the way, I was at the beach over the weekend."	1. Responsiveness 2. Topic maintenance 3. Relevance	"I went skiing." "My girlfriend went, too." "I love weekends!"
Questions	"So how was the dance?"	1. Responsiveness 2. Topic maintenance 3. Relevance 4. Informativeness	"It was OK." "I danced with four or five girls." "I knew most of the dances." "They had a hiphop group."
Requests for repair	"What kind of group?"	1. Responsiveness 2. Adjustment to listener 3. Repair strategies	"A hiphop band." "You know, they play rap music." "Do you know what hiphop is?"
Sources of difficulty	"Can you get that marker for me?" (no marker present)	1. Assertiveness 2. Comprehension monitoring 3. Clarification requests	"There's no marker here." "Did you say *marker*?" "Do you mean a pen?"

Adapted from Brinton, B., & Fujiki, M. (1992). Setting the context for conversational language sampling. In W. Secord (Ed.). *Best practices in school speech-language pathology* (vol 2, pp. 9-19). San Antonio, TX: Psychological Corp, Harcourt Brace Jovanovich.

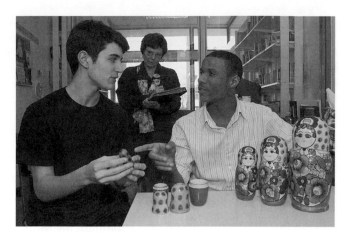

Conversational skill can be assessed in peer interactions.

responses would involve solutions that benefit only one of the characters, that show less awareness of the participants' feelings and desires, and that opt for short-term over long-term solutions.

Register Variation. We can set up role-playing situations similar to those used for children in the L4L stage (Figure 11-6) to look at the ways a student might change the form of speech to fine-tune to the interactive situation. Some examples of situations that can be presented to adolescents for role-playing appear in Figure 13-6. McDonald and Turkstra (1998) also suggested assessing the ability to produce hints. These are indirect requests that do not directly mention their object. For example, a hint for a taste of some fresh-baked cookies might sound like, "Umm, something smells good in here!" Adolescents can be asked to produce a very polite hint in response to hypothetical situations such as hinting to a friend's mother that the student needs a ride home (e.g., "My dad wants me home right after school today.")

Another important aspect of register variation for adolescents is the ability to use slang and in-group language (Rue, 2000; Whitmire, 2000). Cooper and Anderson-Inman (1988) emphasized the importance of the ability to use slang to help teens achieve group identity, to separate themselves from adults and younger children, and to foster peer solidarity. Adolescents with LLD often lack the linguistic facility and flexibility to master the constantly evolving lexicon and subtle pragmatic rules of the slang vernacular.

Assessment of use of slang vernacular can follow procedures used by Nelsen and Rosenbaum (1972). Students can be asked to list all the slang words they know that can be used to talk about a particular topic. Topics such as popular people, unpopular people, dates, sports, money, music, parties, cars, and clothes can be listed on a sheet of paper for the student, who can be asked to list as many slang terms as he or she can think of for each. The clinician also can ask several normally achieving students of the same grade and gender to fill out a similar form. The client's responses can be compared with those of the mainstream students. If the client produces very few slang terms in comparison to peers or produces terms that are different from those given by the typical peers, some difficulty in using in-group language can be inferred. A metapragmatic approach may be used to address this area in intervention (see Chapter 14).

Expressive activities

Have the student role-play producing each speech act in each context. Record the student's utterance and make a judgment as to whether it is appropriate for each context.

Speech act	Context	Student utterance	Appropriate?
Request use of car	1. Father 2. Friend who owns own car 3. Older sister who borrowed parents' car without permission		
Persuade	1. Supervisor to give time off so student can attend party 2. Friend to lend money 3. Teacher to accept late assignment		
Speculate	1. With a friend about what will happen on prom night 2. To teacher about the outcome of a science experiment 3. To parent about what grades will be this term		
Express opinion	1. To parent on appropriate curfew time 2. To teacher on current events topic 3. To friend on best musical group or sports team		

FIGURE 13-6 ✦ An example worksheet for use with role-playing activities to assess register variation skills in adolescents with LLD.

Discourse Genres

Some of the discourse genres we discussed for younger students continue to be a concern for adolescents. These include classroom discourse, which changes to include more formal lecture formats in secondary school; and narratives, whose structures become more complex and elaborated during the adolescent years. Some new discourse genres also come to the fore in secondary school. These include increasing demands for a variety of written forms of expression on the part of the student, as well as the need to process expository text structures in both receptive (e.g., textbooks and reference works) and expressive (essays, oral reports, research reports, laboratory reports) modalities. Let's look at how we can assess some of these discourse structures in adolescents with LLD.

Secondary-School Classroom Discourse. Classroom observation at the secondary level may be more complicated than it was for elementary school students, because adolescents participate in so many different classrooms in the course of a day. In addition, Nelson (1998) pointed out that adolescent students may be very easily embarrassed and would not respond well to a classroom visit by the SLP. Teachers can be asked to audiorecord a class in which the client is enrolled, so that the SLP can get a feel for the rules and expectations of the class and how the student with LLD responds to them. Alternatively, the SLP may interview teachers about the classroom performance of the client, with an eye toward gathering the kind of information that would help identify areas likely to present problems for the student. Box 13-3 presents a sample interview form that might be used to obtain information from teachers about a student's classroom performance.

Reed and Spicer (2003) reported on the communication skills high school teachers consider most important for students to

display. Those receiving the teachers' highest ratings included the following:

- ▶ Narrative skills
- ▶ Logical communication
- ▶ Ability to clarify messages
- ▶ Ability to take another's perspective
- ▶ Appropriate turn-taking

Knowing these teacher priorities can help SLPs focus on helping students improve their classroom performance in areas that teachers consider most important.

Students also can provide information about their own classroom performance. Talking with students about their performance in various classes and asking questions similar to those in Box 13-3 can point the clinician toward the teachers who will be most crucial to interview. We would, of course, want to talk to teachers in whose classes our clients are having difficulty. But it would also be a good idea to interview the teachers with whom the client feels things are going well, or toward whom the client feels especially positive. These interviews can help us assess the accuracy of the client's perceptions about academic work. They also can help us identify environments that are supportive for our students, so we can find ways of extending that support to other settings in which the student needs to function.

One aspect of classroom discourse performance that is especially crucial in the advanced language period is listening skill. Recall that the majority of students' time in secondary classrooms is spent listening. Moreover, the listening demands of the secondary classroom include more than literal comprehension of the verbal material presented. Secondary students need to engage in what Larson and McKinley (1995) called *critical listening*, that is, the ability to differentiate fact from opinion; to

| **BOX 13-3** | **A Sample Interview to Conduct with Teachers of Secondary Students with LLD** |

How is (client) doing academically in your class?

What are (client)'s strengths in your class?

How well-organized is (client)?

How does (client) do at following directions? Answering questions? Completing assignments? Understanding written material? Getting along with peers?

How would you rate (client)'s listening skills? Does he or she understand lectures and classroom conversation?

How would you rate (client)'s vocabulary?

What problems is (client) having in your class?

Are there particular routines in which (client) has trouble "getting with the program?"

Can you describe a recent classroom activity in which (client) took part that will give me an idea of the kinds of trouble he or she has?

What aspects of your curriculum present the greatest stumbling block for (client)?

What changes would you like to see in (client)'s performance in class?

What is your view of (client)'s realistic potential in this class this year?

Adapted from Work, R., Cline, J., Ehren, B., Keiser, D., & Wujek, C. (1993). Adolescent language programs. *Language, Speech, and Hearing Services in Schools, 24*, 43-53; and Nelson, N. (1998). *Childhood language disorders in context: Infancy through adolescence.* Columbus, OH: Merrill.

detect a speaker's intent to persuade the listener or "sell" an object or idea; and to identify false reasoning, bias, or propaganda.

Larson and McKinley (2003a) suggested a two-stage analysis of listening skills for secondary students. The first involves looking at informational or literal-level listening. To examine informational listening, they suggested using a taped lecture—either from one of the client's classes or perhaps a videotape of a lecture from a program on educational television. The student can be shown a 5- to 10-minute segment of the lecture, then asked to give the main idea and several relevant details. For additional dynamic assessment, Larson and McKinley suggested having the student listen to a second portion of the lecture, this time with a printed outline of the segment that lists major topics covered. If the student has difficulty with the unguided listening, but does better when the guide is available, consultation with the teacher can be used to encourage providing such an outline to help the client function in the class.

To assess the second aspect of listening skill, critical listening, Larson and McKinley advised having a student watch a videotape of a commercial or a segment of a political speech. The client is then asked to draw an inference about what the communicative goal, or hidden agenda, of the segment was (to persuade, sell, or encourage listeners to rethink an opinion, etc.). The student can be asked to judge whether the text contained factual material, opinion, or propaganda. The client also can be asked to judge how effectively the intended message was conveyed. Was it convincing? What additional information would be needed to evaluate the claims presented in the segment? Students who are unable to engage effectively in this kind of discussion would benefit from some intervention in critical-listening skill, even if their informational listening abilities are adequate.

Other Discourse Genres

Narrative Text. Rather than assessing story structure in general in secondary students, as we would for elementary students, we want to focus on aspects of narrative that cause the greatest difficulty and are likely to continue to show impairments in adolescents with LLD. A large body of research (summarized by Johnson, 1995; Scott, 1999; Westby, 2005) suggested that these areas include the use and understanding of story-grammar elements relating to characters' internal responses, plans, and motivations; the ability to draw inferences from narrative material and to summarize the story; and the provision of adequate cohesive marking within the text. Use of literate language forms in stories also would be a likely area in which deficits might persist and is one in which we might want to assess adolescents with LLD (Greenhalgh & Strong, 2001).

Normally developing children have acquired a basic story grammar by early school age (Richards & Singer, 2001), and even students with LLD produce narratives containing basic story grammar elements in the secondary school years (Roth & Spekman, 1989; Scott, 2005). However, Stephens (1988) showed that the internal responses of characters, including their intentions, goals, and plans for dealing with the problems central to the story's plot, are the last story grammar elements to emerge in normally developing children. Westby (2005) pointed out

that these elements are particularly difficult for students with LLD. In addition, we should be aware of an important change that takes place in narrative abilities in typical teenagers, as documented by McKeough and Genereux (2003). They found that at about 12 years of age, and increasingly throughout the teen years, students increase in two aspects of narrative ability: structural complexity and interpretive understanding. In terms of structure, they find adolescents increasingly able to embed complete episodes, such as flashbacks, within a narrative. In their use of interpretive understanding, they report a shift during adolescence from understanding behavior in terms of immediate feelings, thoughts, and plans to understanding characters' actions in terms of their personal history and experiences, and long-standing personality traits. As we work with adolescents on narrative tasks, we will want to help guide them toward these more mature perspectives.

We can use curriculum-based assessment to look at students' narrative skills. We can ask the student to choose a story that was read in English class and review the story with the student, having him tell about the main character, asking questions such as the following:

What was _____'s problem?

How did _____ plan to solve it?

What does _____ do to solve the problem?

Do any of the other characters know about the plan? If so, who, and how do they know? If not, why not?

What do other characters in the story think about what _____ is doing to solve the problem?

How does the plan work? Does _____ achieve the goal?

How does _____ feel at the end? Why?

What do other characters feel at the end? Do they feel differently than they did before they know _____'s plan? If so, why?

Asking the student to articulate the internal plans and responses of characters can give us an idea about whether these elements are perceived by the client. Having the client describe any deception the character plays on others in the story is especially helpful for looking at whether the student comprehends the distinction between action and intention that is so important in understanding plans and goals. If students are unable to give adequate accounts of these elements of internal response in stories they read in classroom literature, some work on them in the intervention program will be of use.

We've talked before about the importance of being able to use prior knowledge to "read between the lines" and infer information that is not stated explicitly in a text. Stephens (1988) reported that although normal elementary students are able to draw inferences from stories, inferential questions are more difficult for them than are questions about material that is directly stated. Similarly, Rinaldi (2000) and Roth and Spekman (1989) reported that although students with LLD do make some inferences in comprehending texts, they do not use inferencing as efficiently as a strategy to aid processing and memory as students with normal language development do, and they have more difficulty with drawing inferences from nonliteral language forms. These findings suggest that students with LLD are less adept than their peers with advanced language at going beyond what is on the page both to draw inferences and to organize information for the purpose of providing concise and accurate summaries.

We talked earlier about some ways to assess inferencing skill. To look specifically at inferencing in narrative texts, we've talked about reading students a part of a classroom literature selection, stopping at a crucial point, and asking students to guess what will happen next and tell why they think so. This kind of activity can tell us something about whether the student is able to use information in the text to make a plausible conjecture about where the story may be going. Inferential performance also can be elicited by reading a description of a character in a story and asking the student to infer something about the character from the description. For example, suppose clients are reading *Around the World in Eighty Days* (Verne, 1983) in English class. You might have the students read the following passage describing the main character, Phileas Fogg (pp. 11–12):

> Was Phileas Fogg rich? Undoubtedly. But those who knew him best could not imagine how he had made his fortune, and Mr. Fogg was the last person to whom to apply for the information. He was not lavish, nor, on the contrary, avaricious; for, whenever he knew that money was needed…he supplied it quietly and sometimes anonymously. He was, in short, the least communicative of men. He talked very little, and seemed all the more mysterious for his taciturn manner. His daily habits were quite open to observation; but whatever he did was so exactly the same thing that he had always done before, that the wits of the curious were fairly puzzled.

Students could then be asked to draw some inferences about Mr. Fogg by answering questions, such as the following:

> What would Mr. Fogg do if a street beggar asked him for money?
> What would Mr. Fogg say if you asked him what he did for a living?
> Would Mr. Fogg own a big mansion?
> If Mr. Fogg were alive today, would he go on a TV talk show to tell about his life?
> What did Mr. Fogg's neighbors think about him?
> Did Mr. Fogg like parties?

If students have trouble taking the information in the description and using it to make guesses about some of the character's hypothetical actions in questions like these, they may have problems in inferential comprehension. These problems can be addressed in the intervention program.

Summarizing is a skill that normal children develop during the advanced language period (Stephens, 1988). When we retell a story, we report all the events included in the original narrative, recounting each episode and including all the events and elements that make it up. Summarizing, on the other hand, requires integration and condensation of the material in the story. Johnson (1983) identified six abilities that go into summarizing a narrative:

1. Understanding the individual propositions and events of the story
2. Understanding the connections among the individual propositions of the story
3. Identifying the story grammar elements that organize the story
4. Remembering the sequence of events in the story
5. Selecting the most salient information to be included in the summary
6. Generating a concise and cohesive version of that information

Before we assess the ability to summarize, then, we need to be assured that the student can perform the earlier steps in this sequence. These steps, which comprise what we might call basic, informational, or propositional comprehension, can be assessed using standard reading comprehension instruments. Examples of such tests would include the passage comprehension section of the *Woodcock Reading Mastery Test—Revised* (Woodcock, 1998), the paragraph reading subtest of the *Test of Reading Comprehension—3rd Ed.* (Brown, Hammill, & Wiederholt, 1995), the *Stanford Diagnostic Reading Test—4th Ed.* (Karlsen & Gardner, 2004), or the *Gray Silent Reading Tests (Fourth Edition)* (Wiederholt & Blalock, 2000).

If students perform at primary levels on these measures, they are not ready to address higher-level skills such as summarization. Instead, they need to develop more basic skills in comprehending the literal content of written material. Work addressed at comprehension of both spoken and written information at the L4L level, using techniques like those suggested in Chapter 12, is appropriate for these students. If, on the other hand, clients perform at least at a fourth-grade level on these measures (most of our adolescents with LLD will not be reading on grade level), we can infer that the student has minimally adequate propositional comprehension skills. We can then assess their higher-level summarization skills by asking students to summarize short stories or book chapters they have read in English class or that we present them in the assessment session. It is important to be sure that the material we present them for summarizing is not at a reading level higher than the level they attained on the basic comprehension test. The adequacy of the summary can be judged by evaluating whether:

1. The summary presents an acceptable representation of the sequence of events in the story.
2. The information presented includes the most central elements of the story and excludes minor details.
3. The summary is concise and coherent, so that someone who had not read the text could get the gist of the story.

Students who demonstrate basic comprehension skills but who have trouble providing adequate summaries can be encouraged to develop this skill in an intervention program.

We talked in Chapter 11 about using a procedure based on Liles's (1985) work (Box 11-12) for assessing use of cohesion in narratives produced by elementary students. This procedure also is appropriate for students at advanced language levels. If you collected a narrative sample to look at syntactic production, as discussed earlier, this sample also can be examined for use of cohesive devices, using the scheme in Box 11-12. As we've also discussed, written samples are especially informative in the assessment of students with advanced language. If both a spoken and written narrative were collected for assessing syntactic production, the written narrative is an especially fertile source of information on use of cohesive markers. If a written narrative was not collected as part of the assessment of expressive syntax, it may be useful to collect one to look at these markers of cohesion. If deficits in use of cohesive markers are identified with the assessment suggested in Box 11-12, intervention can focus on improving use of cohesive markers in both spoken and written narratives.

In addition to the categories suggested in Box 11-12, several other types of cohesion identified by Halliday and Hasan (1976) can be examined in the written narratives of adolescents with LLD. These include the use of *lexical cohesion*, *reference*, and *substitution*. Definitions and examples of these markers appear in Box 13-4.

Students who demonstrate appropriate usage of these types of cohesive markers tend to be better writers than students who do not (Strong, 1985). Nelson and Friedman (1988) reported that there was a large decrease in errors of usage related to the first three categories of cohesion between fourth and seventh grades, although even college students made some errors on these markers. Nelson and Friedman found that the error rate for normally achieving secondary students was one or two errors per 100 words in written samples. If a written narrative sample of a secondary student contains more than three or four errors of cohesive markers per 100 words, some problems with the use of cohesion can be inferred. These problems also can be addressed in the intervention program.

In looking at other literary language markers, we can refer to the list of low-frequency, advanced syntactic forms in Table 13-6. If it hasn't already been done, we can analyze a client's written narrative sample for these forms, which are indicators of a literate language style. We also can look for evidence of a literate lexicon. This would include looking for the presence of metalinguistic and metacognitive verbs, as Nippold (1998) suggested. In addition, we can look for the use of adverbs and conjunctions as evidence of a literate language style, as Westby (2005) proposed (Box 11-13).

One additional factor that pertains to both cohesion and a literate language style can be inspected in adolescents' written narrative samples. This is the use of connectives. Connectives are another class of cohesive markers identified by Halliday and Hasan (1976) as a significant means of linking propositions within texts. They also are an important component of the development of literacy and the ability to encode and interpret the connections between propositions in literate discourse (Nippold & Undlin, 1992), and they are considered additional forms of high-level syntax (Scott & Stokes, 1995; see Table 13-6).

BOX 13-4	Some Categories of Cohesive Markers for Assessment at the Advanced Language Stage

Lexical Cohesion

The use of several words at different points in the text to link ideas to the same concept. These would include the use of comparative and superlative markers:

"They were very proud of their team. Still, ours was *better*."

"He eats the most junk food in our family. I eat *the least*."

It also includes the use of more general comparatives such as *same, similar, other, different, else,* and *likewise*:

"Matt thought the student council was too conservative. Mandy held a *similar* opinion."

"There were several dishes on the table. Jesse tried the caviar, and I tried the *others*."

"Jamie's painting won first prize in the contest. I never dreamed he had *such* talent."

Reference

The use of pronouns as well as the use of pro-verbs:

"The plates beneath the earth move. When they *do*, an earthquake can occur."

Substitution

The use of a synonym for a co-referent:

"A goat had attacked our flower bed. When we saw it, we were amazed at the damage the *animal* had done."

Adapted from Halliday, M., & Hasan, R. (1976). *Cohesion in English*. London: Longman.

Connectives include both *conjunctions*, which link propositions within a sentence, and *conjuncts*, which link ideas across sentences. Quirk, Greenbaum, Leech, and Svartvik (1985) provided information on the connectives used in English. A list of these forms appears in Box 13-5. Nippold et al. (2005) found that use of adverbial conjuncts doubled (from .3% to .7%) between the ages of 11 and 17 in students' persuasive writing. We can examine the written narrative samples of adolescent clients for the presence of these connectives as a measure of literate language growth. If samples contain examples of several connectives (Scott's [1988] data suggested a minimum of five different connectives would be expected in a writing sample of 30 to 50 T-units in length), we can assume minimally adequate use of these markers. If connective use is very sparse in the sample, we would probably want to attempt to elicit use of connectives, using a sentence generation procedure ("Make up a sentence with *although* [or *but* or *if* or *unless*] in it"). Alternatively, we might write several conjunctions on cards and provide students with pairs of written sentences to combine by choosing one of the cards and coming up with a complex sentence that uses the conjunction to link the propositions. For example, the student might be given the propositions: "Jeff wanted to ask Megan to the dance" and "Megan had gone to the junior prom with Willie" and the conjunctions *and*, *if*, *when*, *although*, and *until*.

Nippold and Undlin (1992) provided an additional method for testing use of advanced connectives. They gave secondary students a sentence followed by a connective and had students complete the second sentence so that the whole passage made sense. Here's an item from their task (p. 35):

Michael has become an excellent distance runner for the cross-country team. Similarly, _____.

Analogous passages can be constructed to assess other connectives of interest. If students perform adequately on probes like these, further work on connectives may not be necessary. If the students seem unable to use the connectives appropriately, though, we may want to probe their comprehension of these forms. This can be done using a judgment task. Students can be read a list of sentences like those in Box 13-6 and asked to judge whether each "makes sense."

Students who have difficulty with comprehension and production of these advanced connectives can benefit from an intervention program that provides additional exposure to the forms, in literature-based script activities and metalinguistic talk about forms encountered in curriculum-based comprehension and comprehension monitoring work. If comprehension appears adequate and only production is sparse, intervention might focus on activities that encourage sentence combining (see Chapter 14).

At this point you may want to look at Charlie's written sample in Figure 13-3 again and try some of the analyses we've been discussing. My version appears in Appendix 13-3.

Expository Texts. We talked earlier about the role of expository texts in the secondary school curriculum. Much of the curricular material that adolescents encounter, either as orally presented lectures or in written texts, takes an expository form. Conte, Menyuk, and Bashir (1992) showed that adolescents with LLD comprehend expository texts significantly less well than their normally achieving peers, although Scott and Windsor (2000) demonstrated that they are difficult for typically developing students as well.

Nelson (1998) suggested that the best assessment of comprehension of expository texts is the use of curriculum-based activities. We will probably want to look at a student's comprehension of expository texts in a variety of settings. We've talked already about assessing informational comprehension in class lectures. We also might want to look at comprehension of written expository material using a classroom textbook. Sudweeks et al. (2004) recommend that asking students to summarize an expository passage as an assessment technique with empirical support. We can have the student read a passage, summarize it, and answer questions posed by the clinician. Alternatively, we can have students complete assignments regarding the passage, such as answering questions in the review section of the book or demonstrating comprehension by drawing a map or diagram.

Carlisle (1991) advocated comparing students' comprehension of expository texts they read themselves with the same texts read to them. If listening comprehension exceeds comprehension of the same material when read independently, we can consult with teachers to provide taped versions of reading assignments and work with the reading specialist to improve reading comprehension. If comprehension of oral exposition is no better than that of written material, though, we will need to concentrate on improving the student's overall ability to process this kind of text, starting with oral formats and integrating written texts as we go along.

If students have trouble with independent processing of any kind of expository material, we can use some dynamic assessment, providing scaffolding and support to see whether this aid is sufficient to allow them to complete tasks with expository texts. We saw one example of this kind of support for the lecture format: providing an outline to guide comprehension. A similar procedure could be used for written material: providing students with an outline of the written text, listing main headings with lines under each for the students to fill in relevant details. After reading and outlining the passage this way, students can be asked to summarize the passage, recall details, and answer informational questions. If these kinds of scaffolding improve comprehension of the text, then working on getting students to provide themselves with such support using a learning-strategies approach (see Chapter 14) will probably be helpful. Some consultative intervention to encourage teachers to provide such support in their classroom materials also would be beneficial. If dynamic assessment does not demonstrate much improvement of expository text comprehension with scaffolding and support, we may want to work more directly on exposi-

BOX 13-5	**A Sampling of the Connectives in English**

Coordinating Conjunctions

and [then]
or
but
both
neither
either
nor

Subordinating Conjunctions

for
so
that
which(ever)
because
while
if
after
before
who(m)(ever), what(ever), when(ever), where(ever), why, how
though, although
whether
as
since, once
except
until
unless
whereas, whereupon

Conjuncts

Concordant
similarly
moreover
consequently
therefore
furthermore
for example
Discordant
instead
yet
however
contrastively
nevertheless
rather
conversely

Quasicoordinators

as well as
as much as
rather than
more than

Adapted from Quirk, R., Greenbaum, S., Leech, G., & Svartvik, J. (1985). *A comprehensive grammar of the English language*. London: Longman; Nippold, M., & Undlin, R. (1992). Use and understanding of adverbial conjuncts: A developmental study of adolescents and young adults. *Journal of Speech and Hearing Research, 35,* 18-118; and Nippold, M. (1998). *Later language development.* Austin, TX: Pro-Ed.

tory text structure in the intervention program. We'll discuss some approaches to this procedure in the next chapter.

Scott and Windsor (2000) reported that students with LLD produce less mature expository structures, in terms of both form and content, than typically achieving peers. In terms of assessing the production of expository text, Espin et al. (2005) provide guidelines. They propose analyzing students' expository writing for the following elements:

▶ *Premise*: a statement of the writer's position on the topic; stated in an introductory section
▶ *Reason*: an explanation to support or refute the premise
▶ *Elaboration*: an extension or examples of a premise, reason, or conclusion
▶ *Conclusion*: a closing statement

Again, we can look at the student's expository assignments from class work as a way of analyzing these elements. Weak or absent elements can be addressed in an intervention program. Because so many typical students have trouble with expository writing, this is an excellent area for collaborative teaching.

Persuasive and Argumentative Texts. Nippold (1998) and Scott and Erwin (1992) identified persuasion or argumentation as a new discourse genre that confronts secondary students. They suggested that competence with this genre develops even later than exposition, and as such, it may not enter the student's repertoire until late in the adolescent period. We looked at some ways to assess the comprehension of these kinds of texts when we talked about critical listening. Assessment of production of persuasive texts can be examined in oral modes using the role-playing procedures we talked about earlier. We'll look, too, at production of written argumentative texts in the next section as one aspect of the assessment of written communication.

Written Communication. One of the major new demands of the secondary school years is the increasing requirement to produce longer, more elaborated forms of written expression in a variety of discourse genres (Nelson, 1988), and writing has become an especially important area for intervention since the requirement of the No Child Left Behind (NCLB) legislation that requires students in special education to participate in district- and state-wide assessments which invariably include writing (Schumaker & Deschler, 2003). Barry and William (2004) point out that students with learning disabilities are required to pass the same competency exams as students enrolled in general education in order to graduate to new grade levels and to earn a high school diploma. Like most aspects of development, writing acquisition proceeds through a series of phases (Scott, 2005; Silliman, Jimerson, & Wilkinson, 2000). And, as we all would expect, students with LLD show slow progress through these phases and have significant difficulties. Mackie and Dockrell (2004) and Scott (2005) reported that students with LLD produce written texts that are shorter, contain more errors, are rated lower in overall quality, show less sensitivity to audience and genre, and contain less information than writing of typically achieving peers. But writing is difficult for everyone. Normal adolescents take years to master basic skills in effective

---

| **BOX 13-6** | **Sample Sentences for a Judgment Task to Assess Adolescents' Comprehension of Advanced Connectives** |

Instructions: Listen to each sentence and tell me whether it makes sense *(OK)* or is silly *(S)*.

I like heavy metal, so I'll use my birthday money to buy some new discs. *(OK)*

I failed my exam because I gave all the right answers. *(S)*

Our team will have a chance at the state championship if we can get into the play-offs. *(OK)*

After you feel full, you always eat a big sub sandwich. *(S)*

Before you ask someone for a date, ask your folks for the car. *(OK)*

I'll graduate when I pass all my courses. *(OK)*

I'd like to go to the movies, although there's a movie I really want to see. *(S)*

Since you work after school, come home as soon as school lets out. *(S)*

Don't go to the basketball game until you've finished your homework. *(OK)*

I'll get a Super Video system for Christmas unless I get an A in English. *(S)*

I was looking forward to my date with Sam. However, I was worried about his car. *(OK)*

Brian has a history test tomorrow. Nevertheless, he studied hard. *(S)*

Min needs to take his medication at noon every day. Therefore, he never brings his pills to school. *(S)*

Carmen doesn't like to practice the piano. Instead, she works on the instrument at least an hour a day. *(S)*

---

written communication, and adolescents with LLD have even more difficulty (Englert & Raphael, 1988; Schumaker & Deshler, 2003). There are some norm-referenced measures that assess writing ability. These include the *Picture Story Language Test* (Myklebust, 1965), the *Writing Process Test* (Warden & Hutchinson, 1992), and the *Test of Written Language—3* (Hammill & Larsen, 1996). Other standardized batteries for adolescents have written language sections. The *Test of Adolescent and Adult Language—3* (Hammill et al., 1994) and the *Woodcock-Johnson Psycho-educational Battery—Revised* (Woodcock & Johnson, 1990) are two examples. Like all standardized measures, these tests tell us whether an adolescent is different from other students in terms of written language abilities. To establish baseline function and identify intervention targets, we are likely to need to do some criterion-referenced assessment for students who demonstrate written language deficits on standardized instruments.

Scott and Erwin (1992) and Scott (2005) identified a variety of types of writing required of adolescents in school. These include personal experience narratives ("describe the best experience you ever had"), story retelling (book reports), factual retelling ("summarize the passage on the exploration of Antarctica"), fictional stories or guided stories ("write your own myth to explain how we came to have four seasons, as the myth of Ceres does"), expositions on how to do something ("explain how to build a log cabin"), descriptions ("write a description of Massachusetts' main industries"), reporting ("write a report of a sports event you watched"), persuasive pieces ("write an editorial about why students should be allowed to eat lunch at local restaurants instead of the cafeteria"), business letters ("write a letter of application for a job"), and friendly letters ("write a letter to a friend asking him or her to visit during the summer"). When we assess writing in our

students, we want to sample the kinds of writing required by the curriculum. We also want to find out to what extent students have access to, and know how to use, word processors for written assignments. This information will help us to determine whether to emphasize word processing or hand-written work in the intervention program. To the extent that word-processing equipment is available for student writing, it is to our advantage to make use of it, since students who learn this technology in school have an advantage in the transition to employment settings. If word-processing equipment is available, we may want to counsel students to take a keyboarding course to improve typing skills. It is important to be aware, though, that research (Scott, 1999) has shown that computer-produced writing of students with LLD contains more errors than hand-written products, but does not differ in terms of length, structure, or amount of revision. While using a computer may make writing less laborious, it does not automatically improve its quality. In addition, students may need to take high-stakes testing, such as state-wide assessments and SATs by hand. Unless a student's disability qualifies him/her for access to a word processor during such testing, we need to help students practice writing legibly by hand, as well.

Stages of Writing. Jencks (2003) suggested that there are five stages involved in writing. The first two are often referred to as the *writing process* or *planning*. The others can be considered the writing product. These appear in Table 13-8. A major difference between the written work of adolescents with LLD and that of their peers is that good writers spend much more time in the planning and revision processes than do poor writers (Espin et al., 2004). This suggests that assessing these processes may be just as important as evaluating the written product itself for understanding what a student needs to improve written communication.

TABLE 13-8	**Writing Process**	

WRITING PHASES	WRITING STAGES	ELEMENTS IN EACH STAGE
Process	Prewriting	Classroom discussion
		Graphic organizers
		Brainstorming
	Drafting	Free writing
		Concept mapping
		Outlining
Product	Revising	Peer responses
		Teacher conference
	Editing	Sentence combining
		Spelling, punctuation checking
		Peer review
	Publication	Word processing
		Author's theater
		Binding and illustrating

Adapted from Jencks, C. (2003). *Process writing checklist*. ERIC Document No. ED479389.

Assessing the Writing Process. We can assess the planning aspect of writing by asking students to produce a written sample under our observation. When we choose the kind of sample we ask the student to write, again, curricular considerations should be paramount. Box 13-7 provides some questions suggested by Scott and Erwin (1992) for learning about the writing demands of a student's curriculum. We can use the answers to questions like these to guide our choice of a writing assignment to use for process assessment.

Scott and Erwin (1992) discussed using a "Think-aloud Protocol," in which we ask students to verbalize all thoughts about writing as they write. The main goals of this procedure are to find out the following:

▶ Whether the student identifies the goal or purpose of the writing. This decision often includes the choice of the discourse genre to be used in the composition. In many cases, for students, the goal and genre are set by the demands of the assignment. Students may be asked to write an autobiography (narrative), a research or book report (exposition), or an advertisement or editorial (persuasive). When we set the goal by giving the student an assignment, we want to observe whether the student uses the goal as a guide to the writing, chooses the correct genre to fit the goal, and uses self-reminders of the goal throughout the process.

▶ Whether the student takes the audience into account. For students, the audience is often the teacher. We would like to see whether the student takes the teacher's presumed state of knowledge into account by giving the teacher all the necessary background information. On the other hand, often the teacher already possesses much of the information the student is being asked to convey, particularly in expository assignments. In this case, we want to observe whether the student understands the obligation to demonstrate knowledge to the teacher, even though the teacher may already have that knowledge.

▶ Whether the student uses the planning process to revise and refine thinking. This is perhaps the most critical aspect of planning in writing and the reason that many authors claim that they don't know what they think until they write it. *The Writing Process Test* (Warden & Hutchinson, 1992) also can be used in this phase of the assessment.

If students show very poor or limited planning abilities, providing some dynamic assessment through modeling alternative think-aloud procedures, suggesting the use of graphic organizers and outlines, and encouraging students to focus on planning as well as producing written communication can help to determine which elements of writing can best be addressed in the intervention program.

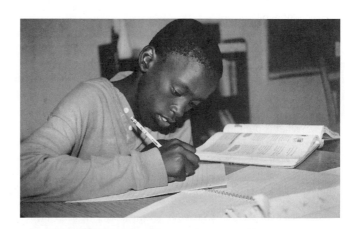

Written language assessment involves both the process and product of writing.

Assessing Written Products. Espin et al. (2004) discussed the various forms of assessing student writing that are in common use. Often, these assessments involve presenting students with a writing "prompt." Example writing prompts appear in Table 13-9. Alternatively, students may be presented with a story starter in the form of a picture or sentence. The four primary methods of assessing writing samples such as these include the following:

▶ *Holistic*: The rater provides a numerical score, based on an overall impression of the writing. The score is norm-referenced in that the rater has in mind what typical writing for a given grade level should look like. This method is most useful for placing writing within a category or level, rather than for evaluation of the writer's instructional needs.

▶ *Primary trait*: The rater measures the sample against predetermined criteria, often in the form of a rubric that provides numerical ratings on a 4-5 point scale, with anchors such as unsatisfactory, minimal, satisfactory, elaborated, superior. This is a criterion-referenced form of assessment, in that it measures the student's writing against a standard rather than against the work of peers.

▶ *Analytic*: Several specific aspects of the writing are each evaluated separately, using a standard evaluation tool. For example, syntax might be rated by using a DSS score, vocabulary might be rated using TTR. This method is usually used with writing elicited through a prompt.

▶ *Curriculum-based measurement* (CBM): A short (3- to 5-minute) timed sample of writing is elicited in response to a curriculum-based topic or story starter. The writing is analyzed according to criteria drawn from the curriculum goals in terms of both form (vocabulary, sentence structure, spelling) and content. Alternatively, writing artifacts collected in a student's portfolio can be analyzed.

Because secondary students are required to produce several varieties of written products, we may want to look at more than one writing sample in doing this assessment. For this purpose, artifact analysis is especially useful. We can ask the student to bring writing samples from several class assignments for us to analyze. We can use the questions in Box 13-7 to guide us as to which kinds of assignments are most important to assess. We would probably want to focus on three or four types of writing that are required most often and that the student perceives as most troublesome.

Scott and Erwin (1992) suggested a hierarchy of approaches to writing assessment that makes use of all Espin et al.'s (2004) methods. The clinician may choose to assess all of these at an initial evaluation; later we may want to track just one or two aspects of writing to assess progress in intervention.

The first element in this hierarchy is *fluency*. Fluency refers to the ability to provide products that are sufficiently long and elaborated for the topic and audience. Malecki and Jewell (2003) report that three analytic measures of fluency are typically used to assess timed writing samples. These are as follows:

▶ The number of words written.
▶ The number of words spelled correctly.
▶ The number of correct word sequences; that is, each pair of adjacent words is examined, and the rater decides if the pair is correct grammatically and in terms of spelling, punctuation, and meaning.

| **BOX 13-7** | **Questions to Determine Writing Demands of Curriculum** |

1. Did you write anything in school this month that was more than a paragraph long? What was the assignment?
2. Do you have homework for chapters in your textbooks that require writing a paragraph or more? What is the wording on these assignments?
3. Do you have essay questions on exams? Can you give me an example of one? How long is your answer? Half a page? A whole page? More?
4. Do you have to write book reports? Research reports? Biographies? Autobiographies? Journals? Lab reports? If so, how are they done? In school or at home? How long are they? Do you write them alone or with other students? Do you have to write more than one draft?
5. Where does the information for your writing come from? Is it all in your textbooks, or do you have to do additional research?
6. What does your teacher think about your writing?
7. What is the longest thing you ever wrote?
8. Do you do any writing on a computer? What kind of writing?
9. Do you take notes in class? Is there anything to copy from the board, or do you write down what you hear?
10. Do you plan before you write? Do you go back over your writing and make changes when you are through?
11. What kinds or writing are easiest for you? What kinds are hardest?

Adapted from Scott, C., & Erwin, D. (1992). Descriptive assessment of writing: Process and products. In W. Secord (Ed.), *Best practices in school speech-language pathology* (vol. II) (pp. 60-73). Austin, TX: Psychological Corp: Harcourt Brace Jovanovich.

| **TABLE 13-9** | **Example Writing Prompts for Secondary Students** |

GENRE	SAMPLE PROMPT
Narrative	Everyone has a frightening experience once in a while. Think about a time when you were very worried or afraid. Write a story about this time. Tell what happened in the order it occurred and tell how it turned out.
Expository	There are many exciting places to visit in the USA. Think about a place you would like to visit. Write about what makes this place special or interesting to you and why you would want to visit there.
Persuasive	Some schools allow teachers or principals to censor the school newspaper and decide if certain articles will be published or not. Write a letter to your principal explaining why you think school newspapers should or should not be censored by teachers.

The first two measures have been shown to be most important for writing at the elementary school level (Malecki & Jewell, 2003). However, many of our students with LLD will be writing below grade level, and these measures give us a way to easily document change over time in students' writing. As such, they can be helpful pre-/post-intervention measures of fluency for secondary students with LLD.

A second aspect of student writing is *lexical maturity*. This can be assessed using a primary trait analysis. A simple method was suggested by Isaacson (1988). We can count the number of words with more than seven letters in a composition. This value has been shown to have a high correlation with scores on achievement tests. Alternatively, we can use the same criteria we talked about earlier in our discussion of the literate lexicon to examine the vocabulary used in the student's writing samples. We could look for the presence of words associated with technical and curriculum topics, metalinguistic and metacognitive verbs, and the use of adverbs and connectives. Scott and Erwin (1992) and Westby and Clauser (2005) suggested further that we look at the use of low-frequency words that add precision and color to the writing. If students produce very few such words in their writing, work on exposing them to such words in literature- and curriculum-based activities and practice in producing written passages with such words may form part of the intervention program.

The third aspect of writing product assessment is to use an analytic approach to examining *sentential syntax*. Here we can use the same procedures we used earlier to look at syntax in the narrative samples we collected to analyze students' oral grammatical production. In examining T-unit length, subordination index, and use of higher level, low-frequency syntactic structures, we want to assess whether the student is using sentences that include the syntactic characteristics of a literate language style. If these forms are lacking in the student's writing, we will want to use literature- and curriculum-based activities to provide intensive exposure to these forms. Practice producing written passages modeled after the ones with complex syntax in the literature-based activities also can be part of the intervention program. An alternative method is to use a measure of the percentage of correct word sequences (CWS), derived from the fluency measure we discussed earlier. The %CWS measure is computed by dividing the number of CWS from

the fluency measure by the total number of possible two-word sequences in the writing sample. Several researchers (Espin et al., 2005; Malecki & Jewell, 2003) have shown this measure to be a valid index of writing accuracy. Moreover, Malecki and Jewell found that it takes less than 2 minutes to compute a %CWS on a writing sample taken from a 3-minute probe. As such the %CWS provides an efficient way to measure change in writing maturity over time.

At our initial evaluation, we may also want to look at students' writing for specific *grammatical and mechanical errors*. Remember that Scott and Windsor (2000) showed that the number of grammatical errors in writing is one of the best ways to distinguish the writing samples of students with LLD from typical peers. In doing grammatical error analysis, we are looking for misuse of tense; poor subject-verb agreement; failure to mark plurals, possessives, and other inflections; and use of nonstandard forms such as *ain't* and *I seen*. If these errors reflect dialect usage, we want to deal with them as "second-dialect" issues, as we discussed in Chapter 5. They may be appropriate speech forms within the home community but are not acceptable in the context of formal writing. Some grammatical errors, however, may be merely "slips of the pen," the result of inattention to details as the student focuses on the composition process. We know (Scott, 1999) that students with LLD make more of these errors than their typically achieving peers. For errors of this type, the function of the editing process must be emphasized in the intervention program. We want to convey the idea that writing is not finished with a first draft and that editing for grammatical and mechanical errors must *always* be part of the writing process.

Mechanical errors include poor legibility and errors in spelling, punctuation, capitalization, and paragraph segmentation. When legibility is very poor, it may be wise to use word-processing equipment instead of insisting students write by hand. This suggestion could be part of the consultation program, when the SLP talks with teachers about curricular modifications for the student with LLD. Other mechanical errors may be "slips of the pen" or they may be the result of incomplete understanding of the rules of writing mechanics. We can determine this by asking students to edit their work and determining whether the student can detect and correct mechanical errors. If not, we should include some work on spelling, punctuation, capitalization, and paragraphing as part of the intervention program, or consult with the LD specialist about including them.

An additional method of writing assessment includes the *holistic* rating (Espin et al., 2004). Here we rate the overall quality and effectiveness of the writing, taking into account its content, organization and macrostructure, cohesion, the transition from thought to thought, and the degree to which the writing accomplishes the intended purpose and provides for the audience's informational needs. Espin et al. (2005) and Jencks (2003) discussed the ways in which holistic assessment can be accomplished. Table 13-10 presents a holistic scoring system adapted from Espin et al. (2005), Malecki and Jewell (2003),

---

TABLE 13-10	**A Sample of Holistic Evaluation Criteria for Assessing Students' Written Products**

SCORE	DESCRIPTION
1. Below basic, inadequate	A below-average paper may present some content; contains errors such as the following: • Omits information or makes only cursory reference to required information, gives insufficient detail or provides irrelevant information; ambiguous or incomplete cohesive marking, meaning is unclear. • Lacks adequate organization. • Contains significant omissions, digressions; may be a disconnected list. • Uses inappropriate tone. • Shows poor control of conventions of standard English; lacks variety in language choice.
2. Basic, but minimal	A low-average paper. It shows most of the following: • Contains sparse number of ideas or propositions, omits important information; some cohesion errors. • Shows some organizational pattern, but has little elaboration. • Rambles; may contain irrelevant details. • Shows limited variety in word and sentence choice. • Shows limited use of conventions of standard English. • Inappropriate tone for purpose and audience.
3. Proficient	An average paper. It may exhibit some of the following: • May imply but not specify certain key information, may lack certain necessary details. • Shows some organization and use of appropriate cohesion, but may be disjointed in moving from one thought to another. Some segments may be out of sequence, omitted, or marked by digressions. • Shows some range of vocabulary and sentence types. • Shows a few errors of standard English usage. • May lack appropriate tone for purpose and audience.
4. Elaborated	A good paper, above average, but not top. • May be less rich in language and detail than a top paper and not so well organized or appropriate, but it is basically well written. • Shows reasoning, clear and useful examples, adequate sentence variety, and general facility with the conventions of standard English.
5. Advanced, superior	A top paper, but not necessarily perfect. It does most of the following: • Includes adequate number of ideas, or propositions; provides sufficient information with adequate details. • Has clear cohesion and organization and moves logically from one paragraph to the next; a clear structure is followed; reader gets a sense of "wholeness"; parts of the composition are related to overall theme or topic. • Shows insightful reasoning, clear and useful examples. • Shows good sentence variety, and general facility with the conventions of standard English. • Uses a consistent and objective tone appropriate to the purpose and audience.

Adapted from Espin, C., Weissenburger, J., & Benson, B. (2004). Assessing the writing performance of students in special education. *Exceptionality, 12,* 55-67; Malecki, C., & Jewell, J. (2003). Developmental, gender, and practical considerations in scoring curriculum-based measurement writing probes. *Psychology in the Schools, 40,* 379-391; Dagenais, D., & Beadle, K. (1984). Written language: When and where to begin. *Topics in Language Disorders, 4,* 59-85; Isaacson, S. (1988). Assessing the writing product: Qualitative and quantitative measures. *Exceptional Children, 54,* 528-534; and Wiig, E. (1995). Assessment of adolescent language. *Seminars in Speech and Language, 16,* 14-31.

Dagenais and Beadle (1984), and Wiig (1995) that can be used to guide the formation of this global judgment.

Westby and Clauser (2005) suggested, in addition, using rubrics, or sets of rules or benchmarks to differentiate among levels of writing performance, and to provide direction for intervention. They provide example rubrics for evaluating various genres of written language, which appear in Appendices 13-4 through 13-7. Figure 13-7 provides a general writing assessment rubric adapted from Popp, Ryan, Thompson, and Behrens (2003). The clinician assigns a level from 0-6 to each element of writing identified, and writes a brief note in the corresponding cell of the form. For example, a clinician might score "ideas" with a mark of 3, and write in the '3' row under ideas "shows some insight."

In addition to assessing writing skills at the beginning of an intervention program, we want to assess changes in writing through the course of the treatment, to decide when objectives have been achieved. Hewitt (2001) advocated using *portfolio assessment* for this purpose. Portfolio assessment involves systematically collecting samples of the student's writing throughout the course of the intervention program and using these samples to evaluate progress. Students are involved in the choice of material to be included in the portfolio and are encouraged to use self-evaluation as well as the teacher's or clinician's judgment to assess their progress. Mitchell, Abernathy, and Gowans (1998) emphasized the importance of clearly defining the focus of the portfolio, so that students know what is being assessed. If the focus is to show progress over a term, students should select materials from beginning, middle, and final periods of time. If it is to showcase the student's "best work," then the student should be clear on the guidelines to use in selection.

Griffith, Dastoli, and Rogers-Adkinson (1994) argued that using student self-evaluation in the context of portfolio assessment helps students reflect on their strengths and weaknesses, set personal goals, appreciate their own progress, and take more ownership of their work. Figure 13-8 provides a form for summarizing the range of writing assessment we have been discussing. A summary form like this can be used with portfolio assessment, and both the clinician and student can evaluate each element in the portfolio. Students can compare their self-assessment with the clinician's and talk about how much progress their writing has shown and what still needs to be improved.

Figure 13-9 presents a writing sample of Crystal's, our client from the beginning of the chapter. You might like to try completing Figure 13-8 with an analysis of her writing. My assessment appears in Appendix 13-8.

ASSESSING THE "METAS"

We've talked a lot about the importance of metalinguistic and metacognitive skills for success in school, and in secondary school this need is even more pronounced. We've already looked at some ways to assess certain advanced language skills at a "meta" level, such as the ability to define words and to edit writing. Let's look at four additional areas we may want to assess in adolescents with LLD to get a picture of "meta" skills: metalinguistic skill, metapragmatic ability, comprehension monitoring, and metacognition.

Metalinguistics

Asking students to edit their own or others' writing samples is, of course, an excellent metalinguistic assessment task, one that

	Ideas	Organization	Voice	Word choice	Sentence fluency	Conventions
0: Unscorable; inadequate						
1: Marginally acceptable; needs improvement						
2: Shows emerging skills						
3: Average for grade level, shows adequate performance						
4: Shows proficiency; basic skills mastered						
5: Above average for grade, well-constructed, shows some insight						
6: Superior, shows insight, logic, varied forms						

FIGURE 13-7 ✦ Example Rubric.
(Adapted from Popp, S., Ryan, J., Thompson, M., & Behrens, J. (2003). *Operationalizing the rubric: The effect of benchmark selection on the assessed quality of writing.* ERIC Document # 481661.)

Student _____ Grade _____

Written assignment _____

	Sample 1	Sample 2	Sample 3
Date of sample:			
Teacher/clinician grade*:			
Student self-assessment grade:			
Number of samples:			
Handwriting:			
Spelling:			
Punctuation:			
Capitalization:			
Paragraphing:			
Grammar:			
Use of literate vocabulary:			
Length of sample (total words):			
Number of different words (NDW):			
Average T-unit length:			
Subordination index:			
Use of low-frequency syntactic forms:			
Number or percent correctly spelled words:			
Number or percent CWS:			
Organization:			
Provides sufficient information:			
Use of appropriate detail:			
Cohesion:			
Tone:			
Holistic evaluation score (1-6) (Table 13-10):			
Rubric scores (1-6) (Fig. 13-7):			

*A = Grade level work;   B = below grade level, but no intervention required;
C = deficits warrant remediation.

FIGURE 13-8 ✦ Worksheet for summarizing information from written language evaluations.
(Adapted from Dagenais, D., & Beadle, K. [1984]. Written language: When and where to begin. *Topics in Language Disorders, 4,* 59-85.)

can provide information on students' ability to focus on the form rather than the content of written language. If we find students having difficulty with editing, we may want to use dynamic assessment to explore further. For example, if we learn that students are unable to detect errors in writing without any scaffolding, we might provide them with a writing sample in which errors have been highlighted but not corrected. We can then see whether guiding the students' selective attention to the error allows them to make appropriate corrections. If so, we might consult with teachers and ask them to return the student's papers with errors highlighted but not corrected so the student can practice making the corrections. Eventually, focus can shift to error detection.

Paraphrasing is another important metalinguistic skill for secondary students. It is needed to write information gathered from library research as they prepare papers and to summarize information from classroom texts. We can assess paraphrasing

ability by asking students to read sentences at their reading level or listen to sentences and restate them. Material for paraphrasing can be drawn from classroom texts or literature materials. Complex sentences, such as "When the pioneers traveled west, they often encountered hardships," will probably be the best sources of paraphrasing activity. Ambiguous sentences, such as those used in proverbs and humor, also are excellent sources. Here the student can be asked to paraphrase a sentence such as "Visiting relatives can be boring." We can then ask, "Can it mean anything else?" If students are unable to detect ambiguity in sentences, some work with ambiguous sentences may be included in the intervention program.

Metapragmatics

We can probe metapragmatic skills by asking students to describe the rules of various interactive situations. Nelson (1998) suggested that, for example, we ask students to describe how the rules for taking a conversational turn politely differ from the rules for taking a turn in an argument. Walker, Schwarz, Nippold, Irvin, and Noell (1994) suggested using video technology to assess pragmatic skills. Students can be shown a videorecorded scenario (such as a student attempting to enter a conversation with other teens; or a student responding to teasing or provocation), then asked to select an appropriate ending from several displayed on the screen or simply to predict an appropriate ending. Since classroom pragmatics are so important for school success, we may wish to focus on student's awareness of the rules for interaction in the classroom. Creaghead (1992) posed a set of specific questions that we can ask students to assess their awareness of the rules of the classrooms of individual teachers. These appear in Box 13-8. In addition, we may want to interview certain teachers to ask them whether the student is aware of classroom rules. We might rephrase each of the questions in Box 13-8. We might ask for example, "Does (client) know when to be quiet?"

Comprehension Monitoring

We talked in Chapter 11 about assessing comprehension monitoring in the L4L period. Barrier games can be used to assess comprehension monitoring in the advanced language stage as they were in the elementary grades. Lloyd (1994) reported that students in secondary grades should be able not only to detect missing information in these games, but to be able to identify what is missing and ask an appropriate, specific question to resolve the problem. Secondary students who are unable to use such strategies in barrier games would benefit from training and practice in monitoring their comprehension and resolving problematic messages in this context. The difference here would be that the material we ask students to process would be more complex. Instead of asking them to "Find the (mumble)," as we did with younger children, we might ask students to "Draw a circular (mumble)," or "Choose the rhomboid shape."

Because so much information is presented in the form of class lectures during this period, it will be very important to assess whether the student can monitor comprehension during classroom presentations. Here curriculum-based assessment,

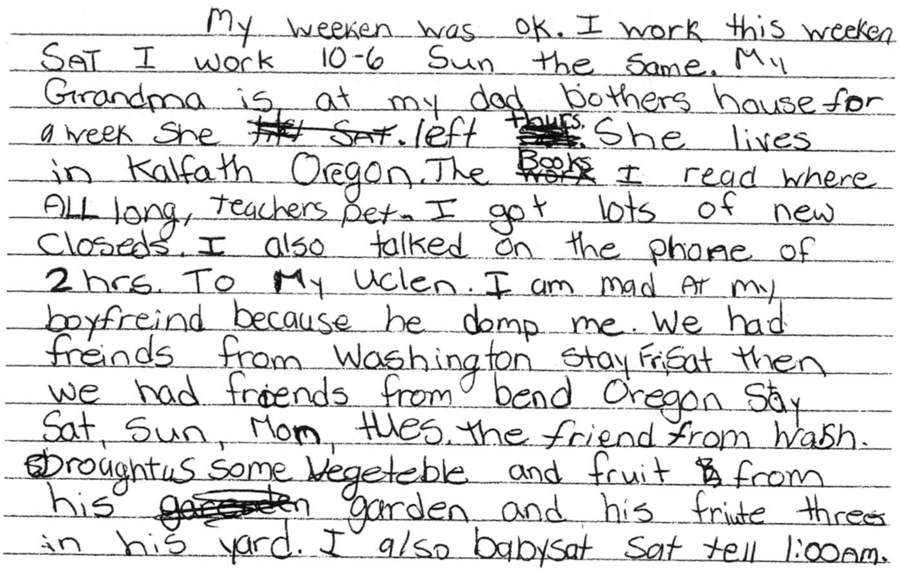

My weeken was OK. I work this weeken Sat I work 10-6 Sun the same. My Grandma is at my dad bothers house for a week She ~~Fit~~ Sat. left ~~thours~~. She lives in Kalfath Oregon. The ~~Books~~ I read where ALL long, teachers pet. I got lots of new Closeds. I also talked on the phone of 2 hrs. To My Uclen. I am mad At my boyfreind because he domp me. We had freinds from Washington stay Fri&Sat then we had froends from bend Oregon Sày Sat, Sun, Mom, tUes. the friend from Wash. Droughtus some Vegeteble and fruit B from his ~~garden~~ garden and his friute threes in his yard. I also babysat Sat tell 1:00Am.

FIGURE 13-9 ✦ Crystal's written language sample (seventh grade).

BOX 13-8 — Questions for Assessing Awareness of Classroom Pragmatic Rules

When is it important to be quiet in this class?

When is talking OK?

When can you talk without raising your hand?

When can you ask questions?

Is it all right in this class to ask another student for help?

What are you supposed to do when you need help?

When are you supposed to give a short answer, and when should you given an elaborated answer?

How important is using correct grammar and spelling when you write for this teacher?

Does this teacher care if you put an "X" when the directions say, "Put a check"?

Adapted from Creaghead, N. (1992). Mutual empowerment through collaboration: A new script for an old problem. In W.A. Secord (Ed.), *Best practices in school speech-language pathology* (vol. II) (pp. 109-116). Austin, TX: Psychological Corporation: Harcourt Brace Jovanovich.

---

using audiotapes of teacher lectures, is useful. This kind of assessment can be integrated with the assessment of basic comprehension that we discussed earlier. After determining whether the student is able to grasp the information presented in the lecture, we might have the student listen again, this time fast-forwarding the tape during a critical piece of information, then continuing the play without comment. We can observe what, if anything, the student does to indicate that some information was missed. If the student fails to indicate a need for further information, we might use a dynamic assessment technique. We can stop the tape, tell the student to be sure to ask if he or she missed anything or needs to hear something again, then repeat the fast-forward procedure. If such cueing helps, we can use a learning-strategies approach to teach the student to provide self-cues to monitor comprehension. If the cueing provided in dynamic assessment does not make a significant change in the student's performance, a more direct approach, like Dollaghan's (1987) method in Chapter 12, may be tried.

In addition to monitoring comprehension of spoken language, our students with LLD need to learn to monitor their reading comprehension. Again, as we did for comprehension of spoken language, we want to assess basic informational comprehension of written material before looking at comprehension monitoring. We can use the standard reading comprehension tests discussed earlier to do this basic-level assessment. If students' basic reading comprehension is above fourth-grade level, we can examine monitoring of reading comprehension. Here we would present photocopies of text material at the student's reading level, or instructions from a board game, a how-to pamphlet, or written instructions for a craft project or homework assignment, with critical words blacked out. If the student does not protest or ask for further information, some deficit in monitoring comprehension in reading can be inferred.

Metacognition

The ability to plan, organize, and reflect on our own cognitive strategies is one of the most important developments of the formal operational period (Westby, 2005). This ability is often referred to as *executive function* (Singer & Bashir, 1999). We can assess metacognitive skill by using "think-aloud protocols" similar to the one we used to assess the planning process in writing. Here we would present students with a task, such as studying a text passage to be tested for recall later, generating an inferential set for a textbook chapter to be read, or planning what might be done to improve a grade in a course. We can ask students to think out loud as they attempt to solve the problem and listen to the strategies used in the thinking. Saldana (2004) suggested supplementing this form of assessment with some dynamic cueing. Here the clinician provides focused assistance, such as reminding the student what the task is, suggesting the use of a new strategy if the student is having difficulty, reminding the student to use the strategy discussed, and so on. If students can take advantage of the model, we may want to continue such modeling and practice in the intervention program. If not, a more structured approach to metacognition, such as the CBM program discussed in Chapter 12, may be a useful addition to the intervention program.

ASSESSING FUNCTIONAL NEEDS IN THE ADVANCED LANGUAGE STAGE

In addition to assessing students' academic communication, we also want to look at their functional communicative skills. This is especially true for older adolescents, at 16 to 21 years of age, who will soon be making the transition from secondary school to higher education or vocational placement, and from family to independent living. As we said when we talked about older clients at the L4L stage, these students will probably already be identified as eligible for services so very little, if any, standardized testing will be needed. Most assessment methods will be observational or criterion-referenced. When we do criterion-referenced or observational assessments for the older, moderate to severely impaired client, we want to use chronologically age-appropriate tasks and materials, of course. We also need to focus on community-referenced assessments.

For students with LLD who are between 16 and 21 years old, Individualized Transition Plans (ITPs), similar to IEPs, are required by the IDEA legislation. A sample from McNamara (2007) appears in Appendix 13-9. They may be developed for students from the age of 14, if appropriate. Generally, the ITP addresses progress toward high school graduation, outlines the post-secondary education or training the student needs,

discusses the community-living support required, and makes preliminary plans to help the student succeed in employment and daily living settings. The communication assessment involved in developing the ITP is community-referenced, as we discussed earlier. If a job or on-the-job-training placement has been decided on during the student's last years in school, the clinician may want to visit the site to do an ecological inventory of the kinds of listening, speaking, reading, and writing demands placed on the student. If college, community college, or vocational training is part of the plan, assessment of the communicative demands of these settings also will be necessary. Lunday (1996) developed a "Communication Checklist" for assessing the communicative demands of post-secondary and vocational settings. This appears in Figure 13-10. These demands can form the basis of the functional communication program designed for the student while still in school.

In addition, we want to talk with the family about their plans for having the student make the transition to independent living. Their input on the student's needs is especially important, since they are most familiar with how the student communicates in everyday life. The family can tell us what they feel are the most important areas in which the student's social communication must improve for an independent-living situation to succeed. Using a checklist such as Bedrosian's (1985) in Figure 11-7 can help parents to focus on the interactive skills with which the student may need additional help to function autonomously. These skills should get high priority in the intervention program during the student's last years in school.

CONCLUSIONS

Assessment of advanced language shares many features with the assessment of students in the L4L stage. Both must focus not only on form and content, but on the way language is used in the unique environment of the classroom. Both must look at how oral language skills support that acquisition of new information from spoken and written material alike. Both must investigate how a student's communicative abilities match the demands of the curriculum and the school environment, and both look beyond the processing of language itself to the ability to focus on metalinguistic and metacognitive activities.

The major difference between the focus of assessment at the L4L stage and that of advanced language is that in assessing advanced language we are working almost exclusively at the literate end of the oral-literate continuum. We are trying to establish the degree to which a student can make sense and make use of the low-frequency, high-density, abstract, and decontextualized language that characterizes literate speech and writing. To do this, we often need to set up special contexts and look not for how often forms are used, but whether they are used at all. And we need to focus even more sharply on the "meta" in assessment, since these skills are essential to success in producing and understanding literate discourse.

Let's look at Mr. Janis's assessment plan for Crystal to see how he would use these principles to guide his selection of evaluation procedures.

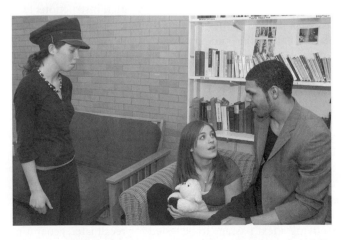

Role playing can be used to assess functional communication skills.

Student: _____ Teacher: _____
Observer: _____ Class: _____
Date: _____ Hour: _____

	Teacher's Expectation			Student's Success		
	yes	no	n/a	pos	+/−	neg

I. Vocabulary

Does the student need to:

	yes	no	n/a	pos	+/−	neg
understand technical terms/jargon?	[ ]	[ ]	[ ]	[ ]	[ ]	[ ]
use technical terms/jargon?	[ ]	[ ]	[ ]	[ ]	[ ]	[ ]
use terms in question form?	[ ]	[ ]	[ ]	[ ]	[ ]	[ ]
comprehend abstract or figurative expressions?	[ ]	[ ]	[ ]	[ ]	[ ]	[ ]
read terms in manuals or textbooks?	[ ]	[ ]	[ ]	[ ]	[ ]	[ ]
read terms on diagrams, charts, and graphs?	[ ]	[ ]	[ ]	[ ]	[ ]	[ ]
write terms in notes, reports, or tests?	[ ]	[ ]	[ ]	[ ]	[ ]	[ ]
spell terms accurately?	[ ]	[ ]	[ ]	[ ]	[ ]	[ ]
summarize project in written report?	[ ]	[ ]	[ ]	[ ]	[ ]	[ ]
identify abbreviations/symbols?	[ ]	[ ]	[ ]	[ ]	[ ]	[ ]

II. Use

Is the student required to:

	yes	no	n/a	pos	+/−	neg
converse with others in group settings?	[ ]	[ ]	[ ]	[ ]	[ ]	[ ]
request tools, supplies, or parts from a stock depot?	[ ]	[ ]	[ ]	[ ]	[ ]	[ ]
follow a step-by-step procedure?	[ ]	[ ]	[ ]	[ ]	[ ]	[ ]
plan or design a schedule/procedure?	[ ]	[ ]	[ ]	[ ]	[ ]	[ ]
explain a procedure to instructor/other student?	[ ]	[ ]	[ ]	[ ]	[ ]	[ ]
ask for specific help?	[ ]	[ ]	[ ]	[ ]	[ ]	[ ]
verbally detail equipment malfunction?	[ ]	[ ]	[ ]	[ ]	[ ]	[ ]
identify and report safety hazards?	[ ]	[ ]	[ ]	[ ]	[ ]	[ ]
orally report assignment/project completion?	[ ]	[ ]	[ ]	[ ]	[ ]	[ ]
attend lecture presentations?	[ ]	[ ]	[ ]	[ ]	[ ]	[ ]
maintain a topic focus?	[ ]	[ ]	[ ]	[ ]	[ ]	[ ]

III. Function

Is the student required to verbally:

	yes	no	n/a	pos	+/−	neg
participate in classroom discussions?	[ ]	[ ]	[ ]	[ ]	[ ]	[ ]
define technical terms?	[ ]	[ ]	[ ]	[ ]	[ ]	[ ]
sequence step-by-step procedures?	[ ]	[ ]	[ ]	[ ]	[ ]	[ ]
report progress?	[ ]	[ ]	[ ]	[ ]	[ ]	[ ]
paraphrase information?	[ ]	[ ]	[ ]	[ ]	[ ]	[ ]
formulate specific questions?	[ ]	[ ]	[ ]	[ ]	[ ]	[ ]
respond to procedural questions?	[ ]	[ ]	[ ]	[ ]	[ ]	[ ]
express/support ideas?	[ ]	[ ]	[ ]	[ ]	[ ]	[ ]
provide suggestions?	[ ]	[ ]	[ ]	[ ]	[ ]	[ ]
give detailed advice?	[ ]	[ ]	[ ]	[ ]	[ ]	[ ]
acknowledge others?	[ ]	[ ]	[ ]	[ ]	[ ]	[ ]

	yes	no	n/a	pos	+/−	neg
describe equipment breakdown?	[ ]	[ ]	[ ]	[ ]	[ ]	[ ]
explain errors?	[ ]	[ ]	[ ]	[ ]	[ ]	[ ]
retrieve previously learned information?	[ ]	[ ]	[ ]	[ ]	[ ]	[ ]

IV. Organization

Does the student need to:

	yes	no	n/a	pos	+/−	neg
keep an organized notebook?	[ ]	[ ]	[ ]	[ ]	[ ]	[ ]
follow prescribed schedule or routine?	[ ]	[ ]	[ ]	[ ]	[ ]	[ ]
anticipate direction from the classroom routine?	[ ]	[ ]	[ ]	[ ]	[ ]	[ ]
manage time based on a syllabus?	[ ]	[ ]	[ ]	[ ]	[ ]	[ ]
use classroom materials independently?	[ ]	[ ]	[ ]	[ ]	[ ]	[ ]

V. Form

Does the student need to:

	yes	no	n/a	pos	+/−	neg
comprehend multilevel directions in complex syntax?	[ ]	[ ]	[ ]	[ ]	[ ]	[ ]
listen for organizational cues or signal words?	[ ]	[ ]	[ ]	[ ]	[ ]	[ ]
decipher complex information?	[ ]	[ ]	[ ]	[ ]	[ ]	[ ]
understand test directions independently?	[ ]	[ ]	[ ]	[ ]	[ ]	[ ]
use writing mechanics correctly?	[ ]	[ ]	[ ]	[ ]	[ ]	[ ]
relate worksheet information to test format?	[ ]	[ ]	[ ]	[ ]	[ ]	[ ]

VI. Pragmatics

Is the student expected to:

	yes	no	n/a	pos	+/−	neg
differentiate speech/register when interacting (e.g., peers, teachers, authority figures, general public)?	[ ]	[ ]	[ ]	[ ]	[ ]	[ ]
use language appropriate to various settings (e.g., classroom, private conversations, group project activities)?	[ ]	[ ]	[ ]	[ ]	[ ]	[ ]
give and react to nonverbal cues?	[ ]	[ ]	[ ]	[ ]	[ ]	[ ]
listen for content importance transmitted by prosody?	[ ]	[ ]	[ ]	[ ]	[ ]	[ ]
modify communication based on feedback?	[ ]	[ ]	[ ]	[ ]	[ ]	[ ]
initiate, take turns, and terminate interactions?	[ ]	[ ]	[ ]	[ ]	[ ]	[ ]
display responsive and appropriate language behavior?	[ ]	[ ]	[ ]	[ ]	[ ]	[ ]
handle concerns and complaints appropriately?	[ ]	[ ]	[ ]	[ ]	[ ]	[ ]
provide and support an opinion?	[ ]	[ ]	[ ]	[ ]	[ ]	[ ]

Other Comments:

FIGURE 13-10 ✦ Checklist of communication skills considered essential to classroom and occupational success. (Reprinted with permission from Lunday, A. [1996]. A collaborative communication skills program for Job Corps centers. *Topics in Language Disorders, 16,* 23-26.)

Mr. Janis met with Crystal to tell her about her score on the CELF-4 screening test, to report to her about her teachers' comments, and to ask her what she thought about her performance in school. He said he would like to do some more testing and talk some more with her teachers to come up with some ideas for helping her improve her grades. He went through the self-assessment form (see Figure 13-1) with her to get some insight into what she considered her strengths and weaknesses. He asked whether it would be OK with her if he asked her teacher to tape some of her classes so he could listen to them later. He said he would call her parents, too, and talk the idea over with them.

Crystal's parents told Mr. Janis on the phone that they knew Crystal was having trouble again, because her first-term grades had been poor and she was starting to say she hated school. They were willing to have Mr. Janis do some more assessment to see whether there were things that could be done to help.

Mr. Janis contacted the school LD specialist, Ms. Naninger, who also had been monitoring Crystal, and called the district reading specialist to plan a transdisciplinary assessment. The reading specialist agreed to assess reading comprehension, and Ms. Naninger arranged to interview Crystal's teachers about her performance. Mr. Janis asked Ms. Naninger to include in her interviews questions from Box 13-3 to get a sense of how her various teachers saw her communication needs and whether there was a consensus among them.

To establish eligibility for services, Mr. Janis gave Crystal the *Test of Adolescent and Adult Language*–3 (TOAL-3; Hammill, Brown, Larsen, & Wiederholt, 1994). Her ranks on all the subtests were below the tenth percentile, with listening a relative strength, and speaking, reading, and writing weaker. Mr. Janis's initial conversation with Crystal had convinced him that she was functioning at an advanced language level; he'd heard few grammatical errors, but did detect some word-finding problems. He found her to be a good conversationalist who was easily engaged in interaction, although she seemed to use an inordinate number of self-corrections and a run-on style in her speech.

He reviewed the information gathered in the teacher interviews by Ms. Naninger. The teachers' comments indicated a consensus that Crystal had trouble with using appropriate vocabulary, planning for and completing assignments, participating in class discussions, writing and note-taking, understanding material presented in texts and lectures, and solving problems with verbal reasoning. All the teachers agreed that Crystal's strengths were in peer interaction. She was popular with other students and had few obvious difficulties interacting with them, despite her somewhat run-on speech style. Crystal's self-assessment also identified writing papers, understanding written material, using a dictionary, organizing and finding main ideas, and participating in class discussion as areas that gave her trouble. The reading specialist's testing showed that Crystal's comprehension was at about a fifth-grade level in most areas.

Mr. Janis decided not to do an assessment of conversational pragmatics at this time, because Crystal's interactive skills were reported to be a strength. He did tell Crystal, though, that if she started to have trouble conversing with peers or understanding their slang, she should let him know and he would look into it. Similarly, he decided not to do a great deal of criterion-referenced assessment of her basic listening skills, since that, too, was a strength, according to

the TOAL. He did want to look at classroom comprehension, though, because of the special demands of that listening situation. Mr. Janis designed the following plan to gather criterion-referenced information on her communication skills:

- Use the *Test of Adolescent/Adult Word Finding* to document word-retrieval problems.
- Conduct a curriculum-based assessment, using passages from her English text, which she said she liked, and her science text, which she said was the most difficult for her. Use the passages to look at her comprehension of advanced vocabulary and word relations, her comprehension of advanced syntax, and reading comprehension monitoring skill. Probe her ability to produce word definitions by asking her to define some of the more unfamiliar words in the passages. Use dynamic assessment to assess expository text comprehension in the science passage. Ask Crystal to read the description of one of the characters in a literature selection in the English text and make inferences about the character.
- Collect a spoken narrative and written narrative sample, each describing an episode of a favorite TV show, to examine T-unit length, subordination index, use of low-frequency forms, %CWS, expression of internal responses, and use of cohesive markers.
- Have Crystal bring a writing sample from an English and a science homework assignment she's completed. Assess her writing in terms of length, lexical maturity, sentential syntax, grammar and mechanics, and overall quality. Assess metalinguistic ability by asking her to edit one of the papers that contains errors.
- Ask Crystal to write a set of instructions on how to knit a sweater (her hobby). Assess planning and metacognitive processes in writing, using a "think-aloud" protocol. Use dynamic assessment to model "thinking out loud" and determine whether the model improves Crystal's performance on subsequent trials.
- Assess Crystal's classroom pragmatic skills by listening to an audiotape of her class performance and noting any problems in Crystal's participation or lack of it. Have Crystal listen to a portion of the lecture and provide a summary. Have her listen to another portion and take notes on it. Ask her to give the main idea of the lecture. Use dynamic assessment, providing a written outline of one portion of the lecture with blank lines for Crystal to fill in with notes. Have her summarize this portion and note differences from the unguided summary. Use the "fast-forward" procedure to assess comprehension monitoring skill.

Although the evaluation process took some time, Mr. Janis was able to use dynamic assessment as a diagnostic teaching procedure, so that he was doing some intervention as he was gathering the data. When he'd collected all his information, he felt in a good position to develop a strong transdisciplinary intervention program that would improve Crystal's chances of successfully completing her schooling.

STUDY GUIDE

I. Language Development in Adolescence
   A. What is meant by advanced language development?
   B. What is formal operational thought?

C. What literate language skills are learned during this period?

D. How does the development of formal operations affect language use?

E. What are some of the new demands of the secondary classroom?

II. Student-Centered Assessment
   A. How can students be involved in the assessment process?
   B. Why is student involvement important?

III. Screening, Case Finding, and Establishing Eligibility with Standardized Tests in the Advanced Language Period
   A. What is the purpose of screening in the advanced language period?
   B. For what populations does screening make most sense?
   C. What other sources of referral are available for adolescents? How can they be accessed?
   D. What is needed to "market" our services to adolescents?
   E. What is the role of standardized testing at the advanced language stage?

IV. Criterion-Referenced Assessment and Behavioral Observation in the Advanced Language Stage
   A. How can we establish that a student is functioning at the advanced language stage?
   B. Discuss methods for assessing the literate lexicon.
   C. How can word-retrieval difficulties be documented in adolescents?
   D. When and how should word definition skill be assessed?
   E. What aspects of word relations can we examine in adolescents? What methods can be used?
   F. How can understanding of figurative language be analyzed?
   G. Discuss procedures for examining semantic integration and verbal reasoning.

H. How would you assess syntactic comprehension in a teenager?

I. Discuss three methods of assessing syntactic production. What sampling context(s) would you use for the assessment?

J. Discuss methods and contexts for evaluating conversational pragmatics in adolescents.

K. How can we assess an adolescent students' classroom discourse performance?

L. Discuss the difference between *informational* and *critical* listening. How can each be evaluated?

M. Discuss narrative analysis at the advanced language level. What will we be looking for? How will we analyze it?

N. Describe methods for assessing understanding of expository text structure.

O. How would you evaluate a student's processing of persuasive texts?

P. Describe methods for assessing the process and products of students' writing.

Q. What are the "meta" skills we can examine in secondary students? How can each be evaluated?

V. Assessing Functional Needs in the Advanced Language Stage
   A. What are Individual Transition Plans? For whom are they done? What do they contain?
   B. What kind of transition planning can be done for a student going directly from high school to employment? To a higher educational setting?
   C. What kinds of assessments are necessary for transition planning?

ANALYSIS OF T-UNIT LENGTH, LOW-FREQUENCY STRUCTURES, AND SUBORDINATION INDEX IN CHARLIE'S ORAL NARRATIVE SAMPLE IN BOX 13-2

APPENDIX
13-1

T-unit Segmentation, Length in Words, Number of Clauses per T-unit

T-UNIT	LENGTH	NO. OF CLAUSES
T1: There was a boy who was about 21 who stole a plane with a woman and champagne in the cockpit,	20	3
T2: (and) then he got court-martialed for that	6	1
T3: (and) then they sent him to a research study.	8	1
T4: It was for monkeys and chimpanzees.	6	1
T5: They taught them how to fly,	6	2
T6: (and) then what they would do is to have three classes.	10	3
T7: White would be a freshman, blue a junior, and red a senior	12	1
T8: (and) they would teach them how to fly.	7	2
T9: Then after they graduated, they took them into this plane.	10	2
T10: There's this one area, called the radiation area	8	2
T11: (and) they put them in a simulator and exposed them to radiation treatment	12	2
T12: (and) they wanted to see how long they would fly until they would die	13	4
T13: (and) so they could see how long humans could fly if they could pilot their missions if the Russians had an attack on us	23	4
T14: (and) then what the boy did is he had a friend, a chimpanzee that knew sign language	16	4
T15: (and) he talked to him	4	1
T16: (and) he taught the other apes	5	1
T17: (and) they were going to kill his friend with the radiation thing.	11	1
T18: There were these people from the Air Force Patrol	9	1
T19: (and) they were watching the studies	5	1
T20: (and) he didn't want them to kill his monkey	8	2
T21: (and so) what he did was he called the lady who taught him sign language	13	4
T22: (and) she came	2	1
T23: (and) they stole a plane with the monkeys in it	9	1
T24: (and) they finally escaped	3	1

Average T-unit length = 226/24 = 9.42.

Subordination index = 46/24 = 1.92.

Use of Low-Frequency Structures

STRUCTURE	FOUND IN T-UNIT
Morphology	T2, T10, T11, T17
Noun phrase postmodification	
With past participles	T10
With present participles	
With infinitives	
With appositives	T14
With relative clauses	T1, T1, T14, T21
With prepositional phrases	T1, T18
Complex verb phrases	
Perfect aspect	
Multiple auxiliaries	
Passive sentence	T2 (less advanced truncated passive form)
Adverbial markers and conjunctions (e.g., *otherwise, instead, after all, only, still, though, anyway, in all, finally, when, because,* etc.)	T9, T12, T13, T24
Complex sentence types	
More than one clause type	T6, T12, T13, T14, T21
Clefting	T6, T14, T21
Left branching	T9

Evaluation: Adequate complexity in speech.

ANALYSIS OF T-UNIT LENGTH, LOW-FREQUENCY STRUCTURES, AND SUBORDINATION INDEX IN CHARLIE'S WRITTEN SAMPLE IN FIGURE 13-3

T-unit Segmentation, Length in Words, Number of Clauses per T-unit

T-UNIT	LENGTH	NO. OF CLAUSES
T1: My best personal quality is that I am very friendly with people and to anyone that needs a friend.	19	3
T2: Where I go to school there are some people that are not nice.	13	3
T3: I don't know that many kids at my school could be nice.	12	2 (Conjunction error)
T4: The people that go to my school could be nice.	10	2
T5: But there are people that are nice to [other] people like me.	12	2
T6: I am very outgoing.	4	1
T7: For example, I like to work on school plays and help the new students around school.	16	3
T8: I am very hardworking at [every thing] that I do.	9	2
T9: For example, I do my homework, [thing] on the computer and [puzzels].	12	1

Average T-unit length = 107/9 = 11.89.
Subordination index = 19/9 = 2.1.

Use of Low-Frequency Structures

STRUCTURE	FOUND IN T-UNIT
Morphology	
Noun phrase postmodification	
With past participles	
With present participles	
With infinitives	
With appositives	
With relative clauses	T1, T2, T4 T5, T8
With prepositional phrases	
Complex verb phrases	
Perfect aspect	
Multiple auxiliaries	
Passive sentence	
Adverbial markers and conjunctions	
(e.g., *otherwise, instead, after all, only, still, though, anyway, in all, finally, when, because, etc.*)	T7, T9 (*not used appropriately*; overused)
Complex sentence types	
More than one clause type	T2
Clefting	T2
Left branching	T4

Evaluation: Adequate T-unit length, subordination, and use of relative clauses. Probe use of adverbials and conjunctions.

T-UNIT	COHESIVE DEVICE	ADEQUATE?
T1: My best personal quality is that *I* am very friendly with people and to *anyone* that needs a friend.	Pronoun Substitution	Yes Yes
T2: Where *I* go to school there are some people that are not nice.	Pronoun	Yes
T3: I don't know that many *kids* at my school could be nice.	Substitution	Yes
T4: The people that go to my school could be nice.		
T5: *But* there are people that are nice to [other] people like me.	Conjunction	Yes
T6: *I* am very outgoing.	Pronoun	Yes
T7: *For example*, I like to work on school plays and help the new students around school.	Conjunct	Yes
T8: *I* am very hardworking at [every thing] that *I* do.	Pronoun	Yes
T9: *For example*, I do my homework, [thing] on the computer and [puzzels].	Conjunct	No

Literate Lexicon

Metalinguistic and metacognitive verbs: *know.*

Adverbs, conjunctions, and connectives: *for example* (overused and used inappropriately), *but.*

Evaluation: Possible difficulty with cohesion; probe in longer sample. Again, probe use of adverbials and connectives.

NARRATIVE RUBRIC

SCORE	SETTING AND MOOD	CHARACTER DEVELOPMENT	PLOT AND NARRATIVE STRUCTURE	VOICE AND TONE
1	The place or time in which the story takes place is unclear or altogether absent	All characters are one-dimensional and stereotypical; little or no background is given on them; little or no relationship between characters or characters who have no relation to the plot; characters do not think or feel	Events are unconnected or contain no conflict; no climax or resolution	Little attention to word choice; emotional atmosphere is not developed; no variety in sentence structure
2	Vague idea of the place and time in which the story is set ("Long ago in a faraway land…")	Physical description of characters is given; actions are displayed by characters	Events are told in sequence, but trivial events are mixed in with important ones; conflict is present but unrelated to characters or significance of conflict is not clearly communicated	Inappropriate word choice at times; very little variety to sentence structure; style is limited to presenting information in a factual manner
3	Enough vivid details are included for the reader to identify or imagine the location, but the setting merely functions as a backdrop to the story or is an unrealistic setting for the story; the details of the setting are told rather than shown	Main characters are identifiable and are given more detail, but lack background information; characters react in stereotypical ways to the plot in which they are placed; characters' thoughts are recorded	Conflict is clear; characters struggle with problems; emotional reactions and outcomes become part of the story; has a familiar plotline in which the reader can guess what will happen next; may not have a resolution	Sentence length and structure is more varied; minimal dialogue; mood is in beginning stages of development
4	Setting is identifiable/imaginable and realistic; some elements of the setting are revealed through the story rather than told by the narrator; sensory information is included	Beginning development of motivations for actions; letting the character speak and interact with others	Conflict is clear and importance to characters told but not demonstrated; characters struggle with problems; relationships between events are demonstrated; there is a logical climax and resolution	Narrator is identifiable but may not have a clear voice; imagery begins to be used; sentence structure is varied; dialogue is predictable

SCORE	SETTING AND MOOD	CHARACTER DEVELOPMENT	PLOT AND NARRATIVE STRUCTURE	VOICE AND TONE
5	Setting is identifiable/imaginable and realistic; many elements of the setting are revealed through the narrative at appropriate junctures	Protagonists and antagonists emerge and interact with one another in believable ways	Conflict is clear and complex and its importance to the characters nearly convincing; characters struggle with problems; story has a logical climax and resolution, although perhaps forced; events of the story flow in chronological order; subplots are introduced although not resolved	Narrator has a clear voice; sentence structure is varied; figurative language and action verbs are used; dialogue becomes more interesting
6	The time and place are incorporated at appropriate turns in the story; the setting provides an overall mood that reflects that of the characters and/or unfolding drama; the world depicted is believable and internally consistent and enhances the narrative; techniques such as foreshadowing are used	Character development is complete; characters behave in ways that seem natural to their development; characters become dynamic and psychologically complex; characters are developed through appearance, action, thoughts, and speech	Conflict is clear and complex and its importance to the characters convincing; series of events are interesting and draw the reader in; characters struggle with problems in interesting and meaningful ways; story has a logical climax and satisfying resolution; techniques such as flashbacks and foreshadowing are used to vary the structure from a straightforward, chronological sequence of events; subplots are introduced and resolved	First person narrative is used; variety in sentence structure matches intentions of story; precise and varied word choices are used; lively language, including the use of similes, metaphors, and analogies, are used; imagery and symbolic language are used; dialogue is interesting and lively

DEVELOPMENTAL RUBRIC—EXPOSITORY WRITING

SCORE	ORGANIZATION (TEXT STRUCTURE)	CONTEXT/THEME (COHERENCE)	WRITTEN LANGUAGE (DEVELOPMENT OF SYNTAX, COHESION STRATEGIES, VOCABULARY)	WRITTEN CONVENTIONS (MECHANICS)	SENSE OF AUDIENCE
1	May be extremely brief or confused	Tendency to write either partially or completely in the narrative mode; associated ideas; much content extraneous to the topic or indirectly related to topic	Use of simple sentences (NVO); sentences juxtaposed; if connectors between sentences are used, they are primarily "and," "then"; may use pronominal reference with numerous ambiguous pronouns (referent not retrievable from text); use of simple vocabulary	Beginning differentiation of drawing and printing; use of recursive letter-like shapes when printing; some phoneme-grapheme awareness for initial sounds; text not readable by others	No sense of audience; writes for self from own perspective; often references based on personal experiences that are not retrievable from text
2	May attempt to structure, attempting to center or chaining ideas, but it may be difficult to determine the structure; many ideas included in one paragraph or each idea written as a paragraph, or the response may be so brief that its organization cannot be evaluated	May have misleading introductions and/or conclusions; first-hand experiences; some content extraneous to the topic; ideas are quite disjointed	Compound subjects; compound predicates; within text pronominal reference; coordinating conjunctions—primarily "and," "then," "but," "because" (used for motivational, not logical reasons); use of adequate vocabulary	Printing/writing recognizable letters; use of invented spelling with most sounds represented; no spacing between words or inconsistent spacing, incomplete sentences; a variety of grammatical errors; errors likely to affect readers' comprehension	Writes with knowledge that others will read text; does not adjust writing for specific audiences
3	Structure is somewhat unclear; centers or chains, but has difficulty doing both; lack of clear opening; some of the support and elaborations are paragraphed correctly; most ideas relate to main topic or issue with no specific connections; may include major rambling from the main topic	Topic knowledge developing; some content extraneous to the topic may be present; may have misleading introductions and conclusions; moderately disjointed; misleading statements	Adverbial subordinate clauses, particularly with conjunctions "when," "while," "because" (now used for logical justification); relative clauses, primarily those that post-modify object nouns; use of appropriate vocabulary	May continue to have some difficulty with handwriting; invented spelling continues; use of capitals on words at beginning of sentences and persons' names, periods, question marks, exclamation points, apostrophes; pronominal reference may be unclear, errors may affect readers' comprehension	Usually writes for teacher; depends on teacher to set organization format

SCORE	ORGANIZATION (TEXT STRUCTURE)	CONTEXT/THEME (COHERENCE)	WRITTEN LANGUAGE (DEVELOPMENT OF SYNTAX, COHESION STRATEGIES, VOCABULARY)	WRITTEN CONVENTIONS (MECHANICS)	SENSE OF AUDIENCE
4	Structure of the paper is clear; coordination of centering and chaining; some clusters of ideas are paragraphed appropriately; planned opening and closing to paper when appropriate; use of specific expository structures (e.g., definitions, comparison/contrast, cause/effect, sequences, problem/solution); ideas relate to the topic without specific connections; may include off-topic material	Development may be uneven with some clusters of ideas elaborated, others not; lacks depth of content	Use of low-frequency adverbials—"though," "although," "even if," "as," "unless," "provided that"; nominal clauses as subjects; use of some precise vocabulary	Handwriting automatized; spelling mostly conventional; developing use of a greater variety of punctuation (comma, colon, semicolon, quotation marks); few run-on sentences; subject/verb agreement and tenses consistent; paragraphing developing	Given an assignment, student begins to select independently the organizational format appropriate to task and audience; may not select the most appropriate format or may not be able to maintain the chosen format
5	Structure of paper is clear; most of the major clusters of ideas are paragraphed effectively; planned opening and closing to paper, if appropriate; coherence may be demonstrated by overall structure (topic sentences in paragraphs); cohesion developed by various methods (pronouns, parallel structure, some repetition); may include minor off-topic material	Main ideas developed with appropriate and varied details; some risks may be taken that are mostly successful; may have minor flaws; progresses logically	Use of concordant conjuncts "similarly," "moreover," "consequently," "therefore," "furthermore," "for example"; and discordant conjuncts "instead," "yet," "however," "nevertheless," "conversely"; use of vocabulary precise and carefully chosen	Spelling mostly automatized and conventional (student self-edits); more consistent use of correct punctuation; appropriate text formatting for different genres; consistently clear pronominal reference	Given an assignment, student begins to select independently the organizational format appropriate to task and audience; selects from several possible structures the one most appropriate for purpose and audience
6	Structure of paper is clear; all of the major points; opening and closing when appropriate; effectively paragraphed; transitional devices used to develop coherence and cohesion; all ideas are presented logically and are interrelated; no off-topic material; use of a wide variety of organizational structures	Main ideas developed with appropriate and varied details; writer may take compositional risks, resulting in effective, vivid response	Use of structures to achieve literary style, e.g., subject-verb split, absolute phrases; use of vocabulary precise and carefully chosen	Errors in spelling, punctuation, grammar, usage are rare	Response has a coherent sense of purpose and audience; careful consideration of organizational structure from a wide variety of organizational structures that best highlight information for a particular audience

Adapted with permission from Westby, C., & Clauser, D. (2005). The right stuff for writing. In H. Catts & A. Kahmi (Eds.). *Language and reading disabilities* (2nd ed., pp. 288-289). Boston, MA: Allyn & Bacon.

Developmental Rubric—Persuasive Writing

ORGANIZATION (TEXT STRUCTURE)	ARGUMENT	CONTENT/ THEME (COHERENCE)	WRITTEN LANGUAGE (DEVELOPMENT OF SYNTAX, COHESION STRATEGIES, VOCABULARY)	WRITTEN CONVENTIONS (MECHANICS)	SENSE OF AUDIENCE
May be extremely brief or confused	No claim is made or claim is made but no reasons are given to support the claim or reasons given are not relevant to the claim	Tendency to write either partially or completely in the narrative mode; some content extraneous to the claim present	Use of simple sentences (N + V + O); sentences juxtaposed; if connectors between sentences are used, they are primarily "and," and "then"; may use pronominal reference with numerous ambiguous pronouns (reference not retrievable from the text); use of simple vocabulary	Displays severe mechanical errors/or may be so brief that knowledge of mechanics can not be determined (errors may interfere with readers' comprehension)	No sense of audience; writes for self from own perspective; often references based on personal experiences that are not retrievable from text
May attempt to structure, but structure is difficult to determine; many ideas included in one paragraph or each idea written as a paragraph, or the response may be so brief that its organization cannot be evaluated	Claim is made and reasons are given to support it, but the self-centered reasons are not developed or are rambling or disjointed	May have misleading introductions and/or conclusions; some content extraneous to the claim is present	Compound subjects, compound predicates; within text pronominal reference; coordinating conjunctions primarily "and," "then," "but"; "because" used for motivational reasons; use of adequate vocabulary	Displays numerous severe errors in mechanics (errors may interfere to a degree with readers' comprehension)	Writes with knowledge that others will read text; does not adjust writing for specific audiences

Adapted from Nippold, M.A, Duthie, J.K., & Larsen, J. (2005). Literacy as a leisure activity: Free-time preferences of older children and young adolescents. *Language, Speech and Hearing Services in Schools. 36, (2)*:93-102; Westby, C., & Clauser, P. (2005). The right stuff for writing: Assessing and facilitating written language. In H. Catts and A. Kahmi (Eds.). *Language and reading disabilities* (2nd ed.). (pp. 288-289). Boston: Allyn & Bacon.

ORGANIZATION (TEXT STRUCTURE)	ARGUMENT	CONTENT/ THEME (COHERENCE)	WRITTEN LANGUAGE (DEVELOPMENT OF SYNTAX, COHESION STRATEGIES, VOCABULARY)	WRITTEN CONVENTIONS (MECHANICS)	SENSE OF AUDIENCE
Structure is somewhat unclear; some of the support and explanations are paragraphed correctly; most ideas related to claim or issue with no specific connections; may include major rambling from the main topic	Claim is made and supported by self-centered reasons to support the claim; some further explanations made but not elaborated; may mention briefly an opposite point of view	May have misleading introductions and/or conclusions; some content extraneous to the claim may be present	Adverbial subordinate clauses, particularly with the conjunctions "when," "while," "because" (now used for logical justification); relative clauses, primarily those that post modify object nouns; use of age-appropriate vocabulary	Displays a pattern or errors in mechanics (errors may interfere with readability)	Increasing ability to assume another's perspective; begins to adjust writing for the audience and to identify problems in own writing that may be difficult for others to understand
Structure of the paper is clear; some clusters or arguments are paragraphed appropriately; planned opening and closing to paper; ideas related to the topic without specific connections; may include minor off-topic material	Claim is made and supported by a non–self-centered reason; at least one explanation included with formal development; may have a brief summary of the opposite point of view	Development may be uneven with some clusters of ideas elaborated, others not	Use of low-frequency adverbials: "though," "although," "even if," "as"; "unless," "provided that"; nominal clauses as subjects; use of some precise vocabulary	May display errors in mechanics but there is no consistent pattern	Can take a third person's perspective; recognizes what might be difficult for a reader to understand; makes appropriate changes

ORGANIZATION (TEXT STRUCTURE)	ARGUMENT	CONTENT/ THEME (COHERENCE)	WRITTEN LANGUAGE (DEVELOPMENT OF SYNTAX, COHESION STRATEGIES, VOCABULARY)	WRITTEN CONVENTIONS (MECHANICS)	SENSE OF AUDIENCE
Structure of the paper is clear; most of the major clusters of ideas are paragraphed effectively; planned opening and closing to paper; coherence may be demonstrated by overall structure (topic sentences in paragraphs); cohesion developed by various methods (pronoun, parallel structure, some repetition); may include minor off-topic material	Claim is made that is supported by general reasons with explanations; includes an attempt to discuss or disprove the opposite point of view	Main ideas developed with appropriate and varied details; some risks may be taken that are mostly successful; may have minor flaws; progresses logically	Use of concordant conjuncts "similarly," "moreover," "consequently," "therefore," "furthermore," "for example"; and discordant conjuncts "instead," "yet," "however," "nevertheless," "conversely"; use of vocabulary precise and carefully chosen	Few errors in mechanics	Considers potential readers' perspective as text is written; presents persuasive information with beliefs and values of readers in mind
Structure of the paper is clear; all of the major points, opening and closing, are appropriately paragraphed; transitional devices used to develop coherence and cohesion, all ideas are presented logically and are interrelated; no off-topic material	Claim is made that is supported by general reasons with explanations, including a thorough discussion and/or refutation of the opposite point of view; summarizes this view and discusses why it is narrow or incorrect	Main ideas developed with appropriate and varied details; writer may take compositional risks resulting in an effective, vivid response	Use of structures to achieve literary style, e.g., subject-verb split, absolute phrases; careful crafting in choice of vocabulary	Minor, if any, errors in mechanics	Able to consider the opposite point of view, presents it, and discusses the reason it is incorrect

The 6+1 Trait® Writing
Scoring Continuum

☼ Wow!

Exceeds expectations

◎ Strong

Shows control and skill in this trait; many strengths present

↓ Effective

On balance, the strengths outweigh the weaknesses; a small amount of revision is needed

→ Developing

Strengths and need for revision are about equal; about half-way home

↑ Emerging

Need for revision outweighs strengths; isolated moments hint at what the writer has in mind

← Not Yet

A bare beginning; writer not yet showing control

▣ Ideas
▣ Organization
▣ Voice
▣ Word Choice
▣ Sentence Fluency
▣ Conventions
▣ Presentation

6+1 Trait® Writing Rubric
Ideas

Ideas: The heart of the message, the content of the piece, the main theme, with details that enrich and develop that theme	
⑤	*This paper is clear and focused. It holds the reader's attention. Relevant anecdotes and details enrich the central theme* A. The topic is narrow and manageable B. Relevant, telling, quality details go beyond the obvious C. Reasonably accurate details D. Writing from knowledge or experience; ideas are fresh and original E. Reader's questions are anticipated and answered F. Insight
③	*The writer is beginning to define the topic, even though development is still basic or general* A. The topic is fairly broad B. Support is attempted C. Ideas are reasonably clear D. Writer has difficulty going from general observations to specifics E. The reader is left with questions F. The writer stays on topic
①	*The paper has no clear sense of purpose or central theme. The reader must make inferences based on sketchy or missing details* A. The writer is still in search of a topic B. Information is limited or unclear or the length is not adequate for development C. The idea is a simple statement or a simple answer to the question D. The writer has not begun to define the topic E. Everything seems as important as everything else F. The text may be repetitious, disconnected, and contains too many random thoughts

6+1 Trait® Writing Rubric
Organization

Organization: The internal structure, the thread of central meaning, the logical and sometimes intriguing pattern of ideas.	
⑤	*The organizational structure of this paper enhances and showcases the central idea or theme of the paper; includes a satisfying introduction and conclusion* A. An inviting introduction draws the reader in; a satisfying conclusion leaves the reader with a sense of closure and resolution B. Thoughtful transitions C. Sequencing is logical and effective D. Pacing is well controlled E. The title, if desired, is original F. Flows so smoothly, the reader hardly thinks about it
③	*The organizational structure is strong enough to move the reader through the text without too much confusion* A. The paper has a recognizable introduction and conclusion B. Transitions often work well C. Sequencing shows some logic, yet structure takes attention away from content D. Pacing is fairly well controlled E. Organization sometimes supports the main point or storyline F. A title (if desired) is present
①	*The writing lacks a clear sense of direction* A. No real lead B. Connections between ideas are confusing C. Sequencing needs work D. Pacing feels awkward E. No title is present (if requested) F. Problems with organization make it hard for the reader to get a grip on the main point or storyline

6+1 Trait® Writing Rubric
Voice

Voice: The unique perspective of the writer coming through in the piece through honesty, conviction, integrity, and believability	
⑤	*The writer of this paper speaks directly to the reader in a manner that is individual, compelling, and respects the purpose and audience for the writing.* A. Adds interest; appropriate of purpose and audience B. The reader feels a strong interaction with the writer C. The writer takes a risk D. Expository or persuasive reflects understanding and commitment to topic E. Narrative writing seems honest, personal, and engaging
③	*The writer seems sincere but not fully engaged or involved. The result is pleasant or even personable, but not compelling.* A. Obvious generalities B. Earnest, pleasing, safe writing C. The voice fades in and out D. Expository or persuasive writing lacks consistent engagement E. Narrative writing is reasonably sincere
①	*The writer seems indifferent, uninvolved, or distanced from the topic and/or the audience.* A. No concern with audience B. Monotone C. Hum-drum and risk-free D. Lifeless or mechanical E. No point of view is present

6+1 Trait® Writing Rubric
Word Choice

Word Choice: The use of rich, colorful, precise language that moves and enlightens the reader	
⑤	*Words convey the intended message in a precise, interesting, and natural way* A. Words are specific and accurate B. Striking words and phrases C. Natural, effective, and appropriate language D. Lively verbs, specific nouns and modifiers E. Language enhances and clarifies meaning
③	*The language is functional, even if it lacks much energy* A. Words are adequate and correct in a general sense B. Familiar words and phrases communicate C. Attempts at colorful language D. Passive verbs, everyday nouns, mundane modifiers E. Functional with one or two fine moments F. Occasionally, the words show refinement and precision
①	*The writer struggles with a limited vocabulary* A. Words are nonspecific or distracting B. Many of the words don't work C. Language is used incorrectly D. Limited vocabulary, misuse of parts of speech E. Words and phrases are unimaginative and lifeless F. Jargon or clichés, persistent redundancy

6+1 Trait® Writing Rubric
Sentence Fluency

Sentence Fluency: The rhythm and flow of the language, the sound of word patterns, the way in which the writing plays to the ear—not just to the eye	
⑤	***The writing has an easy flow, rhythm and cadence. Sentences are well built.*** A. Sentences enhance the meaning. B. Sentences vary in length as well as structure. C. Purposeful and varied sentence beginnings. D. Creative and appropriate connectives. E. The writing has cadence.
③	***The text hums along with a steady beat, but tends to be more pleasant or businesslike than musical.*** A. Sentences get the job done in a routine fashion. B. Sentences are usually constructed correctly. C. Sentence beginnings are not ALL alike; some variety is attempted. D. The reader sometimes has to hunt for clues. E. Parts of the text invite expressive oral reading; others may be stiff, awkward, choppy, or gangly.
①	***The reader has to practice quite a bit in order to give this paper a fair interpretive reading.*** A. Sentences are choppy, incomplete, rambling, or awkward. Phrasing does not sound natural. B. No "sentence sense" present. C. Sentences begin the same way. D. Endless connectives. E. Does not invite expressive oral reading.

6+1 Trait® Writing Rubric
Conventions

Conventions: The mechanical correctness of the piece; spelling, grammar, and usage, paragraphing, use of capitals, and punctuation*	
⑤	***The writer demonstrates a good grasp of standard writing conventions (e.g., spelling, punctuation, capitalization, grammar, usage, paragraphing)*** A. Spelling is generally correct B. Punctuation is accurate C. Capitalization skills are present D. Grammar and usage are correct E. Paragraphing tends to be sound F. The writer may manipulate conventions for stylistic effect; and it works!
③	***The writer shows reasonable control over a limited range of standard writing conventions*** A. Spelling is usually correct or reasonably phonetic on common words B. End punctuation is usually correct C. Most words are capitalized correctly D. Problems with grammar and usage are not serious E. Paragraphing is attempted F. Moderate (a little of this, a little of that) editing
①	***Errors in spelling, punctuation, capitalization, usage and grammar, and/or paragraphing repeatedly distract the reader and make text difficult to read*** A. Spelling errors are frequent B. Punctuation missing or incorrect C. Capitalization is random D. Errors in grammar or usage are very noticeable E. Paragraphing is missing F. The reader must read once to decode, then again for meaning
	* Grades 7 and Up Only: The writing is sufficiently complex to allow the writer to show skill in using a wide range of conventions

© Northwest Regional Educational Laboratory.

Student: _____Crystal_____   Grade _____7_____

Written assignment: _____Write about your weekend_____

	SAMPLE 1	SAMPLE 2	SAMPLE 3
Date of sample:			
Teacher/clinician grade*:			
Student self-assessment grade:			
No. of samples			
Handwriting	B		
Spelling	C		
Punctuation	C		
Capitalization	C		
Paragraphing			
Grammar	B†		
Use of literate vocabulary	C		
Length of sample/total words	14 T-units (B)/117 words		
No. of different words (NDW)	80		
Average T-unit length	8.4 (B)		
Subordination index	1.2 (B)		
Use of low-frequency syntactic forms	2 (1 used incorrectly): C		
Number or % correctly spelled words	87 or 74% (C)		
Number or % CWS	28 or 47% (C)		
Organization	C		
Provides sufficient information	B		
Use of appropriate detail	C		
Cohesion	B		
Tone	B		
Holistic evaluation score (1–6) (Table 13-10)	2–3		
Expository Rubrics (1–6) (Appendix 13-5)	2, 3–4, 2, 3, 1–2		

*A = grade-level work.

B = below-grade level but no intervention required.

C = deficits warrant remediation.

†Some errors may be spelling rather than grammar; e.g., *work/worked*.

TRANSITION PLANNING SUMMARY

1. **Statement of Transition Service Needs for students age 14 and older:** (Must be completed at each annual review following a student's 13th birthday)
   Crystal will benefit from coordination of educational, prevocational and community participation supports to prepare her to function at her optimum capacity in a supported vocational or community experience programs.

2. **Student Preferences/Interests - document the following:** (Sections2, 3, and 4 must be completed at each annual review following a student's 15th birthday)

   a. Was the student invited to attend her/his planning and placement team (PTT) meeting?　　　　**X** Yes　　❑ No

   b. Did the student attend?　　　　**X** Yes　　❑ No

   c. How were the student's preferences/interests, as they relate to planning for transition services, determined?　　X Personal interviews　❑ Informal/formal testing

   X Vocational assesment　　　　❑ Comments at meeting　　　　**X** Other: (specify) *Interview of student's family*

   d. Summarize student preferences/interests as they relate to planning for transition services: ***Crystal has demonstrated an interest in prevocational activities and community experiences that involve consistent routines, physical activity, and opportunities to socialize with others. Activities that Crystal has experienced and responded favorably to include volunteer activities ("Meals on Wheels), landscape work and gardening, and building maintenance. She demonstrated a distinct dislike of sedentary assembly work, unpredictable schedules, and work routines with long periods of inactivity, as evidenced by her verbal and behavioral responses to such experiences.***

3. **Agency participation:**

   a. Were any outside agencies invited to attend the PPT meeting?　　**X** Yes　　　　❑ No (If no, specify reason) _____

   b. If yes, did the agency's representative attend?　　**X** Yes　　　　❑ No

   c. Has any participating agency agreed to provide or pay for services/linkages?　❑ No　　　**X** Yes (specify) *4 hours/week prevocational training and community experience*

4. **Justification statements for transition services not being addressed:**

   a. If an annual goal and related objectives were not developed for independent living or community participation, provide a justification statement.

   NA (goals developed)

   b. If activities/training are <u>not</u> provided in both the <u>community</u> and the <u>classroom,</u> provide a justification statement:

   NA - Activities/training are provided in <u>both</u> locations

5. At least one year prior to reaching age 18, the student must be informed of her/his rights under IDEA, if any, which will transfer to her/him at age 18.

   NA (student will not be 17 within 1 year)

Courtesy of the Connecticut State Department of Education © 2000.

INTERVENTION FOR ADVANCED LANGUAGE

CHAPTER OBJECTIVES

- State a rationale for providing treatment for communication disorders in secondary school students.
- List the appropriate products of intervention at the secondary stage.
- Describe a range of intervention methods for working with students at the advanced language stage.
- Describe connections among oral language, learning, and literacy at the secondary level.

- Discuss the appropriate contexts for intervention at the secondary school level.
- Discuss the process of transition planning for students over the age of 14.
- List appropriate goals and procedures for secondary age students with severe communication disorders.

Michael had been diagnosed with autism when he was 3. At that time, he was not talking at all, was withdrawn and preoccupied with spinning things. He received intervention throughout his preschool years, and by the time he was 6, he was speaking in full sentences. IQ testing at that time showed that his nonverbal IQ was in the superior range. He was able to draw complex, scaled drawings of buildings and memorize train and airplane timetables. He was placed in mainstream classrooms and received supportive services throughout elementary school. Consultative services were provided to his teachers in middle school, to help them adapt their programs to his communicative abilities. He always did well in math and science. His vocabulary was enormous, as one of his hobbies was reading the dictionary. But he had trouble with subjects such as English, history, and geography that required any kind of social understanding. He was perplexed by the feelings described in the literature he read for English class and had a great deal of difficulty understanding the plots of stories. He had a hard time getting along with others, too. Although he no longer spent hours spinning objects, he continued to be preoccupied with his obsessive interests of drawing, map reading, timetables, and dictionary reading. All his attempts at conversation, with peers, teachers, or family, centered on these subjects, and he seemed both mystified by and uninterested in conversing about anything else. Despite his obvious talents in architectural drawing and his superior memory, Michael was unable to use his abilities in a functional way, always falling back into his preoccupations. As he

entered high school, his family's concern about his future increased, and they requested an assessment of his current educational needs, so that some intervention to improve his functional skills could go on during his last years in school.

Michael needs help with several areas of communication to be ready to make the transition from school to higher education or employment. Students like Michael, who have communication abilities at the advanced language level, require help with a variety of skills at the literate end of the oral-literate continuum, as well as with using the skills they have in the most functional manner possible. Let's look at some of the issues we will need to address in designing language intervention programs for adolescents, before we get into our discussion of the intervention itself.

ISSUES IN INTERVENTION AT THE ADVANCED LANGUAGE STAGE

RATIONALE FOR SERVICES TO ADOLESCENTS

It is fair to ask what benefit can be provided to an adolescent like Michael who has received services throughout his school career and will never be "cured" of his disability. Wouldn't he do just as well if left alone to do his best to get through high school without lavishing additional expensive services on him that will probably not make a great deal of difference in his final status at the end of his school years? Although the question is legitimate, there are good reasons for continuing to provide services to adolescents in advanced language stages. Larson and McKinley (2003a) summarized them:

1. The ante is continually "upped" as the student proceeds through the secondary grades. Even if intervention allowed students to function in mainstream settings in elementary school, the more intense demands of the secondary curriculum can often cause students who could "make it" in earlier grades to sink beneath their weight, creating the "porpoise kid" phenomenon (Launer, 1993). The transition from one educational setting to another and from school to work or higher education also places stressful requirements on the shaky communication skills of adolescents with language learning disorders (LLD). Students may need special services in secondary school to allow them to maintain the same level of performance in these new high-demand settings that they were able to achieve in earlier grades.

2. A transition from concrete to formal operational thinking that typically takes place during adolescence is necessary to succeed in the secondary school curriculum. The level of abstract thinking and language use required at this level may not be accessible without support for students with disabilities. The speech-language pathologist (SLP) can provide important linguistic scaffolding to this new level of thinking.

3. Administrators often ask whether the communication needs of students with LLD cannot be managed in the context of the mainstream language arts curriculum, again questioning the need for special services. Here it is important to remember that only academic communication needs are stressed in these settings. Communication skills needed for interaction and functional communication for vocational and independent-living environments are only addressed through services delivered by an SLP, and instruction in these areas is mandated by the 2004 Individuals with Disabilities Education Act (IDEA).

4. Communication programs targeted for adolescents pay off in terms of reduced dropout rates (Larson & McKinley, 2003a). Kaufman, Kwan, Kline, and Chapman (2000) and Rukeyser (1988) have documented that every potential dropout who stays in school saves taxpayers money—in terms of the costs of adult literacy programs, welfare, basic job training, and incarceration—that would have to be spent later if the student dropped out of school. Language services can make the difference for students at risk for leaving school without graduating.

STUDENT-CENTERED INTERVENTION

We've talked before about the importance of engaging the client and fostering a feeling of collaboration between the teen and the clinician to maximize our chances for success. Just as we asked the student to do some self-assessment, we also can involve the student in planning the intervention program. We

can review the assessment results with the student, point out what our testing revealed were strong and weak areas, and ask whether the findings jibe with the student's perception of his or her own problem areas. We can then invite the student to set priorities among the needs identified and choose the skills in which he or she would most like to improve. Adolescent students should be present at the Individualized Educational Plan (IEP) meeting, should discuss service-delivery options with parents and professionals, and should feel a part of the process of determining the intervention program. Adolescent students also should sign the IEP or Individualized Transition Plan (ITP) themselves, along with their parents, to indicate their participation. Myer and Eisenman (2005), in fact, suggest that secondary students should lead the development of their own IEPs, using the planning session as a context for discussion of the students goals, strengths, and needs, allowing the student to choose sections of the IEP that she or he will lead the discussion on in the meeting, and developing a script and role-play activities to prepare the student to present his section of the IEP to the team.

Larson and McKinley (2003a) suggested drawing up a *communication contract* with the adolescent. The contract can state the goals listed in the IEP or ITP and can ask the student to take responsibility for achieving them. By placing responsibility for achieving goals firmly on the student's shoulders, motivation and cooperation are likely to increase. Again, though, it is important to remember that if we expect adolescents to take responsibility for their own goals, we must involve them in the goal-setting process first. Figure 14-1 contains an example of a student communication contract that might be drawn up in collaboration with Michael.

Apel and Swank (1999) and Novak (2002) talked about the importance of developing self-esteem and increasing motivation in our adolescent students. They point out that years of difficulty in school may have led these students to feelings of inadequacy, reduced motivation, and a reluctance to devote effort to additional intervention activities. For this reason, students in the advanced language stage may need counseling, as well as language intervention. Larson and McKinley (2003a) defined counseling in this context as talking with adolescents about their communication problems, giving them information, and providing them with support in facing their feelings about their disability. Adolescence is a turbulent time of life for everyone, and students who are having trouble communicating with others, establishing peer relations, and succeeding in school are likely to be even more frustrated and confused than typical teens. Even if we are offering no direct intervention to an adolescent with LLD and are primarily consulting with teachers and designing curricular adaptations, we can arrange to have a few "chats" with each student. We can talk about how communication is going and where more help is needed, and lend an ear to whatever each student feels a need to tell us. Although it is important to confine our counseling role to issues of communication, we may be able to help direct students to other adults who can help, such as the guidance counselor, school nurse, or another special educator, if additional problems

I _____ hereby agree to complete this contract
  (name)
starting on _____ and ending on _____. I understand
         (date)   (date)
that my overall contract grade for the term will be decided by
averaging the letter grades for each behavioral objective in the
contract.* Grading will be done by the adult who signs the
contract.

  If I do not complete this contract by the date stated, earning an overall grade of at least a C, I will undergo following
consequences:

Have my drawing materials confiscated for 1 week. Give up trips
to the dictionary in the school library for 2 weeks.

_____ _____
Student signature   Professional's signature

Annual goal: improving conversational interaction

Behavioral Objective	Student's grade				
	A	B	C	D	F
Have three conversations with peers about school sports events.	—	—	—	—	—
Make a list of slang terms I hear other students use. Discuss them with (clinician).	—	—	—	—	—
When talking is allowed, ask another student to explain something I don't understand about a story I read in English, at least three different times during the term.	—	—	—	—	—
Make a plan with (clinician) to convince my parents to give me a new privilege. Have a conversation with parents and try to convince them. Discuss conversation with (clinician) to see how it went. Get suggestions for improvement.	—	—	—	—	—

*Make an agreement with the student that full achievement of
the objective will earn an A for that objective, nearly full
achievement a B, and so on.

FIGURE 14-1 ✦ A sample communication contract for Michael. (Adapted from Larson, V., & McKinley, N. (2003a). *Communication Solutions for Older Students.* Eau Claire, WI: Thinking Publications.)

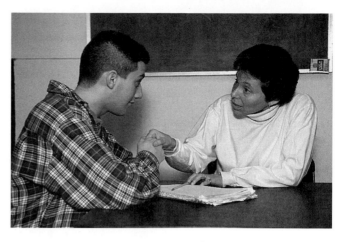

Communication contracts involve students in their intervention planning.

having these "chats," we want to emphasize to students that confidentiality is strictly maintained about any personal information, but if the student tells us about something illegal or dangerous (such as suicidal thoughts), we have to report it.

PRODUCTS OF INTERVENTION IN THE ADVANCED LANGUAGE STAGE

NEW INTERVENTION PURPOSES AT THE ADVANCED LANGUAGE LEVEL

We talked earlier about several different purposes intervention might have. Intervention can attempt to eliminate or "cure" a disorder, change or ameliorate the disorder, or change the way the client responds to the disorder by providing compensatory strategies. In our discussions of intervention up to this point, we have usually identified the purpose of intervention as the second of these choices: changing the disorder. We have had as our purpose the provision of basic communication skills that lessen the client's disability. With adolescents, particularly those in the advanced language stage, however, the third of these purposes also comes into play. That is, for some clients at advanced language stages, who have had years of intervention aimed at changing their disorder, the time has come to help them find ways of compensating for it instead.

  Larson and McKinley (1995) suggested that to succeed at a learning-strategies approach in intervention, students need to function within the average range of intelligence and have reading and oral language skills at least at a fourth-grade level. In other words, students need to be in the advanced language stage as we have defined it here. Students functioning at earlier levels of communicative ability would not be good candidates for this approach because of its reliance on reading and writing skills and its demands for metacognitive capacity. Adolescents who are functioning at language-for-learning (L4L), developing, or emerging language levels should continue to be served with methods appropriate for those levels.

arise. Naturally, we are not psychotherapists, and if a student is having serious emotional problems, referral may be necessary. But very often some understanding remarks from a respected adult and the opportunity to "talk things out" a bit with an accepting listener can be helpful, at least in the short term. In

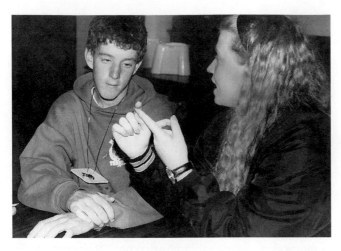

Learning-strategy approaches to intervention are used with students at the advanced language stage.

The advantages of a learning strategies approach, for students for whom it is developmentally appropriate, are that it helps them move toward more independent functioning by teaching them not a basic skill, but a more "meta"-level ability. A learning-strategies approach, as defined by its originators, Allen and Deschler (1979), includes "techniques, principles, or rules that will facilitate the acquisition, manipulation, integration, storage, and retrieval of information across situations and settings." As such, it gives students the tools to improve their own learning abilities, both during the intervention program and after it's over. Ehren (2002) helps to define *strategies* by distinguishing them from *knowledge* and *skills* in the following way:

▶ Knowledge is information we have; for example, vocabulary *knowledge* is having the information to link a referent to a word.

▶ Skills are something we can do; for example, syntactic *skills* allow us to formulate sentences.

▶ Strategies are a deliberate attempt to use the knowledge and skills we have effectively; for example, deciding to summarize a passage we read in order to remember its content is a reading comprehension *strategy.*

Providing students with learning strategies and giving them the opportunity to practice them on curriculum-related material becomes an additional role the SLP can play in intervention for students at the advanced language stage.

THE FUNCTIONAL VERSUS THE ACADEMIC CURRICULUM

A good number of adolescents with LLD will go on to higher education or vocational training after high school. Aune and Friehe (1996) reported that one-third of youth with learning disabilities enrolled in postsecondary school within 5 years of high school graduation. For these students, academic skills continue to be important. We need to address aspects of these students' communication problems that impede their success in the mainstream curriculum. Other students with LLD do

not go on to higher education. And even those who continue in academic settings may have problems with "survival communication," the language skills that allow people to function successfully and autonomously in their homes, jobs, and communities (Novak, 2002). For these reasons, functional language skills need to be part of the intervention program for adolescents with LLD. Functional skills include the ability to ask questions, follow verbal and written instructions, initiate and maintain conversations, use language to initiate and maintain social interactions and relationships, negotiate and solve interpersonal conflicts, gain basic information from writing, use written language to provide basic information on forms, questionnaires, letters, and so on (Novak, 2002). For students with advanced language who need functional communication skill development, a remedial approach, focused on changing the disorder, will probably be necessary. For work directed at improving academic communication, a learning-strategies approach should be at least one aspect of the intervention program.

▌ PROCESSES OF INTERVENTION IN THE ADVANCED LANGUAGE STAGE

Let's talk now about specific processes of intervention for students with LLD in the advanced language stage. As we do, you'll notice that the organizational scheme of the discussion is somewhat different from the one we've been using up to now. Since the purpose of most of our intervention up to this stage has been to provide remediation to change the disorder by alleviating deficits in basic communication skills, we described the process of intervention using the three approaches to this type of remediation that were advanced by Fey (1986): clinician-directed, child-centered, and hybrid. However, in the advanced language stage, we want to look also at intervention aimed not only at remediating deficits but at teaching compensatory strategies. For this reason, we'll organize our discussion of intervention at the advanced language stage along somewhat different lines: we'll talk first about intervention directed at remediating basic deficits in language used for academic and functional contexts, then about intervention using a learning strategies approach. This latter approach is aimed at giving clients the tools for compensating for their difficulties.

BASIC SKILLS APPROACHES TO INTERVENTION IN THE ADVANCED LANGUAGE STAGE

A variety of commercial materials are available for providing basic skill instruction at this level, as are numerous computer software programs. Many suggestions for these materials appeared in Larson and McKinley (2003a). When we use basic skills approaches with adolescents, they can be aimed at both academic and functional skills. Let's look at some of the areas of academic performance for which basic skill intervention is still appropriate. Then we'll talk about some basic skills procedures for improving functional communication in our secondary-school students.

Academic Communication

Semantics. Work on semantic skills in the academic context focuses on words and usages at the literate end of the oral-literate continuum. Jitendra, Edwards, Sacks, and Jacobson (2004) emphasized the close connection between vocabulary knowledge and reading comprehension. They report that students with LLD typically have nonspecific knowledge of word meanings and do not spontaneously use strategies for learning new words from context. They argue that direct instruction in vocabulary is necessary for these individuals. In fact, Beimiller (2003) advocates teaching 300 to 400 new words by direct instruction each year.

The Literate Lexicon. Direct instruction in vocabulary has been found to be highly effective in increasing word knowledge and reading comprehension (Jitendra et al., 2004). Direct instruction involves traditional activities such as giving students lists of words to look up in the dictionary, define orally, use in sentences, find synonyms for, and select correct meanings and uses in multiple choice formats. It is important to remember, however, that if students are required to use a dictionary, they need to be taught how. Explicit explanation of dictionary features, such as alphabetical organization, use of guide words on each page, pronunciation keys, and selection from among several meanings will be necessary. If this instruction has been given in the classroom, the SLP will need to provide reinforcement and practice in the therapeutic setting.

Direct vocabulary instruction can also involve more activity-based methods, such as matching words and meanings in a Concentration game, or "hunting" for words with certain characteristics (roots of *graph, tele*, or prefixes such as *inter-* and *un-*, for example) in assigned texts. Students can also be encouraged to identify unfamiliar words on television shows, newspapers, or curriculum material. They can then be required to find the meaning of these words in a dictionary and teach the meaning to other students in the group. Beck, McKeown, and Omanson (1987) suggested designating students as "Word Wizards" who can earn points by reporting on their own or others' use of new words outside the intervention setting. Moats (2004) suggests using the book *Language! Roots* (Bebko, Alexander, & Ducet, 2001) as a source for sequenced activities involving root words and affixes. Graves (1987) asserted that

games such as Boggle or Scrabble can provide incentives to students to acquire and practice new words. Clinicians can set up tournaments of these games for clients to play among themselves and can use some of the intervention time to provide opportunities for students to work on new vocabulary that they can use to dazzle their opponents in these games. When using direct instructional methods, it is important to remember that practice is necessary to achieve solid knowledge. Hearing, defining, or using a new word only once will not make it a permanent part of the student's lexicon. Clinicians need to provide multiple opportunities for students to interact with their new words. And Bryant, Goodwin, Bryant, and Higgins (2003) reported that students who received some activity-based methods or elaborated exposure along with traditional instruction did better in learning new vocabulary than students who received dictionary instruction alone.

Another way to increase vocabulary knowledge is to expand understanding of words already in students' vocabulary. Elshout-Mohr and van Daalen-Kapteijns (1987) suggested ways to help students consolidate what they know about words and to extend their current meanings. They advocated using Knowledge Rating checklists like the one in Table 12-1 to summarize students' existing knowledge of word meanings drawn from curricular topics. They also suggested having students draw tree diagrams to illustrate how word meanings are connected. Students can choose some related words from a curricular topic, such as a health unit on drug abuse, and work together to construct a tree diagram like the one in Figure 14-2. Fleming and Forester (1997) suggested using materials such as *The Word Kit—Adolescent* (Lanza & Wilson, 1991), *All-Star Vocabulary* (LoGiudice, 2004), *LanguageBurst* (Whiskeyman, 2000), and *Vocabopoly* (Linguisystems, 2002).

Bryant, Goodwin, Bryant, and Higgins (2003) advocate using semantic feature analysis to expand vocabulary knowledge. Here we would present students with a grid, like the one in Table 14-1, with related curriculum words on one axis and a set of attributes relevant to the words on the other. We would first show students a completed grid, like the one in Table 14-1, and discuss the words and attributes. Then students could be given a blank grid and asked to fill it out. New words and attributes can be added to the grid, and new grids developed to work with additional sets of words.

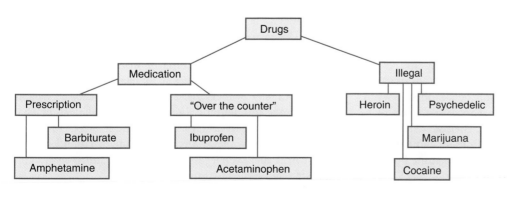

FIGURE 14-2 ✦ Tree diagram for relating word meanings associated with a high school unit on drug abuse. (Adapted from Elshout-Mohr, M., & vanDaalen-Kapteijns, M. [1987]. Cognitive Processes in learning word meanings. In M. McKeown & E. Curtis [Eds.]. *The nature of vocabulary acquisition*. Hillsdale, NJ: Erlbaum.)

TABLE 14-1	A Vocabulary Grid for a Curricular Unit on Prehistoric Biology with Semantic Feature Information

			FEATURE		
WORD	MARINE	EXTINCT	CARNIVOROUS	WINGED	BIPEDAL
Tyrannosaurus	−	+	+	−	+
Stegosaurus	−	+	−	−	−
Crocodile	+	−	+	−	−
Plesiosaur	+	+	+	−	−
Archaeopteryx	−	+	?	+	+
Pterodactyl	−	+	+	+	+

Adapted from Crais, E. (1990). World knowledge to word knowledge. *Topics in Language Disorders, 10,* 45-62.

Gerber (1993) supplied ways to capitalize on the relatedness of words. She advised giving students sets of words that relate in meaning, each on a different card. Students can then be asked to place the cards under related base words. For example,

look	exit
glance	desert
peek	vacate
observe	abandon
glower	depart

The similarities as well as the differences in meaning in these words can be discussed, and students can be encouraged to talk about contexts in which each of the words would be the most appropriate choice. Other techniques for encouraging students to understand the relations among words include visual mapping techniques, like that shown in Figure 14-3. Bryant et al. (2003) showed that visual and graphic organizers were effective in helping students with LLD to acquire new vocabulary. Work on words related by root forms (*clinic, clinician*), using the methods we discussed in Chapter 12, also can be useful for adolescents with LLD, so long as we remember to draw vocabulary items from relevant curriculum topics.

Another way to expand vocabulary knowledge is to work on words with multiple meanings, or *polysemous* words. Vespoor and Lowie (2003) suggested that helping students establish a "core" meaning for each of these words, then elaborating the core with alternate meanings is helpful for improving comprehension and retention. Paul (1992b) suggested one procedure. Students are given, or generate for themselves, a list of words that have multiple meanings and discuss all the meanings they know for each. A dictionary can be used to get additional meanings for the words. Then students write sentences, each containing one of the words used twice, with a different meaning each time. They read their sentences, with "BEEPs" inserted for the target multiple-meaning words. Other students guess what word could be substituted for the BEEP, for example:

I BEEP open this BEEP of beans. (can)

Interactive computer games—such as *Vocabulary Development 2* (Optimum Resource, Inc., 2003), *Accelerated Vocabulary* (Renaissance Learning of Canada, 2002), *WordSmart Software* (Kaplan Writing and Vocabulary Essential Review, Kaplan), *WORDS* (Torgesen & Torgesen, 1985), and *Vocabulary Super Stretch, Set 1 and 2* (Merit Software)—can also be a source of vocabulary development. However, Jitentra et al. in their review of vocabulary instruction (2004) found that results of computer assisted instruction were more mixed than those of direct instruction, so perhaps these methods should be reserved for practice rather than initial introduction of new words.

Finally, an important avenue to learning new words is to encourage students to *ask* about words they do not know. Beimiller (2003) reported that older students benefit from being encouraged to identify and ask for help with unfamiliar words, in an atmosphere that validates and approves their asking.

When working on vocabulary, an important adjunct for older students is attention not only to word meaning and use but also to spelling. Masterson and Crede (1999) pointed out that children with learning disabilities make more frequent spelling errors than age-mates. Scott and Brown (2001) emphasize the importance of ongoing attention to spelling as part of the SLP's role in literacy development. When we work on vocabulary with advanced language students, it is important to remember our principle of integrating oral and written formats. As we call attention to the meaning properties of new words, we also can call attention to their visual (spelled) forms and encourage students to think of words that have related spelling patterns or are derivationally related (e.g., *photograph* is related to *photography*; the short *a* heard in the last syllable of *photograph* can help them remember that *photography* has an *a* in its second-to-last syllable because it is related to this root word. Also, *graph* is a root meaning "writing," seen in other words such as tele*graph*, mono*graph*, and *graph*ic. This root is always spelled with the vowel *a*).

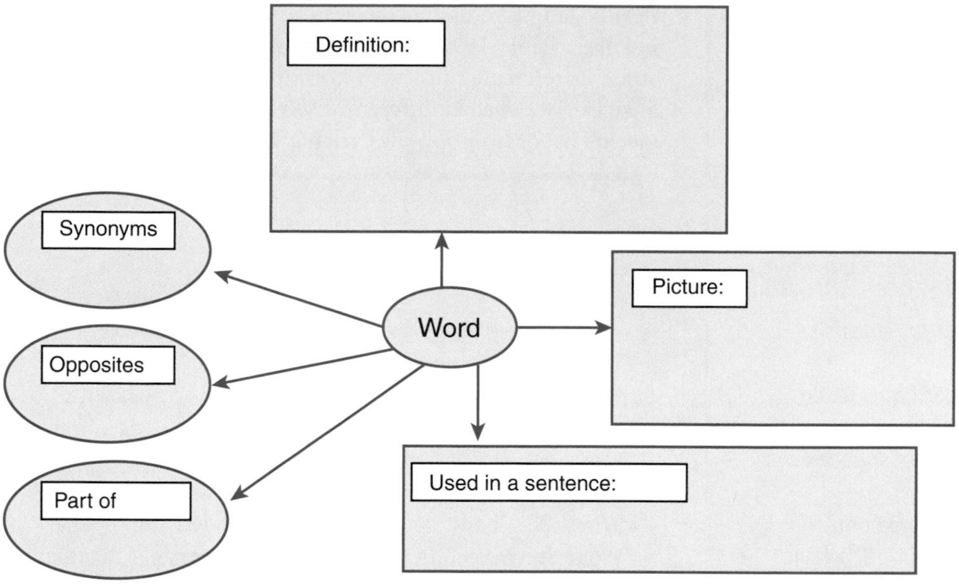

FIGURE 14-3 ✦ Graphic organizer for vocabulary development.

Word Retrieval. Brackenbury and Pye (2005) have argued that a primary semantic difficulty that students with disabilities show is reduced familiarity, and so reduced automaticity of access to words in memory, and reduced number of connections between words. To put it another way, children with language learning disabilities have trouble retrieving words because they know less about the words to begin with, so paths to them are less traveled and less linked to other words and ideas. The implication of this finding is that one way to reduce word retrieval problems is to increase knowledge and connections among the words the student knows. Many of the techniques we discussed in Chapter 12 for addressing word-retrieval problems, including providing elaborated, multiple exposure to deepen word knowledge and build semantic network connections, also are appropriate for adolescents who continue to have word-finding difficulties. Bryant, Goodwin, Bryant, and Higgins (2003) reviewed literature showing that using these kinds of "concept enhancement" approaches to vocabulary acquisition is more effective than instruction through definitions alone.

German (1992) provided additional suggestions for improving word retrieval. She advocated having students stabilize the phonological form of words by practicing saying, then writing the target words several times alone, and then saying and writing each word in five different sentences. While practicing saying the target word, students are told to tap once for each syllable. While writing the word, they are told to draw a line between syllables. Semantic information about target words also can be stabilized. This can be done by having students discuss a group of words within the same semantic category and list the semantic attributes that differentiate them. German emphasized the importance of carrying this work out in groups, rather than in one-to-one settings exclusively, and of providing the intervention in a variety of settings to generalize the program's effects. We also can address these problems through a learning-

strategies approach, by teaching students to consciously invoke both semantic and phonological cues to help recall words. We'll discuss these approaches in the section on learning strategies.

Figurative Language. Norbury (2004) pointed out that the most important aspect of an intervention program on figurative language is repeated exposure. Because of their deficits in reading, students with LLD may not have encountered figurative language as often as their peers; the latter absorb more secondary-level reading material, where figurative language appears more frequently than it does in conversation. It is important for students with LLD to hear figurative language in poetry and literature read to them by teachers and clinicians if they cannot read it themselves. Several books for teens include many examples of these forms. *Not Quite Human: Batteries Not Included* (McEvoy, 1985), *The Phantom Tollbooth* (Juster, 1961), *Ace Hits the Big Time* (Murphy & Wolkoff, 1981), *The Realm of Possibility* (Levithan, 2004), *Bucking the Sarge* (Curtis, 2004), and *Airborn* (Oppel, 2004) are some good examples. Poetry is an especially rich source of figurative language and may be easier for students with LLD, since it is typically short. Collections that might interest adolescents include *Once upon a Poem* (Crossley-Holland, 2004), *Things I Have to Tell You: Poems and Writing by Teenage Girls* (Franco, 2001), and *You Hear Me? Poems and Writing by Teenage Boys* (Franco, 2001). In addition, Palmer and Brookes (2004) provide a list of resources for work on figurative language. These appear in Box 14-1.

Exposure alone, of course, is not enough. Some supportive scaffolding is necessary to help students assimilate the figurative language they hear. Literature selections from English class can be read to students, who can be encouraged to be "detectives" looking for similes and metaphors. Students can be asked to raise a hand whenever they hear one of these figures, so the teacher can write it down for discussion at the end of the selected reading. Advertisements from newspapers or magazines also are good sources of figurative language.

BOX 14-1	**Resources for Teaching Figurative Language**

Cox, J. (1980). *Put your foot in your mouth and other silly sayings*. New York: Random House.

Davis, J., and Davis, L. (2001). Double meanings. *School Library Media Activities Monthly, 18(3)*, 42-22.

Feare, R. (1996). *Everyday idioms: For reference and practice*. New York: Addison-Wesley.

Gravois, M. (2002). *Hands-on activities for learning idioms*. New York: Scholastic.

Terban, M. (1983). *In a pickle and other funny idioms*. New York: Houghton-Mifflin.

Terban, M. (1993). *It figures: Fun figures of speech*. New York: Scholastic.

Terban, M. (1998). *Scholastic dictionary of idioms, phrases, sayings, and expressions*. New York: Scholastic.

Adapted from Palmer, B., & Brooks, M. (2004). Reading until the cows come home: Figurative language and reading comprehension. *Journal of Adolescent and Adult Literacy, 47*, 370-379.

After some period of exposure, Gerber (1993) suggested giving students pairs of words that lend themselves to figurative usage (*eyes* and *stars*, *snake* and *river*) and asking students to use them to construct similes and metaphors, in the context of advertisements for fictitious products or descriptions of people the student knows. Wallach and Miller (1988) suggested further that students be asked then to generate their own lists of word pairs, exchange them with other students, and come up with figurative forms suggested by their peers' sets of words.

Other forms of figurative language, such as idioms and slang, which are common in everyday speech, can be addressed in a similar way. Here students can be asked to keep a notebook, in which they write down every slang or idiomatic expression they hear people using over the course of 1 week. Students can bring their lists to the clinician or to communication class to exchange and discuss with other students. Clinicians can encourage the students to decide which expressions they like and might want to use themselves. They can role-play appropriate contexts for using each expression. Gerber (1993) provided additional suggestions for work on figurative language, and commercial materials, such as Spector's (1997) *Saying One Thing, Meaning Another, Figures of Speech: Multiple Meanings for the Young Adult* (McCarr, 1995), *Slangman Guides* (Burke, 2003), *The Idiom Game* (Wisniewski, 2003), *Idioms* (Paris & Paris, 2005), and *Figurative Language* (Gorman-Gard, 1992) also are helpful.

Humor is another common figurative language vehicle, and students with LLD often have trouble understanding the humor used by peers. Again, students can be asked to collect jokes they hear in a notebook and discuss them with the clinician or communication class. Students also can be guided to produce their own jokes in an effort to help them learn the

flexible language use and awareness of ambiguity that humor involves. Paul (1992b) suggested one procedure for getting students to create puns with homophones (words that sound alike but are spelled differently [*beet* and *beat*]). Students are given a list of homophones, such as:

bow/bough
deer/dear
do/dew
feat/feet

The clinician then gives the students several examples of puns or ambiguous statements that can be created with these words, such as:

My favorite vegetable can't be beet/beat.
What's black and white and re(a)d all over? [newspaper]
What do you call it when a bunch of steers get together on a railroad line? [a track mee(a)t]

Students are then encouraged to come up with their own humorous statements, riddles, or puns using these word pairs. Hamersky's (1995) *Cartoon Cut-Ups* is another useful commercial program for this purpose.

Verbal Reasoning. Masterson and Perry (1999) developed a program that included direct instruction and activities from the school curriculum to train verbal reasoning skills. They reported that students involved in the program showed significant improvement in verbal reasoning relative to peers with LLD who did not receive the training. Their training procedure is outlined in Box 14-2.

Wegerif (2002) demonstrated that using a verbal reasoning program in which students were taught in a group to "talk through" nonverbal problems, such as science or math assignments, resulted in significantly better verbal reasoning test scores for trained than untrained students. This finding suggests that using groups or communication classroom opportunities to help students develop verbal reasoning skills in peer interactive settings can be helpful in addressing this area.

Simon (1991b) also described a program designed to improve verbal reasoning in students with LLD. Activities in this program include, first, helping students differentiate emotional from logical arguments. Students look for "hidden persuaders" in advertising and identify logical, as opposed to emotional, appeals. A second activity involves reading letters to the editor in the local newspaper and identifying the premise and conclusion in the letter. The clinician then helps the student to state the letter's argument as a syllogism ("New taxes are needed if and only if there is no waste in government. There is waste in government; therefore, new taxes are not needed."). Students can then be asked to argue against the letter writer by stating a different syllogism and translating it into a letter to the editor. (Some may even be sent to the local paper, if students use especially cogent reasoning!)

Commercial programs, such as *Analogies for Thinking and Talking* (Nelson & Gillespie, 1992) and *501 Word Analogies*

BOX 14-2	**Masterson and Perry's (1999) Program for Training Verbal Reasoning Skills**

Phase I: Mediated Learning (Sessions 1-5)

Step 1: Define terms and model solution of verbal reasoning problems.

Encoding: Picture each term of the problem and think of a list of attributes for it.

Example: **(A)**horse:[is to] **(B)**foal::[as] **(C)**cow:[is to] **(D)**_____.

I'll picture horse, foal, and cow in my mind, and make a list of features for each, such as:

Horse	Foal	Cow
Animal	Animal	Animal
Adult	Baby	Adult
Eats grass	Eats grass	Eats grass

Inferring: Find the relationship between terms A and B in the problem.

Example: How are horse and foal related? A foal is a baby horse.

Mapping: Use the relationship found for A to B, and find a similar relationship for C and D.

Example: If a foal is a baby horse, then I need to find a baby for the cow.

Applying: Choose an answer that has the same relationship to C as B had to A in the problem.

Example: A foal is a baby horse, and a calf is a baby cow; so calf is the correct answer.

Step 2: Picture analogies. Present problems in the form of pictures. Use group practice, then individual practice on worksheets.

Example: Picture of horse, picture of colt, picture of cow, picture of calf

Step 3: Present analogies in sentence form. Have students read and complete them.

Example: A baseball player makes a home run, just like a soccer player makes a _____.

Step 4: Present paragraphs that contain similes and have students explain the relationship.

Example: Astronauts are like Christopher Columbus because _____.

Then have students construct analogous paragraphs as a group.

Individually complete a worksheet with verbal analogies.

Step 5: After reviewing previous lessons, read a story such as *The Lorax* (Seuss, 1971). Have the students think of real-life situations that are similar to the story. Then have each student generate an analogy from the story and solve each other's analogies.

Phase II: Bridging (Sessions 6–16)

A series of activities is presented that help students use the processes of analogical thinking in everyday activities.

Example: Students are given a recipe that feeds two people and must figure out how to use it to feed 12.

Questions & Answers (LearningExpress, 2002), have been designed to assist students in developing deductive or analogical reasoning skills. Standardized tests students take for college admission have traditionally involved analogical problems, and the books designed to prepare students for these tests frequently contain examples of analogies that students can practice and discuss. Some computer-assisted analogical reasoning programs also are available. *Analogies Tutorial* (Hartley Software, 1992) is one example.

Simon (1991b) also suggested using visual aids to help understand logical relations. For example, students can be given the syllogism, "Ray runs faster than Tim, and Zack runs slower than Tim. Who runs the slowest?" They can then be encouraged to write the initial of each person to represent his position in order to help process the problem:

R

T

Z

Eventually, the clinician can help the students translate these logical problems to symbolic equations by providing examples such as:

$J = H$

Jessica is as tall as Hank.

Marie is as tall as Jessica.

$M = J$

Therefore, Marie is as tall as Hank.

$M = H$

Other logical relationships can be depicted using Venn diagrams, to show how categories are related (Figure 14-4).

Simon also suggested a program on practical logic by Lipman and Sharp (1974), entitled *Harry Stottlemeier's Discovery*, as useful for addressing this area.

Syntax. The goal of syntactic intervention in the advanced language stage is to increase flexibility and help students process and produce language at the literate end of the oral-literate continuum. Nippold, Ward-Lonergan, and Fanning (2005) showed that by age 11, typical students are near adult levels in most aspects of syntax in writing, so that increasing syntactic complexity needs to be part of an intervention program for writers with generally simple sentence structures during the secondary school years. Strong (1986) suggested sentence-combining activities as an effective way to achieve these goals. Students are given sets of simple sentences, drawn from curricular themes or literature selections, and asked to find a variety of ways of combining them into one complex sentence. Gerber (1993) advocated providing sets of sentences that can be combined with a particular syntactic device, such as a relative clause:

> Sound waves strike the eardrum. The eardrum sends vibrations to the middle ear. (Sound waves strike the eardrum, which sends vibrations to the middle ear.)
> The refugees moved away. The community rejected the refugees. (The refugees that the community rejected moved away.)

Later another device, such as the temporal clause, can be introduced:

> The European settlers in North America had friendly relations with Native Americans. Disputes over land and treaties caused conflict. (At first, European settlers in North America had friendly relations with Native Americans, but later disputes over land and treaties caused conflict.)

Killgallon and Killgallon (2000) provided a sequenced program to develop sentence-combining skills, which is outlined in Table 14-2.

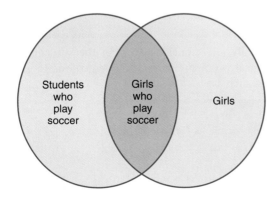

FIGURE 14-4 ✦ Venn diagram.

Gerber also suggested working with sentence manipulation as another avenue to increasing syntactic flexibility. Here, she advocated writing phrases or clauses on cards and having students physically manipulate the cards to arrive at different combinations. For example, the following phrases and clauses could be written, each on a separate card:

> at night
> at our house
> we aren't allowed to watch television
> until we have finished our homework

Students can then be encouraged to see how many different sentences they can make by coming up with different orderings of the phrases and clauses.

Teaching students to combine sentences will move toward increasing two of the indices of syntax that we assessed: T-unit length and the subordination index. To improve students' use of the low-frequency forms listed in Table 13-6 we need to provide exposure to literary language in which the forms appear. If students' reading skills make comprehension of grade-level textbook and literature material difficult, we can encourage parents to read this material to students as part of the students' homework. In addition, we can encourage parents to read other grade-level appropriate literature to the student. If students balk at being read to, parents might try reading the material onto an audiotape and having the student listen to the tape on a personal listening system. Also, many excellent books are available on tape at libraries, and students who refuse to be read to can be assigned to listen to these books on tape as part of their communication-class homework. The school librarian can help the clinician identify grade-appropriate books on tape.

Exposure to literary language is, of course, necessary but not sufficient. Scott (2005) reported that students with LLD show less diversity of sentence types in their writing than typical students do. This suggests that an important intervention activity will be to help students learn to say what they mean in a variety of ways, using a range of sentence forms. Paraphrasing activities are one way to accomplish this. Paraphrasing can be used to encourage students to try out low-frequency forms in their own communication. Here students can choose sentences from textbooks and provide several alternate forms for each one. To increase use of low-frequency forms in this activity, students can be given a list of "dandy language" forms, like the list in Table 13-6. The clinician can discuss the forms with students and work together to identify examples of these forms in the text selection. After some discussion, students can be encouraged, with the clinician's model, to use the forms in some of their paraphrases. Paraphrasing is an important skill to learn, in and of itself, since it helps students in summarizing and in using information from other sources for inclusion in their own writing. Additional suggestions for working on advanced syntax can be found in Haussamen's (2003) *Grammar Alive! A Guide for Teachers.*

Nippold (2000) reminds us of the importance of context in language complexity. Nippold et al. (2005) found use of

TABLE 14-2	**Sequenced Steps for Teaching Syntactic Patterns**	

SYNTACTIC FORM	STEP	EXAMPLE FROM HOLES (SACHAR, 1998)
Prepositional phrases	Define: Direct instruction in target form	A prepositional phrase starts with a preposition (give list of examples) and is followed by a noun and modifiers (give examples). It is used to describe and elaborate the meaning of the word it modifies.
		If you take a bad boy and make him dig a hole every day in the hot sun it will turn him into a good boy.
	Identify: Students find and underline target forms in classroom text	If you take a bad boy and make him dig a hole every day _in the hot sun_ it will turn him _into a good boy_.
	Combine: Students combine given sentences from classroom text by putting the underlined part of the second sentence at the (^) symbol in the first, using the target form, then write the new sentence.	If you take a bad boy and make him dig a hole every day ^ he will turn^; _in the hot sun, into a good boy_.
	Unscramble: Students are given a list of sentence parts from classroom text to unscramble, then write out, underlining the target form in each.	it will turn him and make him dig a hole every day in the hot sun if you take a bad boy into a good boy If you take a bad boy and make him dig a hole every day _in the hot sun_ it will turn him _into a good boy_.
	Expand: Students are given a sentence and told to complete it with a target form where the ^ symbol appears.	If you take a bad boy and make him dig a hole every day ^, it will turn him ^.
	Combine to imitate: Students are given a model sentence from a classroom text, then several related sentences to combine, following the model.	If you take a bad boy and make him dig a hole every day in the hot sun it will turn him into a good boy. There was once a lake there. It was a large lake. That was over a hundred years ago.
	Write your own: Students are given a writing prompt related to the literature selection, and are asked to write a paragraph using a least three examples of the target form.	Everyone feels "cursed" sometimes. Write about a time you did. Use three prepositional phrases.
Participial phrases	Define Identify Combine Unscramble Expand Combine to imitate Write your own	
Compound verbs	Define Identify Combine Unscramble Expand Combine to imitate Write your own	
Adjective clauses	Define Identify Combine Unscramble Expand Combine to imitate Write your own	
Adverbial clauses	Define Identify Combine Unscramble Expand Combine to imitate Write your own	

Adapted from Kilgallon, D., & Kilgallon, J. (2000). *Sentence composing for elementary school: A worktext to build better sentences.* Portsmouth, NH: Heinemann.

significantly more complex syntax in persuasive than in other forms of discourse. This suggests that clinicians should use contexts such as persuasive talks and essays when working on complex syntax. As we do so, we can help students incorporate more complex forms into these discourse situations by reminding them to use introducers such as *in my opinion*, verbal organizers such as *first, next, finally*, conjuncts such as *consequently* and *as a result*, and markers such as *in summary*. Owens (2004) suggests giving students prompt cards like the one in Figure 14-5 and requiring them to use these forms appropriately within their persuasive talk or essay. This can provide an opportunity to help students increase the complexity of their syntax in a pragmatically appropriate way.

Pragmatics

Classroom Discourse. Creaghead (1992) suggested a series of activities that can be used to improve students' ability to function in the secondary classroom. Box 14-3 summarizes an adaptation of Creaghead's program for students at the advanced language stage. Using this approach, students would first be helped to recognize scripts, like those we looked at in Table 12-4 that describe the routines of the classroom with which the student is having trouble. These routines can be identified by the student in consultation with the clinician by reviewing information derived from self-assessments or teacher interviews like the one in Box 13-3.

Norris and Hoffman (1993) suggested using graphic organizers to help students with LLD manage the rules of the classroom. Secondary students can, for example, develop diagrams to summarize classroom rules, and contrast the rules they have to follow in different classes. They can first be asked to list rules for each class, using a script analysis procedure like the one in Box 14-3. They can examine the scripts for each class, noting the similarities and differences. The clinician can then help them to develop a diagram like the one in Figure 14-6 to describe the rules for various classes.

Gallagher (1991) also suggested using peers in informal modeling contexts to improve the classroom communication skills of students with LLD. Many secondary classrooms use some form of cooperative learning, in which students complete assignments by working in groups. These settings provide ideal opportunities for students with LLD to experience peer modeling of cooperative communication. Johnson and Johnson (1990) emphasized the need to develop social skills for cooperative learning to build trust and support within the group and to help students learn to resolve conflicts. This aspect of cooperative learning provides an excellent collaborative intervention opportunity. The SLP can offer to run the first few cooperative learning group sessions, in which students practice these social skills as well as the "rules of the game" for cooperative interaction. Activities that teach social skills and promote bonding within the group benefit the student with LLD and provide peer models of appropriate interaction. These activities also are useful for facilitating cooperative interaction among the mainstream students.

Video modeling is another technique that can be used to improve classroom discourse and social skills. Charlop-Christy,

Instructions: Include the following sections and use at least one suggested form in each section in your persuasive piece:	
Sections	**Suggested forms**
Introduction	In my opinion…
	I believe…
	From my point of view,…
	I think…
Body:	
Connecting words, such as	
	… if…
	… although…
	… even though…
	… although…
	… as a result…
	… consequently…
Counter-opinions, such as	Although…
	However…
	On the other hand…
	To/on the contrary…
	Even though…
Logical organizers, such as	First, next, last…
	For example…
	Most importantly…
	In addition…
Mental words, such as	Think…
	Consider…
	Remember…
	Believe…
	Know…
Conclusion	To summarize…
	In summary…
	In conclusion…
	After considering…

FIGURE 14-5 ✦ Example prompt card to increase complex syntax in persuasive discourse. (Adapted from Owens, R. (2004). *Language disorders: A functional approach to assessment and intervention* (4th ed.). Boston, MA: Allyn & Bacon, p. 406.)

BOX 14-3	A Program for Using Script Analysis to Improve Classroom Discourse Skills in Adolescents with LLD

Step 1: Outline the script

Have the students tell everything they know about the script, including participants, sequence of events, objects needed, and so on. ("Let's list everything that happens when you have to write a composition in English class.")

Step 2: Brainstorm variations

Suggest some variations, and ask students how they would react to each. ("What would you do if the principal came in while the class was writing?")

Step 3: Specify the cues for activating the script

Many students with LLD miss crucial verbal and nonverbal cues given by the teacher during class routines. Encourage students to identify the cues they need to identify. ("What does the teacher do when it's time to stop writing?")

Step 4: Role-play the script

Have students take turns acting out student and teacher roles in this routine. Playing the teacher may help to make students more aware of subtle cues teachers give.

Step 5: Provide strategies for coping with weaknesses

Identify areas in which the student continues to have trouble, and provide reminding systems. Consult with teachers to encourage them to offer similar reminders in the classroom. A teacher might be encouraged to say to the student, for example, "Remember, it's our rule that if you finish your composition before time is up, you should edit your work. Check the editing guide on the board to help you remember where to begin."

Adapted from Creaghead, N. (1992). Mutual empowerment through collaboration: A new script for an old problem. In W.A. Second (Ed.). *Best practices in school speech language pathology* (vol. II, pp. 109-116). Austin, TX: Psychological Corporation: Harcourt Brace Jovanovich.

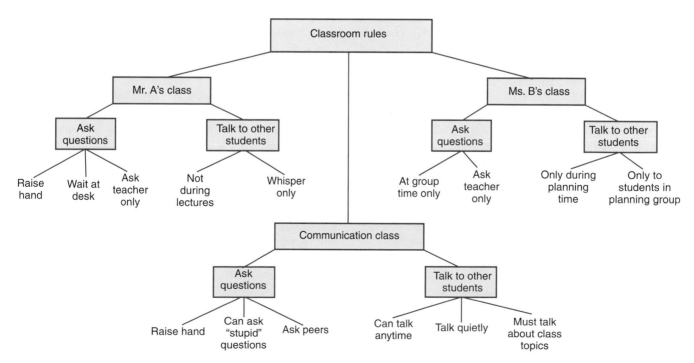

FIGURE 14-6 ✦ Flow chart for comparing classroom rules. (Adapted from Norris, J., & Hoffman, P. [1993]. *Whole language intervention for school-age children.* San Diego, CA: Singular Publishing.)

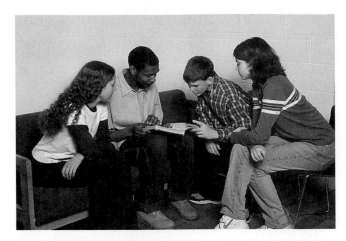

Cooperative learning groups provide opportunities for inclusion of students with LLD.

Le, and Freeman (2000) showed that having children watch peers enact social situations, discuss, and summarize what they had seen, then reenact the scenes themselves resulted in improvement in social functioning. Having several peers act out classroom discourse situations on video can be an additional method of helping students with LLD practice these skills.

Narrative

Comprehension. Basic-skills approaches to narrative comprehension involve, again, exposure to the complex, multiepisode narratives that characterize adolescent and adult literature. Reading and listening to good stories are key here. Again, students whose reading levels preclude independent reading of books like these might listen to parents read them, as homework, or listen to audiotaped readings. *Sarah, Plain and Tall* (MacLachlan, 1985), *Stone Fox* (Gardiner, 1980), *Saving Lenny* (Willey, 1991), *Emako Blue* (Woods, 2004), *Gabriel's Story* (Durham, 2002), *A Northern Light* (Donnelly, 2003), and *Phoenix Rising, or How to Survive Your Life* (Grant, 1989) are some examples of books with these structures that will appeal to teens. The "Reluctant Reader List," published with yearly updates by the American Library Association, provides additional suggestions and is available from school librarians and through public libraries.

Staskowski and Creaghead (2001) provided a sequence of activities that can help children comprehend stories that they hear or read. These include the following:

▶ *Establish a purpose*: Help students decide why reading or hearing this story is important. Reasons might include learning classroom content, answering questions provided by the teacher or clinician, or finding new information of interest to the student.

▶ *Activate prior knowledge*: Help students remember what they already know. For example, in preparing to read Shirley Jackson's *The Lottery*, students can be encouraged to tell what they know about lotteries, share experiences with buying lottery tickets, skim through the story and put "sticky notes" at points where they recognize similarities or differences to the lotteries with which they have had experience.

▶ *Make predictions*: Have students preview the text, pictures, chapter headings, etc. to make guesses about what the story will contain; read one section then have the students predict what may happen next.

▶ *Ask questions*: Have students generate a list of questions, based on their predictions, to be asked during and after reading. Make a chart to record answers.

▶ *Visualize*: Encourage students to 'draw a picture in their mind' of objects and events in the story. Have them describe their image of what characters and scenes from the story look like, or draw pictures to illustrate the story.

Page and Stewart (1985) suggested working on narrative comprehension by having students use inferencing and prediction skills to sequence paragraphs contained in a story or episode. The clinician can photocopy a chapter from a literature selection, cut it into one- to two-paragraph segments, scramble them, and have students put them in correct sequence.

Stanfa and O'Shea (1998) suggested several ways to use drama to enhance students' narrative comprehension. Some examples include the following:

▶ *Use improvisational scenes* to activate a preparatory set before reading. For example, if students are going to read *Romeo and Juliet*, they might talk first about an experience they had of meeting a new boy/girl at a party, and wanting to talk more with the stranger. Students can discuss what they did, what they wish they had done, etc. They can then act out the situation. These improvisations can be recalled during the reading of the literature selection.

▶ *Use improvisations* to explore and enhance understanding of characters in the story. For example, if students are reading a biography of Ben Franklin, they might talk about what kind of person Franklin was, and how he might react to situations such as arriving in a new country or meeting a new person. Students can then act out their impressions and discuss why they had the character act as they did.

▶ *Involve students in writing and acting* in plays to enrich their understanding of stories they read or hear. Students can convert stories or novels they read to plays or adapt literature selections to their own experiences or to contemporary themes and write a new play based on the adaptation. For example, if students read *The War of the Worlds*, they might write a play about what an alien invasion would be like if it happened today. If video equipment is available, the students may tape their play to show to family members.

Activities in which students write or act out fictional interviews, using a book such as *Interview with a Vampire* (Rice, 1976) as a model, can help work on inferencing and character motivation. The clinician might provide students with a list of questions to "ask" their favorite character, and the students must infer or predict what their character would say in response. The clinician can help students refine their answers with probes such as the following:

▶ Why would (character) answer that way?

▶ Does that answer go along with everything else you know about (character)?

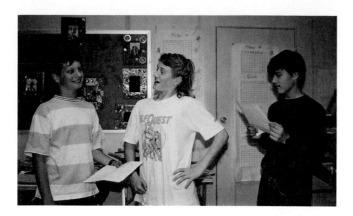

Acting out narratives can deepen students' understanding of this genre.

What happens in your book that makes you think (character) would answer that way?

Work on summarizing is another way to develop narrative comprehension. If students need to write book reports for English class, the clinician can use these as an opportunity to develop summarizing skills with the student. A communication class might also develop its own "Book Review" magazine. With guidance and feedback from the clinician, students would write "reviews" that include a summary of the book's plot and the student's assessment of the book's literary quality and potential appeal for other students. Students also can give "book talks" for younger classes or in the communication class, in which they give similar information orally.

Swanson and De La Paz (1998) suggest teaching story summarizing skills by having students locate story elements in the text and list them on paper, or use a graphic organizer. The list or map can then be transferred to paragraph form. Ae-Hwa, Vaughn, Wanzek, and Shangjin (2004) have shown that using graphic organizers improves reading comprehension for students with LLD.

Westby and Clauser (2005) emphasize the importance, as part of work on narrative comprehension, of helping students understand the "landscape of consciousness;" that is, the way characters' plans, emotions, and intentions govern actions, as well as the way in which point of view determines how events are perceived. Understanding these internal states is crucial to full comprehension of many stories. To address this issue, they suggest using stories such as "The Blind Men and the Elephant," *Voices in the Park* (Brown, 1998), *Passage to Freedom: The Sugihara Story* (Mochizuki, 1997), and *John Brown, Rose, and the Midnight Cat* (Wagner, 1980), all of which tell the same story from several characters' perspectives. Students can then create visual organizers, like the one in Table 14-3, to discuss and describe the various perspectives in the story.

Narrative Production. Narrative writing is also an appropriate target of basic instruction at this level. Larson and McKinley (2003a) reiterate the importance of explicit direct instruction that helps students understand the sequence and cause-effect relationships in stories. They also emphasize the importance of using oral storytelling as a context for addressing some of the oral language difficulties so often seen in students with LLD, such as speech disruptions, syntactic errors, and word-finding problems. Montgomery and Kahn (2003) provide suggestions for teaching students with language learning disabilities using a scaffolded composition process. This process can include the following:

Introduce concept of author: Explain that the author has control of an entire fictional universe with power to make all the decisions about it. Tell students, "You are going to be an author!"

Refer to the aspects of the story, using a poster or graphic organizer:

Setting

Characters

Problem

Attempt

Consequence

Resolution

Assist the student to make a decision about each element in planning the story (e.g., *Adult:* "Who will your characters be?"

TABLE 14-3	Character Perspective Map for *Passage to Freedom: The Sugihara Story* (Mochizuki, 1997)	
STORY EVENT	MR. SUGIHARA'S PERSPECTIVE	PERSPECTIVE OF JEWISH FAMILIES
Outbreak of WWII	Doing his job; obeying orders	Worried, unsure of what will happen
Jewish families arrive from Poland	Torn between duty to superiors and desperate needs of families seeking visas	Desperate to escape deportation
Lithuania is conquered by Russia	Determined to carry his humanitarian efforts as far as possible	Frantic for last chance at escape

Adapted from Westby, C., & Clauser, P. (2005). The right stuff for writing: Assessing and facilitating written language. In H. Catts & A. Kahmi (Eds.). *Language and reading disabilities* (2nd ed.). (pp. 274-340). Boston: Allyn & Bacon.

Student: "I don't know" *Adult:* "They could be teenagers, adults, children, animals, aliens, anybody. You decide." If the student cannot make a decision, suggest teenagers. Continue with a similar process until each element has been addressed).

▶ *Have the student draw a sequence story*: Divide a sheet of paper into six or eight sections, and have the student draw a simple stick figure drawing to outline the story

▶ *Have the student describe the main characters*: Encourage the students to give detailed descriptions of who the characters are, what they look like, what they like and do.

▶ *Use the poster or graphic organizer*: Encourage the student to write or tell each aspect of the story, following their picture sequence and incorporating the information they produced about their characters. Use questions to scaffold the student's production, giving suggestions only when the student refuses or is unable to make a choice.

▶ *Support the student in writing or dictating the story*: Help select words, sentence forms, and spelling. Encourage students to try various forms orally to see how they sound before writing them.

▶ *Revise*: Use the opportunity for incidental teaching about spelling, punctuation, capitalization, and so on, whether the student writes the story himself or dictates it. Encourage the student also to think about word choice and consider alternative wordings, using a dictionary or thesaurus.

When working on producing narratives, we want to talk frequently with students about characters' motivations and internal responses. Using some of the "trickster tales" we discussed in Chapter 12 can be a starting point for younger adolescents. Discussions of all the stories we work on should center on plans, motivations, and internal responses. When students write stories or plays, for example, the clinician can help them focus on making internal response elements explicit by asking questions such as:

Why does (character) do that?
What is (character)'s plan?
How does (character) feel about what happened?

Basic skill instruction in narrative production can also include use of cohesive elements: pronouns, connectives, and other cohesive markers, such as those in Box 13-4. Many of the activities we outlined for working on use of pronouns and conjunctions as cohesive markers in Chapter 12 can be adapted for adolescents by using grade-appropriate materials. Work on conjuncts and other advanced forms of cohesion can begin, again, with exposure. We can explain to students about the use of one or more types of these cohesive markers and give them texts containing marked examples. Students can be asked to explain how the two elements are linked. If students are reading *A Wrinkle in Time* (L'Engle, 1962) in class, for example, we might give them the following pairs of sentences adapted from the story and ask them to identify the cohesive element present in each:

Now they were in the clouds. They could see nothing but drifting whiteness. (lexical cohesion)
In front . . . Charles Wallace sat quietly. Once he turned . . . (pronoun cohesion)
Below them were still rocks . . . but now . . . Meg could see where the mountain at last came to an end. (substitution)
As they moved through the greyness, Meg caught a glimpse of slaglike rocks. Still, there were no traces of trees or bushes. (conjunct)

After talking about the cohesive devices they encounter in their reading, students can be asked to produce several different pairs of sentences, each containing one of the devices discussed. When they have practiced producing series of sentences with different devices, they can write a group story in which each member has the responsibility for including one of the devices studied. Eventually, students can be asked to write individual stories with some of these cohesive elements in them. Jago (2002) presents additional ideas for enhancing cohesion in student writing.

One particularly useful technique for improving cohesive writing is sentence combining (Keen, 2004). Keen showed that encouraging students to combine sentences during rewriting, modeling and prompting the use of grammatical forms such as the subordinate clauses, results in improvements in the coherence of students' writing. This is just another example of the ways in which SLPs, in their legitimate role of helping students expand their grammatical development, can achieve improvements in students' ability to elaborate their meaning and establish cohesion in both speech and writing.

Other Discourse Genres. In addition to work on narrative, basic skills instruction in other written language genres will often be necessary for students at the advanced language stage.

Writing Mechanics. Writing instruction will undoubtedly include mechanics: spelling, punctuation, capitalization, and handwriting. Although these skills have often been taught in the mainstream language arts program and students in secondary school "should" have mastered these basics. Many of our clients with LLD probably did not "get it" the first time around, however. Intelligible writing requires these fundamentals, and students who have trouble with written communication need help with these building blocks, just as a preschooler with unintelligible speech needs help in producing fundamental speech sounds. Delpit (1988) pointed out that many secondary teachers refuse to teach these basics, because they consider it the elementary teacher's job. They tend to concentrate instead on the process and content aspects of writing. That's why it is sometimes necessary for us as language specialists to step into the breach and provide some basic-level instruction in writing mechanics for our older students with LLD. Again, using the revision process as an incidental teaching opportunity for addressing these mechanics helps students see their relevance (Kervin, 2002). Novak (2002) reminded us of the importance of continuing to use multi-modal activities with adolescents with LLD, just as we did for their younger counterparts. Involving a range of sensory and motor behaviors can maximize the chances that information will be retained, and will also be more engaging for students. Van Zile (2003) suggested some multimodal activities that can be used to practice mechanical skills for writing. One appears in Box 14-4.

Moore (1989) presented a concise set of rules for capitalization and punctuation that can be made into posters, "rulebooks," or "crib sheets." Posters with sets of such rules or "crib sheets" for individual students can be used in the communication class. Students can bring writing samples from other classes to the communication class. Work on editing them can proceed through several passes over the document: one for appropriate spelling, one for capitalization, and one for each type of punctuation in turn (period, comma, question mark, apostrophe, quotation mark, etc.). At the beginning of each pass, students can be referred to the rules governing use of the element being examined. In the context of a communication class, a unit on editing might include exercises in which students are given writing samples of the teacher's in which they are to identify errors. As we discussed earlier, these could at first contain cues such as highlighting on sentences that have a mistake for the student to find. Gradually, the cues can be faded.

Handwriting problems can often be addressed by allowing students to use word-processing equipment for written work. This is not always the easy solution it sounds, since students with fine-motor problems that impair handwriting have fine-motor problems on a keyboard, too. And in some contexts keyboarding may not be an option; for example, the new SAT writing test requires handwritten responses. Still, this form of compensatory programming can make it possible for the student's work to be read, even if it remains laborious for the student to produce. Most secondary schools have keyboarding courses, and students using word processors for written work should be encouraged to take these as electives. Using a keyboard for class note-taking, examinations, and assignments is a legitimate accommodation for students with LLD, and can be included on their IEPs.

MacArthur, Haynes, and DeLa Paz (1996) suggested using speech synthesis and word prediction software to help students with poor legibility and spelling. This software is often used to enable students with severe speech disorders to express themselves by "writing out loud," having the software produce spoken versions of what the student spells on the screen. Much of this software includes word prediction capacity; the program "guesses" what word the writer means from the first few letters. If the writer types "po," for example, the program will generate a list of words such as:

Poisonous
Pony
Post
Possible
Possibility
Portent
Potent

The writer then selects the one that he or she intended to spell, and the program pronounces it. While the intention is to speed up message transmission for students with severe speech disorders, this software also can help students with poor spelling abilities to produce correct versions of intended words more quickly, recognize them, and increase their chances of retaining them for later use.

Spelling can also be addressed using the procedures we've already discussed for identifying root words and relations among words that are preserved in spelling (our *clinic-clinician* example, again). In addition, students can be encouraged to create personal dictionaries in which they record frequently used spellings, spellings of new words they learn in the curriculum, and words they come across in their reading that they think might be useful in their own writing. Again, technology can be helpful here. If students use word processors for their writing, they can be taught to use the spelling checker available on most programs. While this is not a substitute for learning to spell, it does reinforce the idea that it is important to check spelling as one aspect of the editing process. Electronic, hand-held spelling aids also are available. Students pursuing an academic curriculum might be encouraged to save up for one.

And beyond these mechanics, we will want to assist students to become more effective writers for a variety of purposes. We will discuss a range of learning strategies that can assist students in this development a bit later. But in a review of writing intervention programs for students with LLD, Gersten and

---

BOX 14-4 | **Multimodal Activity for Practicing Writing Mechanics Skills**

Punctuating Dialogue Cards. Compose five lines of a humorous dialogue. Include interrogative, exclamatory, and declarative sentences. Type one line of dialogue on each of several sheets of pages. Within each sentence create blank spaces to show where punctuation marks belong. Laminate the papers. Place soft-sided pieces of Velcro in the blanks. Use colored paper to make quotation marks, commas, question marks, exclamation points, and periods. Color code the punctuation marks (e.g., use yellow for quotation marks and pink for commas). Cut out and laminate the punctuation marks, and place a rough-sided piece of Velcro on the back. Have students use the cards to practice punctuating dialogue, such as:

( )Eggbert, did you put sardines on Ralphie's sandwich again ( ) ( )asked Ethel ( )

Adapted from Van Zile, S. (2003). Grammar that'll move you! *Instructor, 112,* 32-35.

Baker (2001) found that there were three critical elements that should be part of any instructional program for these students. These elements include the following:

▶ Explicit teaching of the steps in the writing process (planning, composing, revising)
▶ Discussion of purposes and audiences for writing
▶ Scaffolding and feedback on the quality of the writing product, not only from adults but also from peers

Incorporating these components in the intervention we provide for struggling writers will help us maximize the effectiveness of our writing intervention.

Expository and Argumentative Texts. New discourse genres that come to the fore at the secondary level are *expository* texts that explain or relate factual material, and *argumentative* texts that persuade or discuss opinions. These discourse genres will form the bulk of school-sponsored writing during adolescence, and some direct instruction will be presented in the course of classroom English and language arts classes. In fact, many state-required writing assessments, as well as the new SAT writing section, require the production of persuasive essays. These often form a large part of the writing curriculum in secondary grades. As such, these are ideal collaborative intervention opportunities for the SLP, who can work with the teacher to outline, preteach, guest teach, and follow-up instruction in these areas for students with IEPs.

Students are generally expected to use the "Five Paragraph Essay," as the basic structure for much of the expository and persuasive discourse they are required to produce in school. The first paragraph introduces the thesis of the essay and foreshadows the main supporting subtopics. The second through fourth paragraphs are all similar in format. They individually restate the subtopics, and are developed by giving supporting information. The fifth and last paragraph restates the main thesis or idea and reminds the reader of the three main supporting ideas that were developed. Each paragraph begins with a topic sentence that states the paragraph's main idea, and ends with a "clincher" sentence that sums up the paragraph. Basic skills approaches to helping students develop this form in expository and persuasive writing are outlined by Westby and Clauser (2005). These employ three phases of instruction:

▶ *Modeling*: The genre is introduced in the context of curriculum-related material. The communicative function and the structure of the genre are discussed, examples from classroom texts are displayed, and features are pointed out and highlighted.
▶ *Joint construction*: Teachers and students work together to transform information students have collected (from library and Internet research, interviews, videos, field trips, etc.) into an essay. Students do research on a curriculum-related topic in cooperative learning groups. The teacher guides them in summarizing the information; displaying their organization of it into headings and subheadings on the blackboard. Once it is organized, the teacher has students orally dictate individual sentences. These are discussed and critiqued by the group as the teacher records them.

▶ *Independent construction*: Students are given a curriculum-related "writing prompt." For example, after reading *Passage to Freedom* (Mochizuki, 1998), they might be told, "Mr. Sugihara was extremely courageous. Write about someone you admire for courage. Explain why this person deserves to be called courageous." Students write a draft of their essay, referring to the purposes and structures discussed in the earlier lessons. They then consult with a teacher about the draft and receive guiding feedback.

All genres of writing are difficult for students with LLD. However, the persuasive essay is both most difficult (Nippold, 2005) and the one required in the majority of "high stakes" situations, such as school-wide achievement tests and SATs. As such, special attention should be paid to its structure and function when working with struggling writers. Westby and Clauser (2005) outline the three parts that need to be present in making an effective argument:

▶ *Claim*: the basic assertion being made; e.g., students should be allowed to choose their own clothing for school.
▶ *Warrant*: the principles that connect data to the claim; e.g., uniforms don't make students behave better in school.
▶ *Data*: factual information that supports that warrant; e.g., research shows no improvements in behavior or achievement in schools that require uniforms (Brunsma, 1998).

The basic structure of the persuasive essay includes the following:

1. Clear opening statement that expresses the argument, opinion, or position of the writer
2. Development of the argument by supplying three or more reasons, with data and warrants
3. Attempt to influence the audience's opinion by providing a statement of personal belief based on the arguments made, a prediction based on these arguments, or a summary of the major ideas presented

Westby and Clauser (2005) point out that one reason for the difficulty with persuasive texts is that students tend to have less exposure to them than to narratives or exposition. This suggests that one way to improve persuasive writing is to precede writing instruction with work on reading persuasive texts, such as editorials in newspapers and magazines or political advertisements. Having students critique these by identifying their claims and examining how well they are supported by warrants and data, can be helpful in getting students more familiar with the discourse genre.

Nelson and Van Meter (2002) discuss one additional issue that is crucial in improving students' writing. This concerns the need for students to perceive writing as an authentic activity; one that has relevance for their real world and is not important solely for "getting through" school. Fortunately, young people's facility and fascination with the Internet provides an important forum for authentic writing. Many teenagers have discovered the joys of "blogging," creating online journals (Web logs, or "blogs") in which they chronicle their lives and discuss issues of interest to them, as well as read the blogs of others. Many sites, including Blurty.com, Blogger.com, and Blogtext.org, offer free blogging facilities. Clinicians can help students establish blogs, review others' blogs for ideas to respond to, and write and post their own responses to issues being discussed on-line by their peers. Although blogging is more tolerant of misspelling and grammatical errors than more formal writing settings, it provides one opportunity—which clinicians and teachers will augment with other more standard, formal opportunities—to express thoughts in writing for an audience of peers. As such, it can motivate students to try writing as a means of expression that has a part in the big picture of their lives, not just in the small corner of the classroom.

Functional Communication

Conversation. A variety of published programs for helping adolescents improve social and conversational skills are available (Frank & Smith-Rex, 1997; Hanken & Kennedy, 1998; Hazel, Schumaker, Sherman, & Sheldon-Wildgen, 1981; Hoskins, 1999; Kelly, 2001; Jackson, Jackson, & Bennett, 1998; La Greca & Mesibov, 1981; LoGiudice & McConnell, 1998; Marquis & Addy-Trout, 1992; Mayo & Waldo, 1994; Minskoff, 1982; Reese & Challenner, 2001; Schrieber & McKinley, 1995; Walker, Todis, Holmes, & Horton, 1988; Wanat, 1983; Wiig, 1982b). Larson and McKinley (2003a) outline seven crucial elements for social skills instruction:

1. *Introduction*: Tell the students about the skill, what they will learn and why it is important to them. Have students share experiences related to the skill.
2. *Guided instruction*: Lay out the steps to be taught. Define the skill and list the steps involved in accomplishing it.
3. *Modeling*: Demonstrate with role-playing or audio or video recordings the skill to be learned. Model self-talk about thinking through how/when to apply the skill.
4. *Rehearsal*: Students describe verbally the sequence of actions involved in the skill and then role-play with a group of peers.
5. *Feedback*: Provide encouragement for the use of appropriate behaviors and ask students to describe the successful behavior they used; when giving corrective feedback use a positive, nonthreatening way and have students describe the appropriate behavior.
6. *Planning*: Have students discuss how/when/with whom they can use the new skill. Encourage them to use the following formula to help plan future interactions:

   STOP: think before talking, use self-control strategies if necessary

   PLOT: plan ahead and brainstorm options before deciding what to say/do

   GO: choose the best option from brainstorming and implement it

   SO: evaluate. Encourage students to ask themselves how it went, what they did well, what they might *change next time*.
7. *Generalization*: Encourage students to try their new skill at home with family or in class with friends. Have them report back to the clinician to discuss the outcome. If more help is needed, the clinician can discreetly 'sit in' on an interaction in which the student uses the skill with a peer, and give feedback.

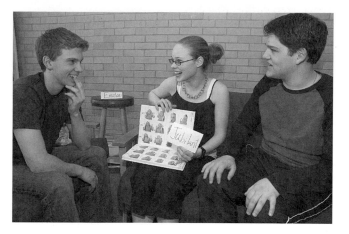

Discussing emotions can be part of social skills training.

Bryan (1986) reported that structured situations in which peers provide models of a target behavior, such as a talk-show format in which the "host" must ask open-ended questions to elicit conversation from the guest, are very effective in eliciting functional communication targets from adolescents with LLD. In general, peer modeling is a tool with demonstrated effectiveness for helping adolescents develop conversational styles that lead to greater acceptance (Paul, 2003). Peers involved in direct instruction can be trained to model positive conversational behaviors. Such behaviors might include appropriate topic initiation and continuation, using open-ended and follow-up questions to keep the conversation moving, and providing affirmative comments on the contributions of the student with LLD. Instruction to peers can be relatively informal or more highly structured. Several programs have provided very structured training, using behavioral technology, to organize the interactions between students with LLD and peer tutors. Gaylord-Ross, Haring, Breen, and Pitts-Conway (1984), for example, used highly structured interactions between students with autism and peers to teach basic communicative skills, such as requesting and offering objects and greeting and elaborating greetings.

Kilman and Negri-Schoultz (1987) described a social-skills program designed for high-functioning autistic students like Michael that can be adapted for use with advanced language students with a variety of disabilities. Their program involved a social "club" for students with disabilities in which the students work with professionals to create a satisfying interactive experience. Professionals plan discussion groups with preset topics, such as the problems of meeting people, the loneliness of being different, and school stress. Students discuss their experiences on these topics with models provided by the professionals. Other meetings involve interactive games, such as charades or "Pictionary," that involve communication and take advantage of nonverbal strengths of the participants. Still others involve planning and preparing refreshments for special events put on by the "club." These might include shows displaying participants' artwork or dances to which members may invite friends. Throughout these activities, careful modeling of appropriate behavior is provided by professionals, and discussion about the effectiveness of the clients' communication, within and outside the "club," goes on. Although this program was designed as "extracurricular," it could be incorporated as a social skills unit within a communication class for secondary students with LLD. Strulovitch and Tagalakis (2003) also provided guidelines for running groups for students with social disabilities. Other approaches derived from the literature on autism include *Pivotal Response Training* (Bregman & Gerdtz, 1997), *The New Social Story Book,* and *Comic Strip Conversations* (Gray, 2000b, 1994), which can be adapted for use with students with other disabilities who need help with functional communication.

Another approach is the *Model, Analyze, Practice* (MAP) program (Hess & Fairchild, 1988). Here students view pairs of peer interactions on videotape, one in which the interaction is successful and one in which it is less so. Students analyze the pairs of interactions for features identified by the clinician to understand why one is more successful. These features include topic initiation, use of questions, appropriate turn-taking, and similar concerns. After analyzing the tapes, students practice using the techniques they identified on the tapes as effective and videotape themselves doing so. They then critique the tapes of their own performance. As we saw, video modeling programs like these have demonstrated efficacy with younger children (Paul, 2003), so they are a reasonable method to try with adolescents who need to develop conversational skills. Such a program could be incorporated as one unit of a communication class.

Walker, Schwartz, Nippold, Irvin, and Noell (1994) discussed the importance of following up activities like these with scaffolded opportunities to apply newly learned skills in natural interactions. They recommended having the clinician structure interactions between clients and normally developing peers. In these interactions, the clinician can act as a "coach," providing cues and prompts first during and later before the interactions. Special student helpers can be designated to provide this coaching at a later point in the program. Clinicians also should establish incentive systems, such as earning days off from homework for successful conversations with peers. Debriefing, or having students relate and analyze their experiences in these scaffolded conversations, also is important to support the students' extension of newly learned skills into their behavioral repertoire. Paul (2003) and Strulovitch and Tagalakis (2003) discussed a variety of social skills training programs aimed primarily at adolescents with autism that can also be adapted for students with other disabilities.

Paul and Sutherland (2003) identified several skills to be taught in these kinds of programs. One is the use of communicative rituals. Rituals are scripted conversational patterns such as greetings ("Hi, how are you?" "Fine, thanks, and you?"). A variety of rituals such as partings, introductions, asking for help, entering conversations, and asking for clarification can be written out in script form, practiced, and memorized. Although these ritualistic interactions are not completely natural, they are often improvements over the unusual behaviors students like Michael may use. Krantz and McClannahan (1998) showed that fading these scripts, by gradually cutting

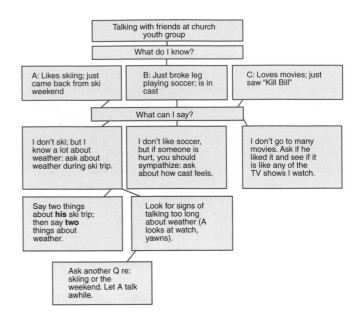

FIGURE 14-7 ✦ Conversational map. (Adapted from Hallenbeck, M. (1996). The cognitive strategy in writing: Welcome relief for adolescents with learning disabilities. *Learning Disabilities Research and Practice, 11,* 107-119.

off increasingly larger segments of the written form, and requiring students to rely on their memory rather than the written script, increased generalization of these procedures to settings outside the therapy context.

A second area conversational programs might address is topic management. Here students can be taught to listen first and talk later, taking time to identify the topic under discussion before entering the conversation. They also can be instructed to check the appropriateness of their topic ("Do you want to talk about a movie I saw?") or to confirm the topic they identify ("Are you talking about last night's game?"). Students with a tendency to "get stuck" on a favorite topic can also be encouraged to say, for example, just three things about their topic, and then offer to switch to a topic of their interlocutor's interest. Conversational maps, like the one in Figure 14-7, can be used to help students think ahead to choose appropriate topics for different partners, based on what they know about each one. Brinton, Robinson, and Fujiki (2004) developed a game called "The Conversation Can" to address these issues. They emphasize that the program took a long period of time before generalized change was achieved, however, so clinicians should not expect changes in these behaviors overnight. The program's basic sequence is as follows:

❱ Brainstorm a list of topics classmates might want to discuss.
❱ Write each on a slip of paper.
❱ Put slips in can.
❱ Take turns pulling out a topic.
❱ Start conversation:
  ❱ Think first: What should I say?
  ❱ Say two things about the topic.
  ❱ Ask interlocutor a question about the topic.
  ❱ Listen while interlocutor answers.

Again, these strategies are somewhat artificial but can help to build skills that will eventually allow more fluid and natural participation in conversations. And again, visual cues and organizers can be helpful. Figure 14-8 provides several examples of visual cues for conversational training.

Mentis (1994) emphasized the importance of access to flexible syntactic forms in the conversational skills of students with LLD. In taking a remedial approach to conversational development, it is important to integrate work on improving conversational ability with the use of linguistic markers that can elaborate discourse. Mentis pointed to adverbial conjuncts, question forms, relative clauses, ellipsis, and other cohesive devices

as being especially important in this regard. As we work on basic conversational skills with students at the advanced language level, we want to adhere to the same principle we've talked about for working on pragmatics with younger clients. That is, we want to use conversational contexts as a means to practice semantic and syntactic forms. By integrating these forms into pragmatic contexts, such as conversation, we have the greatest chance to effect an overall improvement in the student's communication.

Survival Skills. In addition to improving social communication, adolescents with LLD may need help on developing the daily living skills they need to make the transition to adulthood. Work, Cline, Ehren, Keiser, and Wujek (1993)

FIGURE 14-8 ✦ Visual and graphic supports for conversation.

Script

Walk up to a classmate.

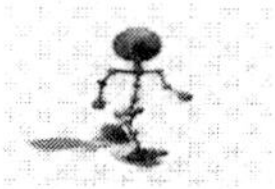

Make eye contact.

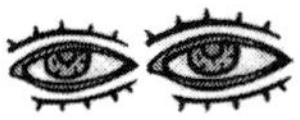

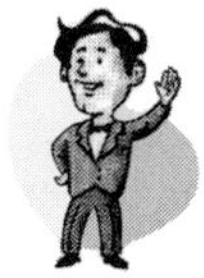

Say, "Hi _____ (their name)."

Checklists

When I had a conversation, did I

look at my friend?_____

stand one arm's length away?_____

appear interested by asking questions and listening?_____

talk about what my friend is interested in?_____

Posters

Important Parts of Conversation:

☺ Topic: Pick something your friend wants to talk about.

? Questions: Use these to keep the back-and-forth going.

" " Comments: Say something new that your friend doesn't know but would find interesting.

FIGURE 14-8 ✦—cont'd

Choice boards

Pick your conversation topic for today:

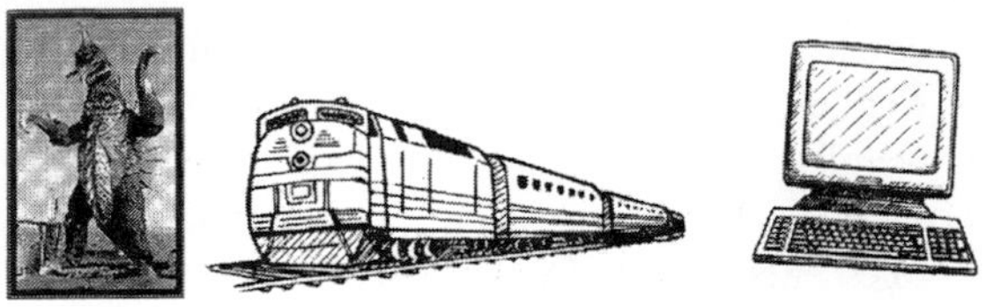

Movie	Trains	Computers

Choice lists

Great Greetings

Yo!

Hey, pal!

High five!

What up!

Hi, how ya doin'!

described several secondary school programs that contain functional communication strands. These programs address skills needed by students to function in home, work, and community contexts.

Vocational skill development can focus on exploring realistic career options. Work et al. described one vocational exploration program in which each student in a communication class is required to research and orally report on two careers in which he or she has a realistic interest. Each student compiles a portfolio on the two careers. The portfolio includes a resume of the student's qualifications for the position, a completed job application form, and information on the training needed for the position. In addition, each student participates in a practice interview for the position, which is videotaped and critiqued by the clinician and classmates. The student can then redo the interview, using suggestions from the critique. Montague and Lund (1991) and Sigler and Fitzpatrick (2000) also provided a commercial program for working on vocationally related communication skills.

Survival skills needed for family or independent living also can be addressed. Here students would be given assignments to research nutrition and meal planning, consumer skills such as label reading and unit pricing, housing searches using news-paper ads for rental units, and similar topics. Students would present the results of their research orally to the class. Role-playing activities, similar to the practice job interview, could be used to rehearse such tasks as applying for an apartment, asking a store manager about sale prices, and planning and shopping for a week's worth of balanced meals. Drug abuse, family planning, and hygiene information also might be part of this unit, with collaboration from the school health teacher. A curriculum such as *Smooth Sailing in the Next Generation* (Plumridge & Hylton, 1987), which discusses prevention of birth defects, also may be an appropriate addition to the func-tional curriculum. Other commercial programs, such as Mannix's *Life Skills Activities for Secondary Students with Special Needs* (2002a), *Social Skills Activities: For Secondary Students with Special Needs* (Mannix, 2002b), *Life Skills: 225 Ready-to-Use Health Activities for Success and Well-being* (McTavish, 2003), and *That's LIFE! Life Skills* (Smith, 1998), also are available.

Larson and McKinley (2003a) and Novak (2002) emphasize another important survival skill for adolescents with LLD: emotional expression. All teenagers experience a wide range of strong emotions; they feel angry at adults who set limits on them, frustrated at their own limitations, anxious about what others think of them, and so on. For students with LLD, their poor communication skills often make it difficult to acknowledge, share, and manage these feelings. The role of the SLP in this area is to provide the words and opportunities to practice talking about these feelings, first in a therapeutic atmosphere, and later in supported naturalistic settings. Gajewski, Hirn, and Mayo (1998) and *Room 28* (LoGiudice & McConnell, 2004) provide materials for practicing communication skills in a variety of social settings and include activities for emotional expression.

LEARNING-STRATEGIES APPROACHES TO INTERVENTION IN THE ADVANCED LANGUAGE STAGE

Learning strategies methods of intervention are essentially "meta" approaches. As such, they conform to one of the basic principles of intervention for school-age clients that we outlined earlier. In addition, they provide the other advantages we discussed for students in the advanced language stage, those with normal intellectual ability and reading skills at a fourth-grade level or higher. That is, they help these students move toward more independent functioning and give them the tools to improve their own learning abilities. Swanson and De La Paz (1998) outlined seven steps that comprise a learning-strategy, or what they call a "self-regulated strategy development" (SRSD), approach. These are given in Box 14-5. In their review of instructional approaches for students with LLD, Vaughn, Gersten, and Chard (2000) found that, along with small group instruction and controlling the difficulty of the task, the use of learning strategies was one of the three key elements that produced the strongest impact on students' learning. When using a learning strategies approach, it is important to remember, as Ehren (2002) pointed out, that strategies should be practiced in curriculum-based material. Instead of tutoring students in the material itself, best practice dictates that we take materials and topics related to the curriculum and use them to teach students how to improve their own mastery of the content. Although we may need to use materials that are below the students' grade level for initial strategy instruction, these materials should still be selected to enhance the students' curricular knowledge. As students become more adept at using the strategies we teach, materials closer to grade level can be added. Let's look again at some of the areas that we assessed in adolescents with LLD and see how we might use these compensatory-strategy approaches to improve academic functioning and increase autonomy in our secondary school students.

Semantics

Several "meta" approaches for increasing *lexical skills* were presented by Crais (1990). The *root word* strategy is one. Here the clinician introduces a root word and helps students identify possible additions of inflectional endings (*-ing, -ed, -s*) and derivational suffixes (*-less, -ly, -tion*) and prefixes (*un-, in-, dis-*). The clinician can discuss how each affix changes the meaning or part of speech of the root word. Students can then be encouraged to hunt for affixed roots in textbooks and

literature selections and to talk about how identifying root words can help to elucidate word meaning. The clinician also might introduce some roots from Greek (e.g., *tele* [distance], *phon* [sound]) and Latin (e.g., *amor* [love], *terra* [earth]) that are relevant to curricular topics. Students can hunt for words containing these roots in their textbooks and talk about how the roots can be used to help identify word meaning. Students can be asked to keep a root-word dictionary, recording new roots as they learn them, listing all the words they know that contain the roots, and adding new entries as they are encountered. The strategy to be taught here is to look for relations among words and to consult prior knowledge when confronted with a new word.

Sternberg and Powell (1983) provided a set of strategies for helping students to use *context* to decipher the meaning of new words. Their approach involves encouraging students to focus on specific cues available in the context to make their guesses. They direct students to use a range of cues including temporal, spatial, descriptive state or function, causal, class membership, grammatical category, and equivalence information. The clinician can start by using sentences containing nonsense words and encouraging students to recognize clues to the word's meaning in the other words in the sentence. For example, we might write on the board:

> At dusk, the cleebs began to appear and twinkled behind the moon in the darkening sky. Their sparkle was reflected in her starry eyes.

The clinician can model using the following cues to detect the word's meaning from the context:

> temporal = dusk
> spatial = behind moon
> descriptive (state or function) = twinkle
> class membership = same as moon; something we see in the sky
> grammatical = -s ending, comes after the; therefore, is probably a noun
> causal = began to appear; therefore, not visible all the time
> equivalence = starry

Students can then be encouraged to find an unfamiliar word in a textbook selection and use as many of the cues as are available to make a stab at its meaning. We might provide the student with a list of the category of cues to complete. For example:

> temporal =
> spatial =
> descriptive (state or function) =
> class membership =
> grammatical =
> causal =
> equivalence =

BOX 14-5	Seven Steps to Teaching Self-Regulated Learning Strategies

Step 1

Describe the strategy. The teacher explains the strategy (e.g., summarizing) and students and teacher review the student's current performance (e.g., on a pretest).

Step 2

Activate background knowledge. Review information students have already learned that is important for learning this strategy (e.g., taking notes; students will use summarizing to help with more efficient note-taking).

Step 3

Review current performance level. Provide feedback to students about their current functioning in this area, and explain benefits of using the strategy to improve performance (e.g., summarizing will make it easier to take notes, remember information for tests, write book reports).

Step 4

Model the strategy and self-instructions. The teacher shows how to use the strategy, using a "think-aloud" procedure to demonstrate each step (e.g., "This paragraph seems to be talking about trade routes to India. Let's see, it says the major routes were [a], [b], and [c] . . .) Self-statements such as "What should I do first?" or "Am I using the strategy?" demonstrate to students how to manage their performance.

Step 5

Collaborative practice. The teacher and students, as a group, model and rehearse the strategy. The teacher provides multiple opportunities for practicing the strategies and self-cues as a class, in small groups, in pairs. The teacher monitors students' progress and provides prompts or re-instruction, when necessary.

Step 6

Independent practice and mastery. Students apply the strategy to materials at a low level of difficulty for them. The teacher provides prompts and corrective feedback, when necessary. Practice sessions are repeated with materials of increasing difficulty. Students and teacher collect data and evaluate their own performance on the materials used.

Step 7

Generalization practice using the strategy on curricular material. The students apply the strategy to textbooks and a variety of regular classroom content. The teacher discusses with students times/situations when the use of the newly learned strategy will be helpful, and provides additional feedback. Strategy use is then tested. Additional instruction and models are provided, if necessary.

Adapted from Seidenberg, P. (1988). Cognitive and academic instructional intervention for learning-disabled adolescents. *Topics in Language Disorders, 8,* 56-71; and Swanson, P., & De La Paz, S. (1998). Teaching effective comprehension strategies to students with learning and reading disabilities. *Intervention in School and Clinic, 33,* 209-218.

Students can then be encouraged to check their guesses by looking up the word in the dictionary. Additional practice can be provided and the importance of using contextual strategies to disambiguate unknown words can be emphasized as we teach the strategy.

Levin et al. (1984) proposed a strategy for helping students retain the meanings of new words or roots, the *keyword method.* Here students are taught to link a new word (for example, *truculent*: fierce and aggressive) or root (*terra* for earth) with a familiar keyword that shares some sound or visual feature; for example, *tear* could be a keyword for *terra*; *truck* could be a keyword for *truculent*. To learn the new word, the students are told to do the following:

- Draw a picture that links the meaning of the keyword and the new word and write the connection underneath ("*Terra* means 'earth'; let's not tear it apart;" "The truck driver was *truculent*" beneath a picture of a truck with a fierce-looking driver.)
- To learn the new word, the student is told to do the following:
  - Say the new word (*truculent*) and think of its keyword (*truck*).

▶ Think of the picture with the keyword in it.

▶ Remember the connection that symbolized the picture (The [fierce] truck driver was *truculent*).

▶ Retrieve the meaning of the new word (*truculent*: fierce and aggressive).

The keyword then becomes a retrieval cue for the new word or root. Terrill, Scruggs, and Mastropieri (2004) showed that using a keyword strategy was more effective than traditional instruction in terms of the number of new words maintained by high school students with LLD.

Word retrieval is another area in which compensatory strategies are especially helpful, since many students with LLD retain word-finding problems throughout their adulthood. We can encourage students to activate consciously all the semantic and phonological information they can about a word they want to retrieve. A variation of the "Password" game is a good first step toward developing these strategies. One student (or the clinician) thinks of a word and gives either a semantic or phonological clue to the partner, whose job it is to guess the password. If the first clue is insufficient for the partner to guess, another is given, until the word is guessed. The game also can be played in teams of two students. The teams alternate turns, with one team member providing clues and the other trying to guess the password from the accumulated clues given by both teams. The first team whose "guesser" gets the password wins. Semantic and phonological clues can be alternated, or the game can be restricted to one type of clue.

After practice with this game, students can be encouraged to give themselves similar clues when they are having trouble finding a word. They might start out by writing down each clue they can give themselves and recording how many they need to find the word. They can keep track of their self-cueing and try to reduce the number of clues they need to give themselves before they retrieve the word. Again, a compensatory-strategy approach is intended to help students learn to cue themselves, rather than depending on the clinician to help them when they get stuck. Teaching students to activate their keyword strategies can also help with word retrieval.

German (1992) provided additional compensatory strategies. She suggested teaching students *reflective pausing*, or the constructive use of pause time to use retrieval strategies and reduce inaccurate competitive responses. Students can be encouraged to "wait and think" when they have trouble finding a word, rather than saying the first competing response that enters their head. Once the ability to use reflective pausing has been established, students can be encouraged to use a variety of self-cueing strategies to try to retrieve the target word. In addition to the phonemic and semantic cues we've already discussed, German suggested teaching students to use graphemic cueing (trying to remember what the word looks like in writing), imagery cueing (revisualizing the referent as a cue to the target word), gesture cueing (motor schemes or actions associated with the target word, such as twisting the lid to retrieve *jar*), and associative cueing (using an intermediate word to cue the target, such as *story* for *book*). German also recommended teaching students that if they cannot retrieve the word they want, they should use an alternate form, such as a synonym or word in the same category to convey their meaning, as a last resort.

Norbury (2004) showed that children with a variety of kinds of communication disorders were less likely than typical peers to use the available context to help them understand *figurative language*. So in this aspect of semantics, too, one of our roles is to help students learn and use a strategic approach when they encounter something they don't understand. Palmer and Brooks (2004) recommend a three-step strategy for improving figurative comprehension:

1. Have the students identify figurative language in passages they read or hear. For each possible nonliteral expression, they can be trained to ask themselves, "Does the writer mean exactly what the words say, or is something else being conveyed?" The clinician can model a think-aloud procedure for deciding this by saying, for example, "Does this make sense here, considering the usual meaning of these words?"

2. For each expression they decide is not literal, students are encouraged to decide what the author is really trying to say. They can use the cues we talked about earlier (temporal, spatial, causal, etc.) to decide what the expression might mean.

3. Finally, students are encouraged to activate everything they know about the words in the figurative expression to attempt to make a connection between the intended meaning and the surface form.

Students can be asked to keep logs of new figurative expressions they decipher using this strategy, for discussion with the clinician and for future reference.

Syntax

Learning strategies approaches to syntax, like those we discussed for semantics, also involve teaching students self-cueing. Much of this self-cueing can go on in the context of editing written work for syntactic accuracy and maturity. Students can be encouraged to make several passes through their writing in the editing process, with one pass dedicated to looking for errors in syntax and how syntax can be improved by using connectives, cohesive devices, and other "dandy language" forms listed in Table 13-6. Students can be encouraged to ask themselves as they edit each paragraph of their writing, "Have I said it clearly? Have I connected the ideas? Have I used a formal style?" If students are writing on word processors, the grammar-checking program in the word processor may help identify sentences that could use rewriting. Alternatively, the clinician can underline sections that could benefit from rewriting. These might be coded with a "C" for providing connectives between ideas, a "CH" for using cohesive devices, and a "D" for writing with "dandy language" forms. Eventually, students can be encouraged to use these codes in editing their own syntax. Scott (2005) showed that students do better at first editing *others'* writing, rather than their own. An initial phase in this instruction then, could be to have students go through each of the steps outlined above on a peer's writing sample. The next phase would involve repeating these steps on their own written product.

Pragmatics

Classroom Discourse. Silliman and Wilkinson (1991) advocated facilitating classroom discourse skills by using what they call "dialogic mentoring." This is a form of supportive prompting that offers verbal cues or choices as external support to students for accessing a solution to a problem or an answer to a question. The goal of this support is to give students a model for doing this scaffolding for themselves. To use dialogic mentoring, it is important that problems posed to students with LLD be within their zone of proximal development, not so easy as to require little cognitive processing and not so hard as to be beyond their current cognitive grasp.

An approach to dialogic modeling was presented by Brown and Campione (1990), which they referred to as *reciprocal teaching*. Reciprocal teaching (RT) is a learning-strategy approach to helping students engage in self-regulated learning within the classroom setting. Brown and Palinscar (1987) outlined four steps in the reciprocal teaching process. The "facilitator" (teacher or clinician) first models each step on a segment of curricular material, such as a lecture, reading selection, or mathematics or science problem. The facilitator then assigns one of the students to use the same series of steps on a related passage or problem. Each student is given a turn to act as facilitator for the group. The student with LLD can serve as facilitator last, to take advantage of the additional modeling provided by the other students. Brown and Palinscar's procedures for RT are outlined in Box 14-6.

Hoskins (1990) provided additional techniques that can be used in conjunction with RT or in other collaborative intervention settings to provide scaffolding for students' learning strategies. She suggested, for example, using *postscript modeling* as an additional approach for increasing students' learning strategies in classroom discourse situations. Here the facilitator provides scaffolding comments about students' remarks in the discussion of the class material. The clinician can provide an accepting but corrected version of a student comment, encourage brainstorming to solve comprehension problems, identify areas of misunderstanding or inadequate skill development (need for instruction in punctuation or capitalization, for example), and provide appropriate instruction as needed. Postscript modeling also can scaffold by taking a student comment to a higher cognitive level. Suppose, for example, that Michael answers a question about how a story character feels with, "She feels sad, she feels sorry her dad is not home." A postscript model would take Michael's answer to a deeper level of character motivation by replying, "Yes, Meg feels sad because her father had been away for some time, and no one knows where he is. Not knowing probably makes her feel worse. How do you think you might feel if someone in your family were gone and you didn't know where he was?"

Vaughn et al.'s (2000) review of effective practices for students with LLD suggests that the use of RT techniques, and other activities that involve interactive dialogue between teacher and student as well as among students, are among the most effective ways of improving both reading and writing skills in students with LLD. All these forms of dialogic mentoring are ideally suited to collaborative intervention settings, in which the teacher presents some curricular material and the clinician follows up the teacher's lecture with a reciprocal teaching session on the same material or provides scaffolding questions to increase students' control of their learning. In our role as SLPs, we can encourage teachers to make use of these highly effective practices, modeling them in collaborative teaching sessions. These techniques also can be used in a communication class setting. We can also use RT approaches in therapeutic oral language activities with students, as a bridge toward helping them acquire skills and strategies they can apply to written language formats. Alternatively, these methodologies can be presented in consultative or in-service training sessions as particularly appropriate techniques to use in classrooms in

---

BOX 14-6	Procedures for Reciprocal Teaching

Predict. Encourage students to examine their prior knowledge on the topic and develop a purpose for reading or listening. Scan headings and boldface print to guide predictions. Have students tell what they already know about the topic and what they expect to learn from the passage.

Generate questions. After reading or listening, ask questions the teacher might ask about the passage.

Summarize the essential information to provide a self-review and deepen comprehension. Paraphrase is an especially useful technique. When students perform this step, take corrective action if incomplete or erroneous comprehension is evidenced in the summary.

Clarify ambiguous or unfamiliar material. Have students identify gaps in their understanding. Guide them in rereading and scanning headings or notes to look for clues within the text to provide needed clarity. If cues cannot be found, guide students in discussion of resources that might be used, such as dictionaries, encyclopedias, maps, and questions to knowledgeable people, to provide the information.

Adapted from Brown, A., & Palinscar, A. (1987). Reciprocal teaching of comprehension strategies. In J. Day & J. Borkowski (Eds.). *Intelligence and exceptionality: New directions for theory, assessment, and instructional practice* (pp. 81-132). Norwood, NJ: Ablex; and Gerber, A. (1993). *Language-related learning disabilities: Their nature and treatment.* Baltimore, MD: Paul H. Brookes.

which students with LLD are placed. We can emphasize that these techniques have been shown to benefit all the students in the classroom (Vaughn et al., 2000).

Conversational Discourse. Most of our intervention for conversational pragmatics is done in the functional strand of our curriculum. We also can, when assessment indicates the need, work on self-cueing approaches to the use of advanced discourse intentions such as persuasion, negotiation, and use of presuppositional devices and flexible speech styles. Here role-playing; barrier games; and when possible, video modeling procedures like those used in the MAP program can be used. After initial practice in persuading, negotiating, presenting adequate information, or using an appropriate speech register in activities like those outlined in Chapter 12, work can "go meta."

Let's take persuasion as an example. Students can talk about what is needed to be persuasive, such as taking the other person's needs and point of view into account. They can read some political speeches or advertising copy and identify elements in the text that are intended to persuade. They can then be asked to write their own advertisement or speech. In doing so, they can be required to list first what they will try to persuade the reader to do, what reader needs they will try to address, and what arguments they will use to address those needs. Hallenbeck (1996) suggested using a "think sheet" like the one

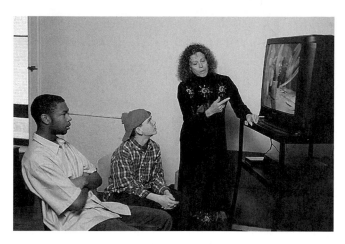

Video modeling helps students learn self-monitoring skills in conversation.

in Figure 14-9 to help students plan these arguments. They can then be assigned to create the ad or speech. Next a role-playing situation might be used in which the student must plan an "attack" on parents to, for example, persuade them to lift their curfew for a special school event. Again, before role-playing the argument, the students should plan their strategy, stating explicitly the parent needs they will address (such as

FIGURE 14-9 ✦ Graphic "think-sheet" for organizing a persuasive piece.

What do I want to argue for?

Whom do I need to convince?

Where and when will I make my argument?

What are the points I will make?

First:

Next:

Third:

Then:

Finally:

How will I sum up?

the need to believe the students are safe and chaperoned), what arguments they will use, and how the arguments will be phrased. Only then will they role-play the situation. After the role-play, they can evaluate their performance and list ways it could be improved. Similar "meta" approaches can be used for other aspects of conversational discourse. Again, the goal of a learning-strategies approach is to encourage conscious planning, self-cueing, and self-monitoring to give students tools for improving their own performance.

Other Discourse Genres

Narrative Texts. Most of the narrative text that students encounter in secondary school will be in literature classes, and perhaps in some work on biography in other subjects. This suggests that English teachers will be ideal collaborative partners for helping students to master these important discourse structures. Vaughn et al. (2000) pointed out that two of the most important interventions for students with LLD are (1) control of the difficulty of the material they must process, so that (2) they persist longer in working on the task. If our students are immature in their narrative abilities, the narratives presented in the typical classroom may be so far "above their head," that they may simply give up. One role the SLP can play is to provide guided practice and feedback in work on narratives with more controlled levels of difficulty, to encourage the student to persist so that eventually she or he can move up toward grade-appropriate material.

Comprehension. Students with LLD typically show poor reading comprehension (Moats, 2004). Helping students improve their understanding of stories they hear and read is an important aspect of our role as SLPs. We can help to shore up this ability by working in both oral and written formats to provide students with strategies they can invoke to help them get more out of what they hear and read. Katim and Harris (1997) suggested using a paraphrasing strategy to help students with story comprehension. Entitled RAP, the strategy entails having students read one paragraph at a time. After each, the strategy instructs the students to:

> Read
> Ask questions
> Put ideas in their own words

If students have difficulty, they are provided with an organizer like the one in Box 14-7. Katim and Harris demonstrated that the use of this strategy improved reading comprehension significantly for both typical students and those with LLD in an inclusive classroom setting.

Scheffel, Shroyer, and Strongin (2003) reviewed literature suggesting that the use of visual maps and organizers improved students' comprehension of narrative material. Other activities they found to be related to improved narrative comprehension included the use of RT techniques applied to narrative texts and the use of preparatory sets such as predicting and foregrounding prior knowledge before reading or listening. Finally, they found the "What I Know," or K-W-H-L, strategy to be effective in improving understanding of stories. This

BOX 14-7	**Steps in the RAP Strategy**

Step 1: Read a paragraph.
Step 2: Ask yourself, "What were the main idea and details of this paragraph?"
Places to look, if you're stumped:
  Look in the first sentence.
  Look for repetitions of the same word or words in the whole paragraph.
Questions to ask yourself, if you're stumped:
  What is the paragraph about?
  This paragraph is about _____.
  What does it tell me about _____?
  It tells me _____.
Step 3: Put the main idea and details into your own words.

Adapted from Katim, D., & Harris, S. (1997). Improving the reading comprehension of middle school students in inclusive classrooms. *Journal of Adolescent and Adult Literacy, 41,* 116-123.

strategy consists of teaching students to use a chart to outline knowledge before and after reading:

- **K** stands for what you already KNOW about the subject.
- **W** stands for what you WANT to learn.
- **H** stands for figuring out HOW you can learn more about the topic.
- **L** stands for what you LEARN as you read.

A graphic organizer for this strategy that might be used for the first chapter of Homer's *Odyssey* is depicted in Table 14-4.

Graves and Montague (1991) suggested a story grammar checklist for this purpose. The students read a story and record events from the story that fill in, or *instantiate*, each aspect of the story grammar. They then check off each aspect as they record it, to indicate that they have identified that element of the story. An example story grammar checklist appears in Table 14-5.

Production. Vallecorsa and deBettencourt (1997) emphasized, though, that story comprehension activities will not necessarily lead to generalized improvements in story production without explicit instruction. It is important, then, to provide students with strategies for both understanding and producing stories. Vallecorsa and deBettencourt suggested using a story map, like the one in Figure 14-10, to help students with narrative production. Students use the map to guide and organize their story production, drawing on the story element structure we have discussed.

Nelson and Van Meter (2002) emphasized the importance of having a real communicative purpose in composing a story, a purpose beyond merely pleasing the clinician or getting a grade. Classroom units on biography and autobiography make ideal contexts for encouraging students to write their own life stories, a topic that cannot help being of vital interest to the

TABLE 14-4	Graphic Organizer for K-W-H-L Strategy for Improving Narrative Comprehension

WHAT DO I ALREADY *KNOW* BEFORE READING?	WHAT DO I *WANT* TO KNOW?	*HOW* CAN I LEARN MORE?	WHAT DID I *LEARN* AFTER READING?
Odysseus is a hero.	Why is the book so long?	Web sites on Trojan War.	Odysseus fought in the Trojan War.
The story is from a very long time ago. It has something to do with the Trojan War.	What does Odysseus have to do with an odyssey? What is an odyssey?	Watch the movie "Troy."	An odyssey is a long trip.
I saw a Simpsons episode that was about this. What happened was…	Why didn't Odysseus just go straight home instead of stopping at all those places?	Review Greek mythology unit from last year's English class.	Odysseus was in trouble with some of the gods, so they made his trip long and hard.

TABLE 14-5	An Example of a Story Grammar Checklist for Dickens' *A Christmas Carol*

STORY GRAMMAR ELEMENT	EVENT FROM STORY	CHECK OFF
Setting		
When	Christmas, over 100 years ago	✓
Where	England	
Who	Mr. Scrooge	
Problem	It's Christmas, a time to be generous, and he is very stingy.	✓
Internal response	Hates Christmas	✓
Plan or attempt	Wants to ignore it	✓
Response	Goes to bed early; a ghost visits him to bring him visions of Christmases past, present, and future	✓
Additional plan or attempt	(Additional episodes in the story can be charted)	
Additional response:		
Resolution or consequence	Mr. Scrooge learns the meaning of the holiday and the joy of giving.	✓

Adapted from Graves, A., & Montague, M. (1991). Using story-grammar cueing to improve the writing of students with learning disabilities. *Learning Disabilities Research and Practice, 6*, 246–250.

author. Again, we can motivate story production by having students write plays for production or videotaping, or by having them produce contemporary versions of literature the students read in class for publication (with the student's permission) in a class literary magazine distributed to friends and family.

Montague, Graves, and Leavell (1991) suggested a learning-strategies approach to producing mature narratives by providing students with "story grammar cue cards." Students can be given a set of index cards, each of which contains a major story grammar element and a set of questions to answer in producing that element in a story. They use the cards as cues as they construct their stories. The cards can be used in the process of writing story summaries for book reports or as a guide to the student's original story compositions. Box 14-8 provides an example of a set of story grammar cue cards that can be given to students. Students should be encouraged not to answer the questions one by one, but instead to include information that will answer the questions within their story. Students can use the cues to guide their production of oral and written summaries for "book talks" given to peers or younger students and "book review" magazines produced in class. Story grammar cue cards also can help increase students' comprehension and summarization of stories they read. They can use the cards as study guides in their reading of curricular literature. Being encouraged to ask themselves the questions on the cards can help them to organize their processing of the story and aid in retention. Again, reciprocal teaching approaches, using visual organizers, and highlighting background knowledge in activities such as K-W-H-L are strategies that can improve narrative expression as well as comprehension. Merritt, Culatta, and Trostle (1998) provide additional suggestions for improving narrative discourse skills.

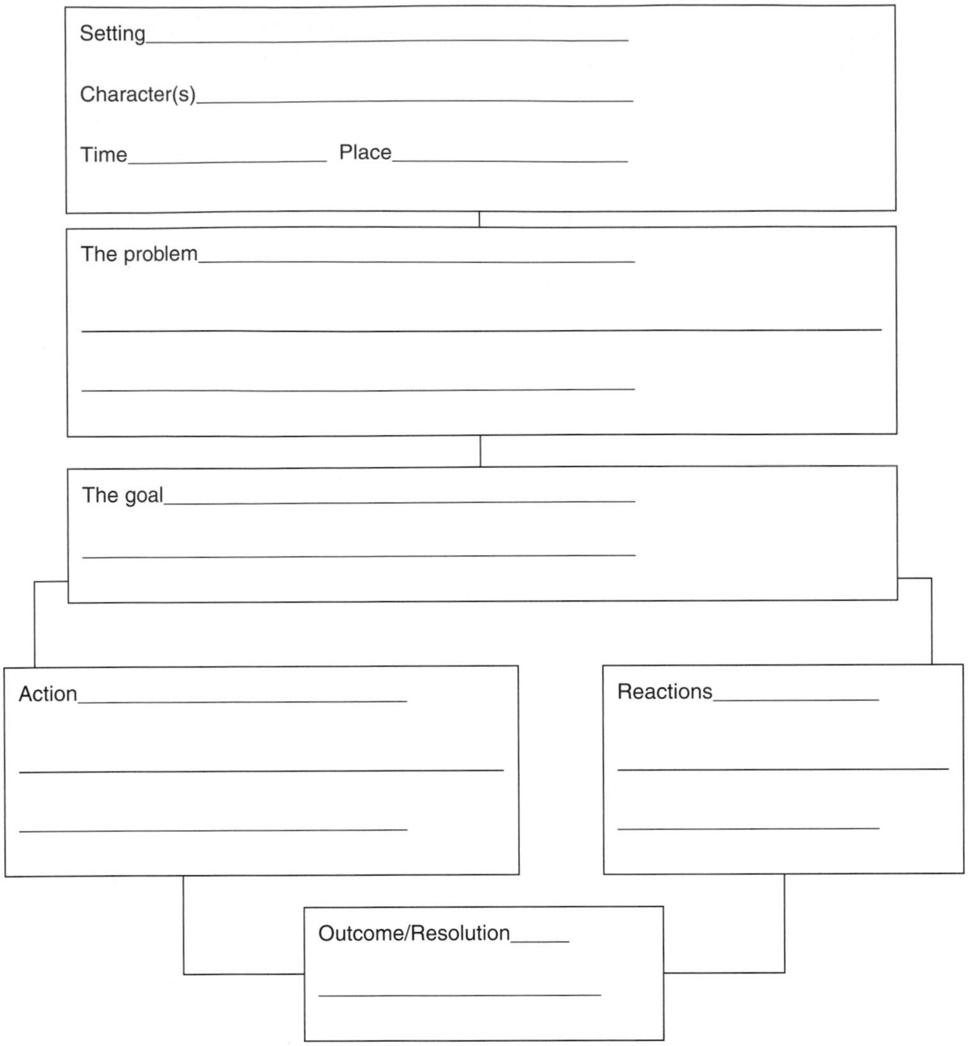

Setting_____

Character(s)_____

Time_____ Place_____

The problem_____

_____

_____

The goal_____

_____

Action_____

_____

_____

Reactions_____

_____

_____

Outcome/Resolution_____

_____

FIGURE 14-10 ✦ Story map for narrative production. (Adapted from Vallecorsa, A., & deBettencourt, L. (1997). Using a mapping procedure to teach reading and writing skills to middle grade students with learning disabilities. *Education and Treatment of Children, 20,* 173-188.)

BOX 14-8	**An Example of a Set of Story Grammar Cue Cards**

Card 1: Setting
Where and when does the story take place? Who are the main characters?

Card 2: Problem
What happens to get the story started? What is the problem the main character must solve?

Card 3: Internal Response
What thoughts or feelings does the main character have about the problem? What makes him or her want to do something about it?

Card 4: Plan
What is the main character's goal? What does he or she plan to do? What are his or her intentions?

Card 5: Attempt
What does the character do to carry out the plan?

Card 6: Consequence
What happens when the character tries to carry out the plan? Is it successful or unsuccessful? How and why? What else happens when the character tries to carry out the plan? Did he or she intend for that to happen?

Card 7: Reaction
How do the characters feel about what happened in the story? What do they think about the problem, the plan, and the result?

Adapted from Montague, M., Graves, A., & Leavell, A. (1991). Planning, procedural facilitation, and narrative composition of junior high students with learning disabilities. *Learning Disabilities Research and Practice, 6,* 219-224.

Expository Texts. Most of the texts students encounter outside of literature classes in secondary school take an expository form. We talked in Chapter 10 about the difficulties inherent in expository texts, especially for our students with LLD. Expository texts include both classroom books and teachers' lectures. Students will be expected both to understand information presented in these formats, and to produce expository speech and writing. Larson and McKinley (2003a) argue that success in school relies on expository text competence. The SLP's role in developing this competence involves helping students acquire strategies for producing and understanding these difficult text structures in both oral and written forms. Vaughn et al. (2000), in reviewing studies addressing expository skills in students with LLD, found there were several elements common to successful programs. These are summarized in Box 14-9.

Let's look at how we can incorporate these effective practices in our work.

Comprehending Expository Text. Vaughn et al. (2000) showed that even when students use strategies successfully to support their understanding of narratives, they don't spontaneously carry these strategies over to expository texts. For this reason, it is important to teach strategies for comprehending expository texts explicitly. A learning-strategies approach to exposition involves, first, helping students identify the macrostructures typically used in this genre (Bakken & Whedon, 2002). Englert and Hiebert (1984) reported on a classification system proposed by Meyer (1975) that includes six basic expository text struc-

tures. Piccolo (1987) suggested using both verbal and visual organizers to help students identify these common expository structures. Westby (2005) gave some examples of verbal organizers that can be helpful. These appear in Table 14-6. The "comprehension cues" in Table 14-6 can be used as study guides, as students prepare to be tested on material with each type of structure. They also are questions students should be taught to consider to guide their processing of expository material and can serve as self-cues to use when writing expository texts with each of the structures they are learning. Examples of visual organizers, following those suggested by Piccolo (1987) and others appear in Figure 14-11.

Identifying these structures is a useful learning strategy because it gives students a set of organizers they can bring to the task of processing new information in expository text formats. We need to remember, though, that these ideal formats are not followed in all expository writing, and much of what students read is not so easily classified into one macrostructure or another. The point of teaching this strategy is not to get bogged down in meticulous identification of text structure, but simply to give students some organizing tools that can help them make more sense and retain more information from the large amount of reading they must do to complete the high school curriculum. Analysis of text structure can easily be combined with other learning strategies approaches, such as RT. The point of expository analysis is simply to give students another tool for aiding their comprehension of this difficult material. Dickson, Simmons, and Kameenui (1995) used comparison/contrast texts as an example to demonstrate the use of notesheets, such as those in Figures 14-12 and 14-13, to aid students in comprehending expository structures.

Bakken and Whedon suggest that, after helping students to identify the structure of a text, the clinician provide a note-taking form specific to that structure. Figure 14-14 presents an example note-taking form that might be given to a selection identified as a Sequence structure. Each structure is practiced on material that is controlled for difficulty until students can take notes on it effectively, then a new structure is introduced. After several structures have been learned in this way, students are encouraged to identify text structures from several possible alternatives, and choose the correct note-taking form for reading each one. Once students can accomplish this successfully on below-grade-level material, texts closer to grade level are gradually introduced.

DiCecco and Gleason (2002) presented an additional strategy-based approach to improving comprehension of expository text in students with LLD. Their approach, presented in an intensive format (daily 40-minute sessions for four weeks), included vocabulary and preparatory set instruction before reading, oral reading by students with literal and inferential questions asked by the teacher, presentation of relationships of ideas within the passage using graphic organizers (GOs) like the ones in Figure 14-15 as a postreading activity, followed by having students write summaries of each text read. Students were taught the following strategy for writing summaries:

▶ List key points.
▶ Combine the points that go together.

BOX 14-9	**Essential Elements in Strategy Instruction**

Expository Text

- Controlling task difficulty by sequencing materials to maintain high levels of success
- Interactive, small group (3 to 10 students) instruction (ideal group size appears to be 6 students)
- Teaching students to generate their own questions as they proceed through material and asking guiding questions that stimulate thinking and invite interactive responses
- Modeling think-alouds to make the process as clear and explicit as possible, and having students think aloud as they complete tasks
- Providing extended practice and feedback from both adults and peers
- Explicit teaching of the steps in comprehending or producing exposition, using "think sheets," mnemonics, visual organizers, and other strategies
- Explicit teaching of text structures

Adapted from Baker, S., Gersten, R., & Graham, S. (2003). Teaching expressive writing to students with learning disabilities: Research-based applications and examples. *Journal of Learning Disabilities, 36,* 109-123.

TABLE 14-6	Verbal Organizers for Identifying Expository Text Structures		
TEXT STRUCTURE	**FUNCTION**	**KEY WORDS**	**COMPREHENSION CUES**
Sequence	To tell what happened or how to do or make something	*First, next, then, second, third, following, finally, subsequently, from here to, before, after, eventually*	Give the steps . . . When did . . . happen?
Enumerative	To give a list of things related to a topic and describe each	*An example, for instance, another, such as, to illustrate*	Give examples . . . Describe and give examples of . . . Give a list of . . .
Cause-effect	To explain or give reasons why something happens or exists	*Because, since, reasons, then, therefore, for this reason, results or effects, consequently, so, in order to, thus, hence, depends on, influences, affects, is a function of, leads to, produces*	Explain . . . Predict . . . Why did . . . happen? How did . . . happen? Give the causes (reasons, effects, results, etc.) of . . .
Descriptive	To tell what something is	*Is called, is, can be defined, can be interpreted, is explained, refers to, is someone who, means*	Define . . . Describe . . . List . . . What is . . . Who is . . .
Problem or solution	To state a problem and offer solutions	*The problem is, a solution is, challenges facing, proposed ways of addressing*	Describe the problem of . . . What are some proposed solutions to . . . ?
Comparison or contrast	To show likenesses and differences	*Different or same, alike or disparate, similar or dissimilar, although, or, however, on the other hand, compared to, contrasted with, rather than, instead of, but, yet, still*	Compare and contrast . . . Discuss similarities and differences . . . How are . . . alike and different?

Adapted from Westby, C. (1998a). Communication refinement in school age and adolescence. In W. Haynes & B. Shulman (Eds.), *Communication development: Foundations, processes and clinical applications* (pp. 311-360). Baltimore, MD: Williams and Wilkins.

▶ Number the points in a logical order.

▶ Reread the list in order.

▶ Write the numbered points into a paragraph.

DiCecco and Gleason were able to show that this combined approach resulted in more improvements in understanding of expository information by students with LLD than did approaches without the intensive, GO-supported instruction.

Another learning-strategy approach to improving students' comprehension of expository text material is the multipass or SQ3R method (Just & Carpenter, 1987; Robinson, 1970; Schumaker, Deshler, Denton, Alley, Clark, & Nolan, 1982), developed during World War II to teach GIs to acquire the specialized job skills needed for the war effort quickly. This procedure can be combined with the identification of expository structure to help students get the most out of their reading of expository material. Here we would teach the students the five SQ3R steps outlined in Box 14-10. This approach can readily be combined with reciprocal teaching. To do this, we would first model the SQ3R method on an expository text passage, then give each student a turn to act as facilitator in guiding the rest of the group through the process. The ultimate goal, of course, is to get students to use the method independently on their classroom material. Lasky (1991) presented a series of strategies that can serve as tools for acquiring and retaining information from texts and lectures. We can follow the steps outlined in Box 14-5 in teaching each of these strategies. We may want to introduce several, then ask students which they would like to concentrate on or which seem most effective to them. We can then provide more intensive instruction in these particular strategies. Let's look at some of Lasky's suggestions.

Verbal mediation involves overt "talking through." Students can be trained to provide themselves with verbal mediation by describing the steps necessary to accomplish a curricular task, such as doing a science experiment. They can be required to say the steps aloud, write them out, then follow their own instructions. Once they can do this kind of mediation overtly, they can be asked to do the mediation covertly, "in their heads." Students can practice covert mediation with a written description of the steps at first. Later the written form can be faded and students can be encouraged to do the same mediation all internally.

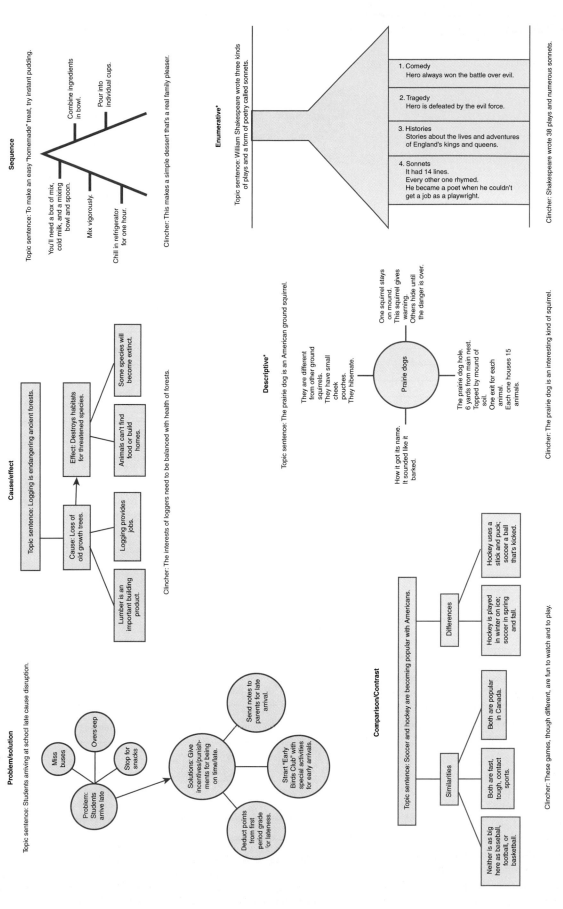

Sequence

Topic sentence: To make an easy "homemade" treat, try instant pudding.

You'll need a box of mix, cold milk, and a mixing bowl and spoon.

Combine ingredients in bowl.

Mix vigorously.

Pour into individual cups.

Chill in refrigerator for one hour.

Clincher: This makes a simple dessert that's a real family pleaser.

Enumerative*

Topic sentence: William Shakespeare wrote three kinds of plays and a form of poetry called sonnets.

1. Comedy
   Hero always won the battle over evil.

2. Tragedy
   Hero is defeated by the evil force.

3. Histories
   Stories about the lives and adventures of England's kings and queens.

4. Sonnets
   It had 14 lines.
   Every other one rhymed.
   He became a poet when he couldn't get a job as a playwright.

Clincher: Shakespeare wrote 38 plays and numerous sonnets.

Cause/effect

Topic sentence: Logging is endangering ancient forests.

Cause: Loss of old growth trees.

Lumber is an important building product.

Logging provides jobs.

Effect: Destroys habitats for threatened species.

Animals can't find food or build homes.

Some species will become extinct.

Clincher: The interests of loggers need to be balanced with health of forests.

Descriptive*

Topic sentence: The prairie dog is an American ground squirrel.

How it got its name.
It sounded like it barked.

They are different from other ground squirrels.
They have small cheek pouches.
They hibernate.

Prairie dogs

One squirrel stays on mound.
This squirrel gives warning.
Others hide until the danger is over.

The prairie dog hole.
6 yards from main nest.
Topped by mound of soil.
One exit for each animal.
Each one houses 15 animals.

Clincher: The prairie dog is an interesting kind of squirrel.

Problem/solution

Topic sentence: Students arriving at school late cause disruption.

Miss buses

Overs eep

Stop for snacks

Problem: Students arrive late

Solutions: Give incentives/punishments for being on time/late.

Send notes to parents for late arrival.

Start "Early Birds Club" with special activities for early arrivals.

Deduct points from first period grade 'or lateness.

Comparison/Contrast

Topic sentence: Soccer and hockey are becoming popular with Americans.

Differences

Hockey is played in winter on ice; soccer in spring and fall.

Hockey uses a stick and puck; soccer a ball that's kicked.

Similarities

Neither is as big here as baseball, football, or basketball.

Both are fast, tough, contact sports.

Both are popular in Canada.

Clincher: These games, though different, are fun to watch and to play.

FIGURE 14-11 ♦ Visual organizers for expository text structures. (Adapted from Calfee, R., & Chambliss, M. [1988]. Beyond decoding: Pictures of expository prose. *Annals of Dyslexia, 38,* 243–257; Meyer, B. [1975]. *The organization of prose and its effects on memory.* Amsterdam: North Holland; Nelson, N. [1993]. *Child language disorders in context: Infancy through adolescence.* Columbus, OH: Merrill; Pehrsson, R., & Denner, P. [1988]. Semantic organizers: Implications for reading and writing. *Topics in Language Disorders, 8,* 24–37; Piccolo, J. [1987]. Expository text structure: Teaching and learning strategies. *The Reading Teacher, 40,* 838–847; Richgels, D., McGee, L., Lomax, R., & Sheard, C. [1987]. Awareness of four text structures: Effects on recall of expository text. *Reading Research Quarterly, 22,*177–196; and Westby, C. [1991]. *Steps to developing and achieving language-based curriculum in the classroom.* Rockville, MD: American Speech-Language-Hearing Association.
*Reprinted with permission from Piccolo, 1987.

Comparison/Contrast Notesheet

Key words

-er words
different
but
like
similarly
in contrast

Questions to ask

1. What is being compared?
2. What features are being compared?
3. How are they alike?
4. How are they different?

Theme:_____

Use **A** if features are alike and **D** if features are different. Use **?** if you cannot tell.

Feature	A	Is alike **a** or is different **d**	B

FIGURE 14-12 ✦ Note sheet for identifying topics and features in comparison/contrast expository texts. (Adapted from Dickson, S., Simmons, D., & Kameenui, E. (1995). Instruction in expository text: A focus on compare/contrast structure. *Learning Disabilities Forum, 20,* 8-15).

Topic: _____

Similarities

_____
_____
_____

Differences

_____
_____
_____

FIGURE 14-13 ✦ Comparison/contrast organization sheet. (Adapted from Dickson, S., Simmons, D., & Kameenui, E. (1995). Instruction in expository text: A focus on compare/contrast structure. *Learning Disabilities Forum, 20,* 8-15).

Rehearsal means repeating information to store it in memory. Students with LLD are less likely than peers with normal language development to use this strategy spontaneously, but show improvement in retention of material when the strategy is used (Wiig, 1984). Students can be encouraged to use active (out-loud) rehearsal for curricular material that needs to be memorized (such as chemistry formulas, countries and capitals, or wars and dates). Written rehearsal, in which students write the information to be learned several times, also can be used. Later, silent rehearsal can be encouraged.

Paraphrasing is a strategy that requires students to transform the information to be learned into their own words and integrate the information with what is already known. It is a good follow-up strategy to verbatim rehearsal, in that it requires deeper levels of processing of the information. Students can

Sequence

General topic: _____

Step	Difference between this and previous step
1._____	_____
2._____	_____
3._____	_____
4._____	_____

FIGURE 14-14 ✦ Sample Note-taking Form for Sequence Expository Text Structure. (Adapted from Bakken, J., & Whedon, C. (2002). Teaching text structure to improve reading comprehension. *Intervention in School and Clinic, 37,* 229-233).

How Technology Influenced Life after WWI

FIGURE 14-15 ✦ Graphic organizer for relating ideas within a passage. (Adapted from DiCecco & Gleason, 2002.)

BOX 14-10	**Five Steps in the SQ3R Learning Strategy**

Survey: Skim the table of contents, headings, boldface print, illustrations, summary sections, and so on to glean the passage's main idea and general organization. Get a preparatory set on the material.

Question: Ask a set of preparatory questions based on the survey of the material to review prior knowledge and set up some purposes for reading.

Read: Read one section of the material and try to answer the preparatory questions developed for that section.

Recite: Give answers to the questions, take notes of main points and details associated with each, and give examples of important ideas contained in the text.

Review: Go over the main points, with the help of the notes. List major subpoints and give details for each. Rehearse to try to remember the main points and subpoints.

Adapted from Just, M., & Carpenter, P. (1987). *The psychology of reading and language comprehension.* Boston: Allyn and Bacon; Robinson, F. (1970). *Effective study.* New York: Harper and Row; and Schumaker, J., Deshler, D., Denton, P., Alley, G., Clark, F., & Nolan, M. (1982). Multipass: A learning strategy for improving reading comprehension. *Learning Disability Quarterly, 5,* 295-304.

---

be encouraged to play the role of teacher explaining material to a student and to imagine themselves as a "teacher" to themselves, as they paraphrase material to be studied and reviewed. The steps in Box 14-7 can be used to help students develop a paraphrasing strategy for both narrative and expository texts.

Visual imagery involves drawing or making a mental picture of information presented. Students can be asked to imagine scenes from history lessons or maps containing a variety of information from geography material. To start, students can put the images on paper. Later they can be encouraged to use mental imaging.

Networking is a strategy in which students use key words or concepts and relate them to something they already know. In this way the student builds a bridge or network from prior knowledge to the new information. Outlining is probably the most familiar form of networking. We can provide students with preconstructed outlines of textbooks or classroom lectures with main headings and some subheads filled in and others left blank. Then we can ask the student to read or listen to the material and fill in the blank lines on the outline. Gradually, students can be asked to fill in larger and larger sections of the outline. When they are proficient at this, they can be asked to scan reading material for headings and boldface type and use these cues to develop a set of main headings for a prereading outline of the passage. They can then read the passage and add subheads and details to the main headings they prepared. Using outlining combined with a prereading scan of the material is a very effective networking strategy. When students are adept at it, we can encourage them to use this strategy on their own as they confront new curricular material.

Systematic retrieval involves teaching students self-questioning strategies. Here students are taught to ask themselves a series of questions about a passage, starting by asking themselves what the main idea of the passage is. They then generate a list of questions they might be asked by the teacher about the material. Lasky (1991) suggested that we encourage students to ask themselves "why" questions in addition to questions about the "who, what, when, where, and how" of the passage. This strategy is especially effective when combined with verbal organizers for expository material (see Table 14-6). If students first identify the form of expository text, they can use the "comprehension questions" that go along with that form as a guide to their self-questions.

Scruggs and Mastropieri (1990) presented some additional mnemonic strategies students can use to aid retention of curricular material. We've talked already about the *keyword* strategy. This cues students to associate a piece of new information with a phonetically or semantically similar word (using *card*, because gambling is illegal in some places, to remember *incarcerate*, for example). The *peg word* strategy encourages students to use rhyming cues to help recall a list of information. Students might be encouraged, for example, to learn state capitals by thinking of rhymes for the first capital of each region of the country, then associating the rest of the capitals in that region with the rhyme.

Acronym strategies also can be used. In these, students use the first letters of each word in a list that needs to be remembered to form a word. The *foil* (*f*irst, *o*uter, *i*nner, *l*ast) acronym is one example. This is used to remember how to multiply algebraic terms of the form $(x + 4)(x + 5)$. The first terms in each set of parentheses are multiplied first (x^2), then the two *outer* terms ($5x$), then the two *inner* terms ($4x$), then the *last* terms in each set of parentheses ($4 \times 5 = 20$). Other mnemonics use sentences in which each word starts with the first letter of one of the items to be memorized. Many communication-disorders students learn the sentence, "*O*ld, *o*ld *T*ed *T*immons *a*bducted *F*rancis *a*cross *G*old *V*alley *A*ncient *H*ighway" to help them memorize the cranial nerves (*o*lfactory, *o*ptic, *t*rochlear, *t*rigeminal, *a*bducens, *f*acial, *a*uditory, *g*lossopharyngeal, *v*agus, *a*ccessory, *h*ypoglossal), for example. Nelson (1998) warned that although teaching mnemonic strategies like these to students with LLD can help them learn to retain information, the mnemonics should not be taught in isolation, but only in the context of other learning strategies that have the purpose of helping students store information for later recall.

Englert and Mariage (1991) developed a metacognitive approach to study skills that combines many of the techniques we've been discussing. Labeled the POSSE strategy, it is used to teach students a sequence of steps, similar to SQ3R, that can be used to maximize their acquisition and retention of curricular material. Students are taught to go through each of the following steps in the POSSE program, one for each letter in its acronym title:

Predict. Students are taught to scan the text for headings, boldface print, pictures, and any other information they can use to invoke a preparatory set, activate background information, and generate prereading questions.

Organize. Students are taught to brainstorm their prereading questions into a set of categories of information that the passage will contain. They might schematize this, using a semantic map or visual organizer.

Search. Students read the passage with their questions and organizer in mind. They look for the information they highlighted in their prereading questions.

Summarize. Students give an oral summary of the passage, stating the main idea, supporting ideas, and most salient details. They ask additional questions.

Evaluate. Students identify gaps in their understanding. They compare what they learned with what they predicted, clarify misunderstandings they encountered, and predict the topic of the next section of the passage.

In addition to these metacognitive strategies, the Kansas Institute for Research in Learning Disabilities (Schumaker & Deshler, 1984) has developed a variety of detailed lesson plans for teaching learning strategies to students with learning disabilities, which are available through the Institute.

Staskowski and Creaghead (2001) summarize the essential components for the SLP to attend to in working toward improving text comprehension in students with LLD. These

appear in Box 14-11. Culatta, Horn, and Merritt (1998) provide additional ideas for facilitating expository text comprehension.

Writing Expository Text. The expository text structures we've been discussing also are good tools for organizing students' production of written reports, research papers, and other content-based writing assignments. After going through each of the text structures, using Piccolo's procedures and practicing with verbal and visual organizers, it might be useful to have students apply the structures to their own writing. We might take a homework assignment, such as writing a report on a particular country, and write it two different ways: once using, say, an enumerative structure, and once using, perhaps, a descriptive format. Exercises like this can help students develop more flexibility and efficiency in their written communication. Strum and Rankin-Erikson (2002) demonstrated that the use of visual supports and graphic organizers like these resulted in significant increases in both length and overall quality of expository writing of students with LLD.

Piccolo suggested starting with sequence structures first, because they are most similar to the time-based organization in narratives, and following the order given in Table 14-6 when introducing expository types to students. She recommended the following series of steps for teaching students to recognize each of the expository macrostructures and provided detailed lesson plans for accomplishing each of these steps:

---

1. Define and label the structure.
2. Have students examine model paragraphs, using verbal and visual organizers to find the critical attributes of each.
3. Write a group paragraph modeling the original paragraph using a visual organizer.
4. Have students compose paragraphs individually, using the visual organizer.
5. Look for the pattern in paragraphs from students' texts.

We talked earlier about the role the SLP can play in helping students master the mechanics of writing. Although we approach these using basic remedial approaches in incidental teaching contexts, as they come up in the course of editing and revision, the process and organizational aspects of writing are best addressed by means of learning-strategies methods. Graham, Harris, and Troia (2000) showed that learning strategies approaches are effective in improving student writing. Let's look first at some strategies we can teach students to aid in the writing process. Then we'll talk about some strategies for improving their written products.

We talked earlier, too, about the basic steps in the writing process: planning, composition, and revision. Wong (2000) suggests referring to these with the acronym POWER: plan, organize, write, edit, revise. For students with LLD the first phase—planning and organizing—is usually a problem. Baker, Gersten, and Graham (2003) point out that a major difficulty for students with LLD is generating ideas for writing. They tend to have a relatively sparse knowledge base to begin with and even then fail to access all their knowledge about a topic when writing. They may forget ideas they do generate because

Essential Elements in the SLP's Approach to Improving Text Comprehension

- Develop background knowledge by providing enriching language experience around reading.
- Develop knowledge of text structure.
- Encourage use of strategies for comprehension by:
  - Determining purpose for comprehension
  - Activating prior knowledge
  - Making predictions
  - Using self-questioning
  - Retelling and summarizing
  - Visualizing and using graphic organizers
  - Self-monitoring and reflecting on comprehension

Adapted from Staskowski, M., & Creaghead, N. (2001). Reading comprehension: A language intervention target from early childhood through adolescence. *Seminars in Speech and Language, 22,* 185-207.

of interference from poorly developed spelling and laborious handwriting, and they terminate the planning process too soon, going on to composition before they develop an adequate plan for their composition. The result is writing that is sparse and unelaborated. Baker et al. found that teaching steps in the planning process explicitly, with think-alouds and encouragement for students to engage in extended dialogue with the teacher and peers during the planning process was effective in improving the writing of students with LLD. Graham and Harris (1999) propose a three-step planning strategy:

1. *Think:* Who will read this?
   Why am I writing it?
   What do I know about this topic?
   What do I want to say?
2. *Plan* what to say, using brainstorming with teacher and peers and an organizing think-sheet (Figs. 14-16 and 14-17).
3. *Write,* then **say more**.

Figure 14-16 provides a brainstorming and organizing think-sheet students can use to aid in the second of these steps, with the example of "Snowboarding" as the topic for writing. After students generate the basic ideas for the piece (the circles surrounding the topic oval), they indicate several supplementary ideas for each basic idea on the lines beside its circle.

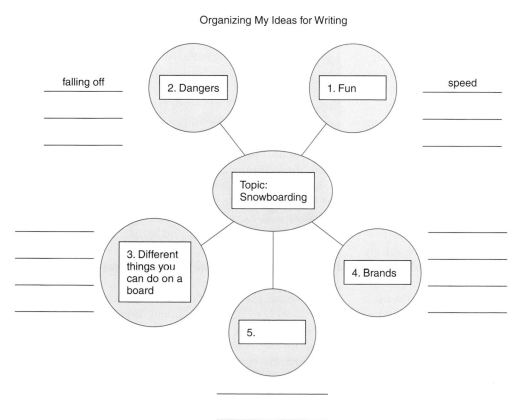

Organizing My Ideas for Writing

FIGURE 14-16 ✦ Sample brainstorming and organization thinksheet. (Based on Hallenbeck, M. (1996). The cognitive strategy in writing: Welcome relief for adolescents with learning disabilities. *Learning Disabilities Research and Practice, 11,* 107-119.

They then number the circles in the order in which they will appear in the composition. An alternative approach is simply to list all the ideas that come to mind about a topic, then use highlighters to color code ideas that should go together in the same paragraph (all the ideas about the dangers of snowboarding can be highlighted in blue; those about the different ways to use the board can be highlighted in yellow, etc.). When one of these processes is completed, students try to add additional ideas (e.g., to fill circle No. 5). Information we gained from our assessment of the writing process (see Chapter 13) can guide in developing this part of the intervention plan. The important point to remember is that encouraging students to make fuller use of the planning phase of writing is a crucial step in producing better written products. And, as Baker et al. point out, another important function of think sheets is to get students to think-aloud, and provide opportunities for extended dialogue and feedback from teachers and peers. In other words, a main function of think-sheets and other visual organizers is to give students something to talk about with others as they plan their writing. Nelson, Van Meter, Chamberlain, and Bahr (2001) remind us that an essential role the SLP can play is to encourage students to use oral language in the planning phase. We can, in collaborative settings or communication classroom settings, work with groups of students containing those with LLD to get them to talk through their planning activities, modeling and eliciting think-alouds from students before they transfer their thoughts to think-sheets and other visual forms. Figure 14-17 provides another example. Graham, Harris, and Troia (2000) provide additional ideas for developing writing skills by means of self-regulatory strategies.

Kerrigan (1974) developed another structured method for teaching students the planning phase in writing. The six steps in this procedure are given in Box 14-12. The steps can be translated into a think-aloud protocol. In using these protocols for intervention, though, we would give students the script for the protocol, based on the steps in Box 14-12, rather than leaving them on their own to develop it. In this way we would be guiding the students' thinking and providing them with a base from which to expand skills in the writing process. And we also want to remember the importance of initially controlling the difficulty of the task so that students experience success that makes them willing to persist, and of providing guided practice, feedback, and interactive questions throughout the activity.

Wiig (1984) presented an additional strategy for getting students into the composition process. She had students first free-associate to a topic, listing words or drawing a picture. Next, the students generated a list of key words about the topic that describe its interesting, unexpected aspects. These key words were then built into simple sentences. The sentences were sequenced to reflect the structure of the topic (temporal, causal, and so on). The simple sentences were then elaborated with missing details, adverbs, and modifier phrases. They were then combined into complex sentences. This process can be carried out on paper or using a word processor with a separate printout for each step in the process. Again, once students have been guided through these steps several times, they are

encouraged to guide themselves and to use similar strategies in independent writing activities.

Gerber (1993) offered some additional questions students might be taught to ask themselves in planning a composition. They include the following:

- What do I know about this topic?
- How do I feel about it?
- What has happened to me in connection with this topic? How have my experiences shaped my beliefs and values?
- What could I explain, show, or prove about this topic?
- What do my classmates know about the topic?
- What do I want them to know?

Of course, following the steps in procedures like these does not lead to the production of great literature. Eventually students have to go beyond these simplistic protocols to produce truly original writing. The advantage of simple systems like these is that they help students take that first step on the long journey toward mature, independent writing. It gets them thinking, planning, and writing, and as Vaughn et al. (2000) note, the best way to improve student writing is to get students to write!

Cochran and Bull (1991) and Nelson et al. (2001) provided ideas for using word processors to enhance the writing process. They suggested that the *Logowriter* software program (Logowriter, 1990) is particularly suited to working with students at advanced language levels. It allows students to create both text and graphics, which can be linked together. These kinds of productions make ideal "newspapers" and "magazines" for publishing student work. Westby and Clauser (1999) suggest *The Amazing Writing Machine* (Broderbund, 1995) and the *Ultimate Writing and Creativity Center* (The Learning Co., 1996), as well. Additional resources include *Secret Writer's Society* (Learning Upgrade LLC, 1999), *Storybook Weaver Deluxe* (The Learning Company, 2004), *Write On! Plus, Author's Toolkit and Literature Series I* (Sunburst, 1997), *Diary Maker* (Tom Snyder Productions, 1994), *The Writer's Companion* (Visions Technology in Education, 2003), and *Composition* (Homeworkhelp.com, 2005). In addition, hypermedia, CD-ROM and Internet resources allow students to produce materials that combine text, graphics, video, and audio information. These applications can allow students to develop exciting materials that incorporate their writing. Landis (2002), MacArthur (2000), and Strum and Koppenhaver (2000) provide additional suggestions for using assistive technology with students with disabilities.

Once students have been guided to plan written compositions, we can attend to the next phase of writing, composition. Here students must turn their raw ideas into literate statements and organize the ideas into a coherent composition. Wong, Butler, Ficzere, and Kuperis (1996) suggest using "prompt cards" to aid students in turning ideas into sentences. These cards remind students of the verbal organizers used in each type of expository writing. Clinicians and students can work together to design prompt cards for each expository category, using the information in Table 14-6 as a guide. A prompt card for cause/effect writing, adapted from Wong

Name _____

Topic: Women in the Civil War

Who: Who am I writing for? my history teacher and the others in my history class.

Why: Why am I writing? to show that it wasn't only the soldiers who took part in the

Civil War.

What: What do I know? It was hard to get clothes and things in the South because all

the factories were in the North.

_____

_____

_____

How: How can I group my ideas?

Nursing		Getting food

_____   _____
_____   _____
_____   _____

Making clothes		Writing letters

_____   _____
_____   _____
_____   _____

How will I organize my writing?

_____ Sequence   _____Comparison/contrast _____ Enumerative

_____ Cause/effect   _____Description   _____ Problem/solution

FIGURE 14-17 ✦ Example planning sheet for expository writing.

BOX 14-12 **Basic Steps in Beginning the Process of Composition**

Step 1: Write a short, simple sentence that states one idea.

Step 2: Write three sentences about the sentence in Step 1. Be sure they relate to the meaning of the entire sentence, not just one part of it. Each of these will be the topic sentence for a new paragraph.

Step 3: Write four or five sentences about each of the three topic sentences in Step 2.

Step 4: Make the sentences in Step 3 as detailed as possible. Try to say a lot about each idea, instead of talking about a lot of different ideas.

Step 5: Start a new paragraph with each topic sentence in Step 2. Follow each of these topic sentences with the detail sentences you wrote in Steps 3 and 4. Make sure that each of the sentences in each paragraph relates to the topic sentence.

Step 6: Make sure each sentence in the composition is related to the sentence that comes before it. Be sure each paragraph is clearly related to the paragraph that comes before it.

Adapted from Kerrigan, W. (1974). *Writing to the point: Six basic steps.* New York: Harcourt, Brace, Jovanovich.

Introductory phrases

This paper explains . . .
We will discuss why . . .
The cause of. . .

Explanatory phrases

The reasons for . . .
For this reason . . .
As a result of. . .
In order to . . .

Concluding phrases

To sum up the reasons for . . .
In conclusion, the explanation for _____ is . . .
As we have seen, the cause of_____ can be considered . . .

FIGURE 14-18 ✦ Prompt card for writing a cause/effect expository structure. (Adapted from Wong, B. [2000]. Writing strategies instruction for expository essays for adolescents with and without learning disabilities. *Topics in Language Disorders, 20[4],* 29-44.)

(2000) is presented in Figure 14-18. When a student decides to use the cause/effect structure for sentence generation, the card can be displayed and the student encouraged to use it to help produce sentences appropriate for that form.

The final step in a writing intervention program is to focus students' attention on the quality of their *written products.*

This attention takes place in the context of *editing* and *revising.* It's a good policy to keep the processes of generating and editing writing distinct. We want students to feel relatively uninhibited by worries about errors during the planning and process stages of writing, so that ideas can flow freely. Once the basic composition has been generated, though, it is legitimate and necessary to edit and revise for clarity, organization, and mechanics. A learning-strategies approach to this aspect of writing requires that we get students to monitor and correct their own written products, rather than correcting them ourselves.

Gerber (1993) suggested that we encourage students to start the editing process by reading their composition aloud. This slows down the reading, allowing more time to detect errors and for the student to hear how the product might sound to others. Wiig (1984) suggested that the first passes through the composition in the editing process should focus on mechanics: spelling, punctuation, capitalization, and paragraph segmentation. This gives us opportunities to supply basic-skill instruction in these areas, if needed, and to emphasize to students the importance of editing their own work for these elements. Once basic skills in writing mechanics are adequate, we can focus on strategies, such as computer-assisted spelling and grammar checkers in word-processing programs as well as careful proofreading, to maximize the accuracy of error identification. It is useful for most students to develop a strategy of making several passes through the composition, each time looking for just one element: spelling, capitalization, or punctuation.

Graham and Harris (1999) cautioned, however, that too many students with LLD think editing means *only* correcting mechanical errors. Students also need to learn that revising is essential in writing. Revising differs from editing in that its aim is to improve the overall quality of the composition rather than just correct mistakes. Graham and Harris (1999) described a strategy for revising that includes a series of self-directed prompts and reported that its use led to a significant increase in meaning-based revisions and overall writing quality in students with LLD. The strategy is summarized in Box 14-13.

The box also gives a strategy for peer revision, in which students work in pairs to provide prompts to each other. Either way, students need to be given practice in focusing on the revision process not only to correct errors but also to make meaning-related changes that enhance the quality of their writing. Westby and Clauser (2005) suggested using a form like the one in Table 14-7 to aid in peer revision activities as well. The form helps peers provide specific comments, rather than vague generalities, like "This is a good paper," on their fellow students' writing.

Baker et al. (2003) suggest an additional possibility at the revision stage: cognitive apprenticeship (CA). CA involves pairing the student with an older or more effective writing mentor and having the mentor think-aloud as she or he goes through the composition, talking through strategies like those in Box 14-13, discussing and questioning the apprentice and demonstrating the ways in which the writing can be improved by changing words, sentences, and organization. This procedure would follow editing for mechanical errors in order to

BOX 14-13   Self- and Peer Prompts for Revising Compositions of Students with LLD at the Advanced Language Stage

Self-Prompts

Read your composition.
Find the sentence that gives the main idea. Is it clear?
Add two sentences to make it clearer or stronger.
SCAN each sentence:
• Does it make *Sense?*
• Is it *Connected* to the rest of the composition?
• Can you *Add* more?
• *Note* errors.
Make necessary changes on your computer or on your paper with a red marker.
Reread the composition. Make any final changes.
Recopy or print out revised version.

Peer Prompts

(Two peers provide suggestions to each other on how to revise their respective writings.)
Listen as your partner reads the piece out loud and read along.
Tell what your partner's paper is about and what you liked best.
Reread your partner's paper and make notes:
• Is everything clear?
• Can any details be added?
Discuss your suggestions with your partner.
Revise your own paper.
Exchange papers and check for errors:
• Capitalization
• Punctuation
• Spelling

Adapted from Graham, S., & Harris, K. (1999). Assessment and intervention in overcoming writing difficulties: An illustration from the self-regulated strategy development model. *Language, Speech, and Hearing Services in Schools, 30,* 255-264.

allow the student to focus on the improvement of tone, meaning, and organization in the writing.

If students are using word processors to write the compositions, the prompts can be used when the first draft has been completed and edited for mechanical errors, and changes can be made on the screen before printing. If students are working on paper, they can make revisions with a different-colored pen.

We also can encourage students to use some of our assessment instruments for self-assessment and as guides to revision. Students can be given, for example, Dagenais and Beadle's (1984) holistic evaluation criteria listed in Table 13-10. The clinician can give guided practice in applying the criteria to work the students are producing for some of their academic classes. They can then be encouraged to use these criteria in revising the writing, attempting to make changes that would result in a higher score. They can be encouraged to focus on one criterion at a time, such as providing sufficient information, giving clear cohesion, or using a literate language tone. Again, they can be taught to make several passes through the writing, each time attending to just one of the criteria and making changes that improve that one element. After several passes, they can be asked to use the criteria to reevaluate their writing sample and see how much they have improved it. As Baker et al. (2003) showed, teaching self-monitoring is an important aspect of improving writing for secondary students with LLD.

Similarly, students can be asked to do a self-assessment of a writing sample using the checklist in Table 13-1. Here they can be encouraged to give themselves a "+" or "−" for each element on the checklist, at first in consultation with the SLP. For each element for which they gave themselves a "−," students can be asked to make one pass through the composition and find ways to improve their performance. After revising for each "−," they can reread their composition and reevaluate it.

As a final step, Graham (1992) suggested having students use a checklist to monitor their completion of all the steps in the writing process. A version of this checklist appears in Figure 14-19. This kind of self-monitoring can help students develop the habit of "double checking" themselves as they complete academic assignments.

The goals of a learning-strategies approach to writing instruction for students with LLD are two. First, we want to help students to get more fluent in the planning process of writing and to learn to devote some time to planning before producing the actual product. Second, we want to impress on them the importance of editing and revising and to help them see these steps as essential in the production of a finished writing product. By giving students some self-prompting and cueing strategies for achieving these steps in the writing process, we are providing the tools they need to develop into independent, literate writers.

Persuasive Text. We talked earlier about the prevalence of persuasive texts in high stakes tests at the secondary level. Once basic skill instruction has been used to familiarize students with the functions and structures of persuasive writing, we can use the same sorts of strategies for helping them learn to evaluate and improve their own persuasive writing as we do for other genres. These strategies include graphic organizers, think-aloud procedures, "think sheets," and so on, geared toward persuasive writing. Figure 14-20 provides an example visual organizer for a persuasive essay.

The Metas

Learning-strategy approaches are ideally suited to working on "meta" skills with students at the advanced language level.

TABLE 14-7	Guidelines for Peer Comments on Expository Writing

GUIDELINE: WHEN YOU WORK WITH A PARTNER TO REVISE YOUR WRITING, ASK YOURSELF, DID I:	EXAMPLE
Praise specific aspects of the writing? Ask questions that guide thinking? Make comments that link to text?	*You gave a vivid description of rainforests in the first paragraph.* *You said the rainforest is endangered. Why? Give three reasons.* *You said tigers are disappearing from the rainforest because of hunting. That surprised me; isn't hunting illegal? Are there other reasons?*
Offer to think together about how to improve the essay.	*I got confused in the second paragraph when you talked about acid rain. Maybe we can figure out a way to make that clearer. What did you mean?*

Adapted from Westby, C., & Clauser, P. (2005.) The right stuff for writing: Assessing and facilitating written language. In H. Catts & A. Kahmi (Eds.) *Language and reading disabilities* (2nd ed.). (pp. 274-340). Boston: Allyn & Bacon.

____ I found a quiet place to work.
____ I read or listened to the teacher's directions carefully.
____ I thought about who would read my paper.
____ I thought about what I know about the subject.
____ I thought about what I wanted my paper to accomplish.
____ I used brainstorming to plan my paper before I wrote.
____ I organized my ideas before I wrote.
____ I got all the information I needed before I wrote.
____ I thought about the reader as I wrote.
____ I thought about what I wanted to accomplish as I wrote.
____ I continued to think and plan as I wrote.
____ I revised the first draft of my paper.
____ I checked to be sure a reader could understand what I meant.
____ I checked to make sure I had accomplished my goals.
____ I checked my paper for spelling, capitalization, and punctuation errors.
____ I reread my paper before turning it in.
____ I asked other students or my parents to read the paper to see what they thought.
____ I rewarded myself when I finished.

FIGURE 14-19 ✦ Self-monitoring checklist for student writing. (Adapted from Graham, S. [1992]. Helping students with LD progress as writers. *Intervention in School and Clinic, 27*, 134-144.)

Since "meta" skills require awareness and conscious attention, they mesh well with learning-strategies approaches that teach students to use planning and self-evaluation. We've already talked about a variety of metalinguistic strategies for the areas of semantics, syntax, and pragmatics. Let's look at the other two areas of "meta" skills we've been discussing, self-regulation and metacognition, and examine some learning-strategies approaches for each.

Self-Regulation. Students need to continually evaluate their own performance in order to decide when to invoke the strategies they have. This aspect of metacognition is often called self-regulation. Like the other strategies we teach our students, instruction in self-regulation strategies, though at a more

"meta" level, requires the same components we have been discussing, which are summarized in Box 14-9. Wong (2000) presents an example of a prompt-sheet that can be used for teaching self-regulatory strategies in the area of curricular writing. This appears in Figure 14-21.

Equally important is students' ability to *monitor their comprehension* of both written and spoken material. When working on comprehension monitoring, the strategies we teach students address both detection of gaps in their understanding and procedures for doing something to fill in those gaps.

Bunce (1991) suggested using a barrier-game format to develop comprehension monitoring skill for spoken material. Here students take turns being speaker and listener, giving and

Visual organizer for persuasive essay in response to prompt: 'In some schools, officials have the right to search students' personal property (lockers, backpacks, purses) without permission. Decide whether you are **for** or **against** officials having this right. Write an essay for the school newspaper to convince other students of your position. Be sure to include supporting details.

Thesis: I think that school officials should/should not have the right to search students' personal property without their permission.

Argument: First,
Warrant:
Data:

Argument: Second,
Warrant:
Data:

Argument: Third,
Warrant:
Data:

Restatement of thesis: In summary,

FIGURE 14-20 ✦ Visual organizer for persuasive essay.

POWER CHECKLIST

Plan

____ Did I complete a think sheet?

____ Did I talk it over with my teacher and other students?

____ Do I have my think sheet with me?

____ Did I put my name, date, and title of the essay on my paper?

Organize

____ Have I chosen an organizational structure for my paper?

____ Did I use a graphic organizer to lay out my ideas?

Write

____ Did I follow my plan?

____ Did I include all the ideas in my graphic organizer?

____ Does the first paragraph state my opinion and give supporting ideas?

____ Do my middle paragraphs elaborate my main idea?

____ Does my last paragraph give a summary and reasons for my conclusion?

Edit

____ Have I checked for spelling mistakes?

____ Have I checked for grammar mistakes?

____ Have I checked for punctuation mistakes?

____ Have I checked for capitalization mistakes?

____ Have I asked a teacher or peer to check over the paper with me?

____ Have I made all the corrections?

Revise

____ Have I read my paper aloud and conferenced with my partner?

____ Have I found ways to make my paper clearer and more mature?

FIGURE 14-21 ✦ Checklist for self-regulation in writing a persuasive essay. (Adapted from Wong, B. (2000). Writing strategies instruction for expository essays for adolescents with and without learning disabilities. *Topics in Language Disorders, 20(4)*, 29-44.)

following a set of directions for, for example, drawing a map from a pattern in the book for a geography assignment. The directions given by each speaker are tape-recorded. After the map has been drawn and the pattern and drawn map compared, students listen together to the tape. They identify areas in the instructions that were unclear or misleading and discuss how the directions could have been given differently to result in a more accurate product. Students can then generate a list of "pointers" for giving clear directions. They can try the exercise again, this time stopping each other at points at which the speaker has failed to follow the "pointers" developed by the partners. Students also can be encouraged to ask specific questions of themselves as they hear each step of the directions. These questions are designed both to detect errors in understanding and to provide a strategy for correcting the problem. Questions such as the following might be used:

• Did I "get" it? What did the instruction tell me to do?
• Can I follow the direction? Do I have everything I need?
• Do I need to ask (student) to repeat the instruction? Part of it?
• Do I need to ask what a word means?
• Do I need to check that I got it right? Shall I repeat what I heard and ask if it's correct?

After some work of this kind in the barrier-game setting, students can be encouraged to apply their strategies to classroom lectures. Here video or audiotaped lectures can be used. Students can be required to listen to a portion of the lecture, take notes, then examine their notes for gaps in their understanding. In the lecture format, unlike in the barrier game, it may not always be acceptable to stop the lecturer to ask for clarification, repetition, or additional background information when a comprehension gap arises. For this reason, students need to learn to give themselves signals in their notes that a problem occurred. A question mark can be placed in the margin, for example, whenever the student detects a gap in comprehension.

Students then need to develop strategies to clarify these points. Students can be asked to brainstorm with the SLP some ways to fill in the gaps. They might, for example, ask a friend after class, stay after class to ask the teacher, look up an unknown word in the dictionary, check a detail on a map, or reread the relevant passage in the textbook.

Knapczyk (1991) developed a program to help students acquire comprehension-monitoring skills in classroom lecture situations. Students begin, again, by listening to taped lectures from the regular curriculum in the resource-room or communication classroom setting. The tape is stopped periodically, and each time it is stopped students are required to ask a question relevant to the material. At the next session, the same tape is played and students are required to stop the tape themselves when they have a question. However, they are required to stop it only at a natural break in the presentation or when the teacher had indicated it was acceptable to ask a question. Several more sessions of a similar kind are given, using different classroom lectures. Finally, students are instructed to use questions in a specified regular classroom setting. Before entering the class, though, they are reminded to identify points in the lecture where it is appropriate to ask a question and to ask relevant questions designed to fill in gaps in their understanding of the material.

The goal of the development of these comprehension-monitoring strategies is to get students to recognize when they fail to understand; to have some options for repairing the difficulty; and to place the responsibility for monitoring comprehension, as well as the ability to do something about it, in their hands.

Strategies for monitoring comprehension of written material have the same goals. Here we want to encourage students to use a strategy such as the SQ3R method, focusing particularly on the development of a preparatory set of questions. Students would use the questions to guide their reading and note any questions they were unable to answer because of difficulties with comprehension. Self-questioning, using queries like the ones we just looked at, is also helpful for getting students to recognize gaps in their understanding. Students can be encouraged to place a small "sticky" note in the margin of the text to indicate a passage, word, or phrase that they did not understand. They might write a quick note to themselves on the "sticky" to indicate what else they need to know, or what preparatory question the passage could answer if they were able to decipher it. Again, we can encourage students to brainstorm a list of ways to fill in their comprehension gaps. Asking classmates or parents (during homework time), getting to class a minute early to ask the teacher, and checking a dictionary or on-line encyclopedia might be ways to start this list. In addition, Thiede and Anderson (2003) showed that asking students to summarize what they read resulted in more accurate comprehension monitoring than occurred without summarizing. Having students use a summarization strategy, then, combined with explicit instructions to ask themselves how well they summarized and how they could improve their summaries can also increase comprehension monitoring.

It is important to note that comprehension monitoring of written material can only take place in the context of understanding most of the material in the text. If students are reading significantly below grade level, they may not be able to monitor reading comprehension adequately because the gaps are too frequent and too extensive. If this is the case, some modification of the material they are required to read may be needed, or accommodations for them to get the information from some source outside classroom texts may be necessary. As we saw, controlling the difficulty of material is crucial to helping students develop effective strategy use.

Metacognition. Metacognition involves, as we've seen, awareness and management of our own thought processes, and reflection on our own and others' thinking as an object of thought, or "thinking about thinking." Kuhn and Dean (2004) call this "critical thinking." In working on learning strategies in the metacognitive area, we are essentially teaching students tactics for becoming critical readers and thinkers. Kuhn and Dean suggested that one way of supporting metacognitive development is to encourage students to reflect on and evaluate their activities: Why are we doing this? What was gained from having done it? Another source of metacognitive development is the internalization that occurs when students learn to ask themselves questions they have been asked often in similar circumstances. If students participate in discourse where they are frequently asked, "How do you know?" or "What makes you say that?" they become more likely to pose such questions to themselves.

Vaughn et al. (2000) reviewed literature that suggests that learning strategies approaches do foster metacognition, especially if they contain the following elements:

▸ Extended practice with feedback from adults and peers
▸ Use of interactive questions

▸ Breaking tasks down into component parts
▸ Using prompts and cues that are gradually faded

CONTEXTS OF INTERVENTION IN THE ADVANCED LANGUAGE STAGE

AGENTS OF INTERVENTION

For students with advanced language, most intervention is delivered by the SLP in collaboration with other special educators and mainstream teachers. One additional agent of intervention at this level, though, is the normally achieving peer. We've talked already about using peers to help our students improve their functional language and classroom communication skills. Peers also can serve as intervention agents to provide content mastery instruction to students with LLD. In this role, they would work as tutors, perhaps during study halls or homeroom periods, to go over homework, share classroom lecture notes, or answer the curricular questions of a student with LLD. Murray-Seegert (1989) described a program in which regular education students, some of whom were at risk for school failure themselves, volunteered to work with students with disabilities to receive course credit for an "Internal Work Experience."

The advantages of using peer tutors to help our clients with content mastery, rather than tutoring them ourselves, are two. First, it involves the client in direct social interaction with peers, which may blossom into friendship and could provide the student with additional *entree* into the peer circle. Choosing a popular peer to act as a tutor can help to facilitate such outcomes. Second, using peers as content mastery tutors frees up the SLP's time to do what we do best: developing programs that improve communication, rather than working with individuals on subject matter in which we may be less than expert. Finally, recent research (summarized by Anderson, Yilmaz, & Wasburn-Moses, 2004) indicates that when peer-tutoring is instituted class-wide, all students show increases in test results, and students with LLD show larger increases than typical students. When consulting with classroom teachers who have students on IEPs in their classrooms, suggesting class-wide peer tutoring is one way to accommodate the student with LLD while benefiting all the students in the classroom.

Larson and McKinley (1987) provided guidelines for recruiting and training peer tutors. They suggested first enlisting the enthusiasm of other teachers and administrators in the program. This can be accomplished by discussing it at in-services, sending out brief newsletters, and talking informally with faculty and administrators. They advocated recruiting tutors through school newspapers and teacher recommendations and suggested making the process of choosing tutors a selective one, involving formal applications and interviews. This both helps to ensure suitability of the tutors and makes them feel they have achieved something merely by being selected over others. Additional incentives, such as course credit or recognition for volunteer service at awards assemblies, also are wise additions to the program.

In using peers to provide content mastery instruction, we also need to provide some training to the tutor. Here it is important to emphasize that the tutor is not to do the work for the client, but to help guide the student's attention and develop learning strategies. If we do some learning-strategy instruction in collaborative lessons in the regular classroom, we can instruct the tutors to use elements of the methods taught in these sessions, such as SQ3R or POSSE, when addressing the curricular area with which they are helping the client. Larson and McKinley also suggested additional guidelines to emphasize to tutors. These include the following:

1. Focus on the client's strength,
2. Work with the student's interests.
3. Listen to the student.
4. Accept the student at his or her level.
5. Help the student learn to pay attention.
6. Help students complete assignments independently.
7. Create challenges for the student.
8. Make sure the student feels comfortable asking questions.

Some books about tutoring also can be recommended to peer tutors and might be kept in the school library. These include *Developing a Successful Tutoring Program* (Koskinen & Wilson, 1982a), *Tutoring: A Guide to Success* (Koskinen & Wilson, 1982b), *A Guide for Student Tutors* (Koskinen & Wilson, 1982c), and *Tutoring Can Be Fun* (Klausmeier, Jetter, & Nelson, 1972).

Nelson (1998) suggested another use of peers as intervention agents. She advocated a "buddy system" in which a normally achieving and a disabled student take notes on classroom lectures, then share their notes afterward. The key to this system is to have the client take the notes, but to examine and compare them after the lecture with those of the peer. The peer's notes can be copied by the student with LLD, but not before the pair has examined the two versions and identified any inconsistencies or gaps in the client's notes. This system not only provides the client with better access to the information presented in the lecture, but supplies a way to improve note-taking skills by learning from detailed comparison with those of an academically successful peer.

Finally, we should think about having the student with LLD serve as a tutor for others. Vaughn et al. (2000) suggested that working with a partner for sustained amounts of time, switching roles between tutor and tutee, was a highly effective practice in working with students with LLD. Moreover, they found that when students with LLD serve in the role of tutor in reading situations, listening to others' accurate oral reading, following along silently, then formulating relevant questions about what the tutee read, positive effects are increased. We may, then want to think about ways in which we can engage students with LLD in "tutoring" younger successful readers, or in exchanging tutor/tutee roles with peers for reading practice.

SERVICE DELIVERY MODELS

Larson and McKinley (2003b) discussed service delivery options for secondary students with LLD and argued that the pull-out or clinical approach has many problems at this level. They observed that students do not want to give up study halls and free periods for therapy and should not be pulled out of regular classes. They also pointed out additional problems, such as the lack of connection to the curriculum, the lack of communication between the SLP and other faculty, and the "patchy" nature of this kind of intervention. They argued that, although a range of service delivery options should be available, the major portion of the intervention program for adolescents with LLD should take place either in special course-for-credit programs designed for these students or in collaborative or consultation formats aimed at helping the student succeed in the mainstream program.

Ehren (2002), in discussing ways in which SLPs can contribute to academic success for secondary students with LLD, emphasized that, even when we are not seeing students on a one-to-one basis, the therapeutic aspect of our interactions with them should be paramount. That is, whether we are seeing students in a clinical setting, communication classroom group, or as part of an in-class collaboration, the same elements are critical to making our efforts effective, and our involvement different from what the student gets from the regular teacher. Intervention should be:

▶ Individualized and responsive, using ongoing, dynamic assessment and constantly modifying the program to meet the student in his current zone of proximal development

▶ Systematic; that is, organized and sequenced into small segments to control for task difficulty, providing instruction that includes explanation, modeling and guided practice that is scaffolded by questions, explanations, and conversations

▶ Intensive, engaging for extended periods of time (more than would be spent in a typical classroom) on guided, interactive activities that are goal-directed and provide opportunities to achieve mastery and generalization

Let's look at our four service delivery options and talk about how we can use them to achieve this kind of intervention at the secondary level.

The Clinical Model

Although pull-out instruction will probably make up only a small part of the intervention at this level, at some times and for some clients a pull-out/sit-in program is appropriate. When using pull-out with secondary students, we want to be sensitive to the students' feelings of embarrassment about needing help and find ways to minimize them. Working with students in small groups, perhaps during "club" or homeroom period, may help. We also want to be sure to use groups rather than individual students so that no one feels singled out. We should limit the duration of the pull-out intervention, using it only to lay the basis for collaborative or consultative work in the classroom. Coming into the classroom to do individual intervention may be just as embarrassing to a student as being pulled out. When we do come into the class, it should be to provide instruction collaboratively to the whole group.

Pull-out/sit-in instruction can be effective in conjunction with collaborative work on study skills or other metacognitive activities in the mainstream classroom. We can "prep" a small group of clients on the SQ3R method, for example, before going into their social studies class to teach it to the group. This gives the clients a "leg up" on the other students in mastering the technique and gives them that extra guided practice they probably need to succeed with it.

The Language-Based Course for Credit

At the advanced language level, most direct instruction to students should take place in a language class offered as an "elective" within the curriculum. Larson and McKinley (2003b) discussed some of the factors needed for its success. First, they emphasized that students must receive credit toward graduation for the course. This entails receiving grades, although grading can be done in a variety of ways. Students may contract to do certain tasks, which, if completed, ensure them a certain grade in the course. Alternatively, the course may be graded on a pass-fail basis. Portfolio grading—that is, grading products of participation in the course rather than testing—is popular in the mainstream curriculum and can be used in the language-based course for credit as well. Initiating language-based courses for credit may require the SLP to lay some groundwork. Administrators may need to be convinced of the efficacy of the courses and that they do not contradict the spirit of inclusion of students with disabilities within the mainstream curriculum. Again, in-service presentations, short newsletters, and prototype programs can be used to help get over these hurdles.

Larson and McKinley (2003b) suggested scheduling classes to conform to the existing structure of other classes in the building. If some courses are offered in 6- or 8-week modules, these can be ideal scheduling vehicles for language-based classes as well. Semester-long or year-long courses also are options. If other classes in the building last 50 minutes, the language-based course should, too. The classes should be scheduled along with other subject areas in as similar a way as possible.

To get students motivated to take these courses, they need to be held in "real" classrooms, not therapy rooms or other stigmatized settings. Since few SLPs in secondary schools have the luxury of their own classrooms, teaching the class in a mainstream setting may require a nomadic existence, in which the SLP moves each period to whatever classroom is available. Larson and McKinley (1995) argued that the benefits of holding the class in regular education areas are worth this inconvenience.

The name of the course also is an important consideration. Larson and McKinley (2003b) suggested avoiding names that might carry a stigma, such as "Remedial Communication," and opting instead for titles that sound supportive and mainstream. Some suggestions include "Effective Communication," "Communication Studies," and "Communication Laboratory."

To whatever extent possible, we want to group students in a class on the basis of shared needs and similar levels of current functioning, although scheduling considerations also come into play here. When choosing students for the class, Larson, McKinley, and Boley (1993) suggested that class size should be in the 3 to 12 range and that there should be no more than a two-grade spread among students in the class. They advocated involving students actively in the planning of goals and objectives for the class and in choosing from among a set of appropriate topics and activities. The purpose of the class should be explained, and the clinician should be as open as possible about the fact that the class is designed to help the students overcome some of the difficulties they have in school.

The content of the communication class is determined to a large extent by the assessment data on individual students. In general, the goal is to focus on cognitive and communicative skills that enable students to function effectively in school, home, vocational, and leisure settings. Virtually all the activities we discussed in the section on processes of intervention are adaptable to the communication classroom setting. An advantage of this setting, too, is that in addition to using activities with mainstream curricular content, the clinician can focus on a few units or themes that are of high interest to the students, and use these as a context for some of the activities we've discussed. Sports, ancient mythology, careers, and issues in local or school politics have been used effectively as themes in communication classrooms for adolescent students. Ehren (2002) suggested a balance of skills and strategy instruction, all of which included the elements of effective intervention outlined above.

Consultation and Collaboration

All the issues involved in collaborative and consultative service delivery models that we discussed in Chapter 12 apply at the advanced language level as well. The success of these models requires scheduled conference time with other faculty and the building of administrative support, for example. Many of the techniques we discussed for achieving these goals in elementary schools can be used effectively in secondary schools as well.

Larson, McKinley, and Boley (1993) pointed out the difficulties of providing consultation and collaboration at the secondary level. These include the fact that teachers are very independent in their development of course material and that they deal with so many students, spending very little time in one-to-one interaction with each. Furthermore, no one teacher has primary responsibility for any student. Larson et al. argued that secondary teachers may need to be "sold" on the idea of the importance of language as a basis for success throughout the curriculum. A yearly in-service presentation on information like that given in Chapter 10 can help get this message across. Written formats also can be an effective way to communicate with secondary teachers. Newsletters alerting them to your willingness to provide consultation and collaboration or brief statements about the importance of language in the classroom might help make your presence and role in the school better known.

Consultation. One of the first obstacles we'll encounter in providing consultation at the secondary level, as we've seen, is finding teachers who will agree to consult with us. It may help to approach several of a student's teachers and ask whether they would be willing to talk with you periodically about some hints for helping the student do better in the class. If the consultation is originally focused on the student rather than the teacher, teachers may be less likely to believe the consultation's object is to "correct" poor teaching. Ehren (2002) suggests asking, "Can you share with me any approaches that especially help Peter," or "Is there something I can do to help Mike succeed in your class," rather than telling the teacher what to do. Additionally, when we do get to making suggestions we can back them up with concrete help such as making overheads or lecture outlines for the teacher, the consultation is more likely to be well-received. As we discussed before, not every teacher will be willing to enter a consultative relationship. We should try to identify first those who are most interested and receptive, and establish relations with these. As success is seen, it will be easier to find new recruits. Larson and McKinley (1995) and Marvin (1990) provided additional suggestions for effective consultation.

Anderson et al. (2004) identified six practices that appeared to be the most effective in helping students with LLD succeed in general education classrooms. As part of our consulting with classroom teachers, we can suggest the following procedures:

▶ *Mnemonic strategy instruction*: We can encourage teachers to present strategies such as Keywords and POSSE, or offer to present them in collaborative teaching sessions.

▶ *Visual and graphic organizers*: Sharing some of the graphic organizers we use with our student with their classroom teachers can encourage them to use these supports, which are valuable to general as well as special education students.

▶ *Guided notes*: We can work with teachers to provide prepared handouts that guide a student through a lecture or discussion with visual cues and spaces for the student to write key facts and concepts. Teachers may choose to provide these to all students, or only to those on IEPs.

▶ *Class-wide peer tutoring*: As we discussed before, this practice helps students take responsibility for their own learning and benefits even top students as well as those with special needs.

▶ *Linking current knowledge to new information*: Using techniques we've discussed, such as creating anticipatory sets and activating background knowledge, facilitates the ability of all students to assimilate new information.

▶ *Reciprocal teaching*: Providing students with problems, procedures, and materials, having them brainstorm ways to use what they have been given to solve the problem after modeling and support from the teacher helps students master concepts through their own thinking and experimenting.

In general, consultation to secondary teachers about adolescents with LLD can have two goals: to modify the presentation of material and to make some accommodations for the student in the classroom. That is, we can try to make some changes in how the teacher presents material to the students, which will benefit the student with LLD and mainstream students as well. We also can provide guidance and assistance in accommodating the kinds of written assignments, tests, note-taking, and so on that the student with LLD must do to participate in the mainstream curriculum.

In consulting to *modify presentation of information* in the classroom, one approach that can be used is to encourage what Nelson (1998) called "mediational teaching" or what Silliman and Wilkinson (1991) called "dialogic mentoring." We talked earlier about some methods for implementing these approaches, including *reciprocal teaching* and *postscript modeling*. An additional technique was suggested by Westby (1998a). It makes use of Bloom's (1956) taxonomy for categorizing levels of thought. Teachers using this approach would, when students reply to questions, use the answer to identify students' current level of thinking ability and then provide a scaffolding question that encourages the student to operate at the next-higher level. Examples of questions at each level are presented in Table 14-8.

When encouraging teachers to use any of these dialogic-mentoring techniques on a consulting basis, it is important to prepare written summaries of the technique and to discuss it with each teacher, giving detailed examples of how it might be used within that teacher's curricular area. Another helpful approach is to offer to teach one class of the teacher's collaboratively, using the technique, to give a chance for the teacher to see it in action. It is also important in working with teachers on their questioning techniques to encourage teachers to make answering a positive experience for students with LLD. Lunday (1996) suggested circulating "tip sheets" to teachers like the one in Box 14-14 to remind them of the importance of the way they use questions in their classes.

Lasky (1991) presented some additional guidelines for modifying the teacher's presentation of information for the benefit of the student with LLD. She suggested, first, that we ask teachers to use a *slow rate of presentation*. This is perhaps one of the simplest modifications teachers can make and can be extremely helpful to students with LLD. Besides just talking more slowly, teachers can be encouraged to insert short (1-second) pauses within long or complex sentences to give students additional processing time. A second suggestion is to ask teachers to provide *redundancy*. Teachers can paraphrase difficult material so that students hear it several different ways. They also can summarize the main points of the material at the end of the presentation. Even verbatim repetition, with modification of the stress and intonation pattern for emphasis, can be an effective rhetorical technique and provides helpful redundancy. Visual and graphic organizers are also very helpful ways of supporting the learning of students with LLD, and we can remind teachers that they will probably be helpful to many students in the class. Lasky also advised us to have teachers *provide contextual cues*. These might include stating the topic to be discussed; using visual aids such as slides, overheads, and charts to reinforce the verbal presentation; putting an outline of the presentation on an overhead or handout; and asking directed questions to focus students' attention on critical points in the presentation and aid in recall. Another suggestion is to *relate new information to*

TABLE 14-8	Sample Questions Based on Bloom's (1956) Taxonomy	
LEVEL	**DEFINITION**	**EXAMPLE**
Knowledge	Remembers and repeats information presented, answers simple questions.	How many electoral college votes does Texas have in presidential elections?
Comprehension	Demonstrates understanding by paraphrasing or restating information in own words.	Explain how the electoral college works.
Application	Uses information, rules, methods, or principles learned in new but similar situations.	How is the electoral college system like a parliamentary system, such as the one we discussed in Israel?
Analysis	Identifies components, gives explanations, identifies problems.	How would an electoral college system work if it were applied to our student government?
Synthesis	Abstracts from previously learned material to generate solutions to new but related problems.	What kinds of problems can arise from an electoral college system of presidential elections?
Evaluation	Compares alternatives, states and justifies opinions, provides evidence for responses.	Discuss how national election policies should be reformed and why.

Adapted from Westby, C. (2005). Assessing and facilitating text comprehension problems. In H. Catts & A. Kahmi (Eds.). *Language and reading disabilities* (2nd ed., pp. 157-232). Boston: Allyn & Bacon.

BOX 14-14	Sample Teacher "Tip Sheet" for Classroom Questions

Asking Questions: Expecting Answers

Teachers ask questions that they expect students to be able to answer. Questioning students helps the learning process. A teacher's response to students' answers can foster this learning process and also protect the student's self-esteem.

Here are a few basic but powerful behaviors:

Provide wait time: Pausing to allow a student more time to answer instead of moving on to the next student when you don't get a response

Dignify responses: Give credit for the correct aspects of an incorrect response

Restating the question: Asking the question a second time

Rephrasing the questions: Using different words that might increase the probability of a correct response

Providing guidance: Giving enough hints and clues so that the student will eventually determine the correct answer

These actions may seem insignificant, but they send a powerful message of acceptance to students. Students who feel accepted become active learners!

---

consulting with teachers on these techniques, we can present them with a simple list of "suggestions for helping students with disabilities 'make it' in your classroom." The list might look like this:

1. Talk slowly.
2. Pause within long sentences.
3. Repeat important information.
4. Provide visual cues.
5. Relate new information to something students already know.

We might give the list to a willing teacher and ask him or her to see what changes might be made. When the teacher identifies some, we can talk about them in more detail, making concrete suggestions and giving examples from the teacher's classroom content.

In addition to giving teachers techniques like these, we also can offer some simple tips for helping our students succeed in the classroom. These might include asking teachers to write all their instructions on the board as they say them. This both slows them down, so directions are easier to process, and provides an additional visual version that students can refer to if they didn't get it the first time or if they forget the instructions. Conversely, we can ask teachers to read written instructions given on tests and homework assignments aloud, again providing an alternate modality for students who may have trouble processing information from printed material. Asking teachers to pause briefly after they ask a question can give the student with LLD additional time to retrieve an answer. If asking for a list of answers (such as three causes of World War I), teachers can, after a pause, ask the student with LLD for an answer first. This gives him or her the opportunity to provide a correct answer, before all the "good" answers are taken. Mainstream

something the students already know. An easy way to do this is to use names of the students in the class in examples the teacher gives. Choosing examples from areas in which students have experience or interest, such as sports, also aids recall. In

students can provide other aspects of the answer (Lavoie, 1989). Ehren (2002) made some additional suggestions, including the following:

▶ Advising teachers to present learning experiences in addition to listening, such as debates or other participatory activities.

▶ Asking teachers to provide greater guidance and support to students with LLD by breaking assignments down into parts, and giving more opportunities for practice.

▶ Suggesting teachers take the time to explain to students with LLD where they have made errors and how they can correct them.

▶ Helping teachers use anticipatory sets to marshal and evaluate their students' background knowledge on curricular topics. If background knowledge gaps are identified, the SLP can help the student find ways to catch up.

▶ Encouraging teachers to use peer-assisted activities such as cooperative learning groups to provide students with LLD opportunities to practice social skills being developed in the communication classroom setting.

▶ Ask teachers to offer choices to students with LLD about how they complete assignments, the topics they write on, etc. Choices help the student feel more involved.

In addition to providing teachers with suggestions for modifying the presentation of language in the classroom, consultation can be used to make other *accommodations for students with disabilities*. Here we may encounter some resistance, even from formerly cooperative consultees. Some teachers may feel it is "not fair" to make accommodations for students with LLD that are not made for others in the class. Why, for example, should only one student get an outline of the lecture or the opportunity to make a detailed map instead of a written report about a country when the others don't get to do the same? Some of these concerns can be addressed by encouraging the teacher to go ahead and give the aid to *every* student. An outline of a lecture, or flexibility of assignments, will no doubt be of help to all.

Other accommodations, though, such as allowing extra time on tests or reducing the number of questions that must be answered, may not be appropriate for mainstream students. In cases like these, we might want to use an example like that presented by Lavoie (1989). We might ask teachers to imagine that one student in the class suddenly chokes on a piece of gum. Let's say the teacher knows how to do the Heimlich maneuver, but as the student chokes, the teacher tells him, "Well, I could do a Heimlich, but it wouldn't be fair if I did one for you and didn't do it for everyone in the class." The point is that most students do not need the accommodations, but if someone does, it is eminently "fair" to provide them, since survival in the classroom for *this* student may depend on them.

The two ways we can provide accommodations for students in secondary classrooms are by modifying curricular materials and by modifying the way students are required to demonstrate knowledge. Larson and McKinley (1995) provided some suggestions for *adapting materials* for students with LLD. They suggested putting students' textbooks on tape (student volunteer service organizations, school volunteers, or senior citizens may be recruited for this work). This way, students with difficulty reading can get the information auditorily. Students with LLD may be given special permission to write in or highlight textbooks or to make photocopies that can be written in or highlighted. Larson and McKinley also suggested color-coding textbooks for the student. That is, certain textbooks can be highlighted by the clinician and recycled each year for LLD students in the appropriate grade. The clinician can highlight main ideas in yellow, details in blue, and vocabulary to be learned in green, for instance. Students in pull-out/sit-in or language-based courses for credit can work with the clinician to highlight books in study skills units, and these can become part of a clinician's collection of highlighted books available for students in later years. Over time, a clinician can develop an extensive library of color-coded books for the use of students with LLD. Beginning the color coding on older, more worn textbooks may help to enlist administrative support. Simon (1998) suggested some additional ways to adapt classroom materials for students with LLD. These include the following:

▶ *Marginal glosses*: Key concepts and vocabulary are highlighted, then notes explaining them are written to the student in the margin or on "sticky" notes placed next to the highlighted portions.

▶ *Cued texts*: Visual cues are used to show relationships among pronouns and their noun referents, or between other elements of text cohesion. For example, the story character's initials can be written above a pronoun referring to that character.

▶ *Structured overviews*: Mini-outlines, story maps, or semantic webs are placed on "sticky" notes at the beginning of a text section to guide students in reading it.

Again, all these cues can be provided by students working with the clinician within the communication classroom, to be used later by other students for whom the clinician is consulting. Additional ideas for modifying curricular materials for students with LLD can be found in DeMier, Wise, and Marcum (1982), the Oklahoma Project (1982), and Project STILE (1979).

In *modifying the way students are required to demonstrate knowledge*, we are working with teachers to accommodate students' special needs in classroom assignments and tests. We've talked already about providing flexibility in assignments. Students with LLD may not be able to produce written work that is as lengthy or mature as that of their peers, especially if the work must be completed within class time. An SLP can work with receptive teachers to develop rigorous but achievable modifications of class assignments for students with LLD.

We talked earlier, too, about portfolio assessment as an alternative to testing. This method samples student work over a semester or year and allows students to demonstrate their progress by a comparison of work done early in the term with that done later. This system is ideal for students with LLD, who will probably not perform on grade level but should nevertheless be able to demonstrate significant improvement in their work. Kratcoski (1998), Valencia (1990), and Wolf (1989) discussed methods of portfolio assessment. Even if teachers are reluctant to use this method of evaluation for mainstream students, it is a reasonable accommodation for students with LLD.

Larson and McKinley (1987) discussed some accommodations that can be made in tests for teachers who are unwilling to use other assessment methods. They suggested administering tests orally to students and allowing students to dictate or audiorecord answers rather than writing them. Wiig and Semel (1984) suggested other modifications of tests, such as having fewer problems or questions per page to avoid overstimulation for distractible students and extending time limits to allow students to demonstrate their knowledge without the pressure of a time constraint. Fagen, Graves, and Tessier-Switlick (1984) provided additional suggestions.

Collaboration. The issues in establishing collaborative relations with teachers at the secondary level are the same as those we face in elementary schools, only more so. Friend and Cook (1990) discussed some critical elements that need to be present for collaboration to succeed. We talked earlier about Montgomery's (1990) suggestions for enlisting administrative support. These sources can be useful in laying the necessary groundwork. Again, the number of teachers with whom this can work is limited. Teachers of resource rooms may be good first bets, if students with LLD spend part of their day there. English or language arts teachers also are good candidates. You may want to make a general offer at the beginning of each school year to work collaboratively in classes that have students with LLD. You might pique teachers' interest by circulating a list of topics you would like to cover in collaborative sessions. Teachers of many subjects would welcome having someone work with them to teach modules such as "Listening Skills," "Effective Study Strategies," "Remember to Use Mnemonics," "Editing Your Writing," or "Do You Know If You Understand?" for example. We talked earlier about doing collaborative intervention for classroom discourse skills in courses that use cooperative learning groups. These also provide excellent opportunities for moving into the classroom. When we get the go-ahead to teach these collaborative units, they provide a good jumping-off point for some pull-out/sit-in sessions with students who are involved in a clinical intervention model. Some of the commercial sources of lessons that we discussed in Chapter 12 also can be appropriate for use in secondary classrooms. Many of the activities we discussed in the Processes of Intervention section make ideal collaborative lessons, particularly those on the "metas," writing, editing, comprehension monitoring, and other high-level language skills that will be difficult for many students in addition to the identified client.

In collaborative planning we need to work closely with teachers to ensure that they don't see us as just "taking over" the class, leaving them without responsibility. On the other hand, we want to be sure that they don't expect us to work as an aide with only the identified client. Again, we'll need to lay some groundwork in conference sessions with the teacher to establish roles, deciding who will do what with whom in the lessons, following the suggestions we discussed in Chapter 12. Using materials such as the planning forms in Appendix 13-2 can be helpful with secondary teachers, as well as those in elementary schools. This groundwork is crucial for achieving the potential of collaborative intervention.

Also, in going into the classroom to provide collaborative sessions, you will want to observe all the courtesies we discussed in Chapter 12. You'll want to provide the teacher with a structured lesson plan, like the one in Box 12-16, for example. You should provide a commercial lesson plan in case you are sick the day the lesson is scheduled. Punctuality and sticking to the class's time limit also are important. So are providing visual aids and follow-up materials. Most important, perhaps, is to practice what we preach about mediational teaching, question procedures, and good classroom communication. Remember the guidelines that we talked about giving teachers in consultation sessions to improve presentation of material to students? Reviewing these can be a good reminder to ourselves about appropriate classroom language style.

TRANSITIONAL INTERVENTION PLANNING

The ITP is the vehicle used to identify the goals we target for students 16 to 21 years of age, who must soon leave school and make a transition to another setting. As we said in Chapter 13, the development of the ITP, like that of the IEP, is a collaborative effort among teachers, parents, and the student.

The National Joint Committee on Learning Disabilities (1994) listed the responsibilities of school personnel in preparing the ITP. These appear in Box 14-15.

Both the student and the family should have an opportunity to discuss their goals and to think about what the best, realistic postsecondary outcome for each individual student will be. Sturomski (1996) emphasized the importance of starting this process early so that students can begin participating in community activities outside of school, making contacts and visiting potential postsecondary settings. He reported that students who use community services while still in school are more likely to use them in adult life, as well.

Much of the program for transitioning from school to independent living takes place in the context of the functional strand of the curriculum for students with LLD. Here, as we discussed, the curriculum focuses on developing vocational and daily living skills and on improving social communication abilities. The functional strand of the curriculum in the latter years of secondary school can be closely tied to the educational and vocational programs that students will be involved with when they graduate. If you can establish links with higher education and vocational training or job settings in which your students are likely to participate, these links will facilitate the transition. Perhaps a counselor from the local community college or a personnel officer from a company that has made an effort to provide employment for people with disabilities can be invited to talk to the functional communication class. A "field trip" to one of these sites would also be a way to expose students to the next stage of life. Madaus (2005) discussed some of the issues in helping students with LLD make the transition to higher education.

Sturomski (1996) stressed the importance of developing not only basic life skills—such as using money, buying and

BOX 14-15	**Responsibilities of Secondary School Personnel in Individualized Transition Planning**

Form a transition team consisting of a coordinator, the student, the family, administrators, teachers, and related service personnel.

Include the student and parents in the entire planning process.

Demonstrate sensitivity to the culture and values of the student and family.

Develop an appropriate packet of materials to document the student's secondary school program and to facilitate service delivery in the postsecondary setting.

Provide administrative support, resources, and time to foster collaboration among team members.

Inform the student about laws, rules, and regulation that ensure his/her rights.

Provide appropriate course selection, counseling, and academic support services.

Ensure competence in literacy and mathematics.

Ensure that the student learns effective studying, time-management, test-preparation, and test-taking strategies.

Help the student use a range of academic accommodations and technological aids.

Help the student evaluate the need for external supports and adjust the level of assistance when appropriate.

Help the student develop appropriate social skills and interpersonal communication abilities.

Help the student to develop self-advocacy skills, including an understanding of his or her disability and how to use this information in communicating with others.

Foster independence through increased responsibility and opportunity for self-management.

Encourage the student to develop extra-curricular interests and participate in community activities.

Inform the student and family about admission procedures for diverse postsecondary settings.

Inform the student and family about services that postsecondary settings provide, such as disability services, academic counseling, etc.

Ensure the timely development of documentation and material to meet application deadlines.

Help the student and family select and apply to postsecondary institutions that will offer both the challenge and the support necessary.

Develop ongoing communication with postsecondary personnel.

Adapted from the January 1994 Position Paper of the National Joint Committee on Learning Disabilities.

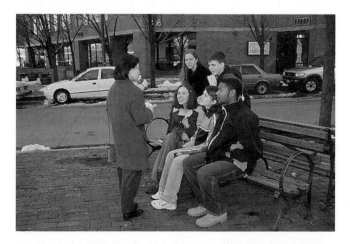

Transition planning includes community referenced skills.

preparing food, using public transportation, securing health care, and participating in recreational activities—but of developing the advocacy skills necessary to secure the accommodations to which our students are entitled. Students need guided practice while they are in school, talking to

employers and neighbors about their disability, explaining its impact, and asking for what will be needed to enable their participation in the community.

As part of the functional strand of the curriculum, the clinician may want to schedule some family conference time, to get parents together with students to talk about what is going to happen after graduation. For students continuing on to higher-education settings, it is an opportunity to discuss whether the student will live at home, on campus, or in an independent-living arrangement. Talking about the realistic pros and cons of each situation with the family can help them focus on how students will achieve their greatest potential. Issues such as cost, the time students must spend on daily living activities as opposed to studying, peer relations, and student preferences must be discussed and weighed.

For students who will go directly to vocational training programs or to the job market, again, living and financial arrangements need to be discussed with the family. Although graduation from high school has traditionally been the time at which adolescents move away from the parental home, more and more mainstream young people are opting for the monetary and emotional support offered by staying under the parents' roof. Some parents want to see their children with disabilities "leave the nest" at the "normal" time. For these families, counseling and referrals to community agencies that can provide some assistance can be given. Other families may feel different, though. In some families, neither the parents nor the client feel ready to make this move. We should not feel that because a student with a disability is supposed to be "mainstreamed," he or she should be denied the option available to other young people—that of remaining within the family for a few more years. When the feeling of the family is to put off a transition to independent living for a while, the clinician can be supportive by making the family aware of agencies and resources that will be available when the client is ready to make the move.

For students at the advanced language level who meet our criteria for using a learning-strategies approach, Sturomski (1996) suggests a strategy they can learn to assist them in solving problems that arise in independent living and vocational situations. This strategy is outlined in Box 14-16. Sturomski reminds us, though, that teaching the strategy is not enough. Students with LLD are likely to forget to use it when they encounter a difficult situation. These students will need repeated practice, role-playing opportunities, and explicit generalization training aimed at getting them to think of how to use the strategies they have learned in new and unfamiliar situations. They also will need repeated reminders to use the strategies they have learned. Teachers need to describe, model, discuss, explain, re-explain, and provide multiple practice opportunities in order to help students use these strategies efficiently in real life. By

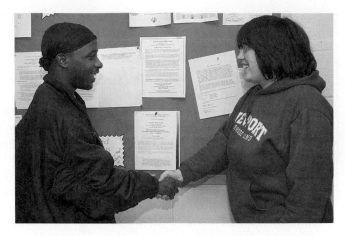

Social skills training is part of transition planning for teens with LLD.

providing this kind of focused instruction, we can prepare our students for a successful transition from secondary school to as large a degree of independence as possible.

For students with severe disabilities, who will be transitioning to adult community programming, perhaps the most important role for the SLP is to insure a viable means of communication that the student can use in community settings. Cascella and McNamara (2005) argue that communication goals for these students be *functional*, aimed toward enabling independent behavior, rather than developmental, or pegged to the child's mental age. Goals such as making a sound to indicate where the student is when called may be more appropriate than working on getting him to say his name. Making sure that the communication modality used by the student works effectively with listeners who may not be familiar with the student is also important. Even for a student who uses speech as the main form of communication, but is unintelligible to people outside his circle, some alternative may need to be introduced to allow for interactions in the community. This can involve taking some "field trips" to try out communication methods in order to find what works best to allow the individual to interact in the community. The main goal of working on communication skills with severely impaired students at the transition level is to maximize the degree of independence and interaction they can achieve, so focusing on functional effective communication in any modality must be our primary objective.

Appendix 14-1 provides an example of an ITP summary.

■ CONCLUSIONS

Planning programs for secondary students with LLD requires thinking about today and thinking about tomorrow. That is, we need to help students perform up to their potential in the school setting now, as well as develop skills that will contribute to a successful adjustment to independent living later. Let's take Michael as our example and look at the kind of intervention program we might develop to address both these sets of needs for a student like him.

BOX 14-16	A Ten-Step Strategy for Independent Living Situations

1. Define the problem.
2. Generate several possible solutions.
3. Evaluate each alternative.
4. Choose the best alternative.
5. Formulate a goal and complete a task analysis to determine the steps you need to take to reach your goal.
6. Complete a task analysis of each of the steps toward your goal.
7. Write a contract with yourself or another adult about achieving each step toward your goal.
8. Begin the steps you need to take toward your goal. Keep a record of your progress and performance.
9. Evaluate the outcome.
10. Revise the contract as necessary, and reward yourself for your achievement.

Adapted from Sturomski, N. (1996). The transition of individuals with learning disabilities into the work setting. *Topics in Language Disorders, 16,* 37-51.

Ms. LaBell was the SLP in Michael's high school. When his parents requested a reevaluation, Ms. LaBell reviewed all his records from throughout his school career. She talked on the phone with the family to discuss their concerns. One of their main ones was that Michael seemed to lack "common sense." Despite his strengths in many areas, he was gullible and easily deceived. They were afraid he would be taken advantage of in some way. He also seemed to have poor judgment, and they were worried about how he could live independently. Ms. LaBell also met with several of his teachers and talked with them about his classroom performance (using the interview format in Box 13-3). Finally, she talked to Michael himself, and had him fill out a self-assessment (Figure 13-1).

Ms. LaBell did some formal testing, but as expected, Michael's scores on standardized tests (she gave him the *Peabody Picture Vocabulary Test–4* and *Test of Adolescent Language*) were within normal limits. His teachers confirmed that his semantic skills, including advanced vocabulary and definitional skills, as well as his syntax were excellent; excessively so, in fact. He often used big words or long, formal-sounding sentences that the other students had trouble understanding, and he just sounded too stiff, even in the classroom situation. The English teacher did note problems with multiple meanings and figurative language, though, when Ms. LaBell asked her specifically about these areas. Ms. LaBell was able to document this deficit using the *Test of Language Competence*. Ms. LaBell asked Michael's permission to observe him during a peer conversation and conducted a conversational analysis (Figure 13-4). There she identified a range of difficulties in conversational interactions. Negotiation skills and register variation were particular problems. She had Michael produce both a spoken and written narrative sample and analyzed them for story grammar, cohesiveness, and use of literate language style. Michael's style in both contained many literate language markers. T-unit length and use of low-frequency structures and connectives were higher than average. But his narratives lacked cohesion and did not contain all the expected story grammar elements. Plans, goals, and internal responses were notably absent. Ms. LaBell looked at his comprehension skills and found he did well with expository texts, like his science book, but had more difficulty with narrative and persuasive or argumentative materials. Informal assessment of "meta" skills and comprehension monitoring showed Michael was aware when he had problems, but had few strategies for correcting them. Analysis of written communication skills showed good performance in writing mechanics and lexical choice, but difficulty with the planning aspect of writing and in providing sufficient information, supplying cohesion, and using appropriate detail. Michael also had a great deal of trouble editing his work. He could identify mechanical errors, but had problems revising other aspects of his writing.

Ms. LaBell had a junior- and senior-level communication class running that year. The academic strand focused on study skills, comprehension monitoring, editing, and vocabulary development. The functional strand concentrated on choice-making, daily living skills, and career development. There were already six students in the class, and Ms. LaBell convinced Michael, with some difficulty, to trade his elective music class for the communication course.

Michael's strong vocabulary skills were an asset in the class. He was assigned to develop a vocabulary list for the unit on ancient mythology that the class was studying. Michael had to preview the material they would read, pick out words that might be hard for the other students, and meet with Ms. LaBell to develop lessons to teach the words. She often added words to his list that had multiple meanings and helped him develop games and lessons on these words. She also encouraged him to involve the class in figurative-language activities using the words.

In the study skills and comprehension-monitoring units, Michael had needs similar to those of the other students in the class. The group engaged in reciprocal teaching activities to improve their reading comprehension. Ms. LaBell was careful to let Michael act as the "facilitator" early in the sessions on expository texts, since he had good command of this type of material. For narrative texts, drawn from their ancient mythology unit, she had Michael act as facilitator only after several other students had modeled the RT. The SQ3R method was also addressed in the study skills unit. For additional narrative development, the group put on a play about their favorite myth, writing the dialogue and acting out various characters. Michael was assigned to a character who needed to show various emotions, and Ms. LaBell talked with him about each emotion he was to portray, why the character felt that way, and when and why Michael himself might have felt that way. Comprehension monitoring was addressed with barrier games and by using audiotapes from lectures given by teachers the students had for other classes. Students were encouraged to use SQ3R as a way to monitor comprehension of material they read.

Because of Michael's strong expository comprehension skills, he helped Ms. LaBell highlight texts for the other students, using color coding to point out main ideas, salient details, and difficult vocabulary. He also made audiotapes of text material that other students who were poorer readers needed to study. To work on negotiation and conversational register skills, Ms. LaBell assigned another student with good conversational skills, Jeffrey, to "tutor" Michael in dyadic conversation. They did role-playing activities, audiotaped them, then listened to the tapes together. Ms. LaBell coached Jeffrey to first critique his own performance, then give Michael some "tips" about his. They then replayed the exercise, and the next time it was Michael's turn to critique first. After they both felt they had gotten it right, Ms. LaBell listened to the tape with them and made further comments.

Ms. LaBell addressed writing and editing by asking students to bring written assignments from other classes and plan and edit them in class. They started the planning process with Hallenbeck's (1996) think-sheet. After producing a draft, students read their drafts aloud to each other and underlined any errors they detected. Ms. LaBell then led them on several passes through the text to detect and correct errors in spelling, capitalization, punctuation, and grammar. In a final pass, they evaluated their writing using Graham and Harris's (1999) self-questions. After going through this process on a few other writing assignments, Ms. LaBell had the students do the activities using reciprocal teaching rather than under her direct instruction. As a final activity, students completed a writing assignment independently, using a checklist to cue them to go through each planning and editing phase. Ms. LaBell also encouraged Michael to check out a blog website and to begin writing about his life there. He found that others responded and even "met" another young man who had a similar disability through the blog site. In addition to having a new "friend" to write to, Michael's resistance to writing decreased as it became a more ordinary activity for him.

In the functional strand of the curriculum, students gave oral reports on jobs that interested them and on job-hunting techniques. They role-played interviewing for an apartment. They did a unit on nutrition and making good nutritional choices, in which the health teacher guest-lectured. This was followed by a unit, taught in conjunction with the school counselor, on self-esteem and making choices to avoid substance abuse. Michael's assignments during this unit involved role-playing situations in which he was invited not only to abuse drugs and alcohol, but to shoplift, and to buy items presented to him at inflated prices. Ms. LaBell emphasized the importance of evaluating options with which students were presented. She used "think-aloud" protocols to get Michael and the others to talk through these choices and arrive at sensible decisions. The class also took a field trip to the local community college and sat in on some classes there. They all talked about what they hoped to do after graduation, and Ms. LaBell encouraged them to consider not only what they wanted but what was realistic for each.

Toward the end of the Michael's sophomore year, Ms. LaBell invited Michael and his parents to a conference to develop his ITP and discuss his future. Michael wanted to attend the flagship branch of the state university, about 3 hours away from his home. Ms. LaBell thought, on the strength of his excellent math and science scores on SATs, that this was a realistic option, but his parents had doubts about his ability to get along on his own there. Michael at first thought he would prefer to be away from home, but after some discussion with Ms. LaBell and role-playing in class about what was involved in dorm living, Michael decided it might be best to stay home for a couple of years after graduation and take courses at the community college. His parents were relieved and felt the decision was best for them all for now. Ms. LaBell gave them the name of a counselor at the community college who would be able to work with Michael to make the transition to the 4-year college when he finished his associate's degree.

STUDY GUIDE

I. Issues in Intervention at the Advanced Language Stage
   A. Suppose you are attempting to convince a high school principal of the need for communication intervention for students with LLD in the school. Give your rationale.
   B. Discuss student-centered intervention at the secondary level.
   C. How can communication contracts be used with secondary students?
   D. Describe the role of counseling with secondary students.
II. Products of Intervention in the Advanced Language Stage
   A. Discuss purposes of intervention at the secondary level.
   B. Define *content mastery* and describe the SLP's role in it at the secondary level.
   C. What are the criteria for including students in a learning-strategies approach to intervention?
   D. Discuss the academic and functional aspects of the communication curriculum for students with LLD.
III. Processes of Intervention in the Advanced Language Stage
   A. Discuss methods for teaching literate lexicon skills to adolescent students with LLD.
   B. How can secondary students' word retrieval be improved?
   C. Describe methods for addressing figurative language skills.
   D. Outline some approaches to teaching verbal reasoning.
   E. Discuss sentence combining and paraphrasing as syntactic intervention methods.
   F. How can students be exposed to literary language at the secondary level?
   G. Discuss basic-skills approaches to improving classroom discourse skills for secondary students with LLD.
   H. What resources are available for exposing teens to advanced narrative structures? Discuss activities that can be used to improve narrative skills in adolescent students with LLD.
   I. Describe activities for increasing appropriate use of cohesive markers.
   J. Discuss basic-skills methods for addressing mechanical problems in the writing of secondary students with LLD.
   K. Describe approaches to improving conversational skills in adolescent clients. How can learning-strategies approaches be used to address conversational skill deficits?
   L. What other skills should be addressed in the functional strand of the curriculum?
   M. Give the steps for teaching a learning strategy.
   N. Discuss some strategy approaches to improving semantic skills in secondary students with LLD.
   O. How can syntactic skills be addressed in the editing process?
   P. Describe some learning-strategy approaches to improving classroom discourse skills.
   Q. Discuss reciprocal teaching and postscript modeling.
   R. Discuss learning-strategy methods for narrative skills.
   S. Describe the use of verbal and visual organizers for improving expository text comprehension.
   T. Discuss additional learning-strategy approaches for expository text material.
   U. How can learning strategies be used to address the writing process?
   V. Discuss the use of the editing process in teaching strategies to improve written products.
   W. Describe methods for teaching comprehension monitoring at the secondary level.

X. What is the relation between reading comprehension skills and monitoring of comprehension of written material?

Y. Discuss metacognitive or study skill instruction at the secondary level.

IV. Contexts of Intervention in the Advanced Language Stage

A. Discuss peer tutoring as an intervention strategy for students with LLD. How should peers be selected and trained? What should the goal of their tutoring be?

B. Discuss the clinical model of intervention at the secondary level. What are its strengths and weaknesses?

C. Describe the language-based course for credit in terms of title, scheduling, content, grading, class composition, and similar issues.

D. What are some special difficulties in providing consultation and collaboration at the secondary level?

E. Discuss some consultation strategies for helping teachers modify the presentation of material to secondary students.

F. Describe methods of modifying curricular materials for students with LLD.

G. What are some ways we can accommodate students with LLD in terms of demonstrating their knowledge on tests and assignments?

H. How can SLPs in secondary schools engage in collaborative classroom intervention?

V. Transitional Intervention Planning

A. Discuss the role of the ITP in intervention planning for students in high school.

B. What are the responsibilities of the school personnel in transition planning?

C. How can the functional strand of the curriculum be used to address transitional intervention planning?

D. How can learning-strategy approaches be used for transition planning for students with LLD?

E. Discuss family conferencing as an aspect of transitional intervention planning.

F. What is self-advocacy, and why is it important for young adults with LLD?

Example of an ITP Summary Form

Transition Planning Summary

Statement of Transition Service Needs for students 14 and older: (Must be completed at each Annual Review following a student's 13th birthday):

Student Preferences/Interests (Sections 2, 3, and 4 must be completed at each Annual Review following a student's 15th birthday):
Was the student invited to attend his/her Planning and Placement Team meeting?
     YES   NO
Did the student attend?
     YES   NO
How were the student's Preferences/Interests, as they relate to planning for Transition Services, determined?
___Personal interview
___Testing
___Vocational assessments
___Comments at meeting
___Interview with family
___Other:
Summarize student Preferences/Interest as they relate to Transitional Services:

Agency Participation:
Were outside agencies involved in the PPT meeting?   YES   NO
(If no, specify reason):
If yes, did the agency's/agencies' representative attend?   YES   NO
(If no, specify reason):
Has any participating agency agreed to provide or pay for services/linkages/transition planning?
NO   YES (Specify):

Justification for Transition Services not being addressed:
If an annual goal and related objectives were not developed for independent living or community participation, provide a justification:

If activities/training are not provided in both the community and the classroom, provide a justification statement:

At least 1 year prior to reaching age 18, the student must be informed of her or his rights under IDEA, if any, which will transfer to her/him at the age.

REFERENCES

Aardema, V. (1975). *Why mosquitoes buzz in people's ears.* New York: Dial.

Abbeduto, L., and Boudreau, D. (2004). Theoretical influences in research on language development and intervention in individuals with mental retardation. *Mental Retardation and Developmental Disabilities Research Reviews, 10,* 184-192.

Abbeduto, L., and Murphy, M. (2004). Language, social cognition, maladaptive behavior and communication in Down syndrome and fragile X syndrome. In M. Rice and S. Warren (Eds.). *Developmental language disorders: From phenotypes to etiology* (pp. 77-98). Mahwah, NJ: Erlbaum.

Accardo, P., and Capute, A. (2005). *The capute scales cognitive adaptive test and clinical linguistic and auditory milestone scale (CAT/CLAMS).* Baltimore: Brookes Publishing.

Accardo, P., and Whitman, B. (Eds., 2002). *Dictionary of developmental disabilities terminology* (2nd ed). Baltimore, MD: Paul H. Brookes.

Achenbach, T., and Edelbrook, C. (2000). *Child behavior checklist.* Burlington, VT: Author.

Achenbach, T.M. (1991). *Manual for the child behavior checklist/4-18 and 1991 profile.* Burlington, VT: Department of Psychiatry, University of Vermont Medical School.

Adams, C. (2001). Clinical diagnostic and intervention studies of children with semantic-pragmatic language disorder. *International Journal of Language and Communication Disorders, 36,* 289-305.

Adams, C. (2002). Practitioner review: The assessment of language pragmatics. *Journal of Child Psychology, Psychiatry, & Allied Disciplines, 43,* 973-988.

Adams, C. (2005). Social communication intervention for school-age children: Rationale and description. *Seminars in Speech and Language, 26,* 181-188.

Adams, C., Baxendale, J., Lloyd, J., and Aldren, C. (2005). Pragmatic language impairment: Case studies of social and pragmatic language therapy. *Child Language Teaching and Therapy, 21,* 227-250.

Adams, C., and Bishop, D. (1989). Conversational characteristics of children with semantic-pragmatic disorder. 2: What features lead to a judgement of inappropriacy. *British Journal of Disorders of Communication, 24,* 241-263.

Adams, C., and Bishop, D. (1990). Conversational characteristics of children with semantic-pragmatic disorder. I: Exchange structure, turn-taking, repairs, and cohesion. *British Journal of Disorders of Communication, 24,* 211-239.

Adams, C., Green, J., Gilchrist, A., and Cox, A. (2002). Conversational behavior of children with Asperger syndrome and conduct disorder. *Journal of Child Psychology and Psychiatry, 43,* 679-690.

Adams, G. (1984). *Comprehensive test of adaptive behavior.* San Antonio, TX: Psychological Corporation.

Adams, M. (1990). *Beginning to read: Thinking and learning about print.* Cambridge, MA: MIT Press.

Adams, M. (1997). The great debate: Then and now. *Annals of Dyslexia, 47,* 265-277.

Adams, M., Foorman, B., Lundberg, I., and Beeler, T. (1998). *Phonological awareness in young children: A classroom curriculum.* Baltimore, MD: Paul H. Brookes.

Adamson, L., and Chance, S. (1998). Coordinating attention to people, objects, and language. In A.M. Wetherby, S.F. Warren, and J. Reichle (Eds.). *Transitions in prelinguistic communication* (pp. 15-37). Baltimore, MD: Paul H. Brookes.

Adler, S. (1990). Multicultural clients: Implications for the SLP. *Language, Speech, and Hearing Services in Schools, 21(3),* 135-139.

Adler, S. (1991). Assessment of language proficiency of limited English proficient speakers: Implications for the speech-language specialist. *Language, Speech, and Hearing Services in Schools, 22(2),* 12-18.

Adler, S. (1993). *Multicultural communication skills in the classroom.* Needham Heights, MA: Allyn & Bacon.

Ae-Hwa Kim, B., Vaughn, S., Wanzek, J., and Shangjin Wei, J. (2004). Graphic organizers and their effects on the reading comprehension of students with LD: A synthesis of research. *Journal of Learning Disabilities, 37,* 105-119.

AGS Publishing. (2005). *Vocabulary with EASE.* Circle Pines, MN: Author.

Ahmed, S.T., Lombardino, L.J., and Leonard, C.M. (2001). Specific language impairment: Definitions, causal mechanisms and neurobiological factors. *Journal of Medical Speech-Language Pathology, 9(1),* 1-15.

Alajouanine, T., and L'hermitte, F. (1965). Acquired aphasia in children. *Brain, 88,* 653-662.

Alexander, R. (2001). *Pediatric feeding and swallowing: Assessment and treatment.* Rockville, MD: ASHA.

Aliki, A. (1966). *Keep your mouth closed, dear.* New York: Dial Press.

Allard, H., and Marshall, J. (1977). *Miss Nelson is missing.* Boston, MA: Houghton Mifflin.

Allen, D.V., and Bliss, L.S. (1987). Concurrent validity of two language screening tests. *Journal of Communication Disorders, 20(4),* 305-317.

Allen, R., and Oliver, J. (1982). The effects of child maltreatment on language development. *Child Abuse and Neglect, 6,* 299-305.

Allen, T. (1994). "Who are the deaf and hard-of-hearing students leaving high school and entering postsecondary education?" Unpublished manuscript, Gallaudet University Center for Assessment and Demographic Studies, Washington, DC.

Alley, G., and Deshler, D. (1979). *Teaching the learning disabled adolesc7ent: Strategies and methods.* Denver, CO: Love Publishing.

Alliance for Excellence in Education (2004). *Reading for the 21st century: Adolescent literacy teaching and learning strategies.* Washington, DC: Author.

Alper, B., and Manno, C. (1996). Dysphagia in infants and children with oral-motor deficits: Assessment and management. *Seminars in Speech and Language, 17,* 283-310.

Alpern, G., Boll, T., and Shearer, M. (1997). *Developmental profile II.* Los Angeles, CA: Western Psychological Services.

Als, H. (1995). *Manual for the naturalistic observation of the newborn (NIDCAP).* Boston, MA: Children's Hospital.

Als, H., Lawhon, G., Duffy, F.H., McAnulty, G.B., Gibes-Grossman, R., and Blickman, J.G. (1994). Individualized development care for the very low-birth-weight preterm infant: Medical and neurofunctional effects. *Journal of the American Medical Association, 272,* 853-858.

Als, H., Lester, B., Tronick, E., and Brazelton, T. (1982). Toward a research instrument for the assessment of preterm infants' behavior (APIB). In H.E. Fitzgerald, B.M. Lester, and M.W. Yogman (Eds.). *Theory and research in behavioral pediatrics* (vol. 1). New York: Plenum Press.

Alsobrook, J., and Pauls, D. (1998). Molecular approaches to child psychopathy. *Human Biology, 70,* 413-432.

Alston, E., and James-Roberts, I. (2005). Home environments of 10 month old infants selected by the WILSTAAR screen for prelanguage difficulties. *International Journal of Language and Communication Disorders, 40,* 123-137.

Alt, M., Plante, E., and Creusere, M. (2004). Semantic features in fast-mapping: Performance of preschoolers with specific language impairment versus preschoolers with normal language. *Journal of Speech, Language, and Hearing Research, 47,* 407-420.

American Academy of Pediatrics. (1982). Joint Committee on Infant Hearing position statement. *Pediatrics, 70,* 496-497.

American Association on Mental Retardation. (2002). *Mental retardation: Definition, classification, and systems of supports* (10th ed.). Annapolis Junction, MD: AAMR Publications.

American Psychiatric Association. (1994). *Diagnostic and statistical manual of mental disorders* (4th ed.). Washington, DC: American Psychiatric Association.

American Speech-Language-Hearing Association. (1981). Guidelines for the employment and utilization of supportive personnel. *American Speech-Language-Hearing Association, 23,* 165-169.

American Speech-Language-Hearing Association. (1982a). Committee on Language, Speech, and Hearing Services in Schools. Definitions: Communicative disorders and variations. *American Speech-Language-Hearing Association, 24,* 949-950.

American Speech-Language-Hearing Association. (1982b). Urban and ethnic perspectives. *American Speech-Language-Hearing Association, 26,* 9-10.

American Speech-Language-Hearing Association. (1984). Committee on Prevention of Speech, Language, and Hearing Problems. Report on status of the profession in prevention. *American Speech-Language-Hearing Association, 26(8).*

American Speech-Language-Hearing Association. (1988). Inside the national office: Office of minority concerns. *American Speech-Language-Hearing Association, 30(8),* 23-25.

American Speech-Language-Hearing Association. (1989). Committee on Language Learning Disorders. Issues in determining eligibility for language intervention. *American Speech-Language-Hearing Association, 31,* 113-118.

American Speech-Language-Hearing Association. (1991). Committee on Prevention of Speech, Language, and Hearing Problems. The prevention of communication disorders tutorial. *American Speech-Language-Hearing Association, 33(9, suppl. 6).*

American Speech-Language-Hearing Association. (1992a). Code of ethics. *American Speech-Language-Hearing Association, 34(3, suppl. 9),* 1-2.

American Speech-Language-Hearing Association. (1992b). *Issues in central auditory processing Disorders: A report from the ASHA Ad Hoc Committee on Central Auditory Processing.* Washington, DC: Author.

American Speech-Language-Hearing Association. (1994). *Admission/discharge criteria in speech-language pathology: Technical report.* Rockville, MD: Author.

American Speech-Language-Hearing Association. (1996). *Practical guide to applying treatment outcomes and efficacy resources.* Rockville, MD: Author.

American Speech-Language-Hearing Association. (1998). Provision of English as a second language instruction by speech-language pathologists in school settings; position statement and technical report. *ASHA Supplement, 18.*

American Speech-Language-Hearing Association (1999). *National outcomes measurement system (NOMS): Pre-kindergarten speech-language pathology training manual.* Rockville, MD: Author.

American Speech-Language-Hearing Association. (2000a). *Schools related resources.* Retrieved February 23, 2005, from http://www.asha.org/members/slp/schools/resources/schools_resources_advocacy

American Speech-Language-Hearing Association. (2000b). *Use and supervision of speech-language pathology assistants in schools.* Rockville, MD: Author.

American Speech-Language-Hearing Association. (2000c). *IDEA and your caseload: A template for eligibility and dismissal criteria for students ages 3-21.* Rockville, MD: Author.

American Speech-Language-Hearing Association. (2001). Roles and responsibilities of speech-language pathologists with respect to reading and writing in children and adolescents (position statement; executive summary of guidelines, technical report). *ASHA Supplement, 21,* 17-27.

American Speech-Language-Hearing Association. (2002). A workload analysis approach for establishing caseload standards in schools: Guidelines. Rockville, MD: Author.

American Speech-Language-Hearing Association. (2003a). Technical report: American English dialects. *ASHA Supplement, 23.*

American Speech-Language-Hearing Association. (2003b). Code of ethics (revised). *ASHA Supplement, 23,* 13-15.

American Speech-Language-Hearing Association (2004a). Admission/discharge criteria in speech-language pathology. *ASHA Supplement, 24,* 65-70.

American Speech-Language-Hearing Association. (2004b). Cochlear implants: Technical report. *ASHA Supplement, 24.*

American Speech-Language-Hearing Association. (2004c). *Preferred practice patterns for the profession of speech-language pathology.* Retrieved from http://www.asha.org/members/deskref-journal/deskref/default

American Speech-Language-Hearing Association. (2004d). *Role of the speech-language pathologists in the neonatal intensive care unit: Technical report.* Rockville, MD: Author.

American Speech-Language-Hearing Association. (2004e). Training, use and supervision of support personnel in speech language pathology: Position statement. *ASHA Supplement, 24.*

American Speech-Language-Hearing Association. (2005a). *Roles and responsibilities of speech-language pathologists in early intervention.* Rockville, MD: Author.

American Speech-Language-Hearing Association. (2005b). *Position statement: Evidence-based practice in communication disorders.* Rockville, MD: Author.

American Speech-Language-Hearing Association. (2005c). *Technical report: (Central) auditory processing disorders.* Retrieved from http://www.asha.org/members/deskref-journals/deskref/default

American Speech-Language-Hearing Association. (2005d). *Curriculum guide to prevention of communication disorders.* Rockville, MD: Author.

American Speech-Language-Hearing Association. (2006). Principles for speech-language pathologists in diagnosis, assessment and treatment of autism spectrum disorders across the life span: Technical report. *ASHA Supplement, 26.*

American Speech-Language-Hearing Association, Audiologic Assessment Panel 1996. (1997). *Guidelines for audiologic screening.* Rockville, MD: Author.

Ammer, J. (1999). *Birth to three checklist of language and learning behaviors.* Austin, TX: Pro-Ed.

Ammer, J., and Bangs, T. (2000). *Birth to three assessment and intervention system—Second edition.* Austin, TX: Pro-Ed.

Andersen, E., Dunlea, A., and Kekelis, L. (1984). Blind children's language: Resolving some differences. *Journal of Child Language, 11,* 645-664.

Andersen, E., Dunlea, A., and Kekelis, L. (1993). The impact of input: Language acquisition in the visually impaired. *First Language, 13(1),* 23-50.

Anderson, G., and Hoshino, Y. (2005) Neurochemical studies of autism. In F. Volkmar, R. Paul, A. Klin, and D. Cohen (Eds.). *Handbook of autism and pervasive developmental disorders* (vol. 1, pp. 453-472). New York: Wiley.

Anderson, R., Miles, M., and Matheny, P. (1963). *Communication evaluation chart from infancy to five years.* Cambridge, MA: Educators Publishing Service.

Anderson, S., Yilmaz, O., and Wasburn-Moses, L. (2004). Middle and high school students with learning disabilities: Practical academic intervention for general education teachers: A review of the literature. *American Secondary Education, 32,* 19-36.

Anderson, S.R., Taras, M., and O'Malley-Cannon, B. (1996). Teaching new skills to young children with autism. In C. Maurice, S. Luce, and G. Green (Eds.). *Behavioral intervention for young children with autism: A manual for parents and professionals* (pp. 181–194). Austin, TX: Pro-Ed.

Anderson, V.A., Morse, S., Catroppa, C., Haritou, F., and Rosenfeld, J. (2004). Thirty month outcome from early childhood head injury: A prospective analysis of neurobehavioural recovery. *Brain, 127,* 2608-2620.

Andreasen, N. (1984). *The broken brain: The biological revolution in psychiatry.* New York: Harper & Row.

Andrews, J., and Andrews, M. (1990). *Family-based treatment in communicative disorders: A systemic approach.* Sandwich, IL: Jannelle Publications.

Andrews, N., and Fey, M. (1986). Analysis of the speech of phonologically impaired children in two sampling conditions. *Language, Speech, and Hearing Services in Schools, 17,* 187-198.

Anglin, J. (1970). *The growth of meaning.* Cambridge, MA: MIT Press.

Aoki, Y., Iseharashi, B., Heller, S., and Bakshi, S. (2002). Parent-infant relationships global assessment scale: A study of its predictive validity. *Psychiatry & Clinical Neurosciences, 56,* 493-497.

Apel, K. (2004). Word study and the speech-language pathologist. *Perspectives on Language Learning and Education, 11(3),* 13-16.

Apel, K., and Masterson, J. (2001). Theory-guided spelling assessment and intervention: A case study. *Language, Speech, and Hearing Services in Schools, 32,* 182-195.

Apel, K., and Masterson, J. (2005). *Assessment and treatment of narrative skills: What's the story?* Rockville, MD: ASHA.

Apel, K., and Swank, L. (1999). Second chances: Improving decoding skills in the older student. *Language, Speech, and Hearing Services in Schools, 30,* 231-242.

Apfel, H., and Provence, S. (2001). *Infant-toddler and family instrument.* Baltimore: Paul H. Brookes.

Apodaca, R. (1987). *PAL oral language dominance measure.* El Paso, TX: El Paso Public Schools.

Appiah, P. (1989). *Tales of an Ashanti father.* Boston, MA: Beacon Press.

Apple Computer Co., Inc. (1989). *HyperCard user's guide* (computer program manual). Cupertino, CA: Apple Computer.

Apple Computer Co., Inc. (1994). *Hypercard 2.2 development kit.* Cupertino, CA: Apple Computer.

Applebee, A. (1978). *The child's concept of a story: Ages 2 to 17.* Chicago, IL: University of Chicago Press.

Aram, D. (1988). Language sequelae of unilateral brain lesions in children. In F. Plum (Ed.). *Language, communication, and the brain* (pp. 171-197). New York: Raven Press.

Aram, D. (1991). Comments on specific language impairment as a clinical category. *Language, Speech, and Hearing Services in Schools, 22,* 84-87.

Aram, D., Ekelman, B., and Nation, J. (1984). Preschoolers with language disorders: Ten years later. *Journal of Speech and Hearing Research, 27,* 232-244.

Aram, D., and Healy, J. (1988). Hyperlexia: A review of extraordinary word recognition. In L.K. Obler and D. Fein (Eds.). *The exceptional brain: Neuropsychology of talent and special abilities* (pp. 70-102). New York: Guilford Press.

Aram, D., and Nation, J. (1975). Patterns of language behavior in children with developmental language disorders. *Journal of Speech and Hearing Research, 18,* 229-241.

Aram, D., and Nation, J. (1980). Preschool language disorders and subsequent language and academic difficulties. *Journal of Communication Disorders, 13,* 159-170.

Aram, D., and Nation, J. (1982). *Child language disorders.* St. Louis, MO: Mosby.

Arnold, D.H., Lonigan, C.J., Whitehurst, G.J., and Epstein, J.N. (1994). Accelerating language development through picture book reading: Replication and extension to a videotape training format. *Journal of Educational Psychology, 86,* 235-243.

Arthur, G. (1969). The Arthur Adaptation of the Leiter International Performance Scale. Washington, DC: Psychological Service Center.

Arvedson, J. (2000). Evaluation of children with feeding and swallowing problems. Language, Speech, and Hearing Services in Schools, 31, 28-41.

Arvedson, J., and Brodsky, L. (1993). Pediatric swallowing and feeding. In M. Wilcox (Ed.). *Early childhood intervention series.* San Diego, CA: Singular Publishing Group.

Arvedson, J., and Lefton-Greif, M. (1996). Anatomy, physiology and development of feeding. *Seminars in Speech and Language, 17,* 261-281.

Arwood, E. (1983). *Pragmaticism: Theory and application.* Rockville, MD: Aspen Publishers.

Aucott, S., Donohue, P., Atkins, E., and Allen, M. (2002). Neurodevelopmental care in the NICU. *Mental Retardation and Developmental Disabilities Research Reviews, 8,* 298-309.

Aune, B., and Friehe, M. (1996). Transition to postsecondary education: Institutional and individual issues. *Topics in Language Disorders, 16,* 1-22.

Bagnato, S., Neisworth, J., and Munson, S. (1997). *Linking assessment and early intervention: An authentic, curriculum-based approach.* Baltimore: Paul H. Brookes.

Bagnato, S., Neisworth, J., Savlia, J., and Hunt, F. (1999). *Temperament and Atypical Behavior Scale (TABS): Early childhood indicators of developmental dysfunction.* Baltimore: Paul H. Brookes.

Bailey, D., Jr., and Simeonsson, R. (1988). *Family assessment in early intervention.* Columbus, OH: Charles E. Merrill.

Baker, S., Gersten, R., and Graham, S. (2003). Teaching expressive writing to students with learning disabilities: Research-based applications and examples. *Journal of Learning Disabilities, 36,* 109-123.

Bakken, J., and Whedon, C. (2002). Teaching text structure to improve reading comprehension. *Intervention in School and Clinic, 37,* 229-233.

Balason, D., and Dollaghan, C. (2002). Grammatical morpheme production in 4-year-old children. *Journal of Speech, Language, and Hearing Research, 45,* 961-969.

Baldwin, D. (2004). A guide to standardized writing assessment. *Educational Leadership, 62,* 72-76.

Baldwin, J. (Ed., 1955). Androcles and the lion. In *Favorite tales of long ago.* New York: J.P. Dutton.

Ball, E., and Blachman, B. (1988). Phoneme segmentation training: Effect on reading readiness. *Annals of Dyslexia, 38,* 28-235.

Ball, E., and Blachman, B. (1991). Does phoneme segmentation in kindergarten make a difference in early word recognition and developmental spelling? *Reading Research Quarterly, 26,* 49-66.

Ball, E., and Blachman, B. (1987, November). A reading readiness program with an emphasis on phoneme segmentation. Paper presented to the Orton Dyslexia Society, San Francisco, CA.

Ball, M.J., and Kent, R.D. (1999). *The new phonologies: Developments in clinical linguistics.* San Diego, CA: Singular Publishing Group.

Baltaxe, C. (2001). Emotional, behavioral, and other psychiatric disorders of childhood associated with communication disorders. In T. Layton, E. Crais, and L. Watson (Eds.). *Handbook of early language impairment in children: Nature* (pp. 63-125). Albany, NY: Delmar Publishers.

Banajee, M., DiCarlo, C., and Stricklin, S. (2003). Core vocabulary determination for toddlers. *Augmentative and Alternative Communication, 19,* 67-73.

Bandstra, E., Vogel, A., Morrow, C., Anthony, J., and Lihua Xue, J. (2004). Severity of prenatal cocaine exposure and child language functioning through age seven years: A longitudinal latent growth curve analysis. *Substance Use & Misuse, 39,* 25-59.

Bangs, T., and Dodson, S. (1979). *Birth to three developmental scales.* Hingham, MA: Teaching Resources.

Banotai, A. (2005). Selective mutism: Creating a therapy program. *Advance, 15,* 6-10.

Barkley, R. (1990). *Attention deficit hyperactivity disorder: A handbook for diagnosis and treatment.* New York: Guilford Press.

Barkley, R. (1995). *Taking charge of ADHD: The complete, authoritative guide for parents.* New York: Guilford Press.

Barkley, R., McMurray, M., and Edelbrock, C. (1990). Side effects of methylphenidate in children with attention deficit hyperactivity disorder: A systematic, placebo-controlled evaluation. *Pediatrics, 86,* 184-192.

Barnes, S., Gutfreund, M., Satterly, D., and Wells, G. (1983). Characteristics of adult speech which predict children's language development. *Journal of Child Language, 10,* 57-65.

Baron-Cohen, S. (1988). Social and pragmatic deficits in autism: Cognitive or affective? *Journal of Autism and Developmental Disorders, 18(3),* 379-402.

Baron-Cohen, S. (1995). *Mindblindness.* Cambridge, MA: MIT Press.

Baron-Cohen, S. (2000). Theory of mind and autism: A fifteen year review. In S. Baron-Cohen, H. Tager-Flusberg, and D. J. Cohen (Eds.). *Understanding other minds: Perspectives from developmental cognitive neuroscience* (pp. 1-20). Oxford University Press.

Baron-Cohen, S., and Swettenham, J. (1997). Theory of mind in autism: Its relationship to executive function and central coherence. In J. Cohen and F. Volkmar (Eds.). *Handbook of autism and pervasive developmental disorders* (pp. 880-894). New York: John Wiley & Sons.

Barr, B. (1982). Teratogenic hearing loss. *Audiology, 21,* 111-127.

Barrie-Blackley, S., Musselwhite, C., and Rogister, S. (1978). *Clinical oral language sampling: A handbook for students and clinicians.* Danville, IL: Interstate Printers and Publishers.

Barry, L., and William, E. (2004). Students with specific learning disabilities can pass state competency exams: Systematic strategy instruction makes a difference. *Preventing School Failure, 48,* 10-17.

Basil, C., and Reyes, S. (2003). Acquisition of literacy skills by children with severe disability. *Child Language Teaching and Therapy, 10,* 28-48.

Basso, K. (1979). *Portraits of "the Whiteman": Linguistic play and cultural symbols among the Western Apache.* London, UK: Cambridge University Press.

Bates, E. (1976). *Language in context: Studies in the acquisition of pragmatics.* New York: Academic Press.

Bates, E. (2003). Explaining and interpreting deficits in language development across clinical groups: Where do we go from here? *Brain and Language, 88,* 248-253.

Bates, E., Bretherton, I., Snyder, L., Shore, C., and Volterra, V. (1980). Vocal and gestural symbols at 13 months. *Merrill-Palmer Quarterly, 26,* 407-423.

Bates, E., and Dick, F. (2002). Language, gesture and the developing brain. *Developmental Psychobiology, 40,* 293-310.

Batshaw, M. (2001). *When your child has a disability: The complete sourcebook of daily and medical care, revised edition.* Baltimore, MD: Paul H. Brookes.

Batshaw, M. (2002a). *Children with disabilities: A medical primer* (5th ed.). Baltimore, MD: Paul H. Brookes.

Batshaw, M. (2002b). Chromosomes and heredity. In M Batshaw (Ed.). *Children with disabilities* (5th ed., p. 326). Baltimore, MD: Paul H. Brookes.

Battle, D. (1996). Language learning and use by African-American children. *Topics in Language Disorders, 16,* 22-37.

Battle, D. (2002a). Communication disorders in a multicultural society. In D.E. Battle (Ed.). *Communication disorders in multicultural populations* (3rd ed., pp. 3-33). Boston: Butterworth-Heinneman.

Battle, D. (Ed.). (2002b). *Communication disorders in multicultural populations* (3rd ed.) Boston: Butterworth-Heinneman.

Bauman, J. (1986). Teaching third-grade students to comprehend anaphoric relationships: The application of a direct instruction model. *Reading Research Quarterly, 21,* 70-90.

Bauman, J., Edwards, E., Font, G., Tereshinski, C., Kameenui, E., and Olejnik, S. (2002). Teaching morphemic and contextual analysis to fifth-grade students. *Reading Research Quarterly, 37,* 150-176.

Bauman-Waengler, J. (2004). *Articulatory and phonological impairments: A clinical focus.* Boston: Allyn & Bacon.

Bavin, E.L., Wilson, P.H., Maruff, P., and Sleeman, F. (2005). Spatio-visual memory of children with specific language impairment: Evidence for generalized processing problems. *International Journal of Language & Communication Disorders, 40(3),* 319-332.

Bayles, K., and Harris, G. (1982). Evaluating speech-language skills in Papago Indian children. *Journal of American Indian Education, 21(2),* 11-20.

Bayley, N. (2005). *Bayley scales of infant development—III.* San Antonio, TX: Harcourt Assessment.

Bear, D., Invernizzi, M., Templeton, S., and Gohnston, F. (2000). Words their way: Word study for phonics vocabulary and spelling instruction (2nd ed.) Englewood Cliffs, NJ: Prentice Hall.

Bear, D., and Templeton, S. (1998). Explorations in developmental spelling. The Reading Teacher, 52, 222-242.

Bebko, A., Alexander, J., and Ducet, R. (2001) *Language! Roots* (2nd ed.). Longmont, CO: Sopris West.

Beck, I., McKeown, M., and Omanson, R. (1987). The effects and uses of diverse vocabulary instructional techniques. In M. McKeown and M. Curtis (Eds.). *The nature of vocabulary acquisition.* Hillsdale, NJ: Erlbaum.

Bedrosian, J. (1985). An approach to developing conversational competence. In D. Ripich and F. Spinelli (Eds.). *School discourse problems.* San Diego, CA: College-Hill Press.

Bedrosian, J. (1997). Language acquisition in young AAC system users. *Augmentative and Alternative Communication, 13,* 179-185.

Bedrosian, J., and Prutting, C. (1978). Communicative performance of mentally retarded adults in four conversational settings. *Journal of Speech and Hearing Research, 21,* 79-95.

Beery, K.E., Buktenica, N.A., and Beery, N.A. (2003). *Beery™-Buktenica Developmental Test of Visual-Motor Integration* (5th ed.). (Beery™ VMI). Eagamn, MN: Pearson Assessments.

Beilinson, J., and Olswang, L. (2003). Facilitating peer-group entry in kindergartners with impairments in social communication. *Language, Speech, and Hearing Services in Schools, 34,* 154-166.

Beitchman, J.H., Hood, J., Rochon, J., Peterson, M., Mantini, T., and Majumdar, S. (1989). Empirical classification of speech/ language impairment in children: I: Identification of speech/language categories. *Journal of the American Academy of Child and Adolescent Psychiatry, 28,* 112-117.

Beliavsky, N. (2003). The sequential acquisition of pronominal reference in narrative discourse. *Word, 54,* 167-189.

Bellman, M., Lingam, S., and Aukett, A. (1996). *Schedule of growing skills— Second edition.* Windsor, UK: NFER-Nelson.

Bellugi, U., Marks, S., Bihrle, A., and Sabo, H. (1998). Dissociation between language and cognitive functions in Williams syndrome. In D. Bishop and K. Mogford (Eds.). *Language development in exceptional circumstances.* Edinburgh, Scotland: Churchill Livingstone.

Benedict, H. (1979). Early lexical development: Comprehension and production. *Journal of Child Language, 6,* 183-200.

Benner, G., Nelson, J., and Epstein, M. (2002). Language skills of children with EBD: A literature review. *Journal of Emotional and Behavioral Disorders, 10,* 43-57.

Bennett, C. (1989). *Referential semantic analysis* (computer program). Woodstock, VA: Teaching Texts.

Bennett, G., Seashore, H., and Wesman, A. (1990). *Differential aptitude tests* (5th ed) San Antonio, TX: Harcourt Assessment.

Benton, A. (1959). Aphasia in children. *Education, 79,* 408-412.

Benton, A. (1964). Developmental aphasia and brain damage. *Cortex, 1,* 40-52.

Berenstain, S., and Berenstain, J. (1968). *Inside, outside, upside down.* New York: Random House.

Berg, E.A., and Grant, D.A. (1980). *The Wisconsin Card Sorting Test (WCST).* Odessa, FL: Psychological Assessment Resources, Inc.

Bernbaum, J., and Batshaw, M. (2002). Born too soon, born too small. In M.L. Batshaw (Ed.). *Children with disabilities* (5th ed., pp. 115-142). Baltimore, MD: Paul H. Brookes.

Berninger, V. (2000). Development of language by hand, and its connections with language by ear, mouth, and eye. *Topics in Language Disorders, 20(4),* 65-85.

Berninger, V., Vermeulen, K., Abbott, R., McCutchen, D., Cotton, S., Cude, J., Dorn, S., and Sharon, T. (2003). Comparison of three approaches to supplementary reading instruction for low-achieving second grade readers. *Language, Speech, and Hearing Services in Schools, 34,* 101-116.

Bernstein, D. (1989). Assessing children with limited English proficiency: Current perspectives. *Topics in Language Disorders, 9(3),* 15-20.

Bernthal, J., and Bankson, N. (2004). *Articulation and phonological disorders* (5th ed.). Boston: Allyn & Bacon.

Berry, P., Groenweg, G., Gibson, D., and Brown, R. (1984). Mental development of adults with Down's syndrome. *American Journal of Mental Deficiency, 89,* 252-256.

Bess, F., and McConnell, F. (1981). *Audiology, education and the hearing impaired child.* St. Louis, MO: Mosby.

Betz, S., and Stoel-Gammon, C. (2005). Measuring articulatory error consistency in children with developmental apraxia of speech. *Clinical Linguistics and Phonetics, 19,* 53-66.

Beukelman, D., and Mirenda, P. (1998). *Augmentative and alternative communication: Management of severe communication disorders in children and adults* (ed. 22nd ed.). Baltimore, MD: Paul H. Brookes.

Beukelman, D., and Mirenda, P. (2005). *Augmentative & alternative communication: Supporting children & adults with complex communication needs* (3rd ed.). Baltimore: Paul H. Brooks Publishing.

Beukelman, D., and Tice, R. (1990). *The vocabulary toolbox* (computer program). Lincoln, NE: University of Nebraska–Lincoln.

Beverly, G., and Williams, C. (2004). Present tense be use in young children with specific language impairment: Less is more. *Journal of Speech, Language, and Hearing Research, 47,* 944-956.

Bhattacharya, A., and Ehri, L. (2004). Graphosyllabic analysis helps adolescent struggling readers read and spell words. *Journal of Learning Disabilities, 37,* 331-348.

Bhutta, A., Cleves, M. Casey, P. Cradock, M., and Anand, K. (2002). Cognitive and behavioral outcomes of school-aged children who were born preterm: A meta-analysis. *Journal of the American Medical Association, 288,* 278-288.

Biemiller, A. (2003). Vocabulary: Needed if more children are to read well. *Reading Psychology, 24,* 323-335.

Biery, K.E. (1982). *Developmental test of visual-motor integration.* Chicago, IL: Follett Publishing Company.

Bigham, D., Portwood, G., and Elliott, L. (1986). *Where in the world is Carmen Sandiego?* (computer program). San Rafael, CA: Broderbund Software.

Biklen, D. (1990). Communication unbound: Autism and praxis. *Harvard Educational Review, 60,* 291-314.

Biklen, D., Morton, M., Gold, D., Berrigan, C., and Swaminathan, S. (1992). Facilitated communication: Implications for individuals with autism. *Topics in Language Disorders, 12(4),* 1-28.

Bird, J., Bishop, D., and Freeman, H. (1995). Phonological awareness and literacy development in children with expressive phonological impairments. *Journal of Speech and Hearing Research, 38,* 446-462.

Bishop, D. (1985). *Automated LARSP* (computer program). Manchester, England: University of Manchester.

Bishop, D. (1992). Language development after focal brain damage. In D. Bishop and K. Mogford (Eds.). *Language development in exceptional circumstances* (pp. 203-219). Hillsdale, NJ: Erlbaum.

Bishop, D. (1997). *Uncommon understanding: Development and disorders of language comprehension in children.* East Sussex, BN 3, 2 FA, UK: Psychology Press Limited.

Bishop, D. (June, 1999). *Genetic and environmental causes of language impairments.* Paper presented to the 20th Symposium on Research in Child Language Disorders, Madison, WI.

Bishop, D. (2000). Pragmatic language impairment: A correlate of SLI, a distinct subgroup, or part of the autistic continuum? In D. Bishop and L. Leonard (Eds.). *Speech and language impairments in children: Causes, characteristics, intervention, and outcome* (pp 99-114). Hove: Psychology Press.

Bishop, D. (2001). Parent and teacher report of pragmatic aspects of communication: Use of the Children's Communication Checklist in a clinical setting. *Developmental Medicine and Child Neurology, 43,* 809-818.

Bishop, D. (2002). The role of genes in the etiology of specific language impairment. *Journal of Communication Disorders, 35(4),* 311-328.

Bishop, D. (2003). *Children's Communication Checklist—2.* London: Harcourt Assessment.

Bishop D. (2005). Individual differences in auditory processing in specific language impairment: A follow-up study using event-related potentials and behavioural thresholds. *Cortex, 41(3),* 327-341.

Bishop, D., Adams, C., and Norbury, C.F. (2006). Distinct genetic influences on grammar and phonological short-term memory: Evidence from 6-year-old twins. *Genes, Brain and Behavior, 5(2),* 158-169.

Bishop, D., and Baird, G. (2001). Parent and teacher report of pragmatic aspects of communication: Use of the Children's Communication Checklist in a clinical setting. *Developmental Medicine and Child Neurology, 43,* 809-818.

Bishop, D., and Bishop, S.J. (1998). Twin language: A risk factor for language impairment. *Journal of Speech, Language, and Hearing Research, 41(1),* 150-160.

Bishop, D., Bishop, S.J., Bright, P., James, C., Delaney, T., and Tallal, P. (1999). Different origin of auditory and phonological processing problems in children with language impairment: Evidence from a twin study. *Journal of Speech, Language, and Hearing Research, 42(1),* 155-168.

Bishop, D., Carlyon, R.P., Deeks, J.M., and Bishop, S.J. (1999). Auditory temporal processing impairment: Neither necessary nor sufficient for causing language impairment in children. *Journal of Speech, Language, and Hearing Research, 42(6),* 1295-1310.

Bishop, D., Chan, J., Adams, C., Hartley, J., and Weir, F. (2000a). Evidence of disproportionate pragmatic difficulties in a subset of children with specific language impairment. *Development and Psychopathology, 12,* 177-199.

Bishop, D., Chan, J., Adams, C., Hartley, J., and Weir, F. (2000b). Conversational responsiveness in specific language impairment. *Development and Psychopathology, 12,* 177-199.

Bishop, D., Chan, J., Hartley, J., and Weir, F. (1998). When a nod is as good as a word: Form-function relationships between questions and their responses. *Applied Psycholinguistics, 19,* 415-432.

Bishop, D., and Edmundson, A. (1986). Is otitis media a major cause of specific developmental language disorders? *British Journal of Disorders of Communication, 21,* 321-338.

Bishop, D., and Edmundson, A. (1987a). Language-impaired 4-year-olds: Distinguishing transient from persistent impairment. *Journal of Speech and Hearing Disorders, 52,* 156-173.

Bishop, D., and Edmundson, A. (1987b). Specific language impairment as a maturational lag: Evidence from longitudinal data on language and motor development. *Developmental Medicine and Child Neurology, 29,* 442-459.

Bishop, D., and McArthur, G.M. (2004). Immature cortical responses to auditory stimuli in specific language impairment: evidence from ERPs to rapid tone sequences. *Developmental Science, 7(4),* F11-F18.

Bishop, D., and Norbury, C. (2002). Exploring the borderlands of autistic disorder and specific language impairment: A study using standardised diagnostic instruments. *Journal of Child Psychology and Psychiatry and Allied Disciplines, 43,* 917-930.

Bishop, D., North, T., and Donlan, C. (1995). Genetic basis of specific language impairment: Evidence from a twin study. *Developmental Medicine and Child Neurology, 37,* 56-71.

Bishop, D., North, T., and Donlan, C. (1996). Non-word repetition as a behavioural marker for inherited language impairment: evidence from a twin study. *Journal of Child Psychology and Psychiatry and Allied Disciplines, 37,* 391-403.

Bishop, D., Price, T., Dale, P., and Plomin, R. (2003). Outcomes of early language delay: II. Etiology of transient and persistent language difficulties. *Journal of Speech, Language, and Hearing Research, 46,* 561-575.

Bishop, D., and Rosenbloom, L. (1987). Classification of childhood language disorders. In W. Yule and M. Rutter (Eds.). *Language development and disorders.* Oxford: MacKeith.

Bishop, D., and Snowling, M.J. (2004). Developmental dyslexia and specific language impairment: Same or different? *Psychological Bulletin, 130(6),* 858-886.

Blachman, B. (1987). An alternative classroom reading program for learning disabled and other low-achieving children. In W. Ellis (Ed.). *Intimacy with language: A forgotten basic in teacher education* (pp. 133-158). Baltimore, MD: The Orton Dyslexia Society.

Blachman, B. (1989). Phonological awareness and word recognition. In A. Kamhi and H. Catts (Eds.). *Reading disabilities: A developmental language perspective.* Boston, MA: College-Hill.

Blachman, B. (1994). What we have learned from longitudinal studies of phonological processing and reading, and some unanswered questions. *Journal of Learning Disabilities, 27,* 287-291.

Blachman, B. (1997). Early intervention and phonological awareness: A cautionary tale. In B. Blachman (Ed.). *Foundations of reading acquisition and dyslexia* (pp. 409-430). Mahway, NJ: Lawrence Erlbaum Associates.

Blachman, B., Ball, E., Black, R., and Tangel, D. (2000). *Road to code.* Baltimore: Paul H. Brookes.

Black, B., and Uhde, T. (1995). Psychiatric characteristics of children with selective mutism: A pilot study. *J Am Academy Child Adolesc Psychiatry, 34,* 847-848.

Blackburn, S. (1978). State organization in the newborn: Implications for caregiving. In K.E. Barnard, S. Blackburn, R. Kang, and A.L. Spietz (Eds.). *Early parent-infant relationships. series 1: The first six hours of life, module 3.* White Plains, NY: The National Foundation/March of Dimes.

Blackstone, S. (1989). ACN's guidelines for teaching literacy skills. *Augmentative Communication News, 3.*

Blagden, C., and McConnell, N. (1984). *Interpersonal language skills assessment.* Moline, IL: LinguiSystems.

Blager, F. (1979). The effect of intervention on the speech and language of abused children. *Child Abuse and Neglect, 5,* 991-996.

Blair, C., and Ramey, C. (1997). Early intervention for low-birth-weight infants and the path to second-generation research. In M.J. Guralnick (Ed.). *The effectiveness of early intervention* (pp. 77-98). Baltimore, MD: Paul H. Brookes.

Blake, J., Quartaro, G., and Onorati, S. (1993). Evaluating quantitative measures of grammatical complexity in spontaneous speech samples. *Journal of Child Language, 20,* 139-152.

Blake, M., and van Sickle, M. (2001). Helping linguistically diverse students share what they know. *Journal of Adolescent and Adult Literacy, 44,* 468-476.

Blakely, R. (2000). *Screening test for developmental apraxia of speech—2nd ed.* Austin, TX: Pro-Ed.

Blanchette, N., Smith, M., King, S., Fernandes-Penney, A., and Read, S. (2002). Cognitive development in school-age children with vertically transmitted HIV infections. *Developmental Neuropsychology, 21,* 223-241.

Blanchowicz, C. (1986). Making connections: Alternatives to the vocabulary notebook. *Journal of Reading, 29,* 643-649.

Bland-Stewart, L. (2005). Difference or deficit in speakers of African American English? *ASHA Leader, 10(6),* 6-30.

Bland-Stewart, L., Seymour, H., Beeghly, M., and Frank, D. (1998). Semantic development of African-American children prenatally exposed to cocaine. *Seminars in Speech and Language, 19,* 167-188.

Blank, M., Rose, S., and Berlin, L. (1978). *The language of learning: The preschool years.* New York: Grune & Stratton.

Blank, M., and White, S. (1986). Questions: A powerful but misused form of classroom exchange. *Topics in Language Disorders, 6(2),* 1-12.

Bleile, K. (1993). The care of children with long-term tracheostomies. San Diego, CA: Singular Publishing Group.

Bleile, K. (2002). Evaluating articulation and phonological disorders when the clock is running. *American Journal of Speech-Language Pathology, 11,* 243-250.

Bleile, K., and Miller, S. (1993). Articulation and phonological disorders in toddlers with medical needs. In J. Bernthal (Ed.). *Articulatory and phonological disorders in special populations* (pp. 81-109). New York: Thieme.

Bligh, S., and Kupperman, P. (1993). Brief report: Facilitated communication evaluation procedure accepted in a court case. *Journal of Autism and Developmental Disorders, 23(3),* 553-558.

Blischak, D., Shah, S., Lombardino, J., and Chiarella, K. (2004). Effects of phonemic awareness instruction on the encoding skills of children whit severe speech impairment. *Disability and Rehabilitation, 26,* 1295-1304.

Bliss, L. (1992). A comparison of tactful messages by children with and without language impairment. *Language, Speech, and Hearing Services in Schools, 23,* 343-347.

Bliss L., and Allen D. (1984). Screening Kit of Language Development: A preschool language screening instrument. *Journal of Communication Disorders, 17,* 133-41.

Bloch, A., Orenstein, W., Wassilak, S., Stetler, H., Turner, P., Amler, R., Bart, K., and Hinman, A. (1986). Epidemiology of measles and its complications. In E. Gruenberg, C. Lewis, and S. Goldston (Eds.). *Vaccinating against brain syndromes.* New York: Oxford University Press.

Blodgett, E., and Cooper, E. (1987). *Analysis of the language of learning: the practical test of metalinguistics.* East Moline, IL: LinguiSystems.

Bloodgood, J., and Pacifici, L. (2004). Bringing word study to intermediate classrooms: Here are four original word study units teachers can easily implement themselves. *The Reading Teacher, 58,* 250-264.

Bloom, L., and Lahey, M. (1978). *Language development and language disorders.* New York: John Wiley & Sons.

Bloom, L., Rocissano, L., and Hood, L. (1976). Adult-child discourse: developmental interaction between information processing and linguistic knowledge. *Cognitive Psychology, 8,* 521-552.

Bloom, N. (1956). *Taxonomy of educational objectives: Handbook 1, Cognitive domain.* New York: Longman.

Bloom, P. (2001). Word learning. *Current Biology, 11,* 5-6.

Blosser, J., and De Pompei, R. (1992, November). *Serving youth with TBI: Circumventing the obstacles to school integration.* Miniseminar presented at the annual convention of the American Speech-Language-Hearing Association, San Antonio, TX.

Blosser, J., and De Pompei, R. (1994). *Pediatric traumatic brain injury: Proactive intervention.* San Diego, CA: Singular Publishing Group.

Blosser, J., and De Pompei, R. (2001). Traumatic brain injury. In T. Layton, E. Crais, and L. Watson (Eds.). *Handbook of early language impairment in children:* Nature (pp. 56-76). Albany, NY: Delmar Publishers.

Blosser, J., and Neidercker, E. (2002). *School programs in speech-language pathology: Organization and service delivery—4th Ed.* Boston: Allyn & Bacon.

Blosser, J.L., and DePompei, R. (2002). *Pediatric traumatic brain injury: Proactive intervention* (2nd ed.). San Diego: Singular.

Blum, N., and Mercugliano, M. (2002). Attention deficit/hyperactivity disorder. In M. Batshaw (Ed.). *Children with disabilities: A medical primer* (5th ed., pp. 449-470). Baltimore, MD: Paul H. Brookes.

Bluma, S., Shearer, M., Frohman, A., and Hilliard, J. (1976). *Portage guide to early education.* Portage, WI: Cooperative Education Service Agency 12.

Boehm, A. (1969). *Boehm test of basic concepts.* New York: Psychological Corporation.

Boehm, A. (1986). *Boehm test of basic concepts—Revised, manual.* New York: Psychological Corporation.

Boehm, A. (1989). *Boehm resource guide for basic concept teaching.* San Antonio, TX: Psychological Corporation.

Boggs, S. (1972). The meaning of questions and narratives to Hawaiian children. In C.B. Cazden, V.P. John, and D. Hymes (Eds.). *Functions of language in the classroom* (pp. 299-330). New York: Teacher's College Press.

Bolitho, R., Carter, R., Hughes, R., Ivanic, R., Masuhara, H., and Tomlinson, B. (2003). Ten questions about language awareness. *English Language Teachers' Journal, 57,* 251-259.

Bolton, S., and Dashiell, S. (1984). *INCH: Interaction checklist for augmentative communication—Revised.* Austin, TX: Pro Ed.

Bondy, A., and Frost, L. (1998). The picture exchange communication system. *Seminars in Speech and Language, 19,* 373-389.

Bondy, A., and Frost, L. (2002). *A picture's worth: PECS and other visual communication strategies in autism.* Bethesda, MD: Woodbine House.

Bondy, A., Tincani, M., and Frost, L. (2004). Multiply controlled verbal operants: An analysis and extension to the Picture Exchange Communication System. *Behavior Analyst, 27,* 247-261.

Bono, M., Daley, T., and Signman, M. (2004). Relations among joint attention, amount of intervention and language gain in autism. *Journal of Autism and Developmental disorders, 34,* 495-506.

Boothroyd, A. (1982). *Hearing impairments in young children.* Englewood Cliffs, NJ: Prentice-Hall.

Bopp, K., Brown, K., and Mirenda, P. (2004). Speech-language pathologists' roles in the delivery of positive behavior support for individuals with developmental disabilities. *American Journal of Speech-Language Pathology, 13,* 5-19.

Bortner, M. (1971). Phrenology, localization, and learning disabilities. *Journal of Special Education, 5,* 23-29.

Botting, N. (2002). Narrative as a tool for the assessment of linguistic and pragmatic impairments. *Child Language Teaching and Therapy, 18,* 1-22.

Botting, N. (2004). Children's Communication Checklist scores in 11 year old child with communication impairments. *International Journal of Language and Communication Disorders, 39,* 215-228.

Botting, N. (2005). Nonverbal cognitive development and language impairment. *Journal of Child Psychology and Psychiatry and Allied Disciplines, 46,* 317-326.

Botting, N., and Conti-Ramsden, G. (2001). Non-word repetition and language development in children with specific language impairment. *International Journal of language and Communication Disorders, 36,* 421-432.

Botting, N., and Conti-Ramsden, G. (2004). Characteristics of children with specific impairment. In L. Verhoeven, and H. van Balkom (Eds.). *Classification of developmental language disorders: Theoretical issues and clinical implications.* Mahwah, NJ: Lawrence Erlbaum Associates.

Boudreau, D. (2006). Narrative abilities in children with language impairments. In R. Paul (Ed.). *Child language disorders from a developmental perspective: Essays in honor of Robin Chapman.* Mahwah, NJ: Erlbaum.

Boudreau, D., and Chapman, R. (2000). The relationship between event representation and linguistic skill in narrative of children and adolescents with Down syndrome. *Journal of Speech, Language, and Hearing Research, 43,* 1146-1159.

Boudreau, D.M., and Hedberg, N.L. (1999). A comparison of early literacy skills in children with specific language impairment and typically developing peers. *American Journal of Speech-Language Pathology, 8,* 248-263.

Boudreau, D. M., and Larsen, J. (2004). Contributing our voice: Speech-language pathologists as members of a literacy team. *Perspectives on Language Learning and Education, 11(3),* 8-12.

Bourassa, D., and Treiman, R. (2001). Spelling development and disability: The importance of linguistic factors. *Language, Speech, and Hearing Services in Schools, 32,* 172-181.

Bowers, L., Barrett, M., Huisingh, R., Orman, S., and LoGiudice, C. (1991). *TOPS—Adolescent: Test of Problem Solving (TOPS).* East Moline, IL: LinguiSystems.

Bowers, L., Barrett, M., Huisingh, R., Orman, S., and LoGiudice, C. (1994). *Test of Problem Solving—Elementary (TOPS-E Revised).* East Moline, IL: LinguiSystems.

Bowers, L., Huisingh, R., LoGiudice, C., and Orman, J. (2002). *Test of Semantic Skills—Primary (TOSS-P).* East Moline, IL: LinguiSystems.

Bowers, P., and Greig, U. (2003). RAN's contribution to reading disabilities. In H. Swanson and K. Harris (Eds.). *Handbook of learning disabilities* (pp. 140-157). New York, US: Guilford Press.

Bowey, J., and Francis, J. (1991). Phonological analysis as a function of age and exposure to reading instruction. *Applied Psycholinguistics, 12,* 91-121.

Boyle, J. (1996). The effect of a cognitive mapping strategy on the literal and inferential comprehension of students with mild disabilities. *Learning Disability Quarterly, 19(2)*, 86-98.

Bracken, B. (1986). *Bracken Concept Development Program.* San Antonio, TX: Psychological Corporation.

Bracken, B.A., and McCallum, R.S. (1998). *Universal Nonverbal Intelligence Test (UNIT).* Itasca, IL: Riverside Publishing.

Brackenbury, T., and Pye, C. (2005). Semantic deficits in children with language impairments: Issues for clinical assessment. *Language, Speech and Hearing Services in School, 36*, 5-16.

Brackett, D. (1997). Intervention for children with hearing impairment in the general education settings. *Language, Speech, and Hearing Services in Schools, 28*, 355-362.

Braddock, J., II, and McPartland, J. (1990). Alternatives to tracking. *Educational Leadership, 47*, 76-79.

Bradley, L. (1988). Rhyme recognition and reading and spelling in young children. In W. Ellis (Ed.). *Intimacy with language: A forgotten basic in teacher education* (pp. 64-73). Baltimore, MD: Orton Dyslexia Society.

Bradley, L., and Bryant, P. (1983). Categorizing sounds and learning to read—A causal connection. *Nature, 30*, 419-421.

Bradley, L., and Bryant, P. (1985). *Rhyme and reason in reading and spelling.* Ann Arbor, MI: University of Michigan Press.

Bradley-Johnson, S., and Johnson, C.M. (2001). *Cognitive Abilities Scale* (2nd ed.). Austin, TX: Pro-Ed.

Bradshaw, M.L. (1998). Efficacy of expansions and cloze procedures in the development of interpretations by preschool children exhibiting delayed language development. *Language, Speech, and Hearing Services in Schools, 29(2)*, 85-95.

Brady, N. (2000). Improved comprehension of object names following voice output communication aid use: Two case studies. *Augmentative & Alternative Communication, 16*, 197-204.

Brady, N., Marquis, J., Fleming, K., and McLean, L. (2004). Prelinguistic predictor of language growth in children with developmental disabilities. *Journal of Speech, Language, and Hearing Research, 47*, 663-677.

Brady, S., and Shankweiler, D. (1991). *Phonological processes in literacy: A tribute to Isabelle Y. Liberman.* Hillsdale, NJ: Lawrence Erlbaum Associates.

Brady, S., Shankweiler, D., and Mann, V. (1983). Speech perception and memory coding in relation to reading ability. *Journal of Experimental Child Psychology, 35*, 345-367.

Bray, C., and Wiig, E. (1987). *Let's talk inventory for children.* San Antonio, TX: Psychological Corporation.

Brazelton, T. (1973). *Neonatal Behavioral Assessment Scale.* Philadelphia, PA: J.B. Lippincott.

Brazelton, T. (1982). Mother-infant reciprocity. In M.H. Klaus, T. Leger, and M.A. Trause (Eds.). *Maternal attachment and mothering disorders. Pediatric round table: 1* (pp. 49-54). Skillman, NJ: Johnson & Johnson Baby Products Company.

Brazelton, T.B., and Nugent, J.K. (1995). *The Neonatal Behavioral Assessment Scale.* Cambridge: Mac Keith Press.

Bregman, J., and Gerdtz, J. (1997). Behavioral interventions. In D. Cohen and F. Volkmar (Eds.). *Handbook of autism and pervasive developmental disorders* (2nd ed., pp. 606-630). New York: John Wiley & Sons.

Bretherton, L., and Holmes, V. (2003). The relationship between auditory temporal processing, phonemic awareness, and reading disability. *Journal of Experimental Child Psychology, 84*, 218-243.

Brice, A. (2002). *The Hispanic child: Speech language, culture and education.* Boston: Allyn & Bacon.

Brice, A., and Roseberry-McKibben, C. (2001). Choice of language in instruction: One language or two. *Teaching Exceptional Children, 33*, 10-16.

Bricker, D. (2002). *Assessment, evaluation, and programming system for infants and children—Second edition.* Baltimore, MD: Paul H. Brookes.

Bricker, D., Capt, B., and Pretti-Frontczak, K. (2002). *Test for birth to three years and three to six years: Assessment, evaluation and programming system for infants and children* (2nd ed.) Baltimore: Paul H. Brookes.

Bricker, D., and Dennison, L. (1978). Training prerequisites to verbal behavior. In *Systematic instruction of the moderately and severely handicapped* (pp. 155-178). Columbus, OH: Charles Merrill.

Bricker, D., and Pretti-Frontczak, K. (2004). *An activity-based approach to early intervention—3rd ed.* Baltimore, MD: Paul H. Brookes.

Bricker, D., and Squires, J. (1999). *Ages and Stages Questionnaire (ASQ): A parent-completed, child monitoring system—Second Edition.* Baltimore, MD: Paul H. Brookes.

Bridges, S., Delsandro, E., Glennen, S., Hewitt, S., Morrell, A., Wolfenden, D., Rossman K. (1999). *Augmentative and alternative communication: Assessment, intervention, facilitation, and funding.* Rockville, MD: ASHA.

Brigance, A.H., and Glascoe, F.P. (2003). *The Brigance Infant and Toddler Screen.* North Billerica, MA: Curriculum Associates.

Brinton, B., and Fujiki, M. (1989). *Conversational management with language-impaired children: Pragmatic assessment and intervention.* Rockville, MD: Aspen Publishers.

Brinton, B., and Fujiki, M. (1992). Setting the context for conversational language sampling. In W. Secord (Ed.). *Best practices in school speech language pathology* (vol. II, pp. 9-19). San Antonio, TX: Psychological Corporation, Harcourt Brace Jovanovich.

Brinton, B., and Fujiki, M. (1994). Ways to teach conversation. In J. Duchan, L. Hewitt, and R. Sonnenmeier (Eds.). *Pragmatics: From theory to practice* (pp. 59-71). Englewood Cliffs, NJ: Prentice-Hall.

Brinton, B., and Fujiki, M. (1995). Conversational intervention with children with specific language impairment. In M.E. Fey, J. Windsor, and S.F. Warren (Eds.). *Language Intervention: Preschool through the elementary years* (vol. 5, pp. 183-212). Baltimore, MD: Paul H. Brookes.

Brinton, B., and Fujiki, M. (1999). Social interactional behaviors of children with specific language impairments. *Topics in Language Disorders, 19*, 49-69.

Brinton, B., and Fujiki, M. (2005). Social competence in children with language impairment: Making connections. *Seminars in Speech and Language, 26*, 151-159.

Brinton, B., Fujiki, M., and Sonnenberg, E. (1988). Responses to requests for clarification by linguistically normal and language-impaired children in conversation. *Journal of Speech and Hearing Research, 53*, 383-391.

Brinton, B., Robinson, L., and Fujiki, M. (2004). Description of a program for social language intervention: "If you can have a conversation, you can have a relationship." *Language, Speech and Hearing Services in Schools, 35*, 283-290.

Broca, P. (1861). Nouvelle observation d'aphémie produite par une lésion de la mortié posterieure des deuxième et troisième circonvolutions frontales. *Bulletin de la Société Anatomique*, 398-407.

Broderbund. (1995). *The amazing writing machine.* Novato, CA: Author.

Bromwich, R., Khokha, E., Fust, L., Baxter, E., Burge, D., and Kass, E. (Ed., 1981). Parent Behavior Progression (PBP) form 1. In R. Bromwich (Ed.). *Working with parents and infants: An interactional approach.* Baltimore, MD: University Park Press.

Brooks, M. (1978). *Your child's speech & language.* Austin, TX: Pro-Ed.

Brooks, M., and Hartung, D. (2000). *Speech and language handouts resource guide, 2nd edition.* Austin, TX: Pro-Ed.

Brown, A., and Campione, J. (1990). Communities of learning and thinking, or a context by any other name. In D. Kuhn (Ed.). *Developmental perspectives on teaching and learning thinking skills* (pp. 108-126). New York: Karger.

Brown, A., and Palinscar, A. (1987). Reciprocal teaching of comprehension strategies. In J. Day and J. Borkowski (Eds.). *Intelligence and exceptionality: New directions for theory, assessment, and instructional practice* (pp. 81-132). Norwood, NJ: Ablex.

Brown, G., Anderson, A., Shillcock, R., and Yule, G. (1984). *Teaching talk.* Cambridge, England: Cambridge University Press.

Brown, L., Sherbenou, R., and Johnsen, S. (1997). *Test of nonverbal intelligence—3.* Austin, TX: Pro-Ed.

Brown, M. (1947). *Stone soup.* New York: Charles Scribner's Sons.

Brown, R. (1973). *A first language: The early stages.* Cambridge, MA: Harvard University Press.

Brown, R., and Hanlon, C. (1970). Derivational complexity and order of acquisition in child speech. In J.R. Hayes (Ed.). *Cognition and the development of language.* New York: John Wiley & Sons.

Brown, V., Hammill, D., and Wiederholt, L. (1995). *Test of Reading Comprehension (TORC).* Austin, TX: Pro-Ed.

Brown, W. (2002). The molecular biology of the fragile X mutation. In R. Hagerman & P. Hagerman (Eds.). *Fragile X syndrome: Diagnosis, treatment and research* (3rd ed, pp. 110-135). Baltimore: Johns Hopkins University Press.

Brown W., and Conroy M. (2002). Promoting peer-related social-communicative competence in preschool children. In H. Goldstein, L. Kaczmarek, and K. English (Eds.). *Promoting social communication* (pp. 173-210). Baltimore: Paul H. Brookes.

Brown, W., Friedman, E., Jenkins, E., Brooks, J., Wisniewski, K., Raguthu, S., and French, J. (1982). Association of fragile X syndrome with autism. *Lancet, 1,* 100.

Browne, B., Jarrett, M., Hvey-Lewis, C., and Freund, M. (1997). *Developmental play group guide.* Austin, TX: Pro-Ed.

Brownell, R. (Ed.). (2000). *Expressive one-word picture vocabulary test—2000 Edition.* Novato, CA: Academic Therapy.

Bruce, B.H., and Watkins, R.V. (1995). Language intervention in a preschool classroom: Implementing a language-focused curriculum. In M.L. Rice and K.A. Wilcox (Eds.). *Building a language focused curriculum for the preschool classroom. A foundation for lifelong communication* (vol 1, pp. 39-72). Baltimore, MD: Paul H. Brookes.

Bruce, M., DiVenere, N., and Bergeron, C. (1998). Preparing students to understand and honor families as partners. *American Journal of Speech-Language Pathology, 7(3),* 85-94.

Bruininks, R., Woodcock, R., Weatherman, R., and Hill, B. (1996). *Scales of independent behavior—Revised.* Itasca, IL: Riverside Publishing.

Bruner, J. (1981). The social context of language acquisition. *Language and Communication, 1,* 155-178.

Bruns, D., and Steeples, T. (2001). Partners from the beginning: Guidelines for encouraging partnerships between parents and NICU and EI professionals. *Infant-Toddler Intervention, 11,* 237-247.

Brunsma, D. (1998). Effects of student uniforms on attendance, behavior problems, substance abuse, and academic achievement. *The Journal of Education Research, 92,* 53-62.

Bryan, T. (1986). A review of studies on learning-disabled children's communicative competence. In R.L. Schiefelbusch (Ed.). *Language competence: Assessment and intervention* (pp. 227-259). Austin, TX: Pro-Ed.

Bryant, B., and Wiederholt, J. (1990). *Gray oral reading tests—Diagnostic.* Austin, TX: Pro-Ed.

Bryant, D., Goodwin, M., Bryant, B., and Higgins, K. (2003). Vocabulary instruction for students with learning disabilities: A review of the research. *Learning Disabilities Quarterly, 26,* 117-128.

Bukendorf, R., Gordon, C., and Goodwyn-Craine, A. (2007). Assessment of the speech mechanism. In R. Paul and P. Cascella (Eds.). *Introduction to clinical methods is communication disorders.* Baltimore: Paul H. Brookes.

Bunce, B. (1991). Referential communication skills: guidelines for therapy. *Language, Speech, and Hearing Services in Schools, 22,* 296-301.

Bunce, B. (1995). *Building a language-focused curriculum for the pre-school classroom: A planning guide* (vol II). Baltimore, MD: Paul H. Brookes.

Burchinal, M., Campbell, F., Bryant., D., Wasik, B., and Ramey, C. (1997). Early intervention and mediating processes. I, Cognitive performance of children of low-income African-American families. *Child Development, 68,* 935-954.

Burgemeister, B., Blum, L., and Lorge, I. (1972). *Columbia mental maturity scale* (3rd ed.). New York: Psychological Corporation.

Burk, D. (2000). *Slangman guides.* CA: Slangman Publishing.

Burt, M., Dulay, H., and Hernandez-Chavez, E. (1975). *Bilingual syntax measure.* San Francisco, CA: Harcourt Brace Jovanovich.

Bus, A., van Ijzendoorn, M., and Pellegrini, A. (1995). Joint book reading makes for success in learning to read: A meta-analysis on intergenerational transmission of literacy. *Review of Educational Research, 65,* 1-21.

Buschbacher, P., and Fox, L. (2003). Understanding and intervening with the challenging behavior of young children with autism spectrum disorder. *Language, Speech and Hearing Services in Schools, 34,* 217-218.

Butler, K., and Silliman, E. (Eds.). (2002). *Speaking, reading, and writing in children with language learning disabilities: New paradigms in research and practice.* Mahwah, NJ: Erlbaum.

Byrne, A., Buckley, S., MacDonald, J., and Bird, G. (1995). Investigating the literacy, language and memory skills of children with Down's syndrome. *Down's Syndrome: Research and Practice, 3,* 53-58.

Byrne, J., Connolly, F., MacLean, S., Beattie., T., Dooley, J., and Gordon, K. (2001). Brain activity and cognitive status in pediatric patients: Development of a clinical assessment protocol. *Journal of Child Neurology, 16,* 325-332.

Bzoch, K., League, R., and Brown, V. (2003). *The receptive expressive emergent language test—Third edition.* Austin, TX: Pro-Ed.

Cain, K. (2003). Text comprehension and its relation to coherence and cohesion in children's fictional narratives. *British Journal of Developmental Psychology, 21,* 335-351.

Cain, K., Oakhill, J., and Elbro, C. (2003). The ability to learn new word meanings from context by school-age children with and without language comprehension difficulties. *Journal of Child Language, 30,* 681-694.

Calculator, S. (1997a). AAC and individuals with severe to profound disabilities. In S.L. Glennen and D.C. DeCoste (Eds.). *Handbook of augmentative and alternative communication.* San Diego, CA: Singular Publishing Group.

Calculator, S. (1997b). Fostering early language acquisition and AAC use. *Alternative and Augmentative Communication, 13,* 149-157.

Calculator, S., and Jorgensen, C. (1991). Integrating AAC instruction into regular education settings: Expounding on best practices. *Augmentative and Alternative Communication, 7,* 204-214.

Calculator, S.N. (1994a). Designing and implementing communicative assessments in inclusive settings. In S.N. Calculator and C.M. Jorgensen (Eds.). *Including severe disabilities in schools: Fostering communication, interaction, and participation* (pp. 113-181). San Diego, CA: Singular Publishing Group.

Calculator, S.N. (1994b). Communicative intervention as a means to successful inclusion. In S.N. Calculator and C.M. Jorgesen (Eds.). *Including students with severe disabilities in schools: Fostering communication, interaction, and participation* (pp. 183-214). San Diego, CA: Singular Publishing Group.

Callanan, C. (1990). *Since Owen: Parent-to-parent guide for care of the disabled child.* Baltimore, MD: The Johns Hopkins University Press.

Camarata, S., and Nelson, K. (2006). Conversational recast intervention with preschool and older children. In R. McCauley and M. Fey (Eds.). *Treatment of language disorders in children.* Baltimore: Paul H. Brookes.

Camarata, S., Nelson, K., and Camarata, M. (1994). A comparison of conversation based to imitation based procedures for training grammatical structures in specifically language impaired children. *Journal of Speech and Hearing Research, 37,* 1414-1423.

Camp, B., and Bash, M. (1981). *Think aloud: Increasing social and cognitive skills—A problem-solving approach.* Champaign, IL: Research Press.

Campbell, T., Dollaghan, C., Needleman, H., and Janosky, J. (1997). Reducing bias in language assessment: Processing-dependent measures. *Journal of Speech, Language, and Hearing Research, 40,* 519-525.

Campbell, T., Dollaghan, C., Rockette, H., Paradise, J., Feldman, H., Shriberg, L., Sabo, D., and Kurs-Lasky, M. (2003). Risk factors for speech delay of unknown origin in 3-year-old children. *Child Development, 74,* 346-357.

Campbell, T.F. (1998). Measurement of functional outcome in preschool children with neurogenic communication disorders. *Seminars in Speech and Language, 19(3),* 223-233.

Canter, L. (1976). *Assertive discipline: A take-charge approach for today's educator.* Seal Beach, CA: Canter and Associates.

Cantlon, T. (1991). *The first four weeks of cooperative learning.* Portland, OR: Prestige Publishers.

Cantwell, D., Baker, L., and Mattison, R. (1979). The prevalence of psychiatric disorder in children with speech and language disorder: an epidemiologic study. *Journal of the American Academy of Child Psychiatry, 18,* 450-461.

Caparulo, B., and Cohen, D. (1983). Developmental language studies in the neuropsychiatric disorders of children. In K.E. Nelson (Ed.). *Children's language 4* (pp. 423-463). Hillsdale, NJ: Erlbaum.

Capone, N., and McGregor, K. (2004). Gesture development: A review for clinical and research practices. *Journal of Speech, Language, and Hearing Research, 47,* 173-187.

Capute, A., Palmer, F., Shapiro, B., Wachtel, R., Schmidt, S., and Ross, A. (1986). Clinical linguistic and auditory milestone scale: Prediction of cognition in infancy. *Developmental Medicine and Child Neurology, 28,* 762-771.

Capute, A., Shapiro, B., Wachtel, R., Gunther, V., and Palmer, F. (1986). The Clinical Linguistic and Auditory Milestone Scale. *American Journal of Diseases in Children, 40,* 694-698.

Carbone, V. (2003). *Promoting speech production skills in children with autism.* Workshop presented at Carbone Clinic, Valley Cottage, NY.

Carey, S. (1978). The child as word learner. In M. Halle, J. Bresnan, and G. Miller (Eds.). *Linguistic theory and psychological reality.* Cambridge, MA: MIT Press.

Carle, E. (1984). *The very busy spider.* New York: Philomel Books.

Carlisle, J. (1991). Planning an assessment of listening and reading comprehension. *Topics in Language Disorders, 12(1),* 17-31.

Carpenter, M., Tomasello, M., and Striano, T. (2005). Role reversal, imitation and language in typically-developing infants and children with autism. *Infancy, 8,* 253-278.

Carpenter, R. (1987). Play scale. In L. Olswang, C. Stoel-Gammon, T. Coggins, and R. Carpenter (Eds.). *Assessing prelinguistic and early behaviors in developmentally young children* (pp. 44-77). Seattle, WA: University of Washington Press.

Carr, E., Binkoff, J., Kologinsky, E., and Eddy, M. (1978). Acquisition of sign language by autistic children: I. Expressive labelling. *Journal of Applied Behavior Analysis, 11,* 489-501.

Carr, E., Dunlap, G., Horner, R.H., Koegel, R.L., Turnbull, A.P., Sailor, W., Anderson, J.L., Albin, R.W., Kern Koegel, L., and Fox, L. (2002). Positive behavior support: Evolution of an applied science. *Journal of Positive Behavior Interventions, 4,* 4-17.

Carr, E., Schriebman, I., and Lovaas, O. (1975). Control of echolalic speech in psychotic children. *Journal of Abnormal Child Psychology, 3,* 331-351.

Carroll, R. (1965). *What whiskers did.* New York: Scholastic Book Service.

Carrow-Woolfolk, E. (1988). *Theory, assessment and intervention in language disorders: An integrative approach.* Philadelphia, PA: Grune & Stratton.

Carrow-Woolfolk, E. (1999a). *Test for auditory comprehension of language—3.* Austin, TX: Pro-Ed.

Carrow-Woolfolk, E. (1999b). *Comprehensive assessment of spoken language.* Circle Pines, MN: AGS Publishing.

Carson, C., Klee, T., Carson, D., and Hime, L. (2003). Phonological profiles of 2-Year-Olds with delayed language development: Predicting clinical outcomes at age 3. *American Journal of Speech-Language Pathology, 12,* 28-40.

Carter, A., Davis, N., Klin, A., and Volkmar, F. (2005). Social development in autism. In F. Volkmar, R. Paul, A. Klin, and D. Cohen (Eds.). *Handbook of autism and pervasive developmental disorders—vol. 1* (pp. 288-311). New York: Wiley.

Carter, J., Lees, J., Murira, G., Gona, J., Neville, B., and Newton, C. (2005). Issues in the development of cross-cultural assessments of speech and language for children. *International Journal of Language and Communication Disorders, 40,* 385-401.

Casati, I., and Lezine, I. (1968). *Les étapes de l'intelligence sensorimotrice.* Paris: Editions de Centre de Psychologie Applique.

Casby, M. (2001). Otitis media and language development: A meta-analysis. *American Journal of Speech-Language Pathology, 10,* 65-80.

Casby, M. (2003a). The development of play in infants, toddlers, and young children. *Communication Disorders Quarterly, 24,* 163-174.

Casby, M. (2003b) Developmental assessment of play: A model for early intervention. *Communication Disorders Quarterly, 24,* 175-183.

Casby, M.W. (1997). Symbolic play of children with language impairment. *Journal of Speech, Language, and Hearing Research, 40,* 468-479.

Cascella, P.W., and McNamara, K. M. (2004, May 11). Practical communication services for high school students with severe disabilities: Collaboration during the transition to adult services. *The ASHA Leader, 6-7,* 18-19.

Casselli, M., and Casadio, P. (1995). *Il primo vocabolario del bambino.* Milano: Franco Angeli.

Cassidy, S. (1997). Prader-Willi syndrome. *Journal of Medical Genetics, 34,* 917-923.

Catroppa, C., and Anderson, V. (2004). Recovery and predictors of language skills two years following pediatric traumatic brain injury. *Brain and Language, 88,* 68-78.

Cattell, P. (1960). *Cattell infant intelligence scale.* New York: Psychological Corporation.

Catts, H. (1986). Speech production/phonological deficits in reading disordered children. *Journal of Learning Disabilities, 19,* 504-508.

Catts, H. (1989). Phonological processing deficits and reading disabilities. In A. Kamhi and H. Catts (Eds.). *Reading disabilities: A developmental language perspective* (pp. 101-132). Boston, MA: College-Hill.

Catts, H. (1991). Facilitating phonological awareness: Role of speech-language pathologists. *Language, Speech, and Hearing Services in Schools, 22,* 196-203.

Catts, H. (1997). The early identification of language-based reading disabilities. *Language, Speech, and Hearing Services in Schools, 28,* 86-89.

Catts, H. (1999a). Phonological awareness: Putting research into practice. *Language, Learning, and Education Newsletter, 6(1),* 26-29.

Catts, H. (1999b). Phonological awareness: Putting research into practice. *Perspectives on Language, Learning, and Education, 7,* 17-19.

Catts, H., Fey, M., Tomblin, B., and Zhang, Z. (2002). A longitudinal investigation of reading outcomes in children with language impairments. *Journal of Speech, Language, and Hearing Research, 45,* 1142-1157.

Catts, H., Fey, M., Zhang, Z., and Tomblin, B. (1999). Language basis of reading and reading disabilities: Evidence from a longitudinal investigation. *Scientific Studies in Reading, 3,* 331-361.

Catts, H., and Kamhi, A. (1986). The linguistic basis for reading disorders: Implications for the speech-language pathologist. *Language, Speech, and Hearing Services in Schools, 17,* 329-341.

Catts, H., and Kamhi, A. (2005a). *Language and reading disabilities—2nd Ed.* Boston: Allyn & Bacon.

Catts, H., and Kamhi, A. (2005b). Causes of reading disabilities. In H. Catts and A. Kamhi (Eds.). *Language and Reading Disabilities—2nd Ed.* (pp. 94-126). Boston: Allyn & Bacon.

Causton-Theoharis, J., and Malmgren, K. (2005). Increasing peer interactions for students with severe disabilities via paraprofessional training. *Exceptional Children, 71,* 431-444.

Cazden, C. (1965). *Environmental assistance to the child's acquisition of grammar.* Unpublished doctoral dissertation, Harvard University, Cambridge, MA.

Cazden, C. (1988). *Classroom discourse: The language of teaching and learning.* Portsmouth, NH: Heinemann.

Cazden, C. (1999). The language of African American students in classroom discourse. In C. Adger, D. Christian, and O. Taylor (Eds.). *Making the connection: Language and academic achievement among African American students in classroom discourse.* Washington, DC: Center for Applied Linguistics.

Cera, R., Vulanich, N., Brady, W., and Blosser, J. (2003). *Traumatic Brain Injury: A family guide to assisting in speech, language, and cognitive rehabilitation.* Austin, TX: Pro Ed.

Chabon, S., Lee-Wilkerson, D., and Green, T. (1992). Drug-exposed infants and children: Living with a lethal legacy. *Clinics in Communication Disorders, 2,* 32-51.

Chaffin, L. (1980). *We be warm till springtime comes.* New York: Macmillan.

Chall, J. (1983). *Stages of reading development.* New York: McGraw-Hill.

Chall, J. (1989). *Learning to read: The great debate 20 years later.* Phi Delta Kappan, 521-538.

Chall, J. (1996). *Learning to read: The great debate* (3rd ed.). New York: McGraw Hill.

Chall, J. (1997). Are reading methods changing again? Annals of Dyslexia, 47, 257-263.

Chan, E., Hopkins, M., Perrin, H., Herrerias, C., and Homer, C. (2005). Diagnostic practices for attention deficit hyperactivity disorder: A national survey of primary care physicians. *Ambulatory Pediatrics, 5,* 201-208.

Chan, S., and Lee, E. (2004). Families with Asian roots. In E. Lynch and M. Hanson (Eds.). *Developing cross-cultural competence* (3rd ed., pp. 219-298). Baltimore, MD: Paul H. Brookes.

Chandler, S., Christie, P., Newson, E., and Prevezer, W. (2002). Developing a diagnostic and intervention package for 2- and 3-year-olds with autism: Outcomes of the Frameworks for Communication Approach. *Autism: The International Journal of Research and Practice, 6,* 47-69.

Chaney, C. (1990). Evaluating the whole language approach to language arts: The pros and cons. *Language, Speech, and Hearing Services in Schools, 21,* 244-249.

Chaney, C., and Estrin, E. (1987, November). *Metalinguistic awareness.* Mini-seminar presented at the annual convention of the American Speech-Language-Hearing Association, New Orleans, LA.

Chaney, C., and Estrin, E. (1989). Stimulating phonological awareness. Unpublished manuscript.

Channell, R. (2003). Automated Developmental Sentence Scoring using Computerized Profiling software. *American Journal of Speech-Language Pathology, 12,* 369-376.

Channell, R., and Johnson, B. (1999). Automated grammatical tagging of child language samples. *Journal of Speech, Language, and Hearing Research, 42(3),* 727-734.

Chapman, R. (1978). Comprehension strategies in children. In J.F. Kavanaugh and W. Strange (Eds.). *Speech and language in the laboratory, school and clinic* (pp. 308-327). Cambridge, MA: MIT Press.

Chapman, R. (1981). Exploring children's communicative intents. In J. Miller (Ed.). *Assessing language production in children* (pp. 111-138). Baltimore, MD: University Park Press.

Chapman, R. (1992). Childtalk: Processes in child language acquisition. St. Louis, MO: Mosby.

Chapman, R. (2000). Children's language learning: An interactionist perspective. *Journal of Child Psychology and Psychiatry, 41,* 33-54.

Chapman, R. (2003). Language and communication in individuals with Down syndrome. In Abbeduto, L. (Ed.). *International review of research in mental retardation, 27.* New York: Academic Press.

Chapman, R., and Hesketh, L. (2000). Behavioral phonotype of individuals with Down syndrome. *Mental Retardation and Developmental Disabilities Research Reviews, 6,* 84-95.

Chapman, R., and Miller, J. (1975). Word order in early two- and three-word utterances: Does production precede comprehension? *Journal of Speech and Hearing Research, 18,* 355-371.

Chapman, R., and Miller, J. (1980). Analyzing language and communication in the child. In R. Schiefelbusch (Ed.). *Nonspeech language and communication: Analysis and intervention.* Baltimore, MD: University Park Press.

Chapman, R., Seung, H., Schwartz, S., and Kay-Raining Bird, E. (1998). Language skills of children and adolescents with Down syndrome. II: Production deficits. *Journal of Speech, Language, and Hearing Research, 41(4),* 861-873.

Chapman, S., McKinnon, L., Levin, H., Song, J., Neier, N., and Chiu, S. (2001). Longitudinal outcome of verbal discourse in children with traumatic brain injury: Three-year follow-up. *Journal of Head Trauma Rehabilitation, 16(5),* 441-455.

Charlop-Christy, M., Carpenter, M., Le, L., Leblanc, L., and Kellet, K. (2002). Using PECS with children with autism. *Journal of Applied Behavior Analysis, 35,* 213-231.

Charlop-Christy, M., and Jones, C. (2006). The picture exchange communication system. In R. McCauley and M. Fey (Eds.). *Treatment of language disorders in children* (pp. 105-122). Baltimore: Paul H. Brookes.

Charlop-Christy, M.H., Le, L., and Freeman, K.A. (2000). A comparison of video modeling with in vivo modeling for teaching children with autism. *Journal of Autism and Developmental Disorders, 30,* 537-552.

Chawarska, K., and Volkmar, F. (2005). Autism in infancy and early childhood. In F. Volkmar, R. Paul, A. Klin, and D. Cohen (Eds.). *Handbook of autism and pervasive developmental disorders—Vol 1* (pp. 223-246). New York: Wiley.

Cheng, L. (1987). Cross-cultural and linguistic considerations in working with Asian populations. *AHSA, 29(6),* 33-41.

Cheng, L. (1989). Service delivery to Asian/Pacific LEP children: A cross-cultural framework. *Topics in Language Disorders, 9(3),* 1-11.

Cheng, L. (1996). Beyond bilingualism: A quest for communicative competence. *Topics in Language Disorders, 16(4),* 9-21.

Cheng, L. (2001). Transcription of English influenced by selected Asian languages. *Communication Disorders Quarterly, 23,* 40-46.

Cheng, L. (2002a). Asian and Pacific-American cultures. In D.E. Battle (Ed.). *Communication disorders in multicultural populations* (3rd ed., pp. 71-112). Boston: Butterworth-Heinneman.

Cheng, L. (2002b). *Assessing Asian language performance* (2nd ed.) Oceanside, CA: Academic Communication Associates.

Cheng, L., Battle, D., Murdoch, B., and Martin, D. (2001). Educating speech-language pathologists for a multicultural world. *Folia Phoniatrica, 53,* 121-127.

Cheseldine, S., and McConkey, R. (1979). Parental speech to young Down's syndrome children: An intervention study. *American Journal of Mental Deficiency, 83,* 612-620.

Child Development Inventories. (1992). *Interagency agreements: A proactive tool for improving the transition from Ireland,* H. Minneapolis, MN: Behavior Science Systems.

Child Development Resources. (1989). *How can we help?* Lightfoot, VA: Child Development Resources.

Children's Defense Fund. (1990). *State of America's children.* Washington, DC: Children's Defense Fund.

Chilosi, A., Pecini, C., Cipriani, P., Brovedani, P. Brizzolara, D., Ferretti, G., Pfanner, L., and Cioni, G. (2005). Atypical language lateralization and early linguistic development in children with focal brain lesions. *Developmental Medicine and Child Neurology, 27,* 725-730.

Chilosi, A.M., Cipriani, P., Bertuccelli, B., Pfanner, L., and Cioni, G. (2001). Early cognitive and communication development in children with focal brain lesions. *Journal of Child Neurology, 16(5),* 309-326.

Chiriboga, C (2003). Fetal alcohol and drug effects. *The Neurologist, 9,* 267-279.

Chomsky, C. (1972). Stages in language development and reading exposure. *Harvard Educational Review, 42,* 1-3.

Chomsky, C. (1980). Reading, writing and phonology. In M. Wolf, M. McQuillain, and E. Radwin (Eds.). *Thought and language/language and reading* (pp. 51-71). Reprint Series #14. Cambridge, MA: Harvard Educational Review.

Chomsky, N. (1957). *Syntactic structures.* Cambridge, MA: MIT Press.

Chomsky, N. (1980). Language without cognition. In M. Piattelli-Palmarini (Ed.). *Language and learning: The debate between Jean Piaget and Noam Chomsky.* Cambridge, MA: Harvard University Press.

Chomsky, N., and Halle, M. (1968). *The sound pattern of English.* New York: Harper & Row.

Christensen, S., and Luckett, C. (1990). Getting into the classroom and making it work! *Language, Speech, and Hearing Services in Schools, 21,* 110-113.

Christie, F. (2003). *Classroom discourse analysis: A functional perspective.* London: Continuum International Publishing Group.

Churchill, J., Beckel-Mitchener, A., Weiler, I., and Greenough, W. (2002). Effects of fragile X syndrome and an FMR1 knockout mouse model on forebrain neuronal cell biology. *Microscopy Research and Technique, 57,* 156-158.

Chute, P., and Nevins, M. (2003). *Candidacy and habilitation of children with cochlear implants.* Rockville, MD: ASHA.

Ciocci, S., and Baran, J. (1998). Use of conversational strategies by children who are deaf. *American Annals of the Deaf, 143,* 235-245.

Cirrin, F. (1989). Issues in determining eligibility for service: Who does what to whom. In A. Kamhi and H. Catts (Eds.). Reading disabilities: A developmental language perspective (pp. 345-368). Boston, MA: College-Hill Press.

Clahsen, H. (1989). *Child language and developmental dysphagia: Linguistic studies of the acquisition of German.* Philadelphia, PA: J. Benjamins Publishing Company.

Clahsen, H. (1991). *Child language and development dysphasia: Linguistic studies of the acquisition of German.* Philadelphia, PA: J. Benjamins Publishing Company.

Clark, D. (1989). Neonates and infants at risk for hearing and speech-language disorders. *Topics in Language Disorders, 10(1),* 1-12.

Clark, J., Jorgensen S., and Blondeau, R. (1995). Investigating the validity of the clinical linguistic auditory milestone scale. *International Journal of Pediatric Otorhinolaryngology, 3,* 63-75.

Clark, M. M., and Plante, E. (1998). Morphology of the inferior frontal gyrus in developmentally language-disordered adults. *Brain and Language, 61,* 288-303.

Clark, T., Morgan, E., and Wilson-Vlotman, A. (1984). *The INSITE model: A parent centered, in-home, sensory intervention, training and educational program.* Logan, UT: Utah State University.

Clark, T., and Watkins, S. (1985). *SKI*HI curriculum manual: Programming for hearing impaired infants through home intervention.* Logan, UT: Utah State University.

Clarke-Klein, S., and Hodson, B.W. (1995). A phonologically based analysis of misspellings of third graders with disordered phonology histories. *Journal of Speech and Hearing Research, 38,* 839-849.

Clarke-Stewart, K. (1973). Interactions between mothers and their young children: Characteristics and consequences. *Monographs of the Society for Research on Child Development, 38*(6-7, serial no. 153).

Clarke-Stewart, K. (1977). *Child care in the family.* New York: Academic Press.

Cleave, P., and Fey, M. (1997). Two approaches to the facilitation of grammar in children with language impairments: Rationale and description. *American Journal of Speech-Language Pathology, 6*, 23-32.

Cleave, P.L., and Rice, M.L. (1997). An examination of the morpheme BE in children with specific language impairment: The role of contractibility and grammatical form class. *Journal of Speech and Hearing Research, 40*, 480-492.

Clezy, G. (1979). *Modification of the mother-child interchange in language, speech, and hearing.* Baltimore, MD: University Park Press.

Cliff, S., Carr, D., Gray, J., Nymann, C., and Redding, S. (1975). *Comprehensive developmental evaluation chart.* El Paso, TX: El Paso Rehabilitation Center.

Clymer, E. (1991). Using hypermedia to develop and deliver assessment or intervention services. *Topics in Language Disorders, 11*, 50-64.

Cobo-Lewis, A., Eilers, R., Pearson, B., and Umbel, V. (2002). Interdependence of Spanish and English knowledge in language and literacy among bilingual children. In D.K. Oller and R.E. Eilers (Eds.). *Language and literacy in bilingual children* (pp. 118-134). Clevedon, England: Multilingual Matters.

Cochran, P., and Bull, G. (1991). Integrating word processing into language intervention. *Topics in Language Disorders, 11*(2), 31-49.

Cochran, P., and Masterson, J. (1995). NOT using a computer in language assessment/intervention: In defense of the reluctant clinician. *Language, Speech, and Hearing Services in Schools, 26*, 213-222.

Coggins, T. (1979). Relational meaning encoded in the two-word utterances of stage I Down's syndrome children. *Journal of Speech and Hearing Research, 22*, 166-178.

Coggins, T. (1991). Bringing context back into assessment. *Topics in Language Disorders, 11*, 43-54.

Coggins, T. (1998). Clinical assessment of emerging language: How to gather evidence and make informed decisions. In A.M. Wetherby, S.F. Warren, and J. Reichle (Eds.). *Transitions in prelinguistic communication* (pp. 233-259). Baltimore, MD: Paul H. Brookes.

Coggins, T., and Carpenter, R. (1981). The communicative intention inventory. *Journal of Applied Psycholinguistics, 2*, 213-234.

Coggins, T., Olswang, L., and Guthrie, J. (1987). Assessing communicative intents in young children: Low-structured or observation tasks? *Journal of Speech and Hearing Disorders, 52*, 44-49.

Cognitive Concepts. (1998). *Earobics Step 2* (computer program). Evanston, IL: Cognitive Concepts, Inc.

Cohen, M. (1997). *The child with multiple birth defects.* New York: Raven Press.

Cohen, N.J., Barwick, M.A., Horodezky, N., and Isaacson, L. (1996). Comorbidity of language and social-emotional disorders: Comparison of psychiatric outpatients and their siblings. *Journal of Clinical and Child Psychology, 25*, 192-200.

Cohen, W., Hodson, A., O'Hare, A., Boyle, J., Durrani, T., McCartney, E., Mattey, M., Naftalin, L., and Watson, J. (2005). Effects of computer-based intervention through acoustically modified speech (Fast ForWord) in severe receptive-expressive language impairment: outcomes from a randomized controlled trial. *Journal of Speech, Language and Hearing Research, 48*(3), 715-729.

Cole, K., and Dale, P. (1986). Direct language instruction and interactive language instruction with language delayed preschool children: A comparison study. *Journal of Speech and Hearing Research, 29*, 206-217.

Cole, K., Maddox, M., and Lim, Y. (2006). Language is the key. In R. McCauley and M. Fey (Eds.). *Treatment of language disorders in children.* Baltimore: Paul H. Brookes.

Cole, K., Mills, P., and Dale, P. (1989). Examination of test-retest and split-half reliability for measures derived from language samples of young handicapped children. *Language, Speech, and Hearing Services in Schools, 20*, 245-258.

Cole, K., Mills, P., and Kelley, D. (1994). Agreement of assessment profiles used in cognitive referencing. *Language, Speech, and Hearing Services in Schools, 25*, 25-31.

Cole, K., Schwartz, I., Notari, A., Dale, P., Mills, P. (1995). Examination of the stability of two methods of defining specific language impairment. *Applied Psycholinguistics, 16*, 103-123.

Cole, L. (1985). *Nonstandard English: Handbook for assessment and instruction.* Silver Spring, MD: L. Cole.

Coleman, T., and McCabe-Smith, L. (2000). Culturally appropriate service delivery: Some considerations. In T. Coleman (Ed.). *Clinical management of communication disorders in culturally diverse children* (pp. 13-30). Boston: Allyn & Bacon.

Coles-White, D. (2004). Negative concord in child African American English: Implications for specific language impairment. *Journal of Speech, Language, and Hearing Research, 47*, 212-222.

Computer Software. (1989). *Early concepts skillbuilder series.* Monterey, CA: Edmark Corporation.

Comrie, J., and Helm, J. (1997). Common feeding problems in the intensive care nursery: Maturation, organization, evaluation, and management strategies. *Seminars in Speech and Language, 18*, 239-262.

Condouris, K., Mayer, E., and Tager-Flusberg, H. (2003). The relationship between standardized measures of language and measures of spontaneous speech in children with autism. *American Journal of Speech-Language Pathology, 12*, 349-359.

Cone-Wesson, B. (2005). Prenatal alcohol and cocaine exposure: Influences on cognition, speech, language, and hearing. *Journal of Communication Disorders, 38*, 279-302.

Connell, P. (1982). On training language rules. *Language, Speech, and Hearing Services in Schools, 13*, 231-248.

Connell, P. (1987). An effect of modeling and imitation teaching procedures on children with and without specific language impairment. *Journal of Speech and Hearing Research, 30*, 105-113.

Connell, P. (1989). Facilitating generalization through induction teaching. In L. McReynolds and J. Spradlin (Eds.). *Generalization strategies in the treatment of communication disorders.* Philadelphia, PA: B.C. Decker.

Connell, P., and Stone, C. (1992). Morpheme learning of children with specific language impairment under controlled instructional conditions. *Journal of Speech and Hearing Research, 34*, 1329-1338.

Constantino, J. (2003). *Social responsiveness scale.* Los Angeles: Western Psychological Service.

Conte, B., Menyuk, P., and Bashir, A. (1992, November). *Text comprehension in normal and language impaired adolescents.* Paper presented at American Speech-Language-Hearing Annual Convention, New Orleans.

Conti-Ramsden, G., and Botting, N. (2004). Social difficulties and victimization in children with SLI at 11 years of age. *Journal of Speech, Language & Hearing Research, 47*(1), 145-161.

Conti-Ramsden, G., Crutchley, A., and Botting, N. (1997). The extent to which psychometric tests differential subgroups of children with SLI. *Journal of Speech, Language and Hearing Research, 40*, 765-777.

Cooper, D., and Anderson-Inman, L. (1988). Language and socialization. In M.A. Nippold (Ed.). *Later language development: Ages nine through nineteen* (pp. 225-245). Austin, TX: Pro-Ed.

Coplan, J. (1993). *Early language milestone scale (ELM Scale-2).* Austin, TX: Pro-Ed.

Coplan, J., and Gleason, J. (1988). Unclear speech: Recognition and significance of unintelligible speech in preschool children. *Pediatrics, 82*, 447-452.

Coplan, J., Gleason, J.R., Ryan, R., Burke, M., and Williams, M. (1982). Validation of an early language milestone scale in a high-risk population. *Pediatrics, 70*, 677-683.

Cordone, I., and Gilkerson, L. (1989). Family administered neonatal activities. *Zero to Three, 10*, 23-28.

Coryell, J., and Holcomb, T. (1997). The use of sign language and sign systems in facilitating the language acquisition and communication of deaf students. *Language, Speech, and Hearing Services in Schools, 28*, 384-394.

Costello, J. (1983). Generalization across settings: Language intervention with children. In J. Miller, D. Yoder, and R. Schiefelbusch (Eds.). *Contemporary issues in language intervention.* Rockville, MD: American Speech-Language-Hearing Association.

Coster, W., and Cicchetti, D. (1993). Research on the communicative development of maltreated children: Clinical implications. *Topics in Language Disorders, 13*(4), 25-38.

Coster, W., Gersten, M., Beeghly, M., and Cicchetti, D. (1989). Communicative functioning in maltreated toddlers. *Developmental Psychology, 25*, 1020-1029.

Coufal, K., Steckelberg, A., and Vasa, S. (1991). Current trends in the training and utilization of paraprofessionals in speech and language programs: A report on an eleven-state survey. *Language, Speech, and Hearing Services in Schools, 22,* 51-59.

Coufal, L. (2002). Technology teaching or mediated learning, Part I: Are computers Skinnerian or Vygotskian? *Topics in Language Disorders, 22,* 1-28.

Council for Exceptional Children. (1969). *Exceptional Children Conference papers: Parent participation in early childhood education.* Reston, VA: Author.

Crabtree, N. (1958). *The Houston test of language development.* Houston, TX: Houston Test Company.

Crago, M., and Cole, E. (1991). Using ethnography to bring children's communicative and cultural worlds into focus. In T.M. Gallagher (Ed.). *Pragmatics of language: Clinical practice issues* (pp. 99-132). San Diego, CA: Singular Publishing Group.

Craig, H. (1983). Applications of pragmatic language models for intervention. In T. Gallagher and C. Prutting (Eds.). *Pragmatic assessment and intervention issues in language* (pp. 101-128). San Diego, CA: College-Hill Press.

Craig, H. (1991). Pragmatic characteristics of the child with specific language impairment: an interactionist perspective. In T. Gallagher (Ed.). *Pragmatics of language: Clinical practice issues* (pp. 163-198). San Diego, CA: Singular Publishing Group.

Craig, H., and Evans, J. (1993). Pragmatics and SLI: Within-group variations in discourse behaviors. *Journal of Speech and Hearing Research, 36,* 777-789.

Craig, H., Thompson, C., Washington, J., and Potter, S. (2003). Phonological features of child African American English. *Journal of Speech, Language and Hearing Research, 46,* 623-635.

Craig, H., and Washington, J. (1995). African-American English and linguistic complexity in preschool discourse: A second look. *Language, Speech, and Hearing Services in Schools, 26,* 87-93.

Craig, H., and Washington, J. (2000). An assessment battery for identifying language impairments in African American children. *Journal of Speech, Language, and Hearing Research, 43,* 366-379.

Craig, H., and Washington, J. (2002). Oral language expectations for African American preschoolers and kindergartners. *American Journal of Speech-Language Pathology, 11,* 59-70.

Craig, H., and Washington, J. (2004a). Grade-related changes in the production of African American English. *Journal of Speech, Language and Hearing Research, 47,* 450-463.

Craig, H., and Washington, J. (2004b). A language screening protocol for use with young African American children in urban settings. *American Journal of Speech-Language Pathology, 13,* 329-340.

Craig, H., and Washington, J. (2005). Oral language expectations for African American children in grades 1 through 5. *American Journal of Speech-Language Pathology, 13,* 119-130.

Crain-Thoreson, C., and Dale, P. S. (1999). Enhancing linguistic performance: Parents and teachers as book reading partners for children with language delays. *Topics in Early Childhood Special Education, 19(1),* 28-40.

Crais, E. (1990). World knowledge to word knowledge. *Topics in Language Disorders, 10(3),* 45-62.

Crais, E. (1991). *A practical guide to embedding family-centered content into existing speech-language-pathology coursework.* Chapel Hill, NC: University of North Carolina.

Crais, E. (1995). Expanding the repertoire of tools and techniques for assessing communication skills for infants and toddlers. *American Journal of Speech-Language Pathology, 4,* 47-59.

Crais, E., and Calculator, S. (1998). Role of caregivers in the assessment process. In A.M. Wetherby, S.F. Warren, and J. Reichle (Eds.). *Transitions in prelinguistic communication* (pp. 261-283). Baltimore, MD: Paul H. Brookes.

Crais, E., and Roberts, J. (1991). Decision making in assessment and early intervention planning. *Language, Speech, and Hearing Services in Schools, 22,* 19-30.

Creaghead, N. (1984). Strategies for evaluating and targeting pragmatic behaviors in young children. *Seminars in Speech and Language, 5,* 241-252.

Creaghead, N. (1990). Mutual empowerment through collaboration: A new script for an old problem. In W. Secord (Ed.). *Best practices in school speech-language pathology* (vol. I, pp. 106-116). San Antonio, TX: Psychological Corporation, Harcourt Brace Jovanovich.

Creaghead, N. (1992). Mutual empowerment through collaboration: a new script for an old problem. In W.A. Second (Ed.). *Best practices in school speech-language pathology* (pp. 109-116). San Antonio, TX: Psychological Corporation, Harcourt Brace Jovanovich.

Creaghead, N. (1994). Collaborative intervention. In D. Ripich and N. Creaghead (Eds.). *School discourse problems* (ed. 22nd ed., pp. 373-386). San Diego, CA: Singular Publishing Group.

Creaghead, N., Newman, P., and Secord, W. (1989). *Assessment and remediation of articulatory and phonological disorders* (2nd ed.). Columbus, OH: Merrill Publishing Company.

Creaghead, N., and Tattershall, S. (1991). Observation and assessment of classroom pragmatic skills. In C.S. Simon (Ed.). *Communication skills and classroom success* (pp. 105-134). San Diego, CA: College-Hill Press.

Cripe, J., and Bricker, D. (1993). *AEPS family interest survey.* Baltimore, MD: Paul H. Brookes.

Crittenden, P. (1981). Abusing, neglecting, problematic, and adequate dyads: Differentiating by patterns of interaction. *Merrill-Palmer Quarterly, 27,* 201-208.

Crittenden, P. (1988). Relationships at risk. In J. Belsky and T. Nezwarski (Eds.). *Clinical implications of attachment* (pp. 136-174). Hillsdale, NJ: Erlbaum.

Cromer, R. (1994). A case study of dissociations between language and cognition. In H. Tager-Flusberg (Ed.). *Constraints in language acquisition: Studies of atypical children.* Hillsdale, NJ: Lawrence Erlbaum Associates Ltd.

Cross, T. (1978). Mothers' speech and its association with rate of syntactic acquisition in young children. In N. Waterson and C. Snow (Eds.). *The development of communication* (pp. 199-216). New York: John Wiley & Sons.

Cross, T. (1984). Habilitating the language-impaired child: Ideas from studies of parent-child interaction. *Topics in Language Disorders, 4,* 1-14.

Crossley, R., and McDonald, A. (1980). *Annie's coming out.* New York: Penguin.

Crossley, R., and Remington-Gurney, J. (1992). Getting the words out: Facilitated communication training. *Topics in Language Disorders, 12,* 29-45.

Crossley-Holland, K. (2004). *Once upon a poem.* Somerset, UK: Chicken House Publishing.

Crowe, T.A. (1997). *Application of counseling in speech language pathology and audiology.* Baltimore, MD: Williams & Wilkins.

Crowley, J. (1983). *Who will be my mother?* Bothell, WA: The Wright Group.

Crystal, D. (1982). *Profiling linguistic disability.* London: Edward Arnold.

Crystal, D., Fletcher, P., and Garman, M. (1976). *The grammatical analysis of language disability: A procedure for assessment and remediation.* London: Arnold.

Culatta, B. (1994). Representational play and story enactments: Formats for language intervention. In J. Duchan, L. Hewitt, and R. Sonnenmeier (Eds.). *Pragmatics: From theory to practice* (pp. 105-119). Englewood Cliffs, NJ: Prentice-Hall.

Culatta, B., Horn, D., and Merritt, D. (1998) Expository text: Facilitating comprehension. In D. Merritt and B. Culatta (Eds.). *Language intervention in the classroom* (pp. 215-276). San Diego, CA: Singular Publishing.

Culp, R., Watkins, R., Lawrence, H., Letts, D., Kelly, D. J., and Rice, M. (1991). Maltreated children's language and speech development: Abused, neglected, and abused and neglected. *First Language, 11,* 377-390.

Cummins, J. (1981). Empirical and theoretical underpinnings of bilingual education. *Journal of Education, 163,* 16-29.

Cunningham, A., and Stanovich, K. (2003). Reading can make you smarter. *Principal, 83,* 34-39.

Cunningham, P., and Cunningham, J. (1992). Making words: Enhancing the invented spelling-decoding connection. *Reading Teacher, 46,* 106-113.

Curenton, S., and Justice, L. (2004). African American and Caucasian Preschoolers' use of decontextualized language: Literate language features in oral narratives. *Language Speech and Hearing Services in Schools, 35,* 240-253.

Curtis, C.P. (2004). *Bucking the Sarge.* New York: Wendy Lamb Books.

Curtiss, S. (1977). *Genie: A psycholinguistic study of a modernday 'wild child'.* London: Academic Press.

Curtiss, S., Prutting, C., and Lowell, E. (1979). Pragmatic and semantic development in young children with impaired hearing. *Journal of Speech and Hearing Research, 22,* 534-552.

Curtiss, S., and Tallal, P. (1985, October). *On the question of subgroups in language impaired children: A first report.* Paper presented at the Tenth Annual Boston University Conference of Language Development.

Dagenais, D., and Beadle, K. (1984). Written language: When and where to begin. *Topics in Language Disorders, 4(2),* 59-85.

Dahl, R. (1970). *Fantastic Mr. Fox.* New York: Knopf.

Dahle, A.J., and Baldwin, R.L. (1992). Audiologic and otolaryngologic concerns. In S.M. Pueschel and J.K. Pueschel (Eds.). *Biomedical concerns in persons with Down syndrome* (pp. 69-80). Baltimore, MD: Paul Brookes.

Dale, P. (1991). The validity of a parent report measure of vocabulary and syntax at 24 months. *Journal of Speech and Hearing Research, 34,* 565-571.

Dale, P. (2005). Commonality and individual differences in vocabulary growth. In. M. Tomasello and D. Slobin (Eds.). *Beyond nature-nurture: Essays in honor of Elizabeth Bates* (pp. 41-78). Mahwah, NJ: Erlbaum.

Dale, P., Bates, E., Reznick, J., and Morisset, C. (1989). The validity of a parent report instrument of child language at twenty months. *Journal of Child Language, 16(2),* 239-249.

Dale, P., Crain-Thoreson, C., Notari-Syverson, A., and Cole, K. (1996). Parent-child story-book reading as an intervention technique for young children with language delays. *Topics in Early Childhood Special Education, 16,* 213-235.

Dale, P., Price, T., Bishop, D., and Plomin, R. (2003). Outcomes of early language delay: I. Predicting persistent and transient language difficulties at 3 and 4 years. *Journal of Speech, Language and Hearing Research, 46,* 544-560.

Damico, J. (1985). Clinical discourse analysis: a functional language assessment technique. In C.S. Simon (Ed.). *Communication skills and classroom success: Assessment of language-learning disabled students* (pp. 165-206). San Diego, CA: College-Hill Press.

Damico, J. (1991). Descriptive assessment of communicative ability in limited English proficient students. In E. Hamayan and J. Damico (Eds.). *Limiting bias in the assessment of bilingual students.* Austin, TX: Pro-Ed.

Damico, J. (1992). Language assessment in adolescents: Addressing critical issues. *Language, Speech, and Hearing Services in Schools, 24(1),* 29-35.

Damico, J. (1993). Language assessment in adolescents: Addressing critical issues. *Language, Speech, and Hearing Services in Schools, 24,* 29-35

Damico, J., and Damico, S. (1993). Language and social skills from a diversity perspective: Considerations for the speech-language pathologist. *Language, Speech, and Hearing Services in Schools, 24(4),* 236-243.

Damico, J., Augustine, L., Hayes, P. (1996). Formulating a functional model of attention deficit hyperactivity disorder for the practicing speech language pathologist. *Seminars in Speech and Language, 17,* 5-20.

Damico, J., Damico, S., and Armstrong, M. (1999). Attention-deficit hyperactivity disorder and communication disorders: Issues and clinical practices. In R. Paul (Ed.). *Child and adolescent psychiatric clinics of North America* (pp. 37-60). Philadelphia, PA: W.B. Saunders Company.

Damico, J., Muller, N., and Ball, M. (2004). Owning up to complexity: A sociocultural orientation to attention deficit hyperactivity disorder. *Seminars in Speech and Language, 25,* 277-285.

Damico, J., and Oller, J. (1980). Pragmatic versus morphological/syntactic criteria for language referrals. *Language, Speech, and Hearing Services in Schools, 11,* 85-94.

Damico, J., Oller, J., and Tetnowski, J. (1999). Investigating the interobserver reliability of a direct observational language assessment technique. *Advances in Speech-Language Pathology, 1(2),* 77-94.

Damico, J., Tetnowski, J., and Nettleton, S. (2004). Emerging issues and trends in attention deficit hyperactivity disorders: An update for the speech-language pathologist. *Seminars in Speech and Language, 25,* 207-214.

Damico, S., and Armstrong, M. (1996). Intervention strategies for students with ADHD: Creating a holistic approach. *Seminars in Speech and Language, 17,* 21-36.

Daniel, D. (2004, May). AAC in the schools: Moving students along a communication continuum. *ASHA Leader, 9,* 16-17.

Danzak, B., and Silliman, E. (2005). Does my identify speak English: A pragmatic approach to the social world of an English language learning with language impairment. *Seminars in Speech and Language, 26,* 189-200.

Darley, F. (1991). A philosophy of appraisal and diagnosis. In F. Darley and D. Spriestersbach (Eds.). *Diagnostic methods in speech pathology* (ed. 22nd ed., pp. 1-23). Prospects Heights, IL: Waveland Press.

Das, J., Kirby, J., and Jarman, R. (1975). Simultaneous and successive synthesis: An alternative model for cognitive abilities. *Psychological Bulletin, 80,* 97-113.

Davis, B. (1988, October). Differential diagnosis of developmental apraxia. In ASHA special interest division newsletter, *Language Learning and Education.*

Davis, B., and Velleman, S. (2000). Differential diagnosis and treatment of developmental apraxia of speech in infants and toddlers. *Infant-Toddler Intervention: The Transdisciplinary Journal, 10,* 177-192.

Davis, Z., and McPherson, M. (1989). Story map instruction: A road map for reading comprehension. *The Reading Teacher, 43,* 232-240.

Dawson, G. (1996). Brief report: Neuropsychology of autism: A report on the state of the science. *Journal of Autism and Developmental Disorders, 26(2),* 179-184.

Dawson, J., Stout, C., and Eyer, J. (2003). *Structured photographic expressive language test* (3rd ed.). DeKalb, IL: Janelle Publications.

De Pompei, R., and Blosser, J. (1987). Strategies for helping head-injured children successfully return to school. *Language, Speech, and Hearing in Schools, 18,* 292-300.

De Santos Loureiro, C., Braga, L., Do Nascimento Souza, L., Filho, G., Queiroz, E., and Dellatolas, G. (2004). Degree of illiteracy and phonological and metaphonological skills in unschooled adults. *Brain and Language, 89,* 499-502.

Deal, J., and Hanuscin, L. (1999). *Barrier games for better communication.* San Antonio, TX: Communication Skill Builders.

DeCoste, D.C. (1997). Augmentative and alternative communication assessment strategies: Motor Access and visual considerations. In S.L. Glennen and D.C. DeCoste (Eds.). *Handbook of augmentative and alternative communication* (pp. 243-282). San Diego, CA: Singular Publishing Group.

DeKemel, K. (2003). *Intervention in the language arts: A practical guide for speech-language pathologists.* Philadelphia: Butterworth-Heinemann.

DeKroon, D., Kyte, C., and Johnson, D. (2002). Partner influences on the social pretend play of children with language impairments. *Language, Speech, and Hearing Services in Schools, 33,* 253-267.

Delacato, C. (1963). *The diagnosis and treatment of speech and reading problems.* Springfield, IL: Thomas.

Delpit, L. (1988). The silenced dialogue: Power and pedagogy in educating other people's children. *Harvard Education Review, 58,* 280-297.

Delprato, D. (2001). Comparison of discrete-trial and normalized behavioral language intervention for young children with autism. *Journal of Autism and Developmental Disorders, 31,* 315-325.

DeMier, D., Wise, B., and Marcum, K. (1982). *Project ACCESS: Adapting current curriculum with essential study skills.* Silverdale, WA: Central Kitsap School District No. 401.

DeMyer, M., Barton, S., and Norton, S. (1972). A comparison of adaptive, verbal, and motor profiles of psychotic and non-psychotic subnormal children. *Journal of Autism and Childhood Schizophrenia, 2,* 359-377.

DeMyer, M., Hingten, J., and Jackson, R. (1981). Infantile autism reviewed: A decade of research. *Schizophrenia Bulletin, 7(3),* 388-451.

Denkla, M. (1985). Motor coordination in dyslexic children: Theoretical and clinical implications. In F. Duffy and N. Geshwind (Eds.). *Dyslexia: A neuroscientific approach to clinical evaluation.* Boston, MA: Little, Brown.

Denman, S.B. (1984). *Denman neuropsychology memory scale.* Charleston, SC: Author.

Department of Health and Human Services. (1990). *Healthy People 2000: National health promotion and disease prevention objectives.* DHHS Publication No. (PHS) 91-50213. Washington, DC: Department of Health and Human Services.

Department of Health and Human Services. (2005). *National health promotion and disease prevention objectives.* Washington, DC: Department of Health and Human Services. Retrieved January 5, 2006, from http://www.cdc.gov/ncbddd/dh/hp2010.htm

DeRivera, C., Girolametto, L. Greenberg, J., and Weitzman, E. (2005). Children's responses to educators' questions in day care play groups. *American Journal of Speech-Language Pathology, 14,* 14-26.

Derr, A. (2003). Growing diversity in our schools: Roles and responsibilities of speech-language pathologists. *Perspectives on Language Learning and Education, 10(2),* 7-12.

Deschler, D. (2000). *Critical dimensions of teaching reading to students with disabilities.* Online Academy, Lawrence, KS: University of Kansas-Center for Research on Learning.

Dewey, M., and Everard, P. (1974). The near normal autistic adolescent. *Journal of Autism and Childhood Schizophrenia, 4,* 348-356.

DiCarlo, C., Stricklin, S., Banajee, M., and Reid, D. (2001). Effects of manual signing on communicative verbalizations by toddlers with and without disabilities in inclusive classrooms. *Journal of the Association for Persons with Severe Handicaps, 26,* 120-126.

DiCecco, V., and Gleason, M. (2002). Using graphic organizers to attain relational knowledge from expository text. *Journal of Learning Disabilities, 35,* 306-320.

Dick, F., Wulfeck, B., Krupa-Kwiatkowski, M., and Bates, E. (2004). The development of complex sentence interpretation in typically developing children compared with children with specific language impairments or early unilateral focal lesions. *Developmental Science, 7(3),* 360-377.

Dickinson, D., Wolf, M., and Stotsky, S. (1993). Words move: the interwoven development of oral and written language. In J.B. Gleason (Ed.). *The development of language* (3rd ed, pp. 369-420). New York: Macmillan.

Dickson, S., Simmons, D., and Kameenui, E. (1995). Instruction in expository text: A focus on compare/contrast structure. *Learning Disabilities Forum, 20,* 8-15.

Dimino, J., Taylor, R., and Gersten, R. (1995). Synthesis of research on story grammar as a means to increase comprehension. *Reading and Writing Quarterly, 11,* 53-72.

Dinnebeil, L., and Hale, L. (2003). Incorporating principles of family-centered practice in early intervention program evaluation. *Zero to Three, 23,* 24-27.

DiSimoni, F. (1989). *Comprehensive apraxia test.* Dalton, PA: Praxis House Publishers.

Dodd, B. (1976). The phonological systems of deaf children. *Journal of Speech and Hearing Disorders, 41,* 185-198.

Dodd, B., and Gillon, G. (2001). Phonological awareness therapy and articulation training approaches (Letter to the Editor). *International Journal of Language and Communication Disorders, 36,* 265-269.

Dodd, V. (2005). Implications of kangaroo care for growth and development in preterm infants. *Journal of Obstetric, Gynecologic and Neonatal Nursing, 34,* 218-232.

Dodge, E. (1992). *The communication lab: A classroom-based collaborative program for the SLP.* Menlo Park, CA: The Pritchard Group.

Dodge, E. (1998). *Communication lab: A classroom communication program.* San Diego, CA: Singular Publishing Group.

Dodici, B., Draper, D., and Peterson, C. (2003). Early parent-child interactions an dearly literacy development. *Topics in Early Childhood Special Education, 23,* 124-136.

Doehring, D., Trites, R., Patel, P., and Fiedorowicz, C. (1981). *Reading disabilities: The interaction of reading, language and neuropsychological deficits.* New York: Academic Press.

Dole, J., Sloan, C., Trathen, W. (1995). Teaching vocabulary within the context of literature. *Journal of Reading, 38,* 452-460.

Dollaghan, C. (1985). Child meets word: "fast mapping" in preschool children. *Journal of Speech and Hearing Research, 28,* 449-454.

Dollaghan, C. (1987). Comprehension monitoring in normal and language-impaired children. *Topics in Language Disorders, 7,* 45-60.

Dollaghan, C. (2003). *Evidence-based practice in pediatric communication disorders: What do we know, and when do we know it?* Presentation at the 13th Annual NIDCE-Sponsored Research Symposium, Outcomes Research and Evidence-Based Practice, Chicago, IL.

Dollaghan, C. (2004a). Evidence-based practice in communication disorders: What do we know and when do we know it? *Journal of Communication Disorders, 37,* 391-400.

Dollaghan, C. (2004b). Evidence-based practice: Myths and realities. *ASHA Leader, 8,* 4-12.

Dollaghan, C., Biber, M.E., and Campbell, T. (1995). Lexical influences on nonword repetition. *Applied Psycholinguistics, 16,* 211-222.

Dollaghan, C., and Campbell, T. (1992). A procedure for classifying disruptions in spontaneous language samples. *Topics in Language Disorders, 12,* 56-68.

Dollaghan, C., and Campbell, T. (1998). Nonword repetition and child language impairment. *Journal of Speech, Language and Hearing Research, 41,* 1136-1146.

Donahue, M. (1994). Differences in classroom discourse styles of students with learning disabilities. In D. Ripich and N. Creaghead (Eds.). *School discourse problems* (2nd ed., pp. 229-262). San Diego, CA: Singular Publishing Group.

Donahue, M., and Bryan, T. (1983). Conversational skills and modeling in learning disabled boys. *Applied Psycholinguistics, 4,* 251-278.

Donahue-Kilburg, G. (1992). *Family-centered early intervention for communication disorders: Prevention and treatment.* Gaithersburg, MD: Aspen Publishers.

Donahue-Kilburg, G. (1993). Family-centered approach to promoting communication wellness. *ASHA, 35,* 45-62.

Donnellan, A., Mirenda, P., Mesaros, R., and Fassbender, L. (1984). Analyzing the communicative functions of aberrant behavior. *Journal of the Association for Persons with Severe Handicaps, 9,* 202-212.

Donnelly, J. (2003). *A northern light.* New York: Harcourt Children's Books.

Donnelly, K., Thomsen, S., Huber, L., and Schoemer, D. (1992). *More than words.* Tucson, AZ: Communication Skill Builders.

Dowden, P., and Marriner, N. (1995). Augmentative and alternative communication: Treatment principles and strategies. *Seminars in Speech and Language, 16,* 140-158.

Downs, M., Walker, D., and Northern, J. (1988). Identification of children with language delays due to recurrent otitis media. In D. Lim, C. Bluestone, J. Klein, and J. Nelson (Eds.). *Recent advances in otitis media* (pp. 382-384). Philadelphia, PA: BC Decker.

Drake, M. (1998). *Take home: Preschool language development.* East Moline, IL: LinguiSystems.

Dubowitz, L., Dubowitz, V., and Mercuri, E. (1999). *Neurological assessment of the preterm and full-term newborn infant—2nd ed.* Clinics in Developmental Medicine, 148. London: MacKeith Press.

Duchan, J. (1982). The elephant is soft and mushy: Problems in assessing children's language. In N. Lass, L. McReynolds, J. Northern, and D. Yoder (Eds.). *Speech, language, and hearing* (pp. 741-760). Philadelphia, PA: W.B. Saunders.

Duchan, J. (1991). Everyday events: Their role in language assessment and intervention. In T. Gallagher (Ed.). *Pragmatics of language: Clinical practice issues* (pp. 43-98). San Diego, CA: Singular Publishing Group.

Duchan, J. (1997). A situated pragmatics approach for supporting children with severe communication disorders. *Topics in Language Disorders, 17,* 1-18.

Dunaway, C. (2004). Attention deficit hyperactivity disorder: An authentic story in the schools and its implications. *Seminars in Speech and Language, 25,* 271-285.

Dunlap, G., and Koegel, R. (1980). Motivating autistic children through stimulus variation. *Journal of Applied Behavior Analysis, 13,* 619-627.

Dunlea, A. (1984). The relationship between concept formation and semantic roles: Some evidence from the blind. In L. Feagans, C. Garvey, and R. Golinkoff (Eds.). *The origins and growth of communication.* Norwood, NJ: Ablex.

Dunlea, A. (1989). *Vision and the emergence of meaning: Blind and sighted children's early language.* New York: Cambridge University Press.

Dunlea, A., and Andersen, E. (1992). The emergence process: Conceptual and linguistic influences on morphological development. *First Language, 12(1),* 95-116.

Dunn, C., and Newton, L. (1986). A comprehensive model for speech development in hearing-impaired. *Topics in Language Disorders, 6(3),* 25-46.

Dunn, L., and Dunn, L. (1997). *Peabody picture vocabulary test—III.* Circle Pines, MN: American Guidance Service.

Dunn, L., and Dunn, L. (2006). *Peabody picture vocabulary test—IV.* Circle Pines, MN: American Guidance Service.

Dunn, L., and Markwardt, F.C., Jr. (1970). *Peabody individual achievement test (PIAT).* Circle Pines, MN: American Guidance Service.

Dunn, L.M., Dunn, L.M., Whetton, C., and Burley, J. (1997). *British picture vocabulary scale: Second edition.* Windsor, UK: NFER-Nelson.

Dunn, M., Flax, J., Sliwinski, M., and Aram, D. (1996). The use of spontaneous language measures as criteria for identifying children with specific language impairment: An attempt to reconcile clinical and research incongruence. *Journal of Speech and Hearing Research, 39,* 643-654.

Dunn Klein, M., ed. (1990). *Parent articles for early intervention.* Austin, TX: Pro-Ed.

Dunst, C. (1980). *A clinical and educational manual for use with the Uzgiris and Hunt scales of infant psychological development.* Austin, TX: Pro-Ed.

Dunst, C. (1986a). *Parent-child play scale.* Unpublished scale, Morganton, NC: Family, Infant, and Preschool Program, Western Carolina Center.

Dunst, C. (1986b). *Caregiver styles of interaction scale.* Unpublished scale, Morganton, NC: Family, Infant, and Preschool Program, Western Carolina Center.

Dunst, C., Boyd, K., Trivette, C., and Hamby, D. (2002). Family-oriented program models and professional helpgiving practices. *Family Relations: Interdisciplinary Journal of Applied Family Studies, 51,* 221-229.

Dunst, C., Cooper, C., Weeldreyer, J., Snyder, K., and Chase, J. (1988). Family Needs Scale. In C. Dunst, C. Trivette, and A. Deal (Eds.). *Enabling and empowering families: Principles and guidelines for practice.* Cambridge, MA: Brookline Books.

Dunst, C., Trivette, C., and Deal, A. (Eds.). (1988). *Enabling and empowering families: Principles and guidelines for practice.* Cambridge, MA: Brookline Books.

Dunst, C.J. (1981). *Infant learning: A cognitive, linguistic intervention strategy.* Allen, TX: DLM/Teaching Resources.

Durham, D.A. (2002). *Gabriel's story.* New York: Anchor.

Durrell, D. (1971). *Analysis of reading difficulty.* New York: Harcourt Brace Jovanovich.

Dykens, E., Hodapp, R., and Leckman, J. (1994). *Behavior and development in fragile X syndrome.* Thousand Oaks, CA: Sage Publications.

Dykes, M., and Erin, J. (1999). *A developmental assessment for students with severe disabilities* (2nd ed.). Austin, TX: Pro-Ed.

Eadie, P., Fey, M., Douglas, J., and Parsons, C. (2002). Profiles of grammatical morphology and sentence imitation in children with specific language impairment and Down syndrome. *Journal of Speech, Language, and Hearing Research, 45,* 720-732.

Early intervention program for infants and toddlers with handicaps: Final regulations (1989, June 22). *Federal Register, 54,* 26306-26348.

Eberlin, M., McConnachie, G., Ibel, S., and Volpe, L. (1993). Facilitated communication: A failure to replicate the phenomenon. *Journal of Autism and Developmental Disorders, 23,* 507-530.

Eckert, P. (1990). Cooperative competition in adolescent "girl talk." *Discourse Processes, 13,* 91-122.

Edmark Corp. (1989). *Early concepts skillbuilder.* Redmond, WA.

Edmonston, N., and Thane, N. (1992). Children's use of comprehension strategies in response to relational words: Implications for assessment. *American Journal of Speech-Language Pathology, 1,* 30-35.

Edmonston, N., and Thane, N. (1999). *Test of relational concepts—Revised.* Washington, DC: Gallaudet University.

Edwards, S., Fletcher, P., Garman, M., Hughes, A., Letts, C., and Sinka, I. (1999). *Reynell developmental language scales—III.* Windsor, UK: NFER-Nelson.

Edwards, W. (2002). *Mental retardation: Definition, classification, and systems of supports.* Washington, DC: AAMR.

Ehren, B. (1989, October). *Learning strategies, approaches to adolescent intervention.* Workshop presented at State Convention of the Oregon Speech-Language and Hearing Association, Eugene, OR.

Ehren, B. (2000a). An intervention focus for inclusionary practice. *Language, Speech, and Hearing Services in Schools, 31,* 219-229.

Ehren, B. (2000b). Maintaining a therapeutic focus and sharing responsibility for student success: Keys to in-classroom speech-language services. *Language, Speech, and Hearing Services in School, 31,* 219-229.

Ehren, B. (2002). Speech-language pathologists contributing significantly to the academic success of high school students: A vision for professional growth. *Topics in Language Disorders, 22(2),* 60-80.

Ehren, B., and Nelson, N. (2005). The responsiveness to intervention approach and language impairment. *Topics in Language Disorders, 25(2),* 120-131.

Ehri, L., Nunes, S., Stahl, S., and Willows, D. (2001). Systematic phonics instruction helps students learn to read: Evidence form the National Reading Panel's meta-analysis. *Review of Educational Research, 71,* 393-447.

Ehri, L., Nunes, S., Willows, D., Schuster, B., Yaghoub-Zadeh, Z., and Shanahan, T. (2001). Phonemic awareness instruction helps children learn to read: Evidence from the National Reading Panel's meta-analysis. *Reading Research Quarterly, 36,* 250-287.

Eicher, P. (2002). Feeding. In M.L. Batshaw (Ed.). *Children with disabilities* (5th ed., pp. 549-566). Baltimore, MD: Paul H. Brookes.

Eigsti, I., and Cicchetti, D. (2004). The impact of child maltreatment on expressive syntax at 60 months. *Developmental Science, 7,* 88-102.

Eikeseth, S., Smith, T., Jahr, E., and Eldevik, S. (2002). Intensive behavioral treatment at school for 4- to 7-year-old children with autism: A 1-year comparison controlled study. *Behavioral Modification, 26(1),* 49-68.

Eimas, P., Miller, J., and Jusczyk, P. (1987). On infant speech perception and the acquisition of language. In S. Harnad (Ed.). *Categorical perception.* Cambridge, England: Cambridge University Press.

Eisenberg, S. (2005). When conversation is not enough: Assessing infinitival complements through elicitation. *American Journal of Speech-Language Pathology, 14(2),* 92-106.

Eisenberg, S., Fersko, R., and Lundgren, C. (2001). The use of MLU for identifying language impairment in preschool children: A review. *American Journal of Speech-Language Pathology, 10,* 323-342.

Eisenmajer, N., Ross, N., and Pratt, C. (2005). Specificity and characteristics of learning disabilities. *Journal of Child Psychology & Psychiatry & Allied Disciplines, 46(10),* 1108-1115.

Eisenson, J. (1972). *Aphasia in children.* New York: Harper & Row.

Elbert, M., and Gierut, J. (1986). *Handbook of clinical phonology: Approaches to assessment and treatment.* San Diego, CA: College-Hill Press.

Elbert, M., Rockman, B., and Saltzman, D. (1980). *Contrasts: The use of minimal pairs in articulation training.* Austin, TX: Pro-Ed.

Elizur, Y., and Perednik, M. (2003). Prevalence and description of selective mutism in immigrant and native families: A controlled study. *Journal of the American Academy of Child and Adolescent Psychiatry, 42,* 1451-1459.

Elkonin, D. (1973). U.S.S.R. In J. Downing (Ed.). *Comparative reading.* New York: MacMillan.

Elksnin, L., and Capilouto, G. (1994). Speech-language specialists' perceptions of integrated service delivery in school settings. *Language, Speech and Hearing Services in Schools, 25,* 248-267.

Elksnin, N., and Elksnin, L. (2001) Adolescents with disabilities: The need for occupational social skills training. *Exceptionality, 9,* 91-105.

Elliot, J. (2003). Dynamic assessment in educational settings: Realizing potential. *Educational Review, 55,* 15-32.

Elliott, J.G. (2000). Dynamic assessment in educational contexts: purpose and promise. In C.S. Lidz and J.G. Elliott (Eds.). *Dynamic assessment: Prevailing models and applications* (pp. 713-740). New York: Elsevier Science.

Elliott-Templeton, K., Van Kleeck, A., Richardson, A., and Imholz, E. (1992, November). *A longitudinal study of mothers, babies and books.* Paper presented at the American Speech-Language-Hearing Association National Convention, San Antonio, TX.

Ellis, L., Schlaudecker, C., and Regimbal, C. (1995). Effectiveness of a collaborative consultation approach to basic concept instruction with kindergarten children. *Speech, Language, and Hearing Services in Schools, 26,* 69-74.

Elshout-Mohr, M., and van Daalen-Kapteijns, M. (1987). Cognitive processes in learning word meanings. In M.G. McKeown and M.E. Curtis (Eds.). *The nature of vocabulary acquisition.* Hillsdale, NJ: Erlbaum.

Encore Software, (N.D.). *Kaplan writing and vocabulary* (computer program). Gardena, CA: Author.

Enderby, V., and Roworth, M. (1984). *Frenchay dysarthria assessment.* San Diego, CA: College-Hill Press.

Englert, C., and Hiebert, E. (1984). Children's developing awareness of text structures in expository material. *Journal of Educational Psychology, 76,* 65-74.

Englert, C., and Mariage, T. (1991). Making students partners in the comprehension process: Organizing the reading "POSSE." *Learning Disability Quarterly, 14,* 123-138.

Englert, C., and Raphael, T. (1988). Constructing well-formed prose: Process, structure, and metacognitive knowledge. *Exceptional Children, 54,* 513-527.

English, K., Goldstein, H., Shafer, K., and Kaczmarek, L. (1997). Promoting interactions among preschoolers with and without disabilities: Effects of a buddy system skills training program. *Exceptional Children, 63,* 229-243.

Ennis, R. (1965). *Cornell deduction tests.* Ithaca, NY: Cornell University.

Ennis, R.H., Gardiner, Guzzetta, J., W.L., Morrow, R., Paulus, D., and Ringel, L. (1964) *Cornell conditional reasoning test.* University of Illinois: Champaign, IL.

Ennis, R.H., Gardiner, W.L., Morrow, R., Paulus, D., and Ringel, L. (1964). *Cornell class reasoning test.* University of Illinois: Champaign, IL.

Ennis, R.H., and Millman, J. (1985). *Cornell critical thinking test, level X.* Critical Thinking Press and Software: Pacific Grove, CA.

Ensher, G., Bobish, B., Garner, J., Michaels, T., Butler, S., Foertsch, R., and Cooper, F. (1997). *Syracuse dynamic assessment for birth to three.* Austin, TX: Pro-Ed.

Erickson, F. (1987). Transformation and school success: The politics and culture of educational achievement. *Anthropology and Educational Quarterly, 18,* 335-357.

Erickson, J. (1987). Analysis of communicative competence. In L. Cole, V. Deal, and V. Rodriquez (Eds.). *Communication disorders in multicultural populations.* Rockville, MD: ASHA.

Erickson, J., and Iglesias, A. (1986). Assessment of communication disorders in non-English proficient children. In O. Taylor (Ed.). *Nature of communication disorders in culturally and linguistically diverse populations.* San Diego, CA: College-Hill Press.

Erikson, K., Koppenhaver, D., Yoder, D., and Nance, J. (1997). Integrated communication and literacy instruction for a child with multiple disabilities. *Focus on Autism and Other Developmental Disabilities, 12,* 142-150.

Erin, J. (1990). Language samples from visually impaired four- and five-year olds. *Journal of Childhood Communication Disorders, 13,* 181-191.

Ertmer, D. (1986). *Language carnival* (computer program). Moline, IL: LinguiSystems.

Ertmer, D. (2002). Challenges in optimizing oral communication in children with cochlear implants. *Language, Speech, and Hearing Services in Schools, 33,* 149-152.

Ertmer, D. Young, N., Grohne, K., Mellon, J., Johnson, C., Corbett, K., and Saindon, K. (2002). Vocal development in young children with cochlear implants: Profiles and implications for intervention. *Language, Speech, and Hearing Services in Schools, 33,* 184-195.

Ertmer, E., Strong, L., and Sadagopan, N. (2003). Beginning to communication after cochlear implantation: Oral language development in a young child. *Journal of Speech, Language, and Hearing Research, 46,* 328-340.

Escalona, S., and Corman, H. (1966). *Albert Einstein scales of sensorimotor development.* Unpublished paper. New York: Albert Einstein College of Medicine, Department of Psychiatry.

Espin, C., La Paz, S., Scierka, B., and Roelofs, L. (2005). Relations between curriculum-based measures in writing expression and quality and completeness of expository writing for middle school students. *Journal of Special Education, 38,* 208-217.

Espin, C., Weissenburger, J., and Benson, B. (2004). Assessing the writing performance of students in special education. *Exceptionality, 12,* 55-67.

Estrin, E., and Chaney, C. (1988). Developing a concept of the WORD. *Childhood Education, 65,* 78-82.

Evans, J. (2000). An emergent account of language impairments in children with SLI: Implications for assessment and intervention. *Journal of Communication Disorders, 34,* 39-54.

Evans, J., Alibali, M., and McNeil, N. (2001). Divergence of verbal expression and embodied knowledge: Evidence from speech and gesture in children with specific language impairment. *Language and Cognitive Processes, 16,* 309-331.

Evans, J., and Craig, H. (1992). Language sample collection and analysis: Interview compared to freeplay assessment contexts. *Journal of Speech and Hearing Research, 35,* 343-353.

Evans, J., and MacWhinney, B. (1999). Sentence processing strategies in children with expressive and expressive-receptive specific language impairments. *International Journal of Language and Communication Disorders, 34,* 117-134.

Evans, J., and Miller, J. (1999). Language sample analysis in the 21st century. *Seminars in Speech and Language, 20,* 101-116.

Ewing, A. (1930). *Aphasia in children.* London, England: Oxford University Press.

Eyer, J., Bedore, L., McGregor, K., Anderson, B., and Viescas, R. (2002). Fast mapping of verbs by children with specific language impairment. *Clinical Linguistics & Phonetics, 16,* 59-77.

Fabiano, G., and Pelham, W. (2002). Comprehensive treatment for attention-deficit/hyperactivity disorders. In D. Marsh and M. Firstad (Eds.). *Handbook of serious emotional disturbance in children and adolescents* (pp. 149-174) Hoboken, NJ: John Wiley & Sons.

Fagen, S., Graves, D., and Tessier-Switlick, D. (1984). *Promoting successful mainstreaming: Reasonable classroom accommodations for language disabled students.* Rockville, MD: Montgomery County Public Schools.

Faircloth, M., and Faircloth, S. (1970). An analysis of the articulatory behavior of a speech defective child in connected speech and isolated word responses. *Journal of Speech and Hearing Disorders, 35,* 51-61.

Falkman, K., Sandberg, A., and Hjelmquist, E. (2002). Preferred communication modes: Prelinguistic and linguistic communication in non-speaking preschool children with cerebral palsy. *International Journal of Language and Communication Disorders, 37,* 59-68.

Falk-Ross, F. (2002). *Classroom-based language and literacy intervention: A programs and case studies approach.* Boston: Allyn & Bacon.

Fallon, K., Light, J., and Paige, T. (2001). Enhancing vocabulary selection for preschoolers who require augmentative and alternative communication. *American Journal of Speech-Language Pathology, 10,* 1058-0360.

Fallon, K., Light, J., McNaughton, D., Drager, K., and Hammer, C. (2004). The effects of direct instruction on the single-word reading skills of children who require augmentative and alternative communication. *Journal of Speech, Language, and Hearing Research, 47,* 1424-1439.

Falvey, M., Grenot-Scheyer, M., and Luddy, E. (1987). Developing and implementing integrated community referenced curricula. In D.J. Cohen and A.M. Donnellan (Eds.). *Handbook of autism and pervasive developmental disorders* (pp. 238-250). New York: John Wiley & Sons.

Fantini, A. (1978). *Language acquisition of a bilingual child: A sociolinguistic perspective.* Putney, VT: Experiment Press.

Farber, J., Denenberg, M., Klyman, S., and Lachman, P. (1992). Language resource room level of service: An urban school district approach to integrative treatment. *Language, Speech, and Hearing Services in Schools, 23,* 293-299.

Farber, J., and Klein, E. (1999). Classroom-based assessment of collaborative intervention program with kindergarten and first-grade students. *Speech, Language, and Hearing Services in Schools, 30,* 83-90.

Farmer, M., and Oliver, A. (2005). Assessment of pragmatic difficulties and socio-emotional adjustment in practice. *International Journal of Language and Communication Disorders, 40,* 403-429.

Farnoff, A., Hack, M., and Walsh, M. (2003). The NICHD neonatal research network; Changes in practice and outcomes during the first 15 years. *Seminars in Perinatology, 27,* 281-287.

Farran, D., Kasari, C., and Jay, S. (1983). *Parent-child interaction scale.* Unpublished instrument, Chapel Hill, NC: Frank Porter Graham Child Development Center, University of North Carolina.

Fay, W. (1969). On the basis of autistic echolalia. *Journal of Communication Disorders, 2,* 38-47.

Fay, W. (1971). On normal and autistic pronouns. *Journal of Speech and Hearing Disorders, 36,* 242-249.

Fay, W. (1992). Infantile autism. In D. Bishop and K. Mogford (Eds.). *Language development in exceptional circumstances* (pp. 190-202). Hillsdale, NJ: Erlbaum.

Fay, W., and Schuler, A. (1980). *Emerging language in autistic children.* Baltimore, MD: University Park Press.

Fazen, L., III, Lovejoy, F., Jr., and Crone, R. (1986). Acute poisoning in a children's hospital: A 2-year experience. *Pediatrics, 77,* 144-151.

Feagans, L., and Applebaum, M. (1986). Validation of language subtypes in learning disabled children. *Journal of Educational Psychology, 78,* 358-364.

Feinberg, C. (1981). The pre-academic language classroom. In A. Gerber and D.N. Bryen (Eds.). *Language and learning disabilities* (pp. 249-268). Baltimore, MD: University Park Press.

Feldman, H., Dale, P., Campbell, T., Colborn, D., Kurs-Lasky, M., Rockette, H., and Paradise, J. (2005). Concurrent and predictive validity of parent reports of child language at age 2 and 3 years. *Child Development, 76,* 856-868.

Felsenfeld, S., and Plomin, R. (1997). Epidemiological and offspring analyses of developmental speech disorders using data from the Colorado Adoption Project. *Journal of Speech, Language, and Hearing Research, 40,* 778-791.

Fenson, L., Dale, P., Reznick, S., Hartung, J., and Burgess, S. (1990, April). *Norms for the MacArthur communicative development inventories.* Poster presented at the International Conference on Infant Studies, Montreal, Quebec.

Fenson, L., Dale, P., Reznick, S., Thal, D., Bates, E., Hartung, J., Pethick, S., and Reilly, J. (1993). *The MacArthur Communicative Development Inventories.* San Diego, CA: Singular Publishing Group.

Fenson, L., Dale, P., Reznick, S., Thal, D., Bates, E., Hartung, J., Pethick, S., and Reilly, J. (2003). *The MacArthur-Bates Communicative Development Inventories.* Baltimore, MD: Paul H. Brookes.

Ferrell, K. (1985). *Reach out and teach.* New York: American Foundation for the Blind.

Fewell, R. (1986). The measurement of family functioning. In L. Bichman and D. Weatherford (Eds.). *Evaluating early intervention programs for severely handicapped children and their families.* Austin, TX: Pro-Ed.

Fewell, R., and Langley, M.B. (1984). *Developmental activities screening inventory (DASI-II).* Austin, TX: Pro-Ed.

Fewell, R., Snyder, P., Sexton, D., Bertrand, S., and Hockless, M. (1991). Implementing IFSPs in Louisiana: Different formats for family-centered practices under Part H. *Topics in Early Childhood Special Education, 11,* 54-65.

Fey, M. (1986). *Language intervention with young children.* San Diego, CA: College-Hill Press.

Fey, M. (2000). Elicited imitation, modeling and recasting in grammar intervention for children with specific language impairments. In D. Bishop and L. Leonard (Eds.). *Specific speech and language disorders in children.* London: Psychology Press.

Fey, M., Catts, H., Proctor-Williams, K., Tomblin, J., and Zhang, X. (2004). Oral and written story composition skills of children with language impairment. *Journal of Speech, Language, and Hearing Research, 47,* 1301-1318.

Fey, M., Cleave, P., Long, S., and Hughes, D. (1993). Two approaches to the facilitation of grammar in children with language impairment: An experimental evaluation. *Journal of Speech and Hearing Research, 36,* 141-157.

Fey, M., and Johnson, B. (1998). Research to practice (and back again) in speech-language intervention. *Topics in Language Disorders, 18,* 23-34.

Fey, M., and Justice, L. (2007). Evidence-based decision making in communication intervention. In R. Paul and P. Cascella (Eds.). *Introduction to clinical methods in communication disorders.* Baltimore: Paul H. Brookes.

Fey, M., and Leonard, L. (1984). Partner age as a variable in the conversational performance of specifically language-impaired and normal-language children. *Journal of Speech and Hearing Research, 27,* 413-423.

Fey, M., and Loeb, D. (2002). An evaluation of the facilitative effects of inverted yes-no questions on the acquisition of auxiliary verbs. *Journal of Speech, Language, and Hearing Research, 45,* 160-174.

Fey, M.E., Long, S.E., and Cleave, P.L. (1994). Reconsideration of IQ criteria in the definition of specific language impairment. In R. Watkins and M. Rice (Eds.). *Specific language impairments in children.* Baltimore, MD: Paul H. Brookes.

Fey, M., Long, S., and Finestack, L. (2003). Ten principles of grammar facilitation for children with specific language impairments. *American Journal of Speech-Language Pathology, 12,* 3-15.

Fey, M., Newhoff, M., and Cole, B. (1978). *Language intervention: effecting changes in mother-child interactions.* Paper presented at the American Speech and Hearing Association Annual Convention, San Francisco, CA.

Fey, M., and Proctor-Williams, K. (2000). Recasting, elicited, imitation and modeling in grammar intervention for children with specific language impairments. In D. Bishop and L. Leonard (Eds.). *Speech and language impairments in children: Causes, characteristics, intervention, and outcome* (pp. 174-194). New York: Psychology Press.

Fiestas, C.E., and Peña, E.D. (2004). Narrative discourse in bilingual children: Language and task effects. *Language, Speech, and Hearing Services in Schools, 35,* 155-68.

Fillmore, L., and Snow, C. (2000). *What teachers need to know about language.* Washington, DC: Office of Educational Research and Improvement. (ERIC Document Reproduction Service No. ED 444 379).

Finn, P., Bothe, A., and Bramlett, R. (2005). Science and pseudoscience in communication disorders: Criteria and applications. *American Journal of Speech-Language Pathology, 14,* 172-186.

Fischler, R., Todd, N., and Feldman, C. (1985). Otitis media and language performance in a cohort of Apache Indian children. *American Journal of Diseases in Children, 139,* 355-360.

Fitts, E. (2001). *Linguistic discrimination: A sociolinguistic perspective.* Houston, TX: ERIC Clearinghouse in Reading, English and Communication (CS512068).

Fleiss, J.L., Levin, B., and Cho Paik, M.C. (2003). *Statistical methods for rates and proportions* (3rd ed.). New York: Wiley.

Fleming, J., and Forester, B. (1997). Infusing language enhancement into the reading curriculum for disadvantaged adolescents. *Language Speech and Hearing Services in Schools, 28,* 177-180.

Fletcher, K., and Ash. B. (2005, Feb. 8). The speech-language pathologist and lactation consultant: The baby's feeding dream team. *The ASHA Leader, 8-9,* 32-33.

Fletcher, P., Chan, C., Wong, P., Stokes, S., Tardif, T., and Leung, S. (2004). The interface between phonetic and lexical abilities in early Cantonese language development. *Clinical Linguistics and Phonetics, 18,* 535-545.

Fletcher, S. (1978). *Diagnosing speech disorders from cleft palate.* New York: Grune & Stratton.

Flexer, C., and Savage, H. (1993). Use of a mild gain amplifier with preschoolers with language delay. *Language, Speech, and Hearing Services in Schools, 24,* 151-155.

Fluharty, N.B. (2000). *Fluharty Preschool Speech and Language Screening Test—Second Edition.* Austin: TX: Pro-Ed.

Flynn, P. (1983). Speech-language pathologists and primary prevention: From ideas to action. *Language, Speech, and Hearing Services in Schools, 14,* 99-104.

Flynt, E., and Cooter, R. (2004). *Flynt-Cooter reading inventory for the classroom.* Columbus, OH: Merrill.

Fokes, J. (1976). *Fokes sentence builder.* New York: Teaching Resources Corporation.

Foley, B. (1993). The development of literacy in individuals with severe congenital speech and motor impairments. *Topics in Language Disorders, 13,* 16-32.

Folger, J., and Chapman, R. (1978). A pragmatic analysis of spontaneous imitations. *Journal of Child Language, 5,* 25-38.

Foorman, B., and Torgesen, J. (2001). Critical elements of classroom and small group instruction promote reading success in all children. *Learning Disabilities Research and Practice, 16,* 203-212.

Forness, S., Youpa, D., Hanna, G., Cantwell, D., and Swanson, J. (1992). Classroom instructional characteristics in attention deficit hyperactivity disorder: Comparison of pure and mixed subgroups. *Behavioral Disorders, 17,* 115-125.

Forrest, K. (2003). Diagnostic criteria of developmental apraxia of speech used by clinical speech-language pathologists. *American Journal of Speech-Language Pathology, 12,* 376-371.

Foster, M. (2002). *Using Call and Response to facilitate language mastery and literacy acquisition among African American students.* Washington, DC: ERIC Clearinghouse on Language and Linguistics (FL027448).

Foster, R., Giddan, J., and Stark, J. (1973). *Assessment of Children's language comprehension.* Austin, TX: Learning Concepts.

Fowler, A. (1988). Determinants of language growth in children with Down syndrome. In L. Nadel (Ed.). *The psychobiology of Down syndrome* (pp. 217-245). Cambridge, MA: MIT Press.

Fowler, A., Doherty, B., and Boynton, L. (1995). The basis of reading skill in young adults with Down syndrome. In L. Nadel and D. Rosenthal (Eds.). *Down syndrome: Living and learning in the community* (pp. 182-196). New York: John Wiley & Sons.

Fox, L., Long, S., and Anglois, A. (1988). Patterns of language comprehension deficit in abused and neglected children. *Journal of Speech and Hearing Disorders, 53,* 239-244.

Fraiberg, S. (1977). *Insights from the blind: Comparative studies of blind and sighted infants.* New York: Basic Books.

Fraiberg, S. (1979). Blind infants and their mothers: An examination of the sign system. In *Before speech: The beginning of interpersonal communication* (pp. 149-169). New York: Cambridge University Press.

Francis, D.J., Fletcher, J.M., Shaywitz, B.A., Shaywitz, S.E., and Rourke, B.P. (1996). Defining learning and language and disabilities: Conceptual and psychometric issues with the use of IQ test. *Language, Speech, and Hearing Services in Schools, 27,* 132-143.

Franco, B. (2001a). *Things I have to tell you: Poems and writing by teenage girls.* Hong Kong: Candlewick.

Franco, B. (2001b). *You hear me? Poems and writing by teenage boys.* Hong Kong: Candlewick.

Frank, K., and Smith-Rex, S. (1997). *Getting with it: A kid's guide to forming good relationships and fitting in.* Minneapolis, MN: Educational Media Corporation.

Frankenburg, W., Dodds, J., and Archer, P. (1990). *Denver II.* Denver, CO: Denver Developmental Materials.

Frankenburg, W., Dodds, J., Archer, P., Bresnick, B., Maschka, P., Edelman, N., and Shapiro, H. (1990). *Denver II: Screening manual.* Denver, CO: Denver Developmental Materials.

Frattali, C.M. (1998). Assessing functional outcomes: An overview. *Seminars in Speech and Language, 19(3),* 209-221.

Frederic, D., Wulfeck, B. Krupa-Kwiatkowski, M., and Bates, E. (2004). The development of complex sentence interpretation in typically developing children compared with children with specific language impairments or early unilateral focal lesions. *Developmental Science, 7(3),* 360-77.

Freedman, E., and Wiig, E. (1995). Classroom management and instruction for adolescents with language disabilities. *Seminars in Speech and Language, 16,* 46-64.

Freeman, S., and Dakes, L. (1996). *Teach me language: A language manual for children with autism, Asperger's syndrome and related disorders.* Langley, Canada: SKF Books.

Friedman, P., and Friedman, K. (1980). Accounting for individual differences when comparing the effectiveness of remedial language teaching methods. *Applied Psycholinguistics, 1,* 151-171.

Fried-Oken, M. (1987). Terminology in augmentative communication. *Language, Speech, and Hearing Services in Schools, 18(2),* 188-190.

Fried-Oken, M., and More, L. (1992). A suggested vocabulary source list for the augmentative and alternative communication of 3- to 6-year-old, preliterate children: Data from environmental and developmental samples. *Augmentative and Alternative Communication, 8,* 41-56.

Friel-Patti, S. (1990). Otitis media with effusion and the development of language: A review of the evidence. *Topics in Language Disorders, 11(1),* 11-22.

Friel-Patti, S., and Finitzo, T. (1990). Language learning in a prospective study of otitis media with effusion in the first two years of life. *Journal of Speech and Hearing Research, 33,* 188-194.

Friel-Patti, S., Finitzo-Hieber, J., Conti, G., and Brown, K. (1982). Language delay in infants associated with middle ear disease and mild, fluctuating hearing impairment. *Clinical Pediatrics, 18,* 205-212.

Friend, M., and Bursuck, W.D. (2002). *Including students with special needs: A practical guide for classroom teachers* (3rd ed.). Boston: Allyn & Bacon.

Friend, M., and Cook, L. (1990). Assessing the climate for collaboration. In W.A. Secord (Ed.). *Best practices in school speech-language pathology* (vol. I, pp. 67-74). San Antonio, TX: Psychological Corporation/Harcourt Brace Jovanovich.

Frome-Loeb, D., and Armstrong, N. (2001). Case studies on the efficacy of expansions and subject-verb-object models in early language intervention. *Child Language Teaching and Therapy, 17,* 35-53.

Frost, L., and Bondy, A. (1994). *The Picture Exchange Communication System training manual.* Cherry Hill, NJ: Pyramid Educational Consultants.

Fucile, S., Gisel, E., and Lau, C. (2005). Effect of an oral stimulation program on sucking skill maturation of preterm infants. *Developmental Medicine and Child Neurology, 47,* 158-162.

Fujiki, M., and Brinton, B. (1991). The verbal noncommunicator: A case study. *Language, Speech, and Hearing Services in Schools, 22,* 322-333.

Fujiki, M., Brinton, B., and Clarke, D. (2002). Emotional regulation in children with specific language impairment. *Language, Speech, and Hearing Services in Schools, 33,* 102-111.

Fujiki, M., Brinton, B., Isaacson, T., and Summers, C. (2001). Social behaviors of children with language impairment on the playground: A pilot study. *Language, Speech, and Hearing Services in Schools, 32,* 101-113.

Fuligni, A., Wen-Jui, H., and Brooks-Gunn, J. (2004). The infant-toddler HOME in the 2nd and 3rd years of life. *Parenting: Science and Practice, 4,* 139-159.

Fulk, B., and Stormont-Spurgin, M. (1995). Fourteen spelling strategies for students with learning disabilities. *Intervention in School and Clinic, 31,* 16-20.

Furey, J., and Watkins, R. (2002). Accuracy of online language sampling: A focus on verbs. *American Journal of Speech-Language Pathology, 11,* 434-439.

Furst, A.L. (1989). Elective mutism: Report of a case successfully treated by a family doctor. *Israel Journal of Psychiatry and Related Science, 26,* 96-102.

Furstenberg, F., Brooks-Gunn, J., and Chase-Lansdale, L. (1989). Teenaged pregnancy and childbearing. *American Psychologist, 44,* 313-320.

Furuno, S., O'Reilly, K., Inatsuka, T., Husaka, C., Allmon, T., and Zeisloft-Falbey, B. (1994). *The Hawaii early learning profile.* Palo Alto, CA: VORT.

Gajewski, N., Hirn, P., and Mayo, P. (1998). *SSS: Social skills strategies* (2nd ed.). Eau Claire, WI: Thinking Publications.

Galaburda, A. M., Sherman, G. F., Rosen, G. D., Aboitiz, F., and Geschwind, N. (1985). Developmental dyslexia: Four consecutive cases with cortical anomalies. *Annals of Neurology, 18,* 222-233.

Galdone, P. (1961). *The house that Jack built.* New York: Whittlesey House.

Galdone, P. (1970). *The three little pigs.* New York: Houghton-Mifflin.

Galdone, P. (1975). *The gingerbread boy.* New York: Seabury Press.

Gall, F. (1825). *On the function of the brain and each of its parts* (vols. 1-6). Phrenological Library. Boston, MA: March, Capen and Lyon.

Gallagher, T. (1983). Pre-assessment: A procedure for accommodating language use variability. In T. Gallagher and C. Prutting (Eds.). *Assessment and intervention issues in language* (pp. 1-28). San Diego, CA: College-Hill Press.

Gallagher, T. (1991). Language and social skills: Implications for assessment and intervention with school-age children. In T.M. Gallagher (Ed.). *Pragmatics of language: Clinical practice issues* (pp. 11-41). San Diego, CA: Singular Publishing Group.

Gallagher, T. (1999). Interrelationships among children's language, behavior, and emotional problems. *Topics in Language Disorders, 19,* 1-15.

Gallagher, T. M. (1993). Language skill and the development of social competence in school-age children. *Language, Speech, and Hearing Services in Schools, 24,* 199-205.

Ganske, K. (2000). *Word journeys: Assessment guided phonics, spelling, and vocabulary instruction.* New York: Guidford.

Gansle, K., Noell, G., Vanderheyden, A., Slider, N., Hoffpauir, L., Whitmarsh, E., and Naquin, G. (2004). An examination of the criterion validity and sensitivity to brief intervention of alternate curriculum-based measures of writing skill. *Psychology in the Schools, 41,* 291-301.

Ganz, J., and Simpson, R. (2004). Effects on communicative requesting and speech development of the Picture Exchange Communication System in children with characteristics of autism. *Journal of Autism and Developmental Disorders, 34,* 395-409.

Gardiner, J. (1980). *Stone fox.* New York: Harper & Row.

Gardner, H. (1983). *Frames of mind: The theory of multiple intelligences.* New York: Basic Books.

Gardner, M. (1986). *Test of visual-motor skills (TVMS) ages 2 years to 13 years.* Burlingame, CA: Psychological and Educational Publications, Inc.

Gardner, M. (1992). *Test of visual motor skills: Upper level adolescents and adults (TVMS: UL) ages 12 years to 40.* Burlingame, CA: Psychological and Educational Publications, Inc.

Garner, J., and Bochna, C. (2004). Transfer of a listening comprehension strategy to independent reading in first grade students. *Early Childhood Education Journal, 32,* 69-74.

Garrett, J. (2002). Supporting multicultural, multilingual families. *Child Care Information Exchange, 147,* 42-44.

Garrison-Harrell, L., Kamps, K., and Kravits, T. (1997). The effects of peer networks on social communication behaviors for students with autism. *Focus on Autism and Other Developmental Disabilities, 12,* 241-254.

Gathercole, S. (1995). Is nonword repetition a test of phonological working memory or long-term knowledge? It all depends on the nonwords. *Memory and Cognition, 23,* 83-94.

Gathercole, S., and Baddeley, A. (1989). Evaluation of the role of phonological STM in the development of vocabulary in children: A longitudinal study. *Journal of Memory and Language, 28,* 200-213.

Gathercole, S., and Baddeley, A. (1990). Phonological memory deficits in language-disordered children: Is there a causal connection? *Journal of Memory and Language, 29,* 336-360.

Gathercole, S., and Baddeley, A. (1996). *Children's test of nonword repetition.* London: The Psychological Corp.

Gaulin, C., and Campbell, T. (1994). Procedure for assessing verbal working memory in normal school-age children: some preliminary data. *Perceptual and Motor Skills, 79*, 55-64.

Gaylord-Ross, R., Haring, T., Breen, C., and Pitts-Conway, V. (1984). The training and generalization of social interactions skills with autistic youth. *Journal of Applied Behavior Analysis, 17*, 229-247.

Gazdag, G., and Warren, S.F. (2000). Effects of adult contingent imitation on development of young children's vocal imitation. *Journal of Early Intervention, 23(1)*, 24-35.

Gebers, J. (2003). *Books are for talking too!* 3rd ed. Austin, TX: Pro-Ed.

Gee, J. (1985). The narrativization of experience in the oral style. *Journal of Education, 167*, 9-35.

Geers, A. (2004). Speech language and reading skills after early cochlear implantation. *Archives of Otolaryngology, Head and Neck Surgery, 130*, 634-638.

Geers, A., and Moog, J. (1989). Factors predictive of the development of literacy in profoundly hearing-impaired adolescents. *The Volta Review, 91*, 69-86.

Geers, A., Nicholas, J., and Sedley, A. (2003). Language skills of children with early cochlear implantation. *Ear and Hearing, 24*, 46-58.

Geisel, T., and Geisel, A. (1963). *Hop on pop.* New York: Random House.

Gentos, J. (1976). *Rotten Ralph.* Boston, MA: Houghton Mifflin.

Gerber, A. (1993). *Language-related learning disabilities: Their nature and treatment.* Baltimore, MD: Paul H. Brookes.

Gerber, S. (1980). *Asphyxia neonatorum and subsequent communicative disorders.* Paper presented at the XVth International Congress of Audiology, Krakow, Poland.

Gerber, S. (1990). *Prevention: The etiology of communicative disorders in children.* Englewood Cliffs, NJ: Prentice-Hall.

Gerber, S., and Kraat, A. (1992). Use of a developmental model of language acquisition: Applications to children using AAC systems. *Augmentative and Alternative Communication, 8*, 19-32.

Gerlach, E.K. (1996). *Autism treatment guide* (revised edition). Eugene, OR: Four Leaf Press.

German, D. (1990). *Test of adolescent/adult word finding.* Austin, TX: Pro-Ed.

German, D. (1991). *Test of word finding in discourse.* Austin, TX: Pro-Ed.

German, D. (1992). Word finding intervention for children and adolescents. *Topics in Language Disorders, 13(1)*, 33-50.

German, D. (1998). *Word finding intervention program.* Austin, TX: Pro-Ed.

German, D. (2000). *Test of word finding—Second edition.* Austin, TX: Pro-Ed.

German, D., and German, A.E. (1993). *Word finding referral checklist.* Chicago, IL: Word Finding Materials.

German, D.J. (2002). A phonologically based strategy to improve word-finding abilities in children. *Communication Disorders Quarterly, 23*, 179-192.

German, D.J. (2005). *Word finding intervention program.* Circle Pines, MN: American Guidance Service.

German, D.J., and Newman, R. (2004). The impact of lexical factors on children's word finding errors. *Journal of Speech, Language, and Hearing Research, 47*, 624-636.

Gerring, J., and Carney, J. (1992). *Head trauma: Strategies for educational reintegration* (2nd ed.). San Diego, CA: Singular Publishing Group.

Gersten, M., Coster, W., Scheider-Rosen, K., Carlson, V., and Cicchetti, D. (1986). The socio-emotional bases of communicative functioning: Quality of attachment, language development, and early maltreatment. In M. Lamb, A. Brown, and B. Rogoff (Eds.). *Advances in developmental psychology* (vol. 4, pp. 105-151). Hillsdale, NJ: Erlbaum.

Gersten, R., and Baker, S. (2001). Teaching expressive writing to students with learning disabilities: A meta-analysis. *The Elementary School Journal, 101*, 251-272.

Gesell, A., and Amatruda, C. (1947). *Developmental diagnosis* (2nd ed.). New York: Hoeber.

Ghere, G., York-Barr J., and Sommerness, J. (2002). *Supporting students with disabilities in inclusive schools: A curriculum for job embedded paraprofessional development.* Minneapolis: University of Minnesota.

Giangreco, M. (2000). Related services research for students with low-incidence disabilities: Implications for the speech-language pathologist. *Language, Speech and Hearing Services in Schools, 31*, 230-239.

Gibson, W. (1960). *The miracle worker.* New York: Samuel French.

Giddan, J. (1991). School children with emotional problems and communication deficits: Implications for speech-language pathologists. *Language, Speech, and Hearing Services in Schools, 22*, 291-295.

Giddan, J., and Milling, L. (1999). Comorbidity of psychiatric and communication disorders in children. In R. Paul (Ed.). *Child and adolescent psychiatric clinics of North America* (pp. 19-36). Philadelphia, PA: W.B. Saunders.

Giddan, J., and Milling, L. (2001). Language disorders and emotional disturbance. In T. Layton, E. Crais, and L. Watson (Eds.). *Handbook of early language impairment in children: Nature* (pp. 126-171). Albany, NY: Delmar Publishers.

Giddan, J., Ross, G., Sechler, L., and Becker, B. (1997). Selective mutism in elementary school: Multidisciplinary interventions. *Language, Speech, and Hearing Services in Schools, 28*, 127-133.

Gierut, J. (1990). Differential learning of phonological oppositions. *Journal of Speech and Hearing Research, 33*, 540-549.

Gierut, J. (2001). Complexity in phonological treatments: Clinical factors. *Language, Speech, and Hearing Services in Schools, 32*, 229-241.

Gilbertson, M., and Bramlett, R. (1998). Phonological awareness screening to identify at-risk readers: Implications for practitioners. *Language, Speech, and Hearing Services in Schools, 29*, 109-116.

Gilkerson, L., Gorski, P., and Panitz, P. (1990). Hospital-based intervention for preterm infants and their families. In S.J. Meisels and J.P. Shonkoff (Eds.). *Handbook of early childhood intervention.* Cambridge, England: Cambridge University Press.

Gillam, R., Loeb, D., and Friel-Patti, S. (2001). Looking back: A summary of five exploratory studies of fast forword. *American Journal of Speech-Language Pathology, 10*, 269-273.

Gillam, R., McFadden, T., and van Kleeck, A. (1995). Improving narrative abilities: Whole language and language and language skills approaches. In M. Fey, J. Windsor, and S.F. Warren (Eds.). *Language intervention: Preschool through the elementary years* (vol. 5, pp. 145-183). Baltimore, MD: Paul H. Brookes.

Gillam, R., and Pearson, N. (2004). *Test of narrative language.* Greenville, SC: SuperDuper Publications.

Gillam, R., Peña, E., and Miller, L. (1999) Dynamic assessment of narrative and expository discourse. *Topics in Language Disorders, 20(1)*, 33-47.

Gillon, G. (2000). The efficacy of phonological awareness intervention for children with spoken language impairment. *Language, Speech and Hearing Services in Schools, 31*, 126-141.

Gillon, G. (2002). Follow-up study investigating the benefits of phonological awareness intervention of children with spoken language impairment. *International Journal of Language and Communication Disorders, 37*, 381-400.

Gillum, H., and Camarata, S. (2004). Importance of treatment efficacy research on language comprehension in MR/DD research. *Mental Retardation and Developmental Disabilities Research Reviews, 10*, 201-207.

Gillum, H., Camarata, S., Nelson, K., and Camarata, M. (2003). A comparison of naturalistic and analog treatment effects in children with expressive language disorder and poor preintervention imitation skills. *Journal of Positive Behavior Interventions, 3*, 171-178.

Gilmour, J., Hill, B., Place, M., and Skuse, D. (2004). Social communication deficits in conduct disorder: A clinical and community survey. *Journal of Child Psychology and Psychiatry and Allied Disciplines, 45*, 967-978.

Girolametto, L. (1997). Development of a parent report measure for profiling the conversational skills of preschool children. *American Journal of Speech-Language Pathology, 6*, 25-33.

Girolametto, L., and Weitzman, E. (2002). Responsiveness of child care providers in interactions with toddlers and preschoolers. *Language, Speech, and Hearing Services in Schools, 33*, 268-281.

Girolametto, L., Greenberg, J., and Manolson, H. (1986). *Developing dialogue skills: The Hanen early language parent program.* New York: Thieme Medical Publishers.

Girolametto, L., Pearce, P., and Weitzman, E. (1996). Effects of lexical intervention on the phonology of late talkers. *Journal of Speech, Language and Hearing Research, 40*, 338-348.

Girolametto, L., and Weitzman, E. (2006). It takes two to talk: The Hanen Program for parents. In R. McCauley and M. Fey (Eds.). *Treatment of language disorders in children* (pp. 77-101). Baltimore: Paul H. Brookes.

Girolametto, L., Weitzman, E., and Greenberg, J. (2003). Training day care staff to facilitate children's language. *American Journal of Speech-Language Pathology, 12,* 299-311.

Girolametto, L., Weitzman, E., Wiigs, M., and Pearce, P. (1999). The relationship between maternal language measures and language development in toddlers with expressive vocabulary delays. *American Journal of Speech-Language Pathology, 8,* 364-374.

Girolametto, L., Wiigs, M., Smyth, R., Weitzman, E., and Pearce, P. (2001). Children with a history of expressive vocabulary delay: Outcomes at 5 years of age. *American Journal of Speech-Language Pathology, 10,* 358-369.

Gleason, J. (2001). *The development of language* (5th ed.). Boston: Allyn & Bacon.

Gleason, M. (1995). Using direct instruction to integrate reading and writing for students with learning disabilities. *Reading and Writing Quarterly, 11,* 91-108.

Glennen, S., and DeCoste, D. (1997). *Handbook of augmentative and alternative communication.* San Diego, CA: Singular Publishing Group.

Glennen, S.L. (1997). Augmentative and alternative communication assessment strategies. In S.L. Glennen and D.C. DeCoste (Eds.). *Handbook of augmentative and alternative communication* (pp. 149-192). San Diego, CA: Singular Publishing Group.

Glos, J., Jariabkova, K., and Szabova, I. (2001). Landau-Kleffner syndrome: A case of a dissociation between spoken and written language. *Bratislavské lekárske listy, 102(12),* 556-61.

Glover, M.E., Sanford, A., and Preminger, J.L. (1995). *Early learning accomplishment profile.* Lewisville, NC: Kaplan Press.

Goble, P. (1988). *Iktomi and the boulder: A plains Indian story.* New York: Orchard Books.

Goble, P. (1990). *Iktomi and the ducks: A plains Indian story.* New York: Orchard Books.

Godar, C., Fields, V., and Schreiber, L. (2004). *Interactive BigBooks: Anterior/posterior contrasts.* Eau Claire, WI: Thinking Publications.

Goffman, L., and Leonard, J. (2000). Growth of language skills in preschool children with specific language impairment: implications for assessment and intervention. *American Journal of Speech-Language Pathology, 9(2),* 151-161.

Goin, R., Nordquist, V., and Twardosz, S. (2004). Parental accounts of home-based literacy processes: Contexts for infants and toddlers with developmental delays. *Early Education and Development, 15,* 187-214.

Goldfield, B., and Snow, C. (1984). Reading books with children: The mechanics of parental influence on children's reading achievement. In J. Flood (Ed.). *Understanding reading comprehension* (pp. 204-218). Newark, DE: International Reading Association.

Goldin-Meadow, S., and Butcher, C. (2003). Pointing toward two-word speech in young children. In K. Sotaro (Ed.). *Pointing: Where language, culture and cognition meet* (pp. 85-107). Mahwah, NJ: Erlbaum.

Goldin-Meadow, S., and Feldman, H. (1977). The development of language-like communication without a language model. *Science, 197,* 401-403.

Goldman, R., and Fristoe, M. (2000). *Goldman-Fristoe test of articulation—Second edition (GFTA-2).* Circle Pines, MN: AGS Publications.

Goldschmid, M., and Bentler, P. (1968). *Goldschmid-Bentler concept assessment kit.* San Diego, CA: Education and Industrial Testing Service.

Goldson, E. (1983). Bronchopulmonary dysplasia: Its relation to two-year developmental functioning in the very low birth weight infants. In T. Field and A. Sostek (Eds.). *Infants born at risk.* New York: Grune & Stratton.

Goldstein, B. (2000). *Cultural and linguistic diversity resource guide for speech-language pathology.* San Diego: Singular Publishing Group.

Goldstein, B. (2001). Transcription of Spanish and Spanish-influenced English. *Communication Disorders Quarterly, 23(1),* 54-60.

Goldstein, B. (Ed.). (2004). *Bilingual language development and disorders in Spanish English speakers.* Baltimore: Brookes.

Goldstein, B., and Iglesias, A. (2006). Issues of cultural and linguistic diversity. In R. Paul and P. Cascella (Eds.). *Introduction to clinical methods in communication disorders—2nd Ed* (pp. 261-280.) Baltimore: Paul H. Brookes.

Goldstein, H. (2002). Communication intervention for children with autism: A review of treatment efficacy. *Journal of Autism and Developmental Disorders, 32,* 373-396.

Goldsworthy, C. (1996). *Developmental reading disabilities: A language based treatment approach.* San Diego, CA: Singular Publishing Group.

Goodman, K. (1976). Reading: a psycholinguistic guessing game. In H. Singer and R.B. Ruddell (Eds.). *Theoretical models and processes of reading.* Newark, DE: International Reading Association.

Goodman, K. (1986). *What's whole in whole language: A parent-teacher guide.* Portsmouth, NH: Heinemann.

Goodman, R. (1997). The strengths and difficulties questionnaire: A research note. *Journal of Child Psychology and Psychiatry and Allied Disciplines, 38,* 581-586.

Goodman, Y. (1986). Children coming to know literacy. In W.H. Teale and E. Sulzby (Eds.). *Emergent literacy: Writing and reading* (pp. 1-14). Norwood, NJ: Ablex.

Goodwyn, S., Acredolo, L., and Brown, C. (2000). Impact of symbolic gesturing on early language development. *Journal of Nonverbal Behavior, 24,* 81-103.

Goosens, C. (1998) *Personal Communication—Modifying piagetian tasks for use with physically challenged individuals.* 20 West 22nd St., New York 10010.

Gopnik, M., and Crago, M.B. (1991). Familial aggregation of developmental language disorder. *Cognition, 39,* 1-50.

Gordon, M. (1983). *The Gordon diagnostic system.* Boulder, CO: Clinical Diagnostic Systems.

Gordon-Brannan, G., & Weiss, C. (2006). *Clinical management of articulatory and phonologic disorders.* Hagerstown, MD: Lippincott, Williams, & Wilkins.

Gordon-Brannan, M. (1994). Assessing intelligibility: Children's expressive phonologies. *Topics in Language Disorders, 14(2),* 17-25.

Gordon-Brannan, M., and Hodson, B. (2000). Intelligibility/severity measures of prekindergarten children's speech. *American Journal of Speech-Language Pathology, 9,* 141-150.

Gorman-Gard, K. (1992). *Figurative language.* Eau Claire, WI: Thinking Publications.

Gorski, P. (1983). Premature infant behavioral/physiological responses to caregiving intervention in the NICU. In J.D. Call, E. Galenson, and R.I. Tyson (Eds.). *Frontiers in infant psychiatry.* New York: Basic Books.

Gorski, P., Davison, M., and Brazelton, B. (1979). Stages of behavioral organization in the high risk neonate: Theoretical and clinical considerations. *Seminars in Perinatology, 3,* 61.

Goswami, U., and Bryant, P. (1990). *Phonological skills and learning to read.* East Sussex, England: Erlbaum.

Gottlieb, G. (1976). *The roles of experience in the development of behavior and the nervous system. Studies on the development of behavior and the nervous system: Neural and behavioral specificity.* New York: Academic Press.

Gough, P., Alford, J., and Holley-Wilcox, P. (1981). Words and contexts. In O.J.L. Tzeng and H. Singer (Eds.). *Perception of print: Reading research in experimental psychology.* Hillsdale, NJ: Erlbaum Associates.

Gough, P., and Tunmer, W. (1986). Decoding, reading, and reading disability. *Remedial and Special Education, 7,* 6-10.

Graham, S. (1992). Helping students with LD progress as writers. *Intervention in School and Clinic, 27,* 134-144.

Graham, S., and Harris, K. (1987). Improving composition skills of inefficient learners with self-instructional strategy training. *Topics in Language Disorders, 7,* 68-77.

Graham, S., and Harris, K. (1999). Assessment and intervention in overcoming writing difficulties: An illustration from the self-regulated strategy development model. *Language Speech and Hearing Services in Schools, 30,* 255-264.

Graham, S., Harris, K., Troia, G. (2000). Self-regulated strategy development revisited: Teaching writing strategies to struggling writers. *Topics in Language Disorders, 20(4),* 1-14.

Grambau, M. (1993). *Study smarter, not harder.* Kent, WA: Classic Printing.

Grandin, T. (1997). A personal perspective on autism. In D. Cohen and F. Volkamr (Eds.). *Handbook of autism and pervasive developmental disorders* (pp. 1032-1042). New York: John Wiley & Sons.

Graner, P., Faggella-Luby, M., and Fritschmann, N. (2005). An overview of responsiveness to intervention: What practitioners ought to know. *Topics in Language Disorders, 25(2),* 93-105.

Grant, C. (1989). *Phoenix rising, or how to survive your life.* New York: Atheneum.

Gravel, J., and Wallace, I. (1992). Listening and language at 4 years of age: Effects of early otitis media. *Journal of Speech and Hearing Research, 35,* 588-595.

Graves, A., and Montague, M. (1991). Using story-grammar cueing to improve the writing of students with learning disabilities. *Learning Disabilities Research and Practice, 6,* 246-250.

Graves, D. (1987). *Writing: Teachers and children at work.* Portsmouth, NH: Heinemann.

Gray, B., and Ryan, B. (1971). *Monterey language program.* Monterey, CA: Monterey Learning Systems.

Gray, C. (1994). *Comic strip conversations.* Arlington, TX: Future Horizons.

Gray, C. (1995a). Teaching children with autism to "read" social situations. In K.A. Quill (Ed.). *Teaching children with autism: Strategies to enhance communication and socialization* (pp. 219-241). Albany, NY: Delmar.

Gray, C. (1995b). *The original social story book.* Arlington, TX: Future Horizons.

Gray, C. (2000a). *Writing social stories.* Arlington, TX: Future Horizons.

Gray, C. (2000b). *The new social story book.* Arlington, TX: Future Horizons.

Gray, S. (2003). Word-learning by preschoolers with specific language impairment: What predicts success. *Journal of Speech, Language, and Hearing Research, 46,* 56-67.

Green, L. (2002). *African American English.* Cambridge: Cambridge University Press.

Greenfield, J. (1978). *A place for Noah.* New York: Pocket Books.

Greenfield, P. (1978). *The structure of communication in early language development.* New York: Academic Press.

Greenfield, P., and Smith, J. (1976). *The structure of communication in early language development.* New York: Academic Press.

Greenhalgh, K., and Strong, C. (2001). Literate language features in spoken narratives of children with typical language and children with language impairments. *Language, Speech and Hearing Services in Schools, 32,* 114-135.

Greensher, J. (1988). Recent advances in injury prevention. *Pediatrics in Review, 8,* 171-177.

Greville, K., Keith, W., and Laven, J. (1985). Performance of children with previous OME on central auditory measures. *Australian Journal of Audiology, 7,* 69-78.

Griffer, M. (2000). Developmental caregiving in the NICU: What speech-language pathologists should know. *Language Learning and Education, 7(1),* 34-35.

Griffin, K., and Hannah, L. (1960). A study of the results of an extremely short instructional unit in listening. *Journal of Communication, 10,* 135-139.

Griffith, C., and Tulbert, B. (1995). The effect of graphic organizers on students' comprehension and recall of expository text: A review of the research and implications for practice. *Reading and Writing Quarterly, 11,* 73-89.

Griffith, P., Dastoli, S., and Rogers-Adkinson, D. (1994). Written language assessment and intervention. In D. Ripich and N. Creaghead (Eds.). *School discourse problems* (2nd ed., pp. 299-342). San Diego, CA: Singular Publishing Group.

Griffiths, R. (1954). *The abilities of babies.* London: University of London Press.

Grigorenko, E.L., Wood, F.B., Meyer, M.S., Hart, L.A., Speed, W.C., Schuster. A., and Pauls, D.L. (1997). Susceptibility loci for distinct components of developmental dyslexia on chromosomes 6 and 15. *American Journal of Human Genetics, 60,* 27-39.

Grigorenko, E.L., Wood, F.B., Meyer, M.S., and Pauls, D.L. (2000). The chromosome 6p influences on different dyslexia-related cognitive processes: Further confirmation. *American Journal of Human Genetics, 66,* 715, 723.

Grove, N., and Dockrell, J. (2000). Multisign combinations by children with intellectual impairments: An analysis of language skills. *Journal of Speech, Language, and Hearing Research, 43,* 309-324.

Gruenewald, L., and Pollack, S. (1990). *Language interaction in curriculum and instruction.* Austin, TX: Pro-Ed.

Grunwell, P. (1981). The development of phonology. *First Language, 2,* 175.

Grunwell, P. (1987). *Clinical phonology* (2nd ed.). Baltimore, MD: Williams & Wilkins.

Guerette, P., Tefft, D., Furumasu, J., and Moy, F. (1999). Development of a cognitive assessment battery for young children with physical impairments. *Infant-Toddler Intervention, 9,* 169-184.

Guess, D., Rutherford, G., and Twichell, A. (1969). Speech acquisition in a mute, visually impaired adolescent. *New Outlook for the Blind, 63,* 8-13.

Guiterrez-Clennen, V., and DeCurtis, L. (2001). Examining the quality of children's stories: Clinical applications. *Seminars in Speech and Language, 22,* 79-88.

Gummersall, D., and Strong, C. (1999). Assessment of complex sentence production in a narrative context. *Language, Speech, and Hearing Services in Schools, 30,* 153-164.

Gunlap, G. (2005). Positive behavior support: An overview. *Perspectives on Language Learning and Education, 12(1),* 3-6.

Guralnick, M. (2000). *Interdisciplinary clinical assessment of young children with developmental disabilities.* Baltimore: Paul H. Brookes.

Guralnick, M., and Paul-Brown, D. (1986). Communicative interactions of mildly delayed and normally developing preschool children: Effects of listener's developmental age. *Journal of Speech and Hearing Research, 29,* 2-10.

Guralnick, M.J. (1997). *The effectiveness of early intervention.* Baltimore, MD: Paul H. Brookes.

Gutierrez-Clellen, V., and Peña, E. (2001). Dynamic assessment of diverse children: A tutorial. *Language, Speech, and Hearing Services in Schools, 32,* 212-224.

Gutierrez-Clennen, V., Restrepo, M., Bedore, L., Peña, E., and Anderson, R. (2000). Language sample analysis in Spanish-speaking children: Methodological considerations. *Language Speech, and Hearing Services in Schools, 31,* 88-98.

Guyette, T.W., and Diedrich, W.M. (1981). A critical review of developmental apraxia of speech. In N.J. Lass (Ed.). *Speech and language: Advances in basic practice* (vol. 5, pp. 1-49). London: Academic Press.

Habib, M., Rey, V., Daffaure, V., Camps, R., Espesser, R., Joly-Pottuz, B., and Demonet, J. (2002). *International Journal of Language and Communication Disorders, 37,* 289-308.

Hadden, D.S., and Fowler, S.A. (2000). Early intervention to preschool special education services. *Young Exceptional Children, 3(4),* 2-7.

Hadley, P. (1998). Language sampling protocols for eliciting text-level discourse. *Language, Speech, and Hearing Services in Schools, 29,* 132-147.

Hadley, P., and Schuele, C.M. (1998). Facilitating peer interaction: Socially relevant objectives for preschool language intervention. *American Journal of Speech-Language Pathology, 7,* 25-36.

Hadley, P., Simmerman, A., Long, M., and Luna, M. (2000). Facilitating language development for inner-city children: Experimental evaluation of a collaborative classroom-based intervention. *Language, Speech, and Hearing Services in Schools, 31,* 280-295.

Hagen, C. (1986). Language disorders in head trauma. In J.M. Costello and A.L. Holland (Eds.). *Handbook of speech and language disorders.* San Diego, CA: College-Hill Press.

Hagerman, R., Altshul-Stark, D., and McBogg, P. (1987). Recurrent otitis media in boys with fragile X syndrome. *American Journal of Diseases of Children, 141,* 184-187.

Hagerman, R., and McBogg, P. (1983). *The fragile X syndrome: Diagnosis, biochemistry, and intervention.* Dillan, CO: Spectra Publishers.

Halford, G. (2004). Information-processing models of development. In U. Goswami (Ed.). *Blackwell handbook of child development* (pp. 555-574). Oxford: Blackwell.

Hall, E. (1983). *The dance of life.* New York: Anchor Press/Doubleday.

Hall, P. (2000). A letter to the parents of a child with developmental apraxia of speech. *Language, Speech, and Hearing Services in Schools, 31,* 169-181.

Hall, P., and Tomblin, J. (1978). A follow-up study of children with articulation and language disorders. *Journal of Speech and Hearing Disorders, 43,* 227-241.

Hall, S., Circello, N., Reed, P., and Hylton, J. (1987). *Considerations for feeding children who have a neuromuscular disorder.* Portland, OR: CDRC Publications.

Halle, J., Brady, N., and Drasgow, E. (2004). Enhancing socially adaptive communicative repairs of beginning communicators with disabilities. *American Journal of Speech-Language Pathology, 13,* 43-54.

Hallenbeck, M. (1996). The cognitive strategy in writing: Welcome relief for adolescents with learning disabilities. *Learning Disabilities Research and Practice, 11,* 107-119.

Halliday, M. (1975). *Learning how to mean: Explorations in the development of language.* New York: Arnold.

Halliday, M., and Hasan, R. (1976). *Cohesion in English.* London: Longmon.

Hamersky, J. (1995). *Cartoon cut-ups.* Eau Claire, WI: Thinking Publications.

Hammer, C. (2004). Parental beliefs about literacy learning in non-majority households: information relevant for the speech-language pathologist. *Perspectives on Language Learning and Education, 11(3),* 17-21.

Hammill, D. (1998). *Detroit test of learning aptitude—4.* Austin, TX: Pro-Ed.

Hammill, D., Brown, V., Larsen, S., and Wiederholt, J. (1994). *Test of adolescent and adult language—3.* Austin, TX: Pro-Ed.

Hammill, D., Hresko, W., Ammer, J., Cronin, M., and Quinby, S. (1998). *Hammill multiability achievement test.* Austin, TX: Pro-Ed.

Hammill, D., and Larsen, S. (1996). *Test of written language—3.* Austin, TX: Pro-Ed.

Hammill, D., Mather, N., and Robers, R. (1968). *Illinois test of psycholinguistic abilities* (3rd ed.). Austin, TX: Pro-Ed.

Hammill, D., and Newcomer, P. (1997). *Test of language development—Intermediate: 3.* Austin, TX: Pro-Ed.

Hammill, D., Pearson, N., and Weiderhold, J.L. (1998). *Comprehensive test of nonverbal intelligence.* Austin, TX: Pro-Ed.

Hancock, T.B., and Kaiser, A.P. (2006). Enhanced milieu teaching. In R. McCauley and M. Fey (Eds.). *Treatment of language disorders in children.* Baltimore: Paul H. Brookes. In press.

Hanen Centre. (2000). *Making the connections that help children communicate.* Toronto, Canada: Author.

Hanken, D., and Kennedy, J. (1998). *Getting to know you! A social skills curriculum, grades 6-9.* Minneapolis, MN: Educational Media Corp.

Hanna, R. M., Lippert, E. A., and Harris, A. B. (1982). *Developmental communication curriculum.* Columbus, OH: Charles E. Merrill.

Hansen, J., and Pearson, P. (1983). An instructional study: Improving the inferential comprehension of good and poor fourth-grade readers. *Journal of Educational Psychology, 75,* 821-829.

Hanson, D., Jackson, A., and Hagerman, R. (1986). Speech disturbances (cluttering) in mildly impaired males with the Martin-Bell fragile X syndrome. *American Journal of Medical Genetics, 23,* 195-206.

Hanson, M. (2004). Ethnic, cultural, and language diversity in service settings. In E. Lynch and M Hanson (Eds.). *Developing cross-cultural competence* (3rd ed., pp. 3-18). Baltimore, MD: Paul H. Brookes.

Hanson, V., and Padden, C. (1989). Interactive video for bilingual ASL/ English instruction of deaf children. *American Annals of the Deaf, 134,* 209-213.

Hanten, G., Zhang, D., Barnes, M., Roberson, G., Archibald, J., Song, J., and Levin, H. (2004). Childhood head injury and metacognitive processed in language and memory. *Developmental Neuropsychology, 25,* 85-106.

Happé, F. (1995). *Autism: An introduction to psychological theory.* Cambridge, MA: Harvard University Press.

Harcherik, D., Cohen, D., Ort, S., Paul, R., Shaywitz, B., Volkmar, F., Rothman, S., and Leckman, J. (1985). Computerized tomographic brain scanning in four neuropsychiatric disorders of childhood. *The American Journal of Psychiatry, 142,* 731-734.

Harcourt Assessment. (1999). *Wechsler abbreviated scale of intelligence (WASI).* San Antonio, TX: Author.

Hargrave, A., and Senechal, M. (2000). Book reading intervention with preschool children who have limited vocabularies: The benefits of regular reading and dialogic reading. *Early Childhood Research Quarterly, 15,* 75-90.

Hargraves, R. (1976). *Mr. Bounce.* New York: Price, Stern, Sloan.

Hargraves, R. (1980a). *Mr. Fussy.* New York: Price, Stern, Sloan.

Hargraves, R. (1980b). *Mr. Happy.* New York: Price, Stern, Sloan.

Hargraves, R. (1980c). *Mr. Worry.* New York: Price, Stern, Sloan.

Harris, D. (1963). *Children's drawings as a measure of intellectual maturity: A revision and extension of the Goodenough Draw-a-Man Test.* New York: Harcourt Brace and World.

Harris, D., and Vanderheiden, G. (1980). Augmentative communication techniques. In R. Schiefelbusch (Ed.). *Nonspeech language and communication: Analysis and intervention.* Baltimore, MD: University Park Press.

Harris, F. (1996). Elective mutism: A tutorial. *Language, Speech, and Hearing Services in Schools, 27,* 10-15.

Harris, G. (1993). American Indian cultures: A lesson in diversity. In D.E. Battle (Ed.). *Communication disorders in multicultural populations* (pp. 78-113). Boston, MA: Andover Medical Publishers.

Harris, M., and Riechle, J. (2004). The impact of aided language stimulation on symbol comprehension and production in children with moderate cognitive disabilities. *American Journal of Speech-Language Pathology, 13,* 155-167.

Harrison, M. (2001). Landau-Kleffner syndrome: Acquired childhood aphasia. In T. Layton, E. Crais, and L. Watson (Eds.). *Handbook of early impairment in children: Nature* (pp. 418-450). Albany, NY: Delmar Publishers.

Harrison, P., Kaufman, A., Kaufman, N., Bruininks, R., Rynders, J., Ilmer, S., Sparrow, C., and Cicchetti, D. (1990). *Early screening profiles.* Circle Pines, MN: American Guidance Service.

Harrison, P., and Oakland, T. (2003). *Adaptive behavior assessment system—2nd. Ed.* San Antonio, TX: Harcourt.

Harris-Schmidt, G., and Noell, E. (1983). Phonology. In C. Wren (Ed.). *Language learning disabilities: Diagnosis and remediation* (pp. 39-84). Rockville, MD: Aspen Publishers.

Hart, B. (1981). Pragmatics: How language is used. *Analytic Intervention in Developmental Disorders, 1,* 299-313.

Hart, B. (2000). A natural history of language experience. *Topics in Early Childhood Special Education, 20,* 28-33.

Hart, B. (2004). What toddlers talk about. *First Language, 24,* 91-106.

Hart, B., and Risley, T. (1975). Incidental teaching of language in the preschool. *Journal of Applied Behavior Analysis, 8,* 411-420.

Hart, B., and Risley, T. (1980). In vivo language intervention: Unanticipated general effects. *Journal of Applied Behavior Analysis, 13,* 407-432.

Hart, K., Fujiki, M., Brinton, B., and Hart, C. (2004). The relationship between social behavior and severity of language impairment. *Journal of Speech, Language, and Hearing Research, 47,* 647-662.

Hartley Software (1992). *Analogies tutorial.* Tucson, AZ: Communication Skill Builders.

Haussamen, B. (2003). *Grammar alive! A guide for teachers.* Urbana, IL: National Council of Teachers of English.

Hayden, D. (1984). The PROMPT system of therapy: Theoretical framework and applications for developmental apraxia of speech. *Seminars in Speech and Language, 3,* 139-156.

Hayes, J., and Flower, L. (1987). On the structure of the writing process. *Topics in Language Disorders, 7(4),* 19-30.

Haynes, W., Moran. M., and Pindzola, R. (1999). *Communication disorders in the classroom: An introduction for professionals in school settings* (3rd ed.). Kendall/Hunt Publishing Company: Dubuque, IA.

Haynes, W., and Pindzola, R. (1998). *Diagnosis and evaluation in speech pathology* (5th ed.). Englewood Cliffs, NJ: Prentice Hall.

Haynes, W., and Shulman, B. (1998a). Ethnic and cultural differences in communication disorders. In W. Haynes and B. Shulman (Eds.). *Communication development: Foundations, processes, and clinical applications* (pp. 387-411). Baltimore, MD: Williams & Wilkins.

Haynes, W., and Shulman, B. (1998b). *Communication development: Foundations, processes, and clinical applications.* Baltimore, MD: Williams & Wilkins.

Hazel, J., Schumaker, J., Sherman, J., and Sheldon-Wildgen, J. (1981). *ASSET: A social skills program for adolescents.* Champaign, IL: Research Press.

Healey, W., Ackerman, B., Chappell, C., Perrin, K., and Stormer, J. (1981). *The prevalence of communicative disorders: A review of the literature.* Rockville, MD: American Speech-Language-Hearing Association.

Heath, S. (1982). What no bedtime story means: Narrative skills at home and school. *Language in Society, 11,* 49-76.

Heath, S. (1986). Talking a cross-cultural look at narratives. *Topics in Language Disorders, 7(1),* 84-94.

Hedrick, D., Prather, E., and Tobin, A. (1995). *Sequenced inventory of communication development—Revised.* Los Angeles, CA: Western Psychological Services.

Hefter, R., Worthington, J., Worthington, S., and Howe, S. (1982). *The Stickybear ABC* (computer program). Middletown, CT: Xerox Education Publications.

Heilmann, J., Weismer, S., Evans, J., and Hollar, C. (2005). Utility of the MacArthur-Bates Communicative Development Inventory in identifying language abilities of late-talking and typically developing toddlers. *American Journal of Speech-Language Pathology, 14,* 40-51.

Heim, M., and Baker-Mills, A. (1996). Early development of symbolic communication and linguistic complexity through augmentative and alternative communication. In S. von Tetzchner and M.H. Jensen (Eds.). *Augmentative and alternative communication: European perspectives* (pp. 232-248). San Diego, CA: Singular Publishing Group.

Heller, M. (1986). How do you know what you know? Metacognitive modeling in the content areas. *Journal of Reading, 29,* 415-422.

Herbert, C. (1977). *Basic inventory of natural language.* San Bernardino, CA: Checkpoint Systems.

Hermann, M. (1986). *Tiger's tales* (computer program). Pleasantville, NY: Sunburst Communications.

Herron, S., Hresko, W., and Peak, P. (1996). *Test of early written language—2.* Austin, TX: Pro-Ed

Hesketh, A. (2004). Early literacy achievement of children with a history of speech problems. *International Journal of Language and Communication Disorders, 39,* 453-468.

Hesketh, A., Adams, C., Nightingale, C., and Hall, R. (2000). Phonological awareness therapy and articulatory training approaches for children with phonological disorders: A comparative outcome study. *International Journal of Language and Communication Disorders, 35,* 337-354.

Hess, L., and Fairchild, J. (1988). Model, analyse, practise (MAP): A language therapy model for learning-disabled adolescents. *Child Language Teaching and Therapy, 4,* 325-338.

Hess, L., Wagner, M., De Wald, B., and Conn, P. (1993). Conversation skill intervention program for adolescents with learning disabilities. *Child Language Teaching and Therapy, 9,* 13-31.

Hester, E. (1996). Narratives of young African-American children. In A. Kamhi, K. Pollock, and J. Harris (Eds.). *Communication development and disorders in African-American children* (pp. 227-246). Baltimore, MD: Paul H. Brookes.

Hetzroni, O., Quist, R., and Lloyd, L. (2002). Translucency and complexity: Effects on Blissymbol learning using computer and teacher presentations. *Language, Speech, and Hearing Services in Schools, 33,* 291-303.

Hetzroni, O., and Schanin, M. (2002). Emergent literacy in children with severe disabilities using interactive multimedia stories. *Journal of Developmental and Physical Disabilities, 14,* 173-190.

Hetzroni, O., and Tannous, J. (2004). Effects of a computer-based intervention program on the communicative functions of children with autism. *Journal of Autism and Developmental Disorders, 34,* 95-113.

Hewitt, G. (2001). The writing portfolio: Assessment starts with A. *Clearing House, 74,* 187-182.

Hewitta, L., Hammer, C., Yont, K., and Tomblin, B. (2005). Language sampling for kindergarten children with and without SLI: Mean length of utterance, IPSyn, and NDW. *Journal of Communication Disorders, 38,* 197-213.

Heyer, J. (1995). The responsibilities of speech-language pathologists toward children with ADHD. *Seminars in Speech and Language, 16,* 275-288.

Hill, E.L. (2001). Non-specific nature of specific language impairment: A review of the literature with regard to concomitant motor impairments. *International Journal of Language and Communication Disorders, 36(2),* 149-171.

Hiskey, M. (1999). *Hiskey-Nebraska test of learning aptitude.* Austin, TX: Pro-Ed.

Hixson, P.K. (1985). *DSS computer program.* Omaha, NE: Computer Language Analysis.

Hoban, R. (1964). *Bread and jam for Frances.* New York: Harper & Row.

Hobbs, F., and Stoops, N. (2002). *Demographic trends in the 20th century.* U.S. Census Bureau, Census 2000 Special Reports, Series CENSR-4. Washington, DC: U.S. Government Printing Office.

Hockey, A., and Crowhurst, J. (1988). Early manifestations of the Martin-Bell syndrome based on a series of both sexes from infancy. *American Journal of Medical Genetics, 30,* 61-71.

Hodgdon, L. (1995). *Visual strategies for improving communication.* Troy, MI: QuirkRoberts Publishing.

Hodge, M. (Oct. 1998). Developmental coordination disorder: A diagnosis with theoretical and clinical implications for developmental apraxia of speech. ASHA special interest division, *Language Learning and Education newsletter.*

Hodson, B. (1994). Helping individuals become intelligible, literate, and articulate: The role of phonology. *Topics in Language Disorders, 14(2),* 1-16.

Hodson, B. (2004). *Hodson assessment of phonological patterns—3rd Ed.* Austin, TX: Pro-Ed.

Hodson, B., and Paden, E. (1991). *Targeting intelligible speech: A phonological approach to remediation* (2nd ed.). Austin, TX: Pro-Ed.

Hof, J., van Dijk, P., Chenault, M., and Anteunis, L. (2005). A two-step scenario for hearing assessment with otoacoustic emissions at compensated middle ear pressure (in children 1–7 years old). *International Journal of Pediatric Otorhinolaryngology, 69,* 649-655.

Hoff, E. (2001). *Language development* (2nd ed.) Stamford, CT: Wadsworth/Thomson Learning.

Hoff-Ginsberg, E. (1987). Topic relations in mother-child conversation. *First Language, 7,* 145-158.

Hoff-Ginsberg, E. (1990). Maternal speech and the child's development of syntax: A further look. *Journal of Child Language, 17,* 85-100.

Hoffman, P., Schuckers, G., and Daniloff, R. (1989). *Children's phonetic disorders: Theory and treatment.* Boston, MA: College-Hill Press.

Hoggan, K., and Strong, C. (1994). The magic of "once upon a time": Narrative teaching strategies. *Language, Speech, and Hearing Services in Schools, 25,* 76-89.

Hohmann, M., Banet, B., and Weikart, D. (1979). *Young children in action: A manual for preschool educators.* Ypsilanti, MI: High/Scope Press.

Holland, A. (Ed.). (1984). *Language disorders in children: Recent advances.* San Diego, CA: College-Hill Press.

Holm, V., and Kunze, L. (1969). Effect of chronic otitis media on language and speech development. *Pediatrics, 43,* 833-839.

Homeworkhelp.com. (2005). *Composition.* Santa Clara, CA: Author.

Hook, P., Macaruso, P., and Jones, S. (2001). Efficacy of FastForWord training on facilitating acquisition of reading skills by children with reading difficulties—A longitudinal study. *Annals of Dyslexia, 51,* 75-96.

Hoover, J.J., and Patton, J.R. (1997). *Curriculum adaptations for students with learning and behavior problems: Principles and practices.* Austin, TX: Pro-Ed.

Hoskins, B. (1987). *Conversations: Language intervention for adolescents.* Allen, TX: DLM.

Hoskins, B. (1990). Language and literacy: Participating in the conversation. *Topics in Language Disorders, 10(2),* 46-62.

Hoskins, B. (1999). *Conversations.* Eau Claire, WI: Thinking Publications.

Hosom, J.P., Shriberg, L., and Green, J. R. (2004). Diagnostic assessment of childhood apraxia of speech using Automatic Speech Recognition (ASR) methods. *Journal of Medical Speech Language Pathology, 12,* 167-171.

Hotz, G., Helm-Estabrooks, N., and Nelson, N.W. (2001). Development of the Pediatric Test of Traumatic Brain Injury. *Journal of Head Trauma Rehabilitation, 16(5),* 426-440.

Howard, J., Sparkman, C., Cohen, H., Green, G., and Stanislaw, H. (2005). A comparison of intensive behavior analytic and eclectic treatments for young children with autism. *Research in Developmental Disabilities, 26,* 359-383.

Howell, C. (2001). Mothers' speech with 12 month old infants: Influences on the amount and complexity of infants' vocalization. *Dissertation Abstracts International Section A: Humanities & Social Sciences, 61 (12-A),* 47-51.

Howlin, P. (2005). Outcomes in autism spectrum disorders. In F. Volkmar, R. Paul, A. Klin, and D. Cohen (Eds.). *Handbook of autism and pervasive developmental disorders—vol. 1* (pp. 201-222). New York: Wiley.

Hoy, E., and McKnight, J. (1977). Communication style and effectiveness in homogeneous and heterogeneous dyads of retarded children. *American Journal of Mental Deficiency, 81,* 587-598.

Hresko, W., Reid, K., and Hammill, D. (1999). *Test of early language development* (3rd ed.). Austin, TX: Pro-Ed.

Hubbard, T., Paradise, J., McWilliams, B., Elster, B., and Taylor, F. (1985). Consequences of unremitting middle-ear disease in early life: Otologic, audiologic, and developmental findings in children with cleft palate. *New England Journal of Medicine, 312,* 1529-1534.

Hubbell, R. (1981). *Children's language disorders: An integrated approach.* Englewood Cliffs, NJ: Prentice-Hall.

Hubbell, R. (1988). *A handbook of English grammar and language sampling.* Englewood Cliffs, NJ: Prentice-Hall.

Huebner, C. (2000). Promoting toddlers' language development through community-based intervention. *Journal of Applied Developmental Psychology, 21,* 513-535.

Huer, M. (1988). *The nonspeech test*. Wauconda, IL: Don Johnston, Inc.

Hughes, D., and Carpenter, R. (1983, Nov.). *Effects of two grammar treatment programs on target generalization to spontaneous language*. Paper presented to the American Speech-Language-Hearing Association annual convention, Cincinnati, OH.

Hughes, D., Fey, M., and Long, S. (1992). Developmental sentence scoring: Still useful after all these years. *Topics in Language Disorders, 12(2)*, 1-12.

Hughes, D., McGillivray, L., and Schmidek, M. (1997). *Guide to narrative language*. Eau Claire, WI: Thinking Publications.

Huisingh, R., Bowers, L., LoGiudice, C., and Orman, J. (2004). *The Word Test—2, Elementary*. East Moline, IL: LinguiSystems.

Huisingh, R., Bowers, L., LoGiudice, C., and Orman, J. (2005). *The Word Test—2, Adolescent*. East Moline, IL: LinguiSystems.

Hulit, L., and Howard, M. (2002). *Born to talk—3rd. Ed*. Boston: Allyn & Bacon.

Hulme, C., and Snowling, M. (1997). *Dyslexia: Biology, cognition, and intervention*. London: Whurr Publishers.

Hunt, K. (1965). *Grammatical structures written at three grade levels* (Research Report No. 3). Urbana, IL: National Council of Teachers of English.

Hutchinson, T.A. (1996). What to look for in the technical manual: Twenty questions for users. *Language Speech and Hearing Services in Schools, 27(2)*, 109-121.

Hwa-Froelich, D., Hodson, B., and Edward, H. (2002). Characteristics of Vietnamese phonology. *American Journal of Speech-Language Pathology, 11*, 264-273.

Hwa-Froelich, D., and Matsuo, H. (2005). Vietnamese children and language-based processing tasks. *Language, Speech, and Hearing Services in Schools, 36*, 230-243.

Hwa-Froelich, D., and Westby, C. (2003). Frameworks of education: Perspectives of southeast Asian parents and head start staff. *Language, Speech, and Hearing Services in Schools, 34*, 299-319.

Hyter, Y., and Westby, C. (1996). Using oral narratives to assess communicative competence. In A. Kamhi, K. Pollock, and J. Harris (Eds.). *Communication development and disorders in African-American children* (pp. 247-284). Baltimore, MD: Paul H. Brookes.

Idol, L., Nevin, A., and Paolucci-Whitcomb, P. (1999). *Models of curriculum-based assessment: A blueprint for learning—3rd ed*. Austin, TX: Pro-Ed.

Iglesias, A. (2001). What test should I use? *Seminars in Speech and Language, 22*, 3-15.

Iglesias, A., and Goldstein, B. (2004). Language and dialectical variations. In J. Bernthal and N. Bankson (Eds.). *Articulation and phonological disorders* (5th ed., pp. 348-375). Boston, MA: Allyn & Bacon.

Illinois Early Learning Project. (2005). *Illinois Early Learning Project Tip Sheets: Language Arts*. Retrieved from http://www.illinoisearlylearning.org/tips.htm#lang

Imhoff, S., and Wigginton, V. (1991). Identifying feeding and swallowing problems in infants and young children. *Clinics in Communication Disorders: Infant Assessment, 1(2)*, 59-68.

Individuals with Disabilities Education Act of 1997, PL 101-336 (1997).

Individuals with Disabilities Education Act of 2004, PL 108-446 (2004).

Infant Health and Development Program. (1990). Enhancing the outcome of low birth weight premature infants: A multi-size random trial. *Journal of the American Medical Association, 263*, 3035.

Ingram, D. (1976). *Phonological disability in children*. New York: Elsevier.

Ingram, D. (1981). The transition from early symbols to syntax. In R. Schiefelbusch and D. Bricker (Eds.). Early language: Acquisition and intervention. Baltimore, MD: University Park Press.

Isaacson, S. (1988). Assessing the writing product: Qualitative and quantitative measures. *Exceptional Children, 54*, 528-534.

Issacs, G. (1996). Persistence of non standard dialect in school-age children. *Journal of Speech and Hearing Research, 39 (2)*, 434-440.

Jabar, C. (1989). *Alice Ann gets ready for school*. Boston, MA: Little, Brown.

Jackson, D.A., Jackson, N.F., & Bennett, M.L. (1998). *Teaching social competence to youth and adults with developmental disabilities: A comprehensive program*. Austin, TX: Pro-Ed.

Jackson, S., and Roberts, J. (2001). Complex syntax production of African American preschoolers. *Journal of Speech, Language, and Hearing Research, 44*, 1083-1096.

Jacobson, J.W., Mulick, J.A., and Swartz, A.A. (1995). A history of facilitated communication: Science, pseudoscience, and antiscience. *American Psychologist, 50*, 750-765.

Jacoby, G., Lee, L., Kummer, A., Levin., L, and Creaghead, N. (2002). The number of individual treatment units necessary to facilitate functional communication improvements in the speech and language of young children. *American Journal of Speech-Language Pathology, 11*, 370–380.

Jaffe, M. (1984). Neurological impairment of speech production: Assessment and treatment. In J. Costello (Ed.). *Speech disorders in children* (pp. 157-186). San Diego, CA: College-Hill Press.

Jaffe, M. (1989). Feeding at-risk infants and toddlers. *Topics in Language Disorders, 10(1)*, 13-25.

Jager Adams, M., Foorman, B.R., Lundberg, I., and Beeler, T. (1998). *Phonemic awareness in young children: A classroom curriculum*. Baltimore, MD: Brookes Publishing Company.

Jago, C. (2002). *Cohesive writing: Why concept is not enough*. Westport, CT: Heinemann.

James, S. (1990). *Normal language acquisition*. Boston, MA: College-Hill Press.

James, S. (1993). Assessing children with language disorders. In D.K. Bernstein and E. (Eds.). *Language and communication disorders in children* (3rd ed., pp. 257-207). Columbus, OH: Merrill/Macmillan.

James, S., and Blachman, B. (1987, November). *Metalinguistic abilities and reading achievement in first through third grades*. Paper presented at the annual convention of the American Speech-Language-Hearing Association, New Orleans, LA.

Jarvey, M and McKeough, A. (2003, April). *Teaching trickster tales: A comparison of instructional approaches in composition*. Paper presented at the Annual General Meeting of the American Educational Research Association, Chicago, IL.

Jelm, J. (1990). *Oral-motor feeding rating scale*. Tucson, AZ: Communication/Therapy Skill Builders.

Jencks, C. (2003). *Process writing checklist*. ERIC Document No. ED479389.

Jenkins, R., and Bowen, L. (1994). Facilitating development of preliterate children's phonological abilities. *Topics in Language Disorders, 14(2)*, 26-39.

Jensen, D., Wallace, S., Kelsay, P. (1994). LATCH: A breastfeeding charting system and documentation tool. *Journal of Obstetric, Gynecologic, and Neonatal Nursing, 23(1)*, 27-32.

Jensen, V., and Sinclair, L. (2002). Treatment of autism in young children: Behavioral intervention and applied behavior analysis. *Infants and Young Children, 14*, 42-52.

Jerger, J. (1962). Scientific writing can be readable. *ASHA, 4*, 101-104.

Jitendra, A., Edwards, L., Sacks, G., and Jacobson, L. (2004). What research says about vocabulary instruction for students with learning disabilities. *Exceptional Children, 70*, 299-322.

Joanisse, M., and Seidenberg, M. (2003). Phonology and syntax in specific language impairment: Evidence from a connectionist model. *Brain and Language, 86*, 40-56.

Joe, J., and Malach, R. (2004). Families with American Indian roots. In E. Lynch and M. Hanson (Eds.). *Developing cross-cultural competence* (3rd ed., pp. 109-140). Baltimore, MD: Paul H. Brookes.

Johnson, A. (1993). *Toning the sweep*. New York: Scholastic.

Johnson, B., McGonigel, M., and Kaufmann, R. (1989). *Guidelines and recommended practices for the individualized family service plan*. Washington, DC: Association for the Care of Children's Health.

Johnson, C. (1995). Expanding norms for narration. *Language, Speech and Hearing Services in Schools, 26*, 326-341.

Johnson, D., and Johnson, R. (1990). Social skills for successful group work. *Educational Leadership, 47(4)*, 29-33.

Johnson, D., and von Hoff Johnson, B. (1986). Highlighting vocabulary in inferential comprehension. *Journal of Reading, 29*, 622-625.

Johnson, J., Baumgart, D., Helmstetter, E., and Curry, C. (1996). *Augmenting basic communication in natural contexts*. Baltimore, MD: Paul H. Brookes.

Johnson, N. (1983). What do you do when you can't tell the whole story? The development of summarization skills. In K.E. Nelson (Ed.). *Children's language* (vol. 4, pp. 315-383). Hillsdale, NJ: Erlbaum.

Johnson, S. (1987). *Cognitive behavior scale*. Vero Beach, FL: The Speech Bin.

Johnson-Martin, N., Hacker, B., and Attermeier, S. (2004). *Carolina curriculum for infants and toddlers with special needs—Third edition.* Baltimore, MD: Paul H. Brookes.

Johnston, E.B., and Johnston, A.V. (1990). *Communication abilities diagnostic test.* Austin, TX: Pro-Ed.

Johnston, J. (1982). Narratives: A new look at communication problems in older language-disordered children. *Language, Speech, and Hearing Services in Schools, 13,* 144-155.

Johnston, J. (1994). Cognitive abilities of children with language impairment. In R. Watkins and M. Rice (Eds.). *Specific language impairments in children* (vol. 4, pp. 107-121). Baltimore, MD: Paul H. Brookes.

Johnston, J., and Ramstad, V. (1978). Cognitive development in pre-adolescent language impaired children. In M. Burns and E.J. Andrews (Eds.). *Selected papers in language and phonology.* Evanston, IL: Institute for Continuing Professional Education.

Johnston, J., and Schery, T. (1976). The use of grammatical morphemes by children with communication disorders. In D.M. Morehead and A.E. Morehead (Eds.). *Normal and deficient child language.* Baltimore, MD: University Park Press.

Johnston, J., Smith, L., and Box, P. (1997). Cognition and communication: Referential strategies used by preschoolers with specific language impairment. *Journal of Speech and Hearing Research, 40,* 964-974.

Johnston, J., and Weismer, S. (1983). Mental rotation abilities in language-disordered children. *Journal of Speech and Hearing Research, 26,* 397-404.

Johnston, J., and Wong, M. (2002). Cultural differences in beliefs and practices concerning talk to children. *Journal of Speech, Language, and Hearing Research, 45,* 916-926.

Johnston, S., Reichle, J., and Evans, J. (2004). Supporting augmentative and alternative communication use by beginning communicators with severe disabilities. *American Journal of Speech-Language Pathology, 13,* 20-30.

Jones, K., Smith, D., Streissguth, A., and Myrianthopoulos, N. (1974). Outcome in offspring of chronic alcoholic women. *Lancet, 1,* 1076-1078.

Joseph, L. (2000). Developing first graders' phonemic awareness, word identification and spelling: A comparison of two contemporary phonic instructional approaches. *Reading Research and Instruction, 39,* 160-169.

Joslin, S. (1961). *What do you do, dear?* New York: Young Scott Books.

Joslin, S. (1986). *What do you say, dear?* New York: Harper Collins.

Juarez, M. (1983). Assessment and treatment of minority-language-handicapped children: The role of the monolingual speech-language pathologist. *Topics in Language Disorders, 3(3),* 57-66.

Junefelt, K. (2004). Identify and development: Lessons learned from a blind child. *Topics in Language Disorders, 24,* 187-100.

Jusczyk, P. (1999). Infant-toddler speech perception. *Journal of Communication Disorders, 22,* 23-29.

Just, M., and Carpenter, P. (1987). *The psychology of reading and language comprehension.* Boston, MA: Allyn & Bacon.

Just, M., Cherkassky, B., Keller, T., and Minshew, N. (2004). Cortical activation and synchronization during sentence comprehension in high-functioning autism: Evidence of underconnectivity. *Brain, 127,* 1811-1821.

Just, M.A., Carpenter, P.A., and Keller, T.A. (1996). The capacity theory of comprehension: New frontiers of evidence and arguments. *Psychological Review, 103(4),* 773-780.

Juster, N. (1961). *The phantom toll booth.* New York: Random House.

Justice, L. (2005). Influence of research and policy on practice in today's schools: Reading, evidence, and speech-language pathology. *Perspectives on Higher Education, 8(2),* 3-6.

Justice, L., Chow, S., Capellini, C., Flanigan, K., and Colton, S. (2003). Emergent literacy intervention for vulnerable preschoolers: Relative effects of two approaches. *American Journal of Speech-Language Pathology, 12,* 320-332.

Justice, L, and Ezell, H. (2002). *The syntax handbook.* Eau Claire, WI: Thinking Publications.

Justice, L., and Ezell, H. (2004). Print referencing: An emergent literacy enhancement strategy and its clinical applications. *Language, Speech, and Hearing Services in Schools, 35,* 185-193.

Justice, L., Invernizzi, M., and Meier, J. (2002). Designing and implementing an early literacy screening protocol: Suggestions for the speech-language pathologist. *Language, Speech and Hearing Services in Schools, 33,* 84-101.

Justice, L., and Kaderavek, J. (2004). Embedded-explicit emergent literacy intervention I: Background and description of approach. *Language, Speech, and Hearing Services in Schools, 35,* 201-211.

Kaderavek, J., and Justice, L. (2002). Shared storybook reading as an intervention context: Practices and potential pitfalls. *American Journal of Speech-Language Pathology, 11,* 395-407.

Kaderavek, J., and Justice, L. (2004). Embedded-explicit emergent literacy intervention II: Goal selection and implementation in the early childhood classroom. *Language, Speech, and Hearing Services in Schools, 35,* 212-228.

Kail, R. (1994). A method for studying the generalized slowing hypothesis in children with specific language impairment. *Journal of Speech and Hearing Research, 37,* 418-421.

Kaiser, A. (1993). Parent-implemented language intervention: An environmental system perspective. In A. Kaiser and D. Gray (Eds.). *Enhancing children's communication: Research foundations for intervention* (vol. 2, pp. 63-84). Baltimore, MD: Paul H. Brookes.

Kaiser, A., and Hemmeter, M. (1996). The effects of teaching parents to use responsive interaction strategies. *Topics in Early Childhood Special Education, 16,* 375-407.

Kamhi, A. (1981). Developmental vs. different theories of mental retardation: A new look. *American Journal of Mental Deficiency, 86,* 1-7.

Kamhi, A. (1987). Metalinguistic abilities in language-impaired children. *Topics in Language Disorders, 7,* 1-12.

Kamhi, A. (1993). Assessing complex behaviors: Problems with reification, quantification, and ranking. *Language, Speech, and Hearing Services in Schools, 24,* 110-113.

Kamhi, A. (1997). Three perspectives on comprehension: Implications for assessing and treating comprehension problems. *Topics in Language Disorders, 17,* 62-74.

Kamhi, A. (1998). Trying to make sense of developmental language disorders. *Language Speech and Hearing Services in Schools, 29,* 35-44.

Kahmi, A. (April 15, 2003). The role of the SLP in improving reading fluency. *The ASHA Leader,* 5-9.

Kamhi, A., Catts, H., Koenig, L., and Lewis, B. (1984). Hypothesis testing and nonlinguistic symbolic activities in language-impaired children. *Journal of Speech and Hearing Disorders, 49,* 169-176.

Kamhi, A., Catts, H., Mauer, D., Apel, K., and Gentry, B. (1988). Phonological and spatial processing abilities in language and reading-impaired children. *Journal of Learning Disabilities, 53,* 316-327.

Kamhi, A., and Catts, H. (1989). *Reading disabilities: A developmental language perspective.* Boston, MA: College-Hill Press.

Kamhi, A., and Catts, H. (2005). Language and reading: Convergences and divergences. In H. Catts and A. Kamhi (Eds.). *Language and Reading Disabilities—2nd ed.* (pp. 1-25). Boston: Allyn & Bacon.

Kamhi, A., and Johnston, J. (1982). Towards an understanding of retarded children's linguistic deficiencies. *Journal of Speech and Hearing Research, 25,* 435-445.

Kamhi, A., and Johnston, J. (1992). Semantic assessment: Determining propositional complexity. In W. Secord (Ed.). *Best practices in school speech-language pathology* (vol. II, pp. 115-122). San Antonio, TX: Psychological Corporation/Harcourt Brace Jovanovich.

Kamhi, A., and Lee, R. (1988). Cognition. In M.A. Nippold (Ed.). *Later language development: Ages nine through nineteen* (pp. 127-158). Austin, TX: Pro-Ed.

Kamhi, A., Pollock, K., and Harris, J. (1996). *Communication development and disorders in African-American children.* Baltimore, MD: Paul H. Brookes.

Kane, D. (1985). *Environmental hazards to young children.* Phoenix, AZ: Oryx Press.

Kannapell, B. (1980). Personal awareness and advocacy in the deaf community. In C. Baker and R. Battison (Eds.). *Sign language and the deaf community.* Washington, DC: National Association for the Deaf.

Kanner, L. (1943). Autistic disturbances of affective contact. *Nervous Child, 2,* 416-426.

Kaplan, R. (1966). Cultural thought patterns in intercultural education. *Language Learning, 16,* 1-2.

Karlsen, B., and Gardner, E. (2004). *Stanford diagnostic reading test* (4th ed.). San Antonio, TX: Harcourt Assessment.

Kasari, C. (2005, December). *Interventions aimed at increasing joint attention.* Paper presented at Yale Child Study Center, New Haven, CT.

Katim, D., and Harris, S. (1997). Improving the reading comprehension of middle school students in inclusive classrooms. *Journal of Adolescent and Adult Literacy, 41,* 116-123.

Kaufman, A., and Kaufman, N. (2004). *Kaufman assessment battery for children* (2nd ed.). Circle Pines, MN: American Guidance Service.

Kaufman, A., and Kaufman, N. (2005). *Kaufman brief intelligence test* (2nd ed.). Circle Pines, MN: American Guidance Service.

Kaufman, P., Kwan, J., Klein, S., and Chapman, C. (2000). Dropout rates in the United States: 1998. *Education Statistics Quarterly, 2(1),* 43-47.

Kavanaugh, J., and Mattingly, I. (1972). *Language by ear and by eye.* Cambridge, MA: MIT Press.

Kavanaugh, J., and Truss, T. (1988). *Learning disabilities: Proceedings of the national conference.* Parkton, MD: York Press.

Kay-Raining Bird, E. (2006). The Case for bilingualism in children with Down syndrome. In R. Paul (Ed.). *Language disorders from a developmental perspective: Essays in honor of Robin Chapman.* Hillsdale, NJ: Erlbaum.

Kayser, H. (1989). Speech and language assessment of Spanish-English speaking children. *Language, Speech, and Hearing Services in Schools, 20(3),* 226-244.

Kayser, H. (1991). Interpreters in speech-language pathology. *Texas Journal of Audiology and Speech Pathology, 17(1),* 28-29.

Kayser, H. (1995). *Bilingual speech-language pathology: An Hispanic focus.* San Diego, CA: Singular Publishing Group.

Kayser, H. (2002). Bilingual language development and language disorders. In D.E. Battle (Ed.). *Communication disorders in multicultural populations* (3rd ed., pp. 205-232). Boston: Butterworth-Heinneman.

Kayser, H. (2004). Biliteracy and second-language learnings. *ASHA Leader, 9,* 5-29.

Keats, E. (1962). *The snowy day.* New York: Viking Press.

Kedesdy, J., and Budd, K. (1998). *Childhood feeding disorders: Biobehavioral assessment and intervention.* Baltimore, MD: Paul H. Brookes.

Keen, D. (2003). Communicative repair strategies and problem behaviours in children with autism. *International Journal of Disability, Development, and Education, 50,* 53-65.

Keen, J. (2004). Sentence-combining and redrafting processes in the writing of secondary school students in the UK. *Linguistics and Education, 15,* 81-98.

Keith, R. (1977). *Central auditory dysfunction.* New York: Grune & Stratton.

Keith, R. (1984). Central auditory dysfunction: A language disorder? *Topics in Language Disorders, 4,* 48-56.

Kekelis, L., Chernus-Mansfield, N., and Hayashi, D. (1984). *Talk to me: A language guide for parents of blind children.* Los Angeles, CA: The Blind Childrens' Center.

Kellman, N. (1982). Noise in the intensive care nursery. *Neonatal Network,* 8-17.

Kelly, A. (2001). *Talkabout: A social communication skills package.* Oxfordshire, UK: Speechmark Publishing Limited.

Kemp, J. (1983). The timing of language intervention for the pediatric population. In J. Miller, D. Yoder, and R. Schiefelbusch (Eds.). *Contemporary issues in language intervention* (pp. 183-195). Rockville, MD: American Speech-Language-Hearing Association.

Kemper, R. (1980). A parent-assisted early childhood environmental language intervention program. *Language, Speech, and Hearing Services in Schools, 11,* 229-235.

Kendall, D. (2005). Social, economic, and environmental influences on disorders of hearing, language, and speech. *Journal of Communication Disorders, 38,* 261-262.

Kennedy, M. (2007). Principles of assessment. In R. Paul and P. Cascella (Eds.). *Introduction to clinical methods is communication disorders.* Baltimore: Paul H. Brookes. In press.

Kent, R., Miolo, G., and Bloedel, S. (1994). The intelligibility of children's speech: A review of evaluation procedures. *American Journal of Speech-Language Pathology: A Journal of Clinical Practice, 3(2),* 81-93.

Kent-Walsh, J., and McNaughton, D. (2005). Communication partner instruction in AAC: Present practice and future directions. *Augmentative and Alternative Communication, 21,* 195-204.

Kephart, N. (1960). *The slow learner in the classroom.* Columbus, OH: Merrill.

Kerrigan, W. (1974). *Writing to the point: Six basic steps.* New York: Harcourt Brace Jovanovich.

Kervin, L. (2002). Proofreading as a strategy for spelling development. *Reading Online,* 39-51.

Kevan, R. (2003). Challenging behaviour and communication difficulties. *British Journal of Learning Disabilities, 31,* 75-80.

Keysor, J., Jette, A., and Haley, S. (2005). Development of the Home and Community Environment instrument. *Journal of Rehabilitation Medicine, 37,* 37-44.

Khan, L., and Lewis, N. (2002). *Khan-Lewis phonological analysis—2nd Ed.* Circle Pines, MN: AGS Publishing.

Kidd, K. (1983). Recent progress on the genetics of stuttering. In C. Ludlow and J. Cooper (Eds.). *Genetic aspects of speech and language disorders* (pp. 197-214). New York: Academic Press.

Kiernan, B., and Gray, S. (1998). Word learning in a supported-learning context by preschool children with specific language impairment. *Journal of Speech, Language, and Hearing Research, 40,* 75-82.

Kiewel, L., and Claeys, T. (1999). *Once upon a sound.* Eau Claire, WI: Thinking Publications.

Kilgallon, D., & Kilgallon, J. (2000). *Sentence composing for elementary school: A worktext to build better sentences.* Portsmouth, NH: Heinemann.

Kilman, B., and Negri-Schoultz, N. (1987). Developing educational programs for working with students with Kanner's autism. In D.J. Cohen and A.M. Donnellan (Eds.). *Handbook of autism and pervasive developmental disorders* (pp. 440-451). New York: John Wiley & Sons.

Kim, Y., Yang, Y., and Hwang, B. (2001). Generalization effects of script-based intervention on language expression of preschool children with language disorders. *Education and Training in Mental Retardation and Developmental disabilities, 36,* 411-423.

Kimmel, E. (1990). *Anansi and the moss-covered rock.* New York: Holiday House.

King, C., and Quigley, S. (1985). *Reading and deafness.* San Diego, CA: College-Hill Press.

King, D., and Goodman, K. (1990). Whole language: Cherishing learners and their language. *Language, Speech, and Hearing Services in Schools, 21,* 221-227.

King, R., Jones, C., and Lasky, E. (1982). In retrospect: A fifteen-year follow-up report of speech-language disordered children. *Language, Speech, and Hearing Services in the Schools, 13,* 24-32.

Kinzler, M., and Johnson, C. (1993). *Joliet 3-minute speech and language screen, revised.* San Antonio, TX: Harcourt Assessment.

Kirchner, D. (1991). Reciprocal book reading: A discourse-based intervention strategy for the child with atypical language development. In T. Gallagher (Ed.). *Pragmatics of language: Clinical practice issues* (pp. 307-332). San Diego, CA: Singular Publishing Group.

Klausmeier, H., Jetter, J., and Nelson, N. (1972). *Tutoring can be fun.* Madison, WI: Wisconsin Research and Development Center for Cognitive Learning.

Klecan-Aker, J., and Hedrick, L. (1985). A study of the syntactic language skills of normal school-age children. *Topics in Language Disorders, 5(3),* 46-54.

Klecan-Aker, J., and Kelty, K. (1990). An investigation of the oral narratives of normal and language-learning disabled children. *Journal of Childhood Communication Disorders, 13,* 207-216.

Klee, T. (1992). Developmental and diagnostic characteristics of quantitative measures of children's language production. *Topics in Language Disorders, 12(2),* 28-41.

Klee, T., Carson, D. Gavin, W., Hall, L., Kent, A., and Reece, S. (1998). Concurrent and predictive validity of an early language screening program. *Journal of Speech, Language, and Hearing Research, 41,* 627-641.

Klee, T., Pearce, K., and Carson, D.K. (2000). Improving the positive predictive value of screening for developmental language disorder. *Journal of Speech, Language, & Hearing Research, 43,* 821-33.

Klee, T., Stokes, S., Wong, A., Fletcher, P., and Gavin, W. (2004). Utterance length and lexical diversity in Cantonese-speaking children with and without specific language impairment. *Journal of Speech, Language, and Hearing Research, 47,* 1396-1410.

Kleiman, K. (2003). *Functional communication scale—Revised.* East Moline, IL: LinguiSystems.

Klein, M., and Briggs, M. (1987). Facilitating mother-infant communicative interactions in mothers of high-risk infants. *Journal of Childhood Communication Disorders, 10(2)*, 95-106.

Klein, S., and Rapin, I. (1992). Intermittent conductive hearing loss and language development. In D. Bishop and K. Mogford (Eds.). *Language development in exceptional circumstances* (pp. 96-109). Hillsdale, NJ: Erlbaum.

Klein-Konigsberg, H. (1984). Semantic integration and language learning disabilities: From research to assessment and intervention. In G.P. Wallach and K.G. Butler (Eds.). *Language learning disabilities in school-age children.* Baltimore, MD: Williams and Wilkins.

Klewe, L. (1993). Brief report: An empirical evaluation of spelling boards as a means of communication for the multihandicapped. *Journal of Autism and Developmental Disorders, 23*, 559-566.

Klin, A., and Volkmar, F. (2003). Asperger syndrome. *Child and Adolescent Psychiatric Clinics of North America, 12* (whole issue).

Klin, A., Volkmar, F., and Sparrow, S. (2000). *Asperger syndrome.* New York: Guilford Press.

Klin, A., Volkmar, F., Sparrow, S., Cicchetti, D., and Rourke, B. (1995). Validity and neuropsychological characterization of Asperger syndrome: Convergence with nonverbal learning disabilities syndrome. *Journal of Child Psychology and Psychiatry, 36*, 1127-1140.

Klink, M., Gerstman, L., Raphael, L., Schlanger, B., and Newsome, L. (1986). Phonological process usage by young EMR children and nonretarded preschool children. *American Journal of Mental Deficiency, 91*, 190-195.

Klug, R. (1983). *Mystery at Pincrest Manor—Microzine No. 3* (computer program). New York: Scholastic.

Knapczyk, D. (1991). Effects of modeling in promoting generalization of student question asking and question answering. *Learning Disabilities Research and Practice, 6*, 75-82.

Knobloch, H., Stevens, F., and Malone, A. (1980). *Manual of developmental diagnosis: The administration and interpretation of the revised Gessell and Armatruda Developmental and Neurologic Examination.* Hagerstown, MA: Harper & Row.

Knutson, J., and Sullivan, P. (1993). Communicative disorders as a risk factor in abuse. *Topics in Language Disorders, 13*, 1-14.

Koegel, R., Klein, E., Koegel, L., Boettcher, M., Brookman-Frazee, L., and Openden, D. (2006). Play dates, social interactions and friendships. In R. Koegel and L. Koegel. *Pivotal response treatments for autism: Communication, social and academic development* (pp. 189-198). Baltimore: Paul H. Brookes Publishers.

Koegel, R., and Koegel, L. (2006). *Pivotal response treatments for autism: Communication, social and academic development.* Baltimore: Paul H. Brookes Publishers.

Koegel, R., Sze, K., Mossman, A., Koegel, L., and Brookman-Frazee, L. (2006). First words: Getting verbal communication started. In R. Koegel and L. Koegel (Eds.). *Pivotal response treatments for autism: Communication, social and academic development* (pp. 141-164). Baltimore: Paul H. Brookes Publishers.

Kohn, A. (1989). Suffer the restless children. *Atlantic, 264(5)*, 90-100.

Kohnert, K., and Windsor, J. (2004). The search for common ground: Part II. Nonlinguistic performance by linguistically diverse learners. *Journal of Speech, Language, and Hearing Research, 47*, 891-903.

Kohnert, K., Yim, D., Nett, K., Kan, P., and Duran, L. (2005). Intervention with linguistically diverse preschool children: A focus on developing home language(s). *Language, Speech, and Hearing Services in Schools, 36*, 251-263.

Kolvin, I., and Fundudis, T. (1981). Elective mute children: psychological development and background factors. *Journal of Child Psychology and Psychiatry, 22*, 219-232.

Koppenhaver, D., Coleman, P., Kalman, S., and Yoder, D. (1991). The implications of emergent literacy research for children with developmental disabilities. *American Journal of Speech-Language Pathology: A Journal of Clinical Practice, 1*, 38-44.

Kosel, M., and Fish, M. (1984). *The factory* (computer program). Pleasantville, New York: Sunburst Communications.

Koskinen, P., and Wilson, R. (1982a). *Developing a successful tutoring program.* New York: Teachers College Press, Columbia University.

Koskinen, P., and Wilson, R. (1982b). *Tutoring: A guide to success.* New York: Teachers College Press, Columbia University.

Koskinen, P., and Wilson, R. (1982c). *A guide for student tutors.* New York: Teachers College Press, Columbia University.

Kouri, T. (2005). Lexical training through modeling and elicitation procedures with late talkers who have specific language impairment and developmental delays. *Journal of Speech, Language, and Hearing Research, 48*, 157-172.

Kovarsky, D., Culatta, N., Franklin, A., and Theadore, G. (2001). "Communication participation" as a way of facilitating and ascertaining communicative outcomes. *Topics in Language Disorders, 21(4)*, 1-20.

Krantz, P., and McClannahan L. (1998). Social interaction skills for children with autism: A script-fading procedure for beginning readers. *Journal of Applied Behavior Analysis, 31*, 191-202.

Krassowski, E., and Plante, E. (1997). IQ variability in children with SLI: Implications for use of cognitive referencing in determining SLI. *Journal of Communication Disorders, 30*, 1-9.

Kratcoski, A. (1998). Guidelines for using portfolios in assessment and evaluation. *Journal of Speech, Language and Hearing Services in Schools, 29*, 3-10.

Kraus, N., McGee, T.J., Carrell, T.D., and Sharma, A. (1995). Neurophysiologic bases of speech discrimination. *Ear and Hearing, 16*, 19-37.

Kraus, R., and Johnson, C. (1945). *The carrot seed.* New York: Harper & Row.

Kravits, T., Kamps, D., Kemmerer, K., and Potucek, J. (2002). Brief report: In creasing communication skills for an elementary-aged student with autism using the Picture Exchange Communication System. *Journal of Autism and Developmental Disorders, 32*, 225-331.

Kretschmer, L., and Kretschmer, R. (2001). Children with hearing impairment. In T. Layton, E. Crais, and L. Watson (Eds.). *Handbook of early language impairment in children: Nature* (pp. 56-84). Albany, NY: Delmar Publishers.

Kretschmer, R. (1997). Issues in the development of school and interpersonal discourse for children who have hearing loss. *Speech, Language, and Hearing Services in Schools, 28*, 374-383.

Kritzinger, A., Louw, B., and Rossetti, L. (2001). A transdisciplinary conceptual framework for the early identification of risks for communication disorders in young children. *South African Journal of Communication Disorders, 48*, 33-44.

Kučera, H., and Francis, W. N. (1967). *Computational analysis of present-day American English.* Providence, RI: Brown University.

Kuder, S. (1997). *Teaching students with language and communication disabilities.* Boston, MA: Allyn & Bacon.

Kuhn, D., and Dean, D. (2004). Metacognition: A bridge between cognitive psychology and educational practice. *Theory Into Practice, 43*, 268-274.

Kuoch, H., and Mirenda, P. (2003). Social story interventions for young children with autism spectrum disorders. *Focus on Autism and Other Developmental Disabilities, 18*, 219-227.

Kussmaul, A. (1877). *Die Stoerungen der Sprache* (p. 211). [Disturbances in linguistic function.] Basel, Germany: Benno Schwabe.

L'Engle, M. (1962). *A wrinkle in time.* New York: Dell Publishing.

La Greca, A., and Mesibov, G. (1981). Facilitating interpersonal functioning with peers in learning disabled children. *Journal of Learning Disabilities, 14*, 197-199.

Lahey, B., Carlson, C., and Frick, P. (1992). Attention deficit disorder without hyperactivity: A review of research relevant to DSM–IV. In T.A. Widiger, A.J. Frances, H.A. Pincus, W. Davis, and M. First (Eds.). *DSM–IV sourcebook* (vol. 1). Washington, DC: American Psychiatric Association.

Lahey, M. (1988). *Language disorders and language development.* New York: Macmillan.

Lahey, M. (1990). Who shall be called language disordered? Some reflections and one perspective. *Journal of Speech and Hearing Disorders, 55*, 612-620.

Lahey, M. (1992). Linguistic and cultural diversity: Further problems for determining who shall be called language disordered. *Journal of Speech and Hearing Research, 35*, 638-641.

Lahey, M., and Bloom, L. (1977). Planning a first lexicon: Which words to teach first. *Journal of Speech and Hearing Disorders, 42*, 340-350.

Lahey, M., and Edwards, J. (1995). Specific language impairment: Preliminary investigation of factors associated with familial history and with patterns of language performance. *Journal of Speech and Hearing Research, 38*, 643-657.

Lahey, M., Liebergott, J., Chesnick, M., Menyuk, P., and Adams, J. (1992). Variability in children's use of grammatical morphemes. *Applied Psycholinguistics, 13*, 373-398.

Laing, S., and Kamhi, A. (2003). Alternative assessment of language and literacy in culturally and linguistically diverse populations. *Language, Speech, and Hearing Services in Schools, 34*, 44-55.

Laird, D.M. (1981). *The three little Hawaiian pigs and the magic shark.* Honolulu, HI: Barnaby Books.

Landa, R., Piven, J. Wzorek, M., Gayle, J., Cloud, D., Chase, G., and Folstein, S. (1992). Social language use in parents of autistic individuals. *Psychological Medicine, 22*, 245.

Landau, B., and Gleitman, L. (1985). *Language and experience: Evidence from the blind child.* Cambridge, MA: Harvard University Press.

Landau, W. (1992). Landau-Kleffner syndrome: An eponymic badge of ignorance. *Archives of Neurology, 49*, 353.

Landau, W., and Kleffner, F. (1957). Syndrome of acquired aphasia with convulsive disorder in children. *Neurology, 7*, 523-530.

Landis, M. (2002). Language and literacy, digitally speaking. *Topics in Language Disorders, 22(4)*, 55-69.

Langdon, H. (2002). Language interpreters and translators. *ASHA Leader, 7(6)*, 14-16.

Langdon, H., and Chen, L. (2002). *Collaborating with interpreters and translators: A guide for communication disorders professionals.* Eau Claire, WI: Thinking Publications.

Lanza, J., and Wilson, C. (1991). *The word kit—adolescent.* Nerang East, Queensland: Pro-Ed Australia.

Lapadat, J. (1991). Pragmatic language skills of students with language and/or learning disabilities: A quantitative synthesis. *Journal of Learning Disabilities, 24*, 147-158.

Larrivee, L., and Catts, H. (1999). Early reading achievement in children with expressive phonological disorders. *American Journal of Speech-Language Pathology, 8*, 118-128.

Larson, V., and McKinley, N. (1987). *Communication assessment and intervention strategies for adolescents.* Eau Claire, WI: Thinking Publications.

Larson, V., and McKinley, N. (1995). *Language disorders in older students.* Eau Claire, WI: Thinking Publications.

Larson, V., and McKinley, N. (2003a). *Communication solutions for older students: Assessment and Intervention Strategies.* Eau Claire, WI: Thinking Publications.

Larson, V., and McKinley, N. (2003b). Service delivery options for secondary students with language disorders. *Seminars in Speech and Language, 24*, 181-198.

Larson, V., McKinley, N., and Boley, D. (1993). Clinical forum: Adolescent language service delivery models for adolescents with language disorders. *Language, Speech, and Hearing Services in Schools, 24*, 36-42.

Lasky, E. (1991). Comprehending and processing of information in clinic and classroom. In C.S. Simon (Ed.). *Communication skills and classroom success* (pp. 113-134). San Diego, CA: College-Hill Press.

Lau v. Nichols. (1974). 94 Supreme Court, 786, CA 414, US563.

Launer, P. (1982). *Acquiring the distinction between related nouns and verbs in ASL.* Ph.D. dissertation, City University of New York.

Launer, P. (1993, March). *A collaboration model for speech-language pathologists in public schools.* Paper presented at the Oregon Speech-Language-Hearing Association, Portland, OR.

Laureate Learning Systems. *The exploring early vocabulary series* (computer program). Burlington, VT: Author.

LaVigna, G. (1987). Non-aversive strategies for managing behavior problems. In D.J. Cohen and A.M. Donnellan (Eds.). *Handbook of autism and pervasive developmental disorders* (pp. 418-429). New York: John Wiley & Sons.

Lavoie, R. (1989). *Understanding learning disabilities: How difficult can this be?* F.A.T. City Workshop. Alexandria, VA: PBS Video.

Law, J., Garrett, Z., and Nye, C. (2004). The efficacy of treatment for children with developmental speech and language delay/disorder: A meta-analysis. *Journal of Speech, Language, and Hearing Research. 47*, 924-943.

Law, J., Garrett, Z., and Nye, C. (2005). *Speech and language therapy interventions for children with primary speech and language delay or disorder* (review). New York: Wiley.

Lawrence, G. (1991). Tips for parents. *Exceptional Parent, 21*, 54.

Laws, G., and Bishop, D. (2004). Pragmatic language impairment and social deficits in Williams syndrome: A comparison with Down's syndrome and specific language impairment. *International Journal of Language and Communication Disorders, 39*, 45-64.

Layton, T. (2001). Young children with Down syndrome. In T. Layton, E. Crais, and L. Watson (Eds.). *Handbook of early language impairment in children: Nature* (pp. 302-360). Albany, NY: Delmar Publishers.

Layton, T., and Watson, L. (1995). Enhancing communication in nonverbal children with autism. In K. Quill (Ed.). *Teaching children with autism* (pp. 73-101). New York: Delmar.

Leadholm, B., and Miller, J. (1992). *Language sample analysis: The Wisconsin guide.* Madison, WI: Wisconsin Department of Public Instruction.

Learning Company. (1996). *The ultimate writing and creativity center.* Cambridge, MA: Author.

Learning Company. (2004). *Storybook weaver deluxe.* Cambridge, MA: Author.

Learning Upgrade LLC. (1999). *Secret writer's society.* San Diego, CA: Author.

LearningExpress. (2002). *501 Word analogies questions & answers.* New York: Author.

Leavell, C. (1996, August). *Central auditory processing and attention in children with learning/behavioral problems.* Paper presented at the 104th Annual Convention of the American Psychological Association, Toronto, Canada.

Lederer, F. (1973). Granulomas and other specific diseases of the ear and temporal bone. In M. Paparella and D. Shumrick (Eds.). *Otolaryngology (vol. 2, Ear).* Philadelphia, PA: W.B. Saunders.

Lederer, S. (2001). Efficacy of parent-child language group intervention for late-talking toddlers. *Infant-Toddler Intervention, 11*, 223-235.

Lee, D., and Allen, R. (1963). *Learning to read through experience.* New York: Appleton-Century-Crofts.

Lee, L. (1966). Developmental sentence types: A method for comparing normal and deviant syntactic development. *Journal of Speech and Hearing Disorders, 31*, 311-330.

Lee, L. (1971). *Northwestern screening syntax test.* Evanston, IL: Northwestern University Press.

Lee, L. (1974). *Developmental sentence analysis.* Evanston, IL: Northwestern University Press.

Lee, L., Koenigsknecht, R., and Mulhern, S. (1975). *Interactive language development teaching.* Evanston, IL: Northwestern University Press.

Leet, H., and Dunst, C. (1988). Family Resource Scale. In C. Dunst, C. Trivette, and A. Deal (Eds.). *Enabling and empowering families: Principles and guidelines for practice.* Cambridge, MA: Brookline Books.

Lefton-Grief, M., and Loughlin, G. (1996). Specialized students in pediatric dysphagia. *Seminars in Speech and Language, 17*, 311-332.

Lehmann, M., Charron, K., Kummer, A., and Keith, R. (1979). The effects of chronic middle ear effusion on speech and language development—a descriptive study. *International Journal of Pediatric Otorhinolaryngology, 1*, 137-144.

Leitao, S., and Fletcher, J. (2004). Literacy outcomes for students with speech impairment: Long-term follow-up. *International Journal of Language and Communication Disorders, 39*, 245-256.

Leonard, C.M., Lombardino, L.J., Walsh, K., Eckert, M.A., Mockler, J.L., Rowe, L.A., Williams, S., and DeBose, C.B. (2002). Anatomical risk factors that distinguish dyslexia from SLI predict reading skill in normal children. *Journal of Communication Disorders, 35*, 501-531.

Leonard, L. (1975a). Modeling as a clinical procedure in language training. *Language, Speech, and Hearing Services in the Schools, 6*, 72-85.

Leonard, L. (1975b). The role of nonlinguistic stimuli and semantic relations in children's acquisition of grammatical utterances. *Journal of Experimental Child Psychology, 19*, 346-357.

Leonard, L. (1981). Facilitating linguistic skills in children with specific language impairment. *Applied Psycholinguistics, 2*, 89-118.

Leonard, L. (1983). Defining the boundaries of language disorders in children. In J. Miller, D. Yoder, and R. Schiefelbusch (Eds.). *Contemporary issues in language intervention.* Rockville, MD: American Speech-Language-Hearing Association.

Leonard, L. (1987). Is specific language impairment a useful construct? In S. Rosenberg (Ed.). *Advances in applied psycholinguistics (vol. 1, Disorders of first language acquisition*, pp. 1-39). New York: Cambridge University Press.

Leonard, L. (1989). Language learnability and specific language impairment in children. *Applied Psycholinguistics, 10,* 179-202.

Leonard, L. (1991). Specific language impairment as a clinical category. *Language, Speech, and Hearing Services in Schools, 22,* 66-68.

Leonard, L. (1994). Some problems facing accounts of morphological deficits in children with specific language impairments. In R. Watkins and M. Rice (Eds.). *Specific language impairments in children* (vol. 4, pp. 91-105). Baltimore, MD: Paul H. Brookes.

Leonard, L. (1995). Prosodic and syntactic bootstrapping and their clinical implications. *American Journal of Speech-Language Pathology, 4,* 66-72.

Leonard, L. (1997). *Children with specific language impairment.* Cambridge, MA: MIT Press.

Leonard, L., and Fey, M. (1991). Facilitating grammatical development: The contribution of pragmatics. In T. Gallagher (Ed.). *Pragmatics of language: Clinical practice issues* (pp. 333-356). San Diego, CA: Singular Publishing Group.

Leonard, L., and Finneran, D. (2003). Grammatical morpheme effects on MLU: "The same can be less" revisited. *Journal of Speech, Language, and Hearing Research, 46,* 878-888.

Leonard, L., and Weiss, A. (1983). Application of nonstandardized assessment procedures to diverse linguistic populations. *Topics in Language Disorders, 3(3),* 35-45.

Leonard, L., Bortolini, U., Caselli, M., McGregor, K., and Sabbadini, L. (1992). Morphological deficits in children with specific language impairment: The status of features in underlying grammar. *Language Acquisition, 2,* 151-180.

Leonard, L., Camarata, S., Rowan, L., and Chapman, K. (1982). The communicative functions of lexical usage by language-impaired children. *Applied Psycholinguistics, 3,* 109-125.

Leonard, L., Cole, B., and Steckol, K. (1979). Lexical usage of retarded children: An examination of informativeness. *American Journal of Mental Deficiency, 84,* 49-54.

LeSieg, T. (1961). *Ten apples up on top.* New York: Random House.

Leslie, L., and Caldwell, J. (2001). *Qualitative Reading Inventory—3.* New York: Addison-Wesley Longman.

Lester, B., LaGasse, L., and Bigsby, R. (1998). Prenatal cocaine exposure and child development: What do we know and what do we do? *Seminars in Speech and Language, 19,* 123-146.

Lester, J. (1990). *Further tales of Uncle Remus: The misadventures of Brer Rabbit, Brer Fox, Brer Wolf, the doodang, and other creatures.* New York: Dial Books.

Letts., C., and Leinonen, E. (2001). Comprehension of inferential meaning in language-impaired and language normal children. *International Journal of Language and Communication Disorders, 36,* 307-328.

Leventhal, T., Selner-O'Hagan, M., Brookes-Gunn, J., Bingenheimer, J., and Earls, F. (2004). The Homelife interview from the Project on Human Development in Chicago Neighborhoods: Assessment of parenting and home environment for 3- to 15-year olds. *Parenting: Science & Practice, 4,* 211-241.

Levett, L., and Muir, J. (1983). Which three year olds need speech therapy? Uses of the Levett-Muir language screening test. *Health Visitor, 56(12),* 454-456.

Levin, H.S., Song, J., Ewing-Cobbs, L., Chapman, S.B., and Mendelsohn, D. (2001). Word fluency in relation to severity of closed head injury, associated frontal brain lesions, and age at injury in children. *Neuropsychologia, 39(2),* 122-131.

Levin, J., Johnson, D., Pittelman, S., Haynes, B., Levin, K., Shriberg, L., and Toms-Bronowski, S. (1984). A comparison of semantic and mnemonic-based vocabulary-learning strategies. *Reading Psychology, 5,* 1-15.

Levine, L. (1988). *Great beginnings™ for early language learning: Nouns 1, nouns 2, concepts, associations, prepositions.* Austin, TX: Pro-Ed.

Levithan, D. (2004). *The realm of possibility.* New York: Knopf Books for Young Readers.

Levitt, H., McGarr, N., and Geffner, D. (1988). *Development of language and communication skills in hearing-impaired children.* ASHA Monographs (No. 26). Rockville, MD: American Speech-Language-Hearing Association.

Lewis, B., and Boucher, T. (1999). *Test of pretend play.* Sydney, Australia: The Psychological Corporation.

Lewis, B., and Thompson, L. (1992). A study of developmental speech and language disorders in twins. *Journal of Speech and Hearing Research, 35,* 1086-1094.

Lewis, B., Ekelman, B., and Aram, D. (1989). A familial study of severe phonological disorders. *Journal of Speech and Hearing Research, 32,* 713-724.

Lewis, B., Freebairn, L., Heeger, S., and Cassidy, S. (2002). Speech and language skills in individuals with Prader-Willi syndrome. *American Journal of Speech-Language Pathology, 11,* 285-294.

Lewis, B., Singer, L., Short, E., Minnes, S., Arendt., R., Weishampel, P., Klein, N., and Min, M. (2004). Four-year language outcomes of children exposed to cocaine in utero. *Neurotoxicology and Teratology, 26,* 617-627.

Lewkowicz, N. (1980). Phonemic awareness training: What to teach and how to teach it. *Journal of Educational Psychology, 72,* 686-700.

Liberman, I. (1985). Should so-called modality preferences determine the nature of instruction for children with reading disabilities? In J. Duffy and N. Geshwind (Eds.). *Dyslexia: A neuroscientific approach to clinical evaluation.* Boston, MA: Little, Brown.

Liberman, I., and Liberman, A. (1990). Whole language vs. code emphasis: Underlying assumptions and their implications for reading instruction. *Annals of Dyslexia, 40,* 51-76.

Lidz, C., and Gindis, B. (2003). Dynamic assessment of evolving cognitive functions in children. In A. Kozulin, B. Gindis, V. Ageyev, and S. Miller (Eds.). *Vygotsky's educational theory in cultural context* (pp. 99-116). New York: Cambridge University Press.

Lidz, C., and Peña, E. (1996). Dynamic assessment: The model, its relevance as a nonbiased approach, and its application to Latino American preschool children. *Language, Speech, and Hearing Services in Schools, 27,* 367-384.

Lieberth, A., and Martin, D. (1995). Authoring and hypermedia. *Language, Speech, and Hearing Services in Schools, 26,* 241-250.

Light, J. (1997). Reflections on the contexts of language learning for children who use aided AAC. *Alternative and Augmentative Communication, 13,* 158-171.

Light, J., and Drager, K. (2002). Improving the design of augmentative and alternative technologies for young children. *Assistive Technology, 14,* 17-32.

Light, J., and McNaughton, D. (1993). Literacy and augmentative and alternative communication (AAC): The expectations and priorities of parents and teachers. *Topics in Language Disorders, 13(2),* 33-46.

Liles, B. (1985). Cohesion in the narratives of normal and language-disordered children. *Journal of Speech and Hearing Research, 28,* 123-133.

Liles, B. (1987). Episode organization and cohesive conjunctions in narratives of children with and without language disorders. *Journal of Speech and Hearing Research, 30,* 185-196.

Liles, B.Z, and Purcell, S. (1987). Departures in the spoken narratives of normal and language disordered children. *Applied Psycholinguistics, 8(2),* 185-202.

Lim, Y.S., and Cole, K.N. (2002). Facilitating first language development in young Korean children through parent training in picture book interactions. *Bilingual Research Journal, 26(2),* 213-227.

Linares, N. (1981). Rules for calculating mean length of utterance in morphemes for Spanish. In J. Erickson and D. Omark (Eds.). *Communication assessment of the bilingual bicultural child* (pp. 291-296). Baltimore, MD: University Park Press.

Lindamood, C., and Lindamood, P. (2004). *Lindamood auditory conceptualization test—Third edition.* Austin, TX: Pro-Ed.

Linder, T. (1993). *Transdisciplinary play-based assessment: A functional approach to working with young children.* Baltimore, MD: Paul H. Brookes.

Lindsay, J. (1973). Profound childhood deafness: Inner ear pathology. *The Annals of Otology, Rhinology, and Laryngology, 82(suppl. 5).*

Ling, D. (1976). *Speech and the hearing-impaired child: Theory and practice.* Washington, DC: A.G. Bell Association for the Deaf.

Ling, D. (1989). *Foundations of spoken language for hearing-impaired children.* Washington, DC: A.G. Bell Association for the Deaf.

Linguisystems, (2002). *VocabOPOLY.* East Moline, IL: Linguisystems.

Linn, R.L., and Miller, M.D. (2005). *Measurement and assessment in teaching* (9th ed.). Upper Saddle River, NJ: Pearson Education.

Lipman, M., and Sharp, A. (1974). *Harry Stottlemeier's discovery.* Upper Montclair, NJ: Institute for Advancement of Philosophy for Children.

Lipsky, D., and Gartner, A. (1997). *Inclusion and school reform: Transforming American classrooms.* Baltimore, MD: Paul H. Brookes.

Lively, M. (1984). Developmental sentence scoring: Common scoring errors. *Language, Speech, and Hearing Services in Schools, 15,* 154-168.

Lloyd, L., Fuller, D., and Arvidson, H. (1997). *Augmentative and alternative communication: A handbook of principles and practices.* Boston: Allyn & Bacon.

Lloyd, P. (1994). Referential communication: Assessment and intervention. *Topics in Language Disorders, 14(3),* 55-69.

Loban, W. (1976). *Language development: Kindergarten through grade twelve.* Urbana, IL: National Council of Teachers of English.

Lobel, A. (1975). *Owl at home.* New York: Harper & Row.

Lobel, A. (1977). *How rooster saved the day.* New York: Greenwillow Books.

Locke, J. (2005). Language and life. *ASHA Leader, 10(10),* 6-26.

Lockhart, B. (1992). Read to me, talk with me. Tucson, AZ: Communication Skill Builders.

LocuTour Multimedia. *Basic Words for Children CD-ROM: Version 2* (computer program). San Luis Obispo, CA: Author.

Loeb, D., Pye, C., Redmond, S., and Richardson, L. (1996). Eliciting verbs from children with specific language impairment. *American Journal of Speech-Language Pathology, 5,* 17-30.

Loeb, D., Stoke, C., and Fey, M. (2001). Language changes associated with Fast ForWord-Language: Evidence from case studies. *American Journal of Speech-Language Pathology, 10,* 216-230.

LoGiudice, C., and LoGiudice, M. (2004). *All-star vocabulary.* East Moline, IL: Linguisystems.

LoGiudice, C., and McConnell, N. (2004). *Room 28.* East Moline, IL: Linguisystems.

Logowriter Computer Systems. (1990). *Logowriter* (computer program). New York: Logo Computer Systems.

London, J. (1963). *The call of the wild and other stories.* New York: Grosset & Dunlap.

Long, C., Blackman, J., Farrell, W., Smolkin, M., and Conaway, M. (2005). A comparison of developmental versus functional assessment in the rehabilitation of young children. *Pediatric Rehabilitation, 8,* 156-161.

Long, S. (1999). Technology applications in the assessment of children's language. *Seminars in Speech and Language, 20,* 117-132.

Long, S. (2001). About time: A comparison of computerized and manual procedures for grammatical and phonological analysis. *Clinical Linguistics and Phonetics, 15,* 399-426.

Long, S., and Channell, R. (2001). Accuracy of four language analysis procedures performed automatically. *American Journal of Speech-Language Pathology, 10,* 180-188.

Long, S., and Fey, M. (2004). *Computerized profiling* (computer program; version 6.9). Milwaukee, WI: Marquette University.

Longhurst, T., and File, J. (1977). *A comparison of developmental sentence scores from Head Start children collected in four conditions.* Unpublished manuscript, Kansas State University, Manhattan, KS.

Lopez, L., and Greenfield, D. (2004). The cross-linguistic transfer of phonological skills of Hispanic Head Start children. *Bilingual Research Journal, 28,* 1-18.

Lord, C. (1985). Autism and the comprehension of language. In E. Schopler and G. Mesibov (Eds.). *Communication problems in autism.* New York: Plenum Press.

Lord, C. (1988). Enhancing communication in adolescents with autism. *Topics in Language Disorders, 9(1),* 72-81.

Lord, C. (1995). Follow-up of two-year-olds referred for possible autism. *Journal of Child Psychology and Psychiatry, 36,* 1365-1382.

Lord, C., and McGee, J. (Eds.). (2001). *Educating children with autism.* Washington, DC: National Academy of Sciences.

Lord, C., and Paul, R. (1997). Language and communication in autism. In D. Cohen and F. Volkmar (Eds.). *Handbook of autism and pervasive developmental disorders* (ed. 22nd ed., pp. 195-225). New York: John Wiley & Sons.

Lord, C., Risi, S., Lambrecht, L., Cook, E., Leventhal, B., DiLavore, P., Pickles, A., and Rutter, M. (2000). The Autism Diagnostic Observation Schedule-Generic: A standard measure of social and communication deficits associated with the spectrum of autism. *Journal of Autism & Developmental Disorders, 30,* 205-223.

Lord, C., Rutter, M., and DiLavore, P.C. (1998). *Autism diagnostic observation schedule—generic.* Unpublished manuscript, University of Chicago, Chicago, IL.

Lord, C., Rutter, M., and LeCouteur, A. (1994). Autism diagnostic interview—revised: A revised version of a diagnostic interview for caregivers of individuals with possible pervasive developmental disorders. *Journal of Autism and Developmental Disorders, 24,* 659-685.

Lord, C., Rutter, M., and Le Couteur, A. (2002). *Autism diagnostic interview.* Los Angeles, CA: Western Psychological Services.

Lord, C., Shulman, C., and DiLavore, P. (2004). Regression and word loss in autistic spectrum disorders. *Journal of Child Psychology and Psychiatry, 45,* 936-955.

Losardo, A., and Notari-Syverson, A. (2001). *Alternative approaches to assessing young children.* Baltimore: Paul H. Brookes.

Louie, A.L. (1982). *Yeh-Shen: A Cinderella story from China.* New York: Philomel Books.

Lovaas, O., Berberich, J., Perloff, B., and Schaeffer, B. (1966). Acquisition of imitative speech by schizophrenic children. *Science, 151,* 701-707.

Lovaas, O.I. (1987). Behavioral treatment and normal educational and intellectual functioning in young autistic children. *Journal of Consulting and Clinical Psychology, 55,* 3-9.

Lowe, M., and Costello, A. (1976). *Manual for the symbolic play test* (experimental ed.). London: NFER-Nelson.

Lowe, M., and Costello, A. (1988). *Symbolic play test—2nd edition.* London: NFER-Nelson.

Lowell, S. (1992). *The three little javelinas.* Flagstaff, AZ: Northland Publishing.

Lowman, D., Murphy, S., and Snell, M. (1999). *The educator's guide to feeding children with disabilities.* Baltimore, MD: Paul H. Brookes.

Lucariello, J. (1990). Freeing talk from the here-and-now: The role of event knowledge and maternal scaffolds. *Topics in Language Disorders, 10(3),* 14-29.

Luckasson, R., Borthwick-Duffy, S., Buntinx, D., Coulter, D., Craig, E., Reeve, A., Schalock, R., Snell, M., Spitalnik, D., Spreat, S., and Tasse, M. (2002). *Mental retardation: Definition, classification, and systems of supports—10th ed.* Washington, DC: American Association for Mental Retardation.

Ludlow, C., and Cooper, J. (1983). Genetic aspects of speech and language disorders: Current status and future directions. In C.L. Ludlow and J.A. Cooper (Eds.). *Genetic aspects of speech and language disorders* (pp. 1-20). New York: Academic Press.

Lund, N., and Duchan, J. (1993). *Assessing children's language in naturalistic contexts* (3rd ed.). Englewood Cliffs, NJ: Prentice-Hall.

Lunday, A. (1996). A collaborative communication skills program for Job Corps centers. *Topics in Language Disorders, 16,* 23-36.

Lundberg, I. (1994). Reading difficulties can be predicted and prevented. In C. Hulme and M. Snowling, (Eds.). *Reading development and dyslexia* (p. 180-199). London: Whurr.

Lundberg, I., Frost, J., and Petersen, O. (1988). Effects of an extensive program for stimulating phonological awareness in preschool children. *Reading Research Quarterly, 23,* 263-285.

Lundgren, K. (1998). Play in children with cocaine exposure: Development and implications for assessment. *Seminars in Speech and Language, 19,* 189-199.

Lynch, E. (2004a). Conceptual framework: From culture shock to cultural learning. In E. Lynch and M. Hanson (Eds.). *Developing cross-cultural competence* (3rd ed., pp. 19-40). Baltimore, MD: Paul H. Brookes Publishing.

Lynch, E. (2004b). Developing cross-cultural competence. In E. Lynch and M. Hanson (Eds.). *Developing cross-cultural competence* (3rd ed., pp. 41-78). Baltimore, MD: Paul H. Brookes Publishing.

Lynch, E., and Hanson, M. (2004a). Children of many songs. In E. Lynch and M. Hanson (Eds.). *Developing cross-cultural competence* (3rd ed., pp. 441-446). Baltimore, MD: Paul H. Brookes.

Lynch, E., and Hanson, M. (2004b). Steps in the right direction: Implications for service providers. In E. Lynch and M. Hanson (Eds.). *Developing cross-cultural competence* (3rd ed., pp. 449-466). Baltimore: Paul H. Brookes Publishing.

Lynch, M., and Roberts, J. (1982). The consequences of child abuse. New York: Academic Press.

Lynch-Fraser, D., and Tiegerman, E. (1987). *Baby signals.* New York: Walker and Co.

Lyon, G., Shaywitz, S., and Shaywitz, B. (2003). A definition of dyslexia. *Annals of Dyslexia, 53,* 1-14.

Lyon, R. (1999). Reading development, reading disorders, and reading instruction. *Language, Learning, and Education Newsletter, 6 (1),* 8-17.

Lyytinen, P., Eklund, K., and Lyytinen, H. (2003). The play and language behavior of mothers with and without dyslexia and its association to their toddlers' language development. *Journal of Learning Disabilities, 36*, 74-86.

Lyytinen, P., Poikkeus, A., Laakso, M., Eklund, K., and Lyytinen, H. (2001). Language development and symbolic play in children with and without familial risk for dyslexia. *Journal of Speech, Language, and Hearing Research, 44*, 873-885.

Maag, J., and Reid, R. (1996). Treatment of attention deficit hyperactivity disorder: A multi-modal model for schools. *Seminars in Speech and Language, 17*, 37-58.

MacArthur, C. (2000). New tools for writing: Assistive technology for students with writing difficulties. *Topics in Language Disorders, 20(4)*, 85-104.

MacArthur, C., Haynes, J., and DeLaPaz, S. (1996). Spelling checkers and students with learning disabilities. *Journal of Learning Disabilities, 30*, 35-57.

MacDonald, J. (1978). *Environmental language inventory.* Columbus, OH: Charles E. Merrill.

MacDonald, J. (1989). *Becoming partners with children: From play to conversation.* San Antonio, TX: Special Press.

MacDonald, J., Blott, J., Gordon, K., Spiegel, B., and Hartmann, M. (1974). An experimental parent-assisted treatment program for preschool language-delayed children. *Journal of Speech and Hearing Disorders, 39*, 395-415.

MacDonald, J., and Carroll, J. (1992). A social partnership model for assessing early communication development: An intervention model for preconversational children. *Language, Speech, and Hearing Services in Schools, 23*, 113-124.

Mackie, C., and Dockrell, J. (2004). The nature of written language deficits in children with SLI. *Journal of Speech, Language, and Hearing Research, 47*, 1469-1483.

MacLachlan, P. (1985). *Sarah, plain and tall.* New York: Harper & Row.

MacWhinney, B. (1987). *CHAT manual* (computer program). Pittsburgh, PA: Carnegie-Mellon University.

MacWhinney, B. (1996). The CHILDES system. *American Journal of Speech-Language Pathology, 5 (1)*, 5-14.

MacWhinney, B. (2000). *The CHILDES project: Tools for analyzing talk. Volume 1: Transcription format and programs. Volume 2: The database.* Mahwah, NJ: Lawrence Erlbaum Associates.

Madison, L., George, C., and Moeschler, J. (1986). Cognitive functioning in the fragile-X syndrome: A study of intellectual, memory, and communication skills. *Journal of Mental Deficiency Research, 30*, 129-148.

Maestas, A., and Erickson, J. (1992). Mexican immigrants mothers' beliefs about disabilities. *American Journal of Speech-Language Pathology: A Journal of Clinical Practice, 1(4)*, 5-10.

Magiati, I., and Howlin, P. (2003). A pilot evaluation study of PECS for children with autism spectrum disorder. *Autism: The International Journal of Research & Practice, 7*, 297-320.

Mahoney, G., and Powell, A. (1986). *Transactional intervention program.* Farmington, CT: Pediatric Research and Training Center, University of Connecticut Health Center.

Mahoney, G., and Spiker, D. (1996). Clinical assessment of parent child interaction: Are professionals ready to implement this practice? *Topics in Early Childhood Special Education, 16*, 43-49.

Malecki, C., and Jewell, J. (2003). Developmental, gender, and practical considerations in scoring curriculum-based measurement writing probes. *Psychology in the Schools, 40*, 379-391.

Malkmus, D. (1989). Community reentry: Cognitive-communicative intervention within a social skill context. *Topics in Language Disorders, 9(2)*, 50-66.

Manhardt, J., and Rescorla, L. (2002). Oral narrative skills of late talkers at ages 8 and 9. *Applied Psycholinguistics, 23*, 1-21.

Mann, V., and Liberman, I. (1984). Phonological awareness and verbal short-term memory. *Journal of Learning Disabilities, 17*, 592-598.

Mann, V., Liberman, I., and Shankweiler, D. (1980). Children's memory for sentences and word strings in relation to reading ability. *Memory and Cognition, 8*, 329-335.

Mannix, D. (2002a). *Life skills activities for secondary students with special needs* (2nd ed.). Indianapolis, IN: Jossey-Bass.

Mannix, D. (2002b). *Social skills activities: For secondary students with special needs.* Indianapolis, IN: Jossey-Bass.

Manolson, A. (1992). *It takes two to talk.* Bisbee, AZ: Imaginart.

Manolson, A. (1995). *You make the difference.* Toronto, Ontario: The Hanen Centre.

March of Dimes (2003). *Perinatal profiles: Statistics for monitoring state maternal and infant health.* Retrieved July 28, 2005, from http://www.marchofdimes.com/peristats/

Marchman, V., and Martinez-Sussmann, C. (2002). Concurrent validity of caregiver/parent report measures of language for children who are learning both English and Spanish. *Journal of Speech, Language, and Hearing Research, 45*, 983-997.

Marcus, G.F., and Fisher, S. (2003). FOXP-2 in focus: What can genes tell us about speech and language? *Trends in Cognitive Sciences, 7(6)*, 257-262.

Mardell-Czudnowski, D., and Goldenberg, D. (1998). *DIAL-3: Developmental indicators for the assessment of learning—Third edition.* Circle Pines, MN: American Guidance Service.

Margalit, M., and Al-Yagon, M. (2002). The loneliness experience of children with learning disabilities. In B.Y.L. Wong and M. Donahue (Eds.). *The social dimensions of learning disabilities: Essays in Honor of Tanis Bryan* (Volume in the Special Education and Exceptionality Series, pp. 53-76). Mahwah, NJ: Erlbaum.

Marge, M. (1984). The prevention of communication disorders. *ASHA, 26*, 29-33.

Marge, M. (1993). Disability prevention: Are we ready for the challenge? *ASHA, 35*, 42-44.

Marinellie, S. (2004). Complex syntax used by school-age children with specific language impairment (SLI) in child-adult conversation. *Journal of Communication Disorders, 37*, 517-533.

Marler, J., Champlin, C., and Gillam, R. (2001). Backward and simultaneous masking measured in children with language-learning impairments who received intervention with Fast ForWord or Laureate Learning Systems software. *American Journal of Speech-Language Pathology, 10*, 258-268.

Marquis, M. (1999a). *Creatures and critters.* San Antonio, TX: Communication Skill Builders.

Marquis, M. (1999b). *Tales and scales.* San Antonio, TX: Communication Skill Builders.

Marquis, M. (2004). *Creatures and critters: Barrier games for referential communication.* Austin, TX: Pro-Ed.

Marquis, M., and Addy-Trout, E. (1992). *Social communication: Activities for improving peer interactions and self-esteem.* Eau Claire, WI: Thinking Publications.

Marquis, M., and Blog, T. (1993). *Barrier games with unisets.* Tucson, AZ.: Communication Skill Builders.

Marschark, M., and West, S. (1985). Creative language abilities of deaf children. *Journal of Speech and Hearing Research, 28*, 73-78.

Marshall, J. (1972). *George and Martha.* Boston, MA: Houghton Mifflin.

Marshall, J. (1988). *Goldilocks and the three bears.* New York: Dial Books for Young Readers.

Marshall, K. (1991). Cognitive behavior modification in the classroom: Theoretical and practical perspectives. In C.S. Simon (Ed.). *Communication skills and classroom success* (pp. 59-78). San Diego, CA: College-Hill.

Martin Luther King Junior Elementary School Children v. Ann Arbor School District Board. (1979). 473 F. Supp. 1371.

Martin, B., and Carle, E. (1995). *Brown bear, brown bear, what do you see?* New York: Holt and Co.

Marton, K. (2005). Social cognition and language in children with specific language impairment. *Journal of Communication Disorders, 38*, 143-163.

Marton, K., Abramoff, B., and Rosenzweig, S. (2005). Social cognition and language in children with specific language impairment (SLI). *Journal of Communication Disorders, 38(2)*, 143-162.

Marvin, C. (1990). Problems in school-based speech-language consultation and collaboration services: Defining the terms and improving the process. In W. Secord (Ed.). *Best practices in school speech-language pathology* (pp. 37-48). San Antonio, TX: Psychological Corporation, Harcourt Brace Jovanovich.

Marx, J. (1975). Cytomegalovirus: A major cause of birth defects. *Science, 190*, 1184-1186.

Masterson, J., and Crede, L. (1999). Learning to spell: Implications for assessment and intervention. *Language, Speech, and Hearing Services in Schools, 30*, 243-254.

Masterson, J., and Perry, C. (1999). Training analogical reasoning skills in children with language disorders. *American Journal of Speech-Language Pathology, 8*, 53-61.

Mastropieri, M., and Scruggs, T. (1997). Best practices in promoting reading comprehension in students with learning disabilities. *Remedial and Special Education, 4*, 197-213.

Mattes, L., and Santiago, G. (1985). *Bilingual language proficiency questionnaire.* oceanside, ca: academic communication associates.

Matthews, T. (1995). *Jump to a conclusion!* Oceanside, CA: Academic Communication Associates.

Maxwell, S., and Wallach, G. (1984). The language-learning disabilities connection: Symptoms of early language disability change over time. In G. Wallach and K. Butler (Eds.). *Language and learning disabilities in school-aged children.* Baltimore, MD: Williams and Wilkins.

Mayer, M. (1967). *A boy, a dog and a frog.* New York: Dial Books for Young Readers.

Mayer, M. (1968). *If I had.* New York: Dial Press.

Mayer, M. (1975). *Just for you.* New York: Golden Press.

Mayer, M. (1976). *Liza Lou.* New York: Four Winds Press.

Mayer, M., and Mayer, M. (1971). *A boy, a dog, a frog, and a friend.* New York: Dial Books.

Mayfield, S. (1983). Language and speech behaviors of children with undue lead absorption: A review of the literature. *Journal of Speech and Hearing Research, 26*, 362-368.

Mayo, P., and Waldo, P. (1994). *Scripting: Social communication for adolescents.* Eau Claire, WI: Thinking Publications.

McArthur, G.M., and Bishop, D.V.M. (2004). Which people with specific language impairment have auditory processing deficits? *Cognitive Neuropsychology, 21(1)*, 79-94.

McBride, J., and Levy, K. (1981). The early academic classroom for children with communication disorders. In A. Gerber and D.N. Bryen (Eds.). *Language and learning disabilities* (pp. 269-294). Baltimore, MD: University Park Press.

McCabe, A. (1989). Differential language learning styles in young children: The importance of context. *Developmental Review, 9*, 1-20.

McCabe, A. (1995). Evaluating narrative discourse skills. In K. Cole, P. Dale, and D. Thal (Eds.). *Assessment of communication and language* (pp. 121-141). Baltimore, MD: Paul H. Brookes.

McCabe, A., and Bliss, L. (2003). *Patterns of narrative discourse: A multicultural lifespan approach.* Boston: Allyn & Bacon.

McCabe, A., and Rollins, P. (1994). Assessment of preschool narrative skills. *The Journal of Speech-Language Pathology, 3(1)*, 45-56.

McCarney, S.B. (1986). *The attention deficit disorders evaluation scale (ADDES).* Columbia, MO: Hawthorne Educational Services, Inc.

McCarr, D. (1995). *Multiple meanings for the young adult.* Austin, TX: Pro-Ed, Inc.

McCarthy, C.F., Mclean, L.K., Miller, J.F., Brown, D.P., Romski, M.A., Rourk, J.D., and Yoder, D.E. (1998). *Communication supports checklist for programs serving individuals with severe disabilities.* Baltimore, MD: Paul H. Brookes.

McCathren, R., Yoder, R., and Warren, S. (1999). The relationship between prelinguistic vocalization and later expressive vocabulary in young children with developmental delay. *Journal of Speech, Language, and Hearing Research, 42*, 915-924.

McCauley, R. (1989). Measurement is a dangerous activity. *Journal of Speech-Language Pathology and Audiology, 13*, 29-32.

McCauley, R. (1996). Familiar strangers: Criterion-referenced measures in communication disorders. *Language, Speech, and Hearing Services in Schools, 27*, 122-131.

McCauley, R., and Fey, M. (2006). Introduction. In R. McCauley and M. Fey (Eds.). *Treatment of language disorders in children* (pp. 1-17). Baltimore: Paul H. Brookes. In press.

McCauley, R., and Swisher, L. (1984a). Psychometric review of language and articulation tests for preschool children. *Journal of Speech and Hearing Disorders, 49*, 34-42.

McCauley, R., and Swisher, L. (1984b). Use and misuse of norm-referenced tests in clinical assessment: A hypothetical case. *Journal of Speech and Hearing Disorders, 49*, 338-348.

McConnell, N., and LoGiudice, C. (1998). *That's LIFE! Social language.* East Moline, IL: Linguisystems.

McCord, J., and Haynes, W. (1988). Discourse errors in students with learning disabilities and their normally achieving peers: Molar versus molecular views. *Journal of Learning Disabilities, 21*, 237-243.

McCormick, L. (1997a). Ecological assessment and planning. In L. McCormick, D. Loeb, and R. Shiefelbusch (Eds.). *Supporting children with communication difficulties in inclusive settings—Second edition* (pp. 235-258). Boston: Allyn & Bacon.

McCormick, L. (1997b). Language intervention and support. In L. McCormick, D. Loeb, and R. Schiefelbusch (Eds.). *Supporting children with communication difficulties in inclusive settings—Second edition* (pp. 259-296). Boston: Allyn & Bacon.

McCormick, L. (1997c). Policies and practices. In L. McCormick, D. Loeb, and R. Schiefelbusch (Eds.). *Supporting children with communication difficulties in inclusive settings—Second edition* (pp. 155-188). Boston: Allyn & Bacon.

McCormick, L. (2003). Ecological assessment and planning. In L. McCormick, D. Loeb, and R. Schiefelbusch (Eds.). *Supporting children with communication difficulties in inclusive settings* (pp. 235-258). Boston: Allyn & Bacon.

McCormick, L., and Goldman, R. (1984). Designing an optimal learning program. In L. McCormick and R. Schiefelbusch (Eds.). *Early language intervention: An introduction* (pp. 201-242). Columbus, OH: Merrill.

McCormick, L., and Loeb, D. (2003). Characteristics of students with language and communication difficulties. In L. McCormick, D. Loeb, and R. Schiefelbusch (Eds.). *Supporting children with communication difficulties in inclusive settings—Second edition* (pp. 71-112). Boston: Allyn & Bacon.

McCormick, L., Loeb, D., and Schiefelbusch, R. (2003). *Supporting children with communication difficulties in inclusive settings—Second Edition.* Boston: Allyn & Bacon.

McCracken, G. (1988). *The long interview.* Newbury Park, CA: Sage Publications.

McCune, L. (1995). A normative study of representational play at the transition to language. *Developmental Psychology, 31*, 200-211.

McCune, L., and Vihman, M. (2001). Early phonetic and lexical development: A productivity approach. *Journal of Speech, Language, and Hearing Research, 44*, 670-684.

McCune-Nicolich, L. (1981). The cognitive bases of relational words in the single word period. *Journal of Child Language, 8*, 15-34.

McCune-Nicolich, L., and Carroll, S. (1981). Development of symbolic play: Implications for the language specialist. *Topics in Language Disorders, 2(1)*, 1-15.

McDermott, G. (1972). *Anansi the spider: A tale from the Ashanti.* New York: Holt, Rinehart & Winston.

McDermott, G. (1993). *Raven: A trickster tale from the Pacific Northwest.* San Diego, CA: Harcourt Brace Jovanovich.

McDermott, G. (1994). *Coyote: A trickstar tale from the Pacific Northwest.* San Diego, CA: Harcourt Brace Jovanovich.

McDonald, S., and Turkstra, L. (1998). Adolescents with traumatic brain injury: Assessing pragmatic function. *Clinical Linguistics and Phonetics, 12*, 237-248.

McEachin, J., Smith, T., and Lovaas, O. (1993). Long-term outcome for children with autism who received early intensive behavioral treatment. *American Journal on Mental Retardation, 97*, 359-372.

McEvoy, S. (1985). *Not quite human: Batteries not included.* New York: Archway.

McFadden, T., and Gillam, R. (1996). An examination of the quality of narratives produced by children with language disorders. *Language, Speech, and Hearing Services in Schools, 27*, 48-56.

McGee, A., and Johnson, H. (2003). The effect of inference training on skilled and less skilled comprehenders. *Educational Psychology, 23*, 49-59.

McGinnis, M. (1963). *Aphasic children.* Washington, DC: Alexander Graham Bell Association.

McGinnis, M., Kleffner, F., and Goldstein, R. (1956). *Teaching aphasic children.* Volta Review, 58, 239-244.

McGowan, J., Bleile, K., Fus, L., and Barnas, E. (1993). Communication disorders. In K. Bleile (Ed.). *The care of children with long-term tracheostomies* (pp. 196-242). San Diego, CA: Singular Publishing Group.

McGowan, J., and Kerwin, M. (1993). Oral motor and feeding problems. In K. Bleile (Ed.). *The care of children with long-term tracheostomies* (pp. 157-195). San Diego, CA: Singular Publishing Group.

McGrath, J., and Braescu, A. (2004). State of the science. *Journal of Perinatal and Neonatal Nursing, 18,* 353-368.

McGregor, K., Newman, R., Reilly, R., and Capone, N. (2002). Semantic representation and naming in children with specific language impairment. *Journal of Speech, Language, and Hearing Research, 45,* 998-1014.

McInnes, A., Fung, D., Manassis, K., Fiksenbaum, L., and Tannock, R. (2004). Narrative skills in children with selective mutism: An exploratory study. *American Journal of Speech-Language Pathology, 13,* 304-315.

McInnes, A., and Manassis, K. (2005). When silence is not golden: An integrated approach to selective mutism. *Seminars in Speech and Language, 26,* 201-210.

McInnes, J.M., and Treffry, J.A. (1982). *Deaf-blind infants and children: A developmental guide.* Toronto, Canada: University of Toronto Press.

McKeough, A., and Genereux, R. (2003). Transformation in narrative thought during adolescence: The structure and content of story compositions. *Journal of Educational Psychology, 95,* 537-552.

McKerns, D., and Motchkavitz, L. (1993). *Therapeutic education for the child with traumatic brain injury: From coma to kindergarten.* Tucson, AZ: Communication Skill Builders.

McKinley, N., and Larson, V. (1989). Students who can't communicate: Speech-language services at the secondary level. *National Association of Secondary School Principals Curriculum Report, 19,* 1-8.

McKinley, N., and Larson, V. (2003). *Communication solutions for older students.* Eau Claire, WI: Thinking Publications.

McKinley, N., and Schwartz, L. (1987). *Make-it yourself barrier activities.* Eau Claire, WI: Thinking Publications.

McKirdy, L., and Blank, M. (1982). Dialogue in deaf and hearing preschoolers. *Journal of Speech and Hearing Research, 25,* 487-499.

McLean, J. (1989). A language-communication intervention model. In D. Bernstein and E. Tiegerman (Eds.). *Language and communication disorders in children* (ed. 22nd ed., pp. 208-228). Columbus, OH: Merrill.

McLean, J., Snyder-McLean, L., Rowland, C., Jacobs, P., and Stremel-Campbell, K. (N.D.). *Generic skills assessment inventory: Experimental edition.* Parsons, KS: University of Kansas, Bureau of Child Research.

McLean, L., and Cripe, J. (1997). The effectiveness of early intervention for children with communication disorders. In M.J. Guralnick (Ed.). *The effectiveness of early intervention* (pp. 349-428). Baltimore, MD: Paul H. Brookes.

McLean, M., Wolery, M., and Bailey, D. (2003). *Assessing infants and preschoolers with special needs* (3rd ed.) Baltimore: Paul H. Brookes.

McLeod, S., van Doorn, J., and Reed, V. (2001). Consonant cluster development in two-year-olds: General trends and individual difference. *Journal of Speech, Language, and Hearing Research, 44,* 1144-1171.

McNamara, K. (2007). Interviewing, Counseling, and Clinical Communication. In R. Paul and P. Cascella (Eds.). *Introduction to clinical methods is communication disorders.* Baltimore: Paul H. Brookes. In press.

McNeilly, L. (2005). HIV and communication. *Journal of Communication Disorders, 387,* 303-310.

McNeilly, L., and Coleman, T. (2000). Early intervention: Working with children within the context of their families and communities. In T. Coleman (Ed.). *Clinical management of communication disorders in culturally diverse children* (pp. 77-100). Boston: Allyn & Bacon.

McPherson, D.L., and Davies, K. (1995). Preliminary observations of binaural hearing in an attention-deficit pediatric population. *Fiziologia Cheloveka, 21,* 47-53.

McPherson, J. (1988). *Battle cry of freedom: The civil war era.* New York: Oxford University Press.

McReynolds, L. (1966). Operant conditioning for investigating speech sound discrimination in aphasic children. *Journal of Speech and Hearing Research, 9,* 519-528.

McReynolds, L., and Kearns, K. (1982). *Single subject experimental designs in communication disorders.* Baltimore, MD: University Park Press.

McTavish, S. (2003). *Life skills: 225 Ready-to-use health activities for success and well-being.* Indianapolis, IN: Jossey-Bass.

McWilliams, R. (1992). *Family-centered intervention planning: A routines-based approach.* Tucson, AZ: Communication/Therapy Skills Builders.

Meador, D. (1984). Effects of color on visual discrimination of geometric symbols by severely and profoundly mentally retarded individuals. *American Journal of Mental Deficiency, 89,* 275-286.

Meadow, K. (1980). *Deafness and child development.* Los Angeles, CA: University of California Press.

Mecham, M. (1971). *Verbal language development scale.* Circle Pines, MN: American Guidance Service.

Mecham, M. (2003). *Utah test of language development—4.* Austin, TX: Pro-Ed.

Mehan, H. (1984). Language and schooling. *Sociology of Education, 5,* 174-183.

Mehrabian, A., and Williams, M. (1971). Piagetian measures of cognitive development for children up to age two. *Journal of Psycholinguistic Research, 1(1),* 113-126.

Meichenbaum, D. (1977). *Cognitive behavior modification: An integrative approach.* New York: Plenum Press.

Meitus, I., and Weinberg, B. (1983). *Diagnosis in speech-language pathology.* Baltimore, MD: University Park Press.

Meline, T., and Brackin, S. (1987). Language-impaired children's awareness of inadequate messages. *Journal of Speech and Hearing Disorders, 52,* 263-270.

Mellon, N. (2005). Educating children with hearing loss in an inclusion model. *ASHA Leader, 10(3),* 6-27.

Mengler, E.D., Hogben, J.H., Michie, P., and Bishop, D.V.M. (2005). Poor frequency discrimination is related to oral language disorder in children: A psychoacoustic study. *Dyslexia, 11(3),* 155-173.

Ment, L., Vohr, B., Allan, W., Katz, K., Schneider, D., Westerveld, M., Duncan, C., and Makuch, R. (2003). Change in cognitive function over time in very low birth weight infants. *Journal of the American Medical Association, 289,* 705-712.

Mentis, M. (1994). Topic management in discourse: Assessment and intervention. *Topics in Language Disorders, 14(3),* 29-54.

Mentis, M. (1998). In utero cocaine exposure and language development. *Seminars in Speech and Language, 19,* 147-166.

Menyuk, P. (1964). Comparison of grammar of children with functionally deviant and normal speech. *Journal of Speech and Hearing Research, 7,* 109-121.

Menyuk, P. (1986). Predicting speech and language problems with persistent otitis media. In J.F. Kavanagh (Ed.). *Otitis media and child development.* Parkton, MD: York Press.

Mercer, J. (1973). *Labeling the mentally retarded.* Berkeley: University of California Press.

Merit Software (N.D.) *Vocabulary super stretch, set 1 and 2* (computer program). New York: Author.

Merrell, A.W., and Plante, E. (1997). Norm-referenced test interpretation in the diagnostic process. *Language Speech and Hearing Services in the Schools, 19(3),* 223-233.

Merritt, D., Culatta, B., and Trostle, S. (1998). Narratives: Implementing a discourse framework. In D. Merritt and B Culatta (Eds.). *Language intervention in the classroom* (pp. 277-330). San Diego, CA: Singular Publishing.

Meyer, B. (1975). *The organization of prose and its effects on memory.* Amsterdam: North Holland.

Meyers, L. (1985). *Programs for early acquisition of language* (PEAL, computer program). Calabases, CA: Peal Software.

Michaels, S., and Collins, J. (1984). Oral discourse styles: Classroom interaction and the acquisition of literacy. In D. Tannen (Ed.). *Coherence in spoken and written discourse.* Norwood, NJ: Ablex.

Millar, D., Light, J., and McNaughton, D. (2004). The effect of direct instruction and writer's workshop on the early writing skills of children who use augmentative and alternative communication. *Augmentative and Alternative communication, 20,* 164-178.

Miller, D. (1975). *Native American families in the city.* San Francisco, CA: Institute for Scientific Analysis.

Miller, J. (1978). Assessing children's language behavior: A developmental process approach. In R.L. Schiefelbusch (Ed.). *Bases of language intervention.* Baltimore, MD: University Park Press.

Miller, J. (1981). *Assessing language production in children.* Boston, MA: Allyn & Bacon.

Miller, J. (1983). Identifying children with language disorders and describing their language performance. In J. Miller, D. Yoder, and R. Schiefelbusch (Eds.). *Contemporary issues in language intervention* (pp. 61-74). Rockville, MD: American Speech-Language-Hearing Association.

Miller, J. (1987). Language and communication characteristics of children with Down syndrome. In S. Pueschel, C. Tingley, J. Rynders, A. Crocker, and D. Crutcher (Eds.). *New perspectives on Down syndrome* (p. 233-262). Baltimore, MD: Paul H. Brookes.

Miller, J. (1996). Progress in assessing, describing, and defining child language disorder. In K.N. Cole, P.S. Dale, and D.J. Thal (Eds.). *Assessment of communication and language*. Baltimore, MD: Paul H. Brookes.

Miller, J. (1998, October). *Communication in Down syndrome*. Lecture given to the Southern Conn. State University Chapter of the National Student Speech-Language-Hearing Association, New Haven, CT.

Miller, J. (2006). Documenting Progress in Language Production: The Evolution of a Computerized Language Analysis System. In R. Paul (Ed.). *Language disorders from a developmental perspective: Essays in honor of Robin Chapman*. Hillsdale, NJ: Erlbaum (In press).

Miller, J., Campbell, T., Chapman, R., and Weismer, S. (1984). Language behavior in acquired childhood aphasia. In A. Holland, (Ed.). *Language disorders in children* (pp. 57-99). San Diego, CA: College-Hill Press.

Miller, J., and Chapman, R. (1984). Disorders of communication: Investigating the development of mentally retarded children. *American Journal of Mental Deficiency, 88*, 536-545.

Miller, J., and Chapman, R. (1998). *MACSALT: systematic analysis of language transcripts for the Apple Macintosh computer* (computer programs to analyze language samples). Madison, WI: Language Analysis Laboratory, Waisman Center, University of Wisconsin–Madison.

Miller, J., and Chapman, R. (2003). *SALT: Systematic analysis of language transcripts v. 8.0* (computer programs to analyze language samples). Madison, WI: Language Analysis Laboratory, Waisman Center, University of Wisconsin–Madison.

Miller, J., Chapman, R., Branston, M., and Reichle, J. (1980). Language comprehension in sensorimotor stages V and VI. *Journal of Speech and Hearing Research, 23*, 284-311.

Miller, J., Freiberg, C., Rolland, M., and Reeves, M. (1992). Implementing computerized language sample analysis in the public school. *Topics in Language Disorders, 12(2)*, 69-82.

Miller, J., and Iglesias, A. (2003-2005). *Systematic analysis of language transcripts (SALT), V8.* (computer software). Madison, WI: Language Analysis Lab, Waisman Center, University of Wisconsin.

Miller, J., Miolo, G., Sedey, A., and Rosin, M. (1990). *Productive language deficits in children with Down syndrome.* Paper presented at the 23rd Annual Gatlinburg Conference on Research and Theory in Mental Retardation, Brainerd, MN.

Miller, J., and Paul, R. (1995). *The clinical assessment of language comprehension.* Baltimore, MD: Paul H. Brookes.

Miller, J., Rosin, M., Pierce, K., Miolo, G., and Sedey, A. (November, 1989). *Language profile stability in children with Down syndrome.* Poster presented at the American Speech-Language-Hearing Association Convention, St. Louis, MO.

Miller, J., and Yoder, D. (1983). *Test of grammatical comprehension.* Madison, WI: University of Wisconsin.

Miller, L., Gilliam, R., and Peña, E. (2001). *Dynamic assessment and intervention: Improving children's narrative abilities.* Austin, TX: Pro-Ed.

Miller, N. (1984). *Bilingualism and language disability: Assessment and remediation.* San Diego, CA: College-Hill Press.

Millikin, C. (1997). Symbol systems and vocabulary selection strategies. In S.L. Glennen and D.C. DeCoste (Eds.). *Handbook of augmentative and alternative communication.* San Diego, CA: Singular Publishing Group.

Mills, A. (Ed., 1983). *Language acquisition in the blind child: Normal and deficient.* San Diego, CA: College-Hill Press.

Mills, A. (1992). Visual handicaps. In D. Bishop and K. Mogford (Eds.). *Language development in exceptional circumstances* (pp. 150-164). Hillsdale, NJ: Erlbaum.

Milne, A. (1926). In which Pooh goes visiting and gets into a tight place. In A. Milne. *Three stories from Winnie-the-Pooh.* New York: E.P. Dutton.

Milosky, L. (1987). Narratives in the classroom. *Seminars in Speech and Language, 8(4)*, 329-343.

Milosky, L. (1990). The role of world knowledge in language comprehension and language intervention. *Topics in Language Disorders, 10(3)*, 1-13.

Milosky, L., and Skarakis-Doyle, E. (2006). What else about comprehension? Examining young children's discourse comprehension abilities. In Paul, R. (Ed.). *Language disorders from a developmental perspective.* Mahwah, NJ: Erlbaum. In press.

Minshew, N., Sweeney, J., Bauman, B., and Webb, S. (2005). Neurologic aspects of autism. In F. Volkmar, R. Paul, A. Klin, and D. Cohen (Eds.). *Handbook of autism and pervasive developmental disorders—vol. 1* (pp. 473-514). New York: Wiley.

Minskoff, E. (1982). Sharpening language skills in secondary LD students. *Academic Therapy, 18(1)*, 53-60.

Mirak, J., and Rescorla, R. (1998). Phonetic skills and vocabulary size in late talkers: Concurrent and predictive relationships. *Applied Psycholinguistics, 19*, 1-17.

Mirenda, P. (2003). Toward functional augmentative and alternative communication for students with autism: Manual signs, graphic symbols, and voice output communication aids. *Language, Speech and Hearing Services in Schools, 34*, 203-217.

Mirenda, P., and Donnellan, A. (1987). Issues in curriculum development. In D. Cohen, A. Donnellan, and R. Paul (Eds.). *Handbook of autism and pervasive developmental disorders* (pp. 211-226). New York: John Wiley & Sons.

Mirenda, P., and Santogrossi, J. (1985). A prompt-free strategy to teach pictorial communication system use. *Augmentative and Alternative Communication, 1*, 143-150.

Mirrett, P., Roberts, J., and Price, J. (2003). Early intervention practices and communication intervention strategies for young males with fragile X syndrome. *Language, Speech, and Hearing Services in Schools, 34*, 320-331.

Mitchell, P. (1997). Prelinguistic vocal development: A clinical primer. *Contemporary Issues In Communication Science and Disorders (CICSD), 24*, 87-92.

Mitchell, P., Abernathy, T., and Gowans, L. (1998). Making sense of literacy portfolios: A four-step plan. *Journal of Adolescent and Adult Literacy, 41*, 384-386.

Mithun, M. (1999). *The language of native North America.* Cambridge: Cambridge University Press.

Moats, L. (2004). Efficacy of a structured, systematic language curriculum for adolescent poor readers. *Reading and Writing Quarterly, 20*, 145-159.

Mody, M., Studdert-Kennedy, M., and Brady, S. (1997). Speech perception deficits in poor readers: Auditory processing or phonological coding? *Journal of Experimental Child Psychology, 64*, 199-231.

Moeller, M., Osberger, M., and Eccarius, M. (1986). Cognitively based strategies for use with hearing-impaired students with comprehension deficits. *Topics in Language Disorders, 6(4)*, 37-50.

Moersch, M., and Schafer, S. (1981). *Developmental programming for infants and young children, Volume 1: Assessment and application* (rev. ed.). Ann Arbor, MI: The University of Michigan Press.

Montague, M., Graves, A., and Leavell, A. (1991). Planning, procedural facilitation, and narrative composition of junior high students with learning disabilities. *Learning Disabilities Research and Practice, 6*, 219-224.

Montague, M., and Lund, K. (1991). *Job-related social skills.* Eau Claire, WI: Thinking Publications.

Montague, M., Maddux, C., and Dereshiwsky, M. (1990). Story grammar and comprehension and production of narrative prose by students with learning disabilities. *Journal of Learning Disabilities, 23*, 190-197.

Montgomery, J. (1990). Building administrative support for collaboration. In W.A. Secord (Ed.). *Best practices in school speech-language pathology* (vol. I, pp. 75-80). San Antonio, TX: Psychological Corporation, Harcourt Brace Jovanovich.

Montgomery, J. (2005). Effects of input rate and age on the real-time language processing of children with specific language impairments. *International Journal of Language and Communication Disorders, 40*, 171-188.

Montgomery, J., and Kahn, N. (2003). You are going to be an author: Adolescent narratives as intervention. *Communication Disorders Quarterly, 24*, 143-152.

Montgomery, J., and Levine, M. (1995). Developmental language impairments: Their transactions with other neurodevelopmental factors during the adolescent years. *Seminars in Speech and Language, 16*, 1-13.

Montgomery, J.W. (2000). Verbal working memory and sentence comprehension in children with specific language impairment. *Journal of Speech, Language, and Hearing Research, 43(2)*, 293-308.

Moore, B. (1989). *Writing for whole language learning.* Ontario, Canada: Pembroke Publishers.

Moore, S., Donovan, B., and Hudson, A. (1993). Brief report: Facilitator-suggested conversational evaluation of facilitated communication. *Journal of Autism and Developmental Disorders, 23(3),* 541-552.

Moore-Brown, B., and Montgomery, J. (2001). *Making a difference for America's children: Speech-language pathologists in public schools.* Eau Claire, WI: Thinking Publications.

Moore-Brown, B., Montgomery, J., Bielinski, H., and Shubin, J. (2005). Responsiveness to intervention: Teaching before testing helps avoid labeling. *Topics in Language Disorders, 25(2),* 148-167.

Moos, R. (1974). *Family environment scale.* Palo Alto, CA: Consulting Psychologists Press.

Moran, M., Money, S., and Leonard, L. (1983, November). *Phonological process analysis in the speech of mentally retarded adults.* Paper presented at the Annual Convention of the American Speech-Language-Hearing Association, Cincinnati, OH.

Mordecai, D., and Palin, M. (1982). *Linguest 1 and 2* (computer program). East Moline, IL: Linguest Software.

Mordecai, D., Palin, M., and Palmer, C. (1985). *Linguest* (computer program). Columbus, OH: Macmillan.

Moreau, M., and Fidrych, M. (1998). *The story grammar marker.* Easthampton, MA: SGM, Inc.

Morey, W. (1965). *Gentle Ben.* New York: Avon.

Morley, M. (1957). *The development and disorders of speech in childhood.* Edinburgh, Scotland: E. & S. Livingstone Ltd.

Morocco, C., and Hindin, A. (2002). Role of conversation in a thematic understanding of literature. *Learning Disabilities Research & Practice, 17,* 144-160.

Morris, H., Spriestersbach, D., and Darley, F. (1961). An articulation test for assessing competency of velopharyngeal closure. *Journal of Speech and Hearing Research, 4,* 48-55.

Morris, N., and Crump, W. (1982). Syntactic and vocabulary development in the written language of learning disabled and nondisabled students at four age levels. *Learning Disability Quarterly, 5,* 163-172.

Morris, S. (1981). Communication/interaction development at mealtimes for the multiply handicapped child: Implications for the use of augmentative communication systems. *Language, Speech, and Hearing Services in Schools, 12,* 216-232.

Morris, S. (1982). *Pre-speech assessment scale.* Clifton, NJ: J.A. Preston.

Morris, S., and Klein, M. (2000). *Pre-feeding skills: A comprehensive resource for mealtime development—Second edition.* San Antonio, TX: Harcourt Assessment.

Morris, S., Wilcox, K., and Schooling, T. (1995). The preschool speech intelligibility measure. *American Journal of Speech -Language Pathology, 4,* 22-28.

Morrison, J., and Shriberg, L. (1992). Articulation testing versus conversational speech sampling. *Journal of Speech and Hearing Research, 35,* 259-273.

Morrow, C., Vogel, A., Anthony, J., Ofir, A., Dausa, A., and Bandstra, E. (2004). Expressive and receptive language functioning in preschool children with prenatal cocaine exposure. *Journal of Pediatric Psychology, 29,* 543-554.

Moses, J. (1992, September). Courts weigh tool enabling autistic youth to "talk." *Wall Street Journal,* p. B3.

Mufwene, S., Rickford, J., Baugh, J., and Bailey, G. (Eds.). (1998). *The structure of African-American English.* London: Routledge.

Muir, N., McCaig, S., Gerylo, K., Gompf, M., Burke, T., and Lumsden, P. (2000). *Talk! Talk! Talk! Tools to facilitate language.* Eau Claire, WI: Thinking Publications.

Mulac, A., and Tomlinson, C. (1977). Generalization of an operant remediation program for syntax with language delayed children. *Journal of Communication Disorders, 10,* 231-243.

Mullen, E. (1995). *Mullen scales of early learning: AGS Edition.* Circle Pines, MN: AGS Publishing.

Muma, J. (1971). Language intervention: Ten techniques. *Language, Speech, and Hearing Services in the Schools, 2,* 7-17.

Muma, J. (1978). *Language handbook: Concepts, assessment intervention.* Englewood Cliffs, NJ: Prentice-Hall.

Mundy, P., and Burnette, C. (2005). Joint Attention and Neurodevelopmental Models of Autism. In F. Volkmar, R. Paul, A., Klin, and D. Cohen (Eds.). *Handbook of autism and pervasive developmental disorders—3rd Ed.* (pp. 650-681). New York: Wiley.

Mundy, P., and Crawson, M. (1997). Joint attention and early social communication: Implications for research on intervention with autism. *Journal of Autism and Developmental Disorders, 27,* 653-676.

Mundy, P., Kasari, C., Signman, M., and Ruskin, E. (1995). Nonverbal communication and early language acquisition in children with Down syndrome and normally developing children. *Journal of Speech and Hearing Research, 38,* 157-167.

Mundy, P., Seibert, J., and Hogan, A. (1985). Communication skills in mentally retarded children. In M. Sigman (Ed.). *Children with emotional disorders and developmental disabilities: Assessment and treatment* (pp. 45-70). Orlando, FL: Grune & Stratton.

Mundy, P., and Sigman, M. (1989). Specifying the nature of the social impairment in autism. In G. Dawson (Ed.). *Autism, nature, diagnosis and treatment* (pp. 3-21). New York: Guilford Press.

Munoz, M., Gillam, R., Pena, E., and Gulley-Faehnle, A. (2003). Measures of language development in fictional narratives of Latino children. *Language, Speech, and Hearing Services in Schools, 34,* 332-342.

Munson, B., Bjorum, E.M., and Windsor, J. (2003). Acoustic and perceptual correlates of stress in nonwords produced by children with suspected developmental apraxia of speech and children with phonological disorder. *Journal of Speech, Language, and Hearing Research, 46(1),* 189-202.

Murdoch, B., and Theodoros, D.G. (2001). *Traumatic brain injury: Associated speech, language, and swallowing disorders.* San Diego: Singular.

Murphy, B., and Wolkoff, J. (1981). *Ace hits the big time.* New York: Dell Publishing.

Murray, S., Feinstein, C., and Blouin, A. (1985). The Token Test for Children: Diagnostic patterns and programming implications. In C.S. Simon (Ed.). *Communication skills and classroom success: Assessment of language-learning disabled students.* San Diego, CA: College-Hill Press.

Murray-Seegert, C. (1989). *Nasty girls, thugs, and humans like us: Social relations between severely disabled and nondisabled students in high school.* Baltimore, MD: Paul H. Brookes.

Myklebust, H. (1954). *Auditory disorders in children: A manual for differential diagnosis.* New York: Grune & Stratton.

Myklebust, H. (1965). *Development and disorders of written language* (vol. 1). Picture Story Language Test. New York: Grune and Stratton.

Myklebust, H. (1971). Childhood aphasia: An evolving concept. In L. Travis (Ed.). *Handbook on speech pathology and audiology* (pp. 1181-1202). Englewood Cliffs, NJ: Prentice-Hall.

Myles, B., and Simpson, R. (1998). *Asperger syndrome: A guide for educators and parents.* Austin, TX: Pro-Ed.

Naglieri, J. (1985). *Matrix analogies test—Short form and expanded form.* San Antonio, TX: Harcourt Assessment.

Naglieri, J. (2003). *Naglieri nonverbal ability test®—Individual administration (NNAT®—individual administration).* San Antonio, TX: Harcourt Assessment.

Naito, M., and Nagayama, K. (2004). Autistic children's use of semantic common sense and theory of mind: A comparison with typical and mentally retarded children. *Journal of Autism & Developmental Disorders, 34(5),* 507-519.

Naremore, R. (1980). Language disorders in children. In T. Hixon, L. Shriberg, and J. Saxman (Eds.). *Introduction to communication disorders* (pp. 137-176). Englewood Cliffs, NJ: Prentice-Hall.

Naremore, R., Densmore, A., and Harman, D. (1995). *Narrative intervention with school-aged children: Conversation, narrative, and text.* San Diego, CA: Singular Publishing Group.

Nation, K., Clarke, P., Marshall, C., and Durand, M. (2004). Hidden language impairments in children: Parallels between poor reading comprehension and specific language impairment? *Journal of Speech, Language, and Hearing Research, 47,* 199-211.

Nation, K., and Hulme, C. (1997). Phonemic segmentation, not onset-rhyme segmentation, predicts early reading and spelling skills. *Reading Research Quarterly, 32,* 154-167.

National Center for Health Statistics. (1985). *Advance report of the final mortality statistics,* 19483. Monthly Vital Statistics Report, 34(6). Supplement DHHS Pub. No. (PHS) 85-1120, Hyattsville, MD: Public Health Service.

National Joint Committee on Learning Disabilities (1994). Position paper. Reprinted in *Topics in Language Disorders, 16 (1996)*, 69-73.

National Joint Committee on Learning Disabilities (March 1999). Learning disabilities: Use of paraprofessionals. *ASHA, 41(suppl. 19)*, 37-46.

National Research Council. (2001). *Educating children with autism.* Washington, DC: Author.

Needleman, H. (1977). Effects of hearing loss from early recurrent otitis media on speech and language development. In B. Jaffe (Ed.). *Hearing loss in children* (pp. 640-649). Baltimore, MD: University Park Press.

Neeley, P., Neeley, R., Justen, J., and Tipton-Sumner, C. (2001). Scripted play as a language intervention strategy for preschoolers with developmental disabilities. *Early Childhood Education Journal, 28*, 243-246.

Negri, N. (1992). Individuals with autism: Language acquisition with restricted social and emotional knowledge. In R.S. Chapman (Ed.). *Processes in language acquisition and disorders* (pp. 279-298). St. Louis, MO: Mosby.

Nelsen, E., and Rosenbaum, E. (1972). Language patterns within the youth subculture: Development of slang vocabulary. *Merrill-Palmer Quarterly, 18*, 273-285.

Nelson, C. (1991). *Practical procedures for children with language disorders.* Austin, TX: Pro-Ed.

Nelson, J., Brenner, G., and Rogers-Adkinson, D. (2003). An investigation of the characteristics of K-12 students with comorbid emotional disturbance and significant language deficits served in public school settings. *Behavioral Disorders, 29*, 25-33.

Nelson, K. (1973). Structure and strategy in learning to talk. *Monographs of the Society for Research in Child Development, 38* (Serial No. 149).

Nelson, K., Camarata, S., Welsh, J., and Butkovsky, L. (1992, November). *Syntax acquisition by SLD and language normal children given controlled input.* Paper presented at the American Speech-Language-Hearing Association National Convention, San Antonio, TX.

Nelson, K., Camarata, S., Welsh, J., Butkovsky, L., and Camarata, M. (1996). Effects of imitative and conversational recasting treatment on the acquisition of grammar in children with specific language impairment and younger language-normal children. *Journal of Speech and Hearing Research, 39*, 850-859.

Nelson, N. (1976). Comprehension of spoken language by normal children as a function of speaking rate, sentence difficulty, and listener age and sex. *Child Development, 47*, 299-303.

Nelson, N. (1988). *Planning individualized speech and language intervention programs* (2nd ed.). Tucson, AZ: Communication Skill Builders.

Nelson, N. (1998). *Childhood language disorders in context: Infancy through adolescence* (2nd ed.). Columbus, OH: Merrill.

Nelson, N. (2000). Basing eligibility on discrepancy criteria: A bad idea whose time has passed. *Language Learning and Education, 7*, 8-12.

Nelson, N. (2005). The context of discourse difficulty in classroom and clinic: An update. *Topics in Language Disorders, 25*, 322-331.

Nelson, N., and Friedman, K. (1988). *Development of the concept of story in narratives written by older children.* Unpublished paper. Kalamazoo, MI: Western Michigan University.

Nelson, N., and Gillespie, L. (1992). *Analogies for thinking and talking.* Tucson, AZ: Communication Skill Builders.

Nelson, N., and Hyter, Y. (2001). Public policies affecting clinical practice. In R. Paul (Ed.). *Introduction to clinical methods in communication disorders* (pp. 219-238). Baltimore: Paul H. Brookes.

Nelson, N., and Van Meter, A. (2002). Assessing curriculum-based reading and writing Samples. *Topics in Language Disorders, 22(2)*, 35-59.

Nelson, N., Van Meter, A., Chamberlain, D., and Bahr, C. (2001). The speech-language pathologist's role in a writing lab approach. *Seminars in Speech and Language, 22*, 209-220.

Nelson, R., and Hawley, H. (2004). Inner control as an operational mechanism in attention deficits hyperactivity disorders. *Seminars in Speech and Language, 25*, 255-262.

Nessel, D. (1989). Do your students think when they read? *Learning, 17*, 55-58.

Netley, C. (1983). Sex chromosome abnormalities and the development of verbal and nonverbal abilities. In C. Ludlow and J. Cooper (Eds.). *Genetic aspects of speech and language disorders.* New York: Academic Press.

Neuman, S. (2004). The effect of print-rich classroom environments on early literacy growth. *Reading Teacher, 58 (1)*, 89-91.

Newborg, J., Stock, J., Wnek, L., Guidubaldi, J., and Svinicki, J. (2004). *Battelle developmental inventory, second edition.* Itasca, IL: Riverside Publishing.

Newbury, D., and Monaco, A. (2002). Molecular genetics of speech and language disorders. *Current Opinion in Pediatrics, 14*, 696-701.

Newcomer, P., and Barenbaum, E. (2003). *Test of phonological awareness skills.* Austin, TX: Pro-Ed.

Newcomer, P., and Hammill, D. (1997). *Test of Language Development—3 Primary.* Austin, TX: Pro-Ed.

Newhoff, M. (1986). Attentional deficit—what it is, what it is not. *The Clinical Connection, 10*, 10-11.

Newman, R. (2003). Prosodic differences in mothers' speech to toddlers in quiet and noisy environments. *Applied Psycholinguistics, 24*, 539-560.

NICHD (2000). *Report of the National Reading Panel: Teaching children to read: An evidence-based assessment of the scientific research literature on reading and its implications for reading instruction: Reports of the subgroups.* Washington, DC: National Institute of Child Health and Human Development.

Nicolich, L. (1977). Beyond sensorimotor intelligence: Assessment of symbolic maturity through analysis of pretend play. *Merrill-Palmer Quarterly, 23*, 89-99.

Nikopoulos, C., and Keenan, M. (2004). Effects of video modeling on social initiations by children with autism. *Journal of Applied Behavior Analysis, 37*, 93-96.

Nippold, M. (1988). The literate lexicon. In M.A. Nippold (Ed.). *Later language development: Ages nine through nineteen* (pp. 29-48). Austin, TX: Pro-Ed.

Nippold, M. (1993). Developmental markers in adolescent language: Syntax, semantics, and pragmatics. *Language, Speech, and Hearing Services in Schools, 24(1)*, 21-28.

Nippold, M. (1994). Persuasive talk in social contexts: Development, assessment, and intervention. *Topics in Language Disorders, 14(3)*, 1-12.

Nippold, M. (1995). School-age children and adolescents: Norms for word definition. *Language, Speech, and Hearing Services in Schools, 26*, 320-325.

Nippold, M. (1998). *Later language development: The school-age and adolescent years.* Austin, TX: Pro-Ed.

Nippold, M. (2000). Language development during the adolescent years: Aspects of pragmatics, syntax, and semantics. *Topics in Language Disorders, 20(2)*, 15-28.

Nippold, M. (2004). Research on later language development: International perspectives (pp. 1-8). In R. Berman (Ed.). *Language development across childhood and adolescence.* Philadelphia: John Benjamins Publishing Co.

Nippold, M., Duthie, J.K., Larsen, J. (2005). Literacy as a leisure activity: Free-time preferences of older children and young adolescents. *Language, Speech and Hearing Services in School, 36, (2)*: 93-102.

Nippold, M., and Haq, F. (1996). Proverb comprehension in youth: The role of concreteness and familiarity. *Journal of Speech and Hearing Research, 39*, 166-176.

Nippold, M., Hegel, S., Sohlberg, M., and Schwarz, I. (1999). Defining abstract entities: Development in pre-adolescents, adolescents, and young adults. *Journal of Speech, Language, and Hearing Research, 42*, 473-481.

Nippold, M., and Martin, S. (1989). Idiom interpretation in isolation versus context: A developmental study with adolescents. *Journal of Speech and Hearing Research, 32*, 59-66.

Nippold, M., Moran, C., and Schwarz, M. (2001). Idiom understanding in preadolescents: Synergy in action. *American Journal of Speech-Language Pathology, 10*, 169-179.

Nippold, M., and Taylor, C. (2002). Judgments of idiom familiarity and transparency: A comparison of children and adolescents. *Journal of Speech, language, and Hearing Research, 45*, 384-391.

Nippold, M., Taylor, C., and Baker, J. (1996). Idiom understanding in Australian youth. *Journal of Speech and Hearing Research, 39*, 442-447.

Nippold, M., and Undlin, R. (1992). Use and understanding of adverbial conjuncts: A developmental study of adolescents and young adults. *Journal of Speech and Hearing Research, 35*, 18-118.

Noble, T. (1979). *The king's tea.* New York: Dial Press.

Noble-Sanderson, G. (1993). *Classroom phonology: A narrative approach to speech sound awareness and remediation.* San Antonio, TX: Psychological Corporation.

Noell, G., VanDerHeyden, A., Gatti, S., and Whitmarsh, E. (2001). Functional assessment of the effects of escape and attention on students' compliance during instruction. *School Psychology Quarterly, 16*, 253-69.

Nohara, M., McKay, S., and Trehub, S. (1995). Analyzing conversations between mothers and their hearing impaired and deaf adolescents. *Volta Review, 97,* 123-134.

Norbury, C. (2004). Factors supporting idiom comprehension in children with communication disorders. *Journal of Speech, Language, and Hearing Research, 47,* 1179-1193.

Norbury, C., and Bishop, D. (2002). Inferential processing and story recall in children with communication problems: A comparison of specific language impairment, pragmatic language impairment and high functioning autism. *International Journal of Language and Communication Disorders, 37,* 227-251.

Norbury, C., and Bishop, D. (2003). Narrative skills of children with communication impairments. *International Journal of Language and Communication Disorders, 38,* 287-313.

Norbury, C., Nash, M., Baird, G., and Bishop, D. (2004). Using a parental checklist to identify diagnostic groups in children with communication impairment: A validation of the Children's Communication Checklist—2. *International Journal of Communication Disorders, 39,* 345-354.

Norris, J. (1994). Issues underlying whole language: Clarifying the debate. *Language, Speech, and Hearing Services in Schools, 25,* 40-44.

Norris, J. (1995). Expanding language norms for school-age children and adolescents: Is it pragmatic? *Language, Speech, and Hearing Services in Schools, 26,* 342-352.

Norris, J., and Damico, J. (1990). Whole language in theory and practice: Implications for language intervention. *Language, Speech, and Hearing Services in Schools, 21,* 212-220.

Norris, J., and Hoffman, P. (1990a). Comparison of adult-initiated vs. child-initiated interaction styles with handicapped pre-language children. *Language, Speech, and Hearing Services in Schools, 21,* 28-36.

Norris, J., and Hoffman, P. (1990b). Language intervention within naturalistic environments. *Language, Speech, and Hearing Services in Schools, 21,* 72-84.

Norris, J., and Hoffman, P. (1993). *Whole language intervention for school-age children.* San Diego, CA: Singular Publishing Group.

Northcott, W. (1973). Parenting a hearing-impaired child. *Hearing and Speech News, 41,* 10-12, 28-29.

Northcott, W. (1977). *Curriculum guide: Hearing-impaired children—Birth to three years—and their parents, revised edition.* Washington, DC: Alexander Graham Bell Association for the Deaf.

Northern, J., and Downs, M. (2002). *Hearing in children* (5th ed). Baltimore: Williams & Wilkins.

Notari, A., Cole, K., and Mills, P. (1992). Cognitive referencing: The (non)relationship between theory and application. *Topics in Early Childhood Special Education, 11,* 22-38.

Novak, J. (2002). Improving communication in adolescents with language/learning disorders: Clinical considerations and adolescent skills. *Contemporary Issues in Communication Sciences and Disorders, 29,* 79-90.

Nover, S., Christensen, K., and Cheng, L. (1998). Development of ASL and English competence for learners who are deaf. *Topics in Language Disorders, 18(4),* 61-72.

Nugent, J., Keefer, C., O'Brien, S., Johnson, L., and Blanchard, Y. (2005). *The newborn behavioral observation system.* Boston, MA: The Brazelton Institute.

Numeroff, L. (1985). *If you give a mouse a cookie.* New York: Harper Collins.

Numeroff, L. (1991). *If you give a moose a muffin.* New York: Harper Collins.

Nungesser, N., and Watkins, R. (2005). Preschool teachers' perceptions and reactions to challenging classroom behavior: Implications for speech-language pathologists. *Language, Speech, and Hearing Services in Schools, 36,* 139-151.

Nunnery, B. (1993). *Songs, rhymes, and fingerplays: Language through action and rhyming.* Tucson, AZ: Communication Skill Builders.

Nyquist, K., Sjoden, P., and Ewald, U. (1999). Preterm infant breastfeeding behavior scale. *Early Human Development, 55,* 247-264.

O'Brien, M., and Nagle, K. (1987). Parents' speech to toddlers: The effect of play context. *Journal of Child Language, 14,* 269-279.

O'Brien, R.C. (1971). *Mrs. Frisby and the rats of NIMH.* New York: Aladdin Books.

O'Connell, P. (1997). *Speech, language and hearing programs in schools: A guide for students and practitioners.* Gaithersburg, MD: Aspen Publishers.

O'Connor, R., and Jenkins, J. (1995). Improving the generalization of sound/symbol knowledge: Teaching spelling to kindergarten children with disabilities. *The Journal of Special Education, 29,* 255-275.

O'Donnell, D. (1999). *A guide for understanding and developing IEPs.* Madison, WI: Wisconsin Department of Public Instruction.

O'Donnell, R., Griffin, W., and Norris, R. (1967). *Syntax of kindergarten and elementary school children: A transformational analysis* (Research Rep. No. 8). Champaign, IL: National Council of Teachers of English.

O'Leary, C. (2004). Fetal alcohol syndrome: Diagnosis, epidemiology, and developmental outcomes. *Journal of Pediatric and Child Health, 40,* 2-7.

Oates, R., Peacock, A., and Forrest, D. (1984). The development of abused children. *Developmental Medicine and Child Neurology, 26,* 649-656.

Ochsner, G. (2003, April). Evidence-based practice. *ASHA Leader, 7,* 27.

Odom, S.L., McConnell, S.R., McEvoy, M.A., Peterson, C., Ostrosky, M., Chandler, L.K., Spicuzza, R.J., Skellenger, A., Creighton, M., and Favazza, P.C. (1999). Relative effects of interventions for supporting the social competence of young children with disabilities. *Topics in Early Childhood Special Education, 19,* 75-92.

Oetting, J., and McDonald, J. (2000). Methods for characterizing participants' nonmainstream dialect use in child language research. *Journal of Speech, Language, and Hearing Research, 45,* 505-518.

Oklahoma Project. (1982). *Exceptions: A handbook for teachers of mainstream students.* Cushing, OK: Project Mainstream in Cooperation with the Oklahoma Child Service Demonstration Center and Developer/Demonstrator Project.

Oller, D.K., Eilers, R., and Basinger, D. (2001). Intuitive identification of infant vocal sounds by parents. *Developmental Science, 4,* 49-61.

Oller, D.K., Levine, S., Cobo-Lewis, A., Eilers, R., Pearson, B. (1998). Vocal precursors to linguistic communication: How babbling is connected to meaningful speech. In R. Paul (Ed.). *Exploring the speech-language connection* (pp. 1-23). Baltimore, MD: Paul H. Brookes.

Oller, K. (2000). *The emergence of speech capacity.* Mahwah, NJ: Erlbaum.

Olley, J. G. (2005). Curriculum and classroom structure. In F. R. Volkmar, R. Paul, A. Klin, D. J. Cohen (Eds.). *Handbook of autism and pervasive developmental disorders* (3rd ed., vol. 2, pp. 863-881). Hoboken, NJ: John Wiley & Sons, Inc.

Ollman, H. (1989). Cause and effect in the real world. *Journal of Reading, 33,* 224-225.

Olson, R., and Gayan, J. (2003). Brains, genes, and environment in reading development. In S. Neuman and D. Dickinson (Eds.). *Handbook of early literacy research* (pp. 81-96). N.Y.: Guilford Press.

Olswang, L. (1996). *Preschool functional communication inventory.* Seattle, WA: University of Washington Speech and Hearing Clinic.

Olswang, L., and Bain, B. (1991). Intervention issues for toddlers with specific language impairments. *Topics in Language Disorders, 11,* 69-86.

Olswang, L., and Bain, B. (1996). Assessment information for predicting upcoming change in language production. *Journal of Speech, Language, and Hearing Research, 39(20),* 414-423.

Olswang, L., Coggins, T., and Timler, G. (2001). Outcome measures for school-age children with social communication problems. *Topics in Language Disorders, 22(1),* 50-73.

Olswang, L., Rodriguez, B., and Timler, G. (1998). Recommending intervention for toddlers with specific language learning difficulties: We may not have all the answers, but we know a lot. *American Journal of Speech-Language Pathology, 7,* 23-32.

Olswang, L., Stoel-Gammon, C., Coggins, T., and Carpenter, R. (1987). *Assessing prelinguistic and early linguistic behaviors in developmentally young children.* Seattle, WA: University of Washington Press.

O'Neill, R.E., Horner, R.H., Albin, R.W., Sprague, J.R., Storey, K., and Newton, J.S. (1997). *Functional assessment and program development for problem behavior.* Pacific Grove, CA: Brooks/Cole.

Oppel, K. (2004). *Airborn.* New York: Eos.

Optimum Resource, (N.D.) *Vocabulary development 2* (computer program). Hilton Head Island, SC: Author.

Ortiz, S. (2001). Assessment of cognitive abilities in Hispanic children. *Seminars in Speech and Language, 22,* 17-38.

Orton, S. (1937). *Reading, writing and speech problems in children: A presentation of certain types of disorders in the development of the language faculty.* New York: W. W. Norton.

Osbourne, S. (Producer) and Templeton, G. (Director, 1994). *Frog, where are you?* (video, available from The Phoenix Learning Group, 2349 Chaffee Drive, St. Louis, MO 63146.)

Osgood, C., and Miron, M. (1963). *Approaches to the study of aphasia.* Urbana, IL: University of Illinois Press.

Otto, W., and White, S. (Eds.). (1982). *Reading expository material.* New York: Academic Press.

Owen, A., and Leonard, L. (2002). Lexical diversity in the spontaneous speech of children with specific language impairment: Application of D. *Journal of Speech, Language, & Hearing Research, 45,* 927-937.

Owens, R. (1997). Mental retardation. In D.K. Bernstein and E. Tiegerman (Eds.). *Language and communication disorders in children* (ed. 4, pp. 366-430). Columbus, OH: Merrill/Macmillan.

Owens, R. (2004). *Language disorders: A functional approach to assessment and intervention* (4th ed.). Boston, MA: Allyn & Bacon.

Owens, R. (2005). *Language development: An introduction* (6th ed.). Boston: Allyn & Bacon.

Owens, R., and MacDonald, J. (1982). Communicative uses of the early speech of nondelayed and Down syndrome children. *American Journal of Mental Deficiency, 86,* 503-510.

Owens, R., Metz, D., and Haas, A. (2003). *Introduction to communication disorders* (2nd ed.) Boston: Allyn & Bacon.

Owens, R., and Robinson, L. (1997). Once upon a time: Use of children's literature in the preschool classroom. *Topics in Language Disorders, 17,* 19-48.

Ozcaliskan, S., and Goldin-Meadow, S. (2005). Gesture is at the cutting edge of early language development. *Cognition, 96,* 101-113.

Ozonoff, S. (1997). Causal mechanisms of autism: Unifying perspectives from an information-processing framework. In J. Cohen and F. Volkmar (Eds.). *Handbook of autism and pervasive developmental disorders* (pp. 868-879). New York: John Wiley & Sons.

PACER Center, Inc. (1990). *A guide for parents to the individual education program (IEP) plan.* Minnesota: PACER.

Padden, C. (1980). The deaf community and the culture of deaf people. In C. Baker and R. Battison (Eds.). *Sign language and the deaf community.* Washington, DC: National Association for the Deaf.

Padden, C., and Ramsey, C. (1998). Reading ability in signing deaf children. *Topics in Language Disorders, 18(4),* 30-46.

Paden, E., Novak, M., and Beiter, A. (1987). Predictors of phonologic inadequacy in young children prone to otitis media. *Journal of Speech and Hearing Disorders, 52,* 232-242.

Page, J., and Stewart, S. (1985). Story grammar skills in school-age children. *Topics in Language Disorders, 5(2),* 16-30.

Palmer, B., and Brooks, M. (2004). Reading until the cows come home: Figurative language and reading comprehension. *Journal of Adolescent and Adult Literacy, 47,* 370-379.

Palmer, M. M., Crawley, K., and Blanco, I. (1993). Neonatal oral-motor assessment scale: A reliability study. *Journal of Perinatology, 13(1),* 28–35.

Paradis, J. (2005). Grammatical morphology in children learning English as a second language: Implications of similarities with specific language impairment. *Language, Speech and Hearing Services in Schools, 36,* 172-187.

Paradise, J. (1997). Otitis media and child development: Should we worry? *Pediatric Infectious Disease Journal, 17,* 1076-1083.

Parette, P., Huer, M., and Wyatt, T. (2002). Young African-American children with disabilities and augmentative and alternative communication issues. *Early Childhood Education Journal, 29,* 201-207.

Paris, J., and Paris, J. (2005). *Idioms.* Hillsboro, OR: Butte Publications.

Parker, F. (1986). *Linguistics for nonlinguists.* Boston, MA: College-Hill Press.

Partington, J., and Sundberg, M. (1998). *Teaching language to children with autism and other developmental disabilities.* Danville, CA: Behavior Analyst.

Patrick, B. (2002). *Native American languages.* Broomall, PA: Mason Crest Publishers.

Patterson, J. (2000). Observed and reported expressive vocabulary and word combinations in bilingual toddlers. *Journal of Speech, Language, and Hearing Research, 43,* 121-129.

Patterson, J., and Westby, C. (1998). The development of play. In W. Haynes and B. (Eds.). *Communication development: Foundations, processes, and clinical applications* (pp. 135-162). Baltimore, MD: Williams & Wilkins.

Paul, R. (1981). Analyzing complex sentence development. In J.F. Miller (Ed.). *Assessing language production in children: Experimental procedures* (pp. 36-40). Needham Heights, MA: Allyn & Bacon.

Paul, R. (1987a). Natural history. In D.J. Cohen and A.M. Donnellan (Eds.). *Handbook of autism and pervasive developmental disorders* (pp. 121-132). New York: John Wiley & Sons.

Paul, R. (1987b). Communication. In D.J. Cohen and A.M. Donnellan (Eds.). *Handbook of autism and pervasive developmental disorders* (pp. 61-84). New York: John Wiley & Sons.

Paul, R. (1990). Comprehension strategies: Interactions between world knowledge and the development of sentence comprehension. *Topics in Language Disorders, 10(3),* 63-75.

Paul, R. (1991a). Profiles of toddlers with slow expressive language development. *Topics in Language Disorders, 11(4),* 1-13.

Paul, R. (1991b). Assessing communication skills in toddlers. *Clinics in Communication Disorders: Infant Assessment, 1(2),* 7-23.

Paul, R. (November, 1991c). *Patterns of development in late-talkers.* Mini-seminar presented at the American Speech-Language-Hearing Association National Convention, Atlanta, GA.

Paul, R. (1992a). Language and speech disorders. In S.R. Hooper, G.W. Hynd, and R.E. Mattison (Eds.). *Developmental disorders: Diagnostic criteria and clinical assessment* (pp. 209-238). Hillsdale, NJ: Lawrence Erlbaum.

Paul, R. (1992b). *Pragmatic activities for language intervention: Semantics, syntax, and emerging literacy.* Tucson, AZ: Communication Skill Builders.

Paul, R. (1992c). Speech language interactions in the talk of young children. In R. Chapman (Ed.). *Child talk: Processes in child/language acquisition* (pp. 235-254). St. Louis, MO: Mosby.

Paul, R. (1993a). Specific developmental language disorders. In R. Michels (Ed.). *Psychiatry.* New York: Lippincott.

Paul, R. (1993b). Patterns of development in late talkers: Preschool years. *Journal of Childhood Communication Disorders, 15,* 7-14.

Paul, R. (1996). Clinical implications of the natural history of slow expressive language development. *American Journal of Speech-Language Pathology, 5,* 5-21.

Paul, R. (1997a). Understanding language delay: A response to van Kleeck, Gillam, and Davis. *American Journal of Speech-Language Pathology, 6,* 41-49.

Paul, R. (1997b). Facilitating transitions in language development from children using AAC. *Alternative and Augmentative, 13,* 141-148.

Paul, R. (1998). Communicative development in augmented modalities: Language without speech? In R. Paul (Ed.). *Exploring the speech-language connection* (pp. 139-161). Baltimore, MD: Paul H. Brookes.

Paul, R. (1999). Predicting outcomes of early expressive language delay. Infant-toddler intervention. *The Transdisciplinary Journal.*

Paul, R. (2000a). Disorders of communication. In M. Lewis (Ed.). *Child and adolescent psychiatry* (3rd ed., pp. 510-519). Baltimore, MD: Williams & Wilkins.

Paul, R. (2000b). Ethical implications of the natural history of slow expressive language development. In D. Bishop and L. Leonard (Eds.). *Proceedings of the Third International Symposium for Aphasic and Speech Impaired Children.* London: Psychology Press.

Paul, R. (2000c). Understanding the "whole" of it: Comprehension assessment. *Seminars in Speech and Language, 21(3),* 10-17.

Paul, R. (2003a). Enhancing social communication in high functioning individuals with autistic spectrum disorders. *Child and Adolescent Psychiatric Clinics of North America, 12,* 87-106.

Paul, R. (2003b). *Beyond MLU: Syntactic analysis for the 21st century.* Invited presentation at the Symposium for Research in Child Language Disorders. Madison, WI.

Paul, R. (2003c). Guest Editor: Asperger syndrome. *Perspectives on Language Learning and Education, 10(2).*

Paul, R. (2005). Assessing communication in autism spectrum disorders. In F. Volkmar, A. Klin, R. Paul, and D. Cohen (Eds.). *Handbook of autism and pervasive developmental disorders—3rd. Ed.,* vol. II (pp. 799-816). New York: Wiley & Sons.

Paul, R., Chawarska, K., Klin, A., and Volkmar, F. (2006). Dissociations in the development of early communication in autism spectrum disorders. In R. Paul (Ed.). *Language disorders from a developmental perspective: Essays in honor of Robin Chapman.* Mahwah, NJ: Erlbaum.

Paul, R., and Cohen, D. (1984). Outcomes of severe disorders of language acquisition. *Journal of Autism and Developmental Disorders, 14,* 405-421.

Paul, R., Cohen, D., Brag, W., Watson, M., and Herman, S. (1984). Fragile X syndrome: Its relation to speech and language disorders. *Journal of Speech and Hearing Disorders, 49,* 328-332.

Paul, R., Cohen, D., and Caparulo, B. (1983). A longitudinal study of patients with severe, specific developmental language disorders. *Journal of American Academy of Child Psychiatry, 22,* 525-534.

Paul, R., Cohen, D., Klin, A., Volkmar, F. (1999). Multiplex developmental disorders: The role of communication in the construction of a self. In R. Paul (Ed.). *Child and adolescent psychiatric clinics of North America* (pp. 189-202). Philadelphia, PA: W.B. Saunders.

Paul, R., and Elwood, T. (1991). Maternal linguistic input to toddlers with slow expressive language development. *Journal of Speech and Hearing Research, 34,* 982-988.

Paul, R., Fisher, M., and Cohen, D. (1988). Sentence comprehension strategies in children with autism and specific language disorders. *Journal of Autism and Developmental Disorders, 18,* 669-679.

Paul, R., and Fountain, R. (1999). Predicting outcomes of early expressive language delay. *Infant Toddler Intervention, 8,* 123-136.

Paul, R., Hernandez, R., Taylor, L., and Johnson, K. (1996). Narrative development in late talkers: Early school age. *Journal of Speech and Hearing Research, 39,* 1295-1303.

Paul, R., and Jennings, P. (1992). Phonological behavior in toddlers with slow expressive language development. *Journal of Speech and Hearing Research, 35,* 99-107.

Paul, R., and Kellog, L. (1997). Temperament in late talkers. *Journal of Child Psychology and Psychiatry, 38,* 803-812.

Paul, R., Laszlo, C., and McFarland, L. (November, 1992). *Emergent literacy skills in late talkers.* Mini-seminar presented at the annual convention of the American Speech-Language-Hearing Association, San Antonio, TX.

Paul, R., Lynn, T., and Lohr-Flanders, M. (1993). History of middle ear involvement and speech/language development in late talkers. *Journal of Speech and Hearing Research, 36,* 1055-1062.

Paul, R., McNamara, K., Reuler, E., Roy, K., and Peterson, F. (2001). *Screening for language delay in five year olds using spontaneous speech sampling.* Paper presented at the National Convention of the American Speech, Language and Hearing Association. Atlanta, GA.

Paul, R., Parent, E., Rubin, E., Romanik, L., Klin, A., Shriberg, L., Carroll, M., Kennedy, M., Marans, W., Volkmar, F., and Cohen, D. (1998). *Communication profiles in autism and Asperger syndrome.* Poster presented at the National Convention of the American Speech-Language-Hearing Association. San Antonio, TX.

Paul, R., and Riback, M. (June, 1993). *Sentence structure development in late talkers.* Poster session presented at the Symposium for Research in Child Language Disorders, Madison, WI.

Paul, R., and Shiffer, M. (1991). Communicative initiations in normal and late-talking toddlers. *Applied Psycholinguistics, 12(4),* 419-431.

Paul, R., and Shriberg, L. (1982). Associations between phonology and syntax in speech-delayed children. *Journal of Speech and Hearing Research, 25,* 536-547.

Paul, R., and Smith, R. (1993). Narrative skills in 4-year-olds with normal, impaired, and late-developing language. *Journal of Speech and Hearing Research, 36,* 592-598.

Paul, R., Spangle-Looney, S., and Dahm, P. (1991). Communication and socialization skills at ages 2 and 3 in "late-talking" young children. *Journal of Speech and Hearing Research, 34,* 858-865.

Paul, R., and Sutherland, D. (2003). Asperger syndrome: The role of the speech-language pathologist. *Perspectives on Language Learning and Education, 10(2),* 9-15.

Paul, R., and Sutherland, D. (2005). Enhancing early language in children with autism spectrum disorders. In F. Volkmar, R. Paul, A. Klin, and D. Cohen (Eds.). *Handbook of autism and pervasive developmental disorders—vol. 2* (pp. 946-976). New York: Wiley.

Paul, R., Tetnowski, J., and Reuler, E. (2007). Communication sampling. In R. Paul and P. Cascella (Eds.). *Introduction to clinical methods is communication disorders.* Baltimore: Paul H. Brookes. In press.

Paul-Brown, D., and Goldberg, L. (2001). Current policies and new directions for speech-language pathology assistants. Language, Speech, and Hearing Services in Schools, 32, 4-17.

Paulsen, G. (1987). Hatchet. New York: Bradbury Press.

Pavri, S., and Fowler, S. (2001). Child find, screening and tracking: Serving culturally and linguistically diverse children and families. Tech. Rpt. Early Childhood Research Institute on Culturally and Linguistically Appropriate Services. Urbana, IL: Illinois University-Urbana.

Pearce, W.M., McCormack, P.F., and James, D.G.H. (2003). Exploring the boundaries of SLI: Findings from morphosyntactic and story grammar analyses. Clinical Linguistics and Phonetics, 17(4/5), 325-334.

Pearl, R. (2002). Students with learning disabilities and their classroom companions. In B.Y.L. Wong and M. Donahue (Eds.). *The social dimensions of learning disabilities: Essays in honor of Tanis Bryan* (Volume in the Special Education and Exceptionality Series, pp. 77-93). Mahwah, NJ: Erlbaum.

Pears, K. (2005). Developmental, cognitive, and neuropsychological functioning in preschool-aged foster children: Associations with prior maltreatment and placement history. *Journal of Developmental & Behavioral Pediatrics, 26,* 112-122.

Pearson, B. (2004). Theoretical and empirical bases for dialect-neutral language assessment: Contributions from theoretical and applied linguistics to communication disorders. *Seminars in Speech and Language, 25(1),* 13-26.

Pease, D., Gleason, J., and Pan, B. (1993). Learning the meaning of words: Semantic development and beyond. In J.B. Gleason (Ed.). *The development of language* (3rd ed., pp. 115-150). New York: Macmillan.

Peck, A., and Scarpati, S. (2004). Using positive behavior support strategies. *Teaching Exceptional Children, 37,* 7-8.

Pelham, W. (2002). Psychosocial interventions for ADHD. In P. Jenson and J. Cooper (Eds.). *Attention deficits hyperactivity disorders: State of the science—Best practices* (pp. 12-16). Kingston, NJ: Civic Research Institute.

Peña, E. (1996). Dynamic assessment: The model and its language applications. In K. Cole, P. Dale, and D. Thal (Eds.). *Assessment of communication and language* (pp. 281-307). Baltimore, MD: Paul H. Brookes.

Peña, E., Iglesias, A., and Lidz, C.S. (2001) Reducing test bias through dynamic assessment of children's word learning ability. *American Journal of Speech-Language Pathology, 10,* 138-154.

Peña, E., and Quinn, R. (2003). Developing effective collaboration teams in speech-language pathology: A case study. *Communication Disorders Quarterly, 24,* 53-63.

Peng, S., Spencer, L., and Tomblin, J.B. (2004). Speech intelligibility of pediatric cochlear implant recipients with 7 years of device experience. *Journal of Speech, Language and Hearing Research, 47,* 1227-1236.

Pennington, B.F, and Lefly, D.L. (2001). Early reading development in children at family risk for dyslexia. *Child Development, 72(3),* 816-833.

Pepper, J., and Weitzman, E. (2004). *It takes two to talk: A practical guide for parents of children with language delays* (3rd ed.). Toronto, Canada: The Hanen Centre.

Pérez-Pereira, M., and Conti-Ramsden, G. (1999). *Language development and social interaction in blind children.* Hove, England: Psychology Press/Taylor & Francis.

Perfetti, C. (1985). *Reading ability.* New York: Oxford University Press.

Perfetti, C. (1994). Psycholinguistics and reading ability. In M.A. Gernsbacher (Ed.). *Handbook of psycholinguistics.* San Diego, CA: Academic Press.

Perfetti, C., and Lesgold, A. (1979). Coding and comprehension in skilled reading and implications for reading instruction. In L.B. Resnick and P.A. Weaver (Eds.). *Theory and practice of early reading* (vol. 1). Hillsdale, NJ: Erlbaum.

Perona, K., Plante, K., and Vance, R. (2005). Diagnostic accuracy of the Structured Photographic Expressive Language Test: 3rd. Ed. (SPELT-3). *Language, Speech, and Hearing Services in Schools, 36,* 103-115.

Perozzi, J. (1985). A pilot study of language facilitation for bilingual, language-handicapped children: Theoretical and intervention implications. *Journal of Speech and Hearing Disorders, 50,* 403-406.

Perozzi, J., and Chavez-Sanchez, M. (1992). The effect of instruction in L1 on receptive acquisition of L2 for bilingual children with language delay. *Language, Speech, and Hearing Services in Schools, 23,* 348-352.

Persaud, T. (1985). Causes of developmental defects. In T.V.N. Persaud, A.E. Chudley, and R.G. Skalko (Eds.). *Basic concepts in teratology.* New York: Alan R. Liss.

Peterson, C., and McCabe, A. (1983). *Developmental psycholinguistics: Three ways of looking at a child's narrative.* New York: Plenum Press.

Peterson, H.A., and Marquardt, T.P. (1994). *Appraisal and diagnosis of speech and language disorders* (3rd ed.). Englewood Cliffs, NJ: Prentice Hall.

Peterson, P. (2004). Naturalistic language teaching procedures for children at risk for language delays. *The Behavior Analyst Today, 5,* 404-424.

Peterson, P., Carta, J., and Greenwood, C. (2005). Teaching enhanced milieu language teaching skills to parents of multiple risk families. *Journal of Early Intervention, 27,* 94-109.

Pharr, A., Ratner, N., and Rescorla, L. (2000). Syllable structure development of toddlers with expressive specific language impairment. *Applied Psycholinguistics, 21,* 429-449.

Phelps, R. (2005). *Defending standardized testing.* Mahwah, NJ: Erlbaum.

Phelps-Terasaki, D., and Phelps-Gunn, T. (1992). *Test of pragmatic language.* Austin, TX: Pro-Ed.

Phillips, S. (1972). Participant structures and communicative competence: Warm Springs children in community and classroom. In C. Cazden, V. John, and D. Hymes (Eds.). *Functions of language in the classroom* (pp. 370-394). New York: Teachers College Press.

Piccolo, J. (1987). Expository text structure: Teaching and learning strategies. *The Reading Teacher, 40,* 838-847.

Pinker, S. (1994). *The language instinct.* London: Penguin Press.

Plante, E. (1998). Criteria for SLI: The Stark and Tallal legacy and beyond. *Journal of Speech Language and Hearing Research, 41,* 951-962.

Plante, E., and Vance, R. (1994). Selection of preschool language tests: A data-based approach. *Language, Speech, and Hearing Services in Schools, 25,* 15-24.

Plourde, L. (1985). *Classroom listening and speaking: K-2.* Tucson, AZ: Communication Skill Builders.

Plourde, L. (1989). *More classroom listening and speaking: K-2.* Tuscon, AZ: Communication Skill Builders.

Plumridge, D., and Hylton, J. (1987). *Smooth sailing into the next generation.* Clackamas County: Association for Retarded Citizens.

Poehlmann, J., and Fiese, B. (2001). Parent-infant interaction as a mediator of the relation between neonatal risk status and 12-month cognitive development. *Infant Behavior and Development, 24,* 171-188.

Polmanteer, K., and Turbiville, V. (2000). Family-responsive individualized family service plans for speech-language pathologists. *Language, Speech and Hearing Services in Schools, 31,* 4-14.

Popp, S., Ryan, J., Thompson, M., and Behrens, J. (2003). *Operationalizing the rubric: The effect of benchmark selection on the assessed quality of writing.* ERIC Document # 481661.

Pore, S., and Reed, K. (1999). *Quick reference to speech-language pathology.* Gaithersburg, MD: Aspen Publishers.

Portage Project (2003). *The Portage guide: Birth to six.* Portage, WI: Author.

Powell, R., and Bishop, D.V.M. (1992). Clumsiness and perceptual problems in children with specific language impairment. *Developmental Medicine and Child Neurology, 34,* 755-765.

Prather, E., Beecher, S., Stafford, M., and Wallace, E. (1980). *Screening test of adolescent language.* Seattle, WA: University of Washington Press.

Pratt, S. (2005). Aural habilitation update. *ASHA Leader, 10(4),* 9-32.

Preisser, D., Hodson, B., and Paden, E. (1988). Developmental phonology: 18-29 Months. *Journal of Speech and Hearing Disorders, 53,* 125-130.

Preissler, M. (2003). *Symbolic understanding of pictures and words in low-functioning children with autism and normally developing 18- and 24-month olds.* Dissertation Abstracts International: Section B: The Science and Engineering, 64, 2423.

Prelock, E., Ford, C., Beasman, J., and Evans, D. (1999). An inclusion model for children with language learning disabilities: Building classroom partnerships. *Topics in Language Disorders, 19,* 1-18.

Prelock, P. (2000). An intervention focus for inclusionary practice. *Language, Speech, and Hearing Services in Schools, 31,* 296-298.

Prelock, P., Beatson, J., Bitner, B., Broder, C., and Ducker, A. (2003). Inter-disciplinary assessment of young children with autism spectrum disorder. *Language, Speech and Hearing Services in Schools, 34,* 194-202.

Prelock, P., Beatson, J., Contompasis, S., and Kirk, K. (1999). A model for family centered interdisciplinary practice in the community. *Topics in Language Disorders, 19,* 19-35.

Prelock, P., Cataland, J., Honchell, C., and Cordonnier, M. (1993, November). *Effective collaborative intervention models for the preschool and home setting.* Poster session presented at National Convention of the American Speech-Language-Hearing Association, Anaheim, CA.

Prelock, P., Miller, B., and Reed, N. (1993). *Working with the classroom curriculum: A guide for analysis and use in speech therapy.* Austin, TX: Pro-Ed.

Prelock, P., Miller, B., and Reed, N. (1995). Collaborative partnerships in language in the classroom program. *Language, Speech, and Hearing Services in Schools, 26,* 286-292.

Prelutsky, J. (1986). *Read-aloud rhymes for the very young.* New York: Knopf Books for Young Readers.

Prendeville, J., and Ross-Allen, J. (2002). The transition process in the early years: Enhancing speech-language pathologists' perspectives. *Language, Speech and Hearing Services in Schools, 33,* 130-136.

Pressley, M. (1998). *Reading instruction that works: The case for balanced teaching.* New York: Guilford Press

Pressley, M., and Wharton-McDonald, R. (1997). Skilled comprehension and its development through instruction. *School Psychology Review, 26,* 448-466.

Pressman, H., and Berkowitz, M. (2003, Oct. 21). Treating children with feeding disorders. *The ASHA Leader, 8(19),* 10-11.

Prinz, P., and Strong, M. (1998). ASL Proficiency and English literacy within a bilingual deaf education model of instruction. *Topics in Language Disorders, 18(4),* 47-60.

Prizant, B. (1982). Gestalt language and gestalt processing in autism. *Topics in Language Disorders, 3,* 16-24.

Prizant, B. (1987). Theoretical and clinical implications of echolalic behavior in autism. In T.L. Layton (Ed.). *Language and treatment of autistic and developmentally disordered children* (pp. 65-88). Springfield, IL: Charles C Thomas.

Prizant, B. (1991). *Early intervention: Focus on communication assessment and enhancement.* Workshop presented in Beaverton, OR.

Prizant, B. (1996). Communication, language, social, and emotional development. *Journal of Autism and Developmental Disorders, 26,* 173-178.

Prizant, B., Audet, L., Burke, G., Hummel, L., Maher, S., and Theadore, G. (1990). Communication disorders and emotional/behavioral disorders in children and adolescents. *Journal of Speech and Hearing Research, 55,* 179-192.

Prizant, B., and Duchan, J. (1981). The functions of immediate echolalia in autistic children. *Journal of Speech and Hearing Disorders, 46,* 241-249.

Prizant, B., and Meyer, E. (1993). Socioemotional aspects of language and social-communication disorders in young children. *American Journal of Speech-Language Pathology: A Journal of Clinical Practice, 2(3),* 56-71.

Prizant, B., and Rydell, P. (1984). Analysis of functions of delayed echolalia in autistic children. *Journal of Speech and Hearing Research, 27,* 183-192.

Prizant, B., and Schuler, A. (1987). Facilitating communication: Theoretical foundations. In D.J. Cohen and A.M. Donnellan (Eds.). *Handbook of autism and pervasive developmental disorders* (pp. 316-332). New York: John Wiley & Sons.

Prizant, B., Schuler, A., Wetherby, A., and Rydell, P. (1997). Enhancing language and communication development: Language approaches. In D. Cohen and F. Volkmar (Eds.). *Handbook of autism and pervasive developmental disorders* (pp. 572-605). New York: John Wiley & Sons.

Prizant, B., and Wetherby, A. (1989). Enhancing communication: From theory to practice. In G. Dawson (Ed.). *Autism: New perspectives on diagnosis, nature and treatment.* New York: Guilford Press.

Prizant, B., and Wetherby, A. (1998). Understanding the continuum of discrete-trial traditional behavioral to social-pragmatic developmental approaches in communication enhancement for young children with autism/PDD. *Seminars in Speech and Language, 19,* 329-354.

Prizant, B., and Wetherby, A. (2005). Critical issues in enhancing communication abilities for persons with autism spectrum disorders. In F. Volkmar, R. Paul, A. Klin, and D. Cohen (Eds.). *Handbook of autism and pervasive developmental disorders* (vol. II, pp. 925-945). New York: Wiley.

Prizant, B., Wetherby, A., Rubin, E., Laurent, A., and Rydell, P. (2006). *The SCERTS model.* Baltimore: Paul H. Brookes Publishers.

Proctor, A. (1989). Stages of normal noncry vocal development in infancy: A protocol for assessment. *Topics in Language Disorders, 10(1),* 26-42.

Proctor, W.J. (1995). *Infant developmental screening scale.* San Antonio, TX: The Psychological Corporation.

Proctor-Williams, K., Fey, M., and Loeb, D. (2001). Parental recasts and production of copulas and articles by children with specific language impairment and typical development. *American Journal of Speech-Language Pathology, 10,* 155-168.

Project STILE, Draft copy. (1979). Lawrence, KS: Lawrence High School.

Prutting, C., Gallagher, T., and Mulac, A. (1975). The expressive portion of the N.S.S.T. compared to a spontaneous language sample. *Journal of Speech and Hearing Disorders, 40,* 40-49.

Prutting, C., and Kirchner, D. (1983). Applied pragmatics. In T.M. Gallagher and C.A. Prutting (Eds.). *Pragmatic assessment and intervention issues in language* (pp. 29-64). San Diego, CA: College-Hill Press.

Pushaw, D. (1976). *Teach your child to talk, revised Ed.* New York: Dantree Press.

Pye, C. (1987). *Pye analysis of language* (computer program). Lawrence: University of Kansas.

Qualls, C., and O'Brien, R. (2003). Contextual variation, familiarity, academic literacy and rural adolescents' idiom knowledge. *Language, Speech and Hearing Services in Schools, 34,* 69-79.

Quick, J., and O'Neal, A. (1997). *Promoting communication in infants and young children.* Vero Beach, FL: The Speech Bin.

Quigley, S., and Kretchmer, R. (1982). *The education of deaf children: Issues, theory and practice.* London: Edward Arnold.

Quigley, S., and Paul, P. (1984). *Language and deafness.* London: Croom Helm.

Quigley, S., Power, D., and Steinkamp, M. (1977). The language structure of deaf children. *Volta Review, 79,* 73-84.

Quigley, S., Smith, N., and Wilbur, R. (1974). Comprehension of relativized sentences by deaf students. *Journal of Speech and Hearing Research, 17,* 325-341.

Quill, K. (1998). Environmental supports to enhance social-communication. *Seminars in Speech and Language, 19,* 407-423.

Quirk, R., Greenbaum, S., Leech, G., and Svartvik, J. (1985). *A comprehensive grammar of the English language.* London: Longman.

Quirk, R., Greenbaum, S., Leech, G., and Svartvik, J. (1990). *A grammar of contemporary English* (rev. ed.). New York: Seminar Press.

Rabren, K., Darch, C., and Eaves, R. (1999). The differential effects of two systematic reading comprehension approaches with students with learning disabilities. *Journal of Learning Disabilities, 32,* 36-47.

Radziewicz, C., and Antonellis, S. (1997). Considerations and implications for habilitation of hearing impaired children. In D.K. Bernstein and E. Tiegerman (Eds.). *Language and communication disorders in children* (ed. 4, pp. 482-514). New York: Macmillan.

Raffaelli, M., and Duckett, E. (1989). "We were just talking...": Conversations in early adolescence. *Journal of Youth and Adolescence, 18,* 567-581.

Rais-Bahrami, K., Short, L., and Batshaw, M. (2002). Premature and small for date infants. In M. Batshaw (Ed.). *Children with disabilities—5th Ed* (pp. 85-106). Baltimore, MD: Paul H. Brookes.

Ramirez, A., and Politzer, R. (1978). Comprehension and production in English as a second language by elementary school children and adolescents. In E.M. Hatch (Ed.). *Second language acquisition* (pp. 313-332). Rowley, MA: Newbury House Publishers.

Raphael, T. (1984). Teaching learners about sources of information for answering comprehension questions. *Journal of Reading, 27,* 303-311.

Rapin, I. (1988). Discussion of developmental language disorders. In J.F. Kavanagh and T.J. Truss, Jr. (Eds.). *Learning disabilities: Proceedings of the national conference* (pp. 273-280). Parkton, MD: York Press.

Rapin, I., and Allen, D. (1983). Developmental language disorders: Nosologic considerations. In U. Kirk (Ed.). *Neuropsychology of language, reading, and spelling.* New York: Academic Press.

Rapin, I., and Allen, D. (1987). *Developmental dysphagia and autism in preschool children: Characteristics and subtypes.* Proceedings of the First International Symposium on Specific Speech and Language Disorders in Children. London: Association for All Speech Impaired Children.

Rapoport, J., and Ismond, D. (1984). *DSM–III training guide for diagnosis of childhood disorders.* New York: Brunner/Mazel.

Ratner, N. (2004). Attention deficit hyperactivity disorder. *Seminars in Speech and Language, 25,* 205-206.

Ratner, N., Parker, B., and Gardner, P. (1993). Joint bookreading as a language scaffolding activity for communicatively impaired children. *Seminars in Speech and Language, 14,* 296-313.

Rauh, V., Achenbach, T., Nurcombe, B., Howell, C., and Teti, D. (1988). Minimizing adverse effects of low birthweight: Four-year results of an early intervention program. *Child Development, 59(3),* 544-553.

Raven, J. (1965). *Raven's coloured and standard progressive matrices.* San Antonio, TX: Psychological Corporation.

Rayner, K., and Pollatsek, A. (1987). Eye movements in reading: A tutorial review. In M. Coltheart (Ed.). *Attention and performance, XII: The psychology of reading.* London: Erlbaum.

Redmond, S. (2002). The use of rating scales with children who have language impairments. *American Journal of Speech-Language Pathology, 11,* 124-138.

Redmond, S. (2003). Children's productions of the affix –ed in past tense and past participle contexts. *Journal of Speech, Language, and Hearing Research, 46,* 1095-1109.

Redmond, S., and Rice, M. (1998). The socioemotional behaviors of children with SLI: Social adaption or social deviance? *Journal of Speech, Language, and Hearing Research, 41,* 688-700.

Redmond, S., and Rice, M. (2001). Detection of irregular verb violations by children with and without SLI. *Journal of Speech, Language, & Hearing Research, 44,* 655-670.

Redmond, S., and Rice, M. (2003). Stability of behavioral ratings of children with SLI. *Journal of Speech, Language, and Hearing Research, 45,* 190-201.

Redmond, S.M., and Johnston, S.S. (2001). Evaluating the morphological competence of children with severe speech and physical impairments. *Journal of Speech, Language & Hearing Research, 44(6),* 1362-1375.

Reed, V., Bradfield, M., and McAllister, L. (1998). The relative importance of selected communication skills for successful adolescent peer interactions. *Clinical Linguistics and Phonetics, 12,* 205-220.

Reed, V., Griffith, F., and Rasmussen, A. (1998). Morphosyntactic structures in the spoken language of older children and adolescents. *Clinical Linguistics and Phonetics, 12,* 163-181.

Reed, V., MacMillan, V., and McLeod, S. (2001). Elucidating the effect of different definitions of utterance on selected syntactic measures of older children's speech samples. *Asia Pacific Journal of Speech, Language, and Hearing, 6,* 39-45.

Reed, V., and Spicer, L. (2003). The relative importance of selected communication skills in for adolescents' interactions with their teachers: High school teachers' opinions. *Language, Speech, and Hearing Services in Schools, 34,* 343-357.

Rees, N., and Shulman, M. (1978). I don't understand what you mean by comprehension. *Journal of Speech and Hearing Disorders, 43,* 208-219.

Reese, P.B., and Challenner, N.C. (2001). *Autism & PDD: Adolescent social skills lessons 5—Book set.* East Moline, IL: Linguisystems.

Reichle, J., Mirenda, P., Locke, P., Piche, L., and Johnson, S. (1991). Beginning augmentative communication systems. In S. Warren and J. Reichle (Eds.). *Causes and effects in communication and language intervention* (pp. 131-156). Baltimore, MD: Paul H. Brookes.

Reid, D.K. (2000). Ebonics and Hispanic, Asian and Native American dialects of English. In K. Fahey and D.K. Reid (Eds.). *Language development, differences, and disorders* (pp. 219-246). Austin, TX: Pro-Ed.

Reilly, J., Losh, M., Bellugi, U., and Wulfeck, B. (2004). "Frog, where are you?" Narratives in children with specific language impairment, early focal brain injury, and Williams syndrome. *Brain and Language, 88,* 229-247.

Reinwein, D. (1982). Treatment of diminished thyroid hormone formation. In D. Reinwein and E. Klein (Eds.). *Diminished thyroid formation: Possible causes and clinical aspects.* Stuttgart: Schattauer Verlag.

Reitan, R., and Boll, T. (1973). Neuropsychological correlates of minimal brain dysfunction. *New York Academy of Science, 205,* 65-88.

Renaissance Learning, (N.D.) *Accelerated vocabulary* (computer program). Wisconsin Rapids, WI: Author.

Renfrew, C. (1991). *The bus story: A test of continuous speech* (ed. 22nd ed.). Old Headington, Oxford, England: C. Renfrew.

Renzaglia, A., Karvonen, M., Drasgow, E., and Stoxen, C. (2003). Promoting a lifetime of inclusion. *Focus on Autism & Other Developmental Disabilities, 18,* 140-149.

Rescorla, L. (1989). The Language Development Survey: A screening tool for delayed language in toddlers. *Journal of Speech and Hearing Disorders, 54,* 587-599.

Rescorla, L. (1990, June). *Outcomes of expressive language delay.* Paper presented at the Symposium for Research in Child Language Disorders, Madison, WI.

Rescorla, L. (2002). Language and reading outcomes to age 9 in late-talking toddlers. *Journal of Speech, Language, and Hearing Research, 45,* 360-371.

Rescorla, L. (2005). Age 13 language and reading outcomes in late-talking toddlers. *Journal of Speech, Language, and Hearing Research, 48,* 459-472.

Rescorla, L., and Achenbach, T. (2002). Use of the Language Development Survey in a national probability sample of children from 18 to 35 months old. *Journal of Speech, Language & Hearing Research, 45,* 1092-4388.

Rescorla, L., and Alley, A. (2001). Validation of the Language Development Survey: A parent report tool for identifying language delay in toddlers. *Journal of Speech, Language, and Hearing Research, 44,* 34-45.

Rescorla, L., Dahlsgaard, K., and Roberts, J. (2000). Late-talking toddlers: MLU and IPSyn outcomes at 3;0 and 4;0. *Journal of Child Language, 27,* 643-664.

Rescorla, L, and Fenchnay, T. (1996). Mother-child synchrony and communicative reciprocity in late-talking toddlers. *Journal of Speech and Hearing Research, 39,* 200-208.

Rescorla, L., and Goossens, M. (1992). Symbolic play development in toddlers with expressive specific language impairment. *Journal of Speech and Hearing Research, 35,* 1290-1302.

Rescorla, L., and Lee, E. (2001). Language impairment in young children. In T. Layton, E. Crais, and L. Watson (Eds.). *Handbook of early language impairment in children: Nature* (pp. 1-55). Albany, New York: Delmar Publishers.

Rescorla, L., Mirak, J., and Singh, L. (2000). Vocabulary growth in late talkers: Lexical development from 2;0 to 3;0. *Journal of Child Language, 27,* 293-311.

Rescorla, L., and Mirren, L. (1998). Communicative intent in late-talking toddlers. *Applied Psycholinguistics, 19,* 393-411.

Rescorla, L., and Paul, R. (November, 1990). *Screening for expressive language delay at age two.* Paper presented at the annual convention of the American Speech-Language-Hearing Association, Seattle, WA.

Rescorla, L., and Ratner, N.B. (1996). Phonetic profiles of toddlers with severe expressive language impairments (SLI-E). *Journal of Speech and Hearing Research, 39,* 153-165.

Rescorla, L, and Roberts, J. (2002). Nominal versus verbal morpheme use in late talkers at ages 3 and 4. *Journal of Speech, Language and Hearing Research, 45,* 1219-1232.

Rescorla, L., Roberts, J., and Dahlsgaard, K. (1997). Late talkers at 2: Outcome at age 3. *Journal of Speech and Hearing Research, 40,* 556-566.

Restrepo, M. (1998). Identification of predominantly Spanish-speaking children with language impairment. *Journal of Speech, Language, and Hearing Research, 41,* 1398-1411.

Restrepo, M. (2005). The case for bilingual intervention for typical and atypical language learners. *Perspectives on Language Learning and Education, 12,* 13-17.

Restrepo, M., and Silverman, S. (2001). Validity of the Spanish Preschool Language Scale—3 for use with bilingual children. *American Journal of Speech-Language Pathology, 10,* 382-393.

Retherford, K. (1992). *Guide applied: Production characteristics of language-impaired children.* Eau Claire, WI: Thinking Publications.

Retherford, K. (2000). *Guide to analysis of language transcripts* (3rd ed.). Eau Claire, WI: Thinking Publications.

Rey, H. (1952). *Curious George rides a bike.* New York: Houghton Mifflin.

Reynell, J. (1979). *The Reynell-Zinkin Scales: Developmental scales for young visually handicapped children.* Windsor, England: NFER Publishing.

Reynell, J., and Gruber, C. (1990). *Reynell developmental language scales* (American Edition). Los Angeles, CA: Western Psychological Services.

Reynolds, C., and Hickman, J. (2004). *Draw-a-person intellectual ability test for children, adolescents, and adults.* Austin, TX: Pro-Ed.

Reynolds, C.R., and Kamphaus, R.W. (2003a). *Reynolds intellectual assessment scales (RIAS).* Lutz, FL: Psychological Assessment Resources.

Reynolds, C.R., and Kamphaus, R.W. (2003b). *Reynolds intellectual screening test (RIST).* Lutz, FL: Psychological Assessment Resources.

Reynolds, R., Want, M., and Walberg, H. (2003). *Early childhood programs for a new century.* Washington, DC: Child Welfare League of America, Inc.

Reznick, S., and Goldsmith, L. (1989). A multiple form word production checklist for assessing early language. *Journal of Child Language, 16,* 91-100.

Rice, A. (1976). *Interview with a vampire.* New York: Knopf.

Rice, M. (1983). Contemporary accounts of the cognition/language relationship: Implications for speech-language clinicians. *Journal of Speech and Hearing Disorders, 48,* 347-359.

Rice, M. (2000). Grammatical symptoms of specific language impairment. In D.V.M. Bishop & L.B. Leonard (Eds.). *Speech and language impairments in children: Causes, characteristics, intervention and outcome* (pp. 17-34). Hove: Psychology Press.

Rice, M. (2004). Growth models of developmental language disorders. In M. Rice & F. Warren (Eds.). *Developmental language disorders: From phenotypes to etiologies* (pp. 207-240). Mahwah, NH: Lawrence Erlbaum.

Rice, M., and Bode, J. (1993). GAPS in the lexicon of children with specific language impairment. *First Language, 13,* 113-132.

Rice, M., Buhr, J., and Nemeth, M. (1990). Fast mapping word-learning abilities of language-delayed preschoolers. *Journal of Speech and Hearing Disorders, 55,* 33-42.

Rice, M., Buhr, J.C., and Oetting, J.B. (1992). Speech-language impaired children's quick incidental learning of words: The effect of a pause. *Journal of Speech and Hearing Research, 35,* 1040-1048.

Rice, M., Sell, M., and Hadley, P. (1990). The social interactive coding system (SICS): An on-line, clinically relevant descriptive tool. *Language, Speech and Hearing Services in Schools, 21,* 2-14.

Rice, M., Warren, S., and Betz, S. (2005). Language symptoms of developmental language disorders: An overview of autism, Down syndrome, fragile X, specific language impairment, and Williams syndrome. *Applied Psycholinguistics, 26,* 7-27.

Rice, M., and Wexler, K. (1996). Toward tense as a clinical marker of specific language impairment in English-speaking children. *Journal of Speech and Hearing Research, 39,* 1239-1257.

Rice, M., Wexler, K., and Cleave, P. (1995). Specific language impairment as a period of extended optional infinitive. *Journal of Speech and Hearing Research, 38,* 850-863.

Rice, M., and Wilcox, K. (1995). *Building a language-focused curriculum for the preschool classroom* (vol. I, A foundation for lifelong communication). Baltimore, MD: Paul H. Brookes.

Richard, G., and Hanner, M. (1995). *The language processing test—Revised (LPT-R).* East Moline, IL: LinguiSystems.

Richards, E., and Singer, M. (2001). Representation of complex goal structures in narrative comprehension. *Discourse Processes, 3,* 11-135.

Rickford, J. (1999). *African American vernacular English.* Oxford, England: Blackwell Publishing.

Ricks, D. (1975). Vocal communication in pre-verbal normal and autistic children. In N. O'Conner (Ed.). *Language, cognitive deficits and retardation.* London: Butterworths.

Riddle, M., Anderson, G., Cicchetti, D., McIntosh, S., and Cohen, D.J. (1991). *Increases with whole brain radiation in childhood leukemia (summary).* Scientific proceedings of the Annual Meeting of the American Academy of Child and Adolescent Psychiatry VII (p. 63).

Rinaldi, W. (2000). Pragmatic comprehension in secondary school-aged students with specific developmental language disorder. *International Journal of Language and Communication Disorders, 35,* 1-29.

Rinaldi, W. (2001). *Social use of language programme-Revised.* Windsor: NFER Nelson.

Rini, D. (2001). Family centered practice. In R. Paul (Ed.). *Introduction to clinical methods in communication disorders* (pp. 317-335). Baltimore: Paul H. Brookes.

Rini, D., and Hindenlang, J. (2006). Family-centered practice. In R. Paul and P. Cascella, (Eds.). *Introduction to clinical methods in communication disorders* (pp. 317-336). Baltimore: Paul H. Brookes.

Rini, D., and Whitney, G. (1999). Family-centered practice for children with communication disorders. In. R. Paul (Ed.). *Child and adolescent psychiatric clinics of North America: Language disorders* (pp. 153-174). Philadelphia, PA: W.B. Saunders.

Ripich, D., and Griffith, P. (1988). Narrative abilities of children with learning disabilities and nondisabled children: Story structure, cohesion and propositions. *Journal of Learning Disabilities, 21,* 165-173.

Ripich, D., and Spinelli, F. (1985). *School discourse problems.* San Diego, CA: College-Hill Press.

Rispoli, M., and Hadley, P. (2001). The leading edge: The significance of sentence disruptions in the development of grammar. *Journal of Speech, language, and Hearing Research, 44,* 1131-1143.

Ritvo, E. (1976). *Autism: Diagnosis, current research, and management.* New York: Spectrum.

Rivara, F., and Barber, M. (1985). Demographic analysis of childhood pedestrian injuries. *Pediatrics, 76,* 375-381.

Roberts, J. (2004). Otitis media, hearing loss, and language learning: Controversies and current research. *Journal of Developmental and Behavioral Pediatrics, 25,* 110-122.

Roberts, J., Burchinal, M., Davis, B., Collier, A., and Henderson, F. (1991). Otitis media in early childhood and later language. *Journal of Speech and Hearing Research, 34,* 1158-1168.

Roberts, J., Burchinal, M., Koch, M., Footo, M., and Henderson, F. (1988). Otitis media in early childhood and its relationship to later speech and language. In D. Lim, C. Bluestone, J. Klein, and J. Nelson (Eds.). *Recent advances in otitis media* (pp. 423-430). Philadelphia, PA: BC Decker.

Roberts, J., Medley, L., Swartzfager, J., and Neebe, E. (1997). Assessing the communication of African-American one-year-olds using the communication and symbolic behavior scales. *American Journal of Speech-Language Pathology, 6,* 59-65.

Roberts, J., Mirrett, P., Anderson, K., Burchinall, M., and Neebe, E. (2002). Early communication, symbolic behavior and social profiles in young males with fragile X syndrome. *American Journal of Speech-Language Pathology, 11,* 295-304.

Roberts, J., Prizant, B., and McWilliam, R.A. (1995). Out-of-class versus in-class service delivery in language intervention: Effects on communication interactions with young children. *American Journal of Speech-Language Pathology, 4,* 87-93.

Roberts, J., Rescorla, L., Giroux, J., and Stevens, L. (1998). Phonological skills of children with specific expressive language impairments: Outcome at age 3. *Journal of Speech, Language, and Hearing Research, 41,* 374-385.

Roberts, J., Sanyni, M., Burchinal, M., Collier, A., Ranney, C., and Henderson, F. (1986). Otitis media in early childhood and its relationship to later verbal and academic performance. *Pediatrics, 78,* 428-430.

Roberts, J., and Schuele, C. (1990). Otitis media and later academic performance: The linkage and implications for intervention. *Topics in Language Disorders, 11(1),* 43-62.

Robertson, C., and Salter, W. (1995). *The phonological awareness profile.* East Moline, IL: LinguiSystems.

Robertson, C., and Salter, W. (1997). *The phonological awareness test.* East Moline, IL: LinguiSystems.

Robertson, S., and Weismer, S. (1999). Effects of treatment on linguistic and social skills in toddlers with delayed language development. *Journal of Speech, Language, and Hearing Research, 42,* 1234-1248.

Robinson, C., Bataillon, K., Fieber, N., Jackson, B., Rasmussen, J. (1985). *Sensorimotor assessment form.* Omaha, NE: Meyer Rehabilitation Center.

Robinson, F. (1970). *Effective study.* New York: Harper & Row.

Robinson, G. (1982). *Raven the trickster: Legends of the North American Indians.* New York: Atheneum.

Robinson, R. (2003). Landau-Kleffner syndrome: Current issues. *Neurology, 19,* 53-56.

Robinson, R.O., Baird, G., Robinson, G., and Simonoff, E. (2001). Landau-Kleffner syndrome: Course and correlates with outcome. *Developmental Medicine and Child Neurology, 43(4),* 243-247.

Robinson-Zanartu, C. (1996). Serving Native American children and families. *Language, Speech, and Hearing Services in Schools, 27,* 373-384.

Rodekohr, R.K., and Haynes W.O. (2001). Differentiating dialect from disorder: A comparison of two processing tasks and a standardized language test. *Journal of Communication Disorders, 34,* 255-272.

Rodriguez, B., and Olswang, B. (2003). Mexican-American and Anglo-American mothers' beliefs and values about child rearing, education and language impairment. *American Journal of Speech-Language Pathology, 12,* 452-462.

Roeser, R. (1988). Cochlear implants and tactile aids for the profoundly deaf student. In R.J. Roeser and M.P. Downs (Eds.). *Auditory disorders in school children* (pp. 260-280). New York: Thieme Medical Publishers.

Rogers, S. (1996). Brief report; Early intervention in autism. *Journal of Autism and Developmental Disorders, 26,* 243-246.

Rogers, S. (2006). Evidence-based intervention for language development in young children with autism. In T. Charman and W. Stone (Eds.). *Social and communication development in autism spectrum disorders: Early identification, diagnosis, and intervention.* New York: Guilford. In press.

Rogers, S., Donovan, C., D'Eugenio, D., Brown, S., Lynch, E., Moersch, M., and Schafer, S. (1981). *Developmental programming for infants and young children, Volume 2: Early intervention developmental profile* (rev. ed.). Ann Arbor, MI: The University of Michigan Press.

Rogers-Warren, A., and Warren, S. (1980). Mands for verbalization: Facilitating the generalization of newly trained language in children. *Behavior Modification, 4,* 230-245.

Roid, G., and Miller, L. (1997). *Leiter international performance scale—Revised.* Wood Dale, IL: Stoelting.

Roid, G., and Miller, L. (1999). *Stoelting brief intelligence test (S–BIT).* Wood Dale, IL: Stoelting.

Roland, P., and Brown, O. (1990). Tympanostomy tubes: A rational clinical treatment for middle ear disease. *Topics in Language Disorders, 11(1),* 23-28.

Romski, M.A., and Sevcik, R.A. (1996). *Breaking the speech barrier: Language development through augmented means.* Baltimore, MD: Paul H. Brookes.

Romski, M., Sevcik, R., Cheslock, M., and Barton, A. (2006). The system for augmenting language. In R. McCauley and M. Fey (Eds.). *Treatment of language disorders in children.* Baltimore: Paul H. Brookes. In press.

Romski, M., Sevcik, R., and Pate, J. (1988). Establishment of symbolic communication in persons with severe retardation. *Journal of Speech and Hearing Disorders, 53,* 94-107.

Roseberry, C., and Connell, P. (1991). The use of an invented language rule in the differentiation of normal and language-impaired Spanish-speaking children. *Journal of Speech and Hearing Research, 34,* 596-603.

Roseberry-McKibben, C. (2002a). *Multicultural students with special language needs* (2nd ed.) Oceanside, CA: Academic Communication Associates.

Roseberry-McKibben, C. (2002b). Principles and strategies in intervention. In A. Brice (Ed.). *The Hispanic child: Speech language, culture and education* (pp. 199-233). Boston: Allyn & Bacon.

Rosen, S. (2003). Auditory processing in dyslexia and specific language impairment: Is there a deficit? What is its nature? Does it explain anything? *Journal of Phonetics, 31/3-4,* 509-527.

Rosenbek, J., and Wertz, R. (1972). A review of 50 cases of developmental apraxia of speech. *Language, Speech, and Hearing Services in Schools, 3,* 23-33.

Rosenquest, B. (2002). Literacy-based planning and pedagogy that supports toddler language development. *Early Childhood Education Journal, 29,* 241-249.

Ross, D. (1986). *Ross information processing assessment.* Austin, TX: Pro-Ed.

Ross, J.D., and Ross, C.M. (1976). *Ross test of higher cognitive processes.* Novata, CA: Academic Therapy Publications.

Rossetti, L. (1986). *High-risk infants: Identification, assessment, and intervention.* Boston, MA: College-Hill Press.

Rossetti, L. (1990). *The Rossetti infant-toddler language scale: A measure of communication and interaction.* East Moline, IL: LinguiSystems.

Rossetti, L. (1992). *Assessment and intervention with high-risk infants and toddlers.* Moline, IL: LinguiSystems.

Rossetti, L. (1993, October). *Neurodevelopmental assessment of infants and toddlers.* Paper presented at State Conference of Oregon, Speech-Language and Hearing Association, Sunriver, OR.

Rossetti, L. (1995). *The Rossetti infant-toddler language scale: A measure of communication and interaction.* East Moline, IL: LinguiSystems.

Rossetti, L. (2001). *Communication intervention: Birth to three—2nd Ed.* San Diego, CA: Singular Publishing Group.

Roswell, F., and Chall, J. (1971). *Roswell-Chall auditory blending test.* New York: Essay Press.

Roth, F. (1986). Oral narrative abilities of learning-disabled students. *Topics in Language Disorders, 7,* 21-30.

Roth, F. (2000). Narrative writing: Development and teaching with children with writing difficulties. *Topics in Language Disorders, 20(4),* 15-28.

Roth, F., and Baden, B. (2001). Investing in emergent literacy intervention: A key role for speech-language pathologists. *Seminars in Speech and Language, 22,* 163-174.

Roth, F., and Spekman, N. (1984a). Assessing the pragmatic abilities of children: Part 1. Organizational framework and assessment parameters. *Journal of Speech and Hearing Disorders, 49,* 2-11.

Roth, F., and Spekman, N. (1984b). Assessing the pragmatic abilities of children: Part 2. Guidelines, considerations, and specific evaluation procedures. *Journal of Speech and Hearing Disorders, 49,* 12-17.

Roth, F., and Spekman, N. (1989). Higher-order language processes and reading disabilities. In A. Kamhi and H. Catts (Eds.). *Reading disabilities: A developmental language perspective* (pp. 159-198). Boston, MA: College-Hill.

Roth, F., and Worthington, C. (2005). *Treatment resource manual for speech-language pathology* (3rd ed.). Clifton, Park, NY: Delmar.

Rothganger, H. (2003). Analysis of the sounds of the child in the first year of age and a comparison to the language. *Early Human Development, 75,* 55-69.

Roulstone, S., Loader, S., Northstone, K., and Beveridge, M. (2002). The speech and language development of children aged 25 months: Descriptive data from the Avon longitudinal study of parents and children. *Early Child Development and Care, 172,* 259-268.

Rourke, B. (1989). *Nonverbal learning disabilities.* New York: Guilford Press.

Rourke, B. (1995). *Syndrome of nonverbal learning disabilities: Neurodevelopmental manifestations.* New York: Guilford Press.

Rourke, B., Ahmad, S., Collins, D., Hayman-Abello, B., Satyman-Abello, S., and Warriner, E. (2002). Child clinical pediatric neuropsychology: Some recent advances. *Annual Reviews of Psychology, 53,* 309-339.

Rowland, C., and Schweigert, P. (1993). *Analyzing the communication environment (ACE): An inventory of ways to encourage communication in functional activities.* Tucson, AZ: Communication Skill Builders.

Rozwell, F., and Chall, J. (1971). *Auditory blending test.* New York: Essay.

Rubin, D. (1987). Divergence and convergence between oral and written communication. *Topics in Language Disorders, 7(4),* 1-18.

Rubin, E. (2004). Asperger syndrome and high functioning autism: Addressing social communication and emotional regulation. *Topics in Language Disorders, 24* (whole issue).

Ruder, K., Bunce, B., and Ruder, C. (1984). Language intervention in a preschool/classroom setting. In L. McCormick and R. Schiefelbusch (Eds.). *Early language intervention* (pp. 267-298). Columbus, OH: Merrill.

Rudin, E. (1982). *The three billy goats gruff.* New York: Western Publishing Company.

Rue, G. (2000). School slang: What does your class have to say? *Writing, 23,* 20-22.

Ruiz-Palaez, J., Charpak, N., and Cuervo, L. (2004). Kangaroo Mother Care: An example to follow from developing countries. *British Medical Journal, 329,* 1179-1182.

Rukeyser, L. (Aug. 30, 1988). U.S. firms make it their business to help ease the dropout dilemma. *Star Tribune,* Minneapolis, Minn (p. 2 D).

Rumelhart, D., and McClelland, J. (1986). *Parallel distributed processing: Explorations in the microstructure of cognition.* Cambridge, MA: Bradford Books.

Russell, N. (1993). Educational considerations in traumatic brain injury: The role of the speech-language pathologist. Language, Speech, and Hearing Services in Schools, 24, 67-75.

Russell, N., and Smith, A. (1961). Post-traumatic amnesia in closed head injury. *Archives of Neurology, 5,* 4-17.

Rutter, M. (1987). Continuities and discontinuities from infancy. In J. Doniger Osofsky (Ed.). *Handbook of infant development* (2nd ed.). New York: John Wiley & Sons.

Rutter, M. (2005). Genetic influences and autism. In F. Volkmar, R. Paul, A. Klin, and D. Cohen (Eds.). *Handbook of autism and pervasive developmental disorders—vol. 1* (pp. 425-452). New York: Wiley.

Rutter, M., Bailey, A., and Lord, C. (2003). *Social communication questionnaire.* Los Angeles, CA: Western Psychological Services.

Rutter, M., Bailey, A., Simonoff, E., and Pickles, A. (1997). Genetic influences of autism. In D. Cohen and F. Volkmar (Eds.). *Handbook of autism and pervasive developmental disorders* (pp. 370-387). New York: John Wiley & Sons.

Rutter, R., Bailey, A., and Lord, C. (1999). *Social communication questionnaire.* Los Angeles: Western Psychological Service.

Rvachew, S., Ohberg, A., Grawburg, M., and Heyding, J. (2003). Phonological awareness and phonemic perception in 4 year old children with delayed expressive phonology skills. *American Journal of Speech-Language Pathology, 12,* 463-471.

Rylant, C. (1982). *When I was young in the mountains.* New York: E.P. Dutton.

Saben, C., and Ingham, J. (1991). The effects of minimal pairs treatment on the speech-sound production of two children with phonological disorders. *Journal of Speech and Hearing Research, 34,* 1023-1040.

Sabers, D.L. (1996). By their tests we will know them. *Language Speech and Hearing Services in Schools, 27(2),* 102-108.

Sachs, J. (1983). Talking about the there and then: The emergence of displaced reference in parent-child discourse. In K.E. Nelson (Ed.). *Children's language* (vol. 4). Hillsdale, NJ: Erlbaum.

Sackett, D.L., Straus, S.E., Richardson, W.S., Rosenberg, W., and Haynes, R.B. (2000). *Evidence-based medicine: How to practice and teach EBM.* Edinburgh: Churchill Livingstone.

Saenz, L., and Fuchs, L. (2002). Examining the reading difficulty of secondary students with learning disabilities: expository versus narrative text. *Remedial and Special Education, 23,* 31-41.

Saldana, D. (2004). Interactive assessment of metacognition: Exploratory study of a procedure for persons with severe mental retardation. *European Journal of Psychology of Education, 19,* 349-365.

Salvia, J., and Ysseldyke, J. (2000). *Assessment in special and remedial education* (8th ed.). Boston, MA: Houghton-Mifflin.

San Souci, R. (1989). *The talking eggs.* New York: Dial.

Sandberg, A.D. (2001). Reading and spelling, phonological awareness, and working memory in children with severe speech impairments: A longitudinal study. *AAC: Augmentative & Alternative Communication, 17(1),* 11-26.

Sanger, D., Moore-Brown, B., Magnuson, G., and Svoboda, N. (2003). Prevalence of language problems among adolescent delinquents. *Communication Disorders Quarterly, 23,* 17-26.

Sansosti, F., Powell-Smith, K., and Kincaid, D. (2004). A research synthesis of social story interventions for children with autism spectrum disorders. *Focus on Autism and Other Developmental Disabilities, 19,* 194-204.

Sarachan-Deily, A. (1985). Written narratives of deaf and hearing students: Story recall and inference. *Journal of Speech and Hearing Research, 28,* 151-159.

Satz, P., and Bullard-Bates, C. (1981). Acquired aphasia in children. In M.T. Sarno (Ed.). *Acquired aphasia.* New York: Academic Press.

Savage, R.C., DePompei, R., Tyler, J., and Lash, M. (2005). Pediatric traumatic brain injury: A review of pertinent issues. *Pediatric Rehabilitation, 8(2),* 92-103.

Sawyer, D. (1987). *Test of awareness of language segments.* Austin, TX: Pro-Ed.

Saxton, M. (2005). 'Recast' in a new light: Insights for practice from typical language studies. *Child Language Teaching and Therapy, 21,* 23-38.

Scarborough, H. (1990). Index of productive syntax. *Applied Psycholinguistics, 11,* 1-22.

Scarborough, H., and Dobrich, W. (1990). Development of children with early language delay. *Journal of Speech and Hearing Disorders, 33,* 70-83.

Scarborough, H.S. (2003). Connecting early language and literacy to later reading (dis)abilities: Evidence, theory, and practice. In S. Neuman and D. Dickinson (Eds.). *Handbook of early literacy research* (pp. 97-110). N.Y.: Guilford Press.

Scharfenaker, S. (1990). The fragile X syndrome. *ASHA, 32,* 45-47.

Schauwers, K., Gillis, S., and Govaerts, P. (2005). Language acquisition in children with a cochlear implant. In P. Fletcher and J. Miller (Eds.). *Developmental theory and language disorders* (pp. 95-120). Philadelphia: John Benjamins Publishing Co.

Scheffel, D., and Ingrisano, D. (2000). Linguistic emphasis in maternal speech to preschool language learners with language impairments: An acoustical perspective. *Infant-Toddler Intervention, 10,* 127-135.

Scheffel, D., Shroyer, J., and Strongin, D. (2003). Significant reading improvement among underachieving adolescents using LANGUAGE! A structured approach. *Reading Improvement, 40(2),* 83-96.

Scheffner Hammer, C., Miccio, A., and Rodriguez, B. (2004). Bilingual language acquisition and the child socialization process. In B. Goldstein (ed.). *Bilingual language development and disorders in Spanish-English speakers* (pp. 21-50). Baltimore: Brookes.

Scherer, N., and Olswang, L. (1984). Role of mothers' expansions in stimulating children's language production. *Journal of Speech and Hearing Research, 27,* 387-396.

Schery, T., and O'Conner, L. (1995). Computers as a context for language intervention. In M. Fey, J. Windsor, and S.F. Warren (Eds.). *Language intervention: Preschool through the elementary years* (vol. 5, pp. 275-314). Baltimore, MD: Paul H. Brookes.

Schery, T., and O'Connor, L. (1997). Language intervention: Computer training for young children with special needs. *British Journal of Educational Technology, 28,* 271-279.

Schery, T., and Wilcoxen, A. (1982). *The initial communication processes scale.* Monterey, CA: CTB/McGraw-Hill.

Schlieper, A., Kisilevsky, H., Mattingly, S., and Yorke, L. (1985). Mild conductive hearing loss and language development: A one year follow-up study. *Developmental Behavioral Pediatrics, 6,* 65-68.

Schmidt, R., and Windsor, J. (1993, June). *The effect of context on language measures for mothers, children with Down syndrome, and children with typical language development.* Poster presented at the 14th annual symposium on research in child language disorders, Madison, WI.

Schneider, P., and Watkins, R. (1996). Applying Vygotskian theory to language intervention. *Language, Speech, and Hearing Services in Schools, 27,* 157-170.

Schoenbrodt, L. (2001a). *Children with traumatic brain injury: A parent's guide.* Bethesda, MD: Woodbine House.

Schoenbrodt, L. (2001b). How TBI affects speech and language. In L. Schoenbrodt (Ed.). *Children with traumatic brain injury: A parent's guide* (pp. 177-204). Bethesda, MD: Woodbine House.

Schoenbrodt, L., Kumin, L., and Sloan, J. (1997). Learning disabilities existing concomitantly with communication disorder. *Journal of Learning Disability, 30,* 264-281.

Schopler, E., Reichler, R., and Renner, B. (1993). *Childhood autism rating scale.* Los Angeles, CA: Western Psychological Services.

Schopmeyer, B., and Lowe, F. (1992). *The fragile X child.* San Diego, CA: Singular Publishing Group.

Schory, M. (1990). Whole language and the speech-language pathologist. *Language, Speech, and Hearing Services in Schools, 21,* 206-211.

Schreibman, L., Stahmer, A.C., and Pierce, K.L. (1996). Alternative applications of pivotal response training: Teaching symbolic play and social interaction skills. In L.K. Koegel, R.L. Koegel, and G. Dunlap (Eds.). *Positive behavioral support: Including people with difficult behavior in the community* (pp. 353-371). Baltimore, MD: Paul H. Brookes.

Schrieber, L., and McKinley, N. (1995). *Daily communication: Strategies for adolescents with language disorders* (2nd ed.). Eau Claire, WI: Thinking Publications.

Schroeder, S., LeBlanc, J., and Mayo, L. (1996). Brief report: A life-span perspective on the development of individuals with autism. *Journal of Autism and Developmental Disorders, 26,* 251-256.

Schuele, C., and van Kleeck, A. (1987). Precursors to literacy: Assessment and intervention. *Topics in Language Disorders, 7,* 32-44.

Schuele, M., and Larrivee, L. (2004). What's my job: Differential diagnosis of the speech-language pathologist's role in literacy learning. *Perspectives on Language Learning and Education, 11(3),* 4-8.

Schuler, A., and Prizant, B. (1987). Facilitating communication: Pre-language approaches. In D.J. Cohen and A.M. Donnellan (Eds.). *Handbook of autism and pervasive developmental disorders* (pp. 301-315). New York: John Wiley & Sons.

Schuler, A., Prizant, B., and Wetherby, A. (1997). Enhancing language and communication development: Prelinguistic approaches. In D. Cohen and F. Volkmar (Eds.). *Handbook of autism and pervasive developmental disorders* (pp. 539-571). New York: John Wiley & Sons.

Schultz, J., Florio, S., and Erickson, R. (1982). Where's the floor? Aspects of the cultural organization of social relationships in communication at home and in school. In P. Gilmore and A. Glatthorn (Eds.). *Children in and out of school: Ethnography and education.* Washington, DC: Center for Applied Linguistics.

Schultz, R., and Robins, D. (2005). Functional neuroimaging studies of autism spectrum disorders. In F. Volkmar, R. Paul, A. Klin, and D. Cohen (Eds.). *Handbook of autism and pervasive developmental disorders—vol. 1* (pp. 512-533). New York: Wiley.

Schumaker, J., and Deshler, D. (1984). Setting demand variables: A major factor in program planning for the LD adolescent. *Topics in Language Disorders, 4(2),* 22-40.

Schumaker, J., and Deshler, D. (2003). Can students with LD become competent writers? *Learning Disability Quarterly, 26(2),* 129-142.

Schumaker, J., Deshler, D., Alley, G., Warner, M., Clark, F., and Nolan, S. (1982). Error monitoring: A learning strategy for improving adolescent academic performance. In W.M. Cruickshank and J.W. Lerner (Eds.). *Best of ACLD* (vol. 3). Syracuse, NY: Syracuse University Press.

Schumaker, J., Deshler, D., Denton, P., Alley, G., Clark, F., and Nolan, M. (1982). Multipass: A learning strategy for improving reading comprehension. *Learning Disability Quarterly, 5,* 295-304.

Schutter, L., and Brinker, R. (1992). Conjuring a new category of disability from prenatal cocaine exposure: Are the infants unique biological or caretaking casualties? *Topics in Early Childhood Special Education, 11(4),* 84-111.

Schwartz, R., Chapman, K., Terrell, B., Prelock, P., and Rowan, L. (1985). Facilitating word combinations in language-impaired children through discourse structure. *Journal of Speech and Hearing Disorders, 50,* 31-39.

Schwartz, R., and Leonard, L. (1982). Do children pick and choose? Phonological selection and avoidance in early lexical acquisition. *Journal of Child Language, 9,* 319-336.

Schwartz, S. (1996). *Choices in deafness.* Bethesda, MD: Woodbine House.

Schwartz-Cowley, R., and Stepanik, M. (1989). Communication disorders and treatment in the acute trauma center setting. *Topics in Language Disorders, 9(2),* 1-14.

Scientific Learning Corporation (2000). *FastForward.* Berkley, CA: Author.

Scieszka, J. (1989). *The true story of the three little pigs.* New York: Viking.

Scott, C. (1984, November). *What happened in that: Structural characteristics of school children's narratives.* Paper presented at the Annual Convention of the American Speech-Language-Hearing Association, San Francisco.

Scott, C. (1988). Spoken and written syntax. In M. Nippold (Ed.). *Later language development* (pp. 49-96). Boston, MA: College-Hill Press.

Scott, C. (1999). Learning to write. In H. Catts and A. Kamhi (Eds.). *Language and reading disabilities* (pp. 224-258). Boston, MA: Allyn & Bacon.

Scott, C. (2000). Principles and methods of spelling instruction: Applications for poor spellers. *Topics in Language Disorders, 20(3),* 66-82.

Scott, C. (2004). Syntactic ability in children and adolescents with language and learning disabilities (pp. 111-134). In R. Berman (Ed.). *Language development across childhood and adolescence.* Philadelphia: John Benjamins Publishing Co.

Scott, C. (2005). Learning to write. In H. Catts and A. Kamhi (Eds.). *Language and reading disabilities* (2nd ed., pp. 233-273). Boston, MA: Allyn & Bacon.

Scott, C., and Brown, S. (2001). Spelling and the speech-language pathologist: There's more than meets the eye. *Seminars in Speech and Language, 22,* 197-208.

Scott, C., and Erwin, D. (1992). Descriptive assessment of writing: Process and products. In W. Secord (Ed.). *Best practices in school speech-language pathology* (vol. II, pp. 60-73). San Antonio, TX: Psychological Corporation, Harcourt Brace Jovanovich.

Scott, C., and Layton, T. (2001). HIV infection in young children. In T. Layton, E. Crais, and L. Watson (Eds.). *Handbook of early language impairment in children: Nature* (pp. 488-540). Albany, New York: Delmar Publishers.

Scott, C., and Rogers, L. (1996). In A. Kamhi, K. Pollock, and J. Harris (Eds.). *Communication development and disorders in African American children* (pp. 307-332). Baltimore, MD: Paul H. Brookes.

Scott, C., and Stokes, S. (1995). Measures of syntax in school-age children and adolescents. *Language, Speech, and Hearing Services in Schools, 26,* 309-317.

Scott, C., and Windsor, J. (2000). General language performance measures in spoken and written narrative and expository discourse of school-age children with language learning disabilities. *Journal of Speech, Language, and Hearing Research, 43,* 324-39.

Scruggs, T., and Mastropieri, M. (1990). Mnemonic instruction for students with learning disabilities: What it is and what it does. *Learning Disability Quarterly, 13,* 271-280.

Secord, W. (1989). The traditional approach to treatment. In N. Creaghead, P. Newman, and W. Secord (Eds.). *Assessment and remediation of articulatory and phonological disorders* (2nd ed., pp. 129-157). Columbus, OH: Merrill Publishing Co.

Secord, W. (1990). *Best practices in school speech-language pathology: Collaborative programs in the schools.* San Antonio, TX: Psychological Corporation.

Secord, W., and Donohue, J. (2000) *Clinical assessment of articulation and phonology.* Greenville, SC: Super Duper, Publications.

Sedey, A., Miolo, G., and Miller, J. (1993). *Optimizing language samples in typically developing children and children with Down syndrome.* Paper presented at the National Convention of the American Speech-Language-Hearing Association. 1993, Anaheim, CA.

Segers, E., and Verhoeven, L. (2004). Computer supported phonological awareness intervention for kindergarten children with specific language impairment. *Language, Speech, and Hearing Services in Schools, 35,* 229-239.

Seidenberg, P. (1988). Cognitive and academic instructional intervention for learning-disabled adolescents. *Topics in Language Disorders, 8(3),* 56-71.

Seitz, S., and Marcus, S. (1976). Mother-child interactions: A foundation for language development. *Exceptional Children, 42,* 445-449.

Selman, R., Beardslee, W., Schultz, L., Krupa, M., and Podorefsky, D. (1986). Assessing adolescent interpersonal negotiation strategies: Toward the integration of structural and functional models. *Developmental Psychology, 22,* 450-459.

Selz, M., and Reitan, R. (1979). Neuropsychological test performance of normal, learning disabled, and brain-damaged older children. *Journal of Nervous and Mental Disorders, 167,* 298-302.

Semel, E., Wiig, E., and Secord, W. (2003). *Clinical evaluation of language fundamentals—4 (CELF–4).* San Antonio, TX: Harcourt Assessment.

Semel, E., Wiig, E., and Secord, W. (2004). *CELF–4 Screening test.* San Antonio, TX: Harcourt Assessment.

Semmel, M., Barritt, L., and Bennett, S. (1970). Performance of EMR and non-retarded children on a modified cloze task. *American Journal of Mental Deficiency, 74,* 681-688.

Semmel, M., and Herzog, B. (1966). The effects of grammatical form class on the recall of Negro and Caucasian educable retarded children. *Studies of Language and Language Behavior, 3,* 1-9.

Semrud-Clikeman, M. (2001). *Traumatic brain injury in children and adolescents: Assessment and intervention.* New York: Guilford Press.

Serpell, R., Sonnenschein, S., Baker, and Ganapathy, H. (2002). Intimate culture of families in early socialization of literacy. *Journal of Family Psychology, 16,* 391-405.

Seuss, Dr. (1956). *Green eggs and ham.* New York: Random House.

Seuss, Dr. (1970). *Mr. Brown can moo, can you?* New York: Random House.

Seuss, Dr. (1971). *The lorax.* New York: Random House.

Seymour, H. (2004). The challenge of language assessment for African American English-speaking children: A historical perspective. *Seminars in Speech and Language, 25,* 3-12.

Seymour, H., and Pearson, B.Z. (Ed.). (2004). Evaluating language variation: Distinguishing dialect and development from disorder. *Seminars in Speech and Language, 25.*

Seymour, H., Roeper, T., and deVilliers, J. (2005). *Diagnostic evaluation of language variation—Norm referenced.* San Antonio, TX: Harcourt Assessment.

Shafer, D. (2005). Research probes optimum age for implants. *ASHA Leader, 10(4),* 5-13.

Shane, H. (1993). The dark side of facilitated communication. *Topics in Language Disorders, 13(4),* 9-14.

Shankweiler, D., Liberman, I., Mark, L., Fowler, C., and Fischer, F. (1979). The speech code and learning to read. *Journal of Experimental Psychology: Human Learning and Memory, 5,* 531-545.

Shapiro, S., McCormick, M., Starfield, B., and Crawley, B. (1983). Changes in infant morbidity associated with decreases in neonatal mortality. *Pediatrics, 72,* 408-414.

Shatz, M., and Gelman, R. (1973). The development of communication skills: Modifications in the speech of young children as a function of the listener. *Monograph of Society for Research in Child Development, 38.*

Shaw, E., Goode, S., Ringwalt, S., and Ayankoya, B. (2005). Minibiliography: Early identification of culturally and linguistically diverse children. *Communication Disorders Quarterly, 26,* 49-54.

Shaywitz, B.A., Fletcher, J.M., and Shaywitz, S.E. (1995). Defining and classifying learning disabilities and attention-deficit/hyperactivity disorder. *Journal of Child Neurology, 10,* S50-S57.

Shaywitz, S., Shaywitz, B., Fletcher, J., and Escobar, M. (1990). Prevalence of reading disability in boys and girls: Results of the Connecticut longitudinal study. *Journal of the American Medical Association, 264,* 998-1002.

Shea, V. (2005). A perspective on the research literature related to early intensive behavioral intervention (Lovaas) for young children with autism. *Communication Disorders Quarterly, 26,* 102-111.

Sheftel, D., Perelman, R., and Farrell, P. (1982). Long-term consequences of hyaline membrane disease. In P. Farrell (Ed.). *Lung development: Biological and clinical perspectives* (vol. II), Neonatal respiratory distress. New York: Academic Press.

Sheinkopf, S.J., and Siegel, B. (1998). Home-based behavioral treatment of young children with autism. *Journal of Autism and Developmental Disorders, 28,* 15-23.

Sheldon, M., and Rush, D. (2001). The ten myths about providing early intervention services in natural environments. *Infants and Young Children, 14(1),* 1-13.

Shelton, T., and Barkley, R. (1994). Critical issues in the assessment of attention deficit disorders in children. *Topics in Language Disorders, 14,* 26-41.

Sheng, L., McGregor, K., and Xu, Y. (2005). Prosodic and lexical syntactic aspects of the therapeutic register. *Clinical Linguistics and Phonetics, 17,* 355-363.

Shepard, N., Davis, J., Gorga, M., and Stelmachowicz, P. (1981). Characteristics of hearing-impaired children in the public schools: Part 1—Demographic data. *Journal of Speech and Hearing Disorders, 46,* 123-129.

Shepard, S. (2005). Linking formative assessment to scaffolding. *Educational Leadership, 63,* 66-75.

Sheppard, J. (1987). Assessment of oral-motor behaviors in cerebral palsy. In E.D. Mysak (Ed.). *Seminars in speech and language.* New York: Thieme-Stratton.

Shipley, K., and McAfee, J. (2004). *Assessment in speech-language pathology: A resource manual* (3rd ed.). Clifton Park: NY: Thomson Delmar Learning.

Shorto, R. (1990). *The untold story of Cinderella.* New York: Dial.

Shprintzen, R. (1997). *Genetics, syndromes, and communication disorders.* San Diego, CA: Singular Publishing Group.

Shriberg, L. (1986). *PEPPER program to examine phonetic and phonological evaluation records* (computer program). San Diego, CA: College-Hill Software.

Shriberg, L. (1987, October). *Phonological assessment.* Paper presented at the meeting of the Oregon-Washington Regional Speech and Hearing Association, Seattle, WA.

Shriberg, L. (1993). Four new speech and prosody-voice measures for genetics research and other studies in developmental phonological disorders. *Journal of Speech and Hearing Research, 36,* 105-140.

Shriberg, L. (1994). Five subtypes of development phonological disorders. *Clinics in Communication Disorders, 4,* 48-53.

Shriberg, L., Aram, D., and Kwiatkowski, J. (1997). Developmental apraxia of speech, III. A subtype marked by inappropriate stress. *Journal of Speech and Hearing Research, 40,* 313-337.

Shriberg, L., and Austin, D. (1998). Comorbidity of speech-language disorder: Implications for a phenotype marker for speech delay. In R. Paul (Ed.). *Exploring the speech-language connection.* Baltimore, MD: Paul H. Brookes.

Shriberg, L., Campbell, T., Karlsson, B., Brown, R., McSweeny, J., and Nadler, C. (2003). A diagnostic marker for childhood apraxia of speech: The lexical stress ratio. *Clinical Linguistics and Phonetics, 17,* 549-556.

Shriberg, L.D., Green, J.R., Campbell, T.F., McSweeny, J.L., and Scheer, A. (2003). A diagnostic marker for childhood apraxia of speech: Coefficient of variation ratio for childhood AOS. *Clinical Linguistics and Phonetics, 17(7),* 575-595.

Shriberg, L., and Kwiatkowski, J. (1980). *Natural process analysis: A procedure for phonological analysis of continuous speech samples.* New York: John Wiley & Sons.

Shriberg, L., and Kwiatkowski, J. (1982a). Phonological disorders, II: A conceptual framework for management. *Journal of Speech and Hearing Disorders, 47,* 242-256.

Shriberg, L., and Kwiatkowski, J. (1982b). Phonological disorders, III: A procedure for assessing severity of involvement. *Journal of Speech and Hearing Disorders, 47,* 256-270.

Shriberg, L., and Kwiatkowski, J. (1986). *Natural process analysis: A procedure for phonological analysis of continuous speech samples.* New York: John Wiley & Sons.

Shriberg, L., and Kwiatkowski, J. (1988). A follow-up study of children with phonological disorders of unknown origin. *Journal of Speech and Hearing Disorders, 53,* 144-155.

Shriberg, L., and Kwiatkowski, J. (1994). Developmental phonological disorders, I: A clinical profile. *Journal of Speech and Hearing Research, 37,* 1100-1126.

Shriberg, L., Kwiatkowski, J., Best, S., Hengst, J., and Terselic-Weber, B. (1986). Characteristics of children with speech delays of unknown origin. *Journal of Speech and Hearing Disorders, 51,* 140-160.

Shriberg, L., Kwiatkowski, J., and Rasmussen, C. (1990). *Prosody-voice screening profile.* Tucson, AZ: Communication Skill Builders.

Shriberg, L., Kwiatkowski, J., and Snyder, T. (1990). Tabletop versus microcomputer-assisted speech management: Response evocation phase. *Journal of Speech and Hearing Disorders, 55,* 635-655.

Shriberg, L., Paul, R., McSweeney, J., Klin, A., Cohen, D., and Volkmar, F. (2001). Speech and prosody characteristics of adolescents and adults with high functioning autism and Asperger syndrome. *Journal of Speech, Language and Hearing Research, 44,* 1097-1115.

Shriberg, L., and Smith, A. (1983). Phonological correlates of middle ear involvement in speech-delayed children: A methodological note. *Journal of Speech and Hearing Research, 26,* 293-297.

Shriberg, L., and Widder, C. (1990). Speech and prosody characteristics of adults with mental retardation. *Journal of Speech and Hearing Research, 33,* 627-653.

Shulman, B. (1986). *Test of pragmatic skills* (rev.). Tucson, AZ: Communication Skill Builders.

Siegel, B. (2005). *Pervasive developmental disorders screening test—II.* San Antonio, TX: Harcourt.

Siegel-Causey, E., and Guess, D. (1989). *Enhancing nonsymbolic communication interactions among learners with severe disabilities.* Baltimore, MD: Paul H. Brookes.

Sieratzki, J.S., Calvert, G.A., Brammer, M., David, A., and Woll, B. (2001). Accessibility of spoken, written, and sign language in Landau-Kleffner syndrome: A linguistic and functional MRI study. *Epileptic Disorders, 3(2),* 79-89.

Sigafoos, J., Didden, R., and O'Reilly, M. (2003). Effects of speech output on maintenance of requesting and frequency of vocalization in three children with developmental disabilities. *Augmentative and Alternative Communication, 19,* 37-47.

Sigafoos, J., Drasgow, E., Reichle, J., O'Reilly, M., Green, V., and Tait, K. (2004). Tutorial: Teaching communicative rejecting to children with severe disabilities. *American Journal of Speech-Language Pathology, 13,* 31-42.

Sigman, M., Dissanayake, C., Arbelle, S., and Ruskin, E. (1997). Cognition and emotion in children and adolescents with autism. In J. Cohen and F. Volkmar (Eds.). *Handbook of autism and pervasive development disorders* (pp. 248-265.) New York: John Wiley & Sons.

Sigman, M., Mundy, P., Sherman, T., and Ungerer, J. (1986). Social interactions of autistic, mentally retarded and normal children and their caregivers. *Journal of Child Psychology and Psychiatry, 27,* 647-656.

Silliman, E. (1987). Individual differences in the classroom performance of language-impaired children. *Seminars in Speech and Language, 8,* 357-373.

Silliman, E., Ford, C.S., Beasman, J., and Evans, D. (1999). An inclusion model for children with language disabilities: Building a classroom partnership. *Topics In Language Disorders, 19,* 1-18.

Silliman, E., Jimerson, T., and Wilkinson, L. (2000). A dynamic systems approach to writing assessment with students with language learning problems. *Topics in Language Disorders, 20(4),* 45-64.

Silliman, E., and Wilkinson, L. (1991). *Communicating for learning: Classroom observation and collaboration.* Gaithersburg, MD: Aspen Publishers.

Silva, P., Kirkland, C., Simpson, A., Stewart, I., and Williams, S. (1982). Some developmental and behavioral problems associated with bilateral otitis media with effusion. *Journal of Learning Disabilities, 15,* 417-421.

Silvaroli, N., and Maynes, J. (1975). *Oral language evaluation.* Clinton, MD: D.A. Lewis Associates.

Simon, C. (1984). Functional-pragmatic evaluation of communication skills in school-aged children. *Language, Speech, and Hearing Services in Schools, 15(2),* 83-97.

Simon, C. (1987). Out of the broom closet and into the classroom: The emerging SLP. Journal of Childhood Communication Disorders, 11, 41-66.

Simon, C. (1991a). *Communication skills and classroom success: Therapy methodologies for language-learning disabled students.* San Diego, CA: College-Hill Press.

Simon, C. (1991b). *Teaching logical thinking and discussion skills. In C.S. Simon (Ed.). Communication skills and classroom success* (pp. 219-241). San Diego, CA: College-Hill Press.

Simon, C. (1994). *Evaluating communicative competence.* Tucson, AZ: Communication Skill Builders.

Simon, C. (1998). When big kids don't learn: Contextual modifications and intervention strategies for age 8-18 at-risk students. *Clinical Linguistics and Phonetics, 12,* 249-280.

Simon, C. (1999a). On being dyslexic: An inside view. *American Speech-Language-Hearing Association, 41(2),* 19-23.

Simon, C. (1999b). *"Teaching kids to play the school game."* Workshop presented at the Connecticut Speech-Language Association State Convention, Weston, CT.

Singer, B., and Bashir, A. (1999). What are executive functions and self-regulation and what do they have to do with language-learning disorders. *Language, Speech and Hearing Services in Schools, 30,* 265-273.

Singleton, J., Supalla, S., Litchfield, S., and Schley, S. (1998). From sign to word: Considering modality constraints in ASL/English bilingual education. Topics in Language Disorders, 18(4), 16-29.

Skarakis-Doyle, E., and Murphy, L. (1995). Discourse-based language intervention: An efficacy study. *Journal of Children's Communication Development, 17,* 11-22.

Skuse, D. (1993). Extreme deprivation in early childhood. In D. Bishop and K. Mogford (Eds.). *Language development in exceptional circumstances* (pp. 29-46). Hillsdale, NJ: Erlbaum.

Sleight, M., and Niman, C. (1984). *Gross motor and oral motor development in children with Down syndrome: Birth through three years.* St. Louis, MO: St. Louis Association for Retarded Citizens.

Slentz, K., and Bricker, D. (1992). Family-guided assessment for IFSP development: Jumping off the family assessment bandwagon. *Journal of Early Intervention, 16(1),* 11-19.

Slentz, K., Walker, B., and Bricker, D. (1989). Supporting involvement in early intervention: A role-taking model. In G. Singer and L. Irvin (Eds.). *Support for caregiving families: Enabling positive adaptation to disability.* Baltimore, MD: Paul H. Brookes.

SLI Consortium. (2002). A genomewide scan identifies two novel loci involved in specific language impairment. *American Journal of Human Genetics, 70,* 384-398.

Slingerland, B. (1971). *A multisensory approach to language arts for specific language disability children: A guide for primary teachers.* Cambridge, MA: Educators Publishing Service.

Slobin, D. (1973). Cognitive prerequisites for the development of grammar. In C. Ferguson and D. Slobin (Eds.). *Studies of child language development.* New York: Holt, Rinehart & Winston.

Slosson, S., Nicholson, C., and Hibpshman, T. (2002). *Slosson intelligence test, revised 3rd Ed.* East Aurora, NY: Slosson.

Smith, F. (1985). *Reading without nonsense* (2nd ed.). New York: Teachers College Press.

Smith, J., Johnstone, S., and Barry, R. (2003). Aiding diagnosis of attention-deficit/hyperactivity disorder and its subtypes: Discriminant function analysis of event-related potential data. *Journal of Child Psychology and Psychiatry and Allied Disciplines, 44,* 1067-1075.

Smith, M.M. (2001). Simply a speech impairment? Literacy challenges for individuals with severe congenital speech impairments. *International Journal of Disability, Development and Education, 48(4),* 331-353.

Smith, P. (1998). *That's LIFE! Life skills.* East Moline, IL: Linguisystems.

Smith, S., Pennington, B., Kimberling, W., and Lubs, H. (1983). A genetic analysis of specific reading disability. In C. Ludlow and J. Cooper (Eds.). *Genetic aspects of speech and language disorders* (pp. 169-178). New York: Academic Press.

Smyer, K., and Westby, C. (2005). Using children's literature to promote positive self-identify in CLD students. *Perspectives in Language Learning and Education, 12,* 22-25.

Snider, V. (1989). Reading comprehension performance of adolescents with learning disabilities. *Learning Disability Quarterly, 12,* 87-96.

Snow, C. (1983). Literacy and language: Relationships during the preschool years. *Harvard Educational Review, 53,* 165-189.

Snow, C. (1999). Facilitating language development promotes literacy learning. In L. Eldering and P. Leseman (Eds.). *Effective early intervention: Cross-cultural perspectives* (pp. 141-161). New York: Falmer.

Snow, C.E. (2002). *Reading for understanding: Toward a research and development program in reading comprehension.* Pittsburgh, PA: RAND.

Snow, C., Burns, S., and Griffin, P. (1998). *Preventing reading difficulties in young children.* Washington, DC: National Academy Press.

Snow, C., and Dickinson, D. (1991). Skills that aren't basic in a new conception of literacy. In A. Purves and E. Jennings (Eds.). *Literate systems and individual lives: Perspectives on literacy and schooling.* Albany, NY: SUNY Press.

Snow, C., and Goldfield, B. (1983). Turn the page please: Situation-specific language learning. *Journal of Child Learning, 10,* 551-570.

Snowling, M. (1996). Developmental dyslexia. In M. Snowling and J. Stackhouse (Eds.). *Dyslexia, speech, and language: A practitioner's handbook* (pp. 1-11). London: Whurr Publishers.

Snowling, M., Adams, J., Bishop, D., and Stothard, S. (2001). Educational attainments of school leavers with a preschool history of speech-language impairments. *International Journal of Language and Communication Disorders, 36,* 173-183.

Snowling, M., and Bishop, D. (2000). Is preschool language impairment a risk factor for dyslexia in adolescence? *Journal of Child Psychology and Psychiatry, 41,* 587-600.

Snowling, M., and Nation, K. (1997). Language, phonology and learning to read. In C. Hulme and M. Snowling (Eds.). *Dyslexia: Biology, cognition, and intervention* (pp. 153-166). London: Whurr Publishers.

Snowling, M., and Stackhouse, J. (1996). *Dyslexia, speech, and language: A practitioner's handbook.* London: Whurr Publishers.

Snowling, M.J., Bishop, D.V.M., and Stothard, S.E. (2000). Is preschool language impairment a risk factor for dyslexia in adolescence? *Journal of Child Psychology and Psychiatry and Allied Disciplines, 41(5),* 587-600.

Sohlberg, M., and Mateer, C. (1989). The assessment of cognitive-communicative functions in head injury. *Topics in Language Disorders, 9(2),* 15-33.

Soliday, S. (2004, October). *Improving service by changing the service model: The 3:1 service model.* Workshop presented at the Iowa Speech and Hearing Association State Convention.

Southwood., F., and Russell, A. (2004). Comparison of conversation freeplay, and story generation as methods of language sample elicitation. *Journal of Speech, Language, and Hearing Research, 47,* 366-376.

Sparks, R., and Holland, A. (1976). Method: Melodic intonation therapy for aphasia. *Journal of Speech and Hearing Disorders, 41,* 287-297.

Sparks, S. (1984). *Birth defects and speech-language disorders.* Boston, MA: College-Hill Press.

Sparks, S. (1989). Assessment and intervention with at-risk infants and toddlers: Guidelines for the speech-language pathologist. *Topics in Language Disorders, 10(1),* 43-56.

Sparks, S. (1993). *Children of prenatal substance abuse.* San Diego, CA: Singular Publishing Group.

Sparks, S. (2001). Prenatal substance use and its impact on young children. In T. Layton, E. Crais, and L. Watson (Eds.). *Handbook of early language impairment in children: Nature* (pp. 451-487). Albany, NY: Delmar Publishers.

Sparrow, S., Cicchetti, D., and Balla, D. (2005). *Vineland adaptive behavior scales—II.* Circle Pines, MN: AGS Publications.

Spatz, D. (2004). Ten steps for promoting and protecting breastfeeding for vulnerable infants. *Journal of Perinatal and Neonatal Nursing, 18,* 385-397.

Spector, C. (1997). *Saying one thing, meaning another.* Eau Claire, WI: Thinking Publications.

Spier, P. (1961). *The fox went out on a chilly night.* New York: Doubleday.

Spinelli, J. (1990). *Maniac Magee.* New York: Scholastic.

Spiridigliozzi, G., Lachiewicz, A., Mirrett, S., and McConkie-Rosell, A. (2001). Fragile X syndrome in young children. In T. Layton, E. Crais, and L. Watson (Eds.). *Handbook of early language impairment in children: Nature* (pp. 258-301). Albany, NY: Delmar Publishers.

Spitz, R.V., Tallel, P., Flax, J., and Benasich, A.A. (1997). Look who's talking: A prospective study of familial transmission of language impairments. *Journal of Speech, Language, and Hearing Research, 40,* 990-1001.

Spradlin, J., and Siegel, G. (1982). Language training in natural and clinical environments. *Journal of Speech and Hearing Disorders, 47,* 2-7.

Spriestersbach, D., Morris, H., and Darley, F. (1991). Examination of the speech mechanism. In F. Darley and D. Spriestersbach (Eds.). *Diagnostic methods in speech pathology* (2nd ed., pp. 111-132). Prospects Heights, IL: Waveland Press.

St. Louis, K., and Ruscello, D. (2000). *Oral speech mechanism screening exam* (3rd ed.). Austin, TX: Pro-Ed.

Stackhouse, J. (1996). Speech, spelling, and reading. In M. Snowling and J. Stackhouse (Eds.). *Dyslexia, speech, and language: A practitioner's handbook* (pp. 12-30). London: Whurr Publishers.

Stackhouse, J., and Wells, B. (1997). How do speech and language problems affect literacy development? In C. Hulme and M. Snowling (Eds.). *Dyslexia: Biology, cognition, and intervention* (pp. 182-211). London: Whurr Publishers.

Stahl, K. (2004). Proof, practice, and promise: Comprehension strategy instruction in the primary grades. *The Reading Teacher, 57,* 598-610.

Stanfa, K., and O'Shea, D. (1998). The play's the thing for reading comprehension. *Teaching Exceptional Children, 31,* 48-54.

Stanovich, K. (1986). Matthew effects in reading: Some consequences of individual differences in the acquisition of literacy. *Reading Research Quarterly, 21,* 360-406.

Stark, R., and Bernstein, L. (1984). Evaluating central auditory processing in children. *Topics in Language Disorders, 4,* 57-70.

Stark, R., and Tallal, P. (1981). Selection of children with specific language deficits. *Journal of Speech and Hearing Disorders, 46,* 114-122.

Staskowski, M., and Creaghead, N. (2001). Reading comprehension: A language intervention target from early childhood through adolescence. *Seminars in Speech and Language, 22,* 185-207.

Steele, M. (2004). Making the case for early identification and intervention for young children at risk for learning disabilities. *Early Childhood Education Journal, 32,* 75-79.

Stein, N., and Glenn, C. (1979). An analysis of story comprehension in elementary school children. In R. Freedle (Ed.). *New directions in discourse processing* (vol. 2, pp. 53-120). Norwood, NJ: Ablex.

Steiner, S., and Larson, V. (1991). Integrating microcomputers into language intervention. *Topics in Language Disorders, 11,* 18-30.

Stephens, M. (1988). Pragmatics. In M.A. Nippold (Ed.). *Later language development* (pp. 247-262). Boston, MA: College-Hill Press.

Steptoe, J. (1987). *Mufaro's beautiful daughters.* New York: Lothrop Lee Shepard.

Sterling-Orth, A. (2005). *Sound reading: Literature lists for phonology & articulation.* Eau Claire, WI: Thinking Publications.

Sternberg, R., and Powell, J. (1983). Comprehending verbal comprehension. *American Psychologist, 38,* 878-893.

Sternberg, R.J. (1987). Most vocabulary is learned from context. In M.G. McKeown and M.E. Curtis (Eds.). *The nature of vocabulary acquisition.* Hillsdale, NJ: Erlbaum.

Stevenson, J., and Richman, N. (1976). The prevalence of language delay in a population of three year old children and its association with general retardation. *Developmental Medicine and Child Neurology, 18,* 431-441.

Stewart, S. (1991). Development of written language proficiency: Methods for teaching text structure. In C.S. Simon (Ed.). *Communication skills and classroom success* (pp. 59-78). San Diego, CA: College-Hill Press.

Stock, C.D. (2002). The effects of responsive caregiver communication on the language development of at-risk preschoolers. *Dissertation Abstracts International Section A: Humanities & Social Sciences, 63(6-A),* 21-25.

Stockman, I. (1996). The promises and pitfalls of language sample analysis as an assessment tool for linguistic minority children. *Language, Speech, and Hearing Services in Schools, 27,* 355-372.

Stockman, I., and Vaughn-Cooke, F. (1986). Implications of semantic category research for the language assessment of nonstandard speakers. *Topics in Language Disorders, 6(4),* 15-25.

Stoel-Gammon, C. (1987). Phonological skills of two-year olds. *Language, Speech, and Hearing Services in Schools, 18,* 323-329.

Stoel-Gammon, C. (1988). Prelinguistic vocalizations of hearing-impaired and normally speaking subjects: A comparison of consonant inventories. *Journal of Speech and Hearing Research, 53,* 302-315.

Stoel-Gammon, C. (1990). Down syndrome. *American Speech-Language-Hearing Association, 32,* 42-44.

Stoel-Gammon, C. (1991). Normal and disordered phonology in two-year olds. *Topics in Language Disorders, 11(4),* 21-32.

Stoel-Gammon, C. (1998). Sounds and words in early language acquisition: The relationship between lexical and phonological development. In R. Paul (Ed.). *Exploring the speech-language connection* (pp. 25-52). Baltimore, MD: Paul H. Brookes.

Stoel-Gammon, C. (2002). Intervocalic consonants in the speech of typically developing children: Emergence and early use. *Clinical Linguistics and Phonetics, 16,* 155-168.

Stone, J. (1992). *The animated alphabet.* La Mesa, CA: J. Stone Creations.

Storkel, H., and Morrisette, M. (2002). The lexicon and phonology: Interactions in language acquisition. *Language, Speech, and Hearing Services in Schools, 33,* 24-37.

Stothard, S., Snowling, M., Bishop, D., Chipchase, B., and Kaplan, C. (1998). Language-impaired preschoolers: A follow-up into adolescence. *Journal of Speech, Language and Hearing Research, 41,* 407-418.

Stott, D., Merricks, M., Bolton, P., and Goodyer, I. (2002). Screening for speech and language disorders: The reliability, validity and accuracy of the General Language Screen. *International Journal of Language and Communication Disorders, 37,* 133-150.

Stout, G., and Windle, J. (1992). *Developmental Approach to Successful Listening II—DASLII.* Denver, CO: Resource Point.

Strand, E. (1995). Treatment of motor speech disorders in children. *Seminars in Speech and Language, 16,* 126-139.

Streissguth, A. (1997). *Fetal alcohol syndrome: A guide for families and communities.* Baltimore, MD: Paul H. Brookes.

Streissguth, A., Aase, J., Clarren, S., Randels, S., La Due, R., and Smith, D. (1991). Fetal alcohol syndrome in adolescents and adults. *Journal of the American Medical Association, 265,* 1961-1967.

Streissguth, A., LaDue, R., and Randels, S. (1988). *A manual on adolescent and adults with fetal alcohol syndrome with special reference to American Indians.* Seattle, WA: University of Washington.

Stromswold, K. (1998). Genetics of spoken language disorders. *Human Biology, 70,* 297-324.

Strong, C. (1998). *Strong narrative assessment procedure.* Eau Claire, WI: Thinking Publications.

Strong, M. (1988). *Language learning and deafness.* New York: Cambridge University Press.

Strong, W. (1985). Linguistics and writing. In B.W. McClelland and T.R. Donovan (Eds.). *Perspectives on research and scholarship in composition* (pp. 68-86). New York: Modern Language Association of America.

Strong, W. (1986). *Creative approaches to sentence combining. Theory and research into practice.* Urbana, IL: ERIC Clearinghouse on Reading and Communication Skills.

Strulovitch, J., and Tagalakis, V. (2003). Social skills groups for adolescents with Asperger syndrome. *Perspectives on Language Learning and Education, 10(2),* 15-18.

Strum, J., and Koppenhaver, D. (2000). Supporting writing development in adolescents with developmental disabilities. *Topics in Language Disorders, 20(2),* 73-96.

Strum. J., and Rankin-Erickson, J. (2002). Effects of hand-drawn and computer-generated concept mapping on the expository writing of middle school students with learning disabilities. *Learning Disabilities Research & Practice, 17,* 124-139.

Studdert-Kennedy, M., and Mody, M. (1995). Auditory temporal perception deficits in the reading-impaired: A critical review of the evidence. *Psychological Bulletin, 2,* 508-514.

Sturm, J., and Clendon, S. (2004). Augmentative and alternative communication, language, and literacy. *Topics in Language Disorders, 24(1),* 76-91

Sturm, J.M. (2003). Writing in AAC. *ASHA Leader, 8(16),* 8-11.

Sturm, J.M., and Clendon, S.A. (2004). Augmentative and alternative communication, language, and literacy. *Topics in Language Disorders, 24(1),* 76-91.

Sturner, R., Layton, T., Evans, A., Heller, J., Funk, S., and Machon, M. (1994). Preschool speech and language screening: A review of currently available tests. *American Journal of Speech-Language Pathology, 3(1),* 25-36.

Sturner, R.A., Funk, S.G., and Green, J.A. (1996). Preschool speech and language screening: Further validation of the sentence repetition screening test. *Journal of Developmental & Behavioral Pediatrics, 17(6),* 405-413.

Sturomski, N. (1996). The transition of individuals with learning disabilities into the work setting. *Topics in Language Disorders, 16,* 37-51.

Stutsman, R. (1948). *Merrill-Palmer scale of mental tests.* New York: Harcourt Brace Jovanovich.

Sudweeks, R., Glissmeyer, C., Morrison, R., and Wilcox, B. (2004). Establishing reliable procedures for rating ELL students' reading comprehension using oral retellings. *Reading Research & Instruction, 43(2),* 65-86.

Sullivan, E.T., Clark, W.W., and Tiegs, E.W. (1961). *California test of mental maturity.* CTB: McGraw-Hill.

Sulman, B.B., and Sherman, T. (1996). Pediatric Language Acquisition Screening Tool for Early Referral—Revised (PLASTER-R): Experimental Edition. Unpublished manuscript.

Sulzby, E. (1980). Word concept development activities. In E.H. Henderson, and J.W. Beers (Eds.). *Developmental and cognitive aspects of learning to spell: A reflection of word knowledge.* Newark, DE: International Reading Association.

Sulzby, E., and Teale, W. (1991). Emergent literacy. In R. Barr, M.L. Kamil, P. Mosenthal, and P.D. Pearson (Eds.). *Handbook of reading research* (vol. II, pp. 727-758). New York: Longman.

Sulzby, E., and Zecker, L. (1991). The oral monologue as a form of emergent reading. In A. McCabe and C. Peterson (Eds.). *Developing narrative structure* (pp. 175-214). Hillsdale, NJ: Erlbaum.

Sulzer-Azaroff, B., and Mayer, G.R. (1991). *Behavior analysis for lasting change.* Fort Worth, TX: Holt, Rinehart & Winston.

Sunburst. (1997a). *Write on!* Plus. Elgin, IL: Author.

Sunburst. (1997b). *Author's toolkit.* Elgin, IL: Author.

Sunburst. (1997c). *Literature series I.* Elgin, IL: Author.

Sundberg, M., and Michael, J. (2001). The benefits of Skinner's analysis of verbal behavior for children with autism. *Behavior Modification, 25,* 698-724.

Sussman, F. (1999). *More than words: Helping parents promote communication and social skills in children with autism spectrum disorder.* Toronto, Canada: The Hanen Centre.

Sutton, A., Soto, G., and Blockberger, S. (2002). Grammatical issues in graphic symbol communication. *Augmentative and Alternative Communication, 18,* 192-205.

Swank, L. (1994). Phonological coding abilities: Identification of impairments related to phonologically based reading problems. *Topics in Language Disorders, 14(2),* 56-71.

Swank, L. (1997). Linguistic influences on the emergence of written word decoding in first grade. *American Journal of Speech-Language Pathology, 6(4),* 62-66.

Swank, L. (1999). Phonological awareness and the role of speech-language pathologists for meeting reading goals. *Language, Learning, and Education Newsletter, 6(1),* 26-29.

Swank, L., and Catts, H. (1994). Phonological awareness and written word decoding. *Language, Speech, and Hearing Services in Schools, 25,* 9-14.

Swank, L., and Larrivee, L. (1999). Phonology, metaphonology and the development of literacy. In R. Paul (Ed.). *Exploring the speech-language connection* (vol. 8, pp. 253-297). Baltimore, MD: Paul H. Brookes.

Swanson, H.L. (1996). *Swanson cognitive abilities scale.* Austin, TX: Pro-Ed.

Swanson, L., Fey, M., Mills, C., and Hood, S. (2005). Use of narrative based language intervention with children who have specific language impairment. *American Journal of Speech-Language Pathology, 14,* 131-143.

Swanson, P., and De La Paz, S. (1998). Teaching effective comprehension strategies to students with learning and reading disabilities. *Intervention in School and Clinic, 33,* 209-218.

Swiecki, M., and Martson, B. (1991). *In plain English.* East Moline, IL: LinguiSystems.

Swisher, L. (1985). Language disorders in children. In J. Darby (Ed.). *Speech and language evaluation in neurology: Childhood disorders.* Orlando, FL: Grune & Stratton.

Tabors, P., Paez, M., and Lopez, L. (2002). *Early childhood study of language and literacy development of Spanish-speaking children.* Paper presented at the National Association of Bilingual Education Conference, Philadelphia.

Tabors, P.O., Snow, C.E., and Dickinson, D.K. (2001). Homes and schools together: Supporting language and literacy development. In K.K. Dickinson and P.O. Tabors (Eds.). *Beginning literacy with language: Young children learning at home and at school* (pp. 313-334). Baltimore: Brookes.

Tager-Flusberg, H. (1981). Sentence comprehension in autistic children. *Applied Psycholinguistics, 2,* 5-24.

Tager-Flusberg, H. (1985). Putting words together: Morphology and syntax in the preschool years. In J. Berko Gleason (Ed.). *The development of language* (pp. 151-194). Columbus, OH: Merrill.

Tager-Flusberg, H. (1995). Dissociations in form and function in the acquisition of language in autistic children. In H. Tager-Flusberg (Ed.). *Constraints on language acquisition: Studies of atypical children* (pp. 175-194). Hillsdale, NJ: Erlbaum.

Tager-Flusberg, H., and Joseph, R. (2003). Identifying neurocognitive phenotypes in autism. *Philosophical Transactions of the Royal Society Series, B, 358,* 303-314.

Tager-Flusberg, H., Paul, R., and Lord, C. (2005). Language and communication in autism. In F. Volkmar, R. Paul, A. Klin, and D. Cohen (Eds.). *Handbook of autism and pervasive developmental disorders—3rd Ed* (pp. 335-364). New York: Wiley.

Tait, K., Sigafoos, J., Woodyatt, G., O'Reilly, M., and Lancioni, G. (2004). Evaluating parent use of functional communication training to replace and enhance prelinguistic behaviors in six children with developmental and physical disabilities. *Disability and Rehabilitation, 26,* 1241-1254.

Tallal, P. (1976). Rapid auditory processing in normal and disordered language development. *Journal of Speech and Hearing Research, 19,* 561-571.

Tallal, P. (1988). Developmental language disorders. In J.F. Kavanagh and T.J. Truss, Jr. (Eds.). *Learning disabilities: Proceedings of the national conference* (pp. 181-272). Parkton, MD: York Press.

Tallal, P. (1990). Fine-grained discrimination in language learning impaired children are specific neither to the auditory modality nor to speech perception. *Journal of Speech and Hearing Research, 33,* 616-617.

Tallal, P. (1999a). Moving research from the laboratory to clinics and class-rooms," In D. Drake (Ed.). *Reading and attention disorders: neurobiological sources of co-morbidity* (pp. 201-264) London: Psychology Press.

Tallal, P. (1999b). *Integrating cognitive neuroscience with remediation.* Paper presented at the Third International Symposium on Child Language Disorders. York, England.

Tallal, P. (2000). Experimental studies of language learning impairments: From research to remediation. In D.V.M. Bishop & L. B. Leonard (Eds.). *Speech and language impairments in children: Causes, characteristics, inter-vention and outcome* (pp. 131-155). Hove, UK: Psychology Press.

Tallal, P. (2003). Language learning disabilities: Integrating research approaches. *Current Directions in Psychological Science, 12,* 206-211.

Tallal, P. (2004). Improving language and literacy is a matter of time. *Nature Reviews Neuroscience, 5,* 721-728.

Tallal, P., Merzenich, M., Burns, M., Gelfond, S., Young, M., Shipley, J., and Polow, N. (November, 1997). *Temporal training for language impaired children: National clinical trial results.* Paper presented to the Annual Convention of the American Speech-Language-Hearing Association, Boston.

Tallal, P., Miller, S., Bedi, G., Byman, G., Wang, X., Nagarajan, S., Schreiner, C., Jenkins, W., and Merzenich, M. (1996). Language comprehension in language learning impaired children improved with acoustically modified speech. *Science, 271,* 81-84.

Tallal, P., Miller, S., and Fitch, R.H. (1993). Neurobiological basis of speech: A case for the pre-eminence of temporal processing. In P. Tallal, A.M. Galaburda, R.R. Llinas, and C. von Euler (Eds.). *Annals of the New York Academy of Sciences: Temporal information processing in the nervous system.* New York: New York Academy of Sciences.

Tallal, P., and Piercy, M. (1975). Developmental aphasia: The perception of brief vowels and extended stop consonants. *Neuropsychologia, 13,* 69-74.

Tallal, P., Ross, R., and Curtiss, S. (1989). Familial aggregation in specific language impairment. *Journal of Speech and Hearing Disorders, 54(2),* 167-173.

Tami, T.A., and Lee, K.C. (1994). Otolaryngologic manifestations of HIV disease. In P.T. Cohen, M.A. Sande, and P.A. Volberding (Eds.). *The AIDS knowledge base: A textbook on HIV disease from the University of California, San Francisco, and the San Francisco General Hospital* (pp. 5.29-1–5.29-25). Boston, MA: Little, Brown.

Tannen, D. (1982). Oral and literate strategies in spoken and written discourse. *Language, 58,* 1-20.

Tannock, R., and Girolametto, L. (1992). Reassessing parent-focused language intervention programs. In S.F. Warren and J. Reichle (Eds.). *Causes and effects in communication and language intervention* (pp. 49-80). Baltimore, MD: Paul H. Brookes.

Tarulli, N. (1998). Using photography to enhance language and learning: A picture can encourage a thousand words. *Language, Speech, and Hearing Services in Schools, 29,* 54-57.

Taylor, G., Burack, C., Holding, P., Lekine, N., and Hack, M. (2002). Sources of variability in sequelae of very low birth weight. *Neuropsychology, Development, and Cognition, 8,* 163-178.

Taylor, J. (1992). *Speech-language pathology services in the schools* (2nd ed.). Needham Heights, MA: Allyn and Bacon.

Taylor, M. (1975). *Roll of thunder, hear my cry.* New York: Dial.

Taylor, O. (1986). A cultural and communicative approach to teaching standard English as a second dialect. In O.L. Taylor (Ed.). *Treatment of communication disorders in culturally and linguistically diverse populations* (pp. 153-178). Austin, TX: Pro-Ed.

Teagle, H., and Moore, J. (2002). School-based services for children with cochlear implants. *Language, Speech, and Hearing Services in Schools, 33,* 162-171.

Teele, D., Klein, J., Rosner, B., and The Greater Boston Otitis Media Study Group. (1984). Otitis media with effusion during the first three years of life and development of speech and language. *Pediatrics, 74,* 282-287.

Temple, E., Deutsch, G., Poldrack, R., Miller, S., Tallal, P. Merzenich, M., and Gabrieli, J. (2003). Neural deficits in children with dyslexia ameliorated by behavioral remediation: Evidence from functional MRI. *Proceedings of the National Academy of Sciences of the USA, 100,* 2860-2865.

Templin, M. (1957). *Certain language skills in children: Their development and inter-relationships.* Minneapolis, MN: University of Minnesota Press.

Terban, M. (1982). *Eight ate: A feast of homonym riddles.* New York: Houghton Mifflin.

Terban, M. (1988). *The dove dove: Funny homograph riddles.* New York: Clarion.

Terpstra, J. (2002). Can I play? Classroom-based interventions for teaching play skills to children with autism. *Focus on Autism and Other Developmental Disabilities, 17,* 119-126.

Terrell, S. (1991). Sickle cell anemia and fetal alcohol syndrome: Two main organic disorders in multicultural populations. *Texas Journal of Audiology and Speech Pathology, 17(1),* 10-12.

Terrell, S., Arensberg, K., and Rosa, M. (1992). Parent-child comparative analysis: A criterion-referenced method for the nondiscriminatory assessment of a child who spoke a relatively uncommon dialect of English. *Language, Speech, and Hearing Services in Schools, 23(1),* 34-42.

Terrell, S., and Jackson, R. (2002). African-Americans in the Americas. In D.E. Battle (Ed.). *Communication disorders in multicultural populations* (3rd ed., pp. 71-113). Boston: Butterworth-Heinneman.

Terrell, S., and Terrell, F. (1983). Effects of speaking Black English upon employment opportunities. *ASHA, 26,* 27-29.

Terrell, S., and Terrell, F. (1996). The importance of psychological and socio-cultural factors for providing clinical services to African American children. In A. Kahmi, K. Pollock, and J. Harris (Eds.). *Communication development and disorders in African American children* (pp. 55-72). Baltimore, MD: Paul H. Brookes.

Terrill, M., Scruggs, T., and Mastropieri, M. (2004). SAT Vocabulary instruction for high school students with learning disabilities. *Intervention in School and Clinic, 39,* 288-294.

Tetnowski, J. (2004). Attention deficit hyperactivity disorders and concomitant communicative disorders. *Seminars in Speech and Language, 25,* 215-224.

Thal, D. (1991). Language and cognition in normal and late-talking toddlers. *Topics in Language Disorders, 11(4),* 33-42.

Thal., D., and Clancy, B. (2001). Brain development and language learning: Implications for nonbiologically based language learning disorders. *Journal of Speech-Language Pathology and Audiology, 25,* 52-76.

Thal, D., and Flores, M. (2001). Development of sentence interpretation strategies by typically developing and late-talking toddlers. *Journal of Child Language, 28,* 173-93.

Thal, D., O'Hanlon, L., Clemmons, M., and Fralin, L. (1999). Validity of a parent report measure of vocabulary and syntax for preschool children with language impairment. *Journal of Speech, Language, and Hearing Research, 42(2),* 482-496.

Thal, D.J., Reilly, J., Seibert, L., Jeffries, R., and Fenson, J. (2004). Language development in children at risk for language impairment: Cross-population comparisons. *Brain & Language, 88(2),* 167-179.

Tharp, R. (1989). Psychocultural variables and constants: Effects on teaching and learning in schools. *American Psychological Association, 44(2),* 1-11.

The Whole Language Teachers Association Newsletter. (1988, Spring). Sudbury, MA.: Whole Language Teachers Association.

Thiede, K., and Anderson, M. (2003). Summarizing can improve metacomprehension accuracy. *Contemporary Educational Psychology, 28,* 129-161.

Thinking Publications. *The deciders take on concepts: Interactive software* (computer program). Eau Claire, WI: Author.

Thomas, M., and Karmiloff-Smith, A. (2003). Modelling language acquisition in atypical phenotypes. *Psychological Review, 110(4),* 647-682.

Thomas, P. (1971). *"Stand back, " said the elephant, "I'm going to sneeze!"* New York: Lothrop, Lee, & Shepard Company.

Thompson, C., Craig, H., and Washington, J. (2004). Variable production of African American English across oracy and literacy contexts. *Language, Speech and Hearing Services in Schools, 35,* 269-282.

Thompson., J., Bryant, B., Campbell, E., Craig, E. Hughes, C., Rotholz, D., Schalock, R., Silverman, W., Tassé, M., and Wehmeyer, M. (2005). *Supports intensity scale.* Washington, DC: American Association for Mental Retardation.

Thompson, L. (1995). *Foreign language assessment in grades K-8: An annotated bibliography of assessment instruments.* McHenry, IL: Delta Systems Co, Inc.

Thompson, R., Rivara, F., and Thompson, D. (1989). A case control study of the effectiveness of bicycle safety helmets. *New England Journal of Medicine, 320,* 1361-1367.

Thordardottir, E. T., and Weismer, S. E. (2001). High frequency verbs and verb diversity in the spontaneous speech of school-age children with specific language impairment. *International Journal of Language and Communication Disorders, 36,* 221-244.

Thorndike, R.M. (2005). *Measurement and evaluation in psychology and education* (7th ed.). Upper Saddle River, NJ: Pearson Education.

Thoyre, S., Shaker, C., and Pridham, K. (2005). The early feeding skills assessment for preterm infants. *Neonatal Network, 24,* 7-16.

Throneburg, R., Calvert, L., Sturm, J., Paramboukas, A., and Paul, P. (2000). A comparison of service delivery models: Effects on curricular vocabulary skills in the school setting. *American Journal of Speech-Language Pathology, 9,* 10-20.

Timler, G., Olswang, L., and Coggins, T. (2005a). Do I know what I need to do? A social communication intervention for children with complex clinical profiles. *Language, Speech, and Hearing Services in Schools, 36,* 73-85.

Timler, G., Olswang, L., and Coggins, T. (2005b). Social communication interventions for preschoolers: Targeting peer interactions during peer group entry and cooperative play. *Seminars in Speech and language, 26,* 170-180.

Tincani, M. (2004). Comparing the Picture Exchange Communication system and Sign Language training for children with autism. *Focus on Autism and Other Developmental Disabilities, 19,* 152-163.

Tingley, S., Kyte, C., Johnson, C., and Beitchman, J. (2003). Single-word and conversational measure of word-finding proficiency. *American Journal of Speech-Language Pathology, 12,* 359-369.

Tom Snyder Productions. (1994). *Diary maker.* Watertown, MA: Author.

Tomasello, M. (2002). Things are what they do: Katherine Nelson's functional approach to language and cognition. *Journal of Cognition and Development 3,* 5-19.

Tomblin, B. (1989). Familial concentration of developmental language impairment. *Journal of Speech and Hearing Disorders, 54,* 587-595.

Tomblin, B. (1991). Examining the cause of specific language impairment. *Language, Speech, and Hearing Services in Schools, 22,* 69-74.

Tomblin, B., and Buckwalter, P.R. (1998). Heredibility of poor language achievement among twins. *Journal of Speech and Hearing Research, 41,* 188-199.

Tomblin, B., Records, N., Bukwalter, P., Zhang, X., Smith, E., and O'Brien, M. (1997). Prevalence of specific language impairment in kindergarten children. *Journal of Speech, Language, and Hearing Research, 40,* 1245-1260.

Tomblin, B., Zhang, X., Buckwalter, P., and O'Brien, M. (2003). The stability of primary language disorder: Four years after kindergarten. *Journal of Speech, Language, and Hearing Research, 46,* 1283-2396.

Tomblin, J. (2000). Perspectives on diagnosis. In J.B. Tomblin and D.C. Spriestersbach (Eds.). *Diagnosis in speech-language pathology* (2nd ed., pp. 2-33). San Diego, CA: Singular.

Tomblin, J., Freese, P., and Records, N. (1992). Diagnosing specific language impairment in adults for the purpose of pedigree analysis. *Journal of Speech and Hearing Research, 35,* 832-843.

Tomblin, J.B., Shriberg, L.D., Nishimura, C., Zhang, X., and Murray, J. (1999, March). *Association of specific language impairments with loci at 7q31.* Poster presented at the Third International Symposium on Speech and Language Impairments: From Theory to Practice, York, United Kingdom.

Tomblin, J.B., Spencer, L., Flock, S., Tyler, R., and Gantz, B. (1999). Language achievement in children with cochlear implants and children using hearing aids. *Journal of Speech, Language, and Hearing Research, 42,* 497-509.

Tomblin, J.B., Zhang, X., and Buckwalter, P. (2003). The stability of primary language disorders: Four years after kindergarten diagnosis. *Journal of Speech, Language and Hearing Research, 46(6),* 1283-1296.

Tomblin, N., Records, N., and Zhang, X. (1996). A system for the diagnosis of specific language impairment in kindergarten children. *Journal of Speech and Hearing Research, 39,* 1284-1294.

Toppelberg, C., Medrano, L., Pena Morgens, L., and Nieto-Castanon, A. (2002). Bilingual children referred for psychiatric services: Associations of language disorders, language skills, and psychopathology. *Journal of the American Academy of Child and Adolescent Psychiatry, 41,* 712-722.

Torgesen, J. (1999). Assessment and instruction for phonemic awareness and word recognition skills. In H. Catts and A. Kamhi (Eds.). *Language and reading disabilities* (pp. 128-153). Needham heights, MA: Allyn & Bacon.

Torgesen, J., and Bryant, P. (2004). *Test of phonological awareness—Second edition.* Austin, TX: Pro-Ed.

Torgesen, J., Otaiba, S., and Grek, M. (2005). Assessment and instruction for phonetic awareness and word recognition skills. In H. Catts and A. Kamhi (Eds.). *Language and reading disabilities* (2nd ed., pp. 127-156). Boston: Allyn & Bacon.

Torgesen, J., and Torgesen, J. (1985). *WORDS* (computer program). Tallahassee, FL: Florida State University.

Toronto, A. (1976). Developmental assessment of Spanish grammar. *Journal of Speech and Hearing Disorders, 41(2),* 150-171.

Tough, J. (1977). *The development of meaning.* New York: Halsted Press.

Treisman, R. (2001). Linguistics and reading. In M. Aronoff and J. Rees-Miller (Eds.). *Blackwell handbook of linguistics* (pp. 664-672). Oxford: Blackwell.

Trickett, P., Aber, J., Carlson, V., and Cicchetti, D. (1991). Relationship of socioeconomic status to the etiology and developmental sequelae of physical child abuse. *Developmental Psychology, 27,* 148-158.

Trivette, C., and Dunst, C. (1988). Inventory of Social Support. In C. Dunst, C. Trivette, and A. Deal (Eds.). *Enabling and empowering families: Principles and guidelines for practice.* Cambridge, MA: Brookline Books.

Trivette, C., and Dunst, C. (2000). Recommended practices in family-based practices. In S. Sandall, M. McLean, and J. Smith (Eds.). *DEC recommended practices in early intervention/early childhood special education* (pp. 39-46). Longmont, CO: Sopris West.

Trivette, C., Dunst, C., and Deal, A. (1988). Family Strengths Profile. In C. Dunst, C. Trivette, and A. Deal (Eds.). *Enabling and empowering families: Principles and guidelines for practice.* Cambridge, MA: Brookline Books.

Troia, G. (2005). Responsiveness to intervention: Roles for speech-language pathologists in the prevention and identification of learning disabilities. *Topics in Language Disorders, 25(2),* 106-119.

Troia, G., and Whitney, S. (2003). A close look at the efficacy of FastForWord™ language for children with academic weaknesses. *Contemporary Educational Psychology, 28,* 465-494.

Trumball, E. (1984). *Metalinguistic skills: Can they be taught?* Unpublished doctoral dissertation, Boston University.

Trybus, R., and Karchmer, M. (1977). School achievement scores of hearing-impaired children: National data on achievement status and growth patterns. *American Annals of the Deaf Directory of Programs and Services, 122,* 62-69.

Tsatsanis, K. (2005). Neuropsychological characteristics in autism and related conditions. In F. Volkmar, R. Paul, A. Klin, and D. Cohen (Eds.). *Handbook of autism and pervasive developmental disorders—vol. 1* (pp. 365-381). New York: Wiley.

Tsatsanis, K.D., Foley, C., and Donehower, C. (2004). Contemporary outcome research and programming guidelines for Asperger syndrome and high-functioning autism. *Topics in Language Disorders, 24(4),* 249-259.

Tsiouri, I., and Greer, R.D. (2003). Inducing vocal verbal behavior in children with severe language delays through rapid motor imitation responding. *Journal of Behavioral Education, 12,* 185-206.

Tuchman, D., and Walter, R. (1993). *Pediatric feeding and swallowing: Pathophysiology, diagnosis, and treatment.* San Diego, CA: Singular Publishing Group.

Tumner, W., and Cole, P. (1991). Learning to read: A metalinguistic act. In C. Simon (Ed.). *Communication skills and classroom success: Therapy methodologies for language-learning disabled students* (2nd ed., pp. 293-314). San Diego, CA: College-Hill Press.

Turstra, L. (2001). Partner effects in adolescent conversations. *Journal of Communication Disorders, 43,* 151-162.

Turstra, L., Ciccia, A., and Seaton, C. (2003). Interactive behaviors in adolescent conversation dyads. *Language, Speech and Hearing Services in Schools, 34,* 117-127.

Tyack, D., and Portnuff Venable, G. (1998). *Language sampling, analysis, and training, 3rd ed. (LSAT-3).* Austin, TX: Pro-Ed.

Tye-Murray, N. (2003). Conversational fluency of children who use cochlear implants. *Ear and Hearing, 24(1 Suppl.),* 82S-89S.

Tyler, A., Lewis, K., Haskill, A., and Tolbert, L. (2002). Efficacy and cross-domain effects of a morphosyntax and a phonology intervention. *Language, Speech and Hearing Services in Schools, 33,* 52-66.

Tyler, A., Lewis, K., Haskill, A., and Tolbert, L. (2003).Outcomes of different speech and language goal attack strategies. *Journal of Speech, Language and Hearing Research, 46,* 1007-1094.

Tyler, A., and Tolbert, L. (2002). Speech-language assessment in the clinical setting. *American Journal of Speech-Language Pathology, 11,* 215-221.

U.S. Department of Education. (1999). *National Center for Education Statistics.* Retrieved from http://nces.ed.gov

U.S. Department of Education. (2003). *English language learner students in U.S. public schools: 1994 and 2000.* Washington, DC: National Center for Education Statistics. Retrieved May 24, 2005, from http://nces.ed.gov/pubs2004/2004035.pdf

U.S. Department of Health and Human Services. (1985). *Report of the secretary's task force on black and minority health (vol. 1): Executive summary* [Pub. no. 491-313/44706]. Washington, DC: Author.

U.S. Department of Health and Human Services. (2000). *National child abuse and neglect data system glossary.* Retrieved from http://ed.gov/ncands

Uchanski, R.M., and Geers, A.E. (2003). Acoustic characteristics of the speech of young cochlear implant users: A comparison with normal-hearing age-mates. *Ear and Hearing, 24(1S),* 90S-105S.

Ukrainetz, T. (1998). Stickwriting stories: A quick and easy narrative representation strategy. *Language, Speech, and Hearing Services in Schools, 29,* 197-206.

Ukrainetz, T., Harpell, S., Walsh, C., and Coyle, C. (2000). A preliminary investigation of dynamic assessment with Native American kindergartners. *Language, Speech, and Hearing Services in Schools, 31,* 142-154.

Ullman, M., and Gopnik, M. (1994). Part tense production: Regular, irregular, and nonsense verbs. *McGill Working Papers in Linguistics, 10,* 81-118.

Ullman, M., and Pierpont, E. (2005). Specific language impairment is not specific to language: The procedural deficit hypothesis. *Cortex, 41,* 399-433.

Urwin, C. (1978). *The development of communication between blind infants and their parents: Some ways into language.* Doctoral dissertation. United Kingdom: University of Cambridge.

Urwin, C. (1984). *Speech development in blind children: Some ways into language.* Paper prepared for Internationales Symposium des Blinden-und-Sehschwachen-Verbandes der DDR. Brussels, Belgium.

Uzgiris, I.C., and Hunt, J. (1989). *Assessment in infancy: Ordinal scales of infant psychological development.* Champaign, IL: University of Illinois Press.

Valencia, S. (1990). A portfolio approach to classroom reading assessment: The whys, whats, and hows. *The Reading Teacher, January,* 338-340.

Vallecorsa, A., and deBettencourt, L. (1997). Using a mapping procedure to teach reading and writing skills to middle grade students with learning disabilities. *Education and Treatment of Children, 20,* 173-188.

Vallett, R. (1981). *Inventory of critical thinking ability.* Novato, CA: Academic Therapy Publications.

Van der Lely, H. (2005). Domain-specific cognitive systems: Insight from grammatical SLI. *Trends in Cognitive Sciences, 9,* 53-59.

Van der Lely, H., Rosen, S., and Adlard, A. (2004). Grammatical language impairment and the specificity of cognitive domains: Relations between auditory and language abilities. *Cognition, 94,* 167-183.

van Dongen, H., and Loonen, M. (1977). Factors related to prognosis of acquired aphasia in children. *Cortex, 13,* 131-136.

van Keulen, J., Weddinton, G., and DeBose, C. (1998). *Speech, language, and learning and the African American child.* Boston: Allyn & Bacon.

Van Kleeck, A. (1990). Emergent literacy: Learning about print before learning to read. *Topics in Language Disorders, 10,* 25-45.

Van Kleeck, A. (1995). Emphasizing form and meaning separately in pre-reading and early reading in first grade. *Topics in Language Disorders, 16,* 27-49.

Van Kleeck, A., Gillam, R, and McFadden, T. (1998). A study of classroom-based phonological awareness training for preschoolers with speech and/or language disorders. *American Journal of Speech-Language Pathology, 7,* 65-76.

Van Kleeck, A., and Richardson, A. (1995). Assessment of speech and language development. In J. Johnson and J. Goldman (Eds.). *Developmental assessment in clinical child psychology: A handbook* (pp. 462-498). New York: Pergamon Press.

Van Kraayenoord, C., and Schonell, E. (2003). By design. *International Journal of Disability, Development and Education, 50,* 115-118.

Van Riper, C., and Emerick, L. (1987). *Speech correction: An introduction to speech pathology and audiology* (7th ed.). Englewood Cliffs, NJ: Prentice-Hall.

Van Slyke, P.A. (2002). Classroom instruction for children with Landau–Kleffner syndrome. *Child Language Teaching & Therapy, 18(1),* 23-42.

Van Zile, S. (2003). Grammar that'll move you! *Instructor, 112,* 32-35.

VanDemark, D. (1964). Misarticulations and listener judgments of speech of individuals with cleft palates. *Cleft Palate Journal, 1,* 232-245.

VandenBerg, K. (1985). Revising the traditional model: An individualized approach to developmental interventions in the intensive care nursery. *Neonatal Network, 4,* 32-56.

VandenBerg, K. (1997). Basic principles of developmental caregiving. *Neonatal Network, 16(7),* 69-71.

Vandenberg, K. A. (1990). Behaviorally supportive care for the extremely premature infant. In L. Gunderson and C. Kenner (Eds.). *Care of the 24-25 week gestational age infant* (small baby protocol, pp. 129–157). San Francisco, CA: Neonatal Network.

Vargha-Khadem, F., Gadian, D.G., Copp, A., and Mishkin, M. (2005). FOXP2 and the neuroanatomy of speech and language. *Nature Reviews Neuroscience, 6,* 131-138.

Vaughn, S., Gersten, R., and Chard, D. (2000). The underlying message in LD intervention research: Findings from research syntheses. *Exceptional Children, 67,* 99-119.

Vaughn-Cooke, F. (1986). The challenge of assessing the language of non-mainstream speakers. In O.L. Taylor (Ed.). *Treatment of communication disorders in culturally and linguistically diverse populations* (pp. 23-48). Austin, TX: Pro-Ed.

Velleman, S. (1998, October). Lexical stress errors in developmental verbal dyspraxia: The problem and some possible solutions. *ASHA special interest division, Language Learning and Education* (newsletter).

Vellutino, F. (1977). Alternative conceptualization of dyslexia: Evidence in support of a verbal-deficit hypothesis. *Harvard University Review, 47,* 334-354.

Vellutino, F. (1979). *Dyslexia: Theory and research.* Cambridge, MA: MIT Press.

Vellutino, F., Fletcher, J., Snowling, M., and Scalon, D. (2004). Specific reading disability (dyslexia): What have we learned in the past four decades? *Journal of Child Psychology and Psychiatry, 45,* 2-40.

Vellutino, F., Scanlon, D., Sipay, E., Small, S., Pratt, A., Chen, R., and Denckla, M. (1996). Cognitive profiles of difficult-to remediate and readily remediated poor readers. *Journal of Educational Psychology, 88,* 601-638.

Venn, M., Wolery, M., Fleming, L., DeCesare, L., Morris, A., and Cuffs, M. (1993). Effects of teaching preschool peers to use the mand-model procedure during snack activities. *American Journal of Speech-Language Pathology: A Journal of Clinical Practice, 2,* 38-46.

Verlarde, P. (1989). *Old grandfather storyteller.* Santa Fe, N.M.: Clear Light Publishers.

Verne, J. (1983). *Around the world in 80 days.* New York: Airmont Publishing.

Vespoor, M., and Lowie, W. (2003). Making sense of polysemous words. *Language Learning, 53,* 547-586.

Vicari, S., Albertoni, A., Chilosi, A.M., Cipriani, P., Cioni, G., and Bates, E. (2000). Plasticity and reorganization during language development in children with early brain injury. *Cortex, 36(1),* 31-46.

Vigil, D., Hodges, J., and Klee, T. (2005). Quantity and quality of parental language input to late-talking toddlers during play. *Child Language Teaching and Therapy, 21,* 107-123.

Vilaseca, R. (2004). Language acquisition by children with Down syndrome: A naturalistic approach to assisting language acquisition. *Child Language Teaching and Therapy, 20,* 163-180.

Viorst, J. (1972). *Alexander and the terrible, horrible, no good, very bad day.* New York: Atheneum.

Visions Technology in Education. (2003). *The writer's companion.* Eugene, OR: Author.

Voeller, K. (2004). Attention-deficit hyperactivity disorder. *Journal of Child Neurology, 19,* 798-814.

Volden, J. (2002). Nonverbal learning disability: What the SLP needs to know. *ASHA Leader, 7(19),* 4-15.

Volden, J. (2004). Nonverbal learning disability: A tutorial for speech-language pathologists. *American Journal of Speech-Language Pathology, 13,* 128-141.

Volkmar, F., Carter, A., Grossman, J., and Klin, A. (1997). Social development in autism. In D. Cohen and F. Volkmar (Eds.). *Handbook of autism and pervasive developmental disorders* (pp. 173-194). New York: John Wiley & Sons.

von Tetzchner, S., and Grove, N. (Eds.). (2003). *Augmentative and alternative communication: Developmental issues.* London, UK: Whurr Publishers.

Voress, J., and Maddox, T. (1999). *Developmental assessment of young children (DAYC).* Austin, TX: Pro-Ed.

Vulpé, S. (1997). *Vulpé assessment battery—Revised.* East Aurora, NY: Slosson Educational Publications.

Vygotsky, L. (1962). *Thought and language.* Cambridge, MA: MIT Press. (Orig. pub. 1934).

Vygotsky, L. (1978). *Mind in society: The development of higher psychological processes.* Cambridge, MA: Harvard University Press.

Waber, B. (1972). *Ira sleeps over.* Boston, MA: Houghton Mifflin.

Wagner, C., Nettelbladt, U., Sahlen, B., Nilholm, C. (2000). Conversation versus narration in pre-school children with language impairment. *International Journal of Language and Communication Disorders, 35,* 83-93.

Wagner, R., Torgesen, J., and Rashotte, C. (1999). *Comprehensive test of phonological processing (CTOPP).* Austin, TX: Pro-Ed.

Waldron, K. (1992). *Teaching students with learning disabilities.* San Diego, CA: Singular Publishing Group.

Walker, H., Schwarz, I., Nippold, M., Irvin, K., and Noell, J. (1994). Social skills in school-age children and youth: Issues and best practices in assessment and intervention. *Topics in Language Disorders, 14(3),* 70-82.

Walker, H.M., Todis, B., Holmes, D., and Horton, G. (1988). *The Walker social skills curriculum: ACCEPTS.* Austin, TX: Pro-Ed.

Wallace, I., Gravel, J., McCarton, C., and Ruben, R. (1988). Otitis media and language development at 1 year of age. *Journal of Speech and Hearing Disorders, 53,* 245-251.

Wallach, G. (speaker, 1989). *Children's reading and writing disorders: The role of the speech-language pathologist* (ASHA Teleconference Tape Series). Rockville, MD: American Speech-Language-Hearing Association.

Wallace, I., and Hammill, D. (2002). *Comprehensive receptive and expressive vocabulary test—2nd Edition.* Austin, TX: Pro-Ed.

Wallach, G. (2004). Over the brink of the millennium: Have we said all we can say about language-based learning disabilities? *Communication Disorders Quarterly, 25,* 44-55.

Wallach, G. (2005). A conceptual framework in language learning disabilities: School-age language disorders. *Topics in Language Disorders, 25,* 292-301.

Wallach, G., and Butler, K. (1994). *Language learning disabilities in school-aged children and adolescents: Some principles and application.* Needham Heights, MA: Allyn & Bacon.

Wallach, G., and Miller, L. (1988). *Language intervention and academic success.* Boston, MA: College-Hill Publications.

Walt Disney Company. (1983). *Walt Disney comic strip maker* (computer program). New York: Bantam Software.

Wanat, P. (1983). Social skills: An awareness program with learning disabled adolescents. *Journal of Learning Disabilities, 16,* 35-38.

Wankoff, L. (2005). *Innovative methods in language intervention: Treatment outcome measures.* Austin, TX: Pro-Ed.

Ward, S. (1999). An investigation into the effectiveness of an early intervention method for delayed language development in young children. *International Journal of Language and Communication Disorders, 34,* 243-265.

Warden, M., and Hutchinson, T. (1992). *The writing process test.* Chicago, IL: Riverside Publishers.

Warren, D. (1984). *Blindness and early childhood development.* New York: Academic Foundation for the Blind.

Warren, S., Bredin-Oja, S., Fairchild, M., Finestack, L., Fey, M., and Brady, N. (2006). Responsivity education/Prelinguistic milieu teaching. In R. McCauley and M. Fey (Eds.). *Treatment of language disorders in children* (pp. 47-75). Baltimore: Paul H. Brookes. In press.

Warren, S., McQuarter, R., and Rogers-Warren, A. (1984). The effects of mands and models on the speech of unresponsive language-delayed preschool children. *Journal of Speech and Hearing Disorders, 49,* 43-52.

Warren, S., and Yoder, D. (1998). Facilitating the transition from preintentional to intentional communication. In A. Wetherny, S. Warren, and J. Reichle (Eds.). *Transitions in prelinguistic communication* (pp. 365-384). Baltimore, MD: Paul H. Brookes.

Warren, S., Yoder, P., and Leew, S. (2002). Promoting social-communicative development in infants and toddlers. In. H. Goldsteinand L. Kaczmarek, (Eds.). *Promoting social communication: Children with developmental disabilities from birth to adolescence* (pp. 121-149). Baltimore: Paul H. Brookes.

Warren-Leubecker, A., and Carter, B. (1988). Reading and growth in metalinguistic awareness: Relations to socio-economic status and reading readiness skills. *Child Development, 59,* 728-742.

Waryas, C., and Stremel-Campbell, K. (1983). *Communication training program.* New York: Teaching Resources.

Washington, J., and Craig, H. (1992). Articulation test performances of low-income, African-American preschoolers with communication impairments. *Language, Speech, and Hearing Services in Schools, 23,* 203-207.

Wasik, B., and Bond, M. (2001). Beyond the pages of a book: Interactive book reading and language development in preschool classrooms. *Journal of Educational Psychology, 93,* 243-50.

Wasserman, G., Green, A., and Allen, R. (1983). Going beyond abuse: Maladaptive patterns of interaction in abusing mother-infant pairs. *Journal of the American Academy of Child Psychiatry, 22,* 245-252.

Watkins, C. (1985). *American heritage dictionary of Indo-European roots.* Boston: Houghton Mifflin.

Watkins, R. (1990). Processing problems and language impairment in children. *Topics in Language Disorders, 11(1),* 63-72.

Watkins, R. (1994). Grammatical challenges for children with specific language impairment. In R. Watkins and M. Rice (Eds.). *Specific language impairments in children* (vol 4, pp. 53-68). Baltimore, MD: Paul H. Brookes.

Watkins, R., Kelly, D., Harbers, H., and Hollis, W. (1995). Measuring children's lexical diversity: Differentiating typical and impaired language learners. *Journal of Speech and Hearing Research, 38,* 476-489.

Watson, L., Layton, T., Pierce, P., and Abraham, L. (1994). Enhancing emerging literacy in a language preschool. *Language, Speech, and Hearing Services in Schools, 25,* 136-145.

Watson, L.R., and Ozonoff, S. (2001). In T. Layton, E. Crais, and L. Watson (Eds.). *Handbook of early language impairment in children: Nature* (pp. 177-257). Albany, NY: Delmar.

Watson, R. (2003). Literacy and oral language: Implications for early literacy acquisition. In S. Neuman and D. Dickinson (Eds.). *Handbook of early literacy research* (pp. 43-53). N.Y.: Guilford Press.

Weaver, C. (1993). Understanding and educating students with attention deficit hyperactivity disorder: Toward a system theory and whole language perspective. *American Journal of Speech-Language Pathology, 2,* 79-89.

Webster, P., and Plante, A. (1992). Effects of phonological impairment on word, syllable, and phoneme segmentation and reading. *Language, Speech, and Hearing Services in Schools, 23,* 176-182.

Webster, R.I., and Shevell, M.I. (2004). Neurobiology of specific language impairment. *Journal of Child Neurology, 19(7),* 471-481.

Wechsler, D. (1981). *Wechsler adult intelligence scale—Revised manual.* New York: Psychological Corporation.

Wechsler, D. (2002). *Wechsler preschool and primary intelligence scale—3rd Ed.* San Antonio, TX: Harcourt Assessment.

Wechsler, D. (2003). *Wechsler intelligence scale for children—4th Ed.* San Antonio, TX: Harcourt Assessment.

Weckerly, J., Wulfeck, B., and Reilly, J. (2004). The development of morphosyntactic ability in atypical populations: The acquisition of tag questions in children with early focal lesions and children with specific-language impairment. *Brain & Language, 88(2),* 190-202.

Weddington, G. (1987). Guidelines for use of standardized tests with minority children. In L. Cole and V. Deal (Eds.). *Communication disorders in multicultural populations* (pp. 21-22). American Speech-Language-Hearing Association.

Wegerif, R. (2002). Walking or dancing? Images of thinking and learning to think in the classroom. *Journal of Interactive Learning Research, 13,* 1-2.

Weiner, F. (1979). *Phonological process analysis.* Baltimore, MD: University Park Press.

Weiner, F. (1981). Treatment of phonological disability using the method of meaningful minimal contrast: Two case studies. *Journal of Speech and Hearing Disorders, 46,* 97-103.

Weiner, F. (1988). *Parrot easy language sample analysis* (computer program). State College, PA: Parrot Software.

Weiner, J. (2002). Friendship and social adjustment of children with learning disabilities. In B.Y.L. Wong and M. Donahue (Eds.). *The social dimensions of learning disabilities: Essays in honor of Tanis Bryan* (Volume in the Special Education and Exceptionality Series, pp. 93-114). Mahwah, NJ: Erlbaum.

Weiner, P. (1985). The value of follow-up studies. *Topics in Language Disorders, 5,* 78-92.

Weir, R. (1962). *Language in the crib.* The Hague, Netherlands: Mouton.

Weise, M. (June, 1998). *A case study in the treatment of elective mutism.* Poster presented at the Symposium of Research in Child Language Disorders. Madison, WI.

Weismer, S. (1996). Capacity limitations in working memory: The impact on lexical and morphological learning by children with language impairment. *Topics in Language Disorders, 17,* 33-44.

Weismer, S. (1998). The impact of emphatic stress on novel word learning by children with specific language impairment. *Journal of Speech, Language, and Hearing Research, 41,* 1444-1458.

Weismer, S. (2000). Intervention for children with developmental language delay. In Bishop, D., and Leonard, L. (Eds.). *Speech and language impairments in children: Causes, characteristics, intervention and outcome* (pp. 157-176). New York: Psychology Press.

Weismer, S., and Evans, J. (2002). The role of processing limitations in early identification of specific language impairment. *Topics in Language Disorders, 22(3),* 15-29.

Weismer, S., Evans, J., and Hesketh, L. (1997). *Evidence of verbal working memory constraints in specific language impairment.* Poster presented at the annual convention of the American Speech-Language-Hearing Association, Boston, MA.

Weismer, S., and Hesketh, L. (1993). The influence of prosodic and gestural cues on novel word acquisition by children with specific language impairment. *Journal of Speech and Hearing Research, 36,* 1013-1025.

Weismer, S., and Hesketh, L. (1996). *Examinations of processing capacity limitations in specific language impairment.* Poster presented at the 16th annual convention of the American Speech-Language-Hearing Association, Boston, MA.

Weismer, S., and Robertson, S. (2006). Focused stimulation approach to language intervention. In R. McCauley and M. Fey (Eds.). *Treatment of language disorders in children.* Baltimore: Paul H. Brookes. In press.

Weismer, S., and Thordardottir, E. (June, 1998). *Limitations in linguistic processing by children with SLI.* Poster presented at the Symposium for Research in Child Language Disorders, Madison, WI.

Weismer, S., Tomblin, J., Zhang, X., Buckwalter, P., Chynoweth, J., and Jones, J. (2000). Nonword repetition performance in school-age children with and without language impairment. *Journal of Speech, Language, and Hearing Research, 43,* 865-878.

Weiss, A. (1986). Classroom discourse and the hearing-impaired child. *Topics in Language Disorders, 6(3),* 60-70.

Weiss, A., and Nakamura, M. (1992). Children with normal language skills in preschool classrooms for children with language impairments: Differences in modeling styles. *Language, Speech, and Hearing Services in Schools, 23,* 64-70.

Weiss, A., Temperly, T., Stierwalt, J., and Robin, D. (1993, November). *Use of cartoons to elicit narrative language samples from children and adolescents with severe TBI.* Paper presented at American Speech-Language-Hearing Annual Convention, Anaheim, CA.

Weiss, B., Weisz, J., and Bromfield, R. (1986). Performance of retarded and non-retarded persons on information-processing tasks: Further tests of the similar structure hypothesis. *Psychological Bulletin, 100,* 157-175.

Weiss, M., Tannock, R. Kratochvil, C., et al. (2005). A randomized, placebo-controlled study of once-daily atomoxetine in the school setting in children with ADHD. *Journal of the American Academy of Child and Adolescent Psychiatry, 44,* 647-655.

Weitzman, E., and Greenbar, J. (2002). *Learning language and loving it* (2nd ed.). Toronto, Canada: The Hanen Centre.

Wellman, H. (1985). The origins of metacognition. In D. Forrest-Pressley, G. MacKinnon, and T. Waller (Eds.). *Metacognition, cognition and human performance* (pp. 1-31). Orlando: Academic Press.

Wells, W., and Peppe, S. (2003). Intonation abilities of children with speech and language impairments. *Journal of Speech, Language, and Hearing Research, 46,* 5-20.

Wepman, J., and Hass, W. (1969). *A spoken word count.* Chicago, IL: Language Resource Association.

Wepman, J., Jones, L., Bock, R., and Van Pelt, D. (1960). Studies in aphasia: Background and theoretical formulations. *Journal of Speech and Hearing Disorders, 25,* 323-332.

Werner, G., Vismara, L., Koegel, R., and Koegel, L. (2006). In R. Koegel, and L. Koegel (Eds.). *Pivotal response treatments for autism: Communication, social and academic development* (pp. 199-216). Baltimore: Paul H. Brookes Publishers.

Wernicke, K. (1874). The symptom-complex of aphasia. In A. Church (Ed.). *Diseases of the nervous system.* New York: Appleton-Century-Crofts. (1908).

Wesseling, R., and Reitsma, P. (2001). Preschool phonological representations and development of reading skills. *Annals of Dyslexia, 51,* 203-229.

Westby, C. (1984). Development of narrative language abilities. In G. Wallach and K. Butler (Eds.). *Language learning disabilities in school-age children* (pp. 103-127). Baltimore, MD: Williams & Wilkins.

Westby, C. (1986). Cultural differences affecting communication development. In L. Cole and V. Deal (Eds.). *Communication disorders in multicultural populations.* Washington, DC: American Speech-Language-Hearing Association.

Westby, C. (1988, November). *Learning how to ask: Preparing to work with families.* Paper presented at the American Speech-Language-Hearing Association Convention, Boston, MA.

Westby, C. (1989a). *Cultural variations in storytelling.* Paper presented at American Speech-Language-Hearing Association Convention, St. Louis, MO.

Westby, C. (1989b). Assessing and remediating text comprehension problems. In A. Kahmi and H. Catts (Eds.). *Reading disabilities: A developmental language perspective.* Boston, MA: Little, Brown.

Westby, C. (1991). Learning to talk—talking to learn: Oral-literate language differences. In C.S. Simon (Ed.). *Communication skills and classroom success* (pp. 181-218). San Diego, CA: College-Hill.

Westby, C. (1994). *Advanced communication development: Foundations, processes, and clinical applications* (pp. 341-384). Englewood Cliffs, NJ: Prentice-Hall.

Westby, C. (1998a). Communicative refinement in school age and adolescence. In W. Hayes and B. Shulman (Eds.). *Communication development: Foundations, processes, and clinical applications* (pp. 311-360). Baltimore, MD: Williams & Wilkins.

Westby, C. (1998b). Social-emotional bases of communication development. In W. Haynes and B. Shulman (Eds.). *Communication development: Foundations, processes, and clinical applications* (pp. 165-204). Baltimore, MD: Williams & Wilkins.

Westby, C. (2005). Assessing and facilitating text comprehension problems. In H. Catts and A. Kahmi (Eds.). *Language and reading disabilities* (2nd ed., pp. 157-232). Boston: Allyn & Bacon.

Westby, C., and Atencio, D. (2002). Computers, culture, and learning. *Topics in Language Disorders, 22(4),* 70-90.

Westby, C., and Clauser, P. (2005). The right stuff for writing: Assessing and facilitating written language. In H. Catts and A. Kahmi (Eds.). *Language and reading disabilities* (2nd ed.). (pp. 274-340). Boston: Allyn & Bacon.

Westby, C., and Rouse, G. (1985). Culture in education and the instruction of language learning-disabled students. *Topics in Language Disorders, 5(4),* 15-28.

Westby, C.E., Stevens Dominguez, M., and Oetter, P. (1996). A performance/competence model of observational assessment. *Language Speech and Hearing Services in Schools, 27(2),* 144-156.

Westby, C., and Vining, C. (2002). Living in harmony: Providing services to native American children and families. In D.E. Battle (Ed.). *Communication disorders in multicultural populations* (3rd ed., pp. 135-178). Boston: Butterworth-Heinneman.

Westby, C., and Watson, S. (2004). Perspectives on attention deficit hyperactivity disorder: executive functions, working memory and language disabilities. *Seminars in Speech and Language, 25(3),* 241-254.

Wetherby, A. (1986). Ontogeny of communicative functions in autism. *Journal of Autism and Developmental Disorders, 16,* 295-316.

Wetherby, A., Allen, L, Cleary, J., Kublin, K., and Goldstein, H. (2002). Validity and reliability of the Communication and Symbolic Behavior Scales Developmental Profile with very young children. *Journal of Speech, Language, and Hearing Research, 45,* 1202-1218.

Wetherby, A., Cain, D., Yonclas, D., and Walker, V. (1988). Analysis of intentional communication of normal children from the prelinguistic to the multiword stage. *Journal of Speech and Hearing Research, 31,* 240-252.

Wetherby, A., and Prizant, B. (1989). The expression of communicative intent: Assessment guidelines. *Seminars in Speech and Language, 10,* 77-91.

Wetherby, A., and Prizant, B. (1991). Profiling young children's communicative competence. In S. Warren and J. Riechle (Eds.). *Causes and effects in communication and language intervention* (pp. 217-254). Baltimore, MD: Paul H. Brookes.

Wetherby, A., and Prizant, B. (1993). *Communication and symbolic behavior scales.* Baltimore, MD: Paul H. Brookes.

Wetherby, A., and Prizant, B. (2003). *Communication and symbolic behavior scales—Developmental profile.* Baltimore: Paul H. Brookes.

Wetherby, A., and Prizant, B. (2005). Enhancing language and communication development in autism spectrum disorders: Assessment and intervention guidelines. In Zager, D. (Ed.). *Autism spectrum disorders: Identification, education and treatment* (3rd ed., pp. 327-365). Mahwah, NJ: Erlbaum.

Wetherby, A., and Prutting, C. (1984). Profiles of communicative and cognitive-social abilities in autistic children. *Journal of Speech and Hearing Research, 27,* 364-377.

Wetherby, A., Schuler, A., and Prizant, B. (1997). Enhancing language and communication development: Theoretical foundations. In D.J. Cohen and F.R. Volkmar (Eds.). *Handbook of autism and pervasive developmental disorders* (2nd ed., pp. 513-538). New York: John Wiley & Sons.

Wetherby, A., Woods, J., Allen, L, Cleary, J., Dickinson, H., and Lord, C. (2004). Early indicators of autism spectrum disorders in the second year of life. *Journal of Autism and Developmental Disorders, 34,* 473-493.

Wetherby, A., Yonclas, D., and Bryan, A. (1989). Communication profiles of preschool children with handicaps: Implications for early identification. *Journal of Speech and Hearing Disorders, 54,* 148-158.

Wheeler, R. (2005). Code-switch to teach standard English. *English Journal, 94,* 108-112.

Wheeler, R.S., and Swords, R. (2004). Codeswitching: Tools of language and culture transform the dialectally diverse classroom. *Language Arts, 81(6),* 470-479.

Whiskeyman, L. (2000). *LanguageBURST.* East Moline, IL: Linguisystems.

Whissell, C. (2003). Pronounceability: A measure of language samples based on children's mastery of the phonemes employed in them. *Perceptual & Motor Skills, 96,* 748-755.

White, E. (1952). *Charlotte's web.* New York: Harper & Row.

White, E. (1974). *Stuart Little.* New York: Harpers Childrens Books.

Whitehurst, G., Falco, F., Lonigan, C., Fischel, J., DeBaryshe, B., Valdez-Menchaea, M., and Caulfield, M. (1988). Accelerating language development through picture-book reading. *Developmental Psychology, 24,* 552-558.

Whitehurst, G., and Fischel, J. (1994). Early developmental language delay: What, if anything, should the clinician do about it? *Journal of Child Psychology and Psychiatry, 35,* 613-648.

Whitehurst, G., Fischel, J., Arnold, D., and Lonigan, C. (1992). Evaluating outcomes with children with expressive language delay. In S. Warren and J. Riechle (Eds.). *Causes and effects in communication and language intervention* (pp. 277-314). Baltimore, MD: Paul H. Brookes.

Whitehurst, G., Fischel, J., Lonigan, C., Valdez-Menchaca, M., Arnold, D., and Smith, M. (1991). Treatment of early expressive language delay: If, when, and how. *Topics in Language Disorders, 11,* 55-68.

Whitehurst, G., and Lonigan, C. (2003). Emergent literacy: Development from prereaders to readers. In S. Neuman and D. Dickinson (Eds.). *Handbook of early literacy research* (pp. 11-29). N.Y.: Guilford Press.

Whitehurst, G., Smith, M., Fischel, J., Arnold, D., and Lonigan, L. (1991). The continuity of babble and speech in children with early expressive language delay. *Journal of Speech and Hearing Research, 34,* 1121-1129.

Whitmire, K. (2000a). Adolescence as a developmental phase: A tutorial. *Topics in Language Disorders, 20(2),* 1-14.

Whitmire, K. (2000b). Cognitive referencing and discrepancy formulae: Comments from ASHA's resources. *Language Learning and Education, 7,* 13-17.

Whitmire, K. (2002). The evolution of school-based speech-language services: A half century of change and a new century of practice. *Communication Disorders Quarterly, 23,* 68-76.

Whitmire, K., and Dublinske, S. (2003). Provision of speech-language services in the schools: Working with the law. *Seminars in Speech and Language, 24,* 147-154.

Wiederholt, J., and Blalock, G. (2000). *Gray silent reading tests* (4th ed.). Austin, TX: Pro-Ed.

Wiederholt, J., and Bryant, B. (1989). *Gray oral reading tests* (3rd ed.). Austin, TX: Pro-Ed.

Wiig, E. (1982a). Language disabilities in school-age children and youth. In G. Shames and E. Wiig (Eds.). *Human communication disorders: An introduction* (2nd ed., pp. 331-379). Columbus, OH: Merrill.

Wiig, E. (1982b). *Let's talk: Developing prosocial communication skills.* Columbus, OH: Merrill/Macmillan.

Wiig, E. (1984). Language disabilities in adolescents: A question of cognitive strategies. *Topics in Language Disorders, 4(2),* 41-58.

Wiig, E. (1987). *Let's talk inventory for adolescents.* San Antonio, TX: Psychological Corporation.

Wiig, E. (1990). Language disabilities in school-age children. In G. Shames and E. Wiig (Eds.). *Human communication disorders* (pp. 193-221). Columbus, OH: Merrill.

Wiig, E. (1995). Assessment of adolescent language. *Seminars in Speech and Language, 16,* 14-31.

Wiig, E., and Secord, W. (1989). *Test of language competence—Expanded edition.* San Antonio, TX: Harcourt Assessment.

Wiig, E., and Secord, W. (1992a). *Test of word knowledge.* San Antonio, TX: Harcourt Assessment.

Wiig, E., and Secord, W. (1992b). *Measurement and assessment: Making sense of test results.* Buffalo, NY: Educom Associates.

Wiig, E., and Semel, E. (1984). *Language assessment and intervention for the learning disabled.* Columbus, OH: Charles E. Merrill.

Wilbur, R., Goodhart, N., and Montandon, E. (1983). Comprehension of nine syntactic structures by hearing-impaired students. *Volta Review, 85,* 328-345.

Wilcox, K., and Morris, S. (1990). *Children's speech intelligibility measure.* Austin, TX: Pro-Ed.

Wilcox, M.J., and Shannon, M.S. (1998). Facilitating the transition from prelinguistic to linguistic communication. In A.M. Wetherby, S.F. Warren, and J. Reichle (Eds.). *Transitions in prelinguistic communication* (pp. 385-416). Baltimore, MD: Paul H. Brookes.

Wilder, L. (1932). *Little house in the big woods.* New York: Harper Trophy.

Wilford, J. (1999, November). Egypt carvings set earlier date for alphabet. *The New York Times,* p. A1.

Wilhelm, J. (2001). Think-alouds: Boost reading comprehension. *Instructor, 111,* 26-28.

Wilkinson, A., Stratta, L., and Dudley, P. (1974). *Schools Council Oracy Project listening comprehension tests.* London: MacMillan Education.

Wilkinson, L., Milosky, L., and Genishi, C. (1986). Second language learners' use of requests and responses in elementary classrooms. *Topics in Language Disorders, 6(2),* 57-70.

Willey, M. (1991). *Saving Lenny.* New York: Bantam.

Williams, A. (2001). Phonological assessment of child speech. In D. Ruscello (Ed.). *Tests and measurements in speech-language pathology* (pp. 31-76). Boston: Butterworth-Heinemann.

Williams, A., and Elbert, M. (2003). A prospective longitudinal study of phonological development in late talkers. *Language, Speech and Hearing Services in Schools, 34,* 138-154.

Williams, B. (1975). *Kevin's grandma.* New York: Dutton.

Williams, K.T. (2006). *Expressive vocabulary test—2.* Circle Pines, MN: American Guidance Service.

Willis, W. (2004). Families with African American roots. In E. Lynch and M. Hanson (Eds.). *Developing cross-cultural competence—3rd ed* (pp. 141-178). Baltimore: Paul H. Brookes

Wilson, M. (1991). *Sequential software for language intervention* (computer program). Burlington, VT: Laureate Learning Systems.

Wilson, M., and Fox, B. (1982-2005). *First words I, first words II and first verbs, sterling editions* (computer program). Burlington, VT: Laureate Learning Systems.

Wilson, M., and Fox, B. *Words and concepts series* (computer program). Burlington, VT: Laureate Learning Systems.

Wilson, M., and Fox, B. (1983). *Microcomputer language assessment and development systems* (Micro-LADS, computer program). Burlington, VT: Laureate Learning Systems.

Wilson, W., Wilson, J., and Coleman, T. (2000). Culturally appropriate assessment: Issues and strategies. In T. Coleman (Ed.). *Clinical management of communication disorders in culturally diverse children* (pp. 101-127). Boston: Allyn & Bacon.

Windfuhr, K., Faragher, B., and Conti-Ramsden, G. (2002). Lexical learning skills in young children with specific language impairment. *International Journal of Language and Communication Disorders, 37,* 415-432.

Windsor, J., Doyle, S., and Siegel, G. (1994). Language acquisition after mutism: A longitudinal case study of autism. *Journal of Speech and Hearing Research, 37,* 96-105.

Windsor, J., Scott, C., and Street, C. (2000). Verb and noun morphology in the spoken and written language of children with language learning disabilities. *Journal of Speech, Language, and Hearing Research, 43,* 1322-1336.

Wing, L., and Gould. J. (1979). Severe impairments of social interaction and associated abnormalities in children: Epidemiology and classification. *Journal of Autism and Developmental Disorders, 9,* 11-29.

Winner, M. (2003). Asperger syndrome across the home and school day. *ASHA Leader, 8(17),* 4-10.

Winterton, W. (1976). *The effects of extending wait-time on selected verbal response characteristics of some Pueblo Indian children.* Thesis. Albuquerque: University of New Mexico.

Wisniewski, D. (2003). *The idiom game.* Moline, IL: LinguiSystems.

Witt, B. (1998). Cognition and the cognitive language relationship. In W. Haynes and B. Witt (Eds.). *Communication development: Foundations, processes, and clinical applications* (pp. 101-133). Baltimore, MD: Williams & Wilkins.

Wolcott, G., Lash, M., and Pearson, S. (1995). *Signs and strategies for educating students with brain injury: A practical guide for teachers and schools.* Houston, TX: HDI Publishers.

Wolf, D. (1989). Portfolio assessment: Sampling student work. *Educational Leadership, April,* 35-39.

Wolf, L., and Glass, R. (1992a). *Feeding and swallowing disorders in infancy: Assessment and management.* Tucson, AZ: Communication Skill Builders.

Wolf, L., and Glass, R. (Eds., 1992b). *Tools of the trade: Nipples, pacifiers, and bottles. In Feeding and swallowing disorders in infancy.* Tucson, AZ: Therapy Skill Builders.

Wolf, M., Bally, H., and Morris, R. (1986). Automaticity, retrieval processes, and reading: A longitudinal investigation of average and impaired readers. *Child Development, 57,* 988-1000.

Wolf, M., and Denckla, M.B. (2005). *Rapid automatized naming and rapid alternating stimulus tests.* Austin, TX: Pro-Ed.

Wolf, M., O'Rourke, A., Gidney, C., Lovett, M., Cirino, P., and Morris, R. (2002). The second deficit: An investigation of the independence of phonological and naming-speed deficits in developmental dyslexia. *Reading & Writing, 15,* 43-72.

Wolf, S., and Gearhart, M. (1994). Writing what you read: Narrative assessment as a learning event. *Language Arts, 71,* 425-444.

Wolfe, V., Presley, C., and Mesaris, J. (2003). The importance of sound identification training in phonological intervention. *American Journal of Speech-Language Pathology, 12,* 282-288.

Wolff, P., Gardner, J., Lappen, J., Paccia, J., and Meryash, D. (1988). Variable expression of the fragile X syndrome in heterozygous females of normal intelligence. *American Journal of Medical Genetics, 30,* 213-225.

Wolfram, W., Hazen, K., and Tamburro, J. (1997). Isolation within isolation: A solitary century of African-American vernacular English. *Journal of Sociolinguistics, 1,* 7-8.

Wolf-Schein, E., Sudhalter, V., Cohen, I., Fisch, G., Hanson, D., Pfadt, A., Hagerman, R., Jenkins, E., and Brown, W.T. (1987). Speech-language and the fragile X syndrome: Initial findings. *ASHA, 29,* 35-38.

Wong, B. (2000). Writing strategies instruction for expository essays for adolescents with and without learning disabilities. *Topics in Language Disorders, 20(4),* 29-44.

Wong, B., Butler, D., Ficzere, S., and Kuperis, S. (1996). Teaching low achievers and students with learning disabilities to plan, write, and revise opinion essays. *Journal of Learning Disabilities, 29,* 197-212.

Wood, A. (1985). *King Bidgood's in the bathtub.* New York: Harcourt Brace Jovanovich.

Wood, A. (1988). *Elbert's bad word.* San Diego, CA: Harcourt Brace Jovanovich.

Wood, L., and Hood, E. (2004). Shared storybook readings with children who have little or no functional speech: A language intervention tool for students who use augmentative and alternative communication. *Perspectives in Education, 22,* 101-114.

Wood, P. (1980). Appreciating the consequences of disease: The classification of impairments, disabilities, and handicaps. *The World Health Organization Chronicle, 34,* 376-380.

Woodcock, R. (1991). *Woodcock language proficiency battery—Revised.* Chicago, IL: Riverside Publishers.

Woodcock, R. (1998). *Woodcock reading mastery tests—Revised-normative update.* Circle Pines, MN: AGS.

Woodcock, R., and Johnson, M. (1990). *Woodcock-Johnson Psycho-educational Battery—Revised.* Itasca, Il: Riverside Publishing Company.

Woodnorth, G. (2004). Assessment and managing medically fragile children: Tracheostomy and ventilatory support. *Language, Speech, and Hearing Services in Schools, 35,* 363-372.

Woodruff, G., and McGonigel, M. (1988). Early intervention team approaches: The transdisciplinary model. In J. Jordan, J. Gallagher, P. Hutinger, and M. Karnes (Eds.). *Early childhood special education: Birth to three* (pp. 163-182). Reston, VA: Council for Exceptional Children and the Division for Early Childhood.

Woods, B. (2004). *Emako Blue.* New York: Putnam Juvenile.

WordSmart, (N.D.). *WordSmart software.* San Diego, CA: Author.

Work, R., Cline, J., Ehren, B., Keiser, D., and Wujek, C. (1993). Adolescent language programs. *Language, Speech, and Hearing Services in Schools, 24,* 43-53.

World Health Organization. (1992). *International code of diseases* (10th ed.). New York: Author.

World Health Organization. (2001). *International classification of functioning, disability and health.* Geneva: Author.

World Health Organization. (2004). *International statistical classification of diseases and related health problems—10th revision* (2nd ed.). Geneva: Author.

Wright, B.A., and Zecker, S.G. (2004). Learning problems, delayed development, and puberty. *Proceedings of the National Academy of Sciences USA, 101,* 9942-9946.

Wright, H., and Newhoff, M. (2001). Narration abilities of children with language learning disabilities in response to oral and written stimuli. *American Journal of Speech-Language Pathology, 10,* 308-319.

Wright, J., and Jacobs, B. (2003). Teaching phonological awareness and metacognitive strategies to children with reading difficulties: A comparison of two instructional methods. *Educational Psychology, 23,* 17-47.

Wulfeck, B., Bates, E., Krupa-Kwiatkowski, M., and Saltzman, D. (2004). Grammaticality sensitivity in children with early focal brain injury and children with specific language impairment. *Brain & Language, 88(2),* 215-228.

Wulz, S., Hall, M., and Klein, M. (1983). A home-centered instructional communication strategy for severely handicapped children. *Journal of Speech and Hearing Disorders, 48,* 2-11.

Wyatt, T. (2002). Assessing the communicative abilities of clients from diverse cultural and language backgrounds. In D. Battle (Ed.). *Communication disorders in multicultural populations—3rd ed.* (pp. 415-459). Boston: Butterworth-Heinneman.

Yarbrough, C. (1981). *Cornrows.* New York: Putnam Publishers.

Yates, J. (1988). Demography as it affects special education. In A.A. Ortiz and B.A. Ramirez (Eds.). *Schools and the culturally diverse exceptional student: Promising practices and future directions.* Reston, VA: Council for Exceptional Children.

Yeates, K., Swift, E., Taylor, H., Wade, S., Drotar, D., Stancin, T., and Minich, N. (2004). Short- and long-term social outcomes following pediatric traumatic brain injury. *Journal of International Neuropsychological Society, 10(3),* 412-426.

Ylvisaker, M., and Szekeres, S. (1989). Metacognitive and executive impairments in head-injured children and adults. *Topics in Language Disorders, 9(2),* 34-49.

Yoder, P. et al. (1995). Predicting children's response to prelinguistic communication intervention. *Journal of Early Intervention, 19(1),* 74-84.

Yoder, P., Davies, B., Bishop, K., and Munson, L. (1994). Effect of adult Wh-questions on conversational participation in children with developmental disabilities. *Journal of Speech and Hearing Research, 37,* 193-204.

Yoder, P., and Warren, S. (1998). Maternal responsivity predicts the prelinguistic communication intervention that facilitates generalized intentional communication. *Journal of Speech, Language, and Hearing Research, 41,* 1207-1219.

Yoder, P., and Warren, S. (2001). Prelinguistic milieu teaching. In H. Goldstein, L., Kaczmarek, and K. English (Eds.). *Promoting social communication: Children with developmental disabilities from birth to adolescence.* Baltimore: Paul H. Brookes.

Yoder, P., and Warren, S. (2002). Effects of prelinguistic milieu teaching and parent responsivity education on dyads involving children with intellectual disabilities. *Journal of Speech, Language, and Hearing Research, 45,* 1158-1175.

Yoder, P., Warren, S., and Hull, L. (1995). Predicting children's response to prelinguistic communication intervention. *Journal of Early Intervention, 19,* 74-84.

Yoder, P., Warren, S., and McCathren, R. (1998). Determining spoken language prognosis in children with developmental disabilities. *American Journal of Speech-Language Pathology, 7,* 77-87.

Yont, K., and Hewitt, L. (2000). A coding system for describing conversational breakdowns in preschool children. *American Journal of Speech-Language Pathology, 9,* 300-309.

Yont, K., Snow, C., and Vernon-Feagans, L. (2001). Early communicative intents expressed by 12-month-old children with and without chronic otitis media. *First Language, 21,* 265-287.

Yopp, H. (1992). Developing phonemic awareness in young children. *Reading Teacher, 45,* 696-703.

Yopp, H., and Yopp, R. (2000). Supporting phonemic awareness development in the classroom. *Reading Teacher, 54,* 130-143.

Yoshinaga-Itano, C., and Downey, D. (1986). A hearing-impaired child's acquisition of schemata: Something's missing. *Topics in Language Disorders, 7,* 45-57.

Yoshinaga-Itano, C., and Snyder, L. (1985). Form and meaning in the written language of hearing-impaired children. In R.R. Kretschmer (Ed.). Learning to write and writing to learn (monograph). *Volta Review, 87(5),* 75-90.

Yoss, K., and Darley, F. (1974). Developmental apraxia of speech in children with defective articulation. *Journal of Speech and Hearing Research, 17,* 399-416.

Young, E. (1989). *Lon Po Po: A Red Riding Hood story from China.* New York: Philomel Books.

Young, E., Diehl, J., Morris, D., Hyman, S., and Bennetto, L. (2005). The use of two language tests to identify pragmatic language problems in children with autism spectrum disorders. *Language Speech, and Hearing Services in Schools, 36,* 62-72.

Young, E., and Perachio, J. (1993). *Patterned elicitation of syntax test with morphophonemic analysis* (rev. ed). Tucson, AZ: Communication Skill Builders.

Young, P. (1987). *Drugs and pregnancy.* New York: Chelsea House.

Young, R. (1967). *English as a second language for Navajos: An overview of certain cultural and linguistic factors.* Navajo Area Office; Division of Education, Bureau of Indian Affairs: Albuquerque, NM.

Zahner, G., and Pauls, D. (1987). Epidemiological surveys of infantile autism. In D. Cohen, A. Donnellan, and R. Paul (Eds.). *Handbook of autism and pervasive developmental disorders* (pp. 199-210). New York: John Wiley & Sons.

Zeece, P., and Churchill, S. (2001). First stories: Emergent literacy in infants and toddlers. *Early Childhood Education Journal, 29,* 101-104.

Ziev, M. (1999). Earliest intervention: Speech-language pathology services in the newborn intensive care unit. *ASHA, 41,* 32-36.

Zimmerman, I., Steiner, V., and Pond, R. (1992). *Preschool language scale—3.* San Antonio, TX: Psychological Corporation.

Zipprich, M. (1995). Teaching web making as a guided planning tool to improve student narrative writing. *Remedial & Special Education, 16,* 13-15.

Zoller, M. (1991). Use of music activities in speech-language therapy. *Language, Speech, and Hearing Services in Schools, 22,* 272-276.

Zuniga, M. (2004). Families with Latino roots. In E. Lynch and M. Hanson (Eds.). *Developing cross-cultural competence* (3rd ed., pp. 179-218). Baltimore, MD: Paul H. Brookes.

Zwitman, D., and Sonderman, J. (1979). A syntax program designed to present base linguistic structures to language-disordered children. *Journal of Communication Disorders, 2,* 323-335.

SUBJECT INDEX

Get more out of this text **with the Companion CD!**

COMPANION CD

LANGUAGE DISORDERS
from INFANCY THROUGH ADOLESCENCE

PAUL

MOSBY
ELSEVIER

ASSESSMENT &INTERVENTION

WIN/MAC

Third EDITION

9996009173

Copyright © 2007, by Elsevier Inc.
All rights reserved.
Produced in the United States of America.

To help you master the diagnosis and treatment of childhood language disorders, this CD-ROM gives you access to...

- **Video clips** linked to your text that further illustrate key points:
  - o Chapter 1: A parent's long-term perspective
  - o Chapter 2: The hard-to-assess child
  - o Chapter 3: The continuum of naturalness in intervention
  - o Chapter 4: Social disability
  - o Chapter 5: Language delay or difference?
  - o Chapter 6: Parent training
  - o Chapter 7: Late-talking toddler
  - o Chapter 8: Language sample for transcription practice
  - o Chapter 9: Mediating social interaction
  - o Chapter 11: Speech sample: Conversation in language learning disorder for analysis practice
  - o Chapter 12: Student-centered intervention planning
  - o Chapter 13: Narrative sample for analysis practice
  - o Chapter 14: Individual transition planning

- **Suggested projects** to help you assimilate the material covered in each chapter

Try it now!